Lasers in Dermatology and Medicine

Keyvan Nouri
(Editor)

Lasers in Dermatology and Medicine

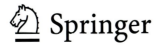

Editor
Keyvan Nouri, MD
Professor of Dermatology and Otolaryngology
Director of Mohs, Dermatologic and Laser Surgery
Director of Surgical Training
Chief of Dermatology at Sylvester Comprehensive
Cancer Center/University of Miami Hospital
and
Clinics, Department of Dermatology and Cutaneous Surgery
University of Miami, Leonard M. Miller School of Medicine
1475 N.W. 12th Avenue
Miami, Florida-33136
USA

ISBN 978-0-85729-280-3 e-ISBN 978-0-85729-281-0
DOI 10.1007/978-0-85729-281-0
Springer London Dordrecht Heidelberg New York

British Library Cataloguing in Publication Data
A catalogue record for this book is available from the British Library

Library of Congress Control Number: 2011922528

© Springer-Verlag London Limited 2011
Apart from any fair dealing for the purposes of research or private study, or criticism or review, as permitted under the Copyright, Designs and Patents Act 1988, this publication may only be reproduced, stored or transmitted, in any form or by any means, with the prior permission in writing of the publishers, or in the case of reprographic reproduction in accordance with the terms of licenses issued by the Copyright Licensing Agency. Enquiries concerning reproduction outside those terms should be sent to the publishers.
The use of registered names, trademarks, etc., in this publication does not imply, even in the absence of a specific statement, that such names are exempt from the relevant laws and regulations and therefore free for general use.
Product liability: The publisher can give no guarantee for information about drug dosage and application thereof contained in this book. In every individual case the respective user must check its accuracy by consulting other pharmaceutical literature.

Cover design: eStudioCalamar, Figueres/Berlin

Printed on acid-free paper

Springer is part of Springer Science+Business Media (www.springer.com)

I dedicate this book to my family and friends who have been there for me in every instance of my life.

I would especially dedicate this book to my wife Dr. Firouzeh Miremadi, and my son Kian Nouri.

I would also like to make a dedication to my mother Mrs. Zohreh Khajavi-Noori, my father Dr. Ali Nouri, my sister Dr. Mahnaz Nouri, my uncle Dr. Farrokh Khajavi, my Grandparents and the rest of my dear family.

I love you all.

Foreword

A refreshing trait of this book about lasers in dermatology is that it is the first in years, to place this topic within the broader perspective of other medical specialties. Almost immediately after the first laser was created in 1960, a handful of visionary physicians recognized that this extremely powerful source of light might have surgical applications. Those pioneers practiced in three organ systems openly accessible for light exposure – ophthalmology, dermatology, laryngology. These are still the specialties that rely heavily on surgical lasers (with the addition of urology, thanks to laser lithotripsy and prostatectomy). By far, dermatologists have a greater variety of therapeutic lasers than any other medical group, while lagging behind in other aspects of laser medicine.

How did we get such a wide, almost dazzling, variety of treatment lasers in dermatology? (*Because, we need them for different uses in various practice settings; lasers are the most tissue-specific surgical tools in existence.*) Do we really need so many? (*Well, we need most all of them. Only a few are interchangeable.*) Are the mechanistic, clinical, safety, ethical and practice-related chapters of this book worthy of study? (*Yes.*) Can't we just learn which buttons to push, in courses provided by the more reputable device manufacturers just after a laser is purchased? (*This approach is foolish beyond words, yet such fools exist. You may encounter them, and some of the patients they have harmed. Even more foolish are those who purchase a used laser and start using it without any training whatsoever.*)

Another asset of this text is its practicality, whether you use lasers or not. If you get hooked on laser dermatology please talk to your colleagues, and attend bona fide laser medical conferences that include your particular clinical interests, in which you are free to ask questions of faculty who are not trying to sell something. Pay close attention to the quality and source of clinical evidence regarding safety and efficacy of a particular laser device. There is no substitute for hands-on training, which cannot be obtained in this book or sitting in a lecture hall. Yet another asset of this book is the breadth of its clinical discussions. Some of the best uses for dermatological lasers are not FDA-labeled indications, and probably never will be. Almost half of my practice with lasers (and with many drugs as well) involves such "off-label" uses. Despite excellent effort by the dedicated people of FDA, clearance of a device for a particular labeled indication, cannot be taken as any assurance that it will work safely and effectively enough to satisfy you and your patients, while lack of FDA clearance for a specific indication cannot be taken as any assurance that it will not work safely and effectively. Many companies and the FDA itself, do not have the resources to keep labeled indications accurately up to date based on clinical evidence. Fortunately, the actual practice of medicine is not part of their mandate. Laser companies are restricted from discussing off-label indications even when these may be a major medical interest. Reading this book is a peer-to-peer event entirely free of such encumbrances!

It is remarkable what lasers can do for our patients. But, we still have a long way to go before the promise of lasers is even close to fulfilled. Diagnostic lasers are heavily used in ophthalmology, yet almost never used in dermatology. The ease and diagnostic confidence of skin biopsies tends to postpone that development, while the difficulty or impossibility of eye biopsies has driven strong development of diagnostic ophthalmic lasers. Ironically, dermatology will end up adopting some amazing laser microscopies from internal organ imaging, e.g. of coronary arteries. In another 50 years, I expect that all medical specialties will rely heavily on laser technologies for both diagnosis and treatments, and that these will in turn become well integrated. Our peculiar use of Mohs surgery is not because skin cancer is the only tumor best removed with microscopic margin control – indeed, skin cancer may be least in need of it. Why, then, are we the only specialty that removes cancer with detailed, microscopic margin control? Because our patients are happily awake during surgery! The glacial pace of Mohs surgery is not tolerable in most operating rooms, and that pace is set by reliance on conventional microscopy. When laser microscopy and laser tissue ablation are finally married, every part of surgical oncology may be affected.

I have been fortunate to play a role in launching several eras of laser dermatology, including some fundamental understanding of skin optics, the concept of selective photothermolysis, lasers specifically designed for dermatological use, permanent laser hair removal, scanning confocal laser microscopy, and more recently, "fractional" laser treatments. We have become fairly good at using lasers to create precise injury, a benevolent form of tissue destruction on the scale that tissue itself is constructed. However, we have barely begun to understand some equally promising therapeutic strategies that may help our patients. Fractional ablative lasers appear to offer a new way for delivery of topical agents, including very high molecular weight macromolecules, and particles. Due to the artificial separation of devices from drugs, of procedural from medical dermatology, we know very little about how to combine lasers with drug treatment. Light-activated drug therapy is one of the oldest known treatments (PUVA arose from treatments dating back about 3500 years), and yet light-activated drugs have never been developed with the high-throughput and targeted approaches routinely used for new drug discovery. Visible and near-infrared light at certain "biostimulating" wavelengths have subtle, poorly understood, but potent effects on cell metabolism. This is particularly the case in settings of hypoxic, ischemic, or oxidative stress. We have just begun to harness the power of light, particularly laser light, in medicine.

Thank you, Dr. Nouri and the many authors involved in this text, for this excellent contribution.

R. Rox Anderson, MD

Preface

Laser technology is quickly evolving with the presence of newer lasers, along with new indications, that are constantly being introduced. The use of lasers has become a major discipline and is currently practiced in Dermatology, Plastic Surgery, Ophthalmology, Cardiology, Gynecology, Otolaryngology, Neurology/Neurosurgery etc. This book offers comprehensive literature covering all the major disciplines in medicine in which lasers are being used.

The authors of *Lasers in Dermatology and Medicine* are well known in their respective fields and have attempted to cover each topic in the most comprehensive, readable, and understandable format. Each chapter consists of an introduction and summary boxes in bulleted formats with up-to-date information highlighting the importance of each respective section, enabling the reader to have an easy approach towards reading and understanding the various topics on lasers. This book has been written with the sincere hope of the editors and the authors to serve as a cornerstone of laser usage in Dermatology and medicine ultimately leading to better patient care and treatments.

Lasers in Dermatology and Plastic Surgery have clearly expanded. The areas or laser treatments include port wine stains, vascular anomalies and lesions, pigmented lesions and tattoos, hair removal and hair re-growth, acne, facial rejuvenation, psoriasis, hypopigmented lesions and vitiligo, and treatment of fat and cellulites, among others. The lasers are also being used for treatment and diagnosis of skin cancers.

Lasers in other fields of medicine have also significantly evolved and expanded significantly. For instance, in Ophthalmology, there are chapters for treatment of anterior segment (i.e. laser vision correction), posterior segments of the eye and control of intraocular pressure.

Furthermore, this book incorporates chapters on the use of lasers in the fields of Cardiology, Gynecology, General Surgery, Anesthesiology, Urology, Neurology and many other specialized branches of medicine making it a unique laser textbook. The expanding knowledge and growing expertise in lasers and light devices makes it necessary for physicians to be up-to-date about the advancements in this field.

We anticipate that this book will be of interest to all the physicians who use or are interested in using lasers in their practice. We are extremely grateful to our contributing authors. This book will serve as a potential study source for dermatologists, plastic surgeons, and laser specialists in different specialties of medicine and surgery.

Miami, Florida   Keyvan Nouri

Acknowledgements

I would like to sincerely thank my family for their support and encouragement throughout my life.

Special thanks to Dr. Lawrence A. Schachner, Chairman of the Department of Dermatology and Cutaneous Surgery at the University of Miami Miller School of Medicine. He has given me great support and has served as a mentor throughout my professional career. His guidance and encouragement over the years have influenced my efforts.

Dr. William H. Eaglestein, former Chairman of Dermatology at the University of Miami School of Medicine, for helping and guiding me since my start in dermatology. I appreciate all of his guidance and support.

Dr. Perry Robins, Dr. Robin Ashinoff, Dr. Vicki Levine, Dr. Seth Orlow, the late Dr. Irvin Freedberg, Dr. Hideko Kamino, and the entire faculty and staff at New York University School of Medicine Department of Dermatology. Thank you all for the wonderful learning and friendship during my surgery fellowship.

I would like to thank the faculty and Dermatology residents, and staff of the Department of Dermatology and Cutaneous Surgery at the University of Miami Miller school of Medicine, for their teaching, expertise, and friendship. Special acknowledgements to the Mohs and Laser Center staff at the Sylvester Cancer Center for their hard work and support on a daily basis. I would also like to thank Maria D. Garcia, my administrative assistant, for her diligence and hard work and the rest of the Mohs staff, including Cathy Mamas, Juana Alonso, Tania Garcia, Veronica Sanchez, Liseth Velasquez, Tatania Carmouze and Lisbeth Napoles, for making my job a pleasure.

Special thanks to my clinical research fellows in Dermatologic Surgery, Dr. Sonal Choudhary, Dr. Mohamed Elsaie and Dr. Voraphol Vejjabhinanta for all their hard work and contributions to this book. Also, I would like to thank Dr. Angela Martins, Dr. Michael Shiman, Angel Leiva and Michael Patrick McLeod for their help in putting this book together.

I would also like to acknowledge the publishing staff Mr. Grant Weston, Ms. Cate Rogers, Ms. Katy Stevens, Ms. Hannah Wilson and the entire Springer Publishing team for having done a superb job with the publication. It has been a pleasure working with them and this excellent project to compile the textbook.

Lastly, I would like to sincerely thank all the authors of this textbook. These individuals are world-renowned in their respective specialties and without their time and energy, writing this book would have not been possible. These individuals have made this a comprehensive, up-to-date, and reliable source on Lasers in Dermatology and Medicine. I truly appreciate their hard work and thank them for their contributions.

Keyvan Nouri, MD

Contents

1 Laser-Tissue Interactions 1
E. Victor Ross and Nathan Uebelhoer

2 Laser Safety: Regulations, Standards and Practice Guidelines 25
Ashley Keyes and Murad Alam

3 Lasers for Treatment of Vascular Lesions 33
Daniel Michael and Suzanne Kilmer

4 Laser for Scars 45
Voraphol Vejjabhinanta, Shalu S. Patel, and Keyvan Nouri

5 Laser Treatment of Leg Veins 53
Robert A. Weiss, Girish S. Munavalli, Sonal Choudhary, Angel Leiva,
and Keyvan Nouri

6 Lasers and Lights for Treating Pigmented Lesions 63
Emmy M. Graber and Jeffrey S. Dover

7 Laser Treatment of Tattoos 83
Voraphol Vejjabhinanta, Caroline V. Caperton, Christopher Wong,
Rawat Charoensawad, and Keyvan Nouri

8 Laser for Hair Removal 91
Voraphol Vejjabhinanta, Keyvan Nouri, Anita Singh, Ran Huo,
and Rawat Charoensawad

9 Lasers for Resurfacing 103
Rungsima Wanitphakdeedecha and Tina S. Alster

10 Fractional Photothermolysis 123
Dieter Manstein and Hans-Joachim Laubach

11 Plasma Resurfacing 149
K. Wade Foster, Edgar F. Fincher, and Ronald L. Moy

12 Sub-Surfacing Lasers 161
Michael H. Gold

13 Non-invasive Rejuvenation/Skin Tightening: Light-Based Devices 175
Javier Ruiz-Esparza

14 Laser and Light Therapies for Acne 187
Voraphol Vejjabhinanta, Anita Singh, Rawat Charoensawad, and Keyvan Nouri

15 Lasers for Psoriasis and Hypopigmentation 193
Aaron M. Bruce and James M. Spencer

16 Lasers and Lights for Adipose Tissue and Cellulite 199
Molly Wanner and Mathew Avram

17 Intense Pulse Light (IPL) 207
Robert A. Weiss, Girish S. Munavalli, Sonal Choudhary, Angel Leiva,
and Keyvan Nouri

18 Photodynamic Therapy 221
Robert Bissonnette

19 Light-Emitting Diode Phototherapy in Dermatological Practice 231
R. Glen Calderhead

20 Laser and Light for Wound Healing Stimulation 267
Navid Bouzari, Mohamed L. Elsaie, and Keyvan Nouri

21 Lasers in Hair Growth and Hair Transplantation 277
Nicole E. Rogers, Joseph Stuto, and Marc R. Avram

22 Reflectance-Mode Confocal Microscopy in Dermatological Oncology 285
Juan Luis Santiago Sánchez-Mateos, Carmen Moreno García del Real,
Pedro Jaén Olasolo, and Salvador González

23 Laser Clinical and Practice Pearls 309
Lori A. Brightman and Roy Geronemus

24 The Selection and Education of Laser Patients 321
Murad Alam and Natalie Kim

25 Anesthesia for Laser Surgery 329
Voraphol Vejjabhinanta, Angela Martins, Ran Huo,
and Keyvan Nouri

26 Laser Application for Ethnic Skin 337
Heather Woolery-Lloyd and Mohamed L. Elsaie

27 Laser Applications in Children 345
Mercedes E. Gonzalez, Michael Shelling, and Elizabeth Alvarez Connelly

28 Dressings/Wound Care for Laser Treatment 359
Stephen C. Davis and Robert Perez

29 Prevention and Treatment of Laser Complications 365
Rachael L. Moore, Juan-Carlos Martinez, and Ken K. Lee

30 Ethical Issues 379
Abel Torres, Tejas Desai, Alpesh Desai, and William Kirby

31 Medicolegal Issues (Documentation/Informed Consent) 383
Abel Torres, Tejas Desai, Alpesh Desai, and William Kirby

32 Psychological Aspects to Consider Within Laser Treatments 387
Dee Anna Glaser

33 Photography of Dermatological Laser Treatment 399
Ashish C. Bhatia, Shraddha Desai, and Doug Roach

34 Online Resources for Dermatologic Laser Therapies 409
Elizabeth E. Uhlenhake, Shraddha Desai, and Ashish C. Bhatia

35 Starting a Laser Practice 413
Vic A. Narurkar

36 Research and Future Directions 417
Fernanda Hidemi Sakamoto and Richard Rox Anderson

37 Laser/Light Applications in Ophthalmology: Visual Refraction 425
Mahnaz Nouri, Amit Todani, and Roberto Pineda

38 Laser/Light Applications in Ophthalmology:
Posterior Segment Applications 435
Amy C. Schefler, Charles C. Wykoff, and Timothy G. Murray

39 Laser/Light Application in Ophthalmology:
Control of Intraocular Pressure 447
Ramez I. Haddadin and Douglas J. Rhee

40 Laser/Light Application in Dental Procedures 463
Steven P.A. Parker

41 Laser/Light Applications in Otolaryngology 495
Vanessa S. Rothholtz and Brian J.F. Wong

42 Laser/Light Applications in Gynecology 523
Cornelia de Riese and Roger Yandell

43 Laser/Light Applications in General Surgery 539
Raymond J. Lanzafame

44 Laser/Light Applications in Urology 561
Nathaniel M. Fried and Brian R. Matlaga

45 Lasers in Cardiology and Cardiothoracic Surgery................ 573
Pritam R. Polkampally, Allyne Topaz, and On Topaz

46 Laser/Light Applications in Neurology and Neurosurgery.......... 583
Marlon S. Mathews, David Abookasis, and Mark E. Linskey

47 Laser/Light Applications in Anesthesiology...................... 597
Julie A. Gayle, Elizabeth A.M. Frost, Clifford Gevirtz,
Sajay B. Churi, and Alan D. Kaye

Index.. 613

Contributors

David Abookasis, PhD Beckman Laser Institute and Medical Clinic, University of California, Irvine, CA, USA

Murad Alam, MD, MSCI Department of Dermatology, Otolaryngology – Head and Neck Surgery, Northwestern University, Chicago, IL, USA

Tina S. Alster, MD Washington Institute of Dermatologic Laser Surgery, Georgetown University Medical Center, Washington, DC, USA

Richard Rox Anderson, MD Professor of Dermatology, Director of the Wellman Center for Photomedicine, Department of Dermatology, Harvard Medical School, Massachusetts General Hospital, Boston, MA, USA

Marc R. Avram, MD Department of Dermatology, Weill Cornell Medical Center, New York, NY, USA

Mathew Avram, MD, JD Department of Dermatology, Massachusetts General Hospital, Harvard Medical School, Boston, MA, USA

Ashish C. Bhatia, MD, FAAD Department of Dermatology, Northwestern University Feinberg School of Medicine, Chicago, IL, USA *and* The Dermatology Institute of DuPage Medical Group, Naperville, IL, USA

Robert Bissonnette, MD Innovaderm Research Inc., Montreal, Quebec, Canada

Navid Bouzari, MD Department of Dermatology, University of Miami, Miller School of Medicine, Miami, FL, USA

Lori A. Brightman, MD Department of Dermatology/Department of Plastic *and* Reconstructive Surgery, New York Eye and Ear Infirmary, New York, NY, USA

Aaron M. Bruce, DO Center for Surgical Dermatology, Westerville, OH, USA

R. Glen Calderhead, MSc PhD(MedSci) FRSM Japan Phototherapy Laboratory, Tsugamachi, Tochigi-ken, Japan

Caroline V. Caperton MSPH University of Miami, Miller School of Medicine, Miami, FL, USA

Rawat Charoensawad, MD Rawat Clinic and Clinical Consultant, Biophile Training Center, Bangkok, Thailand

Sonal Choudhary, MD Department of Dermatology and Cutaneous Surgery, University of Miami, Miller School of Medicine, Miami, FL, USA

Sajay B. Churi, MD, MS Department of Anesthesiology, Tulane University Health Sciences Center, New Orleans, LA, USA

Elizabeth Alvarez Connelly, MD Department of Dermatology and Cutaneous Surgery, University of Miami, Miller School of Medicine, Miami, FL, USA

Stephen C. Davis, BS Department of Dermatology and Cutaneous Surgery, University of Miami, Miller School of Medicine, Miami, FL, USA

Shraddha Desai, MD The Dermatology Institute of DuPage Medical Group, Naperville, IL, USA *and* Loyola University - Stritch School of Medicine, Maywood, IL, USA

Jeffrey S. Dover, MD, FRCPC Department of Dermatology, SkinCare Physicians, Chestnut Hill, MA, USA

Mohamed L. Elsaie, MD, MBA Department of Dermatology and Cutaneous Surgery, University of Miami, Miller School of Medicine, Miami, FL, USA

Edgar F. Fincher, MD, PhD Fincher Dermatology and Cosmetic Surgery, Beverly-Hills, CA, USA

K. Wade Foster, MD, PhD Moy-Fincher Medical Group, Los Angeles, CA, USA

Nathaniel M. Fried, PhD Department of Physics and Optical Science, University of North Carolina, Charlotte, NC, USA

Elizabeth A. M. Frost, MD Mount Sinai Medical Center, New York, NY, USA

Carmen Moreno García del Real Patology Service, Hospital Ramón y Cajal, Alcala University, Madrid, Spain

Julie A. Gayle, MD Department of Anesthesiology, Louisiana Health Sciences Center, New Orleans, LA, USA

Roy Geronemus, MD Laser and Skin Surgery Center of NY, New York, NY, USA

Clifford Gevirtz, MD, MPH Department of Anesthesiology, Louisiana Health Sciences Center, New Orleans, LA, USA

Dee Anna Glaser, MD Department of Dermatology, Saint Louis University School of Medicine, Saint Louis, MO, USA

Michael H. Gold, MD Gold Skin Care Center, Tennessee Clinical Research Center, The Laser Rejuvenation Center, Advanced Aesthetics Medi-Spa, Nashville, TN, USA *and* Department of Dermatology, Vanderbilt University School of Medicine, Vanderbilt University School of Nursing, Nashville, TN, USA

Mercedes E. Gonzalez, MD Department of Dermatology and Cutaneous Surgery, University of Miami, Miller School of Medicine, Miami, FL, USA

Salvador González, MD, PhD Dermatology Service, Memorial Sloan-Kettering Cancer Center, New York, NY, USA *and* Ramón y Cajal Hospital, Alcalá University, Madrid, Spain

Emmy M. Graber, MD Department of Dermatology, Boston University, Director Cosmetic and Laser Center, Boston University, Associate Director, Residency Training Program, Boston, MA, USA

Ramez I. Haddadin Department of Ophthalmology, Massachusetts Eye & Ear Infirmary, Boston, MA, USA

Ran Huo, MD Department of Dermatology and Cutaneous Surgery, University of Miami, Miller School of Medicine, Miami, FL, USA

Alan D. Kaye, MD, PhD Department of Anesthesiology, School of Medicine, Louisiana Health Sciences Center, New Orleans, LA, USA

Ashley Keyes, BA Department of Dermatology, Northwestern University, Feinberg School of Medicine, Chicago, IL, USA

Suzanne Kilmer, MD Department of Dermatology, University of California, Davis, Medical Center, Laser and Skin Surgery Center of Northern California, Sacramento, CA, USA

Natalie Kim, MD Department of Dermatology, Feinberg School of Medicine, Northwestern University, Chicago, IL, USA

Raymond J. Lanzafame, MD, PLLC

Hans-Joachim Laubach, MD Massachusetts General Hospital, Wellman Center for Photomedicine, Harvard Medical School, Boston, MA, USA

Ken K. Lee, MD Dermatologic and Laser Surgery, Oregon Health and Science University, Portland, OR, USA

Angel Leiva Department of Dermatology and Cutaneous Surgery, University of Miami, Miller School of Medicine, Miami, FL, USA

Mark E. Linskey, MD Department of Neurological Surgery, University of California, Irvine, CA, USA

Dieter Manstein, MD, PhD Massachusetts General Hospital, Wellman Center for Photomedicine, Harvard Medical School, Boston, MA, USA

Juan-Carlos Martinez, MD Dermatologic and Laser Surgery, Oregon Health and Science University, Portland, OR, USA

Angela Martins, MD University of Miami, Miller School of Medicine, Miami, Florida, USA

Marlon S. Mathews, MB, BS Department of Neurosurgery, University of California, Irvine, CA, USA

Brian R. Matlaga, MD, MPH Department of Urology, Johns Hopkins University, Baltimore, MD, USA

Daniel Michael, MD, PhD Department of Dermatology, University of California, Davis, Medical Center, Laser and Skin Surgery Center of Northern California, Sacramento, CA, USA

Rachael L. Moore, MD Dermatologic and Laser Surgery, Oregon Health and Science University, Portland, OR, USA

Ronald L. Moy, MD Moy-Fincher Medical Group, Los Angeles, CA, USA

Girish S. Munavalli, MD, MHS Department of Dermatology, Johns Hopkins University, Charlotte, NC, USA

Timothy G. Murray, MD, FACS, MBA Department of Ophthalmology, Bascom Palmer Eye Institute, University of Miami, Miller School of Medicine, FL, USA

Vic A. Narurkar, MD, FAAD Department of Dermatology, California Pacific Medical Center, San Francisco, CA, USA

Keyvan Nouri, MD Professor of Dermatology and Otolaryngology, Director of Mohs, Dermatologic and Laser Surgery, Director of Surgical Training, Chief of Dermatology at Sylvester Comprehensive Cancer Center/University of Miami Hospital and Clinics Department of Dermatology and Cutaneous Surgery, University of Miami, Leonard M. Miller School of Medicine, Miami, FL, USA

Mahnaz Nouri, MD Boston Eye Group, Beacon Street, Brookline, MA, USA

Pedro Jaén Olasolo Dermatology Service, Memorial Sloan-Kettering Cancer Center, New York, NY, USA

Steven P. A. Parker, BDS, LDS, RCS, MFGDP Private Dental Practice, Harrogate, United Kingdom and A.C. Faculty of Medicine, University of Genoa, Italy

Shalu S. Patel, BS Department of Dermatology and Cutaneous Surgery, University of Miami, Miller School of Medicine, Miami, FL, USA

Robert Perez, MD Department of Dermatology and Cutaneous Surgery, University of Miami, Miller School of Medicine, Miami, FL, USA

Roberto Pineda, MD Department of Opthalmology, Massachusetts Ear and Eye Hospital, Boston, MA, USA

Pritam R. Polkampally, MD Department of Cardiology, Virginia Commonwealth University, Richmond, VA, USA

Douglas J. Rhee, MD Department of Ophthalmology, Massachusetts Eye & Ear Infirmary, Boston, MA, USA

Cornelia de Riese, MD, PhD Obstetrics and Gynecology, Texas Tech University Health Sciences Center, Lubbock, TX, USA

Doug Roach, BS University of Miami, Miller School of Medicine, Miami, FL, USA

Nicole E. Rogers, MD Department of Dermatology, Tulane Medical Center, New Orleans, LA, NY, USA

E. Victor Ross, MD Laser and Cosmetic Dermatology, Scripps Clinic, San Diego, CA, USA

Vanessa S. Rothholtz, MD, MSc Department of Otolaryngology – Head and Neck Surgery, University of California, Irvine, CA, USA

Javier Ruiz-Esparza, MD Department of Dermatology, University of California, San Diego, CA, USA

Fernanda Hidemi Sakamoto, MD Instructor in Dermatology, Department of Dermatology, Wellman Center for Photomedicine, Harvard Medical School, Massachusetts General Hospital, Boston, MA, USA

Juan Luis Santiago Sánchez-Mateos Dermatology Service, Hospital Ramón y Cajal, Alcala University, Madrid, Spain

Amy C. Schefler, MD Department of Ophthalmology, Bascom Palmer Eye Institute, Miami, FL, USA

Michael Shelling, MD Department of Dermatology and Cutaneous Surgery, University of Miami, Miller School of Medicine, Miami, FL, USA

Michael Shiman, MD Department of Dermatology and Cutaneous Surgery, University of Miami, Miller School of Medicine, Miami, FL, USA

Anita Singh, MD Montefiore Medical Center, Albert Einstein College of Medicine, Bronx, NY

James M. Spencer, MD, MS Spencer Dermatology & Skin Surgery, St. Petersburgh, FL, USA

Joseph Stuto, BA Department of Dermatology, Weill Cornell Medical Center, New York, NY, USA

Amit Todani, MD Albany Medical Center, Albany, NY, USA

Allyne Topaz, BS School of Medicine, St. George's University, St. George, Grenada, West Indies

On Topaz, MD Duke University School of Medicine, Division of Cardiology, Charles George Veterans Affairs Medical Center, Asheville, NC, USA

Abel Torres, MD, JD Department of Dermatology, Loma Linda University School of Medicine, Loma Linda, CA, USA

Nathan Uebelhoer, MD Naval Medical Center San Diego, San Diego, CA, USA

Elizabeth E. Uhlenhake, BS Northeastern Ohio Universities College of Medicine, Rootstown, OH, USA

Voraphol Vejjabhinanta, MD Department of Dermatology and Cutaneous Surgery, University of Miami, Leonard M. Miller School of Medicine, Miami, FL and Department of Dermatology, Siriraj Hospital, Mahidol University, Bangkok, Thailand

Rungsima Wanitphakdeedecha, MD, MA, MSC Department of Dermatology, Faculty of Medicine Siriraj Hospital, Mahidol University, Bangkok, Thailand

Molly Wanner, MD, MBA Department of Dermatology, Massachusetts General Hospital, Harvard Medical School, Boston, MA, USA

Robert A. Weiss, MD Department of Dermatology, Johns Hopkins University School of Medicine, Hunt Valley, MD, USA

Brian J. F. Wong, MD, PhD, FACS Division of Facial Plastic and Reconstructive Surgery, Department of Otolaryngology Head and Neck Surgery, Department of Biomedical Engineering, Department of Surgery and The Beckman Laser Institute, University of California, Irvine, CA, USA

Christopher Wong, MD University of Miami, Miller School of Medicine, Miami, Florida, USA

Heather Woolery-Lloyd, MD Department of Dermatology and Cutaneous Surgery, University of Miami, Miller School of Medicine, Miami, FL, USA

Charles C. Wykoff, D. Phil., MD Department of Ophthalmology, Bascom Palmer Eye Institute, University of Miami, Miller School of Medicine, Miami, FL, USA

Roger Yandell, MD Obstetrics and Gynecology, Texas Tech University Health Sciences Center, Lubbock, TX, USA

Tejas Desai, DO Associate Professor Clinical Dermatology, Western University of Health Sciences, Pomona, CA, USA and
Associate Professor Clinical Dermatology, University of North Texas, Texas College of Osteopatic Medicine, Ft Worth, TX, USA

Alpesh Desai, DO Program Director for South Texas Dermatology Residency Program, University of North Texas/TCOM, Ft Worth, TX, USA

William Kirby, DO Clinical Assistant Professor, Division of Dermatology, Nova Southeastern University, Ft Lauderdale, FL, USA and
Clinical Assistant Professor of Dermatology, Western University of Health Sciences, Pomona,CA, USA

Laser-Tissue Interactions

E. Victor Ross and Nathan Uebelhoer

The reader should note that although the title of this chapter is "Laser Tissue Interactions", the introduction of many new and diverse technologies make the term somewhat obsolete. We will continue to use the term, but a more appropriate is "electromagnetic radiation (EMR) – tissue interactions". We will use both terms interchangeably in the remainder of the text.

Introduction

1. Light represents one portion of a broader electromagnetic spectrum.
2. Light-tissue interactions involve the complex topics of tissue optics, absorption, heat generation, and heat diffusion
3. Lasers are a special type of light with the characteristics of monochromaticity, directionality, and coherence.
4. Coagulation/denaturation is time and temperature dependent
5. Proper selection of light parameters is based on the color, size, and geometry of the target
6. Wound healing is the final but not least important part of the laser tissue sequence (the epilogue)
7. Laser-tissue interactions are fluid – the operator should closely examine the skin surface during all aspects of the procedure
8. Pulse duration and light doses are often as important as wavelength in predicting tissue responses to laser to irradiation

E. Victor Ross (✉)
Laser and Cosmetic Dermatology, Scripps Clinic,
San Diego, CA, USA
e-mail: ross.edward@scrippshealth.org

The best gauge of laser interactions is the tissue response, and experiment is the most realistic manner to address medical treatment challenges. However, theoretical models are helpful in planning treatment approaches and laser parameters. In this chapter we discuss basics of lasers, their non-laser counterparts, and laser-tissue interactions.[1]

Many physicians choose laser settings out of habit (or reading it off of a label attached to the side of the machine – a "cheat" sheet with skin-type specific parameters), using tissue endpoints to confirm the appropriateness of the parameters. For example, when treating a tattoo with a Q-switched laser, the operator looks for immediate frosty whitening. Like driving a car (where the operator may have no idea about nature of the drive train components), successful laser operation does not demand a complete understanding of the machine or the details of the light-tissue interaction. However, a comprehension of first principles allows for a logical analysis of final clinical outcomes – furthermore, more creative uses of equipment should follow. For example, with an education in laser tissue interactions (LTIs) and tissue cooling, one can deploy the alexandrite (long pulse) laser either as a hair removal device, vascular laser, or to remove lentigines.[2]

Light

Light represents one portion of a much broader electromagnetic spectrum. Light can be divided into the UV (200–400 nm), VIS (400–700 nm), NIR "I" (755–810 nm), NIR "II" (940–1,064 nm), MIR (1.3–3 μm), and Far IR (3 μm and beyond). On a macroscopic level, light is adequately characterized as waves. The amplitude of the wave is perpendicular to the propagation direction. Light waves behave according to our "eyeball" observations in day-to-day life. For example, we are familiar with refraction and reflection. The surface of a pond is a partial mirror (reflection); a fish seen in the pond is actually closer than it appears (refraction).[3] Normally, the percentage of incident light reflected from the skin surface is determined by the index of refraction difference between the skin surface (stratum corneum $n = 1.55$)

K. Nouri (ed.), *Lasers in Dermatology and Medicine*,
DOI: 10.1007/978-0-85729-281-0_1, © Springer-Verlag London Limited 2011

and air ($n = 1$).[4] This regular reflectance is about 4–7% for light incident at right angles to the skin.[3,5] The angle between the light beam and the skin surface determines the % of reflected light. More light is reflected at "grazing" angles of incidence. It follows that, to minimize surface losses, in most laser applications, one should deliver light approximately perpendicular to the skin.[3,6] One can deliberately angle the beam, on the other hand, to decrease penetration depth and also attenuate the surface fluence by "spreading" the beam. One can reduce interface losses by applying an alcohol solution ($n = 1.4$), water ($n = 1.33$), or a sapphire crystal ($n = 1.55$ μm). This allows for optical coupling (vide infra). On the other hand, the surface of dry skin reflects more light because of multiple skin–air interfaces (hence the white appearance of a psoriasis plaque).

Light penetrates into the epidermis according to wavelength dependent absorption and scattering (vide infra).[1,6-8] Because of scattering, much incident light is remitted (remittance refers to the total light returned to the environment due to multiple scattering in the epidermis and dermis, as well as the regular reflection from the surface). In laser surgery, light reflected from the surface is typically "wasted". This "lost" energy varies from 15% to as much as 70% depending on wavelength and skin type. For example, for 1,064 nm, 60% of an incident laser beam may be remitted. One can easily verify this by holding a finger just adjacent to the beam near the skin surface. Warmth can be felt from the remitted portion of the beam.

To describe laser tissue interactions at the molecular/microscopic level, light is considered as a stream of "particles" called photons, where the photon energy depends on the wavelength of light.

$$E_{photon} = hc/\lambda \qquad (1)$$

Where h is Plank's constant (6.6×10^{-34} J-s), and c is the speed of light (3×10^{10} cm/s).[9]

Types of Light Devices

In principle, many non-laser devices could be used for heating skin.[9] Most properties of laser light (i.e., coherence) are unimportant insofar as the way light interacts with tissue in therapeutic applications. And although collimation (lack of divergence) of the incident beam might increase the % of transmitted light with laser versus IPL, the increasing use of filtered flash lamps in dermatology suggests that losses from IPL beam divergence are not critical. In lieu of lasers, some thermal sources can be used in skin surgery (i.e., nitrogen plasma device) for resurfacing (Portrait, Rhytec, MA). The critical features of any device are controlling the device-tissue interaction time to allow for precise heating (vide infra).

Lasers are useful because they allow for precise control of where and how much one heats.[10] There are four properties that are common to all laser types (1) Beam directionality (collimation), (2) Monochromaticity, (3) Spatial and temporal coherence of the beam, and (4) High intensity of the beam.[11] The intensity, directionality, and monochromaticity of laser light allow the beam to be expanded, or focused quite easily. With non-laser sources like flashlamps directed toward the skin surface, the light intensity at the skin surface cannot exceed the brightness of the source lamp. With many lasers, a lamp similar to the intense pulsed light (IPL) flashlamp pumps the laser cavity.[12] The *amplification of light* within the laser cavity sets laser light apart from other sources.

For most visible light applications, laser represents a conversion from lamplight to an amplified monochromatic form.[13] The high power possible with lasers (especially *peak power*) is achieved through *resonance* in the laser cavity. For many dermatology applications requiring ms or longer pulses delivered to large skin areas, IPLs are either adequate or preferable to lasers. The scientific principle on which lasers are based is *stimulated emission*. With spontaneous emission, electrons transition to the lower level in a random process. With stimulated emission, the emission occurs only in the presence of photons of a certain change. The critical point is maintaining a condition where the population of photons in a higher state is larger than that in the lower state. To create this population inversion, a pumping energy must be directed either with electricity, light, or chemical energy.

All lasers contain four main components, the lasing medium, the excitation source, feedback apparatus, and an output coupler. With respect to lasing media, there are diode lasers, solid-state lasers, dye, and gas lasers. Most solid state and dye lasers use optical exciters (lamps), whereas gas and diode lasers use electrical excitation (i.e., CO_2 and RF). The feedback mechanism consists of mirrors where one mirror reflects 100% and the other transmits a small fraction of light.[14] An example of a solid-state laser is the alexandrite laser. A solid-state laser consists of a rod that is pumped by a flashlamp. The lamp pumps the rod for stimulated emission. The rod and lamp assembly must also be designed for adequate cooling. Lasers typically are finicky because all of the components are driven near their damage thresholds (like redlining your car all the time). As an example of this concept, consider the pulsed dye laser (PDL). As the dye degrades, the lamps must work harder to generate higher pulse energies from the dye. Also, mirrors become contaminated over time such that the lamps must work harder and harder. These demands stress the power supply. Thus, eventually, the dye kit, the power supply, lamps, and dye are all working at their maximal output. Often people speak of a tunable dye laser. In fact many dye lasers are tunable; the manufacturers have simply chosen one wavelength. An example of a tunable laser was the Scleroplus pulsed dye laser (tunable from 585 to 600 nm in 5 nm increments) from Candela (Candela, Wayland, MA).

Laser systems differ with regard to duration and power of the emitted laser radiation. In continuous wave lasers (CW mode) with power outputs of up to 10^3 W, the lasing medium is excited continuously. With pulsed lasers, excitation is effected in a single pulse or in on-line pulses (free-running mode). Peak powers of 10^5 W can be developed for a duration of 100 μs–10 ms. Storing the excitation energy and releasing it suddenly (Q-switch mode or mode-locking) leads to a peak power increase of up to 10^{10}–10^{12} W, and a pulse duration of 10 ps–100 ns.[13]

Light emitting diodes (LEDs) are becoming commonplace in dermatology (Fig. 1). Primarily used as a PDT light source, they are also used in biostimulation. LEDs are similar to semiconductor (aka diode) lasers in that they use electrical current placed between two types of semiconductors. However, they lack an amplification process (no mirrors). LEDs do not produce coherent beams but can produce monochromatic light. Semiconductor (diode) lasers contain an LED as the active gain medium. A current passes through a sandwich of two layers consisting of compounds (called p type and n type). Below threshold, there is no oscillation and the semiconductor LASER acts like an LED. This emission is very similar to the visible emission of light emitting diodes. If one adds mirrors it operates as a tiny laser instead of an LED. The overall efficiency of semiconductor lasers is quite high, approximately 30% and among the highest available. Most semiconductor (diode) lasers are operated in CW mode but can be pulsed. New visible semiconductor lasers are available and also laser diode arrays are available where scientists have created large numbers of semiconductor lasers on one substrate. Some diode lasers are housed separate from the handpiece and delivered by fiber optics. Others are configured with the laser diodes in the handpiece as arrays. Modern diode lasers achieve higher powers than in the past, but their peak powers are still lag behind most pulsed solid-state lasers.[14]

Excimer lasers emit UV light and are used for photomodulation of the immune system. They have also been used in surgery. The possible mutagenicity of these lasers has not been well studied. Materials such as the KTP crystal can be used to generate harmonics with lasers. The KTP crystal is used to convert 1,064 nm radiation to 532 green light. Also quality (Q) switching is used for generating short pulses. Much of the electrical energy used to create laser emissions is wasted as heat, which is why water is used for cooling most lasers. Air cooling is used for some high-powered flash lamps and many diode lasers. In the future, free electron lasers might be useful but presently they are too cumbersome and only generate small amounts of energy per unit wavelength.

Intense pulsed light devices are becoming increasingly comparable to lasers that emit ms domain pulses.[15] Absorption spectra of skin chromophores show multiple peaks (HgB) or can be broad (melanin),[16] and therefore a broadband light source is a logical alternative to lasers. Proper filtration of a xenon lamp tailors the output spectrum for a particular application. Some concessions are made with direct use of lamplight. For example, rapid beam divergence obliges that the lamp source be near the skin surface. This subsequent requirement makes for a typically heavier handpiece compared with most lasers (Fig. 2) (the exception being some diode arrays where the light source is also housed in the handpiece-(i.e., Light Sheer, Lumenis, CA)). Also IPL cannot be adapted to fibers for subsurface delivery. High energy short pulses (Q–switched ns pulses) are not possible with flashlamps. They can, however, be used to pump a laser, and some modern IPLs feature a laser attachment where the flashlamp and laser rod are in the handpiece. In general, the size, weight, and cost of both laser and flashlamp technology are steadily decreasing.

Light Device Terminology

Basic parameters for light sources are power, time, and spot size for continuous wave lasers, and for pulsed sources, the energy per pulse, pulse duration, spot size, fluence, repetition rate, and the total number of pulses.[17] Energy is measured in joules (J). The amount of energy delivered per unit area is the fluence, sometimes called the dose or radiant exposure, given in J/cm². The rate of energy delivery is called power, measured in watts (W). One watt is one joule per second (W = J/s). The power delivered per unit area is called the irradiance or power density, usually given in W/cm². Laser exposure duration (called pulsewidth for pulsed lasers) is the time over which energy is delivered. Fluence is equal to the irradiance times the exposure duration.[10] Power density is a critical

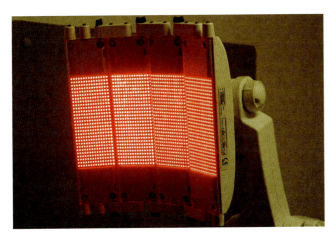

Fig. 1 A *red LED* (OmniLux, Phototherapeutics, Inc.)

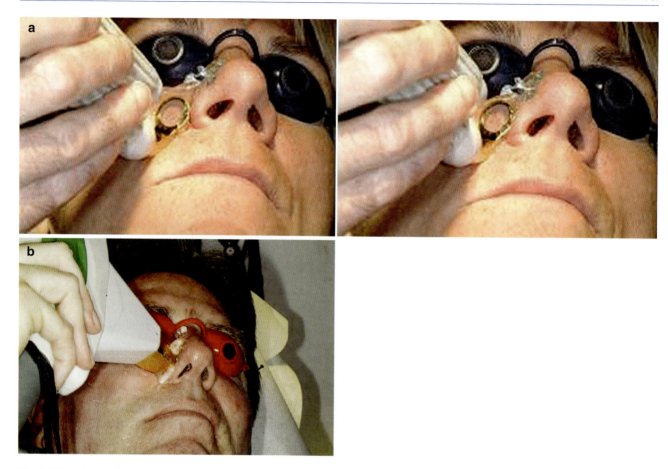

Fig. 2 IPL and *green light laser* – note smaller size of laser handpiece

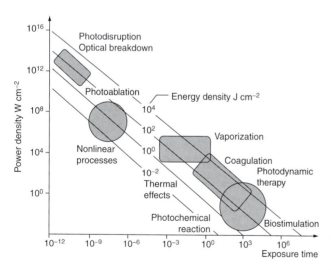

Fig. 3 Different types of laser tissue interactions depend on power density and exposure (From Knappe et al.[18]; Fig. 2)

parameter, for it often determines the action mechanism in cutaneous applications (Fig. 3). For example, a very low irradiance emission (typical range of 2–10 mW/cm²) does not heat tissue and is associated with diagnostic applications, photochemical processes, and biostimulation. On the other extreme, a very short ns pulse can generate high peak power densities associated with shock waves and even plasma formation.[19] Plasma is a "spark" due to ionization of matter.

Another factor is the laser exposure spot size (which greatly affects the beam strength inside the skin). Other characteristics of importance are whether the incident light is convergent, divergent, or diffuse, and the uniformity of irradiance over the exposure area (spatial beam profile). The pulse profile, that is, the character of the pulse shapes in time (instantaneous power versus time) also affects the tissue response.[20]

Many lasers in dermatology are pulsed, and the user interface shows pulse duration, fluence, spot size and fluence. Some multi-wavelength lasers also allow for wavelength selection. Some older lasers, for example a popular CO_2 laser, showed only the pulse energy on the instrument panel, or in continuous wave (CW) mode, the number of watts. In these cases one uses the exposure area and exposure time to calculate the total light dose (fluence).

$$\text{Fluence} = \left(\frac{\text{Power} \times \text{time}}{\text{area}}\right) \quad (2)$$

With the exception of PDT sources and CW CO_2 lasers, most aesthetic lasers create pulsed light. In many CW applications (i.e., wart treatment with a CO_2 laser), the fluence is not of

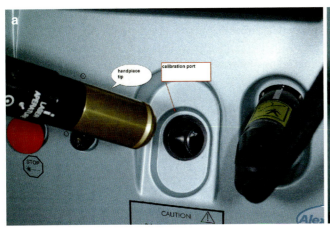 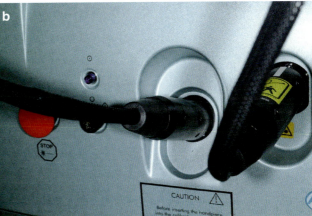

Fig. 4 Figures show handpiece before and during insertion into calibration port of a Q switched alexandrite laser

great importance in characterizing the overall tissue effect. A more important parameter is power density (where higher power densities achieve ablation and lower power densities cause charring), and the physician stops the procedure when an appropriate endpoint is reached. On the other hand, in PDT applications with CW light where the clinical endpoint might be delayed, the total fluence *and* power density are important predictors of the tissue response.

In CW mode, CO_2 lasers are used with a focusing (non-collimated) handpiece such that the physician can control spot size and tissue effects simply by moving the handpiece tip toward or away from the skin. The subsequent rapid changes in power density offer "on the fly" flexibility and control.

A thorough knowledge of a specific laser's operation and quirks is imperative for optimal and "safe" lasering. Vendors are creating lasers that are more intuitive to operate. Increasingly, manufacturers have added touch screen interfaces with application-driven menus and skin-type specific preset parameters. Some devices permit patient laser parameters to be stored for future reference. Most lasers are designed such that the handpiece and instrument panels are electronically interfaced. It follows that the laser control module "knows" what spot size is being used. Typically this "handshake" occurs when one inserts the handpiece into the calibration port, or through a control cable from the handpiece to the laser "main frame". With others, one selects the spotsize on the display, and the laser calculates the fluence accordingly. For example, one of our erbium YAG lasers possesses interchangeable lenses for 1, 3, 5, and 7 mm spots. However, there is no feedback from the handpiece to the laser control board. The user "tells" the laser which lens cell is inserted, and the laser calculates the fluence based on the selected spot and selected pulse energy. In this case, if one changes the spot size (for example, by exchanging the 7 mm for the 3 mm lens cell), the laser still "thinks" the 7 mm spot is being used, and the actual surface fluence is now ~5X the fluence on the panel. The resulting impact on the skin surface (the wound depth and diameter) should alert the enlightened user to reassess his parameter selection.

Most lasers calibrate through a system where the end of the handpiece is placed in a portal on the base unit (Fig. 4). This configuration allows for interrogation of the entire system, from the "pumping" lamps to the fiber/articulated arm to the handpiece optics. For example, if a fiber is damaged, the laser will fail calibration, and an error message appears. Other systems measure the output within the distal end of the handpiece using a small calibration module that "picks off" a portion of the beam.

There are some simple ways to interrogate for system integrity. One can examine the aiming beam as it illuminates a piece of white paper, checking that the beam edges are sharp – this suggests that the treatment beam is also sharp and the profile is according to the manufacturer's specifications. Also, burn paper can be used – here the laser is used with a low energy and the spot is checked for uniformity from beam edge to edge. By checking the impact pattern, one can uncover damaged mirrors in the knuckle of the articulated arm, or a damaged focusing lens that renders the laser unstable or unsafe. Likewise, for scanners, one can ensure that skin coverage will be uniform.

1. LEDs are becoming commonplace in biomedical applications
2. Solid state lasers generally achieve the largest peak powers among laser types
3. The laser operator should know every nook and cranny of a laser's features to optimize patient outcomes and safety
4. Power density determines the mechanism for many LTIs

Beam Profiles: Top Hat Versus Gaussian

Laser beam profiles vary based on intercavity design, lasing medium, and the delivery system. A common profile is Gaussian or bell-shaped. For many lasers, this profile represents the fundamental optimized "mode" of the laser. This shape is usually observed when the beam has been delivered through an articulated arm. For some wavelengths, this is an effective way to deliver energy (CO_2 and erbium). The disadvantage of the rigid arm is limited flexibility, the typically short arm length, the possibility of misalignment from even minor impact, and a tendency for non-uniform heating across the spot.[21] For example, in treating a lentigo with a Q-switched alexandrite laser equipped with a rigid articulated arm, one may observe complete ablation of the epidermis at the center of the "spot", but only whitening at the periphery. On the other hand, sometimes a bell-shaped profile is desirable, for example, when applying a small spot FIR beam with a scanner. In this scenario, the wings of the beam allows for some overlap without delivering "too much" energy at points of overlap.

The Gaussian profile can be modified outside the cavity, which is desirable in many applications. With a fiber equipped delivery system, the beam is mixed within the fiber and can be shaped to be more flat-topped. The lentigo then is more likely to be uniformly heated (so long as the lesion itself if uniformly colored!). Although fiber delivery systems are usually preferred by physicians, some laser beams are difficult to deliver through a fiber. Examples include far IR wavelengths and very short pulses (i.e., few ns with typical Q switched Nd YAG lasers whose high peak power exceeds the damage threshold of most fibers).

Pulse Profiles: Square Versus Spiky

The pulse profile is the temporal shape of the laser pulse (Fig. 5).[22] In many pulsed laser applications, the "macro pulse" is comprised of several shorter micropulses.[23] Depending on the application, the temporal pulse profile may impact the tissue effect. For example, simply by increasing the pulse number from four to six pulselets, the purpura threshold is increased with the PDL. Also, highly energetic spikes tend to increase the epidermal to dermal damage ratio in applications such as laser hair reduction. This is especially true with green-yellow light in vascular applications.

Summary of Wavelength Ranges

In this section we examine wavelength ranges that are useful for cutaneous surgery.

1. UV laser and light sources have been used primarily for treatment of inflammatory skin diseases and/or vitiligo, as well as striae. The presumed action is immunomodulatory. The XeCl excimer laser emits at 308 nm, near the peak action spectrum for psoriasis. Other UV non-laser sources have also been used for hypopigmentation, striae, and various inflammatory diseases.[23,24] Excimer lasers at 193 nm have been used for skin and corneal ablation.

2. Violet IPL emissions, low power 410 nm LED, and fluorescent lamps are used either alone or with ALA. Alone, the devices take advantage of endogenous porphyrins and kill *P. acnes*.[25] After application, of ALA, this wavelength range is highly effective in creating singlet O_2 after absorption by PpIX. Uses include treatment of actinic keratoses, actinic cheilitis, and basal cell carcinomas.[26]

3. *VIS (GY)*. These wavelengths are highly absorbed by HgB and melanin and are especially useful in treating epidermal pigmented lesions and superficial vessels.[27-29] Their relatively poor penetration in skin (and the even poorer penetration in blood – see Table 1) make them poor choices for treatment of *deeper* pigmented lesions or *deeper larger* vessels. Their shallow penetration depths preclude their use in permanent hair reduction (with the possible exception of very large spots (i.e., IPL) that enhance light depth). The effective portions of many IPL spectra include the GY range.

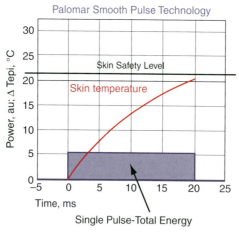
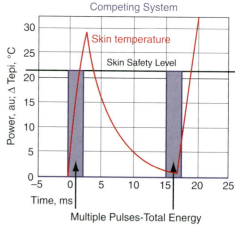

Fig. 5 Figure shows spiky versus smooth pulse and effect on epidermal temperature

Table 1 Absorption coefficients (cm^{-1}) for various chromophores

Wavelength (nm)	410	532	595	694	755	810	940	1,064
Oxy HgB (40% Hct)	1,990	187	35	1.2	2.3	3.6	5.2	2.2
Deoxy HgB	1,296	138	96	6.6	5.2	2.7	3.0	0.6
Melanin[a]	140	56	38	23	17	13	7	5.7
Water	6.7×10^{-5}	0.00044	0.0017	0.005	0.03	0.02	0.27	0.15
Bloodless dermis	10	3	2	1.2	0.8	0.6	0.5	0.4
OPD in skin (μm)	100	350	550	750	1,000	1,200	1,500	1,700

[a](net epidermis) for moderately pigmented adult – 10% mel. volume fraction in epidermis[7,30]

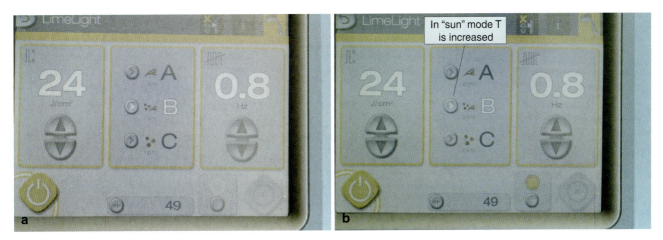

Fig. 6 Figure shows user controllable temperature change with an IPL. By increasing the handpiece tip temperature, pigmented lesion heating is favored over vascular heating

By the proper manipulation a laser delivery device, one can optimize parameters for selective heating of pigmented versus vascular lesions. For example, by applying a compression handpiece without cooling with 595 nm, blood is depleted as a target and pigment is preferentially heated.[31] Also, by (see limelight desert mode – Fig. 6), one can increase or decrease the sapphire window temperature to enhance epidermal versus vascular heating. By reducing the pulsewidth into the nanosecond range, melanosomes are preferentially heated over vessels. For example, extremely short Q-switched 532 nm pulses will cause fine vessels to rupture, but inadequate heat diffusion to the vessel wall precludes long term vessel destruction. On the other hand, melanosomes are sufficiently heated for single-session lentigo destruction. By choosing specific wavelengths with respect to HgB and melanin, one can achieve some degree of selective melanin or HgB heating. For example, if one wanted to avoid HgB in heating a lentigo, 694 nm (ruby) represents a better choice than 532 or 595 nm. This choice might decrease inflammation by unintended heating of normal vessels in the dermis.

There are absorption peaks for PpIX in the green-yellow range, making these wavelengths useful for PDT (i.e., sodium lamp, IPL, frequency doubled Nd YAG, or PDL).[32,33] On the other hand, all visible light can be used for PDT, as the Soret band and smaller "Q-bands" can all create singlet O$_2$ on irradiation of PpIX. Therefore the 532, 595, and IPL devices, when used adjunctively with ALA, can all augment the cosmetic result through both *photothermal* and *photochemical* effects.

4. *Red and Near IR (I) (630, 694, 755, 810 nm)*. Deeply penetrating red light (630 nm) continuous wave devices are efficient activators of PpIX after topical application of ALA. The 694 nm (ruby) laser is optimized for pigment reduction and hair reduction in lighter skin types. The 810 nm diode and 755 nm alexandrite laser, depending on spot size, cooling, pulse duration, and fluence can be configured to optimize outcomes for hair reduction, lentigines, or blood vessels.[34] They are positioned in the absorption spectrum for blood and melanin between the GY wavelengths and 1,064 nm. They will penetrate deeply enough in blood to coagulate vessels up to 2 mm[35-37]; also, they are reasonably tolerant of epidermal pigment in hair reduction (with surface cooling) so long as *very* dark skin is not treated.[38] By decreasing the pulsewidth into the nanosecond range, the alexandrite laser is a first line treatment for many tattoo colors.

5. *Near IR (II). 940 and Nd YAG (1,064 nm)*. These two wavelengths have been used for a broad range of vessel sizes on the leg and face.[39] They occupy a unique place in

the absorption spectrum of our *"big 3"* chromophores, that is *blood, melanin, and water*. Because of the depth of penetration (on the order of mm), they are especially useful for hair reduction and coagulation of deeper blood vessels. By varying fluence and spot size, reticular ectatic veins, as well as those associated with nodular port wine stains or hemangiomas, can be safely targeted. On the other hand, they are not well suited for epidermal-pigmented lesions. Also, although water absorption is poor, it exceeds that of the VIS and near VIS wavelengths. The result is that 940 and 1,064 nm achieve large volume temperature elevation in the skin, and with repeated laser impacts, because of the slow cooling of this volume (large τ – vide infra), catastrophic pan-cutaneous thermal damage is possible. This wavelength (1,064 nm) represents the extreme example of a "what you don't see can hurt you laser"[19] (Fig. 7). The Q-switched YAG laser plays an expanding role in the treatment of tattoos, nevus of Ota, and even melasma.

6. *MIR-lasers and deeply penetrating halogen lamps.* These lasers and lamps heat tissue water. With macrowounding (>1 mm) spot sizes, depending on where we want to heat, we can "choreograph" our laser and/or cooling settings to maximize the skin temperature in certain skin layers. In general, with more deeply penetrating wavelengths, larger volumes are heated. On the other hand, achieving temperature elevations in the volume will require higher fluences than with highly absorbing wavelengths. Without surface cooling, unless very small fluences are applied, a top to bottom thermal injury occurs. The absorption coefficients for the 1,320, 1,450, and 1,540 nm systems are ~3, 20, and 8 cm^{-1} respectively,[40] while the effective scattering coefficients are about 14, 12, and 11 cm^{-1}. The corresponding penetration depths are ~1,500, 300, and 700 μm. It follows that for equal surface cooling and equal fluences, the most superficial heating will occur with the 1,450 nm laser, followed by the 1,540 and 1,320 nm lasers. Newer deeply penetrating lamps have been introduced (Titan, Cutera, Brisbane, CA). They emit light over a 1–2 μm wavelength band with relatively low power densities and long exposures (several seconds). In a typical scenario, the irradiation begins after a roughly two second period of cooling. At this point, a band of tissue from roughly 700 μm–1.5 mm deep in the skin is heated. By varying the fluence, this relatively large volume can be heated to different peak temperatures. As part of each iteration, post pulse cooling is imperative because such a large volume of skin is heated that a "thermal wake" advances toward the skin surface. If one removes the handpiece prematurely, heat accumulates near the skin surface with the risks of pain, dermal thermal injury, and scarring.[41] The 1,320 nm Nd:YAG has been used in the endovenous ablation of the deep saphenous venous system as well as laser liposculpture. Recently the MIR spectral subset has become the mainstay for fractional non-ablative technologies.

7. *Far infrared systems.* The major lasers are the CO_2, erbium YAG, and erbium YSGG (chromium:yttrium-scandium-gallium-garnet) lasers. Overall, the ratio of ablation to heating is much higher with the erbium YAG laser. However, one can enhance the thermal effects of the Er YAG laser by extending the pulse or increasing the repetition rate, and likewise one can decrease residual thermal damage (RTD) of the CO_2 laser by decreasing pw.[42,43] Where precision is required in ablation, Er YAG is preferred. On the other hand, depending on settings, the CO_2 laser enjoys a desirable blend of ablation and heating. The thresholds for ablation for CO_2 and erbium lasers vary inversely with their optical penetration depths in tissue (20 μm and 1 μm respectively). This assumes thermal confinement. It follows that less surface fluence is required for ablation with the erbium laser. The CO_2 laser at typical operating "pulsed" parameters performs self-limited controlled heating of the skin,[44,45] whereas the erbium laser operates in an almost purely ablative regime. The erbium YSGG (2.79 μm) laser has recently been applied to LSR

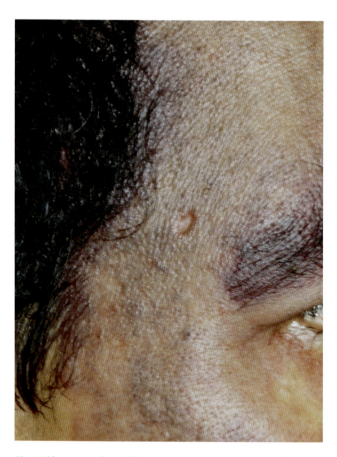

Fig. 7 Note scar after 1,064 nm irradiation of a nodule within a port wine stain

and its absorption coefficient makes it a kind of hybrid between CO_2 and erbium YAG insofar as the ratios of heating to ablation. All three wavelengths (2.79, 2.94, and 10.6 μm) have recently been integrated into fractional delivery systems.

Radiofrequency (RF) Technology

With Radio frequency energy, local heat generation depends on the local electrical resistance and current density. The distribution of the current density is determined by the configuration of the electrodes with respect to the skin anatomy. There are two types of electrode deployments.[46-49] In one scenario, cooled bipolar electrodes are combined with a diode laser, halogen lamp, or intense pulsed light device. In this configuration, there is synergy between the two energy sources.[50] With the bipolar electrode configuration confines the electrical field density is superficially (the field intensity reaches about as deep as one half the distance between the electrodes).

In monopolar configurations, a smaller square electrode placed over the skin "target" is combined with a larger the dispersive electrode is located at a distant point on the body. Monopolar skin rejuvenation systems create large-volume heating. Electrical energy is distributed uniformly over the electrode surface through "capacitive coupling". This type of coupling reduces the natural accumulation of electrical energy at the electrode edge.[51] The first non-ablative RF device (Therma Cool TC, Thermage, Hayward, CA) uses cryogen spray cooling (CSC), where the spray is started before the RF current.

If both positive and negative electrodes are placed in the contact tip (bipolar electrode), current density tends to flow superficially (path of least resistance from electrode to electrode, and therefore temperature elevation is confined to superficial skin). By placing the electrodes further apart, the current density depth will increase. Otherwise, control of the tissue heating is determined by variations in electrode type, power, and cooling times.[50] If one uses "rail" metal type electrodes placed next to a flashlamp crystal, EM field theory predicts that there will be a hot spot near the edge of the electrode. These hot spots can be reduced by electrically coupling the energy into the skin (for example, ensuring that the dry stratum corneum, with high intrinsic impedance, is wetted with an electrolyte solution).

One representative bipolar device (Polaris, Syneron, Richmond Hill, Ontario, Canada) combines RF energy and a 980 diode laser. In this configuration, the local optical energy (fluence) increases the discrete chromophore temperature (i.e., hair, vessel). Localized heating reduces impedance (skin is treated as an electrolyte with decreasing impedance

as a function of increasing temperature) and therefore in higher localized current densities. Thus, there is "synergy" between the optical and electrical parts of the device.[50,52-54] A purported advantage of the treatment is that lower optical energies can be used to selectively heat sub-surface targets than if a light source were used alone (thus enhancing epidermal preservation).

> 1. LTIs are usually based on varying degrees of light absorption by tissue HgB, melanin, and water.
> 2. Wavelength ranges should be chosen to achieve as much specificity as possible in tissue heating.

There are four key components in the sequence of most photothermal laser-tissue interactions (A–D).

(A) Beam Propagation: How the Laser Energy Gets to the Target

Skin optical properties determine the penetration, absorption, and internal dosimetry of laser light. The laser surgeon can divide the skin into two components, (1) the epidermis (primarily an absorber of visible light due to melanin) and (2) The dermis (which can be envisioned as a carton of milk with red dots in it). Light tissue interactions can be broken down into A. The transport of light in tissue, B. Absorption of light and heat generation in tissue, C. Localized temperature elevation in the target tissue (and denaturation of proteins), and D. Heat diffusion away from the target (Fig. 8).[17,55]

The optical properties of the skin mimic a turbid medium intermixed with focal discrete visible and infrared light absorbers (blood, melanin, bilirubin, and dry collagen).[56] The thermal or photochemical effects depend on the *local* energy density at the target. Once the light penetrates the surface, it undergoes a series of absorbing and scattering events. Photons statistically are either scattered or absorbed in a wavelength dependent fashion.[1,57] Scattering is affected by the shape or size of the particle and the index of refraction mismatch between the particle and medium. For most tissues, for $\lambda > 2.5$ μm or less than 250 nm, absorption dominates over scattering. For the remainder of the EM spectrum, scattering is the primary attenuator of light in tissue with the exception of focal discrete absorbers (melanosome, HgB, etc.)

The probabilities of absorption or scattering (designated μ_a and μ_s respectively, Table 1) are determined by experiment. For example, for a μ_a of 0.3 cm^{-1}, the mean free path before absorption is $1/\mu_a$ or 3.3 cm. Generally, light is

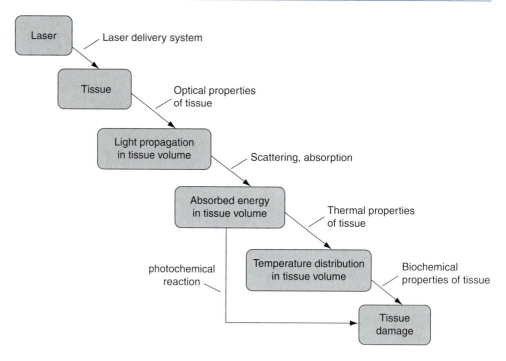

Fig. 8 Interaction between laser light and biological tissue and the resulting effects (From Knappe et al.[18]; Fig. 1)

attenuated as it propagates through tissue. In turbid tissue (i.e., the dermis, where collagen acts as the major scatterer), the fluence attenuation can be described by:

$$I(z) = I_o k e^{(-z/\delta)} \quad (3)$$

where I(z) is the local subsurface fluence at some depth z, k is a constant that accounts for backscattered light and δ is the wavelength dependent optical penetration depth of light, or the depth at which there is attenuation to 37% of the surface value (37% = 1/e, where e = 2.7, the base of the natural logarithm). This depth is determined by absorption and scattering coefficients, as related by the simple equation below[1,57]:

$$\delta = \frac{1}{\sqrt{3\mu_a(\mu_a + \mu_s(1-g))}} \quad (4)$$

Where g is the anisotropy coefficient (a measure of the "mean" direction of the scattered photons). g = 0.9 for the skin. As μ_a and μ_s increase, δ decreases accordingly. For example, for hair removal, based solely on depth of penetration, longer wavelengths such as 800 and 1,064 nm should be preferable to 694 and 755 nm. In the visible light range, this is why red light can penetrate one's hand when shining a flash light on the surface. Scattering decreases roughly proportional to $\lambda^{3/2}$, so that, for example, an 800-nm photon will on average travel about 1.3 times as far in tissue as a 700-nm photon without being scattered. It follows that for "more" scattering wavelengths, there will be greater accumulation of photons near the surface. In addition to scattering, this superficial convergence of photons is based on index of refraction mismatches between air and tissue.[1] Accordingly, light must be deposited more slowly with shorter wavelengths to avoid overheating the superficial tissue.

There is backscattered light that can yield a higher fluence beneath the tissue than at the tissue surface.[58] This paradox of tissue optics is that the internal fluence can actually exceed that at the surface, as below:

$$I = I_o(1 + 6R) \quad (5)$$

Where I is the subsurface energy density, I_o is the surface fluence, R = the surface remittance (0.3, 0.6, and 0.7 for 585, 694, and 1,064 nm respectively). (personal communication from RR Anderson, 1994)

Since neither macromolecules nor water strongly absorb in the red light and near IR (600–1,200 nm) this range allows deeper penetration in most tissues.[10] Various skin pigments can play optical "tricks" on the cutaneous surgeon. For example, poikiloderma appears to be a mix of hyperpigmentation and hypervascularity. In fact, although there is some melanin influence in the red-brown appearance, the dyschromia is by far more a disorder of matted telangiectasia. This is confirmed by the good response of the condition to the PDL, even with aggressive surface cooling that should preclude any impact on superficial cutaneous hyperpigmentation. Additionally, with diascopy, "poikilodermatous" skin often appears no browner than the surrounding apparently normal skin. The explanation is that deoxy-Hb contributes to a "pigmented skin appearance". This finding follows from the absorption spectrum of deoxy-Hb in the 630–700 nm range, which is very similar to the absorption spectrum of epidermal melanin. The size of the vessels in the superficial venous plexus is such that the transmitted light through these vessels is approximately 50% lower than the incident intensity. These vessels therefore appear dark.[59]

In most biological systems, tissue constituents show broad absorption bands with only a few distinct absorption peaks. From 200 to 290 nm (UVC), all biological objects (cells and tissue) absorb energy very strongly. From 290 to 320 (UVB) nm, only a limited number of biomolecules show absorption (aromatic amino acids and nucleic acids). For UVA 320–400 nm, light is weakly absorbed by colorless skin parts. From 400 to 1,000 nm mainly pigments- bilirubin, blood, and melanin absorb light. The heterogeneity of the skin allows for discrete heating over this range, and therefore selective photothermolysis (SPT) is exploited in this band. For >1,100 nm, all biomolecules have specific strong vibrational absorption bands. Tissue water is the primary determiner of the response to laser in this wavelength range.[9]

The absorption coefficient (μ_a) is the relative "probability" per unit path length that a photon at a particular wavelength will be absorbed. It is therefore measured in units of 1/distance and is typically designated μ_a, given as cm^{-1}. The absorption coefficient is chromophore and wavelength dependent. For larger heterogeneous volumes, μ_a can be weighted according to the fraction of a specific chromophore. For example, for a dermis a typical blood fraction (f.blood) is 0.2%, assuming that the blood is uniformly distributed in the skin.[7]

Following the descriptive convention of describing an equivalent average homogeneous f.blood, the net absorption of the dermis, μ_a.derm, is calculated:

$$\mu_a \cdot derm = (f \cdot blood)(\mu_a \cdot blood) \qquad (6)$$
$$+ (1 - f \cdot blood)(\mu_a \cdot skinbaseline)$$

Scattering is responsible for much of light's behavior in skin (beam dispersion, spot size effects, etc.). The dermis appears white because of light scatter. The main scattering wavelengths (relative to absorption) are between 400 and 1,200 nm. Absorption occurs where the laser frequency equals the natural frequency of the free vibrations of the particles (absorption is associated with resonance).[60] Scattering occurs at frequencies not corresponding to those natural frequencies of particles. Scattering is decreased as wavelength increases.[7]

There are four major chromophores (water, blood, tattoo ink, and melanin) in cutaneous laser medicine.[60] *Water* makes up about 65% of the dermis and lower epidermis. There is some water absorption in the UV. Between 400 and 800 nm, water absorption is quite small (which is consistent with our real world experience that light propagates quite readily through a glass of water). Beyond 800 nm, there is a small peak at 980 nm, followed by larger peaks at 1,480 and 10,600 nm. The water absorption maximum is 2,940 nm (erbium YAG).

Hemoglobin: There is a large $HgBO_2$ (oxyhemoglobin) peak at 415 nm, followed by smaller peaks at 540 and 577 nm. An even smaller peak is at 940 nm. For deoxy-hemoglobin (HgB), the peaks are at 430 and 555 nm. The discrete peaks of hemoglobin absorption allow for selective vessel heating. Although the 410 nm peak achieves the greatest theoretical vascular to pigment damage ratio among the other peaks, scattering is too strong for violet light to be a viable option for vascular applications.

Melanin: Most pigmented lesions result from excessive melanin in the epidermis. By choosing almost any wavelength (<800 nm), one can preferentially heat epidermal melanin. Shorter wavelengths will create very high superficial epidermal temperatures, whereas longer wavelengths tend to bypass epidermal melanin (i.e., 1,064 nm).

Fat: Fat shows strong absorption at 1,200 and 1,700 nm.[61] Although the ratios of fat to water absorption are small, the small differences are exploited with the proper choice of parameters. 1,200 nm might represent the best choice due to decreased overall water absorption and therefore increased penetration. Sebum is similar to fat but also is comprised of wax esters and squalene.

Carbon: Carbon is a product of prolonged skin heating. Once carbon is formed at the skin surface, the skin becomes "opaque" to most laser wavelengths (that is, most energy will be absorbed very superficially). It follows that the dynamics of surface heating changes immediately once carbon is formed. This can be used creatively as an advantage. For example, one can convert a deeply penetrating laser to one that would only affect the surface by using a carbon dye. This has been accomplished with a laser peel using a Q Switched Nd YAG laser.

Collagen: Dry collagen has absorption peaks near 6 and 7 μm. With a free electron laser operating at these wavelengths, collagen can be directly heated. Ellis et al. found that this approach might allow for less tissue irradiation and less thermal damage than CO_2 laser.[62]

(B) Heat Generation

Selective Photothermolysis (SPT)

Non-bulk skin heating is based on selective absorption by discrete chromophores of relatively low concentration (i.e., melanin, hemoglobin). Dr. Leon Goldman showed that color contrast allowed for selective damage of dermal targets as early as 1963.[63] However, it was Dr. RR Anderson who elegantly described the concept of selective photothermolysis.[27] Selective photothermolysis offered a mathematically rigorous rationale for tissue-selective lasers. As described by Dr. Anderson, extreme *localized heating* relies on: (1) a wavelength that reaches and is preferentially absorbed by the desired target structures; (2) an exposure

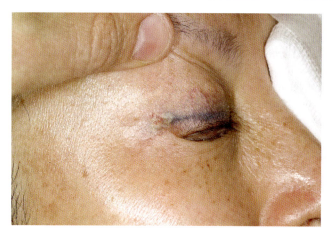

Fig. 9 Figure shows that whitening mirrors profile of tattoo

Table 2 Thermal relaxation time of some potential targets

Erythrocyte – 2 µs
200 µm hair follicle – 40 ms
Melanosome (0.5 µm) – 0.25 µs
Nevus cell (10 µm) – 0.1 ms
0.1 mm diameter vessel – 10 ms
0.4 mm diameter vessel – 80 ms
0.8 mm diameter vessel – 300 ms

duration less than or equal to the time necessary for cooling of the target structures; and (3) sufficient energy to damage the target. The heterogeneity of the skin allows for selective injury in microscopic targets. The focal nature of the heating decreases the likelihood of catastrophic pancutaneous thermal damage. For example, one can apply a 4 mm laser beam and observe only a 1 mm wide tattoo line "whiten" with Q switched Nd YAG laser with a larger round spot (Fig. 9) – the skin outside the tattoo but within the spot will appear normal. Also, a darker lentigo will become white but a lighter lentigo will remain unchanged. The primary areas where SPT is helpful in dermatology is in the treatment of vascular lesions, tattoos, and pigmented lesions. However, even in applications where water is the chromophore, the principles of SPT are useful, as one can design precise heating and ablation protocols based on wavelength and pulse duration.[64]

Thermal Relaxation Time

The thermal relaxation time (τ) is the interval necessary for a target to cool to a certain percentage of its peak temperature.[29] Larger objects require longer times than smaller volumes to cool. For example, a tubful of warm bathwater requires much longer than a thimbleful to cool to room temperature. With laser irradiation, we assume instantaneous heating of the target, so that τ is the time for cooling *after* the pulse. If the pulse is too long, the target cools during the pulse, akin to one pouring water slowly into a leaky bucket. If the water represents heat, one observes that the bucket never fills (akin to a target never becoming very hot). If one wants to spatially confine heating one chooses a short pulse less than τ of the chromophore. For the same volume, a sphere will cool faster than a cylinder, which will cool faster than a slab. When defining thermal relaxation time, the target size and geometry are important. Normally, τ is defined by:

$$\delta^2/g\kappa \quad (7)$$

where δ is the optical penetration depth for homogeneously absorbing layers (such as tissue water for IR applications), and κ is the thermal diffusivity (a measure of heat capacity and conductivity – for tissue, $\kappa \sim 1.3 \times 10^{-3}$ cm^2/s). For discrete absorbers, i.e., the melanosome or a blood vessel, τ is defined in terms of the particle size, and δ represents the diameter of the particle. κ is the thermal diffusivity, a quantity based on the thermal conductivity and specific heat of the medium, and "g" is a constant based on the geometry of the target (slab, cylinder, or sphere).[27] See Table 2 for sample thermal relaxation times for common targets in skin.

The often-used term "thermal relaxation time of the skin" is meaningful only when used for specific wavelengths (or specific skin structures, i.e., the epidermis). With a ubiquitous absorber such as tissue water, τ should be considered within the context of δ and the laser source, not the dimensions of the skin constituents. For example, if one uses the 1,540 nm laser, the entire epidermis and large portions of the dermis are heated, and τ is on the order of seconds, because δ is several hundred µm. So even though τ of the epidermis is about 10 ms based on its thickness, a thicker slab of skin is heated at 1,540 nm, the epidermis will take several seconds to cool because there is no temperature gradient between it and that of the dermis.

For most targets a simple rule can be used: the thermal relaxation time in seconds is about equal to the square of the target dimension in millimeters. Thus a 0.5 µm melanosome (5×10^{-4} mm) should cool in about 25×10^{-8} s, or 250 ns, whereas a 0.1 mm PWS vessel should cool in about 10^{-2} s, or 10 ms. Recall that τ is derived from a solution of a differential equation and does not represent an absolute cooling time, but rather provides approximate pulsewidths for varying degrees of thermal confinement.[13]

Once the local subsurface energy density has been determined 3, heat generation can be predicted by energy balance (conservation of energy), pulse duration, thermal relaxation time, and the wavelength specific absorption for that target.

The temperature increase of a desired target can be roughly calculated by knowing the absorption and scattering coefficients, surface light dose, size of the target, and the length of the pulse, as follows:

$$\Delta T = \frac{F_z \mu_a}{\rho c}\left(\frac{\tau_r}{\tau_r + \tau_p}\right)^{g/2} \qquad (8)$$

where F_z is the local subsurface fluence, ρ is the density, c is the specific heat "g" is a geometric factor ("1" for planes, "2" for cylinders, and "3" for spheres), τ_p is the laser pulse duration, and τ_r is the thermal relaxation time of the target (time for target to cool to 37% of peak temperature), defined by Eq. 7. Thus one can perform some quick algebraic calculations to estimate the peak temperatures of local targets in the skin. The temperature generally decays as a function of diameter and time from the target. For ex, in hair removal the shaft and bulb, heavily invested with melanin, reach high temperatures, and as the wave of heat diffuses from this cylinder, the temperature decreases.

Spatially selective temperature elevation is possible when (1) the absorption coefficient of the target exceeds that of collateral tissue (selective photothermolysis), or (2) when the "innocent bystander" tissues are cooled so their peak temperatures do not exceed some damage threshold or (3) with very small microwounds (fractional). Localized heating, for example, in telangiectasia and lentigines, follows from the concentrations of blood and melanin there, respectively, such that μ_a is focally increased. Verification of the models can be made by real-time measurements, thermocouple needles, thermal cameras, etc.

The geometry (and therefore the microscopic characteristics) of lesions is important – for example in the treatment for a nevus versus a lentigo, the nevus is composed of melanocytes in aggregates as nodules (collectively the nodules are often several hundred μm in diameter) whereas the lentigo is a mere sheet of melanocytes some 10 μm thick. For example, in treating nevus with a long pulsed alexandrite laser with a high fluence, the TRT will approach a second. From the above equation, it follows that thermal confinement will be high, and the peak temperature will rise accordingly. More importantly, the thick slab of melanocytes will take long to cool, such that the will be considerable heat diffusion away from the target. On the other hand, the lentigo represents a slab only tens of microns thick; there will be heat diffusion during the long pulse and rapid cooling after the pulse. Thus, with ms-domain fluences, the nevus case might result in scarring, and a lighter lentigo might not become hot enough for clearance. If one applies ns pulses to the two lesion types, the lentigo shows a good response with possibly complete clearing, whereas the nevus will require multiple sessions, as each laser application will result in heat confined to the most superficial part of the lesion.

Two "offshoots" of SPT are the concepts of *thermal damage time and thermokinetic selectivity (TKS)*.

Thermal damage time. In some applications the immediate absorber and the intended target are not collocated (i.e., hair shaft and hair bulb/bulge). Thermal damage time is defined as the pulsewidth that achieves irreversible target damage with sparing of the surrounding tissue. The thermal damage time represents the interval when the outermost part of the target reaches the target damage temperature through heat diffusion from the heater. In this case the eventual target and the heater (for example, hair shaft) are different and at a considerable distance from each other.[65] Using this model, the thermal damage time can be many times longer than the thermal relaxation time. For example, for laser hair removal, with a 100 μm shaft and 30 μm follicle, the TDT can approach several hundred ms.[65]

Thermokinetic selectivity: Along the same lines is the concept of thermal kinetic selectivity (TKS). Using this principle, one selects larger or smaller targets for heating based on pulse duration. For example, if one wants to damage larger targets while sparing relatively smaller ones, the pulse duration is extended beyond the thermal relaxation time of the smaller target. In this manner, i.e., a melanosome will be heated to a lower temperature than the subjacent vessel.

Molecular Basis of LTI

Most devices for cosmetic rejuvenation are based on photothermal or "electrothermal" mechanisms, that is, the conversion of light or electrical energy to heat. Two fundamental processes govern all interactions of light with matter: absorption and scattering. Absorption and excitation are necessary for all photobiologic effects and laser-tissue interactions. Energy is proportional to frequency and inversely proportional to wavelength. Thus a 532 nm photon (532 nm is the distance between two of the transverse waves in a stream of light) is twice as energetic as a 1,064 nm photon.

Macroscopically, the atomic events in LTIs are not identifiable, but on the molecular level, EMR exchanges energy only in discrete quantities (photons). The molecular basis of LTIs is based on electronic transitions for the ultraviolet (UV) and visible (VIS) wavelengths. For example, hemoglobin is excited to a higher electronic state, followed by a complete relaxation into vibrational modes (internal conversion). However, NIR wavelengths and beyond are absorbed via rotational and vibrational excitations in biomolecules (all of which are hydrocarbons with the exception of pigments). These reactions can be considered a two-step process. In the first the molecule is "pumped" to an excited state. Then, through a process known as non-radiative decay, there are inelastic collisions with nearby molecules.[60] The temperature rise results from the *transfer of photon energy to kinetic energy*.

For thermal reactions to occur, the energy must be randomized with a large ensemble of molecules through statistical processes. With HgB, the electronic excited state gives way to vibrational modes. With longer wavelengths, the quantized energy packets correlate with vibrational transitions from NIR and MIR.

(C) Reaction Types and Effects of Heating

- Photochemical effects (usually 10–1,000 s; 10^{-3}–10 W/cm^2)
- Photothermal effects (1 ms–100 s; 1–10^6 W/cm^2)
- Photomechanical and photoionizing effects (10 ps–100 ns; 10^8–10^{12} W/cm^2)

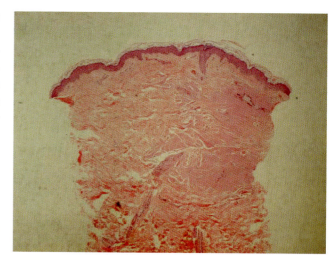

Fig. 10 Figure shows extensive damage from long pulsed 1,064 nm irradiation of tattoo particle

Photothermal effects

Photothermal processes depend on type and degree of heating, from coagulation to vaporization. With a very short pulsewidths (pw), lasers vaporize targets. For example, in treating blood vessels, rapid heating results in acute vessel wall damage and petechial hemorrhage (with Q switched 532 nm).[66-68] With intermediate length pulses (0.1–1.5 ms), one can gently heat targets without immediate rupture of the vessels. Still intravascular thrombosis can create purpura and delayed hemorrhage. With still longer pulses (6–100 ms), the ratio of contraction to thrombosis increases and side effects are less likely. On the other hand, too long pulses with very small targets can create two problems. With highly absorbing targets, (i.e., tattoo inks) –, the heat generation is so great and long-lived that significant diffusion occurs to the surrounding dermis (Fig. 10). On the other hand, using a long pulse YAG for a nevus of Ota results in an insufficient temperature rise as the pigmented nevus cells cool off too fast during the delivery of the pulses (also melanin absorption is much weaker than black ink).

A mild – moderate temperature increase results in denaturation of enzymes and function. If the heating is very fast, a phase change occurs.[60,69] Depending on the rate of energy delivery, photovaporization occurs with or without inertial confinement (vide infra), where time is short compared to the time for pressure relaxation. Here the laser induced pressure causes compressive stresses in tissue. Microcracks in the tissue are the result of these large stress gradients.[13] Whitening after ns irradiation is thought be gas vacuoles with scattering that resolve as the as the "spaces" are refilled with interstitial fluid.

Hemoglobin undergoes a complex set of reactions when heated. Formation of met HgB and deoxy HgB occur during irradiation on the order of ms, representing a real-time change in tissue optics. During the heating phase, hemoglobin absorption undergoes a bathochromic (red) shift of the 580 nm absorption peak (the 540 nm peak does not shift). This has important implications for designing optimal blood vessel protocols. For example, it has been suggested that 585 nm though 600 nm should penetrate deeper than shorter wavelengths and are therefore preferable for treatment. In fact, as the blood temperature rises during laser irradiation, 532 nm light transmission increases and longer wavelength (i.e., 595 nm) transmission decreases.[30,70]

Even after the heating source is removed, whole blood optical properties change. A macroscopic coagulum emerges comprised of denatured HgB, cell membranes of erythrocytes and plasma proteins. Met HgB formation is also important, with absorption peaks near 630–635 nm. With increasing met HgB and deoxy production, 755–1,064 nm lasers penetrate less and will generate more heat in vessels. This is one argument for sequential pulses with 1,064 nm lasers. One potential downside of this is that an abrupt increase in absorption, particularly with 940–1,064 nm, causes too much collateral damage.

Thermal Injury to Cells

There is a range of measurable effects on skin based on temperature. Below 43°C, the skin remains intact, even for very long exposures.[55,71] The first change is a conformational change in the molecular structure that occurs at temperatures from 43° to 50°. After several minutes, there will be tissue necrosis as described by the Arrhenius equation (an equation that quantitatively describes conversion of tissue from a native to denatured state). Thermal denaturation is a rate process: temperature increases the rate at which molecules denature, depending on the specific molecule. For example, at 45°C, cultured human fibroblasts die after about 20 min.

However, the same cells can withstand over $100°C$ for 10^{-3} s. In general, a temperature of $>60°$ lasting for at least six seconds leads to irreversible damage.

Coagulation

Temperature, directly related to the average kinetic energy of molecules, is a critical factor in tissue coagulation. Denaturation depends on time and temperature, and at least for exposures greater than 1 s, conforms to a rate process as described by the Arrhenius equation. The characteristic behavior of the Arrhenius-type kinetic damage model is that, below a threshold temperature, the rate of damage accumulation is negligible; and it increases precipitously when this value is exceeded. An example of coagulation is the cooking of an egg white. Thermal denaturation is both temperature and time dependent, yet it usually shows an all or none like behavior. Most denaturation reactions follow 1st order rate kinetics. For a given heating time there is usually a narrow temperature region above which complete denaturation occurs. As a rule, for denaturation of most proteins, one must increase the temperature by about $10°C$ for every decade of decrease in the heating time to achieve the same amount of thermal coagulation.[13]

An absolute temperature for coagulation-denaturation does not exist. For very short times, higher temperatures than the oft-quoted "62–65°C" should be required. Early signs of microscopic damage are vacuolization, nuclear hyperchromasia and protein denaturation (recognized as a birefringence loss for collagen). Moderate temperature – induced damage phenomena in tissue are difficult to assess with conventional light microscopy. In fact, histology represents and conveys the overall reactions of a complex system and cannot be related to molecular species. Specimens obtained 24 h after irradiation tend to be more sensitive than those obtained immediately after treatment, as often a day is required to show sign of necrosis; also, an inflammatory response might be the most sensitive indicator of injury. Particularly in light of newer large volume low intensity heating devices for rejuvenation, more sensitive tools might be required to characterize subtle thermal effects. Beckham et al.[72] found that over a narrow temperature range, heat shock protein (HSP) expression correlated with laser induced heat stress, and that the HSP production followed the Arrhenius integral. Thus HSP expression (in addition to tissue ultrastructure, i.e., EM) might be an excellent tool to examine low intensity high volume heat injury.

Vaporization

At a certain threshold power density, coagulation gives way to photovaporization (ablation). Water expands as it is converted to steam. Vaporization is beneficial in that much of the heat is carried away from the skin. The evaporation of tissue water acts as a sort of buffer, reducing the peak T to just over $100°C$. When there is vaporization there is also increasing pressure as the water tries to expand in volume. The expansion leads to localized microexplosions. At the surface, particles are ejected at supersonic velocities. At temperatures beyond $100°$ (without further vaporization), carbonization takes place, which is obvious by blackening of adjacent tissue and the escape of smoke. Carbon is the ultimate end product of all living tissues being heated and carbon temperatures often reach up to $300°C$. When treating a wart at low power densities with the CO_2 laser, one can observe almost simultaneously incandescence and combustion. In water free structures, such as char, temperatures can reach $1000°C$, and incandescence can be observed with continued irradiation of char at long pulse cw CO_2 lasers. Normally, this should be avoided, because the depth of tissue injury will extend well beyond the blackened skin surface.[60] This is particularly true, for example, when treating a rhinophyma or performing laser skin resurfacing.

Photomechanical effects

With very short pulses, there is insufficient time for pressure relaxation. Mechanical damage is observed with high-energy, submicrosecond lasers for tattoo and pigmented lesion removal. The time threshold for inertial confinement is predicted by the relation[1]:

$$\delta / v \qquad (9)$$

where δ is the target diameter and v is the velocity of sound in tissue.

Inertially confined ablation occurs when there is high-pressure at constant volume. In a very short pulse, the energy is invested so quickly one that there is no time for the pressure to be relieved. Under these conditions of *inertial confinement*, there's not enough time for material to move – this can lead to the generation of tremendous pressures and relief through shock waves. For example, one can feel the recoil during laser tattoo treatment if one touches the skin surface near the impact site.

Photochemical effects

The absorption of light in tissue does not always generate heat. A term luminescence describes cases where absorbed light causes emission of light of a different color. This occurs after electrons are excited from some lower (ground) state, to an upper level, excited state. If the process is fast, fluorescence occurs. If the is an intermediary reaction and longer decay time, phosphorescence occurs. Most photochemical reactions occur in the UV and violet portion of the spectrum as the electronic transitions demand highly energetic photons.

Photochemical reactions are governed by specific reaction pathways, whereas thermal reactions tend to be non specific. Photochemical reactions include fluorescence, phosphorescence and photodynamic action. The former two involve the reemission of light after absorption at lesser wavelengths. Fluorescence spectra are increasingly used in diagnostic applications. An example is PpIX fluorescence to determine the amount of photosensitizer (PS) in the skin after application of ALA. Fluorescence spectra can also be used to assess collagen content in the skin. Also, keratin fluoresces such that a milium will display a bright yellow color during irradiation with a green light laser. We have occasionally used this technique to distinguish a deep-seated milium from a small pearly BCC. Endogenous fluorescence applications are increasing and have included assays of NADH, collagen, and amino acids[73].

In photodynamic reactions, a photosensitizer (acting as a catalyst) is excited by a certain wavelength of light. The PS then undergoes several sequential decays, forming singlet O_2. In the presence of oxygen, oxygen is transformed from its triplet state, which is its normal ground state, to an excited singlet state. The excited singlet state oxygen reacts with biological molecules and attacks plasma and intracellular membranes (type II PDT reactions). The most common photosensitizer (PS) in dermatology is PpIX. This PS is formed by skin cells by the pro-drug, aminolevulinic acid (ALA). Most photochemical reactions proceed more efficiently with lower power densities, such that for example, the Blu-U light (DUSA, Vahalla, NY) or Omni Lux (Phototherapeutics, CA, USA) will outperform a pulsed source (IPL, KTP, or PDL) for AKs with one treatment. However, largely because most practitioners posses at least one pulsed visible light source, they have been widely used in PDT and shown to be useful in a range of PDT-responsive skin disorders[74,75]. Because pulsed light sources in dermatology do not meet the theoretical PDT saturation threshold (4×10^8 W/m²),[76] in theory there should be significant PDT activity.[77]

Most photochemical activity is observed between 320 and 630 nm. The main absorption peaks for PpIX are 415, 504, 538, 576, and 630 nm. Beyond 800 nm, photochemistry, even with exogenous photosensitizers or pro-drugs, is unlikely. PDT reactions are complex; for example, with ALA, optimization require an understanding of skin pharmacokinetics, conversion kinetics of ALA to PpIX, and proper delivery of light dose (including power density, wavelength, etc.). A new development is a possible role for vascular specific therapy with PDT. Both with hematoporphyrin and benzoporphyrin derivatives, this approach is being investigated for refractory deeper vascular lesions.[78]

Photodisruption or Photodecomposition

This reaction type is usually observed at 10^7–10^8 W/cm² in the UV range. Usually there is little residual thermal damage (RTD).

Rather than heating water directly as their FIR counterparts, these lasers can exceed the bond energies of many organic compounds. Among the available wavelengths (193, 241 and 308 nm) XeCl is more likely to be more thermal because of the lowered energy per photon.

Excimer Laser (308 nm)

The mechanism of action for the excimer laser (XeCl) is thought to be the same as narrow band UV therapy. A reduction in cellular proliferation most likely plays a role in epidermal cellular DNA synthesis and mitosis. In Parrish's original study in 1981, he showed that wavelengths between 300 and 313 nm were most effective.[79] It appears that the excimer laser works through in an immunomodulatory way much like standard non coherent UVB "light boxes". There may be a thermal component as well at fluences >800 mJ/cm².

Biostimulation

Biostimulation belongs to the group of photochemical interactions. Increasingly this field is validated by the number of well-executed investigations. Typical fluences are in the range of one to 10 J/cm², and temperature elevation is absent. Potentially positive reactions include (1) Increase in phagocytic activity (2) Depression in rate of bacteria replication (3) Increase in repair of skin, and (4) Stimulation of wound healing. We should not debunk these applications – certainly they are being studied more and we are witnessing a transition from lab to bedside. One example of a "biostimulation" device is the Gentlewaves LED Photomodulation unit (Light Bio-Science, LLC, Virginia Beach, VA). This device uses 590 nm light in a high repetition rate and low power density to increase collagen synthesis and enhance facial tone. Cell culture work supports this concept.[80] Newer LED devices (800 nm) also support a role for photorejuvenation and even hair growth. It is unknown if any special features of laser light are relevant for biostimulation, although at least one study supports *coherence* as a possible factor in photomodulation. Some investigators have shown that laser showed the best effect while the non-coherent LED light showed the poorest. Coherence does not influence the transmission; rather, because of interference in the scattered light field, coherency influences the microscopic light distribution into tissue.

Plasma Induced Ablation

With very high power densities exceeding 10^8 W/cm², optical breakdown occurs. Plasma removes skin without evidence of mechanical or thermal damage when choosing appropriate parameters. Plasmas are sometimes produced by laser tattoo removal, where one can observe a spark.[13] There is a new resurfacing system that uses plasma created by an RF excited N_2 gas. Unlike laser-induced plasma, this flame heats tissue by direct heat transfer from the plasma edge.

(D) Heat Conduction Away from the Chromophore

This final "physical" step in LTIs in important in characterizing collateral damage. Once heat is generated, heat losses are based on heat conduction, heat convection, or radiation. Radiation can be neglected in most types of laser applications. A good example of heat convection is transfer from blood flow. Heat conduction is the primary mechanism by which heat is transferred to unexposed tissue structures.

Cooling

Surface cooling enhances efficacy and safety in skin laser surgery, especially for visible light technologies, (i.e., green – yellow light sources such as IPL, KTP laser, and PDL) that are popular in cutaneous laser surgery. They are also the wavelength ranges where epidermal damage is most likely. The epidermis is an innocent bystander in cutaneous laser applications where the intended targets, such as hair follicles or blood vessels, are located in the dermis. Specifically, absorption of light by epidermal melanin causes skin surface heating.

The first goal is of surface cooling is preservation of the epidermis. The second and related goal of surface cooling permits higher fluences to the intended target (i.e., the hair bulb and/or bulge or a subsurface blood vessel). Another benefit of surface cooling is analgesia, as almost all cooling strategies will provide some pain relief.[81-90]

The timing of the cooling relative to the laser pulse is important. Cooling can be pre, during the pulse (parallel), or after the pulse (post).[90] Post cooling may prevent retrograde heating (i.e., from the vessel back to the epidermis) from damaging the skin surface. A cooling protection factor (CPF) has been proposed by Dr. Rox Anderson. The cooling protection factor is the ratio of fluence, with and without surface cooling, that spares the epidermis. It is defined by:

$$CPF = \frac{T_c - T_{ic}}{T_c - T_i} \qquad (10)$$

In the above equation, T_{ic} and T_i are basal layer temperatures before laser irradiation with and without cooling, respectively. T_c is the critical temperature at which thermal injury occurs. The detailed calculations described later indicate that if the initial skin temperature is 30°C, contact cooling reduces the temperature of the basal layer to about 20°C. If T_c is assumed to be 60°C (it is actually somewhat higher for the brief laser exposure times in this analysis), this would give the CPF as (60–20)/(60–30) or 1.33. Similarly, cryogen cooling reduces the temperature to about 0°C, thus giving a CPF value as (60–0)/(60–30) or 2.0. Finally, there is *convective air cooling*, where cold air is commonly used in skin chilling. The Zimmer (Cyro5, Zimmer Medizin Systeme, Ulm, Germany) directs −10°C air at the skin at a rapid rate (1,000 L/min). This system proves for good bulk cooling but spatial localization of the cooling is poor. The CPF, depending on the air temperature and nozzle velocity, is near that of contact cooling.

Some Interesting Concepts and Ideas in Laser Tissue Interactions

With Q switched lasers, one might hear a loud "pop" accompanied by a spark-like emission at the skin surface. Normally this is the result of inorganic compounds (make-up) remaining in the skin during irradiation. Thorough cleaning of the skin will remove this distraction. One should ensure that any dark markers are off the skin, especially when using long pulsed visible light technologies. For example, one of our trainees placed a black marking pen to outline an area for a test spot for laser hair removal. During irradiation, the beam was absorbed almost completely by the ink – the hot ink cooled at the expense of the skin surface, such that a very superficial burn occurred.

Also, one should consider oral medications both in the genesis of treatable lesions (i.e., minocycline hyperpigmentation), and in the causation of pigmentation disturbances (i.e., gold). In the case of gold, the medication is sequestered in macrophages of the dermis – the combination of gold and Q-switched lasers produces a photothermal-photochemical conversion such that the gold darkens to a light blue or grey color (Fig. 11). This reaction is a good teaching tool in that it points out the role of pulse duration on the laser tissue interaction.[91,92] As noted earlier, some reactions are dependent on power density – with higher power densities, multi-photon interactions are possible, that is, the energy is condensed into such a short duration, that simultaneous "arrival" of two photons at the same locale can result in two-photon absorption. In the case of gold, the chemical compound structure can be changed (from crystalline to elemental). Once the reaction occurs, one can apply longer pulses to diminish the dyspigmentation (even with the same wavelength!). This reaction also underscores the importance of beam scattering, as the "gold" Q-switched laser reaction extends beyond the diameter of the beam with each pulse.

Focusing the laser beam: A trick to increase the dermal to epidermal damage ratio is use of a convergent lens. This tool

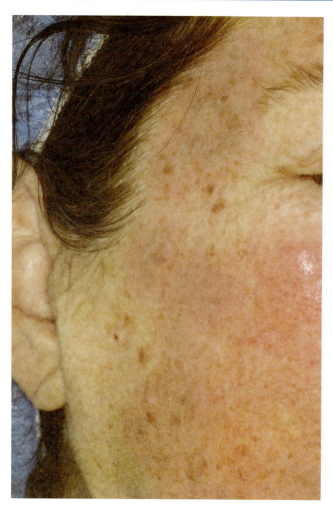

Fig. 11 Note *blue macules*

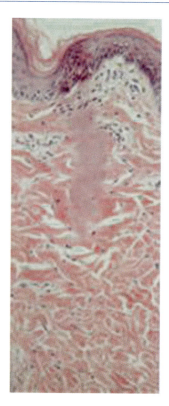

Fig. 12 Note damage pattern with 1,540 nm microbeam

increases the local radiant exposure in the dermis (targeting the hair bulb, a blood vessel, or dermal water). Theoretically, one should be able to use smaller incident fluences, therefore achieving some protection of the epidermis.

Vacuuming the target in the laser beam: A company (Aesthera, Livermore, CA) has created a pneumatic device whereby the skin is vacuumed into the light path such that the light penetration in skin is enhanced. In this way more energetic high frequency photons can be delivered, for example, to the hair follicle, with relative epidermal sparing. By applying suction, the absorption coefficient of the epidermis can be reduced by up to 25%. The technologies have also been used for acne and pain reduction.

By proper timing of the suction with respect to irradiation, selective targeting of various chromophores can be achieved, for example, to increase the dermal blood fraction in pale PWS (and increase the blood vessel diameter). The very small vessels in paler PWS have too small vessel diameters for thermal confinement – that is, the vessels cool too quickly to reach a critical temperature. By applying suction, the blood volume fraction increases, not simply a result of the mechanical force but a physiologic response as well.[93,94]

Pixilated Injury (aka fractional photothermolysis): One can use a "pixilated" injury with water as a chromophore in what is called fractional photothermolysis. Roughly 100 μm spots have been used with 250–500 μm spacing.[95] The tissue can recover from this fractional injury without the widespread epidermal loss observed after traditional resurfacing applications. A number of technologies have been introduced. Despite a wide range of devices, the pitch, wound diameter, wound depth, and other wound features have not been optimized. Ideally one would design devices that maximize downtime while maximizing cosmetic enhancement. One can consider ablative and non ablative approaches. Early evidence suggests that there is a difference between ablative and non ablative wound healing even with similar microvolumes of injury, that is, even when the same total volume is observed, wound healing proceeds differently.

In the most common approach, 75–150 μm wide microwounds are created in the skin (Fig. 12) with densities ranging from 100 to 1,500 microwounds/cm². By spatially confining the micro-lesions, deeper wounds can be created than with a "slab-like" approach, while still managing a larger measure of safety. There are both ablative and nonablative approaches. Ablative devices include the Profractional laser (Sciton), equipped with a scanned microbeam, the Pixel erbium YAG laser from Alma (Alma lasers, Buffalo Grove, IL), and a newly introduced 2,940 nm technology from Palomar. Reliant Technologies is poised to release a newer fractional CO_2 laser system (Re Pair) that creates 125 μm diameter "ablative" wounds as deep as 1 mm. Early investigations have shown immediate superficial skin tightening.

"Macrowound" fractional technologies create wounds greater than 300 μm in diameter. These include the KTP laser with a scanner (with approximately 700 μm wounds) as well as the active FX CO_2 system (Lumenis, Santa Clara, CA), which creates an array of 1.3 mm wounds and covers approximately 60% of the surface area per session. Wound depths range from 80 to 150 μm depending on pulse energy. Fluences with these approaches range from 5 to 15 J/cm^2. The applied fluences are another means (besides wound diameter) to differentiate microwound injuries from macrowound injuries. With ablative microwounds, fluences tends to exceed 30X the ablation threshold, whereas with traditional resurfacing laser applications (CO_2 and erbium) fluences range from 0.8 to 10X ablation threshold per pass.

The original non ablative fractional laser was (Reliant Technologies, Mountain View, CA), deploying a 1,550-nm scanned microbeam that required a surface blue dye for proper tracking along the skin. Recently, Fraxel 2 has replaced this device. The newer technology achieves deeper wounds and does not require the dye. Palomar introduced a fractional 1,540-nm system. This device uses a "stamping" approach, where each 10 mm macro-spot is comprised of 100 beamlets. With progressive passes, an increasing skin surface area is covered. Another nonablative example is a 1,440-nm/1,320 nm Nd YAG laser (Affirm, Cynosure, Chelmsford, MA) that delivers hundreds of beamlets interspersed with a relatively uniform low-fluence background irradiation.

After high-fluence fractional CO_2 and erbium YAG laser (50–200 J/cm^2), one observes microcraters on routine histology. Particularly for the erbium YAG laser, there is immediate water loss through these portals of entry (38), and postoperative discomfort is often severe for an hour after the procedure. Pinpoint bleeding is sometime observed, particularly with higher-pulse energies and shorter pulsed erbium YAG applications.

Optical damping: Replacing air (n = 1.0) with a higher-index medium at the skin surface such as glass (n = 1.5) or sapphire (n = 1.7) tends to spare the epidermis. This effect has nothing to do with heat transfer, but rather is a consequence of optical scattering behavior. At wavelengths from about 600–1,200 nm, most light in Caucasian epidermis is back- and multiply-scattered light. By providing a match to the skin's refractive index, internal reflection of the back-scattered light is greatly reduced, decreasing the natural convergence of photons at the skin surface. This version of optical epidermal sparing requires a physically thick external medium such as a sapphire window or heavy layer of gel.

Compacting the Dermis

One can decrease the depth photons must propagate by applying pressure over the treated area. This maneuver may, for example, decrease the relative depth of the bulb and bulge of the hair follicle up to 30% relative to the skin surface. Disadvantages include variability in the amount of pressure, such that adjacent treatment areas are exposed to different subsurface fluences. Also, it is unclear if compacting the dermis might alter its scattering properties. In theory compression should decrease water content and improve dermal transmission.[96]

Spot diameter: In general the spot size should be 3–4 $X > \delta$, as larger spots make it more likely that photons will be scattered back into the incident collimated beam.[13] Photons scattered out of the beam are essentially wasted. Traveling "alone", they carry insufficient energy to cause macroscopic thermal responses. The consequences of spot size can be explained best on surface to volume arguments. Larger beams (with the same surface fluence as smaller beams) create deeper subsurface cylinders of injury because there is less surface versus volume for photons to escape. Basically, for small beams (narrow), scattered photons are carried out of the beam path after only a few scattering events. As a clinical example of the effect of spot size, we have found for 3 mm vs. 6 mm spots with the YAG laser that roughly ½ the fluence is required with the larger spot for leg vein clearance. For shallow penetrating lasers such as CO_2 and erbium where the $\delta <<$ spotsize (all cases except for fractional devices), the diameter of the beam does not affect the tissue response. That is why equivalent results can be obtained for skin resurfacing using pulsed CO_2 lasers versus scanned, tightly focused cw CO_2 lasers.[45] Although studies suggest that large spots increase the ratio of dermal to epidermal damage (usually desirable, for example, when treating a hair bulb), there are instances where small spots are desirable. For example, when treating a smaller vessel with an Nd YAG laser, a small spot with higher fluence will result in a higher percentage of the energy being invested in vessel heating versus larger spots. For any turbid medium, even if the spot is "top hat", there will be an accumulation of photons near the center of the beam such that a greater clinical effect will often be noted at the center of the spot.

Changing optical properties in real-time: Chromophore concentrations can change during a treatment session. One should never consider each laser tissue interaction as an independent event, but rather a cumulative process where visual endpoints are the most important ally for the physician. Optical properties of the skin are like the weather,[3] and one must accommodate the changes in real–time. For example, the dermal blood fraction increases after one pass of the PDL, such that for a second pass, the skin temperature will increase due to the higher μ_a. The phenomenon will, for example, lower the purpura threshold on a second pass. On the other hand, general anesthesia can decrease the blood flow in PWS and require a higher light dose. A failure to respond to these real-time changes accounts for many laser treatment shortcomings. In treating a PWS, tetracaine, for example, can increase local blood flow, as can applying heating pad or simply placing a patient in Trendelenburg position. One of our patients actually performs jumping jacks prior to her rosacea laser therapy to increase the response.[97]

Most laser tissue interactions are threshold-based, that is, a certain amount of energy must be invested over a specific time to achieve the desired efficacy. For example, to lighten a lentigo on the nose, even ten very–low-fluence passes, so long as the interval between passes is long enough to preclude cumulative heating, will not result in clearance. The analogy is a smallish man trying to push a car up a hill. Even if the man were to arrive every day at 6 AM to push the heavy car, the vehicle will remain stationary. There is no incremental car movement each day. One "laser" exception to this analogy is perhaps tissue tightening and protein denaturation over large volumes with complex molecules (i.e., collagen), where repeated low impact low fluence passes have been shown to increase the percentage of denatured collagen fibers recruited in to the tightening process. Part of this phenomenon might be secondary to differential denaturation temperatures of older versus younger fibers.

When treating vascular lesions, multiple "low" fluence passes can achieve cumulative improvement. For example, a second pass even seconds after an initial pass with the YAG laser or PDL will achieve additional bluing of an angioma. The dynamics of vascular heating is somewhat different than for water and melanin. In vascular applications, dynamic changes in blood properties play a role. Met-HgG is produced by one pass so that additional passes can result in an increase in absorption. Also the partial clot enhances absorption venous red blood.

With pigment lesions, repeated laser pulses delivered over short periods (0.25–1 s) intervals results in progressive graying or darkening of the lesions. On the other hand, repeated passes (after >1 min) will result in cumulative extent.

Both immediate and delayed pigmented darkening (seconds to minute after irradiation) after application is most likely due to optical property changes in melanin as well as erythema deep to the lesions that might add to the darkening perception of (Fig. 13).

Optical clearing with hyperosmolar solutions: Transparency of the skin is enhanced by topical application or intradermal injection of solutions such as glycerin.[98] Water and collagen become less bound such that the effective scattering coefficient of the dermis is reduced. Already this concept has been applied to increase the visibility of blood vessels from the surface. Possible applications include tattoo removal, where particles often are found several mm deep in tissue.

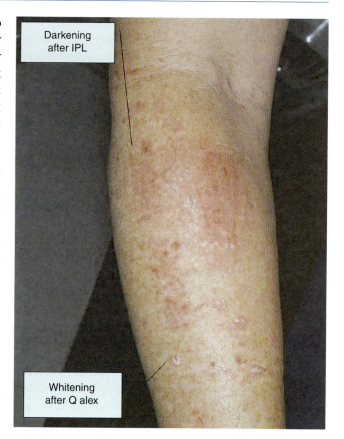

Fig. 13 Figure shows immediate pigment response after IPL and Q switched alexandrite laser

"Carbonization" at the surface: Carbon will cause all wavelengths to increase absorption such that one can convert a deeply penetrating laser to a more superficially penetrating laser by having a fine carbon layer at the surface. For example, one can "convert" a 694 nm ruby laser into a laser with CO_2 laser like effects by applying a fine layer of graphite from a copy machine to the skin surface. In this way the 694 nm laser energy is confined to the surface by the almost 100% absorption by carbon. This fine layer of heated materiel then cools much like a superficial layer of tissue heated by a CO_2 laser alone.

Photon recycling: The remittance of human skin is wavelength dependent (vide supra). These reflected photons are scattered into the environment and "wasted" in surgical laser applications. One can design a simple hemispherical reflector to return reflected light to the incident spot on the skin. In theory the gain in total energy available to skin is a factor of $\frac{1}{(1-R_S R_M)}$, where RS is the skin reflectance, and RM is that of a hemispherical mirror. For example, if RS is 0.7, and RM is 0.9, a gain of $\frac{1}{(1-0.63)}$, or almost threefold, can be achieved.

Photothermal responses in individual cells. Most of our characterization of laser-tissue responses is based on "macroscopic" responses. That is, individual cells are rarely examined during and after laser irradiation. When focal cell damage has been examined, the following considerations are made. (1) Heterogeneity of cell structure can lead to extreme localized light absorption and temperature elevation different from that of a homogenous medium. (2) Localized overheating may cause cell damage, even in the absence of average thermal effects over larger volumes.[99]

After absorption of a laser pulse, non-radiative relaxation of optical energy occurs within 10^{-11} s. Thus heating at the site of absorption is instantaneous. On the other hand, heat diffusion is much slower and characterized by the TRT. In experiment, not unexpectedly, it was found that that temperature fields in cells were more uniform with longer pulses. It follows that short pulses have smaller thermal fields but higher localized T elevations. The shorter the laser pulse, the more the final tissue response will depend on the properties of the local absorbing components. One interesting phenomenon is that on a localized level, an initial thermal field does not provide the maximum amplitude of the integral photothermal response inside a cell. Rather, the T response reaches its maximum as a result of the multiple secondary thermal fields as they emerge.

Using a polarizing lamp to enhance illumination. Laser treatment can be enhanced by using a polarizing lamp during procedures to treat vascular and pigmented lesions.. This is particularly helpful, for ex. when treating PWS in kids using general anesthetic, the lamp is[100] helpful to delineate the edges of the PWS prior to treatment. Also, the visual enhancement tends to result in more complete elimination of vessels, therefore patients are more satisfied.

Selective cell targeting. A process called selected cell targeting has been examined as a way to destroy selected cells. This precise energy deposition is achieved by using laser pulses and light absorbing immunoconjugates tagged to the respective cells. The investigators in one study showed, for example, that lymphocytes could be selectively damaged by attaching iron oxide microparticles absorbing 565 nm radiation at those sites.[101] One can imagine, in the future, using this type of modality to treat T-cell mediated diseases such as atopic dermatitis or psoriasis. In this way, one makes the "bad guy" more noticeable to the laser.

Scatter limited therapy – using small microbeams. Reinisch[102] proposed the use of beam diameter to titrate the depth of penetration, For example, we have studied a fractional (100 μm diameter microbeam and 100 mb/cm²) technology to achieve superficial vessel heating with relative epidermal sparing with just such a device to limit penetration into the dermis. By using the aforementioned spot size arguments, one can exploit the properties of small spots to change the way particular wavelengths behave in the skin. For example, one can tailor a 1,064 nm laser to heat progressively larger depths of skin by increasing the spot size.

Summary

An understanding of the scientific principles in laser applications empowers the physician to optimize the use of this very expensive equipment. At every patient encounter, the physician should craft an approach based on the logical sequence of laser tissue interactions outlined in this chapter. By appropriate choreographing of cooling and heating, the physician can be confidant in predicting the immediate tissue response. However, all approaches should be undertaken within the context of an understanding of wound healing. The physical aspects of the interaction are typically more predictable than the subsequent healing response. If in doubt, test spots are always an option and should be considered for the anxious patient (or physician).

References

1. Jacques SL. Laser-tissue interactions. Photochemical, photothermal, and photomechanical. *Surg Clin North Am.* 1992;72:531-558.
2. Ross E, Anderson R. Laser tissue interactions. In: Goldman M, ed. *Cutaneous and Cosmetic Laser Surgery.* Philadelphia: Elsevier; 2006.
3. Anderson RR, Parrish JA. The optics of human skin. *J Invest Dermatol.* 1981;77:13-19.
4. Grosstweiner L. *The Science of Phototherapy.* Boca Raton: CRC Press; 1994.
5. Wan S, Anderson RR, Parrish JA. Analytical modeling for the optical properties of the skin with in vitro and in vivo applications. *Photochem Photobiol.* 1981;34:493-499.
6. van Gemert MJ, Jacques SL, Sterenborg HJ, et al. Skin optics. *IEEE Trans Biomed Eng.* 1989;36:1146-1154.
7. Jacques S. Skin optics summary. http://www.omlc.ogi.edu/news/jan98/skinoptics.html. Accessed September 2007.
8. Jacques SL, Prahl SA. Modeling optical and thermal distributions in tissue during laser irradiation. *Lasers Surg Med.* 1987;6:494-503.
9. Hillenkamp F. Interaction between laser radiation and biological systems. In: Hillenkamp FRP, Sacchi C, eds. *Lasers in Medicine and Biology*, Series A. New York: Plenum; 1980:37-68.
10. Anderson R, Ross E. Laser-tissue interactions. In: Fitzpatrick R, Goldman M, eds. *Cosmetic Laser Surgery.* St. Louis: Mosby; 2000:1-30.
11. Katzir A. *Lasers and Optical Fibers in Medicine.* San Diego: Academic; 1993.
12. Ross EV. Laser versus intense pulsed light: competing technologies in dermatology. *Lasers Surg Med.* 2006;38:261-272.
13. Anderson R. Laser tissue interactions. In: Goldman M, Fitzparick R, eds. *Cutaneous Laser Surgery-The Art and Science of Selective Photothermolysis.* St. Louis: Mosby; 1994:3-5.
14. Reinisch L. Laser physics and tissue interactions. *Otolaryngol Clin North Am.* 1996;29:893-914.
15. Ross EV, Smirnov M, Pankratov M, ct al. Intense pulsed light and laser treatment of facial telangiectasias and dyspigmentation: some theoretical and practical comparisons. *Dermatol Surg.* 2005;31:1188-1198.
16. Boulnois J. Photophysical processes in recent medical laser developments - a review. *Lasers Med Sci.* 1986;1:47-66.
17. Welch AJ, van Gemert MJ. Overview of optical and thermal interaction and nomenclature. In: Welch AJ, van Gemert MJ, eds.

Optical Thermal Response of Laser-Irradiated Tissue. New York: Plenum; 1995:1-14.

18. Knappe V, Frank F, Rohde E. Principles of lasers and biophotonic effects. *Photomed Laser Surg.* 2004;22:411-417.

19. Fisher JC. Basic biophysical principles of resurfacing of human skin by means of the carbon dioxide laser. *J Clin Laser Med Surg.* 1996;14:193-210.

20. Tanghetti E, Sierra RA, Sherr EA, et al. Evaluation of pulse-duration on purpuric threshold using extended pulse pulsed dye laser (cynosure V-star). *Lasers Surg Med.* 2002;31:363-366.

21. Reinisch L, Ossoff RH. Laser applications in otolaryngology. *Otolaryngol Clin North Am.* 1996;29:891-892.

22. Shafirstein G, Baumler W, Lapidoth M, et al. A new mathematical approach to the diffusion approximation theory for selective photothermolysis modeling and its implication in laser treatment of port-wine stains. *Lasers Surg Med.* 2004;34:335-347.

23. Raulin C, Greve B, Warncke SH, et al. Excimer laser. Treatment of iatrogenic hypopigmentation following skin resurfacing. *Hautarzt.* 2004;55:746-748.

24. Alexiades-Armenakas MR, Bernstein LJ, Friedman PM, et al. The safety and efficacy of the 308-nm excimer laser for pigment correction of hypopigmented scars and striae alba. *Arch Dermatol.* 2004;140:955-960.

25. Gold MH, Goldman MP. 5-aminolevulinic acid photodynamic therapy: where we have been and where we are going. *Dermatol Surg.* 2004;30:1077-1083.

26. Itkin A, Gilchrest BA. delta-Aminolevulinic acid and blue light photodynamic therapy for treatment of multiple basal cell carcinomas in two patients with nevoid basal cell carcinoma syndrome. *Dermatol Surg.* 2004;30:1054-1061.

27. Anderson RR, Parrish JA. Selective photothermolysis: precise microsurgery by selective absorption of pulsed radiation. *Science.* 1983;220:524-527.

28. Anderson RR, Parrish JA. Lasers in dermatology provide a model for exploring new applications in surgical oncology. *Int Adv Surg Oncol.* 1982;5:341-358.

29. Anderson RR, Parrish JA. Microvasculature can be selectively damaged using dye lasers: a basic theory and experimental evidence in human skin. *Lasers Surg Med.* 1981;1:263-276.

30. Black JF, Barton JK. Chemical and structural changes in blood undergoing laser photocoagulation. *Photochem Photobiol.* 2004;80:89-97.

31. Kono T, Manstein D, Chan HH, et al. Q-switched ruby versus long-pulsed dye laser delivered with compression for treatment of facial lentigines in Asians. *Lasers Surg Med.* 2006;38:94-97.

32. Avram DK, Goldman MP. Effectiveness and safety of ALA-IPL in treating actinic keratoses and photodamage. *J Drugs Dermatol.* 2004;3(Suppl 1):S36-S39.

33. Gold MH, Bradshaw VL, Boring MM, et al. The use of a novel intense pulsed light and heat source and ALA-PDT in the treatment of moderate to severe inflammatory acne vulgaris. *J Drugs Dermatol.* 2004;3(Suppl 6):S15-S19.

34. Trafeli JP, Kwan JM, Meehan KJ, et al. Use of a long-pulse alexandrite laser in the treatment of superficial pigmented lesions. *Dermatol Surg.* 2007;33:1477-1482.

35. McDaniel DH, Ash K, Lord J, et al. Laser therapy of spider leg veins: clinical evaluation of a new long pulsed alexandrite laser. *Dermatol Surg.* 1999;25:52-58.

36. Dover JS. New approaches to the laser treatment of vascular lesions. *Australas J Dermatol.* 2000;41:14-18.

37. Kauvar AN, Lou WW. Pulsed alexandrite laser for the treatment of leg telangiectasia and reticular veins. *Arch Dermatol.* 2000;136: 1371-1375.

38. Eremia S, Li C, Umar SH. A side-by-side comparative study of 1064 nm Nd:YAG, 810 nm diode and 755 nm alexandrite lasers for treatment of 0.3-3 mm leg veins. *Dermatol Surg.* 2002;28: 224-230.

39. Passeron T, Olivier V, Duteil L, et al. The new 940-nanometer diode laser: an effective treatment for leg venulectasia. *J Am Acad Dermatol.* 2003;48:768-774.

40. Paithankar DY, Clifford JM, Saleh BA, et al. Subsurface skin renewal by treatment with a 1450-nm laser in combination with dynamic cooling. *J Biomed Opt.* 2003;8:545-551.

41. Zelickson B, Ross V, Kist D, et al. Ultrastructural effects of an infrared handpiece on forehead and abdominal skin. *Dermatol Surg.* 2006;32:897-901.

42. Majaron B, Verkruysse W, Kelly KM, et al. Er:YAG laser skin resurfacing using repetitive long-pulse exposure and cryogen spray cooling: II. Theoretical analysis. *Lasers Surg Med.* 2001;28: 131-138.

43. Majaron B, Kelly KM, Park HB, et al. Er:YAG laser skin resurfacing using repetitive long-pulse exposure and cryogen spray cooling: I. Histological study. *Lasers Surg Med.* 2001;28:121-131.

44. Ross EV, Yashar SS, Naseef GS, et al. A pilot study of in vivo immediate tissue contraction with CO2 skin laser resurfacing in a live farm pig. *Dermatol Surg.* 1999;25:851-856.

45. Ross EV, Grossman MC, Duke D, et al. Long-term results after CO2 laser skin resurfacing: a comparison of scanned and pulsed systems. *J Am Acad Dermatol.* 1997;37:709-718.

46. Carniol PJ, Maas CS. Bipolar radiofrequency resurfacing. *Facial Plast Surg Clin North Am.* 2001;9:337-342.

47. Ruiz-Esparza J, Gomez JB. The medical face lift: a noninvasive, nonsurgical approach to tissue tightening in facial skin using nonablative radiofrequency. *Dermatol Surg.* 2003;29:325-332. discussion 32.

48. Sadick NS. Update on non-ablative light therapy for rejuvenation: a review. *Lasers Surg Med.* 2003;32:120-128.

49. Koch RJ. Radiofrequency nonablative tissue tightening. *Facial Plast Surg Clin North Am.* 2004;12:339-346.

50. Sadick NS, Makino Y. Selective electro-thermolysis in aesthetic medicine: a review. *Lasers Surg Med.* 2004;34:91-97.

51. Zelickson BD, Kist D, Bernstein E, et al. Histological and ultrastructural evaluation of the effects of a radiofrequency-based nonablative dermal remodeling device: a pilot study. *Arch Dermatol.* 2004;140:204-209.

52. Sadick NS, Laughlin SA. Effective epilation of white and blond hair using combined radiofrequency and optical energy. *J Cosmet Laser Ther.* 2004;6:27-31.

53. Sadick NS, Alexiades-Armenakas M, Bitter P Jr, et al. Enhanced full-face skin rejuvenation using synchronous intense pulsed optical and conducted bipolar radiofrequency energy (ELOS): introducing selective radiophotothermolysis. *J Drugs Dermatol.* 2005;4: 181-186.

54. Hammes S, Greve B, Raulin C. Electro-optical synergy (ELOStrade mark) technology for nonablative skin rejuvenation: a preliminary prospective study. *J Eur Acad Dermatol Venereol.* 2006;20: 1070-1075.

55. Pearce J, Thomsen SL. Rate process analysis of theraml damage. In: Welch AJ, van Gemert MJ, eds. *Optical Thermal Response of Laser-Irradiated Tissue.* New York: Plenum; 1995:561-608.

56. Welch AJ, Yoon G, van Gemert MJ. Practical models for light distribution in laser-irradiated tissue. *Lasers Surg Med.* 1987;6: 488-493.

57. Wang L, Jacques S, Zheng L. MCML - Monte Carlo modeling of photon transport in multi-layered tissues. *Comput Meth Programs Biomed.* 1995;47:131.

58. Jacques S. Simple optical theory for light dosimetry during PDT. In: Tuchin V, ed. *Selected Papers on Tissue Optics, MS 102.* Bellingham: SPIE - International Society for Optical Engineering; 1992:655.

59. Stamatas GN, Kollias N. Blood stasis contributions to the perception of skin pigmentation. *J Biomed Opt.* 2004;9:315-322.

60. Niemz M. *Laser-Tissue Interactions.* 2nd ed. Berlin: Springer; 2002.

61. Anderson RR, Farinelli W, Laubach H, et al. Selective photothermolysis of lipid-rich tissues: a free electron laser study. *Lasers Surg Med.* 2006;38:913-919.
62. Ellis DL, Weisberg NK, Chen JS, et al. Free electron laser infrared wavelength specificity for cutaneous contraction. *Lasers Surg Med.* 1999;25:1-7.
63. Goldman L, Rockwell RJ. Laser action at the cellular level. *JAMA.* 1966;198:641-644.
64. Anderson RR. Laser medicine in dermatology. *J Dermatol.* 1996;23:778-782.
65. Altshuler GB, Anderson RR, Manstein D, et al. Extended theory of selective photothermolysis. *Lasers Surg Med.* 2001;29:416-432.
66. Anderson RR, Margolis RJ, Watenabe S, et al. Selective photothermolysis of cutaneous pigmentation by Q-switched Nd: YAG laser pulses at 1064, 532, and 355 nm. *J Invest Dermatol.* 1989;93:28-32.
67. Parrish JA, Anderson RR, Harrist T, et al. Selective thermal effects with pulsed irradiation from lasers: from organ to organelle. *J Invest Dermatol.* 1983;80(Suppl):75s-80s.
68. Anderson RR, Jaenicke KF, Parrish JA. Mechanisms of selective vascular changes caused by dye lasers. *Lasers Surg Med.* 1983;3:211-215.
69. Itzkan I, Izatt J. Medical use of lasers. In: *Encyclopedia of Applied Physics.* Washington, DC: VCH Publishers, Inc. & American Institute of Physics; 1994:33-59.
70. Black JF, Wade N, Barton JK. Mechanistic comparison of blood undergoing laser photocoagulation at 532 and 1, 064 nm. *Lasers Surg Med.* 2005;36:155-165.
71. Polla BS, Anderson RR. Thermal injury by laser pulses: protection by heat shock despite failure to induce heat-shock response. *Lasers Surg Med.* 1987;7:398-404.
72. Beckham JT, Mackanos MA, Crooke C, et al. Assessment of cellular response to thermal laser injury through bioluminescence imaging of heat shock protein 70. *Photochem Photobiol.* 2004;79:76-85.
73. Kollias N, Gillies R, Moran M, et al. Endogenous skin fluorescence includes bands that may serve as quantitative markers of aging and photoaging. *J Invest Dermatol.* 1998;111:776-780.
74. Alexiades-Armenakas MR, Geronemus RG. Laser-mediated photodynamic therapy of actinic cheilitis. *J Drugs Dermatol.* 2004;3: 548-551.
75. Karrer S, Baumler W, Abels C, et al. Long-pulse dye laser for photodynamic therapy: investigations in vitro and in vivo. *Lasers Surg Med.* 1999;25:51-59.
76. Seguchi K, Kawauchi S, Morimoto Y, et al. Critical parameters in the cytotoxicity of photodynamic therapy using a pulsed laser. *Lasers Med Sci.* 2002;17:265-271.
77. Sterenborg HJ, van Gemert MJ. Photodynamic therapy with pulsed light sources: a theoretical analysis. *Phys Med Biol.* 1996;41: 835-849.
78. Smith TK, Choi B, Ramirez-San-Juan JC, et al. Microvascular blood flow dynamics associated with photodynamic therapy, pulsed dye laser irradiation and combined regimens. *Lasers Surg Med.* 2006;38:532-539.
79. Parrish JA, Jaenicke KF. Action spectrum for phototherapy of psoriasis. *J Investig Dermatol.* 1981;76:359-362.
80. Weiss RA, McDaniel DH, Geronemus RG, et al. Clinical trial of a novel non-thermal LED array for reversal of photoaging: clinical, histologic, and surface profilometric results. *Lasers Surg Med.* 2005;36:85-91.
81. Hohenleutner U, Walther T, Wenig M, et al. Leg telangiectasia treatment with a 1.5 ms pulsed dye laser, ice cube cooling of the skin and 595 vs 600 nm: preliminary results. *Lasers Surg Med.* 1998;23:72-78.
82. Greve B, Hammes S, Raulin C. The effect of cold air cooling on 585 nm pulsed dye laser treatment of port-wine stains. *Dermatol Surg.* 2001;27:633-636.
83. Chan HH, Lam LK, Wong DS, et al. Role of skin cooling in improving patient tolerability of Q-switched Alexandrite (QS Alex) laser in nevus of Ota treatment. *Lasers Surg Med.* 2003;32:148-151.
84. Raulin C, Greve B, Hammes S. Cold air in laser therapy: first experiences with a new cooling system. *Lasers Surg Med.* 2000;27:404-410.
85. Huang PS, Chang CJ. Cryogen spray cooling in conjunction with pulse dye laser treatment of port wine stains of the head and neck. *Chang Gung Med J.* 2001;24:469-475.
86. Weiss RA, Sadick NS. Epidermal cooling crystal collar device for improved results and reduced side effects on leg telangiectasias using intense pulsed light. *Dermatol Surg.* 1015;26:1015-1018.
87. Tunnell JW, Nelson JS, Torres JH, et al. Epidermal protection with cryogen spray cooling during high fluence pulsed dye laser irradiation: an ex vivo study. *Lasers Surg Med.* 2000;27:373-383.
88. Kelly KM, Nelson JS, Lask GP, et al. Cryogen spray cooling in combination with nonablative laser treatment of facial rhytides. *Arch Dermatol.* 1999;135:691-694.
89. Weiss RA, Sadick NS. Epidermal cooling crystal collar device for improved results and reduced side effects on leg telangiectasias using intense pulsed light. *Dermatol Surg.* 2000;26:1015-1018.
90. Zenzie HH, Altshuler GB, Smirnov MZ, et al. Evaluation of cooling methods for laser dermatology. *Lasers Surg Med.* 2000;26: 130-144.
91. Almoallim H, Klinkhoff AV, Arthur AB, et al. Laser induced chrysiasis: disfiguring hyperpigmentation following Q-switched laser therapy in a woman previously treated with gold. *J Rheumatol.* 2006;33:620-621.
92. Trotter MJ, Tron VA, Hollingdale J, et al. Localized chrysiasis induced by laser therapy. *Arch Dermatol.* 1995;131:1411-1414.
93. Franco W, Childers M, Nelson JS, et al. Laser surgery of port wine stains using local vacuum [corrected] pressure: changes in calculated energy deposition (Part II). *Lasers Surg Med.* 2007; 39:118-127.
94. Childers MA, Franco W, Nelson JS, et al. Laser surgery of port wine stains using local vacuum pressure: changes in skin morphology and optical properties (Part I). *Lasers Surg Med.* 2007;39:108-117.
95. Manstein D, Herron GS, Sink RK, et al. Fractional photothermolysis: a new concept for cutaneous remodeling using microscopic patterns of thermal injury. *Lasers Surg Med.* 2004;34:426-438.
96. Dierickx CC. Hair removal by lasers and intense pulsed light sources. *Semin Cutan Med Surg.* 2000;19:267-275.
97. Jasim ZF, Handley JM. Treatment of pulsed dye laser-resistant port wine stain birthmarks. *J Am Acad Dermatol.* 2007;57:677-682.
98. Choi B, Tsu L, Chen E, et al. Determination of chemical agent optical clearing potential using in vitro human skin. *Lasers Surg Med.* 2005;36:72-75.
99. Lapotko D, Shnip A, Lukianova E. Photothermal responses of individual cells. *J Biomed Opt.* 2005;10:14006.
100. Anderson RR. Polarized light examination and photography of the skin. *Arch Dermatol.* 1991;127:1000-1005.
101. Pitsillides CM, Joe EK, Wei X, et al. Selective cell targeting with light-absorbing microparticles and nanoparticles. *Biophys J.* 2003;84:4023-4032.
102. Reinisch L. Scatter-limited phototherapy: a model for laser treatment of skin. *Lasers Surg Med.* 2002;30:381-388.

Laser Safety: Regulations, Standards and Practice Guidelines

Ashley Keyes and Murad Alam

Laser Safety

The use of lasers is routine in many medical specialties. In some cases, the particular benefit of lasers has made them desirable alternatives to conventional surgical instruments such as scalpels, electrosurgical units, cryosurgery probes, or microwave devices. The American Society for Laser Medicine and Surgery (ASLMS) outlines several advantages of laser use in clinical practice[1]:

> Lasers allow the surgeon to accomplish more complex tasks, reduce blood loss, decrease postoperative discomfort, reduce the chance of wound infection, decrease the spread of some cancers, minimize the extent of surgery in selected circumstances and result in better wound healing, if used appropriately by a skilled and properly trained surgeon.

Despite these benefits, when misused, lasers can injure both patients and operator. To ensure safety and quality care, guidelines for laser safety have been developed.

Governing Bodies and Professional Organizations

> Many regulatory and professional organizations provide recommendations and guidelines for laser safety. While the American National Standards Institute (ANSI) publishes consensus standards considered to be the standard in laser safety, these standards are recommended practices only. The positions of professional organizations are important to consider in addition to those of ANSI to ensure comprehensive safety standards for laser use are practiced.

A number of regulatory and professional organizations have promulgated and disseminated recommendations for safe laser use. Though there is considerable agreement among professional organizations and regulatory agencies regarding laser safety guidelines, variation among patients, facilities, and state laws ultimately affects how these rules are implemented.

The American National Standards Institute (ANSI) creates and publishes consensus standards for the conduct of business in almost all sectors, including medicine. This chapter will refer to the ANSI Z 136.3, the American National Standard for Safe Use of Lasers in Health Care Facilities, with specific attention to control measures, as it is widely regarded as the standard for laser use. It is important to clarify that these standards are recommended practices rather than rules subject to enforcement, and compliance is both voluntary and dependent on individual organization's specifications.

In addition to the standards set forth by ANSI, medical organizations also set professional standards for their membership. The American Society for Laser Medicine and Surgery (ASLMS), with its multidisciplinary membership, including physicians and surgeons, nurses, and other health professionals, is an umbrella organization for all specialties whose clinical care involves lasers. In addition to formulating standards and guidelines for implementing safe and effective laser practices, ASLMS also makes recommendations to medical laser training programs regarding procedural skill for individuals operating lasers.

The American Academy of Dermatology (AAD), the primary professional organization for practicing dermatologists in the United States, encourages the safe practice of medicine and acknowledges that medical laser is subsumed under the practice of medicine. "The Academy endorses the concept that use of properly trained non-physician office personnel under appropriate supervision allows certain procedures to be performed safely and effectively."[2]

The American Society for Dermatologic Surgery (ASDS), the main professional organization within dermatology for proceduralists, is committed to the development of safe in-office procedures. The ASDS maintains that

---

A. Keyes (✉)
Department of Dermatology, Northwestern University, Feinberg School of Medicine, Chicago, IL, USA
e-mail: ash.keyes@gmail.com

K. Nouri (ed.), *Lasers in Dermatology and Medicine*,
DOI: 10.1007/978-0-85729-281-0_2, © Springer-Verlag London Limited 2011

medical laser use constitutes the practice of medicine, and that non-physicians should use lasers only when delegated do so by physicians who are appropriately supervising them.

Medical laser use is also subject to regulation by the relevant state and by the U.S. Food and Drug Administration (FDA). Laser devices, such as those used for medical application require clearance or premarket approval by the FDA Center for Devices and Radiological Health (CDRH) prior to distribution for commercial use in the United States. The Radiation Control for Health and Safety Act (RCHSA), a standard similar to that of ANSI, is intended to prevent unnecessary or inappropriate access to laser equipment, and to minimize exposure to collateral radiation. Additionally, RCHSA ensures the appropriate performance features and labels are provided by the manufacturer.[2] With respect to laser devices, the FDA is responsible for classifying laser devices based on levels of laser emission. For medical use, lasers are defined as Class III and IV, which require the highest level of regulation for safe use.

Practice Guidelines

> The first tenet to laser safety is the training of physicians, healthcare professionals, and personnel. The American Society for Laser Medicine and Surgery (ASLMS) outlines recommendations for training and credentialing, which are referenced by the ANSI standards.

Procedural Skills

The ASLMS outlines recommendations for the safe use of laser technology, specifically training and credentialing benchmarks, to be used in conjunction with the ANSI Z 136.3 guidelines. Training and credentialing represent distinct issues for laser safety, especially given the escalating debate regarding laser use by non-physicians.

The ANSI Z 136.3 refers to the ASLMS policy "Standards of Training for Physicians for the Use of Lasers in Medicine and Surgery," which was approved by the board of directors on April 3 of 2008, regarding the recommendation for appropriate training for laser privileges. The specific suggestions for training are as follows[3]:

> The initial program should include clinical applications of various wavelengths in the particular specialty field and hands-on practical sessions with lasers and their appropriate surgical or therapeutic delivery systems. A minimum of 8–10 h is suggested by the ANSI standards. A further 40% of the time should be allocated to the practical sessions. However, more time may be required to complete the basic course contents. Usually, basic training is concentrated on one or more wavelengths. Subsequent programs covering different wavelengths or substantially different applications or delivery instruments may require more hours of training of which 50% of the time is allocated to hands-on sessions. A small faculty-student ratio in the range of 1 to 3-5 is optimal.

> It is recommended that an applicant for privileges spend time after the basic training course in a clinical setting with an experienced operator (such programs are often called "preceptorship" training programs or "observation") when appropriate and practical. Several brief visits or a more prolonged period suffices provided that a variety of cases is observed. It is valuable for the novice to perform the laser procedures with supervision by the expert, however, for a variety of reasons, such as hospital privileges, status of patients and insurance coverage of physicians, this is not always possible.

In addition to training recommendations for physicians, ANSI also suggests standards for general laser safety and training programs, with specific attention to nurses and other non-medical personnel. The following summarizes this position[3]:

> Laser safety training for perioperative nursing and support personnel must be compatible with that taught to physicians. A smoothly functioning laser team depends on this, and every effort must be made to eliminate any discrepancies in training materials. Content of this program should stress overall understanding of operation characteristics of equipment, biologic and physical properties of the laser tissue interaction, potential hazards associated with laser use, and procedures and equipment required to ensure a safe laser environment.

ANSI maintains that training in laser safety practices for physicians and non-physicians should be distinguished from training of methods and techniques of laser procedures.

Though the need for operators to be trained in laser use is universally accepted, the process of credentialing physician and/or non-physician operators as competent in laser use is more subject to debate and interpretation. Often strict and multiple criteria bus be simultaneously met to satisfy credentialing rules. In its paper entitled "Procedural Skills for Using Lasers in General Surgery," which was approved on April 6, 2006 by the ASLMS board of directors, the criteria for granting laser privileges are summarized[4]:

A. The physician (attending) must be a diplomat of or be admissible to a specialty Board such as the American Board of Surgery; Orthopedics; Otolaryngology; Ophthalmology; Urology; Dermatology; Plastic Surgery; Cardiovascular Surgery; Neurosurgery; or other medical specialty.

B. The physician must first have been granted appropriate privileges by the facility through the designated certification and facility process. The physician must have privileges to perform requested procedures in the absence of laser use.

C. The physician must have been trained to use laser(s) in a recognized and approved residency program or must have obtained training through an appropriate CME course.

D. Physicians using a laser adapted to an operating microscope or other optical device must demonstrate proficiency in the use of the optical equipment in addition to the laser technology. The physician must already have hospital privileges for the use of these instruments in the performance of procedures with conventional techniques.

E. The user of the laser must be cognizant of the safety hazards of lasers. This knowledge must be obtained either through a residency program or an appropriate CME course. Proof of this training must be supplied in writing to the Laser Usage Committee at the time privileges are requested.

F. Initial approval or use of laser will be provisional until the physician has demonstrated the ability to use lasers to a member of the Medical Staff who has been designated by the facility as being qualified and must have achieved the required standards as previously listed. The criteria for recertification shall be set forth and a yearly review of cases and their outcomes shall be performed.

G. If the applicant requests the use of the laser for investigational purposes, the request must receive approval by the facility's Clinical Investigation Committee (IRB/CIC) as is required for all other research purposes. An appropriate investigational protocol and informed consent process must be in place.

H. Residents involved in the use of lasers may not perform procedures with these instruments until such time as they have attended an in-depth training program or an appropriate CME course recognized to be adequate by the Laser Usage Committee. In addition, residents must be supervised by a laser-certified attending physician during actual utilization of laser technology at all times.

Similarly, ASLMS outlines physician qualifications for proficiency in laser techniques in its policy statement entitled "Procedural Skill and Technique Proficiency for Laser Medicine and Surgery in Dermatology." Approved on November 2, 2005, by the board of directors, the following requirements are relevant to laser use in dermatology[5]:

- Possession of an appropriate medical degree or its equivalent. Candidates must be a Doctor of Medicine (MD) or Doctor of Osteopathy (DO) and complete an ACGME accredited residency in their specialty areas.
- Must possess primary specialty certification from the American Board of Dermatology.
- For a specified period of time (5 years) there will be a practice category for eligibility. Specific criteria for qualifying under this category will be determined and approved by an independent certifying body. Suggested requirements for this category may include the following:
  - (a) Completion of at least 150 h of Category 1 CME including laser safety and physics. At least 20 h of the 150 h must entail hands on workshops proctored by an experienced physician in laser medicine and surgery and a minimum of 50 h in programming approved by the American Society for Laser Medicine and Surgery (ASLMS), American Academy of Dermatology (AAD) or the American Society for Dermatological Surgery (ASDS).
  - (b) Submission of 100 cases with a minimum of 15 sets of before and after photos or videotapes representative of at least four of the nine management areas.
  - (c) Mastery of Standards of Training must be demonstrated by obtaining a passing grade on an examination the content of which will be determined by an independent certifying body.
  - (d) Letters of recommendation attesting to character from at least three practicing physicians in the same specialty.

It is the widely accepted belief of the aforementioned organizations that a necessary precondition for patient safety is the proper training and credentialing of healthcare professionals. As such, despite differences in details, there is minimal, significant variation in the standards by which physicians are assessed with regard to their competence to utilize medical laser devices. Discrepancies arise when considering credentialing of alternative allied health providers, which will be addressed later in this chapter in the section on delegation and regulation by the state.

Administrative Controls

> Administrative controls are essential for the safe operation of lasers within a healthcare facility. These control measures minimize the potential for hazards to operator and patient during laser use. A Laser Safety Officer (LSO) is appointed to ensure the appropriate standards are followed.

The ANSI Z 136.3 is accepted as the standard for guidelines regarding the safe use of laser in health care facilities. Specifically, this document details control measures to minimize the potential hazards of laser use. Though each facility and patient engenders unique safety considerations, the following guidelines address unintended hazards to both patients and personnel.

To ensure administrative control within the health care facility, a Laser Safety Officer (LSO) is appointed to implement the following standards.[3]

4.2.1 Standard Operating Procedures (Class 3B and Class 4). The LSO shall require approved written operating and maintenance SOPs for Class 3B and Class 4 Hospital Care Laser Systems (HCLS). These operating and maintenance SOPs shall be maintained and readily available. The LSO shall require that safety SOPs exist for servicing of the HCLS.

4.2.3 Authorized Personnel-Laser Users and Laser Assistants. Class 3B and Class 4 HCLSs shall be operated by facility-authorized personnel appropriately trained in the safe use of the HCLS.

4.2.5 Procedural Controls. Procedural controls, as determined, by the LSO, shall be used where possible to avoid potential hazards associated with Class 3B and Class 4 HCLSs. These include controls such as:

- (1) Adherence to written safety policies and procedures (SOPs).
- (2) Assignment of a qualified laser assistant, if applicable.
- (3) Maintaining a list of authorized laser users and Health Care Personnel (HCP).
- (4) Requiring storage or disabling (removal of key) of the HCLS where unauthorized operation is of concern.
- (5) Assurance that staff is informed of the location, and w of operating, the emergency stop control provided with each HCLS.

(6) Assurance that the ready function is enabled only when the user is ready to treat the target tissue.
(7) Use of only diffuse reflective materials or instruments with low reflectance in or near the beam path, where feasible.
(8) Taking steps to avoid confusion encountered during surgical procedures when operating with more than one floor pedal.

The specific administrative controls implemented in a health care facility may vary. It is the LSO's responsibility to ensure the appropriate safety measures are in place to accommodate the specific needs of the patient and facility.

Figure 1 illustrates an overview of practice guidelines and to whom they are relevant.

Protective Equipment

> Protective equipment includes warning signs and labels, eye and skin protection, and smoke evacuations to reduce non-beam hazards. Used properly during laser procedures, protective equipment reduces the risk of injury to operator and patient, as well as increasing the overall safety of healthcare facilities in which laser equipment resides.

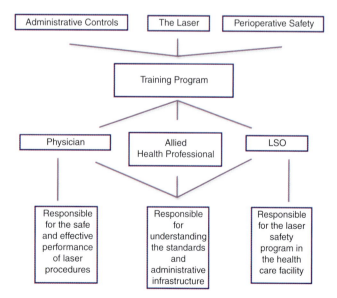

Fig. 1 Three key components of a laser safety program include understanding of administrative controls, knowledge of laser function and use, and guidelines for perioperative safety. Despite variation in responsibilities among physicians, healthcare professionals and the LSO, consensus among practice guidelines is essential to the safe use of medical lasers

Warming Signs and Labels

The Nominal Hazard Zone (NHZ) is the physical space in which levels of radiation, direct, reflected, or scattered, exceed the Maximum Permissible Exposure (MPE), which may be determined by the safety information provided by the manufacturer. While a Class III or Class IV laser is in operation, appropriate warning signs and labels, as well as protective equipment is administratively required for all individuals within the NHZ. Warning signs and labels are provided by the ANSI Z 136.3 in accordance with the Federal Laser Product Performance Standard, including the following[3]:

> 4.7.1 Display of Warning Signs. Warning signs shall be conspicuously displayed on all doors entering the Laser Treatment Controlled Area (LTCA), so as to warn those entering the area of laser use. Warning signs should be covered or removed when the laser is not in use.
>
> 4.7.3 Inclusion of Pertinent Information. Signs and Labels shall conform to the following specifications.
>
> 4.7.3.1 The appropriate signal word (Caution or Danger) shall be located in the upper panel.
>
> 4.7.3.2 Adequate space shall be left on all signs and labels to allow the inclusion of pertinent information. Such information may be included during the printing of the sign or label or may be handwritten in a legible manner, and shall include the following.
>
> (1) At position 1 above the tail of the sunburst, special precautionary instructions or protection action such as "Laser Surgery in Process – Eye Protection Required"
>   a. For Class 2 lasers and laser systems, "Laser Radiation – Do Not Stare into Beam"
>   b. For Class 3 lasers and laser systems where the accessible irradiance does not exceed the appropriate MPE based on a 0.25 s exposure, "Laser Radiation – Do Not Stare into Beam or View with Optical Instruments"
>   c. For all other Class 3R lasers and laser systems, "laser Radiation – Avoid Direct Exposure to Beam"
>   d. For all Class 3B lasers and laser systems, "Laser Radiation – Avoid Direct Exposure to Beam"
>   e. For Class 4 laser and laser systems, "Laser Radiation – Avoid Eye or Skin Exposure to Direct or Scattered Radiation"
> (2) At position 1 above the tail of the sunburst, special precautionary instructions or protective action such as: "laser Surgery in Process – Eye Protection Required"
> (3) At position 2 below the tail of the sunburst, type of laser (Nd: YAG, CO2, etc.) or the emitted wavelength, pulse duration (if appropriate), and maximum output.
> (4) At position 3, the class of the laser or laser system.

Figure 2 shows the appropriate warning signs for (a) Class 2 lasers and (b) Class 3 and 4 lasers.

Eye and Skin Protection

Additional protective measures must be followed to ensure the safety of patients, staff, and operator while in the NHZ. The following recommendations are relevant to eye and skin safety[3]:

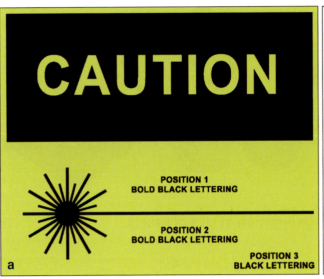 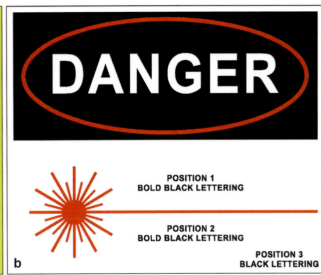

Fig. 2 The distinction between appropriate laser warning signs for (**a**) Class 2 and (**b**) Class 3 and 4 lasers

4.6.2 Protective Eyewear (Class 3B and Class 4). Laser protective eyewear ma include but not be limited to goggles, face shields, spectacles or prescription eyewear using special filter materials or reflective coatings (or a combination of both), which are selected to reduce the potential ocular exposure below the applicable MPE level. Eyewear shall be accompanied by the following information:

(1) Optical density at appropriate wavelengths.
(2) Manufacturer's recommendations on shelf life, storage conditions, and appropriate cleaning methods.

4.6.2.4 Cleaning and Inspection. Periodic cleaning and inspection of protective eyewear shall be made to ensure the maintenance of satisfactory condition. This shall include:

(1) Periodic cleaning of laser eyewear.
(2) Inspection of the attenuation material for pitting, crazing, cracking, discoloration, etc.
(3) Inspection of the frame for mechanical integrity.
(4) Inspection of straps or other retaining devices to ensure that they are not excessively worn or damaged.
(5) Inspection for light leaks and coating damage that would permit hazardous intrabeam viewing.

4.6.3 Laser Protective Barriers and Curtains (Class 3B and Class 4). Facility windows (exterior or interior) or entry ways that are located within the NHZ of a Class 3B or Class 4 laser system, shall be provided with an appropriate filter or barrier which reduces any transmissible radiation to levels below the applicable MPE level.

4.6.3.1 Drapes. Use only wet or nonflammable drapes in the operative field.

4.6.4 Skin Protection (Class 3B and Class 4). The manufacturer of the HCLS or the LSO shall specify the appropriate laser protective equipment by make and model or performance specifications and the locations and conditions for use of the skin protective equipment. Skin protection hall be used whenever there is a potential hazard to HCP.

Though protective equipment is required for all individuals within the NHZ, depending on the nature of the procedure, the protocol for patient eye protection may be different for operator and staff protection. The following specifications are important to consider, especially for procedures performed on the face:

4.4.4 Patient Eye Protection. When the patient's eyes are potentially within the NHZ, they shall be protected from inadvertent exposure by a method approved by the LSO, i.e., suitable protective eye pads or corneal shields adequate to protect the eye from laser exposure.

When facial areas, particularly around the eyes are being treated, e.g., for port wine stains or neoplasia, protective glasses may not be appropriate for shielding the eyes. For treatments on or near the eyelids, appropriate corneal shields are usually required, and the shield shall have appropriate optical properties to reduce exposure below the applicable MPE. Additionally, patient eye protection is not intended to restrict or limit in any way the use of laser radiation intentionally administered for therapeutic or diagnostic purposes.

There is a consensus among professional organizations that laser protective equipment should not only be in good working order, but also meet both local and ANSI standards for protective equipment.

Figure 3 shows a variety of eye protection for both patient and operator.

Non-beam Hazards

Besides direct hazards to the eyes and skin due to laser beam exposure, concerns associated with non-beam hazards present unique laser safety considerations. According to a publication by

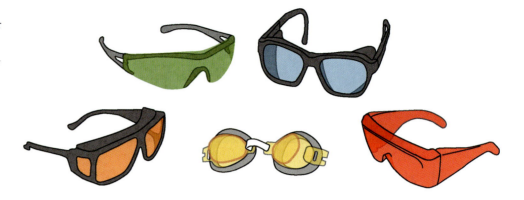

Fig. 3 A selection of eyewear suitable for patient and operator safety. Care should be taken to select the appropriate lenses to protect against various levels of laser emission

the National Institute for Occupational Safety and Health (NIOSH), the plume (smoke byproduct) produced by thermal destruction of tissue can contain toxic gasses or vapors, dead or living cellular material, or even viruses. As a result, control of smoke is essential to minimize health risks to health care personnel, as well as visual interference to the individual performing the procedure. NIOSH recommends the two following methods of ventilation for the management of airborne contaminants[6]:

> Smoke evacuators contain a suction unit (vacuum pump), filter, hose, and an inlet nozzle. The smoke evacuator should have high efficiency in airborne particle reduction and should be used in accordance with the manufacturer's recommendations to achieve maximum efficiency. A capture velocity of about 100 to 150 ft per minute at the inlet nozzle is generally recommended. It is also important to choose a filter that is effective in collecting the contaminants. A High Efficiency Particulate Air (HEPA) filter or equivalent is recommended for trapping particulates. Various filtering and cleaning processes also exist which remove or inactivate airborne gases and vapors. The various filters and absorbers used in smoke evacuators require monitoring and replacement on a regular basis and are considered a possible biohazard requiring proper disposal.
>
> Room suction systems can pull at a much lower rate and were designed primarily to captures liquids rather than particulate or gases. If these systems are used to capture generated smoke, users must install appropriate filters in the line, insure that the line is cleared, and that filters are disposed properly. Generally speaking, the use of smoke evacuators are more effective than room suction systems to control the generated smoke from non-endoscopic laser/electric surgical procedures.

In a statement entitled "Smoking Guns," approved by the Board of Directors of the ASLMS, the aforementioned NIOSH guidelines are referenced; however, the statement highlights that these guidelines stop short of requiring personal respirators for personnel within the operating room. The ANSI Z 136.3 states that currently a suitable half-mask respirator (fitting over the nose and mouth) to exclude laser-generated plume does not exist. As such, the recommendation is that health care facilities rely on appropriate ventilation techniques to protect against laser generated airborne contaminants.[3] It is the unanimous opinion of the aforementioned regulatory organizations that a smoke evacuation apparatus be utilized to protect patient and personnel and to control smoke levels in the operating room.

Delegation of Use of Lasers

> Non-physician use of lasers has been subject to debate in recent years leading to calls for increased regulation regarding delegation of medical procedures to alternative healthcare professionals. While professional organizations maintain their own positions on delegation of medical procedures, state legislature plays a significant role in this determination as well. Regardless of the differences between organizations and states, the consensus is that the physician is ultimately responsible for patient safety.

In recent years, there has been increasing concern regarding frequency and severity of reported adverse events associated with the use of lasers by non-physicians. This has led to calls for increased regulation regarding delegation of medical procedures to non-physicians. Guidelines have been created by professional organizations as well as state medical boards and legislature to delineate who is qualified to safely practice medicine involving lasers.

The ASDS and AAD maintain the position that only active and properly licensed doctors of medicine and osteopathy shall conduct the practice of medicine. But, a physician may delegate certain medical procedures to certified or licensed allied health professionals under the appropriate circumstances. The ASDS Board of Directors approved the following statement in May of 2008.[7]

> The physician must directly supervise the allied health professionals to protect the best interests and welfare of each patient. The supervising physician shall be physically present on-site, immediately available, and able to respond promptly to any question or problem that may occur while the procedure is being performed. It is the responsible physician's obligation to ensure that, with respect to each procedure performed, the allied health professionals possess knowledge of cutaneous medicine, documented training in the procedure, the indications for the procedure, and the pre- and post- operative care involved.

In a position statement approved by the Board of Directors on February 22, 2002, the AAD expressed a similar opinion regarding medical laser use by non-physicians with an additional requirement: "The non-physician office personnel should also be appropriately trained by the delegating physician in cutaneous medicine."[2]

Though the positions of the ASDS and AAD appear clear, delegation remains a controversial issue, especially due to the potential ambiguity that arises from differences in legislation in different states.

In addition to adhering to the standards set forth by their professional organization, physicians must comply with state laws regarding laser use. In this chapter, legislation in California, Florida, Illinois, New York, and Texas will be addressed. The Federation of State Medical Boards last summarized the following regulations for each state on June 5, 2008.

In California, laser regulation adheres closely to the position of the ASDS, with additional stipulations regarding written documentation of supervision protocols and procedures. California also defines which non-physician health professionals may perform laser hair removal[8] (Table 1):

> The Business and Professions Code includes the use of laser devices in the definition of the practice of medicine. Only physicians, dentists, physician assistants and nurses may use laser devices, including intense pulse light devices, with physician supervision within their legal scope of practice. The law requires written protocols and procedures relating to supervision. Laser hair removal may be performed only by a nurse physician or, when working with a physician, registered nurse of physician assistants.

In Florida, however, specifications requiring registration of laser systems with the Department of Health set an additional standard for safety.[8]

> The Board of medicine considers the use of high-powered lasers (all Class IIIa, IIIb, and IV lasers as designated by the FDA) to be the practice of medicine. These may be used only by physicians, or by those exempt from the Medical Practice Act (such as nurses) while acting under the direct supervision of a physician. Florida also requires all high-powered laser systems to be registered with the Department of Health. Failure to do so may be grounds for

disciplinary action against a physician and may result in a criminal penalty.

Additionally, Florida mandates specialty-specific requirements relating to supervision[8]:

> In office setting where supervision not onsite, primary health practitioners limited to supervising four offices in addition to the primary office location; specialty practitioners limited to 2; dermatologists limited to 1.

In Illinois, there are currently two pending articles that could dramatically affect the use of lasers if passed[8]:

> 2007 HB 3679 – Allows a physician to delegate the operation of an intense pulsed light system or laser for the purpose of epilation, photorejuvenation, or other non-medical cosmetic procedures to a physician assistant, advanced practice nurse, registered nurse, electrologist, or other personnel provided those persons have adequate training.
>
> 2008 HB 4667 – States that a board certified plastic surgeon shall be the only individuals permitted to perform laser surgeries, Botox injections, or chemical peels on patients. The Board – certified plastic surgeon may not delegate the performance of any of these procedures to any other individual.

The second statute is controversial as it poses the risk of establishing a hierarchy among physicians, potentially eroding inter-specialty collegiality. Though the interest of the patient is the motivation for strict regulation, this policy could ultimately be detrimental to patient care by restricting the number of qualified physicians allowed to perform laser procedures.

The Board of Medicine in New York regulates the use of lasers for hair removal in a similar manner as California[8]:

> In August 2002, the NY State Board of Medicine passed a resolution recommending that the sue of lasers and intense pulsed light for hair removal to be considered the practice of medicine and thus be performed by a physician or under direct physician supervision.

To ensure compliance with these regulations, the New York Education Law defines the following two statutes as professional misconduct[8]:

Table 1 State regulation of laser use

California	Florida	Illinois	New York	Texas
Lasers constitute practice of medicine	Class III and IV lasers to be used by physicians or under physician supervision	Pending legislation to further restrict who may perform laser procedures	Laser hair removal constitutes practice of medicine; to be performed by physicians or under physician supervision	Physician supervision is defined as physically present in the same building
Written protocol and procedures regarding delegation and supervision	High powered laser systems to be registered with the department of health		Delegation to incompetent healthcare providers is considered professional misconduct	The use of lasers for ablative procedures may only be performed by physicians
Laser hair removal restricted to nurse physicians, RNs or PAs				

(24) Practicing beyond the scope of practice permitted by state law and performing professional responsibilities a licensee knows he/she is not competent to perform.

(25) Delegating professional responsibilities to a person when the licensee delegating such responsibilities knows or has reason to know that such person is not qualified, by training, experience or by licensure to perform.

Though New York law does not address new issues, it strengthens the responsibility of the physician by including regulations on delegation prominently within its code of professional misconduct.

In Texas, the State Board provides a few detailed clarifications the previous states do not. In the position statements on laser regulation, on-site supervision is defined as continuous supervision with the individual in the same building.[8] Further, the State Board explicitly distinguishes practice guidelines for ablative and non-ablative procedures[8]:

(2) The use of lasers/pulsed light devices for non-ablative procedures cannot be delegated to nonphysicians delegates, other than an advanced health care practitioner without the delegating physician being on site and immediately available.

(3) The use of lasers/pulsed light devices for ablative procedures may only be performed by a physician.

The Texas Board also maintains that a physician may not delegate health care procedures that require the exercise of independent medical judgment.

Though the aforementioned guidelines demonstrate some variability, the consensus remains that ultimate responsibility for performing any medical procedure resides with the physician.

Conclusion

Guidelines and regulations for medical lasers are essential for their safe and effective use. As previously noted, there is no single, finite standard of practice, therefore consultation with the appropriate governing bodies and professional organizations is necessary to ensure the quality of care provided and the safety of the laser patient, staff and operator.

References

1. The Laser Revolution – Laser Skin Surgery. Approved by the Board of Directors, American Society for Laser Medicine and Surgery, Inc; October 1, 2007.
2. The Use of Lasers, Pulsed Light, Radio Frequency, and Microwave Devices. Approved by the Board of Directors, American Academy of Dermatology, Inc; February 22, 2002.
3. American National Standards Institute. *American National Standard for Safe Use of Lasers in Health Care Facilities: ANSI Z 136.3 (2005).* Orlando: Laser Institute of America; 2005.
4. Lanzafame RJ. Procedural Skills for Using Lasers in General Surgery. Approved by the Board Directors, American Society for Laser Medicine and Surgery, Inc; April 6, 2006.
5. Procedural Skill and Technique Proficiency for Laser Medicine and Surgery in Dermatology. Approved by the Board of Directors, American Society for Laser Medicine and Surgery, Inc; November 2, 2005.
6. Control of Smoke from Laser/Electric Surgical Procedures. Hazards Controls, HC 11, DHHS (NIOSH) Publication 96-128; 1996.
7. Position Statement on Non-Physician Practice of Medicine and Use of Non-Physician Office Personnel May 2008. [Online American Society for Dermatologic Surgery news room]. Retrieved from http://www.asds.net/PositionStatementonNonPhysicianPracticeOfMedicineAndUseOfNonPhysicianOfficePersonnel.aspx
8. Use of Lasers/Delegation of Medical Functions Regulation by State, Federation of State Medical Boards; June 5, 2008.

Lasers for Treatment of Vascular Lesions

Daniel Michael and Suzanne Kilmer

- Lasers for the treatment of vascular lesions are continually improving using the principles of selective photothermolysis.
- Important variables to consider in the treatment of vascular lesions are size, depth, and composition.
- Effective treatment of vascular lesions requires tailoring the light wavelength, fluence, and pulse duration to the specifics of the targeted lesion.

Introduction

- Lasers can be used to target and destroy vascular lesions.
- Diverse arrays of lasers effective in treatment are currently available.

A large number of lasers and intense non-coherent pulsed light devices are available for the treatment of vascular lesions. They provide for the resolution or improvement of vascular lesions that were previously untreatable. New devices have been developed and existing devices are continually being improved to increase their ability to target vessels while decreasing the risk of adverse reactions. We review here vascular lesions and the lasers commonly utilized for their treatment.

D. Michael (✉)
Department of Dermatology, University of California, Davis, Medical Center, Sacramento, CA, USA
e-mail: dan.michael@ucdmc.ucdavis.edu

Principles of Laser Treatment for Vascular Lasers

- Selective photothermolysis describes the selective interaction of light energy with selected targets within the skin.
  - Chromophores are molecules or structures that preferentially absorb specific wavelengths of light.
  - Thermal relaxation time is the time it takes for a target structure to dissipate 50% of the absorbed energy into surrounding tissue and is an important consideration during the selection of treatment parameters.
  - In the visible and near-visible spectrum, increasing depth of penetration into tissue correlates with increasing wavelengths
- Pulse duration affects selectivity of treatment as well as depth and risk of adverse results.
- Epidermal cooling helps to minimize collateral thermal damage, but has to be tailored to the treatment parameters and lesion location to prevent cryogenic damage or pain.

Selective Photothermolysis

In 1983, Richard Rox Anderson and John Parrish proposed the theory of Selective Photothermolysis.[1] The selective destruction of vascular lesions with light energy is based on this principle. This effect requires a wavelength of light to penetrate to at least the depth of the target and be absorbed significantly more by that target than the surrounding chromophores that are also in the light path. In addition, the target must absorb enough energy to

K. Nouri (ed.), *Lasers in Dermatology and Medicine*,
DOI: 10.1007/978-0-85729-281-0_3, © Springer-Verlag London Limited 2011

irreversibly damage it, but cool quickly enough so that the heated target does not cause thermal damage to the surrounding tissue. The target (chromophore) for vascular lasers is hemoglobin. The wavelength of light that it preferentially absorbed depends on whether it is bound to oxygen or not and whether the ferrous iron in the heme group is oxidized to ferric iron or not.

Lasers available today for the treatment of vascular lesions span a large spectrum of individual wavelengths from 532 to 1,064 nm with non-coherent pulsed light sources spanning a larger spectrum. Choosing the appropriate wavelength involves selecting a wavelength with deep enough penetration that is primarily absorbed by the vascular target. Within this range, shorter wavelengths scatter more quickly and penetrate less deeply than longer wavelengths which can reach several millimeters into the dermis before loss to scattering renders it useless. Oxygenated hemoglobin (oxyhemoglobin) is normally the most abundant form of hemoglobin and has three peaks of absorption (418, 542 and 577 nm). Deoxygenated hemoglobin (deoxyhemoglobin) has an absorption peak of 755 nm that is well targeted by the 755 nm wavelength alexandrite laser. The major chromophores competing for absorption in the skin are melanin, water, and fat.

Melanin is primarily present in the epidermis and may absorb incident laser light. This may reduce the effective energy delivered to the vascular target and possibly cause direct thermal damage to the epidermis. Occurring between 532 and 1,064 nm, absorption by melanin decreases with longer wavelengths from ultraviolet (<400 nm) through the visible (400–760 nm) spectrum (Fig. 1). Longer visible and near infra-red wavelengths are absorbed less by epidermal melanin and penetrate deeper into the dermis and blood than shorter visible and ultraviolet wavelengths.[2]

Pulse Duration

As developed in the theory of selective photothermolysis, Anderson and Parrish describe the selective targeting of a chromophore based on the target size which determines the optimal length of the laser pulse. The thermal relaxation time was defined as the time it takes for a target structure to dissipate 50% of the absorbed energy into surrounding tissue. This can be approximated by the square of the diameter of the target structure. High enough fluences with pulse durations short enough to limit diffusion of heat from the target vessels will cause photocoagulation.[3] Excessively long pulse durations, longer than the thermal relaxation time, can lead to diffusion of thermal damage to surrounding tissue. In contrast, excessively short durations can cause focal boiling of the blood which may lead to cavitation-induced vessel disruption. This can produce excessive purpura without necessarily causing elimination of the vessel.

Epidermal Temperature Control

The epidermis is particularly sensitive to thermal damage. Heat transfer to the epidermis during laser therapy can occur by several mechanisms: direct absorption of light energy, back scatter of light from deeper tissue, and conduction of heat produced in the dermis. Selective cooling of the epidermis before, during, and/or after treatment allows for production of higher temperatures in the target structures without damage to the epidermis. Current methods include: direct contact (conduction), forced cold air (convection), and cryogen spray (conduction and evaporation).

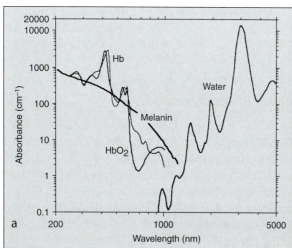 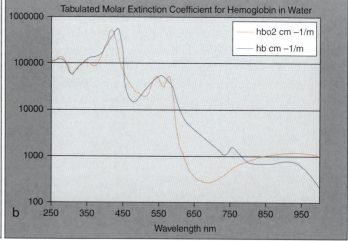

Fig. 1 Absorption curve for (**a**) hemoglobin, melanin and water, and (**b**) for oxygenated and deoxygenated hemoglobin

Lasers for Treatment of Vascular Lasers

- The frequency-doubled Nd:YAG, KTP filtered laser produces laser light of 532 nm and can be used to target very superficial vessels.
- Pulsed dye lasers produce light that penetrates deeper than frequency-doubled Nd:YAG and is more selectively absorbed by hemoglobin. These lasers have become a mainstay of vascular lesion treatment.
- Alexandrite lasers produce 755 nm wavelengths light that can better target deoxygenated hemoglobin.
- Neodymium:Yttrium-Aluminum-Garnet lasers can be used to treat vascular lesions, but are less selective and have a higher risk of causing dermal damage.
- A combination of PDL and Nd:YAG laser has been developed that may more selectively target vessels that have both superficial and deep components.
- Intense pulsed light devices produce high-energy broad spectrum non-coherent light that can be selectively filtered to target vascular lesions.

Frequency-Doubled Nd:YAG (Potassium-Titanyl-Phosphate [KTP])

Frequency-doubled neodymium:yttrium-aluminum-garnet lasers (Nd:YAG) use potassium-titanyl-phosphate (KTP) crystals to double the frequency, which halves the wavelength from 1,064 to 532 nm. Oxygenated hemoglobin absorbs the light of this wavelength about as well as it absorbs the light of 585 nm wavelength (Fig. 1). The shorter wavelength is effective for destruction of the most superficial vessels though melanin also absorbs this wavelength well. Efficient epidermal cooling is necessary when using these devices, especially in darker skin types where epidermal melanin is more of an issue.

Pulsed Dye Lasers (PDL)

The flash lamp-pumped pulsed dye laser (PDL) was the first laser developed for selective photothermolysis of vascular lesions.[1,4] It was initially designed to produce 577 nm light to correspond with one of the oxyhemoglobin peaks[5] (Fig. 1). The wavelength was increased to 585 nm to increase depth of penetration, improving efficacy for the treatment of deeper vessels. The original pulsed dye lasers had short pulse widths of 0.45 ms, whereas the next generation of PDLs had the ability to deliver high frequency pulses that could be combined into longer combined pulse widths of 1.5 ms. The longer pulse widths allow treatment of larger vessels with less extravasation of blood and therefore less purpura. Although longer wavelengths allow deeper penetration, Hb absorption begins to drop off rapidly. The next generation of PDLs is also able to produce light with wavelengths of 585, 590, 595, or 600 nm. The most recent versions of pulsed dye lasers have only the 595 nm wavelength but have adjustable pulse widths ranging from 0.45 to 40 ms to provide optimal treatment parameters for various vessel sizes.

Alexandrite Laser

Bluish vascular lesions often extend deeper and contain more deoxyhemoglobin. PDLs are not very effective against these lesions, because their wavelengths often do not penetrate deeply enough and are not absorbed by deoxygenated hemoglobin as well as they are by oxygenated hemoglobin. One of the most recent advancements in the development of vascular lasers is the utilization of a deoxygenated hemoglobin absorbance peak at 755 nm by the long pulsed alexandrite laser.[6] Initially, the long pulsed alexandrite laser was used for hair removal, but was found to be effective against violaceous deeper vascular lesions.[7] This is because, in addition to being well absorbed by deoxygenated hemoglobin, long pulsed alexandrite lasers produce a longer wavelength over longer pulse widths that allow the light to penetrate further and to target larger vessels.

Neodymium:Yttrium–Aluminum–Garnet (Nd:YAG)

Neodymium:yttrium-aluminum-garnet (Nd:YAG) lasers produce light at 1,064 nm which penetrates deeper than shorter wavelengths. However, at this wavelength, oxyhemoglobin no longer absorbs the energy better than the surrounding dermis. These lasers can be effective, but risk of scarring is significant at fluences high enough to effect vascular damage so these lasers are less often used.[8] Fluences and pulse width used at this wavelength are dependent on vessel size, location, and the oxygenation of hemoglobin. Vessels with larger diameters require longer pulse widths. Conversely, small vessels need shorter pulse widths, but require higher fluences, as there is less chromophore (Hb) present.

Combination PDL and Nd:YAG Laser

Methemoglobin is hemoglobin in which the ferrous iron of the heme group has oxidized to ferric iron. Unlike oxyhemoglobin and melanin, methemoglobin has increased absorption with increasing wavelength from 700 to 1,000 nm and is well targeted by Nd:YAG laser light[reference/spectrum]. It has been shown that pulsed dye lasers are able to induce the transformation of oxyhemoglobin to methemoglobin resulting in a more selective target for an Nd:YAG laser.[9] Recently, a device combining a PDL (595 nm) and Nd:YAG (1,064 nm) was developed utilizing this concept.

In addition, the thrombus that can be formed by PDL energy also absorbs 1,064 nm light better.[9,10] Because of the increased absorption of 1,064 nm by the methemoglobin and thrombus, lower fluences of the Nd:YAG produce vessel specific damage with decreased thermal damage to surrounding tissue.

PDL light only penetrates approximately 0.75 mm into the skin so. For lesions with deeper components, it is necessary to allow the PDL formed products time to flow deeper into the lesion before illumination with the deeper penetrating Nd:YAG laser. The combination therapy works best for superficial discrete telangiectasias with vessels in the 0.2–1.2 mm diameter range. Though PDL remains the treatment of choice for vascular birthmarks, the PDL/Nd:YAG combination may be helpful for lesions resistant to PDL alone. As we get more proficient with the use of the dual wavelength modality, we can use it more efficaciously.

Intense Pulsed Light (IPL)

Intense Pulsed Light (IPL) devices produce high-energy, non-coherent light. Their output covers a broad range of the light spectrum, often ranging from near 500 nm to around 1,200 nm with pulse widths of several milliseconds. Cut-off filters are used to limit the spectrum of the incident light to the desired wavelengths. For treatment of vascular lesions, wavelengths shorter than 580–590 nm are generally filtered out.[11] Newer devices filter out the longer infra-red wavelengths, reducing many of the adverse effects of earlier devices.[11] These devices usually have larger application tips which cover larger surface areas and are well suited to broader treatment areas.

Output varies by wavelength and by device so parameters tend to be device-specific. IPL devices can be effective against capillary malformations, telangiectasias, and small cherry angiomas.[12] Adverse effects include post-inflammatory hyper- or hypopigmentation, blistering, and scarring.

Vascular Lesions and Laser Treatment Options

- Congenital capillary malformations (e.g., port wine stains) are the most common type of vascular malformation and can often be effectively treated with lasers.
- Hemangiomas are vascular neoplasms that often partially resolve, but can cause functional and developmental problems in addition to leaving lasting scars.
- Telangiectasias represent small superficial dilated capillaries and post-capillary venules with thickened walls.
- Venous lakes are late developing venous ectasias that can vary greatly in size and depth. Laser treatment is often effective, but needs to be tailored to the depth and size of the lesion.

Capillary Malformations (e.g., Port Wine Stains or Nevus Flammeus)

Capillary malformations are the most common type of vascular malformation. Also called a port wine stain (PWS) or nevus flammeus, they represent congenital developmental malformations of the superficial dermal capillaries. They are present at birth, grow as the child grows, and do not involve.

Treatment of port wine stains (PWSs) was initially performed with the continuous wave 488–514 nm argon laser.[13,14] The excess heat deposition from this laser often leads to dyspigmentation and scarring. One of the main problems with the argon laser was that the pulse width could not be controlled. This often led to scarring from excess heat deposition. A laser with a longer wavelength and a controllable pulse width was needed. In an effort to overcome the inadequacies of the argon laser for treating these lesions, Richard Rox Anderson and John Parrish developed the theory of selective photothermolysis. This led to the PDL becoming the treatment of choice for these lesions. The PDL in its current reincarnation remains the gold standard.[18] This laser selectively targets hemoglobin, and the pulse width is more closely matched to the thermal relaxation time of the targeted vessels in PWSs.[15,16]

Most PWSs start as pink macules with tiny vessels, but with time these lesions, usually found as hypertrophy and in the vessels, become larger and tortuous.[17] In addition, more of the hemoglobin in larger, older lesions tends to be deoxygenated and are not targeted as well by PDLs. For these reasons PWSs are generally best treated with PDLs earlier in the pink macular stage, as often seen in infants. More mature hypertrophic bluish PWSs often require longer pulse-widths and even longer wavelengths. Successful treatment generally requires repeated treatments especially for larger lesions and those on the distal extremities.[18] As discussed above, longer wavelength PDLs can treat deeper vessels in the lesion and may show improved rates of clearance, though the decreased absorption by hemoglobin necessitates higher fluences which may be more likely to produce post-inflammatory pigment changes.

Most patients see significant improvement, but total removal of the lesion is often not possible. Lesions in newborns tend to respond faster and more completely than those in older patients. There is much less melanin in neonatal skin competing as a chromophore for the absorption of the laser and the lesions tend to be thinner and much smaller than they will often become. All these features make PDLs more effective against earlier lesions than they are against later lesions.

Pink macular PWSs are best treated using 585–595 nm wavelengths with a short pulse-width in the 0.45–1.5 ms range (Fig. 2). The spot size and energy used is dependent on the specific PDL used, but for 10 mm spot size, 7.5 J/cm^2 is often effective and for 12 mm spot size, 7 J/cm^2 is often needed, which may be the maximum output available. For more resistant PWSs, when higher energies are needed, we found that the 7 mm spot size may be needed to deliver 8–10 J/cm^2. As higher energy levels are used, the risk of purpura or ulceration increases and these settings should be used with caution. For PWS composed of larger vessels, the pulse width may need to be lengthened. With longer pulse widths, it becomes very important not to exceed the ability of the cooling to protect the epidermis. It is important to reiterate that as with all lasers, appropriate cooling is important to protect the epidermis while delivering sufficient heat to effectively target the vasculature.

For hypertrophic PWSs, the PDL can be used at 595 nm with similar settings as above, however, increasing the pulse width may improve outcome (Fig. 3). In addition, the absorption peak of deoxygenated hemoglobin near 755 nm allows the long pulse Alexandrite laser (which is more commonly used for hair removal) to take advantage of the deoxygenated nature of the larger vessels. In this case, we typically use 12 mm spot size, 35–40 J/cm^2 with cooling set at 50 ms (Fig. 4). Care must be taken to not overlap these pulses. The 1,064 nm wavelength of the Nd:YAG laser has been used, but it is the most treacherous of the three lasers as selective hemoglobin absorption at this wavelength is somewhat unpredictable and ulcerations have occurred.

Frequency-doubled Nd:YAG (Nd:YAG/KTP) lasers produce sequential nanosecond length pulses at a high frequency (>20,000 Hz) to produce semi-continuous pulses in the 2–20 ms range. The 532 nm wavelength does not penetrate deeply, but has been shown to be effective against the superficial components of PWSs.[19-21]

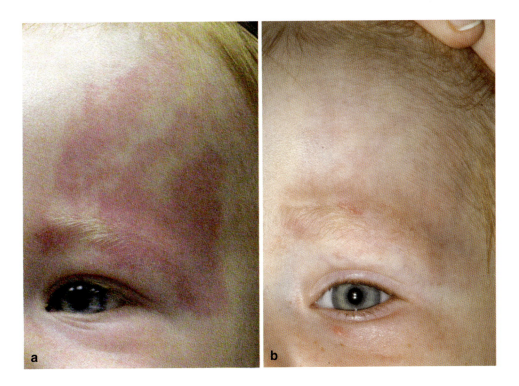

Fig. 2 Young boy with pink macular PWS (**a**) before and (**b**) after ten PDL treatments

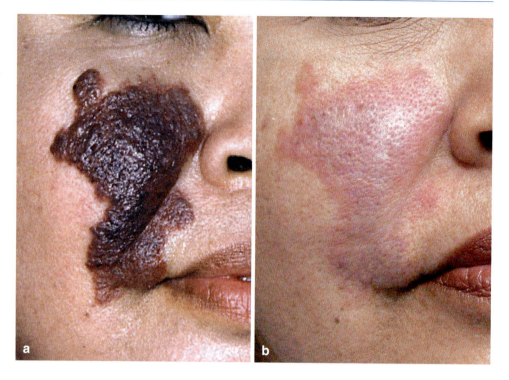

Fig. 3 Hypertrophic violaceous PWS (**a**) before and (**b**) after three long pulsed alexandrite laser treatments with 40 J/cm^2, 12 mm spot size, 3 ms and 50 ms of cryogen spray cooling. The PWS is now pink and was subsequently treated with PDL laser

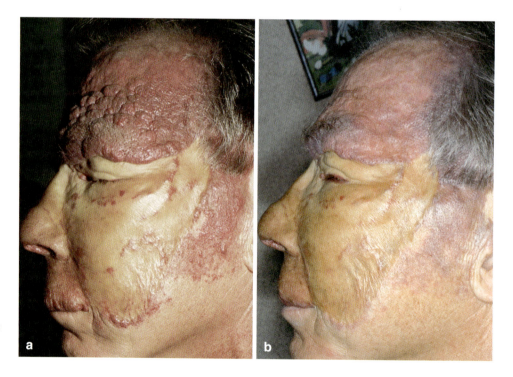

Fig. 4 Sixty-one year old man with PWS (**a**) before and (**b**) after multiple treatments with alexandrite and Nd:YAG. Patient treated with skin graft to mid-face prior to laser treatment

Hypertrophic bluish PWSs have more tortuous dilated vessels and slower blood flow resulting in more deoxygenated hemoglobin. They are therefore better targeted by the 755 nm wavelength of alexandrite lasers. We often find settings of 35–40 J/cm^2 with 12 mm spot size and 3 ms pulse width with 50 ms of spray cooling safe and effective.

Nd:YAG lasers have also been shown to be effective against capillary malformations though there is a greater risk of scarring. For this reason, in infants or young children, we rarely use this wavelength. In a more mature PWS, 60–70 J/cm^2 with a 10–12 mm spot size and 3 ms pulse width have improved resolution in those recalcitrant to previous treatments.

Most recently, the 595 nm wavelengths has been used in combination with the 1,064 nm wavelength to take advantage of the improved absorption of 1,064 nm by methylated hemoglobin so that less energy at 1,064 nm is needed and is therefore safer. PDL and Nd:YAG lasers, when used in combination (Cynosure's Cynergy), are generally set lower than either would be if used alone. Fluences used generally range between 6 and 10 J/cm^2 for the PDL and between 40 and 80 J/cm^2 for the Nd:YAG. However, starting with the PDL set for 7–8 J/cm^2 at 10 ms and the Nd:YAG set for 40 J/cm^2 at 15 ms is often appropriate.

The earlier these lesions are treated, the better the results.[22,23] Not only do they clear better, but the treatments are better tolerated. It is often possible to achieve effective treatment before 6 months of age. Treatment intervals are typically 4–6 weeks apart though there is little documentation establishing the optimal interval. In fact, for resistant PWSs, 2 week intervals have resulted in dramatic improvement without increasing complication rates.[24] This may be because more frequent treatments may prevent neovascularization that would otherwise occur before the next treatment.

Multiple factors influence effectiveness of treatment, including thickness, patient age, and location of the lesion. Treatment response decreases with age and thickness of the lesion.[25] In addition, lesions involving V_2 distribution of the trigeminal nerve as well as those in the V_1 distribution over the nose respond less well than those superior or inferior to those regions.[26,27]

The most common adverse effect of PDL treatment is purpura, though this is becoming less common with newer lasers. It used to be thought that production of purpura is necessary for successful treatment and therefore the lowest energy settings that produce purpura were used. More recently we and others have found that these lesions can be successfully treated without inducing purpura.

Hemangiomas

Infantile hemangiomas, in contrast to vascular malformations, are true neoplasms composed of endothelial cells. They usually develop soon after birth, but almost a third are present at birth.[28] They are more common in Caucasians (~10% of births) and are more likely in infants that are premature, of very low birth weight (<1.5 kg), born to mothers who had chorionic villus sampling, or those with a first-degree relative who have a vascular anomaly.[29] Hemangiomas express placental antigens and are more unpredictable in their natural history.

Though medical students often learn the mnemonic "50% resolve by 5 years, 70% resolve by 7 years, 90% resolve by 9 years" this refers to a resolution that often leaves telangiectatic and atrophic skin.

Infantile hemangiomas can grow rapidly in size, but generally involute spontaneously. For this reason their treatment has been very controversial. However, end-stage or involuted hemangiomas often have residual superficial telangiectasias with saggy appearing skin (atrophic epidermis). In addition, depending on location, function can be permanently affected if left untreated.

Periocular, perineal, and perioral lesions are most likely to have an adverse effect on normal form and function. If periocular lesions obstruct the patient's vision, the loss of vision, temporary though it may be, can impair visual cortex development leading to persistent blindness. Perioral lesions may frequently hemorrhage and can impair feeding ability possibly leading to failure-to-thrive. Perineal lesions often ulcerate and can be very painful. Laser treatment can accelerate re-epithelialization and restore skin integrity and comfort (Fig. 5).

Hemangiomas frequently have a stronger response to laser treatment and need to be handled more carefully to avoid iatrogenic ulceration. Though deep components of the hemangioma will not be treated by the 595 nm lasers, selective elimination of the more superficial component of the hemangioma will preserve superficial skin architecture. Once the deep component regresses, a more normal appearing epidermis is more likely to remain (Fig. 6). In comparison to treatment of PWSs, we typically start more conservatively using settings approximately 1 J/cm^2 lower and then evaluate the response. In addition, these lesions require more frequent monitoring with shorter treatment intervals and careful adjustments made to treatment settings based on evaluation of the response from the previous visits.

Other treatment options may be combined with laser therapy to improve results and are often necessary for larger or complex hemangiomas, especially if they involve deeper or multiple structures such as in diffuse neonatal hemangiomatosis. Intralesional steroid injections may be used in conjunction with laser therapy and their effect has been found to be synergistic with the laser treatments.[30] Intralesional steroids in the treatment of periocular lesions are controversial because of the risk of thrombosis. Systemic prednisone is the mainstay of treatment for the proliferative stage of infantile hemangiomas, but laser treatment of the superficial component can prevent hemorrhage and allow for easier care of the involved skin. In addition, interferon alpha-2a, interferon alpha-2b, and embolization have been used in combination therapies and more recently, propranalol has shown great promise.[31]

Spider Angiomas

Spider Angiomas consist of a central arteriole directly supplying a radiating network of dilated superficial capillaries. Spider angiomas are common among people with lighter

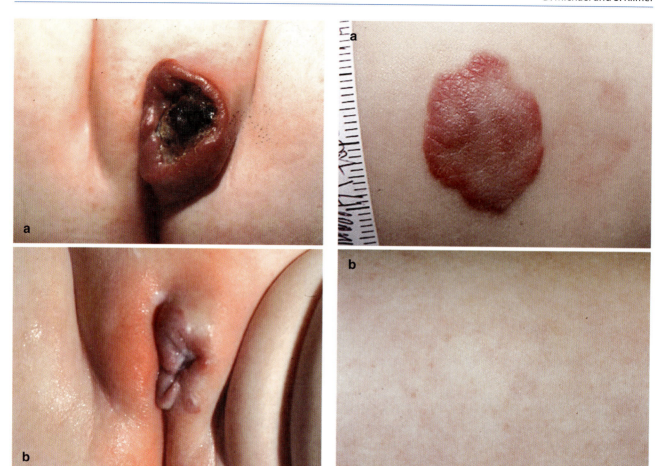

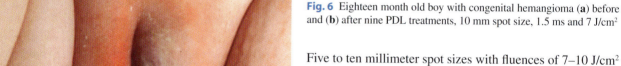

Fig. 6 Eighteen month old boy with congenital hemangioma (a) before and (b) after nine PDL treatments, 10 mm spot size, 1.5 ms and 7 J/cm²

Five to ten millimeter spot sizes with fluences of 7–10 J/cm² are often effective after one to two treatments.

Telangiectasias

Facial telangiectasias are one of the most common complaints encountered by the cosmetic dermatologist. They are more common in people with lighter skin types and are associated with a history of sun exposure. Although people with rosacea frequently develop facial telangiectasias, they are often not the result of rosacea. They represent dilated capillaries and post-capillary venules with thickened walls. They are superficial (200–250 μm deep) and have small cross-sections (200–500 μm in diameter).[32]

PDL continues to be the most effective treatment option, but this laser used to be associated with higher rates of purpura.[32] Current opinion is that telangiectasias can be treated with longer pulse widths in the 6–10 ms range utilizing pulse stacking where two to four pulses are "stacked" immediately one on top of the other until vessel clearing is noted[33] (Fig. 7). In fact, even longer pulse widths in the 20–40 ms range may

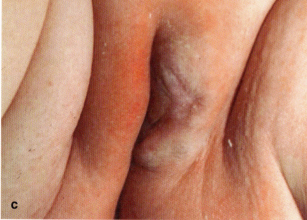

Fig. 5 Ulcerated congenital hemangioma (a) at presentation, (b) after PDL treatment treatment (c) Resolved lesion

skin and are often localized to areas of sun exposure, such as the face, neck, and upper chest. They are also associated with portal hypertension and Hereditary Hemorrhagic Telangiectasia syndrome.

PDLs are the light source of choice for the treatment of spider angiomas. Treatment is aimed at destruction of the central "feeder" vessel which can then be followed by destruction of the peripheral capillaries. Diascopy can be used to target the feeder vessel by blanching the draining capillaries.

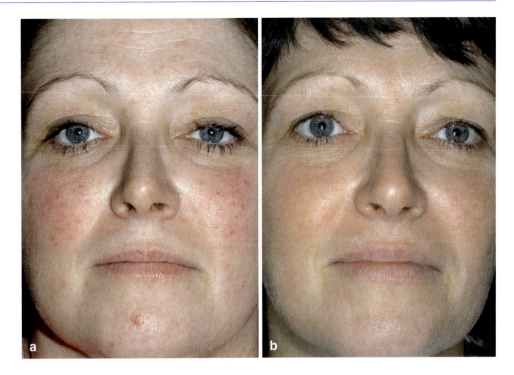

Fig. 7 Fifty year old woman with rosacea (a) before and (b) after two PDL treatments, 10 mm spot size, 6 ms and 7.5 J/cm^2

be effective. Treatment using fluences between 7 and 10 J/cm^2 and spot sizes of 5–10 mm are often effective with pulse widths ranging from 6 to 10 ms. For the combined Cynergy device, the PDL at 7–8 J/cm^2 with a pulse width of 10–20 ms and with a short or medium delay before the Nd:YAG at 30–40 ms with pulse width of 15 ms is often effective. Immediate coagulation/graying that quickly clears is the desired endpoint. Purpura may be more likely to develop in patients taking anti-coagulants (e.g., ASA, Coumadin, vitamin E, etc.).

IPLs have also been shown to be effective against telangiectasias and have a lower risk of inducing purpura and generally induce a mild erythema. Effective fluences range from 32 to 40 J/cm^2 with pulse widths of around 20 ms.[32] While PDLs continue to be the treatment of choice for focal telangiectasias, IPLs may be more tolerable for some patients with larger matted telangiectasias and the diffuse erythema associated with rosacea.

Venous Lakes

Venous lakes are venous ectasias that usually develop after the age of 50 and may enlarge over time.[17] The size and depth can vary greatly. Laser therapy is often effective and needs to be tailored to the depth of the target. PDL is often effective for superficial venous lakes, but the longer wavelengths of diode (800–900 nm), alexandrite (755 nm), or Nd:YAG (1064 nm) lasers are necessary for thicker or deeper lesions. Fluences of 80 J/cm^2, pulse durations of 60 ms or longer, and 10–12 mm tips are often required which puts the epidermis at risk of being thermally damaged. Appropriate cooling is therefore very important. In addition, there can be significant heat return to the epidermis with the longer pulse widths which makes post-laser cooling an important consideration.

The aim with a PDL is to produce mild purpura and edema. With diode and Nd:YAG lasers the goal is reduction in lesion thickness and clearance of the ectatic vessel. For the larger and deeper lesions an Nd:YAG laser with a spot size of 3 mm, pulse widths of 30–100 ms and fluences of up to 150 J/cm^2 may be needed.[32] (Fig. 8).

Other Vascular Anomalies

In addition to the above mentioned vascular lesions, there are a variety of other less common vascular anomalies for which surgery used to be the mainstay of treatment. These lesions can now be treated successfully with laser therapy. Larger more violaceous lesions can be treated with lasers and settings now used for hemangiomas and venous lakes. For example, the lesions of Blue Rubber Bleb Nevus syndrome, which are typically cutaneous venous malformations of varying sizes that enlarge with age, respond well to long pulse alexandrite laser with settings of 40 J/cm^2 with a spot size of 12 mm and efficient cooling (Fig. 9). The long pulse Nd:YAG laser can also be utilized with settings starting at 80 J/cm^2 at 60 ms. Again, appropriate cooling is extremely important. Lymphangioma can also be targeted by vascular lasers when the concentration hemoglobin is high enough to provide a sufficient target for these vascular lasers. More violaceous lesions are best treated with either the long pulsed alexandrite or Nd:YAG.

Fig. 8 (**a**) Before and (**b**) after single pulse with Nd:YAG 80, 60

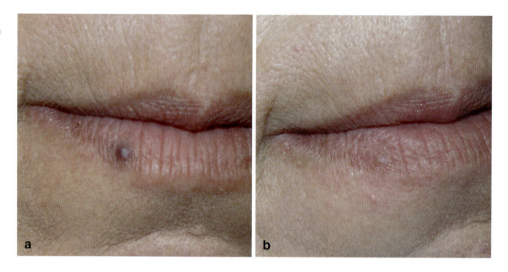

Fig. 9 (**a**) Before and (**b**) after two treatments GentleLase 12 mm, 40 J, 3 ms with 50 ms cryogen spray cooling

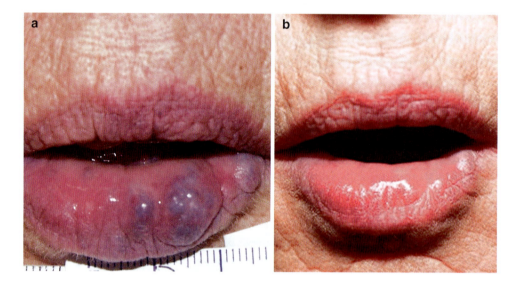

Conclusion

The introduction of lasers in cutaneous medicine and the development of the theory of selective thermolysis have provided clinicians with effective therapies for the treatment of vascular lesions. Understanding the tissue-light interaction and the risks associated with these therapies has allowed for improved end results. The diverse range of devices available require a more in depth understanding of these lasers and intense pulsed light devices to provide our patients with the most effective and appropriate options.

References

1. Anderson RR, Parrish JA. Microvasculature can be selectively damaged using dye lasers: a basic theory and experimental evidence in human skin. *Lasers Surg Med*. 1981;1(3):263-276.
2. Dai T et al. Comparison of human skin opto-thermal response to near-infrared and visible laser irradiations: a theoretical investigation. *Phys Med Biol*. 2004;49(21):4861-4877.
3. Kimel S et al. Vascular response to laser photothermolysis as a function of pulse duration, vessel type, and diameter: implications for port wine stain laser therapy. *Lasers Surg Med*. 2002;30(2): 160-169.
4. Anderson RR, Parrish JA. Selective photothermolysis: precise microsurgery by selective absorption of pulsed radiation. *Science*. 1983;220(4596):524-527.
5. Glassberg E et al. The flashlamp-pumped 577-nm pulsed tunable dye laser: clinical efficacy and in vitro studies. *J Dermatol Surg Oncol*. 1988;14(11):1200-1208.
6. No D et al. Pulsed alexandrite laser treatment of bulky vascular malformations. *Lasers Surg Med*. 2003;32(S15):1.
7. Li L et al. Comparison study of a long-pulse pulsed dye laser and a long-pulse pulsed alexandrite laser in the treatment of port wine stains. *J Cosmet Laser Ther*. 2008;10(1):12-15.
8. Eremia S, Li CY. Treatment of face veins with a cryogen spray variable pulse width 1064 nm Nd:YAG Laser: a prospective study of 17 patients. *Dermatol Surg*. 2002;28(3):244-247.
9. Randeberg LL et al. Methemoglobin formation during laser induced photothermolysis of vascular skin lesions. *Lasers Surg Med*. 2004; 34(5):414-419.

10. Barton JK et al. Cooperative phenomena in two-pulse, two-color laser photocoagulation of cutaneous blood vessels. *Photochem Photobiol*. 2001;73(6):642-650.

11. Bahmer F et al. Recommendation for laser and intense pulsed light (IPL) therapy in dermatology. *J Dtsch Dermatol Ges*. 2007;5(11):1036-1042.

12. Bjerring P, Christiansen K, Troilius A. Intense pulsed light source for treatment of facial telangiectasias. *J Cosmet Laser Ther*. 2001;3(4):169-173.

13. Silver L. Argon laser photocoagulation of port wine stain hemangiomas. *Lasers Surg Med*. 1986;6(1):24-8, 52-5.

14. Dixon JA, Rotering RH, Huether SE. Patient's evaluation of argon laser therapy of port wine stain, decorative tattoo, and essential telangiectasia. *Lasers Surg Med*. 1984;4(2):181-190.

15. Tan OT, Murray S, Kurban AK. Action spectrum of vascular specific injury using pulsed irradiation. *J Invest Dermatol*. 1989;92(6):868-871.

16. Dierickx CC et al. Thermal relaxation of port-wine stain vessels probed in vivo: the need for 1–10-millisecond laser pulse treatment. *J Invest Dermatol*. 1995;105(5):709-714.

17. Bolognia JL et al. *Dermatology*, vol. 2. 2nd ed. St. Louis: Mosby Incorporated; 2008.

18. Kauvar A. Laser treatment of vascular lesion. In: Goldman M, Weiss R, eds. *Advanced Techniques in Dermatologic Surgery*. New York: Taylor & Francis; 2006:185-200.

19. Adrian RM, Tanghetti EA. Long pulse 532-nm laser treatment of facial telangiectasia. *Dermatol Surg*. 1998;24(1):71-74.

20. Apfelberg DB, Bailin P, Rosenberg H. Preliminary investigation of KTP/532 laser light in the treatment of hemangiomas and tattoos. *Lasers Surg Med*. 1986;6(1):38-42, 56-7.

21. Dummer R et al. Treatment of vascular lesions using the VersaPulse variable pulse width frequency doubled neodymium:YAG laser. *Dermatology*. 1998;197(2):158-161.

22. Kohout MP et al. Arteriovenous malformations of the head and neck: natural history and management. *Plast Reconstr Surg*. 1998;102(3):643-654.

23. Morelli JG, Weston WL. Pulsed dye laser treatment of hemangiomas. In: Tan OT, ed. *Management and Treatment of Benign Cutaneous Vascular Lesions*. Philadelphia: Lea & Febiger; 1992.

24. Tomson N et al. The treatment of port-wine stains with the pulsed-dye laser at 2-week and 6-week intervals: a comparative study. *Br J Dermatol*. 2006;154(4):676-679.

25. Yohn JJ et al. Lesion size is a factor for determining the rate of port-wine stain clearing following pulsed dye laser treatment in adults. *Cutis*. 1997;59(5):267-270.

26. Orten SS et al. Port-wine stains. An assessment of 5 years of treatment. *Arch Otolaryngol Head Neck Surg*. 1996;122(11):1174-1179.

27. Renfro L, Geronemus RG. Anatomical differences of port-wine stains in response to treatment with the pulsed dye laser. *Arch Dermatol*. 1993;129(2):182-188.

28. Fishman SJ, Mulliken JB. Hemangiomas and vascular malformations of infancy and childhood. *Pediatr Clin North Am*. 1993;40(6):1177-1200.

29. Haggstrom AN et al. Prospective study of infantile hemangiomas: demographic, prenatal, and perinatal characteristics. *J Pediatr*. 2007;150(3):291-294.

30. Williams EF III et al. Hemangiomas in infants and children. An algorithm for intervention. *Arch Facial Plast Surg*. 2000;2(2):103-111.

31. Leaute-Labreze C et al. Propranolol for severe hemangiomas of infancy. *N Engl J Med*. 2008;358(24):2649-2651.

32. Astner S, Anderson RR. Treating vascular lesions. *Dermatol Ther*. 2005;18(3):267-281.

33. Uebelhoer NS et al. Comparison of stacked pulses versus double-pass treatments of facial acne with a 1, 450-nm laser. *Dermatol Surg*. 2007;33(5):552-559.

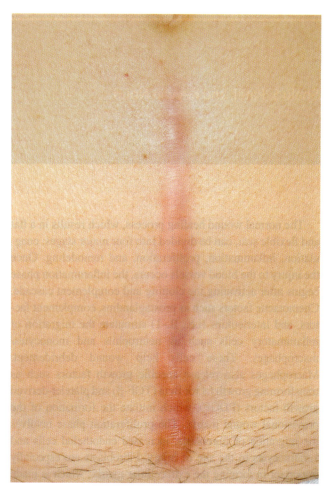

Fig. 1 A well-circumscribed linear hypertrophic scar at lower abdomen after a gynecologic surgery

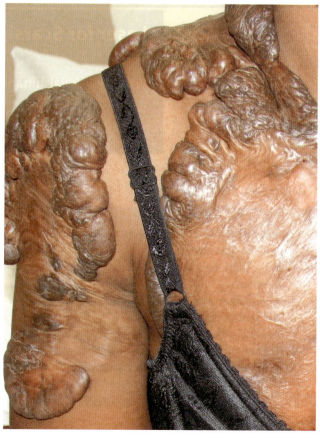

Fig. 2 Multiple keloids at the right arm, shoulder and chest wall of an African American woman

African-Americans, Chinese, and Hispanics. Patients in their second to third decade of life are more commonly affected, with the same prevalence in both sexes.[1-3]

Hypertrophic scars are red, raised, and firm, and usually appear within 1 month at the injury site, especially sites under pressure or frequent movement. Keloids, which can often be disfiguring, are purple/red nodules that are often found beyond the original injury site. Unlike hypertrophic scars, these appear within weeks or even years from the initial injury. Keloids frequently are found on the earlobes, anterior chest, shoulders and upper back. Common processes that may lead to keloid formation are ear piercings, tattoos, infections, vaccination, burns, and inflammatory acne.

The treatment of hypertrophic scars and keloids is challenging due to high recurrence rates and adverse side effects. Previous methods for treatment have included surgery, cryotherapy, electrocautery and desiccation, dermabrasion, intralesional corticosteroids, 5-fluorouracil, and radiation. In terms of lasers, Ablative CO_2 and Erbium:YAG lasers were used for hypertrophic scars but then discontinued. The pulsed dye laser (PDL) is currently the laser of choice for hypertrophic scars, which have yielded more successful results compared to keloids. It works via the principle of selective photothermolysis, in which the laser targets blood vessels, with the 585 nm wavelength specifically absorbed by hemoglobin. It is suggested that the microvascular destruction causes subsequent ischemia and reduction of scarring.

To appropriately treat hypertrophic scars and keloids, a thorough understanding of the processes by which they form is essential.

Indications and Contraindications

- Indications for treatment include side effects, functional impairment, and aesthetics.
- It is important to take into account the patient's skin type and lesion type prior to therapy.

Laser for Scars

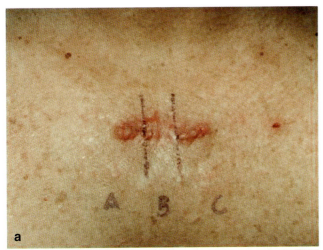

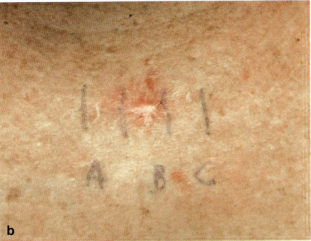

Fig. 3 (**a**) A linear surgical scar on anterior mid upper chest. The right section received 585 nm PDL with pulse duration of 450 μs, the middle remained as a control, and the left section received 585 nm PDL with pulse duration of 1.5 ms. (**b**) One month after the third PDL treatment. There was a significant clinical difference between treated and untreated sites

Patients typically seek medical help due to cosmetic issues or associated symptoms. Thus, indications for treatment of hypertrophic scars include functional impairment, cosmetic appearance, and pruritis and dysesthesias. The typical outcome of laser treatment is reduction of the redness and height of the scar, improvement of pliability, and symptomatic relief of pruritis.

Factors that need to be taken into consideration before treatment include patient skin type and lesion type. Fair skinned individuals (Fitzpatrick skin types I to III) tend to have a better response and fewer side effects to treatment. Patients with Fitzpatrick skin types IV to VI have an increased risk of laser light absorption by epidermal melanin, therefore less effective targeting of the skin and increased risk of postoperative hypo- or hyperpigmentation. It is suggested that in these patients, a test spot is done to predict any potential side effects. Lesion type also plays a role in the success of laser treatment. Lesions that have formed in less than a year and those that are red and raised have proved to be ideal for laser therapy.

Lasers have been found to be useful as a preventative measure as well. The 585 nm PDL was found to be effective in preventing the formation of hypertrophic scars in burn wounds. Further, treating surgical scars starting on the day of suture removal has yielded optimal results (Figs. 3a and b).

Techniques

- Pre-operative management includes obtaining a detailed history and exam of the patient's scars, and if any prior therapy has been done. The area for treatment should be cleaned thoroughly and topical anesthetic may be used for comfort. It is important to take a picture of the scar before therapy to track its progress and note any side effects that may occur.
- Laser therapy involves appropriately calibrating and setting the laser parameters. It may be used alone or in conjunction with intralesional medical therapy. Multiple treatments are needed to obtain better results.
- Post-operatively, the patient should avoid the sun and keep the treatment area clean and protected.

Pre-operative Management

It is important to get a good patient history before laser treatment. The history of the scar or keloid in terms of age, evolution, and previous treatments is helpful in determining treatment prognosis. It is ideal to treat hypertrophic scars early, possibly within the first few months of appearance. This is because of the numerous blood vessels present at this time. Previous treatments, such as cryotherapy, may cause increased fibrosis, and thus adjustments of laser parameters and treatment sessions may need to be made. Location of the scar is also important to note. Dierickx et al. have found that facial scars respond better to treatment.[4] Nouri et al. agree and have found that facial, shoulder, and arm scars respond better than those on the anterior chest wall.[5] However, Alster and Nanni found no relation between scar location and response to treatment.[6]

The PDL treatment for hypertrophic scars and keloids is an outpatient procedure. It typically does not require anesthesia unless requested by the patient. If so, a topical anesthetic cream may be applied 30–60 min before the procedure. Make-up any other creams must be removed from the treatment area with soap and water. In assessing the lesion, the physician should note its size, color, height, pliability, and associated symptoms. A picture should be taken prior to treatment for comparative purposes. It should be taken with the same camera, lighting, and distance. The patient and physician should be wearing eye protection at all times during the procedure.

Description of the Technique

The physician must first calibrate the laser and set parameters to be used. The ideal setting is 585 nm PDL at 450 μs pulse duration, using a spot size of 7–10 mm, with the fluence ranging from 3.5 to 7.5 J/cm^2. When using a smaller spot size, the fluence should be increased; however, initial treatments should all begin with a lower fluence. In ethnic skin, we prefer using a lower fluence (3–3.5 J/cm^2 with a 10 mm spot size) in order to reduce any complications from this procedure.

Once set, the physician should place the handpiece over one end of the scar and start applying the laser pulses over the entire scar surface in a continuous pattern until reaching the opposite end. A 10% overlap is generally accepted.

Laser treatment may be used alone or in combination therapy with intralesional corticosteroids or 5-FU. Alster compared PDL treatment alone with laser therapy combined with intralesional corticosteroid treatment and found that both were similarly effective with no significant difference.[7] It is important to remember, however, that if using intralesional corticosteroids, the injections should be done following the laser procedure. If done before, blanching of the lesion occurs and there is substantial risk of losing the laser target. An average of 10–40 mg/mL immediately after laser treatment can be used.

Post-operative Management

Post-operative management includes strict sun avoidance to avoid pigmentation alterations. The treated area should be cleansed as normal with soap and water. Trauma to the site should be avoided. Subsequent treatments may be done within 4–6 weeks.

Side Effects/Complications and Their Management and Prevention

A typical complaint from laser treatment is pain similar to that of a rubber band snapping against one's skin. A burning or itching sensation in the treated area is common as well, but subsides within a couple days if not sooner. Purpura is the most commonly expected side effect, appearing immediately after the procedure and lasting 7–10 days. Pigmentation alteration may also occur. If hyperpigmentation occurs, a bleaching cream may be used. Also, subsequent treatments may need to be deferred to ensure effective laser targeting of the scar.

Rare complications include crusting, oozing, and vesiculation of the lesion. In these cases, the area should be kept moist with ointment and may be covered with non-occlusive dressing to avoid contact. Subsequent treatments must be postponed until complete healing of the site. Also, the physician must reconsider the settings used to prevent further complications.

Laser for Atrophic Scar

- Atrophic scars resulting from acne, chicken pox, trauma, or even striae can be treated with laser therapy. The three main categories of therapy include ablative resurfacing, nonablative resurfacing, and fractional resurfacing.
- Ablative resurfacing offers effective therapy, but side effects and adverse events post-operatively limit its use.
- Nonablative resurfacing is considered safe, but may not be as effective as ablative resurfacing.
- Fractional resurfacing offers the effectiveness of ablative resurfacing and the safety of nonablative resurfacing. Studies have achieved improved results with this method, though a small percentage of patients experienced side effects.

Atrophic scarring (such as those from acne, chicken pox, or even striae) is depression of the skin due to the destruction of normal dermal or subcutaneous tissue architecture by inflammation, infection, or trauma.

There are many treatment modalities for this condition including topical vitamin A acid application, focal or regional chemical peeling, subcission, punch grafting, injection of fillers, dermabrasion, and laser resurfacing.

Nowadays, laser resurfacing for acne scar can be classified into three main categories:

1. Ablative resurfacing
2. Non-ablative resurfacing
3. Fractional resurfacing

Ablative Laser Resurfacing

The most common devices used for this technique are the carbon dioxide laser and Erbium YAG laser. Both of them are considered the gold standard treatment for acne scars and offer promising results after treatment. However, this method can be quite complicated and can have multiple drawbacks including:

- The need for antibiotic prophylaxis for bacterial-viral-fungal superimposed infections.
- The need for adequate anesthesia and sedation (some are systemic administration in combination with local anesthesia injection).
- The need for complicated post-operative care such as analgesia and dressing, along with post-operative antibiotic coverage.
- The risk for post-operative bleeding when using Erbium YAG laser because it has a high water absorption and thus cannot penetrate deeply (compared with the CO_2 laser), preventing enough heat production to ligate blood vessels.
- A high tendency for post-operative erythema or pigmentary alteration, which may prolong downtime, especially for individuals with skin of color who experience post-inflammatory hyperpigmentation and/or permanent hypopigmentation.

In an effort to reduce these drawbacks, some modalities that have been introduced are pre-operative bleaching agents, combination topical anesthesia with regional nerve block, and oral analgesic and sedation. Further, the following devices were introduced to decrease complications:

- The high energy-short pulsed CO_2 laser, which offers low tissue damage when compared with the conventional continuous mode CO_2 laser.
- The variable pulsed or dual-mode Erbium YAG laser, because the long pulse duration allows it to penetrate deeper than the short pulse duration alone, resulting in an optimal reaction for stimulating skin regeneration and ligation of blood vessels to diminish bleeding.[8,9]
- The combined-mode Erbium YAG/CO_2 laser system, which offers the dual benefit of having the ablative effect of the Erbium YAG laser and the coagulation effect of the CO_2 laser.[10]

Nonablative Laser Resurfacing

This is another modality that was quite popular at the turn of the century due to low complication rates and very low to almost no downtime when compared with ablative resurfacing, chemical peeling or dermabrasion. Some laser devices that demonstrated improvement of acne scars include:

- The 1,064 nm Q-switched Nd:YAG Laser[11]
- The 1,064 nm Long pulse Nd:YAG Laser[12,13]
- The 1,320 Nd:YAG Laser[14,15]
- The 1,450 nm diode Laser[16]
- The 1,540-nm erbium-doped phosphate glass Laser[17]
- The 585 nm flash lamp-pumped pulsed dye laser and Intense pulse light system also show benefit for post acne erythema[18,19]

These lasers are alternatives for people who may desire a less aggressive form of treatment; however, patients must be informed of the cost of treatment, that they may require multiple sessions, and to hold realistic expectations of their outcome.

Fractional Resurfacing

Both physicians and patients have tolerated the high complication rate of ablative laser resurfacing and low efficacy of non-ablative laser resurfacing, but fractional resurfacing is a recently introduced alternative that may the best of both devices. It particularly excels in offering promising results for facial rejuvenation, melasma, and acne scars. This system uses the concept of fractional photothermolysis by creating numerous microscopic thermal injury zones of controlled width, depth and density that are surrounded by normal skin which serves as a reservoir for rapid tissue healing.[20]

The benefits of this system are less downtime and side effects than the conventional ablative laser has, and an increased efficacy of tissue regeneration than the nonablative method offers. There are many devices launched in the market now, the most popular being the Erbium-doped, Erbium:YAG, CO_2 and Xenon lights.

There are many studies that have demonstrated the efficacy of the 1,550 laser system for acne scar treatment. Alster et al. used the 1,550 nm erbium-doped fiber, with fluences of 8–16 J/cm^2 at a density of 125–250 MTZ/cm^2 in 8–10 passes on 53 patients (Fitzpatrick skin types I–IV) with atrophic acne scars. They found that nearly 90% of patients achieved clinical improvement averaging 51–75%; however, multiple treatments were necessary.[21] Lee et al. treated 27 Asian patients (Fitzpatrick skin types IV–V) with moderate to severe facial acne scars. Each patient received three to five sessions of 3–4 weeks apart. At 3 months after the final treatment, eight patients (30%) assessed themselves as having excellent improvement, 16 patients (59%) assessed themselves as having significant improvement, and the final three patients (11%) assessed themselves as having moderate improvement. Adverse events were limited to transient pain, erythema and edema.[22] Emmy at el reviewed 961 patients who were treated with 1,550 nm erbium doped laser. They found that 73 (7.6%) patients developed complications.

The most frequent complications were acneiform eruptions (1.87%) and herpes simplex virus outbreaks (1.77%). Other rare complications include erosions, postinflammatory hyperpigmentation, prolonged erythema, prolonged edema, dermatitis, impetigo, and purpura.[23]

Other fractional laser systems such as the fractional CO_2 laser and fractional Erbium YAG laser are, by theory, more ablative than the 1,550 erbium-doped laser. However, the optimal treatment parameters for achieving a successful acne scar treatment with minimal side effects need to be studied.

Future Directions

- Future directions in scar management include attempting to prevent scar formation at the start by using PDL or intralesional medical therapy.
- These methods, however, do not come without their own side effects. Combination lasers may provide optimal results for laser scar therapy in the future.

Prevention of surgical scar formation is important. An effective way to do this is to use PDL routinely after suture removal. For new, red, hypertrophic scars, combination therapy with intralesional corticosteroids and 5-FU may be effective. However, for older scars that are not red, PDL treatment may not be warranted. These lesions may be treated with intralesional steroids and/or 5-FU. Triamcinolone (TAC) is one of the most commonly used steroids for intralesional injection of keloids and hypertrophic scars. It can be administered (10–40 mg/mL) every 4–6 weeks until resolution. 5-FU (45–50 mg/mL) may be injected a few times per week to once per month depending on the quality of the lesion. Corticosteroids work by inhibiting migration of inflammatory cells, vasoconstriction, and inhibition of fibroblast and keratinocyte proliferation. The mechanism of 5-FU is primarily inhibition of fibroblast proliferation. Both of these methods, though effective, can cause pain at the injection site and side effects such as pruritis and purpura. Studies combining these with PDL treatment are promising.

Further studies, possibly combining various lasers such as short-pulse and long-pulse, may offer interesting results and a potential frontier for scar treatment.

Conclusion

The mechanisms of hypertrophic scar and keloid formation are interesting and important in identifying optimal treatments. Various treatment options are available, and lasers

provide a novel and efficacious approach to therapy. While the 585 nm PDL seems to be the optimal laser, recent results of the fractional laser resurfacings promising. Abnormalities in wound healing remain a challenging topic. Patients suffer physical and emotional consequences. Addressing and managing these factors with minimal side effects in all patients should be the goal of future studies.

References

1. Taylor SC. Epidemiology of skin diseases in people of color. *Cutis.* 2003;71(4):271-275.
2. Alhady SM, Sivanantharajah K. Keloids in various races. A review of 175 cases. *Plast Reconstr Surg.* 1969;44(6):564-566.
3. Oluwasanmi JO. Keloids in the African. *Clin Plast Surg.* 1974;1(1):179-195.
4. Dierickx C, Goldman MP, Fitzpatrick RE. Laser treatment of erythematous/hypertrophic and pigmented scars in 26 patients. *Plast Reconstr Surg.* 1995;95(1):84-90.
5. Nouri K, Jimenez GP, Harrison-Balestra C, et al. 585 nm pulsed dye laser in the treatment of surgical scars starting on the suture removal day. *Dermatol Surg.* 2003;29:65-73.
6. Alster TS, Nanni CA. Pulsed dye laser treatment of hypertrophic burn scars. *Plast Reconstr Surg.* 1998;102(6):2190-2195. Click here to read Links.
7. Alster T. Laser scar revision: comparison study of 585-nm pulsed dye laser with and without intralesional corticosteroids. *Dermatol Surg.* 2003;29(1):25-29.
8. Pozner JM, Goldberg DJ. Histologic effect of a variable pulsed Er:YAG laser. *Dermatol Surg.* 2000;26(8):733-736.
9. Tanzi EL, Alster TS. Treatment of atrophic facial acne scars with a dual-mode Er:YAG laser. *Dermatol Surg.* 2002;28(7):551-555.
10. Goldman MP, Marchell N, Fitzpatrick RE. Laser skin resurfacing of the face with a combined CO2/Er:YAG laser. *Dermatol Surg.* 2000;26(2):102-104.
11. Friedman PM, Jih MH, Skover GR, Payonk GS, Kimyai-Asadi A, Geronemus RG. Treatment of atrophic facial acne scars with the 1064-nm Q-switched Nd:YAG laser: six-month follow-up study. *Arch Dermatol.* 2004;140(11):1337-1341.
12. Keller R, Belda Júnior W, Valente NY, Rodrigues CJ. Nonablative 1,064-nm Nd:YAG laser for treating atrophic facial acne scars: histologic and clinical analysis. *Dermatol Surg.* 2007;33(12):1470-1476.
13. Yaghmai D, Garden JM, Bakus AD, Massa MC. Comparison of a 1,064 nm laser and a 1,320 nm laser for the nonablative treatment of acne scars. *Dermatol Surg.* 2005;31(8 Pt 1):903-909.
14. Rogachefsky AS, Hussain M, Goldberg DJ. Atrophic and a mixed pattern of acne scars improved with a 1320-nm Nd:YAG laser. *Dermatol Surg.* 2003;29(9):904-908.
15. Sadick NS, Schecter AK. A preliminary study of utilization of the 1320-nm Nd:YAG laser for the treatment of acne scarring. *Dermatol Surg.* 2004;30(7):995-1000.
16. Chua SH, Ang P, Khoo LS, Goh CL. Nonablative 1450-nm diode laser in the treatment of facial atrophic acne scars in type IV to V Asian skin. *Dermatol Surg.* 2004;30(10):1287-1291.
17. Lupton JR, Williams CM, Alster TS. Nonablative laser skin resurfacing using a 1540 nm erbium glass laser: a clinical and histologic analysis. *Dermatol Surg.* 2002;28(9):833-835.
18. Alster TS, McMeekin TO. Improvement of facial acne scars by the 585 nm flashlamp-pumped pulsed dye laser. *J Am Acad Dermatol.* 1996;35(1):79-81.
19. Cartier H. Use of intense pulsed light in the treatment of scars. *J Cosmet Dermatol.* 2005;4(1):34-40.
20. Jih MH, Kimyai-Asadi A. Fractional photothermolysis: a review and update. *Semin Cutan Med Surg.* 2008;27(1):63-71.

21. Alster TS, Tanzi EL, Lazarus M. The use of fractional laser photothermolysis for the treatment of atrophic scars. *Dermatol Surg.* 2007;33(3):295-299.

22. Lee HS, Lee JH, Ahn GY, et al. Fractional photothermolysis for the treatment of acne scars: a report of 27 Korean patients. *J Dermatol Treat.* 2008;19(1):45-49.

23. Graber EM, Tanzi EL, Alster TS. Side effects and complications of fractional laser photothermolysis: experience with 961 treatments. *Dermatol Surg.* 2008;34(3):301-305.

Laser Treatment of Leg Veins

Robert A. Weiss, Girish S. Munavalli, Sonal Choudhary, Angel Leiva, and Keyvan Nouri

- Damaged venous valves result in varicose or spider vein formation. Commonly, venous obstruction is caused by increased pressure of reverse blood flow within the superficial venous valve or from direct traumatic injury to the vein.
- Venous valve failure creates high pressure within the venous system which causes other valves to fail. Venous valve failure causes dilation within the entire venous system.
- Venous thrombosis obstructs outflow and eventually destroys the valves within the venous system.

Introduction

Varicose veins and spider veins are normal veins that have dilated under the influence of increased venous pressure.

There are three kinds of veins in the legs- the superficial veins, which lie closest to the skin, the deep veins, which lie in groups of muscles and perforating veins, which connect the superficial veins to the deep veins. The deep veins lead to the inferior vena cava, which runs directly to the heart. In normal veins, one-way valves direct the flow of venous blood upward and inward as the leg veins must work against gravity to return blood to the heart. Varicose veins occur in the superficial veins in the legs.

One-way valves, in the veins keep blood flowing in the right direction. When the leg muscles contract, the valves inside the veins open. When the legs relax, the valves close. This prevents blood from flowing in reverse, back down the legs. The entire process is also called the venous pump.

Deep veins and perforating veins are usually able to withstand short periods of increased pressures. However, in a susceptible individual, the veins can stretch if one repeatedly sits or stands for a long time. This stretching can sometimes weaken the walls of the veins and damage the valves resulting in Varicose veins or their milder form, Spider veins.

In patients with dialysis shunts or with spontaneous arteriovenous malformations, normal veins may dilate and become tortuous in response to continued high pressure. Deep vein thrombosis initially produces an obstruction to outflow, but in most cases the thrombosed vessel eventually recanalizes and becomes a valve-less channel delivering high pressures from above downward.

Most commonly, superficial venous valve failure results from excessive dilatation of a vein from high pressure of reverse flow within the superficial venous system. Valve failure can also result from direct trauma or from thrombotic valve injury. When exposed to high pressure for a long enough periods, superficial veins dilate so much that their delicate valve leaflets are no longer able to meet.

The most common situation is that a single venous valve fails and creates a high-pressure leak between the deep and superficial systems. High pressure within the superficial system causes local dilatation leading to sequential failure (through over-stretching) of other nearby valves in the superficial veins. After a series of valves have failed, the involved veins are no longer capable of directing blood upward and inward. Without functioning valves, venous blood flows in the direction of the pressure gradient: outward and downward into an already congested leg.

Recruitment phenomena may occur, increasing the number of failing valves and communicating the high pressure into a widening network of dilated superficial veins. This may lead to a large numbers of incompetent superficial veins with the typical dilated and tortuous appearance of varicosities, over a period of time.

The deeper veins that are confined within the fascial planes remain invisible despite the fact that they can carry massive amounts of blood at high pressures. On the other hand, even a small increase in pressure can eventually produce massive dilatation of an otherwise normal superficial

R.A. Weiss (✉)
Department of Dermatology, Johns Hopkins University
School of Medicine, Hunt Valley, MD, USA
e-mail: rweiss@mdlsv.com

K. Nouri (ed.), *Lasers in Dermatology and Medicine*,
DOI: 10.1007/978-0-85729-281-0_5, © Springer-Verlag London Limited 2011

vein that carries very little flow. Therefore, visible varicosities are not reliable indicators of venous reflux.

The etiology of varicose veins can be classified as the following three groups:

- Primary: Valvular insufficiency of the superficial veins, most commonly at the saphenofemoral junction.
- Secondary
  - Mainly caused by deep vein thrombosis (DVT) that leads to chronic deep venous obstruction or valvular insufficiency. Long-term clinical sequelae from this have been called the postthrombotic syndrome.
  - Catheter-associated DVTs are also included.
  - Pregnancy-induced and progesterone-induced venous wall and valve weakness worsened by expanded circulating blood volume and enlarged uterus compresses the inferior vena cava and venous return from the lower extremities.
  - Trauma
- Congenital: This includes any venous malformations. A few examples are listed as follows:
  - Klippel-Trenaunay variants
  - Avalvulia
- High serum levels of estradiol are associated with clinical evidence of varicose veins in women. The hormonal changes during pregnancy may render the vein wall and valves more pliable. The sudden appearance of new dilated varicosities during pregnancy still warrants a full evaluation because of the possibility that these may be new bypass pathways related to acute deep vein thrombosis.

The relationship between serum sex steroid hormones and varicose veins in men is unclear. In a study by Kendler et al., elevated serum estradiol and testosterone levels were detected in men with varicose veins and reflux in the Great Saphenous vein (GSV) compared with the patient's own arm veins.[1] Enzymes and hormonal receptors involved in steroid metabolism were down-regulated in patients with GSV reflux and varicose veins, suggestive of a negative feedback regulation. These data support the notion of a possible causal relationship between sex steroids and varicose veins in men. The sequelae of venous insufficiency are related to the venous pressure and to the volume of venous blood that is carried in a retrograde direction through incompetent veins.

Patients may have a host of symptoms, but they are usually caused by venous hypertension rather than the varicose veins themselves. Often patients desire treatment of the unsightly nature of the tortuous, dilated varicosities only due to cosmetic reasons. Complaints of pain, soreness, burning, aching, throbbing, heavy legs, cramping, muscle fatigue, pruritus, night cramps, and "restless legs" are usually secondary to the venous hypertension. Pain and other symptoms may worsen with the menstrual cycle, with pregnancy, and in response to exogenous hormonal therapy (e.g., oral contraceptives).

On physical examination, besides, the visible palpable dilated tortuous veins, pigmentary changes may appear on the skin known as lipodermatosclerosis which results from extravasated blood. Erythematous dermatitis, which may progress to blistering, weeping, or scaling eruption of the skin of the leg or Eczema may be present and ulcers of the medial ankle most likely are the result of underlying venous insufficiency. Palpation of an area of leg pain or tenderness may reveal a firm, thickened, thrombosed vein. These palpable thrombosed vessels are superficial veins, but an associated DVT may exist in a large percentage of patients with superficial phlebitis.

The modalities available for the management of leg veins can be divided as follows:

- Surgical open technique – GSV saphenectomy, Small saphenous vein (SSV) saphenectomy, Stab or ambulatory phlebectomy
- Endovascular Techniques – Endovascular lasers and radiofrequency ablation
- Minimally invasive techniques – Cutaneous electrodessication, Sclerotherapy

---

- During the 1980s, lasers for leg vein treatments became available with the use of argon, though poor results were obtained due to the absence of selective photothermolysis.
- The development of selective photothermolysis, site-specific controlled thermal injury of tissue targets, used to treat facial telangiectasias and port-wine stains has been made available through the use of pulsed dye laser systems.
- Laser treatment for leg veins and telangiectasias can be selected more effectively than sclerotherapy by targeting vessels less than 1–2 mm in diameter.
- Ablation of the varicose pathways with the use of lasers increases the overall venous circulation.
- Patients with obstructed venous pathways should not undergo ablation since blood flow bypasses the obstructed areas.
- Longer pulse durations are used to treat large port-wine stains.
- Epidermal cooling devices appropriate for specified wavelength include the cryogen spray cooling system.

Lasers for Treatment of Leg Veins

In the 1980s, leg vein treatment using lasers involved argon lasers (488 and 518 nm). The disadvantage of this laser was its strong absorption by melanin and its continuous wave nature that did not allow for selective heating of vessels, causing scarring.[2,3] Continuous running Nd:YAG lasers were also tried for leg veins but poor results owing to non-specific heating of surrounding water and large depth of penetration, were observed.[4,5] With the development of the principles of selective photothermolysis, the design of pulsed dye laser (PDL) came into being which effectively treated facial telangiectesias and port-wine stains.[6] Longer wavelength, second generation of PDLs (595 nm) which also had longer pulse duration (1.5 ms) was launched in 1996. These PDLs had deeper penetration, yet were only effective for vessels up to 1 mm in depth and 1 mm in width.[7] To overcome this, near-infrared lasers with a bandwidth of from 750 to 1,100 nm have been used to penetrate further. The longer wavelength alexandrite, diode and Nd:YAG permit sufficient energy to heat deeper leg veins up to 3 mm wide.

Indications

Many patients benefit from a combination of treatments because external lasers and light sources do not effectively treat associated reticular and varicose veins. Although sclerotherapy remains the standard treatment of leg veins and telangiectasias, lasers can be effective in treating vessels less than 1–2 mm in diameter resistant to sclerotherapy and telangiectatic matting which can occur post-sclerotherapy.

Elevated venous pressure most often is the result of venous insufficiency due to valve incompetence in the deep or superficial veins. Varicose veins are the undesirable pathways by which venous blood refluxes back into the congested extremity. Ablation of the varicose pathways invariably improves overall venous circulation.

Chronically increased venous pressure can also be caused by outflow obstruction, either from intravascular thrombosis or from extrinsic compression. In patients with outflow obstruction, varicosities must not be ablated because they are an important bypass pathway allowing blood to flow around the obstruction. Specific diagnostic tests can distinguish between patients who will benefit from ablation of dilated superficial veins and those who will be harmed by the same procedure.

An increasing popularity of lasers for treatment of leg veins has come about due to many reasons,[8] especially due to its use in:

- Non-cannulizable microtelangiectasias
- Vessels that are refractory to conventional sclerotherapy treatments
- Zones of caution such as the ankles and feet where a high incidence of complications such as hyperpigmentation and ulceration occur

- Vessels that arise from prior surgical or sclerotherapy treatment (telangiectatic matting or angiogenic flushing)
- Needle phobic patients
- Most recently, non-surgical eradication of the greater or lesser saphenous vein (GSV and LSV, respectively).[9]

Contraindications

Patients with venous outflow obstruction should not have their varicosities ablated because they are important bypass pathways that allow blood to flow around the obstruction.

Technology

The laser treatment of leg veins is based on the treatment of selective photothermolysis which can be described as the production of site-specific, controlled, thermal injury of microscopic pigmented tissue targets by selectively absorbed pulses of radiation.[10] It takes into account three concepts:

1. A wavelength chosen for preferential absorption by the intended tissue chromophore.
2. Pulse duration shorter than the thermal relaxation time (TRT). (Thermal relaxation time is defined as the time required for the target tissue to cool to half of its peak temperature after being irradiated.)
3. Fluence high enough to cause thermal injury to the desired skin structure should be used.

As the target chromophore for laser in treating vascular lesions is oxyhemoglobin, its absorption peaks of 418, 542 and 577 nm is of importance. Also, there is a less selective peak in the range of 750–1,100 nm.[11] This allows the use of PDL and IPL in treating leg veins. The longer wavelengths (700–1,100 nm) although less selective, have better penetration into the dermis, heating the entire vessel circumference and vein closure. Shorter wavelengths, on the other hand, only heat the anterior vessel wall leading to incomplete thrombosis.[12] But, it is also important to keep in mind that, wavelengths greater than 900 nm could target water due to low specificity and thus a higher fluence may be needed. This could cause damage to surrounding tissues.

In order to heat leg veins, longer pulse durations than those that are used to treat port-wine stains are required as the former are comparatively larger in diameter. As most abnormal veins are 0.1–4 mm in diameter and a typical 1-mm vessel has a TRT of 360 ms, any pulse duration less than 180 ms could be used. Since a leg vein is a non-uniform target, pulse duration longer than the TRT will be needed (Altshuler's extended theory of selective photothermolysis).[13] In clinical practice, pulse durations of 10–100 ms are used. Longer pulse durations are less likely to induce vessel rupture and side effects. The early hypothesis was that by heating the blood so that the steam bubbles formed and then collapsed causing vessel rupture, also known as Cavitation. The current hypothesis believes that the vessel damage can occur either by vessel contraction secondary to collagen shrinkage or by thrombosis followed by inflammation and fibrosis.[12] Heat shock protein and transforming growth factor β (TGF-β) may be mediators of collagen remodeling, fibrosis and ultimately vessel destruction. Heating of blood vessel induces formation of methemoglobin (met-Hb) in blood due to oxidative changes, and met-Hb could result from both oxygenated hemoglobin (Hb-O$_2$) and deoxygenated hemoglobin (Hb).[14-16] Once the met-Hb forms, heme protein has distorted formation and thus protein denaturation occurs. Met-Hb formation leads to change in blood absorption after laser irradiation, the maximum being at 72°C. Met-Hb has an absorbance of 4.75 times higher than that of Hb-O$_2$ and 20 times more than that of Hb. It has been demonstrated that a series of nonuniform laser pulses with subthreshold fluences when used for closing leg veins, the first pulse induces Met-Hb formation thus leading to improved absorption by the following two pulses.[17] In a study by Black et al., it was demonstrated a conformational change of the red blood cells to spheroid shape and presence of Met-Hb in blood irradiated with 1,064 nm laser at therapeutic fluences.[18]

Spot sizes determine how much energy reaches the desired target. Larger spot sizes cause less scatter and more energy can be available for heating the target tissue. Thus with longer wavelength, smaller spot sizes are adequate and safer. The beam diameter or spot size should be matched to the vessel diameter to maximize absorption by the vessel and minimize side effects.

Epidermal cooling techniques appropriate for each wavelength and device should always be used during laser treatment of leg veins. Various modalities can be employed such as contact cooling with a sapphire window or copper plate, cryogen spray cooling, convection air cooling, cold gels etc. These help lower the epidermal temperature while allowing the development of a peak temperature in the dermal vessels.

Lasers for Leg Vein Treatment

Potassium Titanyl Phosphate Laser (KTP Laser)

The KTP laser is a great choice for vascular lesions, especially for bright red vessels. Five hundred and thirty-two nanometer wavelength is well-absorbed by oxygenated hemoglobin and its penetration depth is not more than 0.75 mm. This appears to be great for treating superficial capillaries. But, its absorption by melanin led to frequent hyper- and hypo- pigmentation. KTP laser has showed moderate efficacy in treating veins less than 0.7 mm in width with 33% having complete response, 40% showing visible decrease in vessel diameter and 27% showing no change. Larger diameter vessels did not respond.[19] The KTP laser is effective for fine-caliber vessels, with their dyspigmentation causing ability in mind. Larger spot sizes (3–5 mm) and longer pulse durations of 10–50 ms at fluences of 14–20 J/cm,[2] have achieved better results.[20]

To use the KTP laser for leg vein treatment, a fluence of 12–20 J/cm^2 and with a spot size of 3–5 mm in diameter is required, to deliver a series of pulses over the vessel until spasm or thrombosis occurs. For leg veins smaller than 1 mm in diameter that are not directly connected to a feeding reticular and with a tip chilled to 4°C to protect the epidermis, this can be an effective method. Two to three treatments may be necessary for maximal vessel improvement. Patients with darker or tanned skin may have a relatively high risk of temporary hyperpigmentation or hypopigmentation.

Long Pulsed Dye Laser

As already mentioned in brief, the 595 nm PDL was developed to overcome the limitations of the original PDL to treat the leg veins. Purpura encountered with this PDL was reduced by using its modification of a longer pulse width. Doubling the number of subpulses within each pulse led to eight consecutive subpulses that would stretch over 40 ms. On the basis of the studies performed, it is known that great results can be achieved with PDL to treat leg veins and the commonly noted side effects were edema, purpura and erythema.[21] Small vessels demonstrate better results.[22] Long PDL using multipass technique was tried by Tanghetti and Sherr who concluded that purpuric doses of PDL were required for the effective treatment of leg veins and hyperpigmentaion was noted in more than half of the patients treated.[23]

Thus, the 595 nm PDL is an effective treatment for smaller caliber (<1 mm) vessels, and the new longer pulsed systems may be even more efficacious. The major disadvantages of this laser is the inability to treat larger veins and its side effects of hyperpigmentation and purpura.

Long Pulsed 755 nm Alexandrite Laser

Long pulsed alexandrite laser in its application for leg vein treatment, provides deeper penetration into tissue and has the ability to treat larger diameter and deeply located vessels. Although this wavelength is less absorbed by hemoglobin when compared to 532 nm and 595 nm wavelengths, a sufficient level of photocoagulation of a wide range of vessel sizes can be achieved using higher fluences.

Mc Daniel et al. investigated this laser without cooling and used various parameters in 28 patients.[24] According to them, the ideal fluence was 20 J/cm^2 and pulse duration of 20 ms. After three sessions of 4 weekly treatments, medium vessels ranging from 0.4 to 1 mm achieved clearance of 48%. Telangiectasias less than 0.4 mm responded poorly and side effects such as bruising, erythema, crusting and hypopigmentation were noted.

In another study by Kauvar and Lou with the aim to examine the safety and efficacy of a pulsed alexandrite laser for treatment of leg telangiectasia and reticular veins, cryogen cooling was added to the protocol.[25] This produced excellent clearance of telangiectasia and reticular veins of the leg with minimal adverse effects.

It can be understood that cooling devices may enable higher fluences to be used with the alexandrite laser and provide a good option for the treatment of medium vessels in the patients with lighter skin types. Severe and persistent telangiectatic matting has been reported as adverse effects.[26]

Diode Lasers

Diode lasers generate coherent monochromatic light through excitation of small diodes. These systems offer true continuous pulses of energy up to 250 ms long. Their near-infrared wavelength corresponds to the tertiary hemoglobin peak and in comparison to the yellow light, it has a deeper penetration. Also, it is less absorbed by melanin and thus can be used to treat larger leg veins.

This information can be supported by the study conducted by Trelles et al., where they used an 800 nm diode with pulse stacking (five to eight stacked pulses, pulse duration 50 ms and delay 50 ms) to treat leg veins in ten female patients.[27] More than half the patients achieved 50–74% clearances. Best results were obtained in vessels of 3–4 mm in diameter located on the thigh, and in patients with phototype III skin. Telangiectatic matting and hyperpigmentation were noted side effects. Pulse stacking was identified as the reason for reduced pain felt by patients.

In another study 35 female patients with spider leg veins were treated twice with a pulsed diode laser (810 nm; spot size 12 mm, frequency 2–4 Hz, pulse width 60 ms, fluence 80–100 Jcm^2) at 2 week interval.[28] After the first treatment 15 patients showed a complete disappearance of spider leg veins. After 6 months of follow-up complete resolution was seen in six patients. The effect was almost completely stable

during 1 year of follow-up. The examination of histological specimens before and after laser treatment showed no cellular inflammatory reaction. The mean vascular area was significantly reduced after the first ($p < 0.05$) and after the second ($p < 0.05$) laser treatment. Spectral analysis showed a marked decrease of peaks for oxygenized hemoglobin immediately after laser treatment and during the follow-up. Safety profile was excellent without purpuric reaction or pigmentary changes. Mild scarring was observed in two patients at the end of follow-up.

A combination of diode laser with Radiofrequency (RF) has also been tried in leg vein treatment. Following the selective heating achieved with the laser component, the RF energy is preferentially absorbed by the blood vessel as a result of the increased tissue temperature (brought about by the laser) as well as the high electrical conductivity of blood.[29]

In a study, 900 nm diode was combined with RF to treat leg veins in 40 patients.[30] Results were assessed after each treatment and at 2 and 6 months after the final session. Treatments showed greater efficacy on thicker vessels and in the darker skin types.

Nd:YAG Laser

The 1,064 nm wavelength of the Nd:YAG laser converts hemoglobin to the more spherically shaped met-hemoglobin which has a four times higher absorption coefficient.[12,31] After initial irradiation, further energy is more effective at heating blood and the surrounding vessel.[32]

The Nd:YAG laser has been used to treat leg veins up to 3 mm in size, as this wavelength (1,064 nm) can reach deep and treat larger veins. Combining it with cooling devices makes it much safer to use. Studies have demonstrated great results with this laser using single[33] and multiple[34] treatments.

As of date, no standard protocol for the parameters has been developed and different combinations are being tried based on clinical experience. A mathematical model for the treatment of leg veins was developed by Baumler et al., who used this for treating 1.5 mm deep leg veins of various diameters. Maximal efficiency was achieved with pulse durations of 10–100 ms.[35] In another experiment, Parlette et al. investigate a range of pulse durations to determine an optimal pulse duration for clearance of leg veins.[36] The optimal pulse duration was defined as that pulse duration which resulted in the most complete clearance of vessels with the least side effects. Shorter pulse durations (≤ 20 ms) were associated with occasional spot sized purpura and spot sized post-inflammatory hyperpigmentation. Longer pulse durations (40–60 ms) achieved superior vessel elimination with less post-inflammatory hyperpigmentation. With a single laser treatment, 71% of the treated vessels cleared.

Synchronized pulsing with Nd:YAG laser was studied by Weiss and Weiss in 30 patients.[37] Immediate effects on the targeted vessels were quite apparent. Immediate contraction or shrinkage of vein diameter was a frequently observed phenomenon. This was followed by urtication and visible total vessel closure, as indicated by absence of blanching and visual elimination of the vessel border. Hyperpigmentation was common and often followed total disruption of the vessel, with bruising that occurred in 50% of treated sites.

Spot size and fluence should be chosen to reach the endpoint of immediate vessel disappearance (vessel constriction) or bluing(vessel thrombosis). Interestingly, lower fluences of 100–200 J/cm^2 work best for the coagulation of larger vessels (1.5–3 mm) and higher fluences of 250–400 J/cm^2 are required for smaller vessels (1.5 mm).[38]

It is critical to use protective eyewear while using the long pulsed Nd:YAG laser as it is one of the most penetrating lasers and can damage the retina. The treatment with this laser is painful, making it necessary to use cooling. Anesthesia – topical or local may be used in some cases. When targeting a larger reticular vein with 1,064 nm laser, slight pressure may be used to minimize the total diameter of the vein to allow greater penetration and less total heat accumulation by reducing target size. This may help to reduce the pain somewhat. Small caliber vessels often demonstrate immediate disappearance but large caliber vessels may only undergo spasm.

In another method, the off skin technique, a defocused beam or a divergent collimated beam is used for treatment. A small layer of gel is placed on the skin and the crystal or the fiber delivering the laser energy is held 1–3 cm off the skin. There is sudden change in interface from air to water causing more lateral spread than deep heating. Cryogen may be sued immediately, before and/or after the use of 1,064 nm laser to improve patient comfort and reduce the pain. But, care needs to be invested to prevent potential cryogen burns due to excessive cooling. The best way to perform a safe procedure is by separating two pulses by 2–3 mm and by keeping cumulative cryogen time to less than 40 ms (Figures 1a ,1b, 2a and 2b).

Intense Pulsed Light (IPL)

IPL devices emit a noncoherent broadband of light ranging from 500 to 1,000 nm. Filters may be used to make IPL devices more specific for use in different indications by cutting-off lower wavelengths. The principle behind the development and use of this device is that broadband light provides both superficial and deep tissue penetration and absorption by both oxygenated and deoxygenated Hb. In practice, IPL

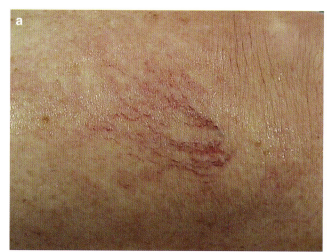
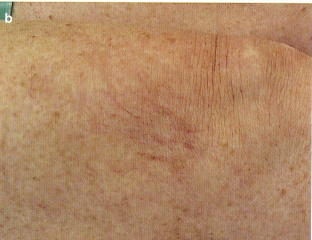

Fig. 1 (**a**) Patient 1 before leg vein treatment (**b**) Patient 1 after leg vein treatment with 1064 nm Nd:YAG laser

devices are used with the 550- and 570 nm filters to deliver primarily yellow and red light and a minor component of near-infrared light.

In a multicenter trial of an IPL device, vessels <0.2 mm, 0.2 mm and 0.5 mm in 159 patients were treated.[39] Light skinned subjects were treated with a 550 nm filter and darker skinned individuals with 570 or 590 nm filter.

Vessels less than 0.2 mm in diameter were treated with a single pulse at 22 J/cm^2 or a double pulse at 40 J/cm^2 with a l0-ms delay. Vessels 0.2–0.5 mm in diameter were treated with double pulses at 40 J/cm^2 with a l0 ms delay or double pulses at 35 J/cm^2 with a 20-ms delay. Vessels 0.5–1 mm in diameter were treated with triple pulses at 50 J/cm^2 with 20 ms delays or fluences of 55–60 J/cm^2 with 30 ms delays. An overall clearance rate of 79% was achieved. Occasional crusting, hyperpigmentation and hypopigmentation were observed. Blistering and superficial erosions developed in darkly pigmented or suntanned skin.

Another study with the same device was conducted where the patients underwent prior surgical excision or sclerotherapy

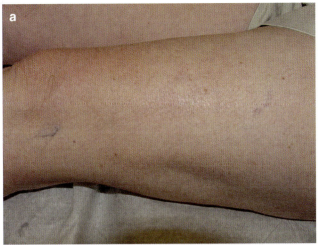

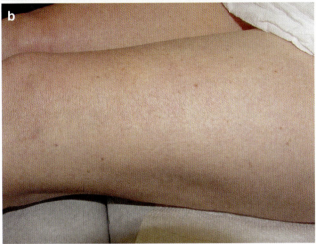

Fig. 2 (a) Patient 2 before leg vein treatment (b) Patient 2 after leg vein treatment with 1064 nm Nd:YAG laser

of larger feeding/refluxing vessels.[40] Excellent clearance of leg telangiectasias (up to 1 mm in diameter) was noted. But an acceptable level of adverse effects was reported by Green with the use of same device, though other parameters were variable.[41]

Standard parameters are difficult to define thus making such assessments difficult to define thus making such assessments difficult.

IPL seems to be most effective for superficial, red telangiectasias <1 mm; most common side-effects being erythema, edema, mild burning, purpura and dyspigmentation.

When using older IPL devices a thicker layer of gel should be used, as the crystal is placed over the target area, also termed as floating the crystal.

Newer IPL devices have a thermokinetically cooled sapphire crystal which requires contact with the skin and a minimal amount of clear coupling gel between the crystal and epidermis. It is very desirable that IPL devices have a built-in skin cooling when used for treatment of leg veins. To minimize rectangular foot-printing, a 10% overlap of pulse placement is used or a second pass may be performed with the direction perpendicular from the original direction.

Clinical Endpoints

For effective treatment and to avoid complications related to device usage, the physician should be vigilant and observe the immediate visual endpoint darkening of the targeted vessel, followed by urtication within 10 min and loss of visual vessel margins. The 1,064 nm laser may demonstrate immediate transient vessel contraction, but in most lasers urtications continue to evolve for as long as 30 min. In any case, blanching needs to be avoided which may be a result of overtreating the vessels with multiple unnecessary passes or excessively high fluences. Most commonly, epidermal injuries may be seen with IPL devices.

One should avoid overlap with 1,064 nm laser as because lateral spread of the heat energy within the vessel wall to nearby connecting vessels is observed and pulses should be spaced more than 1 mm apart while for the other lasers as many as three passes may be performed over the treated areas.

Strict sun-protection is very important for 3–4 weeks following treatment to minimize the appearance of post-inflammatory hyperpigmentation.

Postoperative Results

Seldom, pain may be experienced post-operatively, but not to the extent of requiring pain medications.

As far as seeing results of the treatment goes, although smaller vessels may disappear immediately following treatment while the larger spider veins and reticular veins usually do not disappear following treatment and they may even darken as the blood vessel coagulates.

Mild edema or surrounding the treatment site may be seen with 1,064 nm laser which may resolve rapidly and compression for a certain period may be helpful in achieving maximal benefit, though not mandatory.

If larger veins are treated, patients are advised to wear thigh-high compression stockings, and immediately after procedure, to walk for 10–30 min. They should continue to wear stockings 24 h/day for 2 weeks. Regular exercise, a high-fiber diet, and maintaining a healthy weight are recommended long term to help discourage new visible vein formation.

Post-treatment hyperpigmentation is often seen for 1–3 months and should be discussed with patients as an expected occurrence prior to treatment. The incidence of hyperpigmentation increases with the size of the treated vessel.

Sclerotherapy and Lasers

Several studies comparing sclerotherapy and lasers for treatment of leg veins have been conducted. Coles et al. compared the use of a long pulsed Nd:YAG laser with contact cooling to sclerotherapy with sodium tetradecyl sulfate in 20 patients. The vessels ranged from 0.25 to 3 mm at two comparable sites. One site was treated with long pulsed Nd:YAG laser and the other received sotradecol sclerotherapy. The patients followed up at 8 weeks for another possible laser retreatment and 3 months following the last treatment. Photographs were taken pre- and post-operatively and at each follow-up visit and used for objective comparative analysis. Improvement was tabulated from the photographic assessment on an improvement scale from 0 (no change) to 4 (greater than 75% clearing). The laser treated areas averaged 2.50 and sclerotherapy treated sites averaged 2.30. Patient surveys show 35% preferred laser and 45% choose sclerotherapy; indicating that long pulse Nd:YAG laser can yield results similar to sclerotherapy in the treatment of small leg veins.[5] Levy et al. also could not find a statistical difference when comparing Nd:YAG laser treatment with sclerotherapy.[42]

Unlike sclerotherapy which may require one to two treatments to clear a blood vessel, laser therapy often requires three or more treatments to achieve a similar degree of improvement.

Complications

In patients with darker skin types, postoperative pigmentary changes may occur and usually resolve within 4–6 months.

In the malleolar region, careful use of laser is advised such as reducing the fluence by 20% because of the reflection from the periosteum and the dermis being thin and stretched. Posttreatment, patients with severe inflammation may be given fluticasone proprionate cream 0.05% to apply twice daily for up to 1 week.

If skin breakdown or ulceration occurs, conservative daily wound care is recommended with moist dressings and counseling of the patients is required. They should be told that the ulcers may take 6–10 weeks to heal and will most likely leave a hypopigmented scar. Occlusive hydrocolloid dressings can be used and are left in place for 48–96 h at a time and debridement of necrotic tissue performed gently facilitates re-epithilialization.

Conclusion

Currently laser therapy is preferred for isolated, nonarborizing, superficial telangiectasia of the legs less than 0.3 mm in diameter and postsclerotherapy telangiectatic matting.

Because the 1,064-nm Nd:YAG works for almost all vessel sizes (up to 3 mm in diameter) and is safe in most skin types, it is a popular first choice.

Pain can sometimes be an issue with larger veins, and the Zimmer air-cooling device may be helpful. Topical anesthetic creams can also be used.

Medium-sized blue veins around the ankles are best eliminated with the alexandrite laser, which is considerably less painful than the Nd:YAG would be in this area.[43]

Tiny red spider veins in fair skin are reliably eliminated with a long PDL in combination with cryogen cooling.

Sclerotherapy still remains to be the standard of treatment for leg veins and optimal results can be achieved with sclerotherapy followed by laser or IPL.

Telangiectatic matting secondary to previous therapy should be watched, as most spontaneously resolve. If matting persists, Kauvar recommends the central feeder first be treated with sclerotherapy or a 1,064-nm Nd:YAG, then the remaining matting can be treated with a PDL, alexandrite, 595-nm Nd:YAG, or IPL.[43]

According to Sumner, if patients develop varicosities during pregnancy, it is recommended to wait 6–12 weeks after delivery to allow varices to regress.[44]

Patients known to develop telangiectatic matting may consider temporarily stopping oral contraceptives or hormone replacement therapy for the duration of treatment.

References

1. Kendler M, Makrantonaki E, Kratzsch J, Anderegg U, Wetzig T, Zouboulis C, Simon JC. Elevated sex steroid hormones in great saphenous veins in men. *J Vasc Surg.;* December 31, 2009 [Epub ahead of print].
2. Apfelberg DB, Maser MR, Lash H, White DN, Flores JT. Use of the argon and carbon dioxide lasers for treatment of superficial venous varicosities of the lower extremity. *Lasers Surg Med.* 1984;4(3):221-231.
3. Apfelberg DB, Maser MR, Lash H. Argon laser management of cutaneous vascular deformities. A preliminary report. *West J Med.* 1976;124(2):99-101.
4. Pflugbeil G, Stühler R, von Sommoggy S, Dörrler J, Maurer PC. Ablation of venous valves with Nd-Yag laser – an alternative to conventional valvulotomy? *Vasa.* 1993;22(1):53-56.
5. Coles CM, Werner RS, Zelickson BD. Comparative pilot study evaluating the treatment of leg veins with a long pulse ND:YAG laser and sclerotherapy. *Lasers Surg Med.* 2002;30(2):154-159.
6. Tan OT, Murray S, Kurban AK. Action spectrum of vascular specific injury using pulsed irradiation. *J Invest Dermatol.* 1989;92(6):868-871.
7. Reichert D. Evaluation of the long-pulse dye laser for the treatment of leg telangiectasias. *Dermatol Surg.* 1998;24:737-740.
8. Sadick NS. Laser treatment of leg veins. *Skin Therapy Lett.* 2004;9(9):6-9.
9. Dover JS, Sadick NS, Goldman MP. The role of lasers and light sources in the treatment of leg veins. *Dermatol Surg.* 1999;25(4):328-335; discussion 335–336.
10. Anderson RR, Parrish JA. Selective photothermolysis: precise microsurgery by selective absorption of pulsed radiation. *Science.* 1983;220(4596):524-527.

11. Kauvar ANB, Khrom T. Laser treatment of leg veins. *Semin Cutan Med Surg.* 2005;24:184-192.
12. Ross EV, Domankevitz Y. Laser treatment of leg veins: physical mechanisms and theoretical considerations. *Lasers Surg Med.* 2005;36(2):105-116.
13. Altshuler GB, Anderson RR, Manstein D, Zenzie HH, Smirnov MZ. Extended theory of selective photothermolysis. *Lasers Surg Med.* 2001;29(5):416-432.
14. Alves OC, Wajnberg E. Heat denaturation of metHb and HbNO: e.p.r. evidence for the existence of a new hemichrome. *Int J Biol Macromol.* 1993;15(5):273-279.
15. Seto Y, Kataoka M, Tsuge K. Stability of blood carbon monoxide and hemoglobins during heating. *Forensic Sci Int.* 2001;121(1–2): 144-150.
16. Barton JK, Frangineas G, Pummer H, Black JF. Cooperative phenomena in two-pulse, two-color laser photocoagulation of cutaneous blood vessels. *Photochem Photobiol.* 2001;73(6):642-650.
17. Mordon S, Brisot D, Fournier N. Using a "non uniform pulse sequence" can improve selective coagulation with a Nd:YAG laser (1.06 microm) thanks to Met-hemoglobin absorption: a clinical study on blue leg veins. *Lasers Surg Med.* 2003;32(2):160-170.
18. Black JF, Wade N, Barton JK. Mechanistic comparison of blood undergoing laser photocoagulation at 532 and 1, 064 nm. *Lasers Surg Med.* 2005;36(2):155-165.
19. Spendel S, Prandl EC, Schintler MV, et al. Treatment of spider leg veins with the KTP (532 nm) laser–a prospective study. *Lasers Surg Med.* 2002;31(3):194-201.
20. Bernstein EF, Kornbluth S, Brown DB, Black J. Treatment of spider veins using a 10 millisecond pulse-duration frequency-doubled neodymium YAG laser. *Dermatol Surg.* 1999;25(4):316-320.
21. Bernstein EF. The new-generation, high-energy, 595-nm, long pulse-duration pulsed-dye laser improves the appearance of photodamaged skin. *Lasers Surg Med.* 2007;39(2):157-163.
22. Kono T, Yamaki T, Erçöçen AR, Fujiwara O, Nozaki M. Treatment of leg veins with the long pulse dye laser using variable pulse durations and energy fluences. *Lasers Surg Med.* 2004;35(1):62-67.
23. Tanghetti E, Sherr E. Treatment of telangiectasia using the multipass technique with the extended pulse width, pulsed dye laser (Cynosure V-Star). *J Cosmet Laser Ther.* 2003;5(2):71-75.
24. McDaniel DH, Ash K, Lord J, Newman J, Adrian RM, Zukowski M. Laser therapy of spider leg veins: clinical evaluation of a new long pulsed alexandrite laser. *Dermatol Surg.* 1999;25(1):52-58.
25. Kauvar AN, Lou WW. Pulsed alexandrite laser for the treatment of leg telangiectasia and reticular veins. *Arch Dermatol.* 2000; 136(11):1371-1375.
26. Eremia S, Li C, Umar SH. A side-by-side comparative study of 1064 nm Nd:YAG, 810 nm diode and 755 nm alexandrite lasers for treatment of 0.3-3 mm leg veins. *Dermatol Surg.* 2002;28(3):224-230.
27. Trelles MA, Allones I, Alvarez J, et al. The 800-nm diode laser in the treatment of leg veins: assessment at 6 months. *J Am Acad Dermatol.* 2006;54(2):282-289.
28. Wollina U, Konrad H, Schmidt WD, Haroske G, Astafeva LG, Fassler D. Response of spider leg veins to pulsed diode laser (810 nm): a clinical, histological and remission spectroscopy study. *J Cosmet Laser Ther.* 2003;5(3–4):154-162.
29. Sadick NS, Trelles MA. A clinical, histological, and computer-based assessment of the Polaris LV, combination diode, and radiofrequency system, for leg vein treatment. *Lasers Surg Med.* 2005; 36(2):98-104.
30. Trelles MA, Martín-Vázquez M, Trelles OR, Mordon SR. Treatment effects of combined radio-frequency current and a 900 nm diode laser on leg blood vessels. *Lasers Surg Med.* 2006;38(3):185-195.
31. Black JF, Barton JK. Chemical and structural changes in blood undergoing laser photocoagulation. *Photochem Photobiol.* 2004;80:89-97.
32. Randeberg LL, Bonesrønning JH, Dalaker M, Nelson JS, Svaasand LO. Methemoglobin formation during laser induced photothermolysis of vascular skin lesions. *Lasers Surg Med.* 2004;34(5):414-419.
33. Omura NE, Dover JS, Arndt KA, Kauvar AN. Treatment of reticular leg veins with a 1064 nm long-pulsed Nd:YAG laser. *J Am Acad Dermatol.* 2003;48(1):76-81.
34. Rogachefsky AS, Silapunt S, Goldberg DJ. Nd:YAG laser (1064 nm) irradiation for lower extremity telangiectases and small reticular veins: efficacy as measured by vessel color and size. *Dermatol Surg.* 2002;28(3):220-223.
35. Bäumler W, Ulrich H, Hartl A, Landthaler M, Shafirstein G. Optimal parameters for the treatment of leg veins using Nd:YAG lasers at 1064 nm. *Br J Dermatol.* 2006;155(2):364-371.
36. Parlette EC, Groff WF, Kinshella MJ, Domankevitz Y, O'Neill J, Ross EV. Optimal pulse durations for the treatment of leg telangiectasias with a neodymium YAG laser. *Lasers Surg Med.* 2006;38(2):98-105.
37. Weiss RA, Weiss MA. Early clinical results with a multiple synchronized pulse 1064 NM laser for leg telangiectasias and reticular veins. *Dermatol Surg.* 1999;25(5):399-402.
38. Lupton JR, Alster TS, Romero P. Clinical comparison of sclerotherapy versus long-pulsed Nd:YAG laser treatment for lower extremity telangiectases. *Dermatol Surg.* 2002;28(8):694.
39. Goldman MP, Eckhouse S. Photothermal sclerosis of leg veins. *Dermatol Surg.* 1996;22:323-330.
40. Schroeter CA, Neumann HAM. An intense light source: the photoderm VL-flashlamp as a new treatment possibility for vascular lesions. *Dermatol Surg.* 1998;24:743-748.
41. Green D. Photothermal removal telangiectasias of the lower extremities with the photoderm VL. *J Am Acad Dermatol.* 1998;38:61-68.
42. Levy JL, Elbahr C, Jouve E, Mordon S. Comparison and sequential study of long pulsed Nd:YAG 1, 064 nm laser and sclerotherapy in leg telangiectasias treatment. *Lasers Surg Med.* 2004;34(3):273-276.
43. Krivda MS. The latest approaches to treating leg veins. *Skin Aging.* 2005;13:72-77.
44. Sumner DS. Venous dynamics: varicosities. *Clin Obstet Gynecol.* 1981;24:743.

Lasers and Lights for Treating Pigmented Lesions*

Emmy M. Graber and Jeffrey S. Dover

Outline

Introduction
  History
  • Pigmented lesions were initially treated with destructive non-selective lasers.
  • Now pigment selective Q-switched lasers used.
  Epidemiology
  • Pigmented skin lesions are exceedingly common.
  Basic Science
  • Selective destruction of pigmented lesions relies on the theory of selective photothermolysis.
  • Melanin has a broad absorption spectrum with absorption steadily decreasing with increasing wavelength.
  • Several Q-switched lasers fall within the melanin absorption spectrum. Their nanosecond pulse duration is effective since it is shorter than the thermal relaxation time of melanin.
Indications and Contraindications
  Epidermal Pigmented Lesions
  • Lentigines, Café au lait macules, and ephelides are common epidermal pigmented lesions that respond to laser treatment.
  • Shorter laser wavelengths may suffice as deep tissue penetration is not necessary.
  • Multiple treatments are often needed for complete removal.
  Dermal Pigmented Lesions
  • Melanocytic nevi, nevus of Ota, melasma, post-inflammatory hyperpigmentation, and drug induced pigmentation are dermal pigmented lesions that can be treated with lasers.
  • Longer wavelengths may be needed to reach the pigment.

  • Multiple treatments are necessary.
  • Anesthesia is often needed.
Techniques
  Pre-operative Management
  • It is important to obtain a medical history prior to treatment and to educate patients about the potential outcomes.
  • Anesthesia may be needed for larger or dermal pigmented lesions.
  • Appropriate protective eyewear should be on all persons in the room.
  Description of Technique
  • Laser parameters depend on the particular laser, the patient's skin phototype, and the type of lesion.
  • Adequate fluence should result in an immediate uniform ash white color.
  Post-operative Management
  • An occlusive ointment should be applied and patients should be educated on the healing process.
Adverse Events
  Side Effects/Complications
  • Post-inflammatory hyperpigmentation, an inadequate response and recurrence of the lesion are the most common side effects.
  Prevention and Treatment of Side Effects/Complications
  • Using the appropriate laser and fluence can reduce side effects.
  • Educating patients so that there are realistic expectations can also help to reduce patient frustration and complications.
Future Directions
  • Pico (10^{-12}) and femto second (10^{-15}) domain lasers are being developed.
Conclusions

J.S. Dover (✉)
Department of Dermatology, SkinCare Physicians,
1244 Boylston Street, Chestnut Hill, MA, USA
e-mail: jdover@skincarephysicians.net

*Modified from: Kaminer, M.S., Dover, J.S., and Arndt, K.A. *Atlas of Cosmetic Surgery*. 2002. W.B. Saunders Company.

K. Nouri (ed.), *Lasers in Dermatology and Medicine*,
DOI: 10.1007/978-0-85729-281-0_6, © Springer-Verlag London Limited 2011

Introduction

- Pigmented lesions were initially treated with destructive non-selective lasers.
- Now pigment selective Q-switched lasers used.
- Pigmented skin lesions are exceedingly common.
- Selective destruction of pigmented lesions relies on the theory of selective photothermolysis.
- Melanin has a broad absorption spectrum with absorption steadily decreasing with increasing wavelength.
- Several Q-switched lasers fall within the melanin absorption spectrum. Their nanosecond pulse duration is effective since it is shorter than the thermal relaxation time of melanin.

History

The application of lasers for pigmented lesions began in 1963 when Leon Goldman and colleagues found that 0.5 ms pulses of ruby laser radiation was selectively absorbed by pigmented skin.[1] These investigators also discovered that the threshold radiant exposure for epidermal damage was 10–100 times lower for a quality switched (Q-switched) ruby laser (QSRL) with a pulse duration of 50 ns.[2] Despite these early findings, the ability of the QSRL to selectively target pigment was not initially appreciated. Instead, for many years, pigmented lesions were treated with nonselective continuous wave sources such as the argon[3] and carbon dioxide lasers.[4] After using these more tissue destructive devices, the selective Q-switched lasers at wavelengths other than 694 nm were found to target melanin. In the late 1980s Anderson et al. demonstrated that Q-switched Nd:YAG laser pulses at 1,064, 532, and 355 nm selectively diminished melanin. This group also showed that the longer wavelengths (which are less well-absorbed by melanin) required a higher energy fluence to be effective. Over the last 20 years, after further investigation, pulsed lasers and intense pulsed light sources have become the treatment of choice for epidermal, and, pulsed lasers the choice for dermal pigmented lesions and tattoos.

Epidemiology

Pigmented skin lesions are exceedingly common in all races. Some pigmented lesions are congenital while many are acquired. With increasing sun exposure, pigmented lesions become more prevalent. In a quest to reverse photoaging, there are countless patients that desire lightening or removal of these lesions. For some patients, there appears to also be a cultural influence to correct dyspigmentation.

Basic Science

Laser-Tissue Interactions in Pigmented Skin

The ability of laser and light sources to diminish pigmented lesions is based on the principle of selective photothermolysis. Described in 1983 by Anderson and Parrish, selective photothermolysis predicts that there can be selective thermal damage to an absorbing target using appropriate laser parameters and pulse characteristics. This principle requires: (1) the use of a wavelength that is well absorbed by the target, (2) a pulse duration that is shorter than the thermal relaxation time (the time required for a heated target to cool by 50%), (3) a sufficiently high energy density to achieve the desired tissue effect. Selective photothermolysis was originally applied to the treatment of vascular lesions with oxyhemoglobin as the target chromophore. Thereafter selective photothermolysis was applied to pigmented lesions by targeting endogenous melanin and exogenous carbon particles as target chromophores.

As a target chromophore, melanin has a broad absorption spectrum within the ultraviolet, visible and near-infrared light range (Fig. 1). However, light absorption in melanin decreases steadily with increasing wavelength.[5] Melanocytes contain intracytoplasmic organelles, melanosomes, which are the sites of melanin biosynthesis (Fig. 2). After formation in the melanocytes, melanosomes and their melanin are transferred to surrounding keratinocytes. These melanin containing melanosomes are 1 mm in diameter and are predicted to have a thermal relaxation time between 50 and 500 ns.[5,6] Based on the principle of selective photothermolysis, for this short thermal relaxation time, an extremely short pulse duration should be used to effectively target melanosomes. The delivery of an extremely high energy laser pulse within a very short time span results in rapid heating of the target melanosome (estimated at 10 million degrees per second), causing it to explode.[7]

While electron microscopy has confirmed highly selective destruction of melanosomes within melanocytes and melanized keratinocytes, it is not know precisely how the pigment-containing cells are destroyed. It is believed that destruction of melanocytes and melanized keratinocytes are destroyed due to mechanical damage from acoustic waves that emanate from the absorbing melanosome.[8,9] Damage to these cells results in vacuolization and

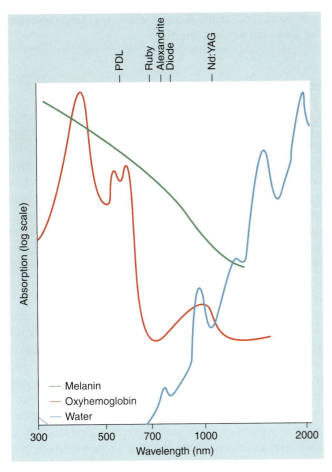

Fig. 1 Absorption curves of melanin, oxyhemoglobin and water (From Bolognia et al. *Dermatology*. 2003)[100]

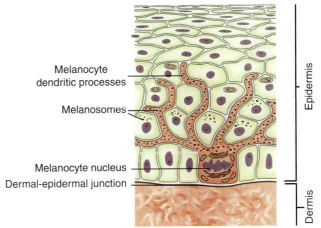

Fig. 2 Melanocyte residing within the epidermis. Melanosomes extend throughout the dendritic processes and are transferred to neighboring keratinocytes (Modified from www.freethought-forum.com)

deposition of pigment and nuclear material at the cellular periphery. In addition, subepidermal vesiculation may occur at the level of the lamina lucida. Following damage, repigmentation results from migration of residual melanocytes from either adnexal structures or adjacent unirradiated skin.

When treating pigmented lesions, Q-switched lasers generate an immediate ash-white color at the site of impact. The cause of this tissue response is due to heat induced steam cavities in melanosomes which cause a scattering of visible light, producing a white color.[10] Well demarcated, circular, highly reflective structures of 1–30 μm within melanosomes have been identified by confocal microscopy, electron microscopy, and optical coherence tomography (Fig. 3). These circular structures are presumed to be gas bubbles and gradually disappear over 20 min, correlating to the disappearance of the clinical ash-white color over the same period of time.[12] The exact content of the gas bubbles is not know, but may be water vapor, nitrogen, or other gases. The adequate laser exposure dose for melanosome damage correlates well with the clinical threshold for immediate skin whitening. In other words, if the clinical ash-white color is not visible, the laser exposure dose is not sufficient. Darker skin has a lower threshold for whitening due to a higher epidermal melanin content.[12] With increasing wavelengths, melanin absorption decreases, and the required threshold laser exposure dose increases.[13,14] Subthreshold fluences appear to actually stimulate melanogenesis because of activation of epidermal melanocytes after non-lethal injury (Fig. 4).[15]

Q-Switched and Pulsed Lasers and Light Sources

Selective damage to melanosomes in human skin was first demonstrated with a 351 nm XeF excimer laser delivering 20 ns pulses.[16] Although light at 351 nm is well absorbed by melanin, this short wavelength only penetrates less than 100 μm into the skin due to light scattering.[17] It was subsequently found that selective melanosome damage could be produced by also the pulsed tunable dye laser[13,18] (wavelength 435–750 nm, pulse width 300–750 ns), Q-switched ruby laser[6] (wavelength 694 nm, pulse width 40 ns) and the Q-switched neodymium:YAG laser[14] (wavelength 355, 532, and 1,064 nm, pulse width 10–12 ns). While shorter wavelengths, such as 351 nm are better at absorbing melanin, longer wavelengths penetrate deeper into the skin, increasing their ability to reach deeper melanosomes (Fig. 5).

Several lasers can be used today to treat pigmented skin lesions (Table 1). These include lasers that are: (1) pigment

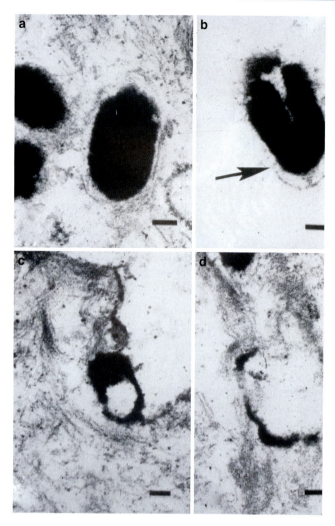

Fig. 3 Electron micrograph obtained immediately after Q-switched ruby laser irradiation. The targeted melanosome shows membrane disruption with disorganization of its internal contents (a) prior to irradiation; (b) immediately after irradiation showing early melanosome disruption; (c) more disruption; (d) almost complete disruption of a melanosome immediately after irradiation (From Ardnt et al.[11])

nonselective, (2) highly pigment selective, (3) and those that are somewhat pigment selective.

Pigment Nonselective Lasers

The carbon dioxide[4,19] (10,600 nm), erbium-YAG (2,940 nm) and Erbium xxx (1,540 nm) and yttrium scandium gallium garnet (YSGG) (2,790 nm) lasers are pigment nonselective lasers that remove epidermal pigment because of their ability to target water and ablate the entire epidermis, including melanocytes and melanized keratinocytes. Earlier devices removed a relatively uniform layer of the epidermis and with the epidermis went the associated pigment. Newer fractionated laser technologies damage columns of the epidermis and dermis while leaving interspersed areas unaffected. In this manner, there is faster healing as the surrounding normal tissue heals each light column of damage (Fig. 6). The fractionated CO_2 and fractionated erbium:YAG lasers work in the same manner as their non-fractionated counterparts but deliver the light in many small columns. Because only fractions of the pigmented epidermis are affected, it stands to reason that a series of treatments is necessary to achieve the desired result and at least some of the original pigmented epidermal lesion would remain even after a series of treatments resulting in incomplete lesion removal.

The YSGG laser is a non fractional device that targets epidermal water and indirectly associated melanin. Plasma skin resurfacing is not a laser but is a device that utilizes radiofrequency energy to convert nitrogen gas into plasma. The plasma gives up energy to the skin and there is rapid heating of the skin into the dermis. Depending on the amount of energy delivered a thinner or thicker layer of the epidermis and adjacent dermis is affected by the treatment. Over

Fig. 4 Histologic appearance of black guinea pig skin immediately after irradiation with the Q-switched ruby laser. (a) Characteristic "ring cell" formation in the basal lamina, representing melanocytes and keratinocytes with condensed nuclear and pigment material at their peripheries. (b) Similar changes in a hair follicle (From Ardnt et al.[11])

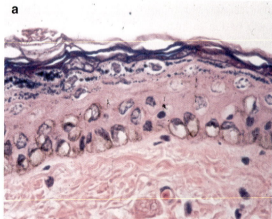
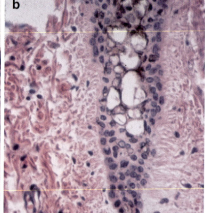

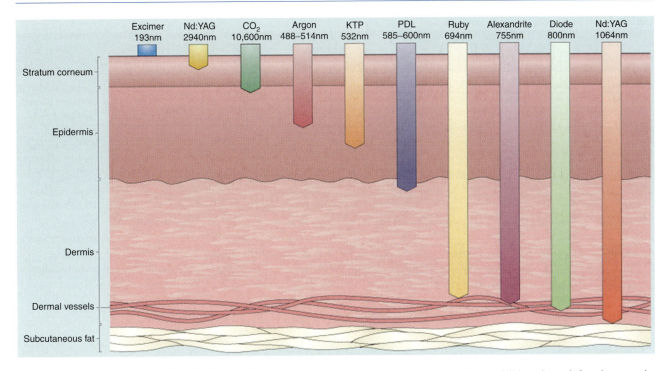

Fig. 5 Laser depth of penetration. Depth of penetration for lasers of varying wavelengths. For lasers in the visible and near infrared ranges, the depth of penetration increases as the wavelength increases (From Bolognia, et al. *Dermatology*. 2003)

24–48 h the epidermis is shed, including melanocytes and pigment laden keratinocytes, and is then regenerated, leaving behind a new epidermis with less unwanted sun induced pigment.

Highly Pigment Selective Lasers

Older technologies, such as continuous wave (CW) and quasi-CW visible light lasers, including the argon laser (488, 514 nm), copper vapor laser (511 nm), and krypton laser (521, 530 nm), can be used to selectively remove epidermal pigmented lesions. However, spatial thermal injury confinement is not possible and unaffected adjacent skin may also be damaged. The risk/benefit ratio is higher with these CW and quasi-CW devices.

There are three short-pulsed, pigment selective lasers that are widely used today: (1) the Q-switched ruby laser (QSRL) (694 nm), (2) the Q-switched alexandrite laser (755 nm), and (3) the Q-switched neodymium:YAG (Nd:YAG and KTP) laser (1,064, 532 nm). These lasers selectively target melanin by delivering high-intensity, short-pulsed radiation at varying wavelengths. "Q-switched" is an abbreviation for "quality-switched" and refers to lasers which release an extremely high powered pulse (10^9 W) with an ultra-short pulse duration. Through the use of an optical shutter, these lasers store large amounts of energy in the laser cavity and then release the stored energy when the laser fires.

The QSRL emits red light at a wavelength of 694 nm and a pulse duration of 28–40 ns (Table 1). Light is delivered through a mirrored articulated arm at a spot size of 5 or 6.5 mm and a repetition rate of 2 Hz. The Q-switched alexandrite laser has a near infrared wavelength of 755 nm, pulse duration of 50–100 ns, spot size of 2–4 mm, and a repetition rate up to 10 Hz. Depending on the exact device, light is delivered either through an articulated arm or through a semi-flexible fiber optic cable. The Q-switched Nd:YAG laser emits infrared light at 1,064 nm. The wavelength can be halved by placing a frequency-doubling KTP (potassium-titanyl-phosphate) crystal in the laser beam's path. Dye-impregnated handpieces can convert the 532 nm wavelength to either 585 nm (yellow) or 650 nm (red). An articulated arm delivers pulses with a spot size to 1.5–8 mm, a pulse duration of 5–10 ns, and a repetition rate up to 10 Hz.

Long-pulsed (millisecond rather than nanosecond domain) 532 nm (KTP) Nd:YAG lasers and 595 nm pulsed-dye lasers, which are traditionally used to treat vascular lesions, can also be used to treat superficial pigmented lesions. However, the long pulse width of these lasers is close to the thermal relaxation time of the entire epidermis (about 10 ms)[21] and therefore does not allow for selective

Table 1 Lasers in the treatment of pigmented lesion

Device	Manufacturer	Laser type	Wavelength (nm)	Pulse duration	Spot size (mm)	Maximum repetition rate(Hz)	Comments
Spectrum RD-1200	Palomar	QS Ruby	694	28 ns	5, 6.5	0.8	Large spot size promotes deeper penetration
EpiTouch	Lumenis	QS Ruby	694	25 ns	5	0.8	Long pulse mode available for hair removal
Sinon	Wavelight	QS Ruby	694	15–40 ns	3–9	20	Long pulse mode available for hair removal
AlexLAZR	Candela	QS alexandrite	755	50 ns	2, 3, 4	5	Fiberoptic delivery system
VersaPulse VPC	Lumenis	FD Nd:YAG	532	2–50 ms	2–10	6	Four lasers within one box
		QS FD Nd:YAG	532	4 ns	2–6	10	
		QS Nd:YAG	1,064	5 ns	2–6	10	
		QS alexandrite	755	45 ns	2–6	10	
Medlite C6	HOYA	QS FD Nd:YAG	532	5–20 ns	2, 3, 4, 6	10	Handpiece converts λ to 585 and 650 nm
	ConBio	QS Nd:YAG	1,064	5–20 ns	3, 4, 6, 8	10	
Alex	Candela	QS FD Nd:YAG	532	50 ns	2, 3, 5	5	
TriVantage		QS alexandrite	755		2, 3, 4	5	
		QS Nd:YAG	1,064		2, 3, 5	5	
SkinClear	Sybaritic	QS FD Nd:YAG	532	10 ns	1, 2, 3		
		QS Nd:YAG	1,064	10 ns	1, 2, 3		
Naturalase	Focus	QS FD Nd:YAG	532	10–20 ns	7		
	Medical	QS Nd:YAG	1,064	10–20 ns	7		

QS Q-switched, *FD* frequency doubled

damage to melanosomes. Because of their longer pulse width, millisecond domain lasers produce a purely thermal effect on their target, unlike the photomechanical effect of Q-switched lasers. The target in this case may in fact be melanocytes rather than melanosomes. Regardless, these longer pulse duration devices, just like intense pulsed light devices are highly effective in removing unwanted epidermal pigment. These lasers are not suitable for treating dermal pigmented lesions because of the limited penetration depth.[22] Although no longer manufactured, a pigmented lesion pulsed dye laser (non-Q-switched) used a xenon flashlamp to pump a coumarin-containing dye that expelled

pulses of green light at 510 nm. Although this laser was useful for epidermal lesions, its shallow penetration made it much less effective on dermal lesions.

The Q-switched ruby, alexandrite and Nd:YAG lasers also have long-pulsed counterparts with the same wavelengths that operate in a normal (non-Q-switched) mode. These normal mode lasers are often used for laser hair removal because their higher fluences and longer pulse durations target large pigmented structures such as hair follicles or nests of cells rather than individual melanosomes or pigmented cells.[23] Normal mode lasers have been shown to be effective in the removal of epidermal pigmented lesions but

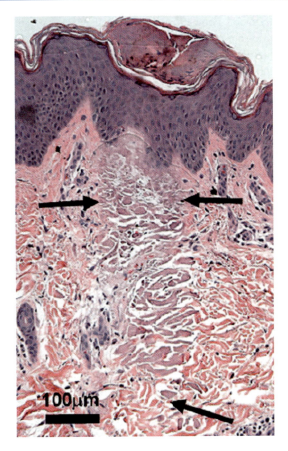

Fig. 6 Fractionated erbium glass laser causing tissue coagulation in a narrow microthermal zone of injury (From Vikramaditya et al.[20])

Indications and Contraindications

- Ephelides, lentigines, and café au lait macules, are common epidermal pigmented lesions that respond to laser and light treatment.
- Melanocytic nevi, nevus of Ota and other dermal melanocytoses, melasma, post-inflammatory hyperpigmentation, and drug induced pigmentation are dermal pigmented lesions that can be treated with lasers. Of these, only nevus of Ota and other dermal melanocytoses respond predictably and favorably.
- Shorter laser wavelengths may suffice for epidermal lesions as deep tissue penetration is not necessary.
- Long wavelengths are required for dermal pigmented lesions.
- Multiple treatments are often needed for complete removal.
- Anesthesia may be needed for larger or dermal lesions.

are not ideal because damage may be imparted on surrounding tissue.

Non-coherent light sources (intense pulsed light or IPL) can also be used for pigment removal. Polychromatic light is emitted ranging from 515 to 1,200 nm (visible to infrared) and filters are used to cut off the light above or below predetermined wavelengths. Since melanin exhibits a broad absorption spectrum, monochromatic laser devices are not necessary to target superficial melanin. The shorter wavelengths emitted by IPL devices are highly absorbed by melanin. IPL devices release light as a series of single, double, or triple pulses (millisecond domain). Like the millisecond domain lasers, the millisecond pulse width of IPL devices approximates the thermal relaxation time of the epidermis (10 ms) and produces a photothermal, not photomechanical effect, on its target. To avoid damage to normal surrounding epidermis, most IPL devices have skin cooling during treatment to protect the epidermis from excessive thermal injury. The IPL devices should not be used for dermal pigmented lesions.

Epidermal Pigmented Lesions

Many clinical studies have proven the efficacy and safety of Q-switched lasers[24-26] and the 510 nm pulsed dye laser[27] in the treatment of various epidermal pigmented lesions, including: ephelides, lentigines, Café au lait macules, seborrheic keratoses, nevi spilus, and Becker's nevi. Since pigment in epidermal lesions is found superficially, shorter-wavelength devices can be used successfully despite their limited penetration depth. For example, the 510 nm wavelength of the pigmented lesion pulsed dye laser and 532 nm pulsed lasers are highly absorbed by melanin but penetrates only about 250 μm into the skin.[17] The Q-switched ruby and alexandrite lasers effectively treat both epidermal and dermal pigmented lesions since their wavelengths are still within the melanin absorption spectrum and they penetrate deeply into the dermis. The Nd:YAG (1,064 nm) laser penetrates deeply but is poorly absorbed by melanin, making the 532 nm wavelength preferable for epidermal lesions. When using the 510 nm and 532 nm wavelengths, hemoglobin competes with melanin for absorption of light. Nanosecond pulses at these wavelengths causes rupture of superficial blood vessels, manifesting clinically as purpura.[13]

Lentigines

Lentigines are extremely common hyperpigmented macules that are most often due to chronic sun exposure and are then referred to as solar lentigines. On pathology lentigines display increased single melanocytes along the basal layer with elongation of club-shaped rete ridges. In addition to solar lentigines, there are lentigines associated with a syndrome (e.g., Peutz-Jeghers (Fig. 7)) and labial melanotic macules (labial lentigines). All three Q-switched lasers are highly effective for treating all types of lentigines.[28,29] Both 35% trichloroacetic acid peels and cryotherapy are inferior to Q-switched lasers in the treatment of lentigines.[30,31] With one treatment using a Q-switched laser, at least 50% clearing of lentigines is expected, and additional treatments may be utilized to remove remaining pigment (Figs. 8 and 9). Although less selective, non Q-switched (millisecond domain) KTP, 595 nm pulsed-dye, ruby, alexandrite, and diode lasers may also be used to treat lentigines. A study of Asian patients with lentigines found a long-pulsed KTP (532 nm) laser (without skin cooling) to be as effective as a 532 nm Q-switched Nd:YAG laser, and with less risk of post-inflammatory hyperpigmentation. Additionally, a study using a 595 nm pulsed-dye laser on lentigines in Asian patients showed a mean of 82% improvement in lentigines by reflectance spectrometry.[22] Several studies have also demonstrated the effectiveness of broad band light sources (Intense Pulsed Light) in clearing lentigines. Adjunctive use of 5-aminolevulinic acid (5-ALA) with IPL provides greater improvement of epidermal pigment than with IPL alone.[32-34]

Café Au Lait Macules

Café au lait macules (CALMs) are well circumscribed, homogenous light brown macules that occur as isolated lesions in the general population. Their prevalence varies amongst ethnicities but ranges from 0.2% to 18%.[35] Café au lait macules may also be found as multiple lesions in association with a syndrome (e.g., neurofibromatosis, Noonan syndrome). Histologically, there is an increase in melanocytes along the basal layer, hypermelanosis of melanocytes and keratinocytes,

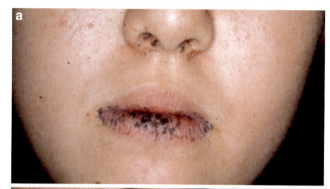

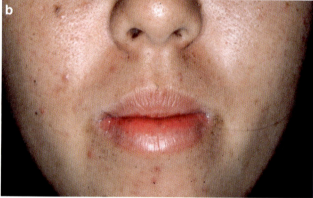

Fig. 7 (**a**) A patient with Peutz-Jeghers syndrome with extensive macular pigmented lesions over the lip prior to treatment. (**b**) After two treatments with the Q-switched ruby laser, the lesions are completely cleared (Courtesy Tadashi Tezuka, MD)

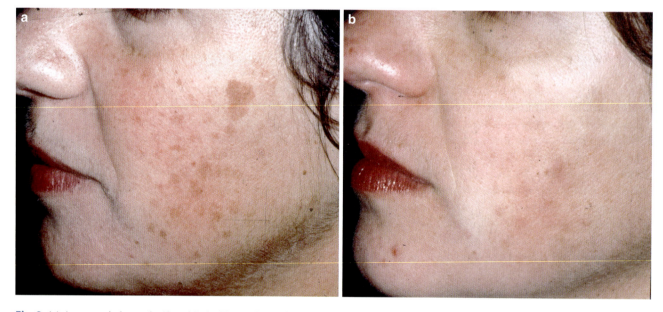

Fig. 8 (**a**) A woman in her early 40 s with significant photoaging and numerous lentigines prior to treatment. (**b**) Six weeks after one single treatment with a Q-switched ruby laser. There is about 70% improvement of the lesion. No further treatments were requested by the patient

Lasers and Lights for Treating Pigmented Lesions

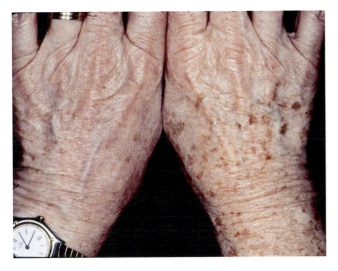

Fig. 9 A patient's right hand with copious solar lentigines and the patient's left hand with significantly fewer solar lentigines after two Q-switched alexandrite treatments

and giant melanin granules. Treatment of CALMs with lasers is minimally successful and often unpredictable.[36] Temporary lightening or clearing can be achieved after multiple treatments (Fig. 10). However, recurrences are seen in up to 50% of treated lesions, even when clearing is initially achieved. Post-inflammatory hyperpigmentation is frequent following laser treatment of CALMs, especially in patients with darker skin types. Alster demonstrated complete elimination of most CALMs after an average of 8.4 treatment sessions with the 510 nm pulsed dye laser, indicating that multiple treatments are needed for complete resolution.[37,38] Er:YAG resurfacing has also been shown to eliminate CALMs.[38]

Other Epidermal Lesions

Ephelides (freckles) are hyperpigmented small macules located on sun-exposed skin and become darker in the summer and lighter in the winter. There is no increase in the number of melanocytes on pathology, but there is an increase in melanin. Ephelides respond well to Q-switched laser treatment (Fig. 11). Another common lesion, seborrheic keratoses, may respond to laser treatment. In general, thinner seborrheic keratoses respond better to laser treatment than thick lesions.[27] Cryotherapy or cryotherapy in combination with laser treatment is preferred to laser treatment alone for thick seborrheic keratoses. A nevus spilus (speckled lentiginous nevus) consists of a background CALM and scattered nests of nevi cells. Successful clearing of the darker nevocellular component has been reported with the QSRL, but the CALM component tends to recur.[24] A Becker's nevus is a hyperpigmented, hair-bearing plaque that most commonly occurs on the upper trunk or shoulder of males. These lesions may also be associated with a dermal smooth muscle hamartoma. The hyperpigmented component of Becker's nevi respond similarly to laser treatment as CALMs, having frequent recurrences (within 6–12 months) and post-inflammatory hyperpigmentation.[39]

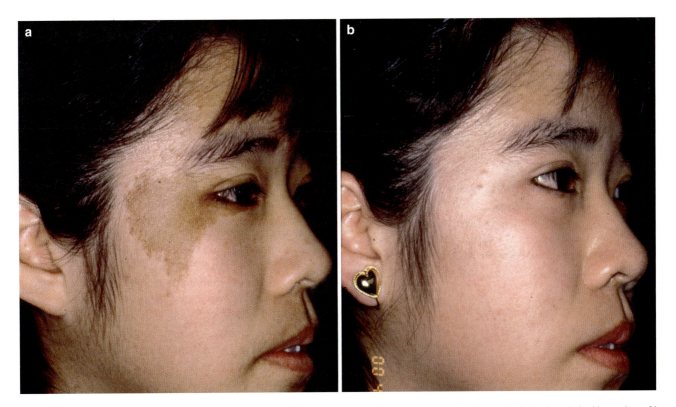

Fig. 10 (a) A young Asian patient with a café au lait macule on her right cheek. (b) After a series of treatments with the Q-switched laser, the café au lait macule has cleared markedly

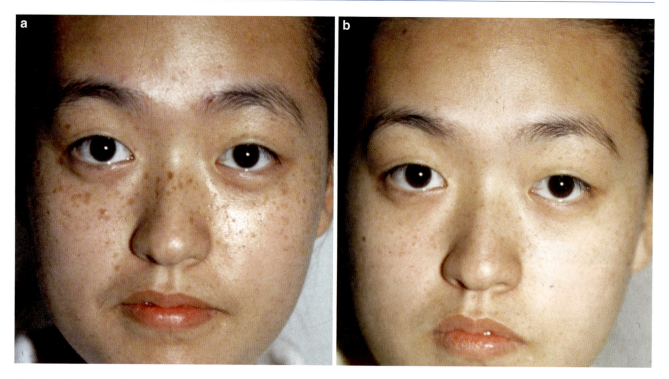

Fig. 11 (a) Japanese male with extensive numbers of freckles prior to treatment. (b) After treatment with a Q-switched ruby laser, the freckles are entirely clear (Courtesy of T.K. Lee, MD)

Dermal Pigmented Lesions

Q-switched lasers have revolutionized the treatment of dermal pigmented lesions including: melanocytic nevi, nevus of Ota, and melasma. Prior to the advent of Q-switched lasers, these lesions were treated with nonspecific destructive means such as excision,[40,41] dermabrasion,[42] salabrasion,[43] cryotherapy,[44] solid carbon dioxide ice,[45] or continuous wave laser ablation.[46] These older methods were ineffective and often caused scarring or dyspigmentation. By selectively targeting dermal melanin, Q-switched lasers provide effective treatment of these lesions without risking textural or pigment alteration. The Q-switched ruby, alexandrite and 1,064 nm Nd:YAG are the most commonly used lasers. All of these lasers are still within the absorption spectrum of melanin yet also have wavelengths that are long enough to penetrate into the dermis. Broad band light sources (such as IPL) lack wavelength specificity and have longer (ms range rather than nanosecond range) pulse durations, making them unsuitable for treating dermal pigmented lesions.

Melanocytic Nevi

Laser treatment of melanocytic nevi is controversial since it is unclear whether laser irradiation has any potential to induce malignant change in nevus cells. In vitro studies of melanoma cells treated with Q-switched lasers have found changes in cell surface integrin expression, with subsequent alteration of cell migration.[47] Another in vitro study found a significant increase in p16INK4a in p16 positive cell lines following irradiation with Q-switched laser light and suggested that sub-lethal laser damage may increase DNA damage leading to an increase in p16 expression.[48] In clinical practice, benign appearing nevi that tend to recur following laser treatment may show newfound clinical and histologic atypia, referred to as pseudomelanoma.[49] Despite this, there has never been a report of true malignant transformation of a benign pigmented lesion following laser treatment.[50] Theoretically, laser treatment of melanocytic lesions may decrease the risk of malignant transformation of a benign pigmented lesion simply by reducing the population of existing potentially premalignant cells. One study reported that no significant malignant markers (such as proliferation cell nuclear antigen, pyrimidine dimers, 8-OhdG, and p53) were found following treatment of nevi with Q-switched lasers.[51] While these findings are notable, additional study is needed to assess the outcome of Q-switched laser treatment of nevi. Until more is known, it is prudent to perform a biopsy prior to laser treatment to confirm the benign nature of the nevus. Laser treatment should not be performed on nevi in patients with a personal or family history of malignant melanoma.

The Q-switched ruby, alexandrite, and 1,064 nm Nd:YAG lasers all have some efficacy in removing flat or slightly raised acquired nevi.[52-54] Lighter nevi respond best to shorter wavelengths that maximize melanin absorption, while darker nevi typically respond to any wavelength within the melanin absorption spectrum. Multiple treatments are frequently necessary for optimal lightening. Clinical lightening is also associated with the development of a subtle microscopic scar up to 1 mm thick that obscures residual nevus cells. It is often unfeasible to attain complete resolution of nevi,[54] and recurrence after laser treatment is common. There may be persistence of nevus cells containing little pigment located in the deeper dermis that are shielded from laser radiation by the more pigmented superficial cells.[52] Q-switched laser radiation does not penetrate sufficiently to effectively treat thicker papillated or dome-shaped dermal nevi. The short pulsed erbium:YAG laser has been reported to be quite effective in removing flat or slightly palpable melanocytic nevi. Single pulses of 5.2–14 J/cm^2 were found to clear 27 of 28 nevi on follow-up and histological examination.[55] The QSRL has been reported to successfully eliminate flat blue nevi.[56]

Although Q-switched lasers may effectively lighten congenital nevi, there is frequently repigmentation due to persistence of nevus cells within the deeper reticular dermis and within adnexae.[50,57] In a split nevus study on 15 patients, Kono et al. showed greater clearing with combined Q-switched and normal-mode ruby laser (NMRL) than in NMRL alone. They also showed a marked decrease in nevus nests at the dermal-epidermal junction, papillary and reticular dermis. In theory, millisecond-domain pulses are more appropriate than Q-switched pulses for treating thick lesions such as congenital nevi because they produce less selective thermal damage, destroying entire nests of cells rather than individual pigmented cells. Japanese investigators have reported impressive long-term clearing of congenital nevi treated with the millisecond-domain normal-mode ruby laser.[23,58] However, other investigators have reported poor results treating congenital nevi with both Q-switched and normal mode ruby lasers.[59] Long-pulse ruby lasers also offer the potential to reduce the amount of hair within congenital nevi. In Japanese studies, no histological or clinical evidence of malignancy has been demonstrated up to 8 years after normal-mode ruby laser treatment.[23,58] However, since congenital nevi have the potential to transform into malignant melanoma, and residual nevus cells persist in the dermis after laser treatment, cautious long-term follow-up of nevi treated with lasers is required.

Both continuous wave lasers[60,61] and the QSRL[62] have been used to treat lentigo maligna. Nonetheless, there are several reports of lentigo maligna recurring following laser treatment, probably due to persistence of melanocytes within deeper adnexal structures.[63,64] Laser treatment of lentigo maligna should be reserved for extreme situations where surgical excision is not feasible due to large lesion size, advanced patient age, or underlying medical condition. Close follow-up to detect any early recurrence is critical.

Nevus of Ota

Nevus of Ota (also known as oculodermal melanoma or nevus fuscoceruleus ophthalmomaxillaris) is a mottled, blue-grey macule that is usually located unilaterally within the distribution of the first and second branches of the trigeminal nerve. Lesions usually occur in a 5:1 female to male ratio. Asians are most commonly affected, with an incidence of 1 in 500 reported in Japan.[65] Nevus of Ota is congenital in about 50% of cases, with others appearing by the second decade of life. Nevus of Ota may affect mucosal surfaces such as cornea, sclera, nasal and buccal mucosa, and tympanic membrane. Histologically, elongated dendritic melanocytes are scattered within the upper dermis. The occurrence of melanoma within nevus of Ota has been reported[66] but is rare.

Q-switched lasers are extremely helpful in treating Nevus of Ota. The degree of lightening is usually directly proportional to the number of treatments performed. Lightening of 70% or more has been reported in the majority of patients treated four or five times with the QSRL[57] (Fig. 12). Post-treatment dyspigmentation occurs occasionally, although textural change has not been reported. Post-treatment biopsies have revealed disintegration of melanocytes up to a depth of 1.5 mm from the skin surface.[57] While the QSRL has been most widely used,[57,67-70] the Q-switched alexandrite[71] and Nd:YAG[25] lasers seem as effective. Large-scale comparative trials between these lasers have not been performed.

Acquired nevus of Ota-like macules (also known as Hori's nevus) differ from the classic nevus of Ota in that they are bilateral, spare mucosa, and occur later in life. Various Q-switched lasers have been reported effective in treating nevus of Ota-like macules.[72-74] Mauskiatti et al. demonstrated greater clearing of bilateral nevus of Ota like macules with a combination carbon dioxide (CO_2) and Q-switched ruby laser (QSRL) treatment than with QSRL alone.[75] Laser treatment of any pigmented lesion is often complicated by post-inflammatory hyperpigmentation. A recent study of Q-switched Nd:YAG treatment for acquired nevus of Ota-like macules suggests that epidermal cooling may be associated with an increased risk of post-inflammatory hyperpigmentation.[76]

Melasma and Post-inflammatory Hyperpigmentation

Melasma is a common acquired hyperpigmentation, most often affecting adult females with skin type III or higher. It occurs as brown to blue-grey macules most frequently on the cheeks, forehead, upper lip, nose, and chin. It is associated

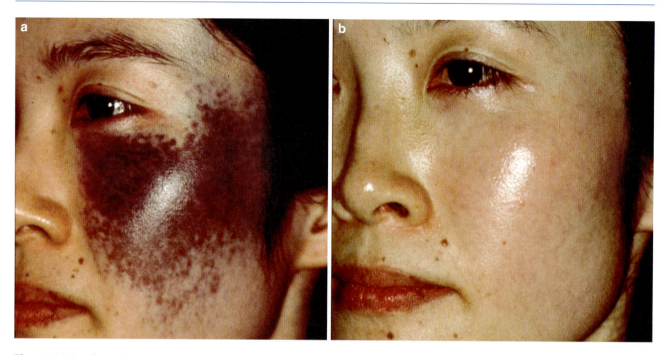

Fig. 12 (**a**) A patient with a dark nevus of Ota extending over a significant portion of the face prior to treatment. (**b**) After a series of treatments with the Q-switched ruby laser, there is impressive lightening of the lesion with no textural change

with sun exposure, pregnancy, and use of oral contraceptives, although it can also be seen in patients without any predisposing factor. Melasma can have increased melanin in either the epidermis, dermis or both. Initial management consists of discontinuing any oral contraceptives or hormonal replacement, and strict sun avoidance. Hydroquinone alone or in combination with topical corticosteroids or retinoids is the mainstay of treatment. Azeleic acid, kojic acid, and superficial chemical peels also provide some benefit. Melasma with dermal melanin is the most difficult to treat. Post inflammatory hyperpigmentation has a similar clinical and histology morphology as melasma, but develops following cutaneous injury or inflammatory process. Studies have shown that Q-switched lasers are largely ineffective in the treatment of melasma and post-inflammatory hyperpigmentation.[25,77] Q-switched laser treatment may actually cause an increase in dermal melanophages and worsening of hyperpigmentation. Carbon dioxide[78] or erbium:YAG[79] laser resurfacing provides an alternative treatment modality for melasma, but post-inflammatory hyperpigmentation is extremely frequent in the postoperative period and as a result these treatment modalities are not recommended. Some of the newer laser technologies, such as the fractionated erbium fiber laser (Fraxel), can be useful in treating melasma.[80,81] A study of ten patients showed 75–100% clearing of melasma in 60% of patients treated with the fractionated erbium fiber laser (Fraxel).[82] These patients were treated at a low fluence but a high density of microthermal zones. Fractionated laser treatment may work by expelling columns of microscopic epidermal debris that contains melanin.

Infraorbital hyperpigmentation (dark circles) may result from a variety of causes, including dermal melanin deposition, post-inflammatory hyperpigmentation from atopic or allergic contact dermatitis, prominent superficial blood vessels, and shadowing from skin laxity and infraorbital swelling[71] The QSRL has been reported to effectively treat infraorbital hyperpigmentation when due to deposition of dermal melanin.[83] The other Q-switched lasers, especially the Q-switched alexandrite laser, are also effective treatments. Improvement of this condition has also been reported following carbon dioxide laser resurfacing[84] and the combination of carbon dioxide laser followed by Q-switched Alexandrite laser. In one study, a striking 75–100% clearing of periorbital hyperpigmentation was noted using a combined CO_2 resurfacing followed immediately by Q-switched alexandrite laser treatment.[85] Blepharoplasty may be indicated when infraorbital darkening is due to excessive skin laxity. Soft tissue augmentation with fillers may be beneficial if there is shadowing due to a hollow in the tear trough.

Drug Induced Pigmentation

Minocycline therapy may cause localized or diffuse mucocutaneous pigmentation. Minocycline-induced pigmentation occurs in approximately 5% of acne vulgaris patients treated with the drug after prolonged use.[86] Three patterns of pigmentation have been reported. In type I, focal blue-gray pigmentation occurs in inflamed or scarred skin, often in acne scars. Histologic studies show pigment within dermal macrophages

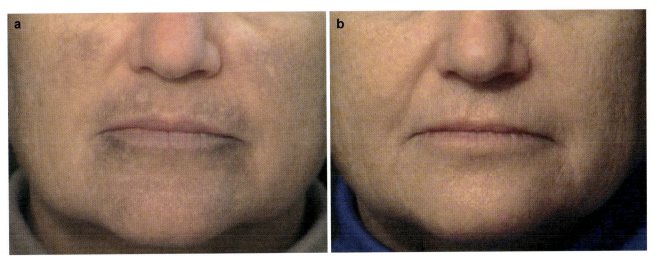

Fig. 13 (**a**) Minocycline pigmentation on the cheeks, upper lip, and chin. (**b**) Removal of pigmentation was achieved after four Q-switched alexandrite laser treatments (From Alster et al.[92])

that stains positively for melanin and iron.[87] Types II and III consist of blue to brown discoloration that is more prominent on the anterior shins and sun-exposed areas, respectively. Histologically, epidermal and superficial dermal pigment is present that stains for both melanin and iron in type II only for melanin[87] in type III. Pigmentation will gradually fade after discontinuation of minocycline, but may take years. The Q-switched ruby laser is effective in treating minocycline-induced pigmentation, with clearing occurring after one to four treatment sessions.[88-90] Successful treatment has also been reported with the Q-switched 532 nm, Q-switched alexandrite,[91] (Fig. 13) and 1,064 nm Nd:YAG laser,[93,94] although the latter wavelength has not proved effective in several reports.[90,93] Amiodarone (an antiarrhythmic) and imipramine (an antidepressant) can also induce hyperpigmentation and have been treated effectively with the Q-switched ruby laser[95,96] In order to prevent recurrences, laser treatment of these conditions should be deferred until the offending medication has been discontinued and sufficient time has elapsed to allow most of the pigmentation to resolve spontaneously.

Q-switched laser treatment may induce paradoxical hyperpigmentation in patients receiving certain medications. In one report, localized chrysiasis developed in a patient on parenteral gold therapy who underwent treatment with a Q-switched ruby laser for post inflammatory hyperpigmentation.[97] This phenomenon is due to a laser-induced alteration in the physiochemical properties of dermal gold deposits. In the reported case, it was found that the induction of this change in pigmentation is irradiance-dependent, i.e., related to the power delivered per unit area (W/cm^2) rather than fluence-dependent. It was concluded that any millisecond laser emitting between 550–850 nm should clear this pigment, and subsequent treatment with a normal mode (3 ms) ruby laser resulted in substantial clearing.[98]

Techniques

- It is important to obtain a medical history prior to treatment and to educate patients about the potential outcomes.
- Anesthesia may be needed for larger or dermal pigmented lesions.
- Appropriate protective eyewear should be on all persons in the room.
- Laser parameters depend on the particular laser, the patient's skin phototype, and the type of lesion.
- Adequate fluence will result in an immediate uniform ash white color.
- Appropriate wound care is essential to ensuring good outcomes. An occlusive ointment should be applied and patients should be educated on the healing process.

Pre-operative Management

Patient Evaluation

A general medical history should be obtained prior to treatment, including medication history, information on wound healing (specifically a history of keloids), any bleeding diatheses, or history of infectious diseases, particularly hepatitis and HIV infection. Patients with a recent history of isotretinoin use or a history of hypertrophic or keloidal scarring should be treated with caution because they may have a higher risk of scarring after laser treatment.

Before treating any pigmented lesion, it is imperative to correctly diagnose the lesion in question. A pre-treatment biopsy should be performed if there is any possibility of atypia in a pigmented lesion or if the diagnosis is at all in question. Once the correct diagnosis has been established, the appropriate laser can be selected based on the probable depth and type of pigment in the skin and on the patient's skin phototype.

Many patients are ill informed and harbor unrealistic expectations about the capabilities of laser surgery. Patients should be fully informed of what to expect from each treatment and the potential side effects. It is vital that patients understand that it will most likely take multiple treatments and that the lesion may not clear entirely. Pre-treatment photographs are essential to document lesions prior to treatment.

Anesthesia

The need for anesthesia when treating pigmented lesions depends on the location, size and depth of the lesion as well as the pain threshold of the patient. The sensation of a laser pulse at the low fluences which are used for epidermal pigmented lesions such as lentigines has been likened to a rubber band snapping against the skin surface. The higher fluences used in the treatment of dermal pigmented lesions such as nevus of Ota produce more discomfort and are more likely to require some type of anesthesia. When limited areas are treated, such as scattered lentigines, many patients require no anesthesia at all. For the treatment of larger pigmented lesions, one or more of the following anesthetic techniques may be required: topical anesthesia (e.g., LMX-5 cream), local infiltration of lidocaine with or without epinephrine, regional nerve block, or oral or intramuscular sedation. In many children and rarely in adults, intravenous sedation or general anesthesia may be necessary.

Safety

Laser safety concerns can be divided into beam hazards, which are related to direct beam impact, and non-beam hazards, such as plume hazards. Beam hazards can include fire, thermal burns, and ocular damage. The room should be designed in such a way that all reflective surfaces and windows are covered, the door is locked from the inside, appropriate signs are posted, and no flammable materials or anesthetics are present. Flammability can occur when the laser is used in the presence of oxygen (e.g., nasal cannula). Drapes, towels and sponges may also be flammable and to avoid this wet or non-flammable material should be used. A nonflammable, water-based lubricant such as Surgilube or K-Y Jelly should be applied to the eyebrows to avoid singeing the hair.

Ocular risks may be encountered when the eye is exposed directly in the laser beam's path or indirectly by a reflected beam. Recalling basic geometric optics, a parallel beam of light (i.e., a laser) that enters a convex element, such as the cornea, will be focused down to a smaller geometric point. This of course concentrates all the power in the beam into a much smaller spot, and results in an infinite irradiance causing more damage. Laser light in the visible to near infrared spectrum (i.e., 400–1,400 nm) can cause damage to the retina that is painless at the time of injury. For this reason, this spectrum of light is also known as the "retinal hazard region". Without eye protection, observing a laser beam in the visible spectrum of light is detected as a bright color flash of the emitted wavelength and an after-image of its complementary color (e.g., a green 532 nm laser light would produce a green flash followed by a red after-image). When the retina is affected, there may be difficulty in detecting blue or green colors secondary to cone damage, and pigmentation of the retina may be detected. Exposure to the Q-switched Nd:YAG laser beam (1,064 nm) is especially hazardous and may initially go undetected because the beam is invisible (in the near-infrared spectrum) and the retina lacks pain sensory nerves. Photoacoustic retinal damage may be associated with an audible "pop" at the time of exposure. Visual disorientation due to retinal damage may not be apparent to the operator until considerable thermal damage has occurred. Laser light in the far infrared (1,400–10,600 nm) spectrum can cause damage to the cornea and/or to the lens because of its preferential absorption of water. Exposure to the invisible carbon dioxide laser beam (10,600 nm) can be detected by a burning pain at the site of exposure on the cornea or sclera.

All persons in the room should wear protective goggles with the correct optical density for the specific laser wavelength. When treating the face, the patient should wear snug metal goggles. If the immediate periocular area is to be treated, protective metal eye shields should be inserted over the conjunctiva after application of a topical ophthalmic anesthetic agent.

Q-switched laser pulses may produce a significant amount of blood and tissue splatter, especially the 1,064 nm Nd:YAG laser. Use of universal precautions is mandatory, including use of gloves, goggles, and laser masks. The protective plastic cone provided with most Q-switched lasers should always be attached to the handpiece before use to minimize tissue splatter and keep tissue debris off the handpiece lens. The plastic cone must be placed in direct contact with the skin to efficiently trap tissue debris. To minimize tissue splatter, pulses may be delivered through a clear hydrogel dressing (e.g., Tegaderm, Second Skin) placed on the skin, although this reduces transmission of light into the skin and raises the risk of ocular injury from reflection of light off the dressing surface. Vacuum suction is useless at capturing tissue splatter because it leaves the surface of the skin far too rapidly – faster than the speed of sound. Although there have been no cases of transmission, the presence of HIV proviral DNA has been demonstrated in the laser plume generated by carbon dioxide laser irradiation of HIV-infected tissue culture.[99]

All makeup and sunscreen should be removed from the area to be treated, as these products will prevent transmission of light to the skin surface. Furthermore, many of these products contain metal-based salts and oxides (such as titanium dioxide) that may ignite following exposure to Q-switched laser pulses.

Description of the Technique

Q-switched lasers should always be calibrated prior to treatment and should be placed in standby mode until ready for use. The laser handpiece should be held perpendicular to the skin with the attached plastic cone or guide resting on the skin to ensure that the laser beam is focused on the area to be treated. Exact parameters vary depending on the particular laser, the patient's Fitzpatrick skin type, and the type of lesion (Table 2). In general, lower fluence is used for dark lesions that contain larger amounts of absorbing chromophore.

One or two laser pulses should be fired at the lesion to ensure that a threshold response occurs, which is defined as immediate whitening of the lesion. The optimal tissue end point is uniform but faint immediate whitening without epidermal disruption. The lowest fluence required to invoke this response should be used. When the fluence is too low, the whitening will be barely noticeable. If using subthreshold fluences, post-inflammatory hyperpigmentation due to stimulation of melanogenesis can result. If the fluence is too high, whitening is a confluent bright white, and epidermal damage with bleeding may occur. This may result in tissue sloughing, prolonged healing, and also a greater likelihood of post-inflammatory hyperpigmentation or hypopigmentation or textural changes. After the optimal fluence is determined, pulses can be delivered rapidly (up to 10 Hz, depending on the laser), with overlapping of about 10% to ensure confluent whitening.

In most cases, additional treatment sessions may be safely performed 6 weeks after the original treatment. While some pigmented lesions (e.g., lentigines) may require only one to two treatments, other lesions (e.g., Café au lait macules) may need multiple treatments.

Unlike dermal pigmented lesions, epidermal pigmented lesions can be treated with millisecond domain lasers and intense pulsed light devices. The clinical endpoint of treatment with these devices is significantly different from that seen after Q-switched laser treatment. Immediately after treatment there is a slight darkening of lentigines, although lighter lentigines may remain unchanged. A faint erythema may also be observed at the periphery of darker lentigines. After treatment, pigmented lesions develop a slight dark scale, which flakes away in a few days. Active skin cooling is used during

Table 2 Standard treatment parameters for pigmented lesions

Lesion	Laser	Spot size (mm)	Fluence (J/cm^2)	Retreatment interval (weeks)
Lentigines	QS ruby	6.5	2.0–4.0	4–8 weeks
	QS Nd:YAG (532 nm)	3	0.7–1.0	
	QS alexandrite	4	3.5–5.5	
	Pulsed dye (510 nm)	3	2.5	
Café au lait macules	QS ruby	6.5	3.0–4.5	4–8 weeks
	QS Nd:YAG (532 nm)	3	1.0–1.5	
	QS alexandrite	4	2.5–4.5	
	Pulsed dye (510 nm)	5	2.0–3.5	
Becker's nevus	QS ruby	6.5	3.0–4.5	4–8 weeks
	QS Nd:YAG (532 nm)	3	1.5–1.8	
	QS Nd:YAG (1,064 nm)	3	4.0–5.0	
	QS alexandrite	4	3.5–5.0	
Nevus spilus	QS ruby	6.5	3.0–4.5	4–8 weeks
	QS Nd:YAG (532 nm)	3	1.5–2.0	
	QS Nd:YAG (1,064 nm)	3	4.0–4.4	
	QS alexandrite	3	5.0–6.0	
Nevus of Ota	QS ruby	6.5	5.0–6.0	6–12 weeks
	QS Nd:YAG (1,064 nm)	3	4.0–7.0	
	QS alexandrite	3	5.5–6.5	

QS Q-switched

treatment with most IPL devices to protect the epidermis from excessive thermal injury. Multiple treatment sessions with IPL are required for optimal clearing of epidermal pigmented lesions. Lighter lentigines, which contain less of the melanin chromophore, may be more resistant to IPL treatment and may respond better to Q-switched laser treatment.

In general, dermal lesions require higher fluences than epidermal lesions. Larger spot sizes have a greater depth of penetration, and are preferred to smaller ones. To achieve the same effect in the dermis, a larger spot size will require lower energy and therefore be gentler on the epidermis and dermal-epidermal junction.

Lower fluences should be used in the treatment of patients with darker skin types, since the threshold response will likely occur at a lower fluence. When treating both epidermal and dermal pigmented lesions, patients with darker skin are at greater risk for postoperative hyperpigmentation or hypopigmentation. It may be preferable to use a longer wavelength device, such as the 1,064 nm Nd:YAG laser, since longer wavelengths penetrate more deeply than shorter wavelengths and produce relatively less epidermal damage for the same dermal effect. Patients with "suntans" should not be treated because they are at risk of spotty hypopigmentation, which can last for weeks to months after treatment.

Post-operative Management

The white tissue reaction that occurs immediately after Q-switched laser treatment fades within 20 min. An urticarial reaction, causing erythema, edema, itching, and stinging, may develop in and around the treated area. This may last for several hours and can be treated, but not prevented, by taking an antihistamine preoperatively. In all patients, the treated lesions appear darker for several days then develop a thin crust that flakes off in 7–10 days. The amount of crusting that occurs depends on the aggressiveness of treatment. Overly aggressive treatment may result in vesiculation or frank blistering. The risk of blistering is highest when shorter wavelength devices (e.g., QSRL) are used to treat patients with dark skin phototypes. Following treatment with the Q-switched 532 nm Nd:YAG, purpura usually develops after skin whitening has faded. This occurs because these wavelengths are well absorbed by both melanin and hemoglobin, causing rupture of blood vessels. Purpura lasts for 5–10 days, and is a notable disadvantage of treatment with the above devices. Purpura can be minimized by treating through a microscope slide held firmly against the skin to compress blood vessels and remove hemoglobin as a target.

Postoperative discomfort may be treated with application of cold water-soaked gauze, ice packs, or a hydroocclusive dressing such as Second Skin or Vigilon. Analgesics are

usually not needed. Antihistamines may be given if the patient has an urticarial reaction. Patients should be instructed to gently wash the treated area with mild soap and apply an occlusive ointment (e.g., petrolatum or Aquaphor Healing Ointment) twice a day. Any crusting should be allowed to slough spontaneously. To minimize the risk of hyperpigmentation and recurrence, patients should avoid excessive sun exposure and use a broad-spectrum sunscreen of SPF 30 or higher for several months after treatment.

Because dermal lesions typically require the use of higher fluences, postoperative changes are more apparent. In addition to the whitening response, erythema and swelling are usually seen in the immediate postoperative period, especially in the periorbital region.

Future Directions

- Pico (10^{-12}) and femto second (10^{-15}) domain lasers are being developed.
- Enhanced effectiveness with less side effects in treating pigmented disorders in patients of color.

Manufacturers and scientists continue to refine and optimize the current laser systems to enhance outcomes with less side effects. By adding cooling to many treatments systems the risk of problems of pigmentation after treatment have decreased. Encouraging work is presently being done on lasers with even shorter pulse durations than typical Q-switched lasers. Pulse durations in the pico (10^{-12}) and femto second (10^{-15}) domains may be more effective in dicusting pigment in restnat tattoos than the typically used shorter pulse durations.

Adverse Events

- Post-inflammatory hyperpigmentation, hypopigmentation, an inadequate response and recurrence of the lesion are the most common side effects.
- Using the appropriate laser and fluence can reduce side effects.
- Educating patients regarding realistic expectations can help to reduce patient frustration and complications.

Side Effects/Complications

Post-inflammatory hyperpigmentation is not a rare side effect when treating pigmented lesions, and is especially common in treating darker skin types. Subthreshold fluences can stimulate melanogenesis in dark skinned patients. While post-inflammatory hyperpigmentation is benign, it can last several months and can be cosmetically bothersome. Topical hydroquinone containing creams are usually effective in lightening the hyperpigmentation.

Although less common than post-inflammatory hyperpigmentation, hypopigmentation can also occur, particularly when treating tanned patients. For this reason, tanned patients should not be treated.

A sub-optimal response to laser treatment is another unwelcome outcome. Most pigmented lesions require multiple treatments and some are prone to recurrence.

Prevention and Treatment of Side Effects/Complications

Hyperpigmentation and hypopigmentation can be avoided by treating with appropriately high fluences and by not treating tanned patients, respectively. For many reasons, it is important to take quality pre-treatment photographs from multiple angles. Photographs can be used to judge improvement, document baseline findings, and may have medico legal importance. It is important for patients to have a realistic understanding of potential outcomes prior to beginning laser treatment. Potential laser candidates should be educated regarding the need for multiple treatments and should be made aware of possible side effects. This patient education should be documented in the patient chart. Side effects and expectations should be reinforced in writing on the consent form.

Conclusions

Pigmented lesions are an exceedingly common occurrence, and often are cosmetically disturbing to the patient. Topical treatment options are ineffective for almost all of these conditions and surgical treatment options often produce unacceptable results. Laser and light therapy is often the preferred manner to diminish a variety of pigmented lesions and disorders of pigmentation. In order to obtain the optimal outcome, the physician needs to select the proper light source, the correct patient and skin characteristics and provide appropriate wound care to achieve optimal results. Thought should be given to the depth of the lesion, the patient's skin phototype, and the laser or light device parameters. Despite the efficacy of laser and light treatments, they are not without potential side effects and complications. Prior to beginning treatment, both the physician and the patient should be well aware of the limitations and disadvantages of laser therapy.

Nevertheless, with a thoughtful treatment plan and adequate patient education, treating pigmented lesions with laser therapy can result in a successful outcome.

References

1. Goldman L, Blaney DJ, Kindel DJ, Franke EK. Effect of the laser beam on the skin: preliminary report. *J Invest Dermatol*. 1963;40:121-122.
2. Goldman L, Wilson RG, Hornby P, Meyer RG. Radiation from a Q-switched ruby laser: effect of repeated impacts of power output of 10 megawatts on a tattoo of man. *J Invest Dermatol*. 1965;44:69-71.
3. Ohshiro T, Maruyama Y. The ruby and argon lasers in the treatment of naevi. *Ann Acad Med*. 1983;12:388-395.
4. Dover JS, Smoller BR, Stein RS, et al. Low-fluence carbon dioxide laser irradiation of lentigines. *Arch Dermatol*. 1988;124:1219-1224.
5. Anderson RR, Parrish JA. Selective photothermolysis: precise microsurgery by selective absorption of pulsed radiation. *Science*. 1983;220:524-527.
6. Polla LL, Margolis RJ, Dover JS, et al. Melanosomes are a primary target of Q-switched ruby laser irradiation in guinea pig skin. *J Invest Dermatol*. 1987;89:281-286.
7. Levins PC, Anderson RR. Q-switched ruby laser for the treatment of pigmented lesions and tattoos. *Clin Dermatol*. 1995;13:75-79.
8. Taylor CR, Anderson RR, Gange RW, et al. Light and electron microscopic analysis of tattoos treated by Q-switched ruby laser. *J Invest Dermatol*. 1991;97:131-136.
9. Ara G, Anderson RR, Mandel KG, et al. Irradiation of pigmented melanoma cells with high intensity pulsed radiation generates acoustic waves and kills cells. *Lasers Surg Med*. 1990;10:52-59.
10. Dover JS, Margolis RJ, Polla LL, et al. Pigmented guinea pig skin irradiated with Q-switched ruby laser pulses. *Arch Dermatol*. 1989;125:43-49.
11. Ardnt KA, Dover JS, Olbricht SM. *Lasers in Cutaneous and Aesthetic Surgery*. Philadelphia: Lippincott-Raven; 1997.
12. Kossida T, Farinelli W, Flotte T, et al. Mechanism of immediate whitening during tattoo Removal. *Lasers Surg Med*. 2006;18:70.
13. Margolis RJ, Dover JS, Polla LL, et al. Visible action spectrum for melanin-specific selective photothermolysis. *Lasers Surg Med*. 1989;9:389-397.
14. Anderson RR, Margolis RJ, Watenabe S, et al. Selective photothermolysis of cutaneous pigmentation by Q-switched Nd:YAG laser pulses at 1064, 532, and 355 nm. *J Invest Dermatol*. 1989;93: 28-32.
15. Hruza GJ, Dover JS, Flotte TJ, et al. Q-switched ruby laser irradiation of normal human skin. *Arch Dermatol*. 1991;127:1799-1805.
16. Murphy GF, Shepard RS, Paul BS, et al. Organelle-specific injury to melanin-containing cells in human skin by pulsed laser irradiation. *Lab Invest*. 1983;49:680-685.
17. Anderson RR, Parrish JA. The optics of human skin. *J Invest Dermatol*. 1981;77:13-19.
18. Sherwood KA, Murray S, Kurban AK, Tan OT. Effect of wavelength on cutaneous pigment using pulsed irradiation. *J Invest Dermatol*. 1989;92:717-720.
19. Nakamura Y, Hossain M, Hirayama K, Matsumoto K. A clinical study on the removal of gingival melanin pigmentation with the CO_2 laser. *Lasers Surg Med*. 1999;25:140-147.
20. Vikramaditya P, Bedi MS, et al. The effects of pulse energy variations on the dimensions of microscopic thermal treatment zones in nonablative fractional resurfacing. *Lasers Surg Med*. 2007;39: 145-155.
21. Ross EV, Ladin Z, Kreindel M, Dierickx C. Theoretical considerations in laser hair removal. *Dermatol Clin*. 1999;17:333-355.

22. Kono T, Manstein D, Chan HH. Q-switched ruby versus long-pulsed dye laser delivered with compression for treatment of facial lentigines in Asians. *Lasers Surg Med*. 2006;38(2):94-97.

23. Ueda S, Imayama S. Normal-mode ruby laser for treating congenital nevi. *Arch Dermatol*. 1997;133:355-359.

24. Taylor CR, Anderson RR. Treatment of benign pigmented epidermal lesions by Q-switched ruby laser. *Int J Dermatol*. 1993;32:908-912.

25. Tse Y, Levine VJ, McClain SA, Ashinoff R. The removal of cutaneous pigmented lesions with the Q-switched ruby laser and the Q-switched neodymium:yttrium-aluminum-garnet laser. *J Dermatol Surg Oncol*. 1994;20:795-800.

26. Kilmer SL, Wheeland RG, Goldberg DJ, Anderson RR. Treatment of epidermal pigmented lesions with the frequency-doubled Q-switched Nd:YAG laser. *Arch Dermatol*. 1994;130:1515-1519.

27. Fitzpatrick RE, Goldman MP, Ruiz-Esparza J. Laser treatment of benign pigmented epidermal lesions using a 300 nsecond pulse and 510 nm wavelength. *J Dermatol Surg Oncol*. 1993;18:341-347.

28. Ashinoff R, Geronemus RG. Q-switched ruby laser treatment of labial lentigos. *J Am Acad Dermatol*. 1992;27:809-811.

29. Gupta G, MacKay IR, MacKie RM. Q-switched ruby laser in the treatment of labial melanotic macules. *Lasers Surg Med*. 1999; 25:219-222.

30. Yung-Tsai L, Kao-Chia Y. Comparison of the frequency-doubled Q-switched Nd:YAG laser and 35% trichloroacetic acid for the treatment of face lentigines. *Dermatol Surg*. 1999;25:202-204.

31. Todd M, Rallis T, Hata T. A comparison of three lasers and liquid nitrogen in the treatment of solar lentigines: a randomized, controlled, comparative trial. *Arch Dermatol*. 2000;50:536-540.

32. Alster TS, Tanzi EL, Welsh EC. Photorejuvenation of facial skin with topical 20% 5-aminolevulinic acid and intense pulsed light treatment: a split-face comparison study. *J Drugs Dermatol*. 2005; 4:35-38.

33. Dover J et al. Adjunctive use of topical aminolevulinic acid with intense pulsed light in the treatment of photoaging. *J Am Acad Dermatol*. 2005;52:795-803.

34. Gold MH et al. Split-face comparison of photodynamic therapy with 5-aminolevulinic acid and intense pulsed light versus intense pulsed light alone for photodamage. *Dermatol Surg*. 2006;32(6):795-801.

35. Tekin M, Bodurtha JN, Riccardi VM. Café au lait spots: the pediatrician's perspective. *Pediatr Rev*. 2001;22:82-90.

36. Grossman MC, Anderson RR, Farinelli W, et al. Treatment of cafe au lait macules with lasers: a clinicopathologic correlation. *Arch Dermatol*. 1995;131:1416-1420.

37. Alster TS. Complete elimination of large cafe-au-lait birthmarks by the 510-nm pulsed dye laser. *Plast Reconstr Surg*. 1995;96:1660.

38. Alora MB, Arndt KA. Successful treatment of a cafe-au-lait macule with the erbium:YAG laser. *J Am Acad Dermatol*. 2001;45(4):566-568.

39. Goldberg DJ. Benign pigmented lesions of the skin. *J Dermatol Surg Oncol*. 1993;19:376-379.

40. Rosio TJ. Techniques for tattoo removal. In: Wheeland RG, ed. *Cutaneous Surgery*. Philadelphia: WB Saunders; 1994:982-997.

41. Kobayashi T. Microsurgical treatment of nevus of Ota. *J Dermatol Surg Oncol*. 1991;17:936-941.

42. Clabaugh WA. Tattoo removal by superficial dermabrasion: five year experience. *Plast Reconstr Surg*. 1975;55:401-405.

43. Koerber WA, Price NM. Salabrasion of tattoos: a correlation of the clinical and histological results. *Arch Dermatol*. 1978;114:884-888.

44. Dvir E, Hirshowitz B. Tattoo removal by cryosurgery. *Plast Reconstr Surg*. 1980;66:373-378.

45. Cosman B, Apfelberg DB, Drucker D. An effective cosmetic treatment for Ota's nevus. *Ann Plast Surg*. 1989;22:36-42.

46. Reid R, Muller S. Tattoo removal by CO_2 laser dermabrasion. *Plast Reconstr Surg*. 1980;65:717-728.

47. van Leeuwen RL, Dekker SW, Byers HR, et al. Modulation of $\alpha4\beta1$ and $\alpha5\beta1$ integrin expression: heterogenous effects of Q-switched ruby, Nd:YAG, and alexandrite lasers on melanoma cells in vitro. *Lasers Surg Med*. 1996;18:63-71.

48. Chan HH, Xiang K, Leung L, et al. In vitro study examining the effect of sub-lethal QS 755 nm lasers on the expression of p161nk4a on melanoma cell lines. *Lasers Surg Med*. 2003;32(2):88-93.

49. Dummer R, Kempf W, Burg G. Pseudo-melanoma after laser therapy. *Dermatology*. 1998;197:71-73.

50. Grevelink JM, van Leeuwen RL, Anderson RR, Byers R. Clinical and histological responses of congenital melanocytic nevi after single treatment with Q-switched lasers. *Arch Dermatol*. 1997;133: 349-353.

51. Goldberg DJ, Zeichner JA, Hodulik SG, et al. Q-switched laser irradiation of pigmented nevi: analysis of markers for malignant transformation. *Lasers Surg Med*. 2006;18:18.

52. Vibhagool C, Byers R, Grevelink JM. Treatment of small nevomelanocytic nevi with a Q-switched ruby laser. *J Am Acad Dermatol*. 1997;36:738-741.

53. Rosenbach A, Williams CM, Alster TS. Comparison of the Q-switched alexandrite (755 nm) and Q-switched Nd:YAG (1064 nm) lasers in the treatment of benign melanocytic nevi. *Dermatol Surg*. 1997;23:239-245.

54. Duke D, Byers R, Sober AJ, et al. Treatment of benign and atypical nevi with the normal-mode ruby laser and the Q-switched ruby laser: clinical improvement but failure to completely eliminate nevomelanocytes. *Arch Dermatol*. 1999;135:290-296.

55. Baba M, Bal N. Efficacy and safety of the short-pulse erbium:YAG laser in the treatment of acquired melanocytic nevi. *Dermatol Surg*. 2006;32:256-260.

56. Milgraum SS, Cohen ME, Auletta MJ. Treatment of blue nevi with the Q-switched ruby laser. *J Am Acad Dermatol*. 1995;32:307-310.

57. Watanabe S, Takahashi H. Treatment of nevus of Ota with the Q-switched ruby laser. *N Engl J Med*. 1994;331:1745-1750.

58. Imayama S, Ueda S. Long- and short-term histological observations of congenital nevi treated with the normal-mode ruby laser. *Arch Dermatol*. 1999;135:1211-1218.

59. Helsing P, Mork G, Sveen B. Ruby laser treatment of congenital melanocytic nevi – a pessimistic view. *Acta Derm Venereol*. 2006;86(3):235-237.

60. Arndt KA. Argon laser treatment of lentigo maligna. *J Am Acad Dermatol*. 1984;10:953-957.

61. Kopera D. Treatment of lentigo maligna with the carbon dioxide laser. *Arch Dermatol*. 1995;131:735-736.

62. Thissen M, Westerhof W. Lentigo maligna treated with ruby laser. *Acta Derm Venereol*. 1997;77:163.

63. Arndt KA. New pigmented macule appearing 4 years after argon laser treatment of lentigo maligna. *J Am Acad Dermatol*. 1986; 14:1092.

64. Lee PK, Rosenberg CN, Tsao H, Sober AJ. Failure of Q-switched ruby laser to eradicate atypical-appearing solar lentigo: report of two cases. *J Am Acad Dermatol*. 1998;38:314-317.

65. Hidano A, Kajama H, Ikeda S, et al. Natural history of nevus of Ota. *Arch Dermatol*. 1967;95:187-195.

66. Jay B. Malignant melanoma of the orbit in a case of oculodermal melanocytosis (nevus of Ota). *Br J Ophthalmol*. 1965;49:359.

67. Geronemus RG. Q-switched ruby laser therapy of nevus of Ota. *Arch Dermatol*. 1992;128:1618-1622.

68. Lowe NJ, Wieder JM, Sawcer D, et al. Nevus of Ota: treatment with high energy fluences of the Q-switched ruby laser. *J Am Acad Dermatol*. 1993;29:997-1001.

69. Taylor CR, Flotte TJ, Gange W, Anderson RR. Treatment of nevus of Ota by Q-switched ruby laser. *J Am Acad Dermatol*. 1994;30: 743-751.

70. Chang CJ, Nelson JS, Achauer BM. Q-switched ruby laser treatment of oculodermal melanosis (nevus of Ota). *Plast Reconstr Surg*. 1996;98:784-790.

71. Alster TS, Williams CM. Treatment of nevus of Ota by the Q-switched alexandrite laser. *Dermatol Surg*. 1995;21:592-596.

72. Lam AY et al. A retrospective study on the efficacy and complications of Q-switched alexandretie laser in the treatment of acquired

bilateral nevus of Ota-like macules. *Dermatol Surg.* 2001;27(11): 937-942.

73. Manuskiatti W et al. Treatment of acquired bilateral nevus of Ota-like macules (Hori's nevus) using a combination of scanned carbon dioxide laser followed by Q-switched ruby laser. *J Am Acad Dermatol.* 2003;48(4):584-591.

74. Polnikorn N et al. Treatment of Hori's nevus with the Q-switched Nd.YAG laser. *Dermatol Surg.* 2000;26(5):477-480.

75. Manuskiatte W, Sivayathorn A, Leelaudomlipi P, Fitzpatrick RE. Treatment of acquired bilateral nevua of Ota-like maculess (Hori's nevus) using a combination of scanned carbon dioxide laser followed by Q-switched ruby laser. *J Am Acad Dermatol.* 2003;48(4):584-591.

76. Manuskiatti W et al. Effect of cold air cooling on the incidence of postinflammatory hyperpigmentation after Q-switched Nd:YAG laser treatment of acquired bilateral nevus of Ota-like macules. *Arch Dermatol.* 2007;143(9):1139-1143.

77. Taylor CR, Anderson RR. Ineffective treatment of refractory melasma and postinflammatory hyperpigmentation by Q-switched ruby laser. *J Dermatol Surg Oncol.* 1994;20:592-597.

78. Nouri K, Bowes L, Chartier T, et al. Combination treatment of melasma with pulsed CO_2 laser followed by Q-switched alexandrite laser: a pilot study. *Dermatol Surg.* 1999;25:494-497.

79. Manaloto RMP, Alster T. Erbium:YAG laser resurfacing for refractory melasma. *Dermatol Surg.* 1999;25:121-123.

80. Narurkar VA. Skin rejuvenation with microthermal fractional photothermolysis. *Dermatol Ther.* 2007;20:S10-S13.

81. Tannous Z, Astner S. Utilizing fractional resurfacing in the treatment of therapy resistant melasma. *J Cosmet Laser Ther.* 2005;7:39-43.

82. Rokhsar CK, Fitzpatrick RE. The treatment of melasma with fractional photothermolysis: a pilot study. *Dermatol Surg.* 2005;32:1 645-1650.

83. Lowe NJ, Wieder JM, Shorr N, et al. Infraorbital pigmented skin: preliminary observations of laser therapy. *Dermatol Surg.* 1995;21: 767-770.

84. West TB, Alster TS. Improvement of infraorbital hyperpigmentation following carbon dioxide laser resurfacing. *Dermatol Surg.* 1998;24:615-616.

85. Manuskiatti W, Fitzpatrick RE, Goldman MP. Red ink tattoo reactions: successful treatment with the Q-switched 532 nm Nd:YAG laser. *Dermatol Surg.* 2000;26(2):113-120.

86. Dwyer CM, Cuddihy AM, Kerr REI, et al. Skin pigmentation due to minocycline treatment of facial dermatoses. *Br J Dermatol.* 1993; 129:158-162.

87. Argenyi ZB, Finelli L, Bergfeld WF, et al. Minocycline-related cutaneous hyperpigmentation as demonstrated by light microscopy, electron microscopy and X-ray energy spectroscopy. *J Cutan Pathol.* 1987;14:176-180.

88. Collins P, Cotterill JA. Minocycline-induced pigmentation resolves after treatment with the Q-switched ruby laser. *Br J Dermatol.* 1996;135:317-319.

89. Knocll KA, Milgraum SS, Kutenplon M. Q-switched ruby laser treatment of minocycline-induced cutaneous hyperpigmentation. *Arch Dermatol.* 1996;132:1251-1253.

90. Tsao H, Dover JS. Treatment of minocycline-induced hyperpigmentation with the Q-switched ruby laser. *Arch Dermatol.* 1996;132:1250-1251.

91. Alster TS, Gupta SN. Minocycline-induced hyperpigmentation treated with a 755-nm Q-switched alexandrite laser. *Dermatol Surg.* 2004;30(9):1201-1204.

92. Alster TS, Gupta SN. Minocycline-induced hyperpigmentation treated with a 755-nm Q-switched alexandrite laser. *Dermatol Surg.* 2004;30(9):1201-4.

93. Wilde JL, English JC, Finley EM. Minocycline-induced hyperpigmentation: treatment with the neodymium:YAG laser. *Arch Dermatol.* 1997;133:1344-1346.

94. Greve B, Schonermark MP, Raulin C. Minocycline-induced hyperpigmentation: treatment with the Q-switched Nd:YAG laser. *Lasers Surg Med.* 1998;22:223-227.

95. Karrer S, Hohenleutner U, Szeimies RM, Landthaler M. Amiodarone-induced pigmentation resolves after treatment with the Q-switched ruby laser. *Arch Dermatol.* 1999;135: 251-253.

96. Atkins DH, Fitzpatrick RE. Laser treatment of imipramine-induced hyperpigmentation. *J Am Acad Dermatol.* 2000;43(1):77-80.

97. Trotter MJ, Tron VA, Hollingdale J, Rivers JK. Localized chrysiasis induced by laser therapy. *Arch Dermatol.* 1995;131:1411-1414.

98. Yun PK, Arndt KA, Anderson RR. Q-switched laser-induced chrysiasis treated with long-pulsed laser. *Arch Dermatol.* 2002;138: 1012-1014.

99. Baggish MS, Poiesz BJ, Joret D, et al. Presence of human immunodeficiency virus DNA in laser smoke. *Lasers Surg Med.* 1991;11:197-203.

100. Hirsch RJ, Anderson RR. Principles of Laser-Skin Interactions. In chapter 136, page 2148 in: *Dermatology* (ed.) Bolognia JL, Jorizzo JL, and Rapini RP. 1st edition, 2003.

Laser Treatment of Tattoos

Voraphol Vejjabhinanta, Caroline V. Caperton, Christopher Wong, Rawat Charoensawad, and Keyvan Nouri

- Tattoos are a long-standing part of human culture.
- Techniques used in tattooing have evolved over the centuries.
- Although 24% of Americans between the ages of 18–50 years have at least one tattoo, 28% of people who get tattoos regret the decision within the first month.
- The three lasers most commonly used are the Q-switched Nd:YAG, Q-switched Ruby, and Q-switched Alexandrite.
- Potential side effects of using lasers in the removal of tattoos include discoloration, redness, scarring, and rarely, stimulating allergic reactions.

Introduction

A tattoo is a mark created by pigments that permanently reside in the dermal layer of the skin. The word tattoo has roots from the Polynesian word "ta" which means "to strike" and the Tahitian word "tatau" which means "to mark." The techniques of tattooing have changed over the years, but the basic principle remains the same. Dyes are manually applied through breaks in the skin. By embedding the various pigments below the epidermis, the pigments resist sloughing due to the natural growth cycle of the skin, thus offering permanence. In the older methods, dye-tipped needles were gently struck by stones and hammers to introduce the dye into the skin. Today, electrical tattoo machines utilize high-speed needle injections that minimize time and pain.

In the United States, an estimated 7–20 million people have at least one tattoo.[1] In a recent study, the prevalence of tattoos among Americans aged 18–50 years old was found to be 24%.[2] Reasons for tattoo application include: fashion, peer pressure, rebelliousness, and romance. For some individuals, regret appears as quickly as the initial decision to get a tattoo. Approximately 28% of people who get tattoos regret the decision within the first month. While the minimum age to obtain a tattoo is 18 years old, 71% of people requesting tattoo removal have had the ink applied when they were under the minimum age. The most common reason to seek tattoo removal was to further enhance self-esteem by freeing oneself from the stigmatizing lesion that was the source of many years of regret. In addition, tattoo owners felt their marks were socially discrediting, perceived pressure by family members to remove them, and believed improvement in employment opportunities would result after removal.[3] On average, actual tattoo removal occurred 14 years later. Much of the delay can be attributed to perceived high financial costs, physical pain, and risk of permanent disfigurement associated with removal. Also, many potential patients admit that they were unaware of the availability of treatment options to remove their tattoo.[4]

Historical Perspectives

As evidenced by "Ötzi the Ice Man," a 5,000-year-old man bearing 57 tattoos whose body was discovered in 1991, tattoos have been a part of human culture for a very long time. Some anthropologists even speculate that the art of tattooing began as early as 12000 B.C. The purpose of tattoos has varied from perceived therapeutic benefits and religious or tribal identification symbols to self-expressions of uniqueness and impulse. Regardless of their age or purpose, tattoos are a large part of human culture today and are becoming more and more popular.

The first tattoos from thousands of years ago were created in a rough manner. During bereavement ceremonies as signs of grief, primitive humans of the Stone Age (12000 B.C.) slashed their skin and rubbed ash into the wounds.[5] It is highly unlikely that the detail of the designs resembled anything near the tattoos that we see today – although a few

V. Vejjabhinanta (✉)
Department of Dermatology and Cutaneous Surgery,
University of Miami, Leonard M. Miller School of Medicine,
Miami, FL and
Department of Dermatology, Siriraj Hospital, Mahidol University,
Bangkok, Thailand
e-mail: vvoraphol@gmail.com

K. Nouri (ed.), *Lasers in Dermatology and Medicine*,
DOI: 10.1007/978-0-85729-281-0_7, © Springer-Verlag London Limited 2011

amateurs come close. The discovery of crude needles and pigment bowls in caves in France, Spain, and Portugal provide circumstantial evidence that decorative tattooing can be traced back to the Bronze Age (8000 B.C.). More well known older techniques were practiced elsewhere in the Ancient world. The Japanese utilized a hand-based tattooing technique that involved elaborate needle-tipped bamboo handles. Samoans, among many other Pacific cultures, used wooden hand tools such as a bone-tipped rake and a striking stick. The ancient Thai employed a tool that closely resembles the electric tattoo devices of today. They used a long brass tube with a sliding pointed rod that ran down the center.

Thomas Alva Edison, the famous inventor of the light bulb, played an unexpected role in the development of the tattoo. In 1891, Samuel O'Reilly modified Edison's autographic printer to become the electric tattoo machine of today. It was a steel instrument that utilized needles that traveled in a vertical direction to pierce the skin at a rate up to 3,000 times/min.

Techniques of Tattooing

- In order for a tattoo to be permanent, the dye must be placed at a certain location within the dermis – too superficial and it will be sloughed off in the epidermis; too deep and it will be taken up by lymphatics.
- Risks of unsterile tattooing techniques include transmission of bacteria, hepatitis B, hepatitis C, syphilis, and HIV.

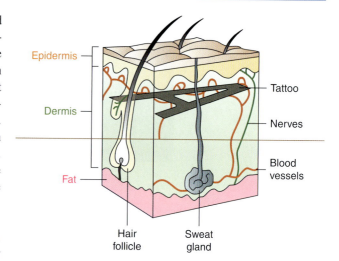

Fig. 1 Placement of tattoo ink within the dermis

The tattoo is actually the appearance through the epidermis of the ink located in the dermis. During the tattoo process, needles are dipped in various inks. The electric tattoo device injects ink particles from the epidermis to a constant depth (usually 1 mm) below the dermal-epidermal junction (Fig. 1). As part of the skin's natural growth cycle, the epidermis is continually sloughed off. In the layers of the dermis, macrophages recognize the dye particles as foreign and attempt to remove the molecules. However, most of dye is captured or ignored and remains in the dermis. Therefore, it is essential that the dye reach the dermis in order to become a permanent mark.

In addition, it is important that the dye not be injected too deeply into the dermis. More commonly reached by amateur-level tattoo artists, these greater depths will increase the likelihood of the dye being carried away by body fluids or for the tattoo to be accompanied by scarring. This can lead to blurring of the tattoo and reduction of its visualization.

Obtaining a tattoo carries with it inherent risks. There have been reports that non-sterile tattooing practices have led to the transmission of infectious organisms such as bacteria, syphilis and hepatitis B; furthermore, there is also the potential for transmission of other blood-borne pathogens such as HIV and hepatitis C.[6]

Allergenicity

- Additives such as PPD can be mixed with tattoo dye, causing allergic reactions in patients.
- Allergic or pruritic reactions to tattoos can be linked to certain colors used in the design.
- No dye used in tattooing is FDA approved for deposition into the dermis.

Some patients have allergic reactions to either the pigments in the tattoo or to the additives that can be mixed in with the dye. Even though 2001 marked the first report of an adverse reaction following the application of a "black" henna tattoo darkened with paraphenylenediamine (PPD)-based chemicals, the notoriety of PPD had been previously established. In the 1930s, the practice of tinting the eyelashes and eyebrows with PPD dye was common. Many adverse reactions to PPD became apparent, with some women suffering serious blistering reactions, blindness, and even death, most notably to the product "Lash Lure." Since there were no laws in place to regulate these products, cosmetic companies were not liable. By 1938, the Food, Drug, and Cosmetic Act was initiated with the first mandate: to remove "Lash Lure" from the American market and ban the use of PPD on skin.[7]

Other allergic reactions associated with tattoos can be linked to the specific color of pigment that was injected into the skin. There have been numerous reports of patients with

Table 1 Tattoo pigments and their common ingredients

Dye color	Dye content
Black	Carbon
Red	Mercury sulfide
Blue	Cobalt aluminate
Brown	Hydrate of iron oxide
Green	Chromium oxide
Lilac	Magnesium
White	Titanium oxide
Yellow	Cadmium sulfide

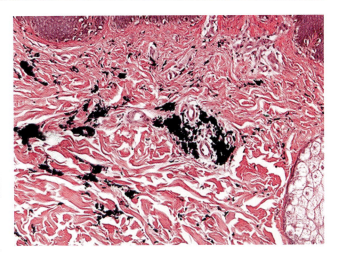

Fig. 2 Tattoo granules present in the dermis prior to treatment

known allergies to mercury or cobalt experiencing type IV hypersensitivity allergic reactions in areas tattooed with red or blue pigment, respectively.[8] There are many common allergenic substances included in common tattoo dyes (Table 1).

It is important to note that tattoo pigments have not FDA approved for intradermal injection. Nevertheless, there have been dramatic advances in the industry of body art, including the development of a biodegradable and bioabsorbable organic dye encapsulated in synthetic polymer. The tattoo is permanent; yet, when targeted with a laser, the beads disintegrate, exposing the ink to be resorbed into the body, thereby completely removing the tattoo.[9]

Methods of Removal

- The most common medical techniques currently used for tattoo removal are laser surgery, surgical excision, and dermabrasion.
- Complications of these procedures, though rare, include discoloration, incomplete removal, scarring, or infection.
- Topical products that lighten naturally pigmented skin are generally not meant for tattoo removal, although current research is ongoing.

Prior to current medical technologies, there was not much available to the patient requesting removal of their tattoo. The patient was offered the choice of harsh exfoliation techniques, chemical peels, thermal means, cryosurgery, or surgical resection. In lieu of medical treatment, many patients today still opt for covering up the tattoo with concealing makeup, or even voluntarily obtaining more tattoos in an attempt to modify or camouflage the original tattoo into a new, often larger design.

Each tattoo is unique; so must each removal technique match the demands of each individual situation. Tattoos that are professionally applied tend to penetrate the deeper layers of the skin at uniform levels (Fig. 2). This uniformity allows dermal surgeons to use techniques that remove broader areas of inked skin at the same depth.

Currently, the most common tattoo removal techniques employed by dermatological professionals are laser surgery, surgical excision, and dermabrasion.

- *Laser surgery*
  The tattoo is treated by targeting selective pigments with a high-intensity laser beam. The type of laser used generally depends upon the colors to be removed. This modality offers a highly effective approach with minimal side effects, although frequently necessitates several treatments for complete removal.
- *Surgical excision*
  The tattoo is cut out and either sutured or allowed to heal, depending on size. The efficacy of this technique is highly dependent upon the individual surgeon, the size of the area to be resected, the tension of the skin in the area, and the individual's tendencies toward scarring or developing a keloid.
- *Dermabrasion*
  The tattoo is gradually removed via exfoliation of the surface and middle layers of pigment by machines, laser or salt. The upper layer of skin is abraded or "sanded," and the underlying layers of skin replace the damaged layers, allowing the pigment to leach out of the skin. Side effects and complications of this procedure are skin discoloration (hyperpigmentation or hypopigmentation) at the treatment site, infection of the tattoo site, incomplete pigment removal, or scarring, even 3–6 months after the tattoo is removed.[10]

It is important to make the distinction between residual tattoo and post inflammatory hyperpigmentation. Post inflammatory hyperpigmentation is different from tattooing in that it is mainly a result of melanocyte stimulation and is exacerbated by exposure to ultra-violet radiation. Tattoos, on the other hand, are not associated with melanocytes, but are rather made up of dyes, which in contrast often fade with sun exposure as the pigment is oxidized and always confined within the previous tattoo position.

There are products available on the market that purport to lighten skin. Products containing hydroquinone are used to treat hyperpigmentation of the skin by reversibly depigmenting the skin. This is accomplished by inhibiting the oxidation of tyrosine to 3, 4-dihydroxyphenyalanine(DOPA) and other melanocyte metabolic processes.

Recent data from Solis et al. demonstrated a significant reduction of tattoo pigment in a guinea pig model. Researchers treated the animals' recent tattoos with imiquimod. After 1 week, the tattoos were no longer detectible either clinically or histopathologically.[11] Although no human models have demonstrated these results, imiquimod remains an attractive non-invasive therapy for the treatment of tattoos. Ricotti and colleagues investigated whether imiquimod in conjunction with laser therapy would be more efficacious in tattoo removal than laser alone. The authors concluded that, in addition to having more adverse reactions than placebo, imiquimod was not an ineffective adjunct to laser treatment of tattoos.[12]

Lasers

- Lasers are commonly used in various medical and cosmetic procedures, including treatment of vascular lesions, scars, dermal remodeling, hair removal, and removal of pigmented lesions.
- Potential side effects of using lasers in the removal of tattoos include discoloration, redness, scarring, and rarely, allergic reactions. These should be discussed with the patient so that an informed decision may be made.
- Specific lasers and wavelengths are better suited for targeted removal of certain colors of pigment than others.
- The Q-switched lasers with pulse durations in nanosecond range are the mainstay devices for tattoo removal.
- Q-switched Ruby (694 nm) is generally used in the removal of black, blue and green tattoos in individuals with fair skin.
- Q-switched Alexandrite (755 nm) is best for removing the green ink.
- Q-switched Nd:YAG (1,064 nm) is useful for treatment black and blue ink in individuals with darkly pigmented skin.
- Q-switched Nd:YAG (532 nm) is useful for treatment red and orange ink.

Laser is an acronym for Light Amplification by Stimulated Emission of Radiation. The first patient for the laser was obtained by Gordon Gould in 1977, although his work on light lasers dated back to 1958. The first medical application of a laser was in 1987, when ophthalmologist Steven Trokel performed refractive surgery on a patient's eyes. Originally designed to precisely cut glass and metal, lasers have revolutionalized the field of medicine with its numerous applications and possibilities.

There are many dermatologic uses of lasers, including treatment of vascular lesions, hypertrophic or keloid scars, striae, acne, hair removal, removal of pigmented lesions, and nonablative dermal remodeling, to name a few. Lasers have become widespread for use in the field for both medical and cosmetic applications.

Due to the ability by some lasers to produce pressure waves significant enough to penetrate the stratum corneum, lasers have become attractive new methods for transdermal drug delivery.[13]

The first use of lasers for the treatment of tattoos was in the 1970s.[14,15] Carbon dioxide lasers, which emit a wavelength of 10,600 nm and target water in the skin, and argon lasers, which emit a continuous wavelength of either 488 or 514 nm, were used non-selectively in an attempt to remove tattoo pigment from the dermis. The CO_2 laser ablates the top layer of skin and often results in scarring when used at a depth necessary for tattoo removal. The argon lasers, due to their continuous energy emitted, transmit heat to other tissue areas, also resulting in hyperpigmented skin, incomplete removal of the pigment, and scarring.

Modern lasers have become paramount in the treatment and removal of tattoos. By selective photothermolysis, lasers allow dermatologists to selectively remove target pigments without destroying the surrounding skin or tissue architecture dramatically. The short-pulse (nanosecond or picosecond) lasers are optimal for tattoo removal without significant scarring. The most commonly used lasers for this purpose include the Q-switched neodymium:yttrium–aluminum–garnet(Nd:YAG), alexandrite, and ruby lasers.[16] Q-switching refers to a switch that allows the release of energy in one pulse such that the target is heated so quickly (within nanoseconds or picoseconds) that it shatters, allowing for selective photothermolysis.

Depending on the wavelength used, the laser is able to target the tattoo pigment while sparing other chromophores in the skin, such as melanin. Due to its primary purpose of absorbing damaging ultraviolet rays, melanin absorbs light, which can be detrimental when attempting to use light to remove a tattoo. Nevertheless, this absorptive property of melanin decreases with longer wavelengths, allowing targeted removal of pigment by lasers without interference or refraction. The biophysics underlying the mechanism by which lasers are able to dissolve tattoos is not well understood, but the accepted theory is that the pulse of light from the laser breaks up the tattoo pigment into smaller components to be digested by macrophages, taken up by scavenger cells, or eliminated transepidermally.[17]

Laser Treatment of Tattoos

How efficacious the laser treatment is in the complete removal of the tattoo depends on multiple factors, including size, length of time since application, depth of pigment, colors used, and patient's skin type. Laser removal of pigment is highly color dependent, since the lasers used emit certain wavelengths that are better able to target certain colors.

The three lasers most commonly used are the Q-switched Ruby, Q-switched Alexandrite, and Q-switched Nd:YAG.

- *Q-switched Ruby* (694 nm)
  Light from this laser is red. Because light is absorbed by its opposite color and reflected by its same color, this laser removes most ink colors well, except red. It is generally used in the removal of blue and black tattoos. It is especially effective in the removal of amateur and traumatic tattoos. This was the first laser to be used in the treatment of tattoos and pigmented lesions.[18,19]
- *Q-switched Alexandrite* (755 nm)
  This laser emits a purple/red light and is therefore best for removing blue, black, and green ink. This laser offers an advantage over older models in that is reliable, with faster repetition rates, and is the laser of choice in the removal of green pigment.
- *Q-switched Nd:YAG* (1,064 nm)
  This laser emits light in the infrared range. It removes black and blue ink best. Because this wavelength is not well absorbed by melanocytes, it is useful for treatment in individuals with darkly pigmented skin (Figs. 3 and 4).
- *Q-switched Nd:YAG* (532 nm)
  This is an alteration of the 1,064 nm Nd:YAG laser made possible by using a potassium-titanyl-phosphate crystal to double the frequency, thus halving the wavelength to 532 nm. This laser emits a green light and removes red and orange ink. This wavelength is absorbed by hemoglobin and thus, may result in temporary purpura after laser treatment.

Amateur tattoos are generally easier to remove since they usually contain only black or blue ink and more superficial. Unfortunately, some amateurs may tattoo too deeply, making the pigment deposition irregular and difficult to target. Professional tattoo artists often mix colors for a gradation effect, which is also more difficult to remove, but will tattoo no deeper than the dermis and at a consistent depth throughout the tattoo.

A minimum interval of 4 weeks is generally required between laser sessions to allow the treatment area adequate

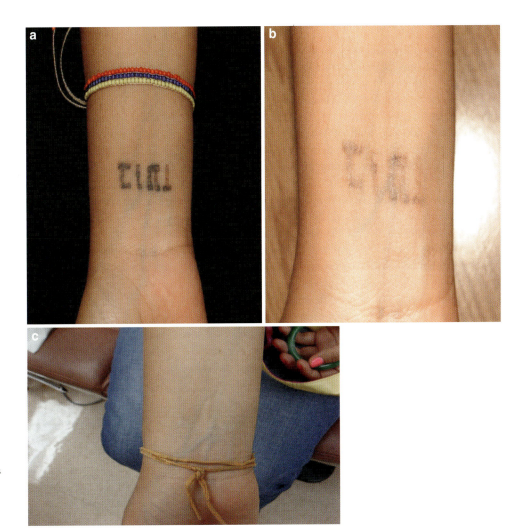

Fig. 3 Laser tattoo removal at the right wrist with Q-switches Nd:YaG. (**a**) before treatment (**b**) two month after the first treatment (**c**) after three treatments

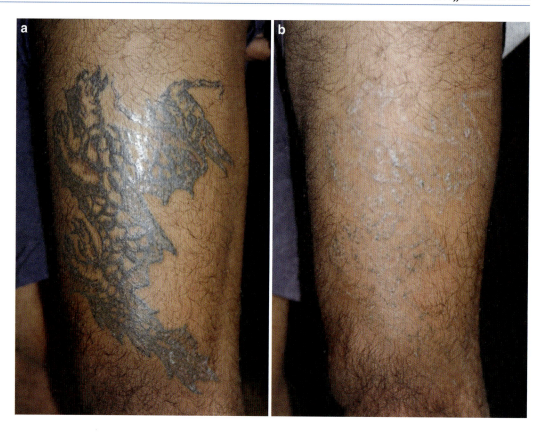

Fig. 4 (**a**) Before treatment and (**b**) the result after seven treatments with Q-Switched Nd:YAG laser

time to heal and the immune system a sufficient period for macrophages to phagocytize the broken pigment molecules.[20] An average tattoo with a surface area of 2 in.[2] requires 6–7 months to be removed, on average, with sessions scheduled every 6–8 weeks.[16]

The absorption spectrum of tattoos is unknown, with some colors responding better than others. As a result, a combination of laser systems may be used in stages for a single tattoo (Table 2).

Although Q-switched lasers are now the mainstay of treatment for the removal of tattoos, it is important to note that there may be unwanted complications associated with the practice. Most commonly, patients experience hyper- or hypopigmentation reactions or immediate erythema at the treatment site that generally subsides within minutes of treatment.[22] Some patients may experience scarring. Some patients, however, may experience hypersensitivity reactions, especially if they had previously experienced allergic reactions upon application of the tattoo pigment.[23] A rare and controversial topic of debate is whether or not laser removal of certain pigments may be associated with the generation of carcinogenic or hazardous compounds.[24]

There are significant costs associated with laser treatments of tattoos, which are not often covered by health insurance companies. Most tattoos require multiple sessions for reasonably anticipated pigment removal, which should be communicated with the patient beforehand to ensure the patient possesses adequate expectations about the outcome of the treatment. More than half of all patients experience a 75–95% reduction of tattoo pigment with a conventional series of three to four laser treatments.[16] These issues should be discussed with the patient in order for an informed decision to be made about his or her treatment and to ensure that realistic expectations are set.

Conclusion

The information presented herein presents a background on the history of tattooing, the methods of removal currently available, and a scientifically-based rationale for why photothermolysis via laser has become implemented into mainstream treatment. Tattoos are widely varied based on the individual patient, the method used in injecting the pigment into the skin, size of tattoo, spectrum of colors used in the design, the duration of time that the patient has had the

Table 2 Choice of laser for removal of tattoo by ink color[21]

Laser	Black	Blue	Green	Red
Alexandrite 755 nm	X	X	XX	
Ruby 694 nm	X	X	X	
Nd:YAG 1,064 nm	X	X		
Nd:YAG 532 nm				X

tattoo, as well as any underlying conditions the patient may have that could affect healing or immune response to therapy. All of these conditions must been taken into consideration when selecting an individualized treatment tailored to not only each patient, but also to each patient's specific tattoo that has been selected for removal. Very recently developed Freedom-2 ink technology uses microencapsulated polymer beads of biodegradable ink to allow complete clearance with just one laser treatment. Whether or not the tattoo is being removed out of necessity (employment requirements, social situations, familial pressures, etc.), it is important for the physician to have an appreciation that the patient may experience some degree of anxiety about becoming detached from a personal symbol which was undoubtedly expected to be embedded within him or her indefinitely. On the other hand, it is a paramount achievement for medicine that we are now able to safely remove tattoos and skin markings that hold negative connotations, that are regarded with regret, or which have become irrelevant in the patient's current life setting.

References

1. Anderson RR. Tattooing should be regulated. *N Engl J Med.* 1992; 326(3):207.
2. Laumann AE, Derick AJ. Tattoos and body piercings in the United States: a national data set. *J Am Acad Dermatol.* 2006;55(3):413-421.
3. Armstrong ML, Stuppy DJ, Gabriel DC, et al. Motivation for tattoo removal. *Arch Dermatol.* 1996;132(4):412-416.
4. Varma S, Lanigan SW. Reasons for requesting laser removal of unwanted tattoos. *Br J Dermatol.* 1999;140(3):483-485.
5. Kilmer SL, Fitzpatrick RE, Goldman MP. Treatment of tattoos. In: Goldman MP, Fitzpatrick RE, eds. *Cutaneous Laser Surgery.* St. Louis: Mosby; 1999:213-252.
6. American Academy of Dermatology. *Position Statement on Tattooing.* Approved by the Board of Directors; October 24, 1998.
7. Jacob SE, Caperton CV. Allergen focus: focus on T.R.U.E. Test allergen #16: black rubber mix. *Skin Aging.* 2006;13(6):20-24.
8. Kazandjieva J, Tsankov N. Tattoos: dermatological complications. *Clin Dermatol.* 2007;25(4):375-382.
9. Schmidt RM, Armstrong ML. Tattooing and body piercing. In: UpToDate, Rose, BD (ed), *UpToDate,* Waltham, MA, 2007.
10. American Society for Dermatologic Surgery. Accessible online: http://www.asds.net/TattooRemovalInformation.aspx.
11. Solis RR, Diven DG, Colome-Grimmer MI, Snyder N IV, Wagner RF Jr. Experimental nonsurgical tattoo removal in a guinea pig model with topical imiquimod and tretinoin. *Dermatol Surg.* 2002;28(1):83-86; discussion 86-87.
12. Ricotti CA, Colaco SM, Shamma HN, Trevino J, Palmer G, Heaphy MR Jr. Laser-assisted tattoo removal with topical 5% imiquimod cream. *Dermatol Surg.* 2007;33(9):1082-1091.
13. Fox LP, Merk HF, Bickers DR. Dermatological pharmacology. In: Brunton LL, ed. *Goodman & Gilman's the Pharmacological Basis of Therapeutics.* 11th ed. New York: McGraw-Hill; 2006: 1679-1704.
14. Apfelberg DB, Maser MR, Lash H. Argon laser treatment of decorative tattoos. *Br J Plast Surg.* 1979;32:141-144.
15. Brady SC, Blokmanis A, Jewett L. Tattoo removal with the carbon dioxide laser. *Ann Plast Surg.* 1978;2:482-490.
16. Bernstein EF. Laser treatment of tattoos. *Clin Dermatol.* 2006;24: 43-55.
17. Ho DD, London R, Zimmerman GB, Young DA. Laser-tattoo removal—a study of the mechanism and the optimal treatment strategy via computer simulations. *Lasers Surg Med.* 2002;30:389.
18. Goldman L, Blaney DJ, Kindel DJ Jr, Richfield D, Franke EK. Pathology of the effect of the laser beam on the skin. *Nature.* 1965;197:912.
19. Goldman L, Wilson RG, Hormby P, Meyer RG. Radiation from a Q-switched ruby laser. Effect of repeated impacts of power output of 10 megawatts on a tattoo of man. *J Invest Dermatol.* 1965;44:69-71.
20. Pfirrmann G, Karsai S, Roos S, Hammes S, Raulin C. Tattoo removal—state of the art. *J Dtsch Dermatol Ges.* 2007;5(10):889-897.
21. Mariwalla K, Dover JS. The use of lasers for decorative tattoo removal. *Skin Therapy Lett.* 2006;11(5):8-11.
22. Burris K, Kim K. Tattoo removal. *Clin Dermatol.* 2007;25:388-392.
23. Ashinoff R, Levine VJ, Soter NA. Allergic reactions to tattoo pigment after laser treatment. *Dermatol Surg.* 1995;21:291.
24. Vasold R, Naarmann N, Ulrich H, et al. Tattoo pigments are cleaved by laser light – the chemical analysis in vitro provide evidence for hazardous compounds. *Photochem Photobiol.* 2004;80:185.

Laser for Hair Removal

Voraphol Vejjabhinanta, Keyvan Nouri, Anita Singh, Ran Huo, and Rawat Charoensawad

- Lasers for hair removal are a fast-growing area in cosmetic dermatology.
- Selective photothermolysis allows for targeting of specific chromophores while minimizing cutaneous damage.
- Treatment of individuals should be individualized based on anatomical area, skin and hair color, by varying the wavelength, fluence, pulse duration, spot size, and cooling technique of the laser.
- Adverse events to laser hair removal include post-treatment erythema, edema, blistering, hypo/hyperpigmentation, scarring, and skin infections.
- Further standardized, well-controlled, and long-term studies are needed to establish the optimal treatment parameters for each laser for each patient demographic.

Introduction

- Laser hair removal is the second most common nonsurgical procedure performed in the U.S.
- Patients and physicians need to have realistic expectations of results for laser hair removal. The level of hair reduction may vary widely amongst individuals.
- Lasers are advantageous because they are fast, safe, and effective when used appropriately.
- Complete hair loss is defined as a lack of regrowing hairs but can be temporary or permanent.
- The mechanism of selective photothermolysis allows lasers to target specific cutaneous chromophores while protecting the outer tissue.
- Active cooling devices, such as cryogen sprays and contact cooling devices help to minimize injury to the epidermis.

The use of lasers for hair removal, or photoepilation, is becoming an increasingly popular trend in the arena of cosmetic dermatology. According to the American Society for Aesthetic Plastic Surgery (ASAPS), 1,566,909 laser hair removal procedures were performed in 2005, increased from 1,411,899 procedures just a year earlier.[1,2] Only Botox injections are pe rformed more frequently for both women and men, according to the ASAPS's list of the top five most popular nonsurgical procedures among Americans. Although there has been a decrease in total nonsurgical procedures among women and men from 2004 to 2005, laser hair removal was an exception with a 1.1% increase in women and about a 1.2% increase in men. Men accounted for about 15% of the total laser hair removal procedures that were performed. Furthermore, laser hair removal was listed by the ASAPS as the top nonsurgical procedure for people 18 and under and for

V. Vejjabhinanta (✉)
Department of Dermatology and Cutaneous Surgery,
University of Miami, Leonard M. Miller School of Medicine,
Miami, FL and
Department of Dermatology, Siriraj Hospital, Mahidol University,
Bangkok, Thailand
e-mail: vvoraphol@gmail.com

K. Nouri (ed.), *Lasers in Dermatology and Medicine*,
DOI: 10.1007/978-0-85729-281-0_8, © Springer-Verlag London Limited 2011

people between 19 and 34 years old. Hair removal has historically been of great interest because excess hair, especially in patients with hypertrichosis or hirsutism, can be troubling both socially and psychologically.[3] Past and present options for hair removal have included shaving, epilation, depilatories, electrolysis and now most currently, lasers.[4] All methods for hair removal have side effects, but lasers are advantageous because they are fast, safe, and effective when used appropriately. With the increased desire for and availability of laser hair reduction around the world, it is necessary to evaluate the current indications and potential side effects of each laser.

The concept of hair removal was defined in 1998 by the US Food and Drug Administration (FDA), which allowed some manufacturers of hair removal lasers and flash lamps used for hair removal to use the term "permanent hair *reduction*." The agency defined permanent hair reduction as, "The long-term, stable reduction in the number of hairs regrowing after a treatment regime. The number of hairs regrowing must be stable over a time greater than the duration of the complete growth cycle of hair follicles, which varies from 4 to 12 months according to body location. Permanent hair reduction does not necessarily imply the elimination of all hairs in the treatment area."[5] In addition, there needs to be a distinction made between permanent and complete hair loss. Complete hair loss is defined as a lack of regrowing hairs, but may be either temporary or permanent. Permanent hair loss is defined as a lack of regrowing hairs indefinitely. Hair removal with lasers usually produces complete but temporary hair loss for 1–3 months. After this time period, there is usually partial but permanent hair loss.[6]

The theory of selective photothermolysis dictates the process of laser hair removal. By varying specific parameters (wavelength, pulse duration, and fluence), specific cutaneous chromophores may be targeted while protecting the outer lying tissue.[7,8] Applying this theory to laser hair removal, the wavelength should be the same as the target chromophore, the pulse duration should be less than the chromophore's thermal relaxation time (TRT), and the fluence must be great enough to sufficiently destroy the chromophore.

In laser hair removal, the specific target is the endogenous chromophore melanin. Melanin is found in the bulb, bulge, and hair shaft of anagen hair. Lasers for hair removal must emit light within the absorption spectrum of melanin, 250–1,200 nm, to be effective.[9] In addition, vascular reduction has also been proposed as a mechanism for long-term epilation.[10] One obstacle to laser hair removal is that melanin resides in the epidermis as well. This is a twofold problem because epidermal melanin not only interferes with the laser's treatment capabilities by detracting some of the laser's energy, but can also cause damage to the epidermis. Because pigmentation of the hair and skin vary to such a great extent among patients, this is a difficult problem to resolve.

Active cooling is an excellent method to minimize injury to the epidermis. Many lasers today are equipped with cooling devices such as cryogen sprays or contact cooling devices. For example, the long-pulsed 694 nm ruby lasers have a cooling hand piece that is applied during treatment to lower the temperature of the skin and spare it from injury. This integrated cooling device pre-cools the skin prior to laser pulse delivery. The long-pulsed 755 nm alexandrite lasers utilize a variety of cooling mechanisms. These mechanisms include a cooling hand piece that allows a continuous flow of chilled air to the treatment area, and a dynamic cooling device that uses short (5–100 ms) cryogen spurts that is delivered to the skin surface through an electronically controlled valve. The 800 nm diode lasers use a sapphire-cooled handpiece that is placed in direct contact with the skin to cool the area. The 1,064 nm Nd:YAG lasers uses a variety of cooling mechanisms and is based on the laser used; currently available options include a chill tip cooling device, pulsed cryogen delivery to the skin, contact pre-cooling and air cooling. Finally, intense pulsed light uses a chilled handpiece that cools the skin and a transparent gel that provides optical coupling, as well as additional cooling.[6] In addition to these methods, ice and refrigerated gels can also provide relief.[11]

Another way to limit thermal injury to the epidermis, in keeping with the theory of selective photothermolysis, is to use a pulse duration between the TRT of the epidermis (3–10 ms) and that of the hair follicle (10–100 ms).[4,11] However, recent studies have sparked a reconsideration of the original theory suggesting a modification whereby the target isn't destroyed by direct heating, but by diffusion from the pigmented area.[11,12] This requires long pulses upwards of 100 ms known as *superpulses*. These *superpulses* would also damage other crucial targets, such as stem cells, which may be another factor for permanent hair reduction.[9]

The current market for laser hair reduction is growing so rapidly that the FDA has not maintained an up-to-date listing of all approved laser devices. Currently used lasers fall into one of four categories: the long-pulsed ruby laser (694 nm), the long-pulsed alexandrite laser (755 nm), the long-pulsed semiconductor diode laser (800–810 nm), and the long-pulsed Nd:YAG laser (1,064 nm). Additionally, the Intense Pulsed Light (IPL) system (515–1,200 nm) is approved as a safe and effective method for hair reduction (Table 1).

Indications/Contraindications

- Unwanted hair is a very common problem affecting individuals from all demographics.
- The ideal candidate for laser hair removal is a person with fair skin and dark terminal hair.
- Some contraindications include active cutaneous infections, history of keloid or hypertrophic scarring, history of recurrent infections, and active vitiligo and psoriasis in targeted areas.

Table 1 Laser and intense pulsed light systems for hair removal

Laser	Method of hair removal	Example	Skin type	Hair color	Hair diameter	Type of hair removal	Hair reduction	Side effects
Long-pulsed ruby lasers (694 nm)	Photothermal destruction	E2000 Epitouch Ruby Ruby Star Sinon	I–III	Dark to light brown	Fine and coarse	Long term hair removal	38–49% hair reduction	Treatment pain, erythema, edema, hypopigmentation, hyperpigmentation, blistering, crusting, erosions, purpura, folliculitis
Long-pulsed alexandrite lasers (755 nm)	Photothermal destruction	Apogee Gentelase Epitouch ALEX Ultrawave II/III Epicare Arion	I–IV	Dark to light brown	Fine and coarse	Long term hair removal	74–78% hair reduction	Treatment pain, erythema, edema, hypopigmentation, hyperpigmentation, blistering, crusting, erosions, purpura, folliculitis
Pulsed diode laser (800 nm)	Photothermal destruction	LightSheer Apex-800 SLP1000 MedioStar F1 Diode Laser	I–IV	Dark to light brown	Coarse	Long term hair removal	70–84% hair reduction	Treatment pain, erythema, edema, hypopigmentation, hyperpigmentation, blistering, crusting, erosions, purpura, folliculitis
Long pulsed Nd:YAG lasers (1,064 nm)	Photothermal destruction	CoolGlide Lyra Ultrawave I/II/III Athos Gentle Yag Varia Acclaim 7000 Smartepil II Dualis Vasculight Elite Profile Mydon	I–VI	Dark	Coarse	Long term hair removal	29–53% hair reduction	Treatment pain, erythema, edema, hypopigmentation, hyperpigmentation, blistering, crusting, erosions, purpura, folliculitis
Intense pulsed light source (515–1,200 nm)	Photothermal destruction	EpiLight Quantum HR Ellipse PhotoLight Estelux ProLite Spatouch Quadra Q4 SpectraPulse	I–VI	Dark to light brown	Coarse	Long term hair removal	49–90% hair reduction	Treatment pain, erythema, edema, hypopigmentation, hyperpigmentation, blistering, crusting, erosions, purpura, folliculitis
Q-switched Nd:YAG lasers	Photomechanical destruction	Softlight MedLite C6	I–VI	Dark to light brown	Fine and coarse	Temporary hair removal	50–66% hair reduction	Treatment pain, erythema, edema, hypopigmentation, hyperpigmentation, blistering, crusting, erosions, purpura, folliculitis

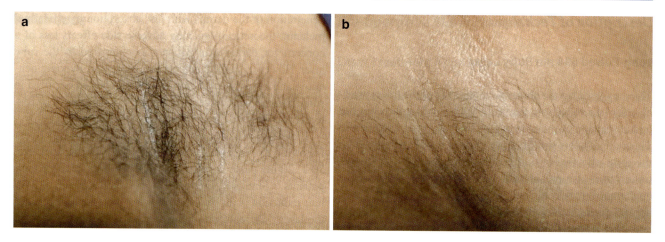

Fig. 2 (**a**) Pretreatment of right axillary area with coarse hair. (**b**) Only fine hair exist after 3 months and five treatments with 1,064 Nd:YAG laser

and found that the alexandrite and diode lasers have similar efficacy.[31] The authors partially attribute the success of their results to the use of relatively high fluences, which they were able to use by carefully selecting patients who were untanned. Tanning increases the chance of epidermal damage and also lowers the laser's effectiveness. Another study found similar results between three treatments of either the alexandrite laser or diode laser. However, in this study, the hair reduction was about 37–46% for the two lasers. Patients from the study reported that the diode laser was more painful and had greater side effects, particularly hyperpigmentation and blistering, as compared with the alexandrite laser.[16,32]

A study comparing various spot sizes (8, 10, and 14 mm) found that after three treatments and at a 3 month follow-up, there was not a significant difference in hair reduction.[16,33] However, as with the ruby laser and the alexandrite laser, two treatments with the diode laser resulted in a greater hair reduction (35–53%) than one treatment (28–33%) after an average 2-month follow-up. Also in this study, the diode laser lead to a significant hair reduction as compared to shaving (13–36% vs −7%).[16,34]

A recent study testing the efficacy of a newer 810 nm diode laser on patients with Fitzpatrick skin types II–IV found histological and clinical evidence of hair reduction (70%) at 6 months follow-up.[35]

1,064 nm Nd:YAG Laser

The 1,064 nm Nd:YAG has the longest wavelength and deepest penetration amongst the aforementioned laser systems available. It is not very well absorbed by melanin, but is sufficient in achieving selective photothermolysis and has superior penetration.[36] The Nd:YAG is able to penetrate the skin 5–7 mm, a depth at which most of the target structures lay. Furthermore, the combination of a low melanin absorption and deep penetration leads to less collateral damage to the melanin-containing epidermis (Fig. 2a, b). These characteristics make this system the safest choice for tanned or darker skinned patients.[9,36] While this laser may be the safest method to treat all skin types, it is not necessarily the most effective. Bouzari et al. compared hair reduction by the long-pulsed Nd:YAG, alexandrite, and diode lasers and found that after 3 months, the Nd:YAG was the least effective of the three.[31] An interesting aspect of their study was that the best results were seen in five patients who underwent combination laser therapy that included treatment with all three systems. They hypothesize that using a variety of wavelengths, they are able to damage hairs at different ranges in the skin; longer wavelengths would damage the deeper hairs and the shorter wavelengths would damage the more superficial hairs. This is analogous to laser tattoo removal which incorporates a combination of lasers to remove the multitude of pigments found in a given tattoo.

A study determining the safety and efficacy of the long-pulsed Nd:YAG laser for all skin types found that the treatments were more successful (46–53% depending on location) in darker skin patients (types V–VI). At 6 months, patients with skin types I–II obtained a 41–43% hair reduction, depending on location, while patients with skin types III–IV obtained a 44–48% hair reduction.[37] Another study comparing fluence levels found similar hair reductions for fluences of 50, 80, and 100 J/cm^2 (29%, 29%, and 27% respectively) in patients with skin types II–IV.[38]

Intense Pulsed Light

The Intense Pulsed Light (IPL) system is not technically a laser, but has recently entered the hair removal arena as a competent contender. In fact, it has been used for virtually all of the same indications as laser systems (Fig. 3a, b). Unlike lasers which emit monochromatic light, IPL systems have

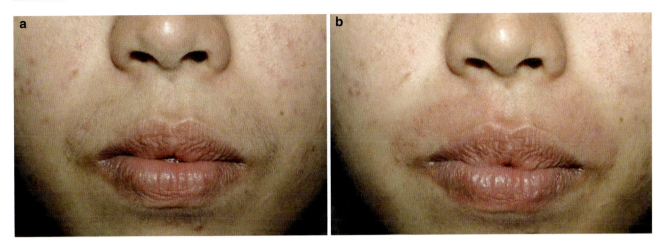

Fig. 3 (**a**) Pretreatment of perioral area. (**b**) Immediately after treatment with IPL system, with perifollicular erythema and edema, as well as burning of hair shaft

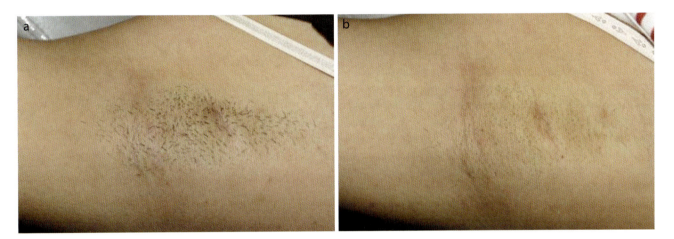

Fig. 4 (**a**) Pretreatment of right axillary area. (**b**) Three months after three treatments with IPL system patient has fine hair and delaying of hair growth

flash lamps which produce non-coherent light in the 515–1,200 nm spectrum.[39] IPL systems work very similarly to lasers and rely on the principle of selective photothermolysis. The IPL systems generally use millisecond pulse duration that is lower than the thermal relaxation times of the targeted chromophores. IPL systems, unlike lasers, use a polychromatic light that can be used to simultaneously treat both pigmented and vascular lesions. Polychromatic light irradiates multiple chromophores with both major and minor absorption peaks, allowing for greater selective energy absorption.[6]

Results using this system have been comparable to the more conventional lasers mentioned (Fig. 4a, b). Similarly to lasers, dark-haired patients responded better to IPL treatment than did blonde or gray-haired patients, who also required more treatment sessions.[40] IPL is not capable of achieving permanent hair removal, but long-term hair reduction with few side effects is possible.[41] Schroeter et al. followed the long-term effects of this laser on hirsute women and reported very good results with 87% mean hair reduction after an average of 27.4 months and eight treatments. Positive results correlated with the number of given treatments. Side-effects reported were mild and transient.[42]

One randomized controlled trial compared the effects of one treatment of IPL with one treatment using the long-pulsed Nd:YAG laser in patients with skin types IV–VI and found no significance in hair reduction after 6-weeks follow-up. However, the IPL treatment resulted in post inflammatory pigmentation (45%) while the Nd:YAG laser did not.[16,43] A nonrandomized controlled trial which compared three treatments of IPL with three treatments using a ruby laser found that in skin types II–IV, 94% of patients obtained an average 49% hair reduction using the IPL system at 6-month follow-up, as compared with only 55% of patients obtaining an average of 21% hair reduction with the ruby laser.[16,44] However, McGill et al. found that the IPL system was not effective as the alexandrite laser in a randomized, split-face comparison of six treatments with both systems with up to 6 months follow-up, the alexandrite laser showed a significantly longer hair-free interval, larger reduction in hair counts, and greater patient satisfaction than the IPL.[45]

Radiofrequency Combinations

Radiofrequency devices have been combined with both IPL and diode lasers to provide optimal hair removal treatments to a wider range of skin types. The combinations are considered safe for patients with darker skin types because the radiofrequency energy is not absorbed by melanin in the epidermis. This technology, termed electro-optical synergy, or ELOS, has a dual mechanism of heating the hair follicle with electrical energy (namely radiofrequency) and heating the hair shaft with optical energy.

The newest evolution in photoepilation involves removing nonpigmented hairs such as "peach fuzz" which the previous lasers fail to remove. A combination of radiofrequency (RF) and lasers have been used for white or blonde hair, but with low efficacy. In recent studies, the combined use of RF and optical energy has been found to be successful, though various mechanisms have been proposed to explain the success.[46-49] Some claims of widespread safety have been made because RF energy is not readily absorbed by the melanin abundantly found in the epidermis of darker skin types, theoretically sparing it from damage. However, a low efficacy of this new technology has been reported so far. Results have indicated that the majority of subjects achieved less than 50% hair reduction after 3 months.[47] In two other studies, average clearances of 48%[48] and 75%[49] were seen at 18-months follow-up. Because this is a relatively new technology, more studies are clearly necessary to provide more reliable results for those with nonpigmented hair or with darker skin types.

Other Removal Methods for Nonpigmented Hair

Meladine, a topical melanin chromophore, has been studied in Europe with interesting results. The liposome solution dye, which is sprayed on, is selectively absorbed by the hair follicle and not the skin. This gives the follicles a temporary boost of melanin to optimize laser hair removal treatments. Clinical studies in Europe have shown vast permanent hair reduction in patients who used Meladine prior to treatment. However, other studies have found Meladine to only offer a delay of hair growth as opposed to permanent hair reduction.[6] Sand et al. used a similar topical liposomal melanin compound in a randomized, controlled, double-blind study with blond and white hair patients, and found that the substance made almost no difference in treatment outcomes for the patients.[50]

Photodynamic therapy may be an effective option for those with nonpigmented or light-colored hair. Because of the lack or diminished amount of a natural chromophore in the hair follicle, a topical photosensitizer 5-aminolevulinic acid (5-ALA) is used. Light exposure activates 5-ALA, which subsequently creates reactive oxygen and allows for destruction of the hair follicle.[6]

Post-operative Management

Post-operatively, ice packs can be used to reduce pain and minimize edema. Analgesics are rarely needed. Mild topical steroid creams may be given to the patient to decrease post-treatment erythema and edema. If any epidermal injury occurs during the procedure, a topical antibiotic can be given to the patient. The patient should be notified that they must use sun block and avoid direct sun exposure.[6]

Adverse Events

- Some of the reported adverse events have included post-treatment erythema, edema, crusting, blistering, paradoxical hair growth, hypo/hyperpigmentation, scarring, and skin infections.
- Methods to decrease the risk of adverse events include effective epidermal cooling, long pulse duration, longer wavelength lasers, ice packs, analgesics, steroid creams, topical antibiotics, and avoidance of sun exposure

Side Effects/Complications

Patients should be warned before the laser procedure that they may experience some discomfort during and after the procedure. Reported adverse events have included post-treatment erythema, edema, crusting, blistering, hypopigmentation, hyperpigmentation, and scarring (Fig. 5a, b). Other complications include herpes simplex outbreaks in patients with a previous history of outbreaks, folliculitis in patients who sweat excessively or swim, transient and permanent pigmentary changes, temporary or permanent leucotrichia, loss of freckles or lightening of tattoos, livedo reticularis, intense pruritus, and urticaria.[6]

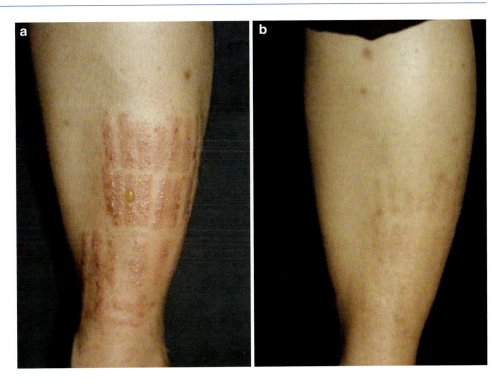

Fig. 5 (**a**) Blister formation, a complication of IPL treatment 3 days after treatment. (**b**) Residual hyperpigmentation is still noticed 9 months after blister formation

In some cases, laser treatment has actually been reported to induce hair growth, particularly on the face and neck. For example, in one study, this was noted in young females of Mediterranean and Middle Eastern descent and with darker skin types (III or IV).[51] The induction of hair growth occurred regardless of the fluency or type of laser used for both intense pulsed light and long-pulsed alexandrite laser. Because neogenesis of hair follicles after birth does not occur, it is likely that the mechanism behind laser-induced hair growth is that local vellus hair follicles transform into terminal pigmented hair follicles.[51] Another theory is that the laser induces synchronization of hair growth cycles by direct light stimulation.[52]

Prevention and Treatment of Side Effects/Complications

Dark-skinned patients are more prone to the adverse effects aforementioned. Several factors may assist in minimizing these side effects. Effective epidermal cooling can reduce epidermal damage from the laser treatment. A long pulse duration allows the hair follicle to be heated effectively while the effect of epidermal cooling is at its peak. In addition, longer wavelength lasers are associated with a lower degree of epidermal damage. Ice packs, analgesics, and mild topical steroid creams can be used post-operatively to reduce pain and minimize erythema and edema. In cases of epidermal injury, a topical antibiotic can be given to the patient. The patient should be advised to avoid sun exposure after the procedure.

In a prospective, randomized, placebo-controlled study, Akinturk et al. showed that piroxicam gel provided adequate pain relief and lowered inflammation after Nd:YAG laser hair removal in patients as compared to placebo control.[53]

Future Directions

- The FDA has approved lasers for permanent hair reduction.
- Strong data from standardized, well-controlled, long-term studies are needed to establish the optimal treatment parameters for each laser.

Currently, the FDA has not approved lasers to be marketed as a permanent hair removal option, although manufacturers have been allowed to claim permanent hair *reduction* based on safety and efficacy. Permanent hair reduction involves the stable reduction in the total amount of hair in a given area over the long-term. To achieve the title of permanent hair removal, future studies should be concerned with the long-term efficacy of these lasers. In general, the ruby laser can be used for skin types I and II, although the alexandrite laser and the diode laser are generally safer with less side effects for skin types III–IV. The Nd:YAG laser is ideal for tanned skin and skin types IV, V and VI, but has a lower efficacy in lighter skin types. Current studies are beginning to investigate the safety and efficacy of specific and newer lasers for various skin types. This is important because as the popularity of photoepilation continues to grow, so will the population of patients interested in this procedure. The challenge ahead lies in gathering strong data from standardized, long-term studies so that optimal parameters can be established.

It must be noted that current trends in laser treatment choice and research have moved away from ruby lasers and to the longer wavelength systems such as the Alexandrite, diode and Nd:YAG lasers, which allow for deeper penetration to the level of hair bulbs.[54]

Conclusion

Excess hair is an extremely common condition affecting both men and women of all ages. Many of the previous options for people seeking to remove or lessen the presence of hair have been painful or have only resulted in short-term effects. With the advent of laser technology, the new generation nonablative lasers and light systems have become some of the most popular procedures in all of cosmetic dermatology. Although lasers are not yet a permanent solution for hair removal, they are able to provide a safe, fast, and effective method for hair reduction.

References

1. The American Society for Aesthetic Plastic Surgery. ASAPS 2005 Cosmetic Surgery National Data Bank statistics. 2005. http://www.surgery.org/download/2005stats.pdf. Accessed March 28, 2006.
2. The American Society for Aesthetic Plastic Surgery. ASAPS 2004 Cosmetic Surgery National Data Bank statistics. 2004. http://www.surgery.org/download/2004-stats.pdf. Accessed March 28, 2006.
3. Nouri K, Trent JT. Lasers. In: Nouri K, Leal-Khouri S, eds. *Techniques in Dermatologic Surgery*, vol. 29. St. Louis: Mosby; 2003:245-258.
4. Olsen EA. Methods of hair removal. *J Am Acad Dermatol*. 1999; 40:143-155.
5. FDA Docket K980517. July 21, 1998. Summary of Safety and Effectiveness for the EpiLaser Normal Mode Ruby Laser. www.accessdata.fda.gov/cdrh_docs/pdf/K980517.pdf. Accessed January 31, 2011.
6. Dierickx C, Grossman M. Laser hair removal. In: Goldberg DJ, ed. *Laser and Lights*, vol. 2. China: Elsevier Saunders; 2005:61-76.
7. Anderson RR, Parrish JA. Selective photothermolysis: precise microsurgery by selective absorption of pulsed radiation. *Science*. 1983;220:524-527.
8. Dierickx C, Alora MB, Dover JS. A clinical overview of hair removal using lasers and light sources. *Dermatol Clin*. 1999;17:357-366.
9. Battle EF, Hobbs LM. Laser-assisted hair removal for darker skin types. *Dermatol Ther*. 2004;17:177-183.
10. Adrian RM. Vascular mechanisms in laser hair removal. *J Cutan Laser Ther*. 2000;2(1):49-50.
11. Tanzi EL, Lupton JR, Alster TS. Lasers in dermatology: four decades of progress. *J Am Acad Dermatol*. 2003;49:1-31.

12. Rogachefsky AS, Silapunt S, Goldberg DJ. Evaluation of a new super-long-pulsed 810 nm diode laser for the removal of unwanted hair: the concept of thermal damage time. *Dermatol Surg*. 2002;28:410-414.
13. Nanni CA, Alster TS. Laser-assisted hair removal: side effects of Q-switched Nd:YAG, long-pulsed ruby, and alexandrite lasers. *J Am Acad Dermatol*. 1999;41:165-171.
14. Campos VB, Dierickx CC, Farinelli WA, Lin TY, Manuskiatti W, Anderson RR. Ruby laser hair removal: evaluation of long-term efficacy and side effects. *Lasers Surg Med*. 2000;26:177-185.
15. Lanigan SW. Incidence of side effects after laser hair removal. *J Am Acad Dermatol*. 2003;49:882-886.
16. Haedersdal M, Wulf HC. Evidence-based review of hair removal using lasers and light sources. *J Eur Acad Dermatol Venereol*. 2006;20:9-20.
17. Elman M, Klein A, Slatkine M. Dark skin tissue reaction in laser assisted hair removal with a long-pulse ruby laser. *J Cutan Laser Ther*. 2000;26:240-243.
18. Polderman MC, Pavel S, Le Cessie S, Grevelink JM, van Leeuwen RL. Efficacy, tolerability, and safety of a long-pulsed ruby laser system in the removal of unwanted hair. *Dermatol Surg*. 2000;26:240-243.
19. Wimmershoff MB, Scherer K, Lorenz S, Landthaler M, Hohenleutner U. Hair removal using a 5-msec long-pulsed ruby laser. *Dermatol Surg*. 2000;26:205-209.
20. Allison KP, Kiernan MN, Waters RA, Clement RM. Evaluation of the ruby 694 chromos for hair removal in various skin sites. *Lasers Med Sci*. 2003;18:165-170.
21. Sommer S, Render C, Sheehan-Dare RA. Facial hirsutism treated with the normal-mode ruby laser: results of a 12-month follow-up study. *J Am Acad Dermatol*. 1999;41:974-979.
22. Lloyd JR, Mirkov M. Long-term evaluation of the long-pulsed alexandrite laser for the removal of bikini hair at shortened treatment intervals. *Dermatol Surg*. 2000;26:633-637.
23. Eremia S, Li CY, Umar SH, Newman N. Laser hair removal: long-term results with a 755 nm alexandrite laser. *Dermatol Surg*. 2001;27:920-924.
24. Nouri K, Chen H, Saghari S, Ricotti CA. Comparing 18- versus 12-mm spot size in hair removal using a Gentlease 755-nm alexandrite laser. *Dermatol Surg*. 2004;30:494-497.
25. Boss WK, Usal H, Thompson RC, Fiorillo MA. A comparison of the long-pulse and short-pulse alexandrite laser hair removal systems. *Ann Plast Surg*. 1999;42:381-384.
26. Goldberg DJ, Akhami R. Evaluation comparing multiple treatments with a 2-msec and 10-msec alexandrite laser for hair removal. *Lasers Surg Med*. 1999;25:223-228.
27. Hussain M, Polnikorn N, Goldberg DJ. Laser-assisted hair removal in Asian skin: efficacy, complications, and the effect of single versus multiple treatments. *Dermatol Surg*. 2003;29:249-247.
28. Görgü M, Aslan G, Aköz T, Erdogan B. Comparison of alexandrite laser and electrolysis for hair removal. *Dermatol Surg*. 2000;26:37-41.
29. Sadighha A, Zahed MG. Meta-analysis of hair removal laser trials. *Lasers Med Sci*. 2007;24(1):21-25 [Epub November 20, 2007].
30. Eremia S, Li C, Newman N. Laser hair removal with alexandrite versus diode laser using four treatment sessions: 1-year results. *Dermatol Surg*. 2001;27:925-930.
31. Bouzari N, Tabatabai H, Abbasi Z, Firooz A, Dowlati Y. Laser hair removal: comparison of long-pulsed Nd:YAG, long-pulsed alexandrite, and long-pulsed diode lasers. *Dermatol Surg*. 2004;30:498-502.
32. Handrick C, Alster TS. Comparison of long-pulsed diode and long-pulsed alexandrite lasers for hair removal: a long-term clinical and histologic study. *Dermatol Surg*. 2001;27:622-626.
33. Bäumler W, Scherer K, Abels C, et al. The effect of different spot sizes on the efficacy of hair removal using a long-pulse diode laser. *Dermatol Surg*. 2002;28:118-121.
34. Lou WW, Quintana AP, Geronemus RG, Grossman MC. Prospective study of hair reduction by diode laser (800 nm) with long-term follow-up. *Dermatol Surg*. 2000;26:428-434.

35. Sadick NS, Prieto VG. The use of a new diode laser for hair removal. *Dermatol Surg*. 2003;29:30-34.
36. Lorenz S, Brunnberg S, Landthaler M, Hohenleutner U. Hair removal with the long pulsed Nd:YAG Laser: a prospective study with one year follow-up. *Lasers Surg Med*. 2002;30:127-134.
37. Tanzi EL, Alster TS. Long-pulsed 1064-nm Nd:YAG laser-assisted hair removal in all skin types. *Dermatol Surg*. 2004;30:13-17.
38. Goldberg DJ, Silapunt S. Hair removal using a long-pulsed Nd:YAG laser: comparison at fluences of 50, 80, and 100 J/cm². *Dermatol Surg*. 2001;27:434-436.
39. Raulin C, Greve B, Grema H. IPL technology: a review. *Lasers Surg Med*. 2003;32:78-87.
40. Schroeter CA, Groenewegen JS, Reineke T, Neumann HA. Hair reduction using intense pulsed light source. *Dermatol Surg*. 2004;30:168-173.
41. Marayiannis KB, Vlachos SP, Savva MP, Kontoes PP. Efficacy of long- and short pulse alexandrite lasers compared with an intense pulsed light source for epilation: a study on 532 sites in 389 patients. *J Cosmet Laser Ther*. 2003;5:140-145.
42. Moreno-Arias GA, Castelo-Branco C, Ferrando J. Side-effects after IPL photodepilation. *Dermatol Surg*. 2002;28:1131-1134.
43. Goh CL. Comparative study on a single treatment response to long pulse Nd:YAG lasers and intense pulse light therapy for hair removal on skin types IV to VI – is longer wavelengths lasers preferred over shorter wavelengths lights for assisted hair removal? *J Dermatol Treat*. 2003;14:243-247.
44. Bjerring P, Cramers M, Egekvist H, Christiansen K, Troilius A. Hair reduction using a new intense pulsed light irradiator and a normal mode ruby laser. *J Cutan Laser Ther*. 2000;2:63-71.
45. McGill DJ, Hutchison C, McKenzie E, McSherry E, Mackay IR. A randomised, split-face comparison of facial hair removal with the alexandrite laser and intense pulsed light system. *Lasers Surg Med*. 2007;39(10):767-772.
46. Goldberg DJ, Marmur ES, Hussain M. Treatment of terminal and vellus non-pigmented hairs with an optical/bipolar radiofrequency energy source—with and without pre-treatment using topical aminolevulinic acid. *J Cosmet Laser Ther*. 2005; 7:25-28.
47. Yaghmai D, Garden JM, Bakus AD, Spenceri EA, Hruza GJ, Kilmer SL. Hair removal using a combination radio-frequency and intense pulsed light source. *J Cosmet Laser Ther*. 2004;6:201-207.
48. Sadick NS, Laughlin SA. Effective epilation of white and blond hair using combined radiofrequency and optical energy. *J Cosmet Laser Ther*. 2004;6:27-31.
49. Sadick NS, Shaoul J. Hair removal using a combination of conducted radiofrequency and optical energies–an 18-month follow-up. *J Cosmet Laser Ther*. 2004;6:21-26.
50. Sand M, Bechara FG, Sand D, Altmeyer P, Hoffmann K. A randomized, controlled, double-blind study evaluating melanin-encapsulated liposomes as a chromophore for laser hair removal of blond, white, and gray hair. *Ann Plast Surg*. 2007;58(5): 551-554.
51. Kontoes P, Vlachos S, Konstantinos M, Anastasia L, Myrto S. Hair induction after laser-assisted hair removal and its treatment. *J Am Acad Dermatol*. 2006;54(1):64-67 [Epub December 2, 2005].
52. Lolis MS, Marmur ES. Paradoxical effects of hair removal systems: a review. *J Cosmet Dermatol*. 2006;5(4):274-276.
53. Gold MH. Lasers and light sources for the removal of unwanted hair. *Clin Dermatol*. 2007;25:443-453.
54. Akinturk S, Eroglu A. Effect of piroxicam gel for pain control and inflammation in Nd:YAG 1064-nm laser hair removal. *J Eur Acad Dermatol Venereol*. 2007;21(3):380-383.

Lasers for Resurfacing

Rungsima Wanitphakdeedecha and Tina S. Alster

- Many signs of cutaneous photodamage are amenable to treatment with a variety of ablative and non-ablative lasers, light sources, and fractional photothermolysis.
- Ablative laser skin resurfacing offers the most substantial clinical improvement, but is associated with several weeks of postoperative recovery.
- Severe side effects and complications after ablative laser skin resurfacing can be minimized by careful patient selection, proper surgical technique, and meticulous postoperative care.
- Non-ablative laser skin remodeling is a good alternative for patients who desire modest improvement of photodamaged skin without significant post-treatment recovery.
- The noninvasive nature of fractional photothermolysis treatment, coupled with an excellent side effect profile, makes it an attractive alternative to ablative laser techniques.
- Good candidates for non-ablative laser and light-source treatments are patients with cutaneous photodamage and realistic clinical expectations.
- With ongoing advancements in laser technology and techniques, improved clinical outcomes with minimal postoperative recovery will be realized.

Introduction

- A wide variety of lasers and light-based sources is available to treat cutaneous photodamage including ablative and non-ablative lasers, light sources, and fractional photothermolysis.

Years of damaging ultraviolet (UV) light exposure manifests clinically as a sallow complexion with roughened surface texture and variable degrees of dyspigmentation, telangiectasias, wrinkling, and skin laxity.[1,2] Histologically, these extrinsic aging effects are usually limited to the epidermis and upper papillary dermis and are therefore amenable to treatment with a variety of ablative and non-ablative lasers and light-sources.[3]

History of Procedures

- Selective photothermolysis theory of laser-tissue interaction is used to create thermal destruction of target tissue without unwanted conduction of heat to surrounding structures by selecting the appropriate laser wavelength and pulse duration.
- The first system specifically developed for cutaneous laser resurfacing was the pulsed carbon dioxide (CO_2) laser.
- The short-pulsed erbium:yttrium–aluminum–garnet (Er:YAG) laser was subsequently used as an alternative to the CO_2 laser to minimize the recovery period and limit side effects while maintaining clinical benefit.

R. Wanitphakdeedecha (✉)
Department of Dermatology, Faculty of Medicine Siriraj Hospital,
Mahidol University, Bangkok, Thailand
e-mail: sirwn@mahidol.ac.th

K. Nouri (ed.), *Lasers in Dermatology and Medicine*,
DOI: 10.1007/978-0-85729-281-0_9, © Springer-Verlag London Limited 2011

Although dermatologic laser surgery is nearly five decades old, the field was revolutionized in 1983 when Anderson and Parrish elucidated the principles of selective photo-thermolysis.[4] This basic theory of laser-tissue interaction explains how selective tissue destruction is possible. In order to effect precise thermal destruction of target tissue without unwanted conduction of heat to surrounding structures, the proper laser wavelength must be selected for preferential absorption by the intended tissue chromophore. Furthermore, the pulse duration of laser emission must be shorter than the thermal relaxation time of the target–thermal relaxation time (T_R) being defined as the amount of time necessary for the targeted structure to cool to one-half of its peak temperature immediately after laser irradiation. The delivered fluence (energy density) must also be sufficiently high to cause the desired degree of thermal injury to the skin. Thus, the laser wavelength, pulse duration, and fluence each must be carefully chosen to achieve maximal target ablation while minimizing surrounding tissue damage.

The first system specifically developed for cutaneous laser resurfacing was the pulsed carbon dioxide (CO_2) laser, which was approved by the Food and Drug Administration (FDA) in 1996. Earlier CO_2 systems were continuous-wave (CW) lasers which were effective for gross lesional destruction,[5,6] but were unable to reliably ablate fine layers of tissue because of excessive tissue heating which produced unacceptably high rates of scarring and pigmentary alteration.[7-9] The unpredictable nature of the CW lasers prevented their widespread use in facial resurfacing procedures. With the subsequent development of high-energy, pulsed lasers it became possible to safely apply higher energy densities with exposure times that were shorter than the thermal relaxation time of water-containing tissue, thus lowering the risk of thermal injury to surrounding non-targeted structures.[3,10]

The short-pulsed erbium:yttrium–aluminum–garnet (Er:YAG) laser was subsequently FDA-approved for cutaneous resurfacing as an alternative to the CO_2 laser in an attempt to minimize the recovery period and limit side effects while maintaining clinical benefit.

In response to growing public interest in minimally-invasive treatment modalities, non-ablative laser and light source technology was later developed. Rapid advances in non-ablative technology have produced several lasers and light-based sources capable of improving fine facial rhytides, dyspigmentation, and telangiectasia associated with cutaneous photodamage.

The armamentarium of lasers and light-based sources currently available to treat cutaneous photodamage is larger than ever before (Table 1). The most appropriate technique depends upon the severity of photodamage and rhytides, the

Table 1 Lasers and light sources for skin resurfacing

	Laser type	Wavelength (nm)
Ablative	CO_2 (pulsed)	10,600
	Er:YAG (pulsed)	2,940
Non-ablative	Pulsed dye	585–595
	Nd:YAG, Q-switched	1,064
	Nd:YAG, long-pulsed	1,320
	Diode, long-pulsed	1,450
	Er:glass, long-pulsed	1,540
	Intense pulsed light source	515–1,200
Fractional	Er-doped fiber	1,550

Er erbium, *Nd* neodymium, *Q-switched* quality-switched, *YAG* yttrium–aluminum–garnet

expertise of the laser surgeon, and the expectations and lifestyle of the individual patient.

Ablative Laser Skin Resurfacing

Indications and Contraindications

- Indications
  - Mild-to-moderate rhytides, preferably in non-movement-associated areas.
  - Other signs of photodamage (e.g., dyspigmentation and keratoses).
  - Shallow atrophic scars.
  - Superficial skin lesions.
- Contraindications
  - Patients with unrealistic expectations.
  - Patients with perpetual sun exposure.
  - Active bacterial, viral, fungal infection or inflammatory skin conditions involving the skin areas to be treated.
  - Patients with prior lower blepharoplasties using an external approach are at greater risk of ectropion formation after infraorbital ablative laser treatment.
  - Patients with darker skin tones (skin phototype IV–VI) have a high incidence of postoperative hyperpigmentation.
  - Concomitant isotretinoin use could potentially lead to an increased risk of hypertrophic scarring.
  - Patients with a propensity to scar will be at greater risk for postoperative scarring.

Lasers for Resurfacing

Table 2 Ablative laser resurfacing: patient selection, risks, and precautions

Preoperative patient evaluation
• Are the lesions amenable to ablative laser skin resurfacing? All suspicious lesions require biopsy before treatment
• Has the patient ever had the areas treated before? Ablative laser resurfacing can unmask hypopigmentation or fibrosis produced by prior dermabrasion, cryosurgery, or phenol peels. Patients with prior lower blepharoplasties using an external approach are at greater risk of ectropion formation after infraorbital ablative laser treatment
• What is the patient's skin phototype? Patients with paler skin tones (skin phototype I or II) have a lower incidence of postoperative hyperpigmentation than do patients with darker skin tones
• Does the patient have a history of herpes labialis? All patients should be treated with prophylactic antiviral medication before perioral treatment, because reactivation and/or dissemination of prior herpes simplex infection can occur. The de-epithelialized skin is also particularly susceptible to primary inoculation by herpes simplex virus
• Does the patient have an autoimmune disease or other immunologic deficiency? Intact immunologic function and collagen repair mechanisms are necessary to optimize the tissue-healing response due to the prolonged recovery associated with ablative resurfacing
• Is the patient taking any medications that are contraindicated? Concomitant isotretinoin use could potentially lead to an increased risk of postoperative hypertrophic scar formation due to its detrimental effect on wound healing and collagenesis. A safe interval between the use of oral retinoids and ablative laser skin resurfacing is difficult to determine; however, most advocate a delay in treatment for at least 6 months after discontinuation of the drug
• Does the patient have a tendency to form hypertrophic scars or keloids? Patients with a propensity to scar will be at greater risk of scar formation after treatment, independent of the laser's selectivity and the operator's expertise
• Does the patient have realistic expectations of the procedure and adhere to postoperative instructions? Patients who cannot physically or emotionally handle the prolonged postoperative course should be dissuaded from pursuing ablative laser skin treatment

The ideal patient for ablative laser skin resurfacing has a fair complexion (skin phototype I or II), exhibits cutaneous lesions that are amenable to treatment, and has realistic expectations of the resurfacing procedure. Adequate preoperative patient evaluation and education are absolute essentials to avoid pitfalls and optimize the clinical outcome (Table 2). Proper patient selection is paramount as ablative laser resurfacing can be complicated by a prolonged postoperative recovery, pigmentary alteration, or unexpected scarring. The patient's emotional ability to tolerate an extended convalescence is an important factor in determining the most appropriate choice of laser. Although CO_2 and modulated Er:YAG lasers often produce the most dramatic clinical results, some patients may be unable to tolerate the intensive recovery period. For patients unable or unwilling to withstand extended postoperative healing, a short-pulsed Er:YAG laser or application of a non-ablative or fractional laser procedure may be a more suitable choice.

Techniques

Preoperative Management

> • Adequate preoperative patient evaluation and education.
> • Oral antibiotic prophylaxis as indicated.

There is no consensus among laser experts regarding the most appropriate preoperative regimen for ablative laser skin resurfacing. The use of topical retinoic acid compounds, hydroquinone bleaching agents, or α-hydroxy acids for several weeks before laser treatment has been touted as a means of speeding recovery and decreasing the incidence of postinflammatory hyperpigmentation.[11] Topical tretinoin enhances penetration of chemicals through the skin and has been shown to accelerate postoperative re-epithelialization after dermabrasion or deep chemical peels.[12] However, because ablative laser-induced wounds are intrinsically different from those created by physically destructive methods, laser skin penetration is not typically affected by the topical application of any of these medications. In addition, being that postinflammatory hyperpigmentation is relatively common after ablative cutaneous laser resurfacing, many laser surgeons originally believed that the prophylactic use of topical bleaching agents would reduce the incidence of this side effect, but investigators subsequently demonstrated that the preoperative use of topical tretinoin, hydroquinone, or glycolic acid had no effect on the incidence of postablative laser hyperpigmentation.[13]

Due to the moist, de-epithelialized state of ablative laser-resurfaced skin and the possibility of bacterial contamination and overgrowth, many laser surgeons advocate oral antibiotic prophylaxis; however, this practice remains controversial due to the results of a controlled study that demonstrated no significant change in post-laser resurfacing infection rate in patients treated with prophylactic antibiotics.[14] The most common infectious complication is a reactivation of labial herpes simplex virus (HSV), most likely caused by the thermal tissue injury and epidermal disruption produced by the laser.[15,16] Any patient undergoing full-face or perioral ablative resurfacing should receive antiviral prophylaxis even when a history of HSV is denied. It is impossible to predict who will develop HSV reactivation, because a negative cold sore history is an unreliable method to determine risk and many patients do not remember having had an outbreak or are asymptomatic HSV carriers. Oral antiviral agents, such as acyclovir, famciclovir, and valacyclovir are effective agents against HSV infection, although severe (disseminated) cases may require intravenous therapy. Patients should begin prophylaxis by the day of surgery and continue for 7–10 days postoperatively.

Description of the Technique

Carbon Dioxide (CO_2) Laser

> * Areas with thinner skin (e.g., periorbital) require fewer laser passes.
> * Non-facial (e.g., neck, chest) areas should be avoided due to paucity of pilosebaceous units with diminished capacity for re-epithelialization.
> * Avoidance of pulse stacking in order to decrease risk of scarring.

The Ultrapulse (Lumenis Corp, Yokeam, Israel), one of the first high-energy, pulsed CO_2 laser systems developed, emits individual high energy pulses (peak energy densities of 500 mJ in 600 μs–1 ms). Its earliest competitor, the SilkTouch (Lumenis Corp, Yokeam, Israel), was a continuous-wave CO_2 system with a microprocessor scanner that continuously moved the laser beam so that light did not dwell on any one area for more than 1 ms. The peak fluences delivered per pulse or scan ranged from 4 to 5 J/cm^2, which were the energy densities determined to be necessary for complete tissue vaporization.[7,17-19] Studies with these and other pulsed or scanned CO_2 laser systems showed that after a typical skin resurfacing procedure, water-containing tissue was vaporized to a depth of approximately 20–60 μm, producing a zone of thermal damage ranging 20–150 μm.[7,18,20-22]

The depth of ablation correlates directly with the number of passes performed and usually is confined to the epidermis and upper papillary dermis; however, stacking of laser pulses by treating an area with multiple passes in rapid succession or by using a high overlap setting on a scanning device can lead to excessive thermal injury with subsequent increased risk of scarring.[15,23,24] An ablative plateau is reached with less

effective tissue ablation and accumulation of thermal injury. This effect is most likely caused by reduced tissue water content after initial desiccation, resulting in less selective absorption of energy.[24] The avoidance of pulse stacking and incomplete removal of partially desiccated tissue is paramount to prevention of excessive thermal accumulation with any laser system.

The objective of ablative laser skin resurfacing is to vaporize tissue to the papillary dermis. Limiting the depth of penetration decreases the risk for scarring and permanent pigmentary alteration. When choosing treatment parameters, the surgeon must consider factors such as the anatomic location to be resurfaced, the skin phototype of the patient, and previous treatments delivered to the area.[17,25] In general, areas with thinner skin (e.g., periorbital) require fewer laser passes and non-facial (e.g., neck, chest) laser resurfacing should be avoided due to the relative paucity of pilosebaceous units in these areas.[25] To reduce the risk of excessive thermal injury, partially desiccated tissue should be removed manually with wet gauze after each laser pass to expose the underlying dermis.[24]

The clinical and histologic benefits of cutaneous laser resurfacing are numerous. With the CO_2 laser, most studies have shown at least a 50% improvement over baseline in overall skin tone and wrinkle severity (Fig. 1a, b).[10,26-30] The biggest advantages associated with CO_2 laser skin resurfacing are the excellent tissue contraction, hemostasis, prolonged neocollagenesis and collagen remodeling that it provides. Histologic examination of laser-treated skin demonstrates replacement of epidermal cellular atypia and dyplasia with normal, healthy epidermal cells from adjacent follicular adnexal structures.[7,21] The most profound effects occur in the papillary dermis, where coagulation of disorganized masses of actinically-induced elastotic material are replaced with normal compact collagen bundles arranged in parallel to the skin's surface.[31,32] Immediately after CO_2 laser treatment, a normal inflammatory response is initiated, with granulation tissue formation, neovascularization, and increased production of macrophages and fibroblasts.[21]

Persistent collagen shrinkage and dermal remodeling are responsible for much of the continued clinical benefits observed after CO_2 resurfacing and are influenced by several factors.[33,34] Thermal effects of laser irradiation of skin produce collagen fiber contraction at temperatures ranging from 55°C to 62°C through disruption of interpeptide bonds resulting in a conformational change to the collagen's basic triple helical structure.[35,36] The collagen molecule is thereby shortened to approximately one third of its normal length. The laser-induced shrinkage of collagen fibers may act as the contracted scaffold for neocollagenesis, leading to subsequent production of the newly shortened form. In turn, fibroblasts that migrate into laser

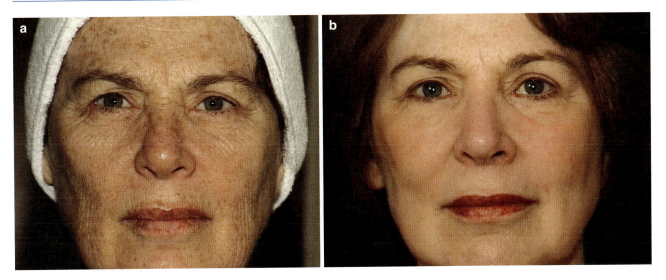

Fig. 1 CO_2 laser resurfacing (**a**) before and (**b**) after

wounds after resurfacing may up-regulate the expression of immune modulating factors that serve to enhance continued collagen shrinkage.[37]

The CO_2 resurfacing laser is a most effective tool for improving photo-induced facial rhytides; however, dynamic rhytides are not as amenable to laser treatment. Many patients experience recurrence of movement-associated rhytides (particularly in the glabellar region) within 6–12 months postoperatively. Thus, cosmetic denervation with intramuscular injections of botulinum toxin type A is often used concomitantly with laser resurfacing to provide prolonged clinical improvement.[38]

Absolute contraindications to CO_2 laser skin resurfacing include active bacterial, viral, or fungal infection or an inflammatory skin condition involving the skin areas to be treated. Isotretinoin use within the preceding 6–month period or history of keloids also are considered contraindications to CO_2 laser treatment because of the unpredictable tissue healing response and greater risk for scarring.[39,40]

In an attempt to address many of the difficulties associated with the use of multiple-pass CO_2 laser skin resurfacing, refinements in surgical technique were subsequently developed. Single-pass CO_2 laser treatment was shown to effect faster re-epithelialization and an improved side effect profile.[41] Rather than remove partially desiccated tissue (as was typical with multiple-pass procedures), the lased skin was left intact to serve as a biologic wound dressing. Additional laser passes could then be applied focally in areas with more severe photodamage in order to limit unnecessary thermal and mechanical trauma to uninvolved skin. Subsequent reports have substantiated the improved side effect profile of this less aggressive procedure.[42-44]

Erbium:Yttrium–Aluminum–Garnet (Er:YAG) Laser

- Typical fluences range from 5 to 15 J/cm^2, depending on the degree of photodamage and anatomic location.
- When lower fluences are applied, it is often necessary to perform multiple passes to ablate the entire epidermis.
- Shorter pulse durations are used for tissue ablation and longer pulses are used to effect coagulation and expand zones of thermal injury.

The Er:YAG laser is a more ablative tool that emits light at 2,940 nm, corresponding well to the 3,000 nm absorption peak of water. The absorption coefficient of the Er:YAG is 12,800 cm^{-1} (compared with 800 cm^{-1} for the CO_2 laser), making it 12–18 times more efficiently absorbed by water-containing tissue than is the CO_2 laser.[45] The pulse duration (averaging 250 μs) is also much shorter than that of the CO_2 laser, resulting in decreased thermal diffusion, less effective hemostasis, and increased intraoperative bleeding which can hamper deeper dermal treatment. Because of limited thermal skin injury, the amount of collagen contraction is also reduced with Er:YAG treatment (1–4%) compared to that observed with CO_2 laser irradiation.[11,46]

The erbium's efficient rate of absorption, short exposure duration, and direct relationship between fluence delivered and amount of tissue ablated leads to 2–4 μm of tissue vaporization per Joule per square centimeter, producing a shallow level of tissue ablation. Much narrower zones of thermal necrosis, averaging only 20–50 μm, are therefore produced.[45,47-49] Laser-induced ejection of desiccated tissue from the target site typically produces a distinctive popping sound. Thermal energy is confined to the selected tissue, with minimal collateral thermal damage. Because little tissue necrosis is produced with each pass of the laser, manual removal of desiccated tissue is often unnecessary.

The short-pulsed erbium laser fluences used most often range from 5 to 15 J/cm², depending on the degree of photodamage and anatomic location. When lower fluences are used, it is often necessary to perform multiple passes to ablate the entire epidermis. The ablation depth with the short-pulsed Er:YAG does not diminish with successive passes, because the amount of thermal necrosis is minimal with each pass. It takes three to four times as many passes with the short-pulsed Er:YAG laser to achieve similar depths of penetration as with one pass of the CO_2 laser at typical treatment parameters.[3,11] To ablate the entire epidermis with the short-pulsed Er:YAG laser at 5 J/cm², at least two or three passes must be used which increases the possibility of uneven tissue penetration. Deeper dermal lesions or areas of the face with extreme photodamage and extensive dermal elastosis may require up to nine or ten passes of the short-pulsed Er:YAG laser, whereas the CO_2 laser would effect similar levels of tissue ablation in two or three passes.[7,18,45]

Pinpoint bleeding caused by inadequate hemostasis and tissue color change with multiple Er:YAG passes can impede adequate clinical assessment of wound depth. Irradiated areas whiten immediately after treatment and then quickly fade. These factors renders far more difficult for the surgeon to determine treatment endpoints and thus requires extensive knowledge of laser–tissue interaction.

Conditions amenable to short-pulsed Er:YAG laser resurfacing include superficial epidermal or dermal lesions, mild photodamage and subtle dyspigmentation. The major advantage of short-pulsed Er:YAG laser treatment is its shorter recovery period. Re-epithelialization is completed within an average of 5.5 days, compared with 8.5 days for multiple-pass CO_2 procedures.[18,47] Postoperative pain and duration of erythema are reduced after short-pulsed Er:YAG laser resurfacing, with postoperative erythema resolving within 3–4 weeks. Because there is less thermal injury and trauma to the skin, the risk of pigmentary disturbance is also decreased, making the short-pulsed Er:YAG laser a good alternative in patients with darker skin phototypes.[3,50] The major disadvantages of the short-pulsed Er:YAG laser are its limited ability to effect significant collagen shrinkage and its failure to induce new and continued collagen formation postoperatively.[3,47,51] The final clinical result is typically less impressive than that produced by CO_2 laser skin resurfacing for deeper rhytides. However, for mild photodamage, improvement of approximately 50% is typical (Fig. 2a, b). Although clinical and histologic effects are less impressive than those produced with the CO_2 laser, short-pulsed Er:YAG laser skin resurfacing still affords modest improvement of photodamaged skin with a shorter recovery time.[17,47]

To address the limitations of the short-pulsed Er:YAG laser, modulated Er:YAG lasers systems were developed to improve hemostasis and increase the amount of collagen shrinkage and remodeling effected. The Er:YAG–CO_2 hybrid laser system delivers both ablative Er:YAG and coagulative CO_2 laser pulses. The Er:YAG component generates fluences up to 28 J/cm² with a 350 μs pulse duration, while excellent hemostasis is provided by the CO_2 component which can be programmed to deliver 1–100 ms pulses at 1–10 W power. Zones

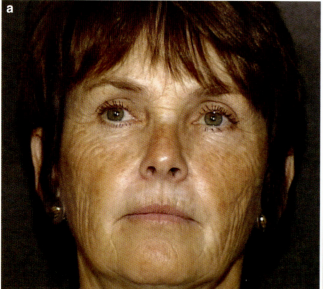 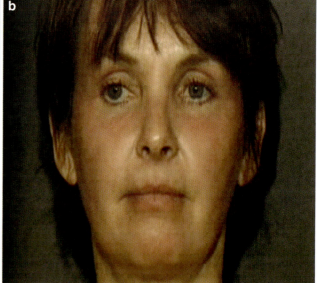

Fig. 2 Erbium:YAG laser resurfacing (**a**) before and (**b**) after

of thermal necrosis measuring as much as 50 μm have been observed depending on the treatment parameters used and significant increase in collagen thickness has been noted 3 months after four passes with this hybrid technology.[52] Another modulated Er:YAG device is a dual-mode Er:YAG laser that emits a combination of short (200–300 μs) pulses and long coagulative pulses to achieve tissue ablation depths of up to 200 μm per pass. The output from the two Er:YAG laser heads are combined into a single stream in a process called optical multiplexing.[53] The desired depth of ablation and coagulation can be programmed by the laser surgeon into the touch-screen control panel. Several investigators have studied the histologic effects of dual-mode Er:YAG laser resurfacing and found a close correlation between the programmed and actual measured depths of ablation.[54,55] The actual zones of thermal injury correlate well to the first pass with decreasing coagulative efficiency on subsequent passes. The variable-pulsed Er:YAG laser system delivers pulse durations ranging 500 μs–10 ms. Shorter pulse durations are used for tissue ablation and longer pulses are used to effect coagulation and zones of thermal injury similar to the CO_2 laser.[53,56]

Since the modulated Er:YAG lasers were developed to produce a greater thermal effect and tissue contraction than their short-pulsed predecessors, investigators compared collagen tightening induced by the CO_2 laser with that of the CO_2–Er:YAG hybrid laser system.[57] Intraoperative contraction of approximately 43% was produced after three passes of the CO_2 laser, compared with 12% contraction following Er:YAG irradiation. At 4 weeks; however, the CO_2 and Er:YAG laser treated sites were contracted to the same degree, highlighting the different mechanisms of tissue tightening observed after laser treatment. Immediate thermal-induced collagen tightening was the predominant response seen after CO_2 irradiation, whereas modulated Er:YAG laser resurfacing did not produce immediate intraoperative contraction but instead induced slow collagen tightening.[53,57]

Postoperative Management

- During the re-epithelialization process, an open- or closed-wound technique can be used.
- Ice pack application, anti-inflammatory and pain medications should be prescribed.
- Early recognition and treatment of side effects (e.g., topical bleaching creams for hyperpigmentation).

Wound care during the immediate postoperative period is vital to the successful recovery of ablative laser-resurfaced skin. During the re-epithelialization process, an open- or closed-wound technique can be prescribed. Partial-thickness cutaneous wounds heal more efficiently and with a reduced risk of scarring when maintained in a moist environment because the presence of a dry crust or scab impedes keratinocyte migration.[58] Although there is consensus on this principle, disagreement exists regarding the optimal dressing for the laser-ablated wound. The "open" technique involves frequent application of a thick healing ointment to the de-epithelialized skin surface; whereas occlusive or semi-occlusive dressings are placed directly on the lased skin in the "closed" technique. While the open technique facilitates easy wound visualization, the closed technique requires less patient involvement and may also decrease postoperative pain. Proposed advantages of a closed wound care regimen include increased patient comfort, decreased erythema and edema, increased rate of re-epithelialization, and decreased patient involvement in wound management.[58,59] On the other hand, additional expense and a higher risk of infection have been associated with the use of these dressings.[3,60,61]

In addition to postoperative wound care, ice pack application and anti-inflammatory medications should be prescribed during this time. Furthermore, pain medication is particularly important for ablative laser-resurfaced patients during the first few postoperative days.

Adverse Events

- Side Effects/Complications
  - Mild: Prolonged erythema, milia, acne, contact dermatitis.
  - Moderate: Infection (bacterial, viral, fungal), hyperpigmentation.
  - Severe: Hypopigmentation, hypertrophic scarring, ectropion.
- Prevention and Treatment
  - Adequate preoperative patient evaluation and education are absolute essentials to avoid pitfalls and optimize clinical outcomes.
  - Preoperative examination to determine eyelid skin laxity/elasticity to prevent ectropion.
  - Avoidance of pulse stacking, scan overlapping, and incomplete removal of partially desiccated tissue to prevent hypertrophic scarring.
  - Topical agents such as retinoic acid derivatives, glycolic acid, salicylic acid, fragrance-containing or chemical-containing cosmetics and sunscreens should be strictly avoided in the early postoperative period until substantial healing has occurred.

- Oral antibiotics may be prescribed for acne flares that do not respond to topical preparations.
- Any patient undergoing full-face or perioral ablative resurfacing should receive antiviral prophylaxis, even if a history of HSV is denied.
- Postinflammatory hyperpigmentation can be hastened with the postoperative use of a variety of topical agents, including hydroquinone, retinoic, azeleic, and glycolic acid.
- Regular sunscreen use is important during the healing process to prevent further skin darkening.

Side effects associated with ablative laser skin resurfacing vary and are related to the expertise of the laser surgeon, the body area treated, and the skin phototype of the patient (Table 3). Certain tissue reactions, such as erythema and edema, are expected in the immediate postoperative period and are not considered adverse events. Erythema can be intense and may persist for several months after the procedure. The degree of erythema correlates directly with the depth of ablation and the number of laser passes performed.[3,16] It may also be aggravated by underlying rosacea or dermatitis. Postoperative erythema resolves spontaneously but can be reduced with the application of topical ascorbic acid which may serve to decrease the degree of inflammation.[62,63] Its use should be reserved for at least 4 weeks after the procedure in order to avoid irritation. Similarly, other topical agents such as retinoic acid derivatives, glycolic acid, fragrance-containing or chemical-containing cosmetics and sunscreens should be strictly avoided in the early postoperative period until substantial healing has occurred.[16] Adequate preoperative patient evaluation and education are absolute essentials to avoid pitfalls and to optimize clinical outcomes.

Mild side effects of laser resurfacing include milia formation and acne exacerbation which may be caused by the use of occlusive dressings and ointments during the postoperative period, particularly in patients who are prone to

acne.[15,16,25,60] Milia and acne usually resolve spontaneously as healing progresses and the application of thick emollient creams and occlusive dressings ceases. Oral antibiotics may be prescribed for acne flares that do not respond to topical preparations.[16,30,60] Contact allergies, irritant or allergic, can also develop from various topical medications, soaps, and moisturizers used postoperatively. Most of these reactions are irritant in nature due to decreased barrier function of the newly resurfaced skin.[16,64]

Wound infections associated with ablative laser resurfacing include *Staphylococcus*, *Pseudomonas*, or cutaneous candidiasis and should be treated aggressively with an appropriate systemic antibiotic or antifungal agent.[61] The use of prophylactic antibiotics remains controversial.[14] After CO_2 resurfacing, approximately 7% of patients develop a localized or disseminated form of HSV.[16] These infections develop within the first postoperative week and can present as erosions without intact vesicles because of the denuded condition of newly lased skin. Even with appropriate prophylaxis, a herpetic outbreak still can occur in up to 10% of patients and must be treated aggressively.[17] In order to prevent this complication, patients should begin prophylaxis by the day of surgery and continue for 7–10 days postoperatively.

The most severe complications associated with ablative cutaneous laser resurfacing include hypertrophic scar and ectropion formation.[15,16] Although the risk of scarring has been significantly reduced with pulsed laser technology (compared to the continuous wave systems), inadvertent pulse stacking or scan overlapping, as well as incomplete removal of desiccated tissue between laser passes can cause excessive thermal injury that could increase the development of fibrosis. Focal areas of bright erythema, with pruritus, particularly along the mandible, may signal impending scar formation.[25,65] Ultrapotent (class I) topical corticosteroid preparations should be applied to decrease the inflammatory response. A pulsed dye laser also can be used to improve the appearance and symptoms of laser-induced burn scars.[65]

Ectropion of the lower eyelid after periorbital laser skin resurfacing is rarely seen, but if encountered, usually requires surgical correction.[25] It is more likely to occur in patients who have had previous lower blepharoplasty or other surgical manipulation of the periorbital region. Preoperative examination is essential to determine eyelid laxity and skin elasticity. If the infraorbital skin does not return briskly to its normal resting position after a manual downward pull (snap test), then ablative laser treatment near the lower eyelid margin should be avoided. In general, lower fluences and fewer laser passes should be applied in the periorbital area to decrease the risk of lid eversion.

Hyperpigmentation is one of the more common side effects of cutaneous laser resurfacing and occurs to some degree in all patients with darker skin tones (Fig. 3).[16,25] The reaction is transient, but its resolution can be hastened with

Table 3 Side effects and complications of ablative laser skin resurfacing

Expected side effects	Complications		
	Mild	Moderate	Severe
Erythema	Prolonged erythema	Infection (bacterial, viral, fungal)	Permanent hypopigmentation
Edema	Milia	Transient hyperpigmentation	Hypertrophic scarring
Pruritus	Acne Dermatitis		Ectropion

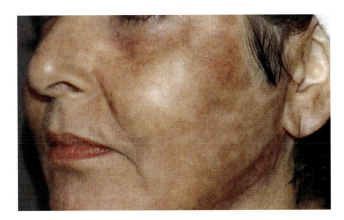

Fig. 3 Postinflammatory hyperpigmention following ablative laser resurfacing

the postoperative use of a variety of topical agents, including hydroquinone, retinoic, azeleic, and glycolic acid. Regular sunscreen use is also important during the healing process to prevent further skin darkening. The prophylactic use of these products preoperatively, however, has not been shown to decrease the incidence of post-treatment hyperpigmentation.[13] Postoperative hypopigmentation, on the other hand, is often not observed for several months and is particularly difficult because of its tendency to be intractable to treatment. The use of an excimer laser or topical photochemotherapy to stimulate repigmentation has proven successful in some patients.[66,67]

Side effects and complications following Er:YAG laser irradiation are similar to those observed after CO_2 laser treatment, but they differ in respect to duration, incidence, and severity.[50,68,69] Although greater postoperative erythema is seen after modulated Er:YAG laser treatment than is usually produced with a short-pulsed Er:YAG system, the side effect profile and recovery period after modulated Er:YAG laser irradiation remain more favorable than after multiple-pass CO_2 laser treatment. In an extended evaluation of 50 patients, investigators reported complete re-epithelialization in an average of 5 days after dual-mode Er:YAG laser skin resurfacing with only three patients having prolonged erythema beyond 4 weeks.[68] In a split-face comparison of 16 patients after pulsed CO_2 and variable-pulsed Er:YAG laser skin resurfacing, other investigators reported decreased erythema, less edema, and faster healing on the Er:YAG laser-treated facial half.[70]

Postinflammatory hyperpigmentation is not uncommon after any cutaneous laser resurfacing procedure. While hyperpigmentation following modulated Er:YAG laser skin resurfacing (mean, 10.4 weeks) can last longer than after treatment with a short-pulsed Er:YAG laser, it is not as persistent as that observed after multiple-pass CO_2 laser resurfacing (mean, 16 weeks).[69] However, when comparing the most current trends in ablative cutaneous laser resurfacing – *single*-pass CO_2 versus multiple-pass, long-pulsed Er:YAG laser skin resurfacing – postoperative healing times and complication profiles are comparable, even in patients with darker skin phototypes. In a retrospective review and analysis of 100 consecutive patients, Tanzi and Alster[44] showed average time to re-epithelialization was 5.5 days with single-pass CO_2 and 5.1 days with long-pulsed Er:YAG laser resurfacing. Postoperative erythema was observed in all patients, lasting an average of 4.5 weeks after single-pass CO_2 laser treatment and 3.6 weeks after long-pulsed Er:YAG laser treatment. Hyperpigmentation was seen in 46% of patients treated with single-pass CO_2 and 42% of patients treated with the long-pulsed Er:YAG laser (average duration 12.7 and 11.4 weeks, respectively). Delayed-onset permanent hypopigmentation – a serious complication that has been observed several months after multiple-pass CO_2 laser skin resurfacing – has not yet been reported following single-pass treatment. To date, only three cases of hypopigmentation after modulated Er:YAG laser skin resurfacing have been reported.[71,72] Since it is possible for hypopigmentation to present several years postoperatively, clinical studies are ongoing to determine its true incidence following either single-pass CO_2 or modulated Er:YAG laser skin resurfacing.

Non-ablative Laser Skin Resurfacing

Indications and Contraindications

- Indications
  - Mild facial rhytides, atrophic scars, and photo damage.
- Contraindications
  - Patients with unrealistic expectations.
  - Patients with darker skin tones (skin phototype IV–VI) have a high incidence of postoperative hyperpigmentation.
  - Patients with perpetual sun exposure.
  - Patients with history of herpes labialis may require prophylactic oral antiviral medications.

Proper patient selection is critical to the success of non-ablative laser skin remodeling. Patients with mild-to-moderate facial photodamage or atrophic scars with realistic expectations of treatment are the best candidates for non-ablative procedures. Patients seeking immediate improvement in photodamaged skin or those who desire a dramatic result may be less than satisfied with the overall clinical outcome.

Techniques

Preoperative Management

> - Adequate preoperative patient evaluation and education.
> - Oral antiviral prophylaxis in patients with history of herpes labialis.

Adequate preoperative patient evaluation and education are absolute essentials (Table 4). For patients with a strong history of herpes labialis, prophylactic oral antiviral medications should be considered when treating the perioral skin. Reactivation of prior herpes simplex infection can occur after non-ablative laser treatment due to the intense heat produced by the laser or light source.

Prior to non-ablative laser procedures, sun exposure should be avoided, particularly when using shorter-wavelength systems such as the pulsed dye laser or intense pulsed-light source. Unwanted absorption of irradiation by activated epidermal melanocytes can increase the risk of side effects, including crusting, blistering, and dyspigmentation.

Description of the Technique

> - Infrared light (1,000–1,500 nm) creates a dermal wound without epidermal injury.
> - Epidermis is preserved during treatment by tissue cooling.

Most of the non-ablative laser systems emit light within the infrared portion of the electromagnetic spectrum (1,000–1,500 nm). At these wavelengths, absorption by superficial water-containing tissue is relatively weak, thereby effecting deeper tissue penetration.[73] Since non-ablative remodeling involves creation of a dermal wound without epidermal injury, all of these laser systems employ unique methods to ensure epidermal preservation during treatment. These methods typically include contact cooling handpieces or dynamic cryogen devices capable of delivering variable duration spray cooling spurts either before, during, and/or after laser irradiation. Since laser beam penetration and dermal wounding must be targeted to the relatively superficial portion of the dermis, contact cooling devices that theoretically lead to excessive dermal cooling may affect the level or degree of energy deposition in the skin. As such, there remains no general consensus concerning which method of cooling is most efficacious during treatment.

In general, treatment of facial photodamage with non-ablative technology does not produce results comparable to those of ablative CO_2 and Er:YAG lasers; however, many patients are willing to accept modest clinical improvement in exchange for fewer associated risks and shorter recovery times.

Pulsed Dye Laser (PDL)

> - Five hundred and eighty-five nanometer and 595 nm pulsed dye laser (PDL) can reduce mild facial rhytides with few side effects.
> - Side effects include mild edema, purpura, and transient postinflammatory hyperpigmentation.

Table 4 Non-ablative laser resurfacing: patient selection, risks, and precautions

Preoperative patient evaluation
- Is the amount of photodamage amenable to non-ablative laser skin remodeling? Patients with mild-to-moderate facial photodamage are the best candidates for non-ablative procedures. Patients with severe rhytides and skin laxity may be disappointed with the overall clinical outcome
- Does the patient have a history of herpes labialis? Reactivation of prior herpes simplex infection can occur with perioral non-ablative laser skin modeling due to the intense heat produced by the laser. Patients with a strong history of herpes simplex labialis may require prophylactic oral antiviral medication to avoid a postoperative outbreak
- What is the patient's skin phototype? Although the majority of current non-ablative systems used are within the mid-infrared range of the electromagnetic spectrum and not avidly absorbed by epidermal melanin, patients with darker skin phototypes may develop postinflammatory hyperpigmentation after non-ablative treatment. This temporary reaction may develop due to inflammation created by concomitant cryogen spray epidermal cooling
- Does the patient have realistic expectations? Patients seeking immediate gratification after a single non-ablative treatment are not good candidates as clinical improvement typically occurs after multiple sequential treatments (usually three to five) and is often delayed 3–6 months after the final session. Moreover, patients seeking dramatic results following non-ablative laser skin techniques should be dissuaded from treatment as clinical improvement may be subtle

Clinical studies have demonstrated the ability of 585 and 595 nm pulsed dye laser (PDL) to reduce mild facial rhytides with few side effects.[74] The most common side effects of PDL treatment include mild edema, purpura, and transient postinflammatory hyperpigmentation. Although increased extracellular matrix proteins and types I and III collagen and procollagen have been detected after PDL treatment, the exact mechanism whereby wrinkle improvement is effected remains unknown.[75] One theory states that vascular endothelial cells damaged by the yellow laser light release mediators that stimulate fibroblasts to produce new collagen fibers.[76]

Intense Pulsed Light (IPL) Source

- The IPL source emits a broad, continuous spectrum of light in the range of 515–1,200 nm.
- Cut-off filters are used to eliminate shorter wavelengths depending on the clinical application, with shorter filters favoring heating of melanin and hemoglobin.
- Treatment is delivered by using the fluences of 30–50 J/cm^2.

Several investigators have shown successful rejuvenation of photodamaged skin after intense pulsed light (IPL) treatment.[77,78] The IPL source emits a broad, continuous spectrum of light in the range of 515–1,200 nm. Cut-off filters are used to eliminate shorter wavelengths depending on the clinical application, with shorter filters favoring heating of melanin and hemoglobin. Bitter[78] showed improvement in wrinkling, skin coarseness, irregular pigmentation, pore size, and telangiectasia in the majority of 49 patients treated with a series of IPL treatments (fluences 30–50 J/cm^2). In a retrospective review of 80 patients with skin phototypes I–IV, Weiss and colleagues[79] reported signs of photoaging, including telangiectasias and mottled pigmentation of the face, neck, and chest, improved by a series of IPL treatments. While substantial clinical improvement of dyspigmentation and telangiectasia associated with cutaneous photodamage is often seen, neocollagenesis and dermal collagen remodeling with subsequent improvement in rhytides following IPL treatment has been minimal. The effect on dermal collagen is thought to be induced by heat diffusion from the vasculature with subsequent release of inflammatory mediators stimulated by vessel heating.[80]

1,064 nm Q-Switched (QS) Neodymium:YAG (Nd:YAG) Laser

- Although absorption of energy by tissue water is relatively weak at the 1,064 nm wavelength, it was possible to achieve dermal penetrative depths that could potentially induce neocollagenesis.
- The nanosecond range pulse duration of the QS Nd:YAG laser was also determined to limit significant thermal diffusion to surrounding structures, thereby making it suitable for non-ablative rejuvenation.
- Treatment is delivered by using the fluences of 2–6 J/cm^2 with 3–7 mm spot size and pulse duration, ranging 6–20 ns.

The 1,064 nm quality-switched (QS) neodymium:YAG (Nd:YAG) laser was the first mid-infrared laser system used for non-ablative cutaneous remodeling. Although absorption of energy by tissue water is relatively weak at the 1,064 nm wavelength, it was possible to achieve dermal penetrative depths that could potentially induce neocollagenesis. The nanosecond range pulse duration of the QS Nd:YAG laser was also determined to limit significant thermal diffusion to surrounding structures, thereby making it suitable for non-ablative rejuvenation.

In 1997, Goldberg and Whitworth[81] published their experience using a 1,064 nm Nd:YAG laser for facial rhytide reduction. Eleven patients (skin phototypes I, II) with mild to moderate periorbital or perioral rhytides underwent treatment on one side of the face with a QS Nd:YAG laser at a fluence of 5.5 J/cm^2 (3 mm spot size) and CO_2 laser ablation on the contralateral side for comparison purposes. Pinpoint bleeding was used as the clinical endpoint of QS Nd:YAG treatment. Not unexpectedly, all of the CO_2-laser irradiated sites demonstrated significant rhytide improvement, whereas only three QS Nd:YAG laser-treated patients demonstrated improvement. These patients also developed prolonged post-treatment erythema (lasting up to 1 month), suggesting that the amount of dermal wounding (with subsequent collagen remodeling) was directly related to the degree of cutaneous injury. Another study using the QS Nd:YAG laser for rhytide reduction in 61 patients (242 sites) was conducted using a topical carbon solution for improved optical penetration of the 1,064 nm light.[82] Patients underwent a series of three monthly QS Nd:YAG laser treatment sessions at a fluence of 2.5 J/cm^2, 7 mm spot size, and pulse durations, ranging 6–20 ns. At least slight improvement was seen in 97% of class I rhytides and 86% of the class II rhytides. Side effects of treatment were mild and limited, including transient erythema, purpura, and postinflammatory hyperpigmentation.

Long-pulsed Nd:YAG laser treatment has more recently been advocated for skin photorejuvenation. Lee [83] evaluated a combination technique using a long-pulsed 1,064 Nd:YAG laser and long-pulsed 532 nm potassium-titanyl-phosphate (KTP) laser, both separately and combined, for non-invasive photorejuvenation in 150 patients with skin phototypes I through V. Patients treated with the combined laser approach showed at least 70% improvement in erythema and pigmentation and 30–40% improvement in fine rhytides. In the patient groups treated with monotherapy, patient satisfaction was greater with KTP laser treatment than with the Nd:YAG laser primarily due to a reduction in dyspigmentation and telangiectasias.

1,320 nm Nd:YAG Laser

- The 1,320 nm wavelength is associated with a high scattering coefficient that allows for dispersion of laser irradiation throughout the dermis.
- A thermal feedback sensor should be used intraoperatively to select appropriate treatment fluences delivered to the individual patient's cutaneous temperature, thereby maximizing dermal temperatures that effectively lead to collagen reformation.
- In order to prevent unwanted sequelae (e.g., blistering) from excessive heat production, it is imperative that epidermal temperatures be kept lower than 50°C.

A long-pulsed 1,320 nm Nd:YAG laser was the first commercially available system marketed solely for the purpose of non-ablative laser skin remodeling. The 1,320 nm wavelength is associated with a high scattering coefficient that allows for dispersion of laser irradiation throughout the dermis. Later models are capable of delivering energy densities up to 24 J/cm^2 with a pulse duration of 350 μs through a 10-mm handpiece. The 1,320 nm Nd:YAG laser handpiece contains three portals: the laser beam itself, a thermal feedback sensor that registers skin surface temperature, and a dynamic cryogen spray apparatus used for epidermal cooling. When skin surface temperatures are maintained at 40–45°C, dermal temperatures reach 60–65°C during laser irradiation, thereby effecting collagen contraction and neocollagenesis. In order to prevent unwanted sequelae (e.g., blistering) from excessive heat production, it is imperative that epidermal temperatures be kept lower than 50°C.

A series of three or more treatment sessions are scheduled at regular intervals (typically once a month) for optimal mitigation of fine rhytides.[73] Side effects of treatment are generally mild and include transient erythema and edema.

Menaker et al.[84] reported effective rhytide reduction in an early study using a prototype 1,320 nm Nd:YAG laser. Ten patients with periocular rhytides received three consecutive laser treatments at bi-weekly intervals. Triple 300 μs pulses were delivered at 100 Hz and fluence of 32 J/cm^2 with a 5 mm handpiece. Epidermal protection was achieved with application of a 20 ms cooling spray after a 10 ms preset delay. Patients were evaluated at 1 and 3 months post-treatment. Although four of the ten patients showed clinical improvement in rhytide severity by end-study, these findings were not statistically significant. Similarly, the slight homogenization of collagen noted on histology at 1 and 3 months following treatment was not statistically significant and inconsistent with the clinical findings.

In another study, Kelly et al.[85] treated 35 patients with mild, moderate, and severe rhytides using a 1,320 nm Nd:YAG laser. Three treatments were delivered at 2-week intervals using fluences ranging 28–36 J/cm^2 with a 5 mm spot size. Cryogen spray cooling was applied in 20–40 ms spurts with 10 ms delays. Patients were evaluated at 12 and 24 weeks following treatment with statistically significant improvement noted in all clinical grades after 12 weeks. Only the most severe rhytides; however, showed persistent improvement 24 weeks following treatment.

Goldberg devised two similar studies to examine the effectiveness of the 1,320 nm Nd:YAG laser for the treatment of facial rhytides. In the first study, ten patients with skin types I–II and class I–II rhytides in the periorbital, perioral, and cheek areas were treated.[86] Four treatments were administered over a 16-week period using fluences of 28–38 J/cm^2 with a 30% overlap and a 5 mm spot size. One or two laser passes were applied to achieve the treatment endpoint of mild erythema. Skin surface temperatures were limited to 40–48°C using the aforementioned dynamic cooling spray in order to provide epidermal protection, whilst effecting dermal temperatures ranging 60–70°C. Six months after treatment, two patients showed no clinical improvement, six showed "some" improvement, and two showed "substantial" improvement. This study emphasized several key points in non-ablative laser resurfacing. It suggested a thermal feedback sensor is best used intraoperatively with this technology in order for appropriate treatment fluences to be selected based upon the individual patient's cutaneous temperature, thereby maximizing dermal temperatures that effectively lead to collagen reformation. Furthermore, longer follow-up periods are usually required to fully appreciate the effect of serial treatment sessions on dermal collagen stimulation. In the second study, ten patients underwent full-face treatments with the 1,320 nm Nd:YAG laser at 3–4 week intervals.[87] As with the first study, treatment results were inconsistent – four patients showed no improvement, four showed some improvement, and two showed substantial improvement in facial rhytides and overall skin tone.

Others also studied the 1,320 nm Nd:YAG laser for treatment of facial rhytides in ten women.[88] Full-face treatment was administered to three patients, whereas two patients had periorbital treatment, and five patients received perioral treatment. Laser fluences of 30–35 J/cm^2 were delivered in triple 300 μs pulses at a repetition rate of 100 Hz. Dynamic cryogen spray cooling was used with a 30 ms spurt and a 40 ms delay between cryogen delivery and laser irradiation. A thermal sensor was also used to maintain peak surface temperatures in the range of 42–45°C in order to avoid excessive tissue heating. Treatments were administered twice a week over a period of 4 weeks for a total of eight treatment sessions. Only two out of ten patients expressed satisfaction with their final result despite clinician evaluations showing significant improvement in five of ten patients and fair improvements in another three. Moreover, there was no correlation between histologic changes and the degree of subjective clinical improvement as judged by the patients.

A more recent study by Fatemi et al.[89] demonstrated that the 1,320 nm Nd:YAG laser produced mild subclinical epidermal injury that could potentially lead to enhanced skin texture and new papillary collagen synthesis by stimulation of cytokines and other inflammatory mediators. Thus, the long-term histologic improvement seen in photodamaged skin may not be based solely on direct laser heating of collagen, but through stimulation of cytokine release by heating the superficial vasculature. In addition, the histologic findings suggested that multiple passes with fluence and cooling adjusted to a T_{max} of 45–48°C can yield improved clinical results, as compared to those specimens in which epidermal temperatures above 45°C were not achieved.

1,450 nm Diode Laser

> - The fluences ranging 10–20 J/cm^2 should be applied in a single nonoverlapping pass with 6-mm spot size.

The 1,450 nm mid-infrared wavelength diode laser targets dermal water and penetrates the skin to an approximate depth of 500 μm. This low-power laser system achieves peak powers in the 10–15 W range with relatively long pulse durations of 150–250 ms. Because of these long exposure times, epidermal cooling must be delivered in sequence during the application of laser energy in order to avoid excessive thermal buildup within the superficial layers of the skin.

Goldberg et al.[90] reported on the effects of 1,450 nm diode laser irradiation in 20 patients with class I–II rhytides. Two to four treatment sessions were delivered with 6-month follow-up evaluation. Patients were treated with laser and cryogen spray cooling on one facial half and cryogen spray cooling alone on the contralateral side. On the laser-treated facial halves, seven did not demonstrate any improvement, ten showed mild improvement, and three had moderate improvement. None of the sites treated with cryogen alone showed any improvement after 6 months. Side effects of treatment were mild and included transient erythema, edematous papules, and one case of post inflammatory hyperpigmentation persisting for 6 months. The authors concluded that the 1,450 nm diode laser was effective for treatment of mild to moderate facial rhytides with minimal morbidity. Additionally, their study demonstrated that non-ablative laser treatment alone was responsible for the clinical improvements and that the non-specific injury induced by cryogen spray cooling could not effect the changes seen.

Hardaway and colleagues[91] demonstrated statistically significant mean wrinkle improvement of 2.3 (range 0–4, with four representing severe wrinkling) at baseline to 1.8 at 6 months following a series of three 1,450 nm diode laser treatments. They concluded that although the 1,450 nm diode laser is capable of targeting dermal collagen and stimulating fibrosis, clinical improvement of rhytides was mild and did not correlate well with the degree of histologic change noted in previous studies.

In a controlled clinical and histologic study, Tanzi and Alster[92] demonstrated improvement in mild to moderate perioral or periorbital rhytides in 25 patients treated with four consecutive 1,450 nm diode laser treatments using fluences ranging 15–20 J/cm^2 with a 4 mm spot size. Peak clinical improvement was seen 6 months after the series of laser treatments. The periorbital area was more responsive to laser treatment than the perioral area – a finding consistent with results obtained using other non-ablative laser systems (Fig. 4a, b). Side effects were limited to transient erythema, edema, and postinflammatory hyperpigmentation. In a separate controlled study performed by the same group, 20 patients with transverse neck lines received three consecutive monthly treatments using a long-pulsed 1,450 nm diode laser.[93] Modest improvements in appearance and texture of the transverse neck lines was reported, as measured by blinded clinical assessments and through three-dimensional in vivo microtopography (PRIMOS Imaging System; GFM, Germany). Mean fluences of 11.6 J/cm^2 were used with a 6 mm spot size and 50 ms total cryogen.

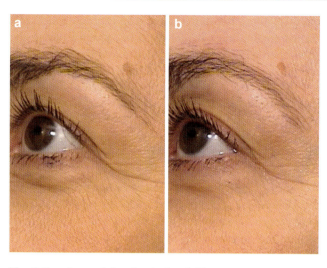

Fig. 4 One thousand four hundred and fifty nanometer long-pulsed diode laser (**a**) before and (**b**) after

Due to the marked dermal remodeling effect of the long-pulsed 1,320-nm Nd:YAG and 1,450-nm diode lasers, Tanzi and Alster[94] reported the long-term clinical and histologic results of these systems on atrophic facial acne scars in 20 patients. Facial halves were randomly assigned to received three consecutive monthly treatments with a 1,320-nm Nd:YAG laser (CoolTouch; CoolTouch Corp., Auburn, CA) on one side and a 1,450-nm diode (SmoothBeam; Candela Corp., Wayland, MA) on the contralateral. The 1,450-nm diode laser was used at fluences ranging 9–14 J/cm^2 (average 11.8 J/cm^2, 6-mm spot size) in a single nonoverlapping pass; whereas, the 1,320-nm Nd:YAG laser was used of fluences ranging 12–17 J/cm^2 (average 14.8 J/cm^2, 10-mm spot size) in two passes. Mild to moderate clinical improvement was observed in the majority of patients. Patient satisfaction scores and *in vivo* microtopography measurements paralleled the photographic and histopathologic changes seen without significant side effects or complications. The 1,450-nm diode laser showed greater clinical scar response at the parameters studied.

1,540 nm Erbium:Glass Laser

- The treatment should be performed on a monthly basis for three to five sessions using a 4 mm spot size, 10 J/cm^2 fluence, and 3.5 ms pulse duration.
- Epidermal protection was achieved with concomitant application of a contact sapphire lens cooled to 5°C.

The 1,540 nm erbium-doped phosphate glass laser is another mid-infrared range laser that has been used for amelioration of fine facial rhytides and atrophic facial scars. Similar to other infrared laser systems, the erbium:glass laser targets intracellular water and penetrates tissue to a depth of 0.4–2 mm.[73] The 1,540 nm wavelength exerts less effect on epidermal melanin as do the 1,320 and 1,450 nm lasers – a potential advantage of this system when treating tanned or darker-skinned patients. Mordon et al.[95] studied the 1,540 nm erbium:glass laser on hairless rat abdominal skin with pulse train irradiation (1.1 J, 3 Hz, 30 pulses) and varying cooling temperatures (+5°C, 0°C, −5°C). Biopsies obtained after 1, 3, and 7 days following treatment demonstrated fibroblast proliferation and new collagen synthesis as early as the third day. The authors concluded that the erbium glass system held promise for treating facial rhytides because of its high water absorption and reduced tissue scattering effect that limits energy deposition to the upper dermis where most solar elastosis is evident.

Ross et al.[96] studied the effect of the 1,540 nm erbium:glass laser with a sapphire cooling handpiece on the preauricular skin of nine patients. A 5 mm collimated beam was used to deliver fluences of 400–1,200 mJ/cm^2. Epidermal necrosis and scar formation were noted at the highest pulse energies. Several key points were illustrated by this study; namely, that denatured collagen located deep in the dermis (more than 600 μm) is associated with granuloma formation and that the peaks of heating and cooling with non-ablative laser remodeling are in proximity, by necessity, since maximum wrinkle reduction may be achieved by a zone of thermal injury 100–400 μm beneath the skin surface.

Lupton et al.[97] reported their use of a 1,540 nm erbium:glass laser to treat 24 patients with fine periorbital and perioral rhytides. Patients underwent a series of three treatments on a monthly basis using a 4 mm spot size, 10 J/cm^2 fluence, and 3.5 ms pulse duration. Epidermal protection was achieved with concomitant application of a contact sapphire lens cooled to 5°C. Histologic specimens demonstrated increased dermal fibroplasia at 6 months after the series of laser treatments. Average clinical scores were improved at 1 and 6 months following the third treatment session with slightly better results observed in the periorbital regions. Side effects of treatment were mild and included transient erythema and edema.

Fournier and colleagues[98] subsequently treated 42 patients (skin phototypes I–IV) with five consecutive 1,540 nm diode laser treatments at 6-week intervals. Patients were evaluated using clinical data, patient satisfaction surveys, digital photography, ultrasound imaging, and profilometry data from silicone imprints. The majority of patients demonstrated modest improvement in objective and subjective measurements which remained stable throughout the 14-month evaluation period.

Radiofrequency (RF) Device

- The treatment should be delivered at the fluences ranging 90–150 J/cm³ in a single, nonoverlapping pass.
- When combining treatment with other lasers or light sources, the fluences of RF can be reduced.

A monopolar radiofrequency device (ThermaCool TC; Thermage Inc, Hayward, CA) has also been studied for deep dermal heating with subsequent tightening of photodamaged skin. Unlike a laser in which light energy is converted into heat, the radiofrequency device generates electric current which produces heat through dermal resistance. The energy is delivered to the skin through a specialized treatment tip with a capacitive coupling membrane which allows for uniform delivery of heat over the entire treatment area. Epidermal protection is provided by simultaneous cryogen cooling within the contact treatment tip. Using this technique, a reverse thermal gradient is generated. The depth of heat penetration is dependent upon the size and specifics of the detachable treatment tip and can be changed according to the clinical application. Preliminary animal studies demonstrated selective dermal heating at the levels of the papillary dermis and as deep as the subcutaneous fat.[80] Ruiz-Esparza and Gomez[99] reported facial tissue tightening in 14 of 15 patients 3 months after a single radiofrequency treatment with minimal side effects.

Alster and Tanzi[100] demonstrated significant improvement in cheek and neck skin laxity in 50 patients received one treatment with a radiofrequency device (ThermaCool; Thermage Corp., Hayward, CA) at fluences ranging 97–144 J/cm³ (level of 13.6–16; average of 130 J/cm²) on the cheeks and 74–134 J/cm³ (average 110 J/cm³) on the neck in a single, nonoverlapping pass. Patient satisfaction scores paralleled the clinical improvement observed with side effects limited to transient erythema, edema, and rare dysesthesia. The tightening continued to be evident 6 months after a single treatment.

Another RF device, Polaris WR™ (Syneron Medical Ltd, Israel), which combines bipolar RF and diode laser energies has been developed in an attempt to address both facial rhytides and skin laxity. Doshi and Alster[101] demonstrated modest clinical improvement of facial rhytides and skin laxity in 20 patients by using optical energies of 32–40 J/cm² (mean 36.4 J/cm²) and radiofrequencies of 50–85 J/cm³ (mean 67.4 J/cm³) for three treatments at 3-week intervals. Side effects were mild and limited to transient erythema and edema. No scarring or pigmentary alteration was seen.

Postoperative Management

- Minimal to no care except sun avoidance.

Since the epidermis remains intact following non-ablative laser skin remodeling, postoperative care is minimal. Some patients experience mild erythema and edema lasting less than 24 h.

Adverse Events

- Side Effects/Complications
    - Transient postinflammatory hyperpigmentation in patients with darker skin phototypes or tans.
- Prevention and Treatment
    - Topical bleaching agents and light glycolic acid peels can hasten the resolution of postinflammatory hyperpigmentation.

Rarely, postoperative hyperpigmentation can develop several weeks after non-ablative skin remodeling and is more likely to be experienced by patients with darker skin tones and/or tans. In some cases, investigators demonstrated an association of post-treatment hyperpigmentation with excess intraoperative epidermal cryogen cooling.[92] Although always transient, topical bleaching agents and light glycolic acid peels can hasten the resolution of postinflammatory hyperpigmentation.

In the weeks following a series of non-ablative laser procedures, in-office visits can help identify patient concerns and increase the overall satisfaction with treatment. Clinical improvements after a series of non-ablative laser procedures may take weeks to realize, thus reassurance by the laser surgeon regarding the patient's progress can be particularly important.

Fractional Photothermolysis

Indications and Contraindications

- Indications
  - Mild to moderate facial rhytides and photo-damage
  - Atrophic scars
  - Superficial lesions
  - Melasma
- Contraindications
  - Patients with unrealistic expectations.
  - Patients with darker skin tones (skin phototype IV–VI) at greater risk of postoperative hyperpigmentation.
  - Patients with perpetual sun exposure.
  - Patients with active bacterial, viral, fungal infection or inflammatory skin conditions involving treatment areas.
  - Patients with history of herpes labialis may require prophylactic oral antiviral medications.
  - Concomitant isotretinoin use could potentially lead to an increased risk of hypertrophic scarring.

Over the past few years, a novel approach in skin resurfacing termed fractional photothermolysis has been developed to address the shortcomings associated with skin rejuvenation using ablative and non-ablative lasers and light sources.[102] Although dramatic clinical improvement can be achieved with ablative lasers, patients are often hesitant to pursue this treatment option because of the extended postoperative recovery period and inherent risks of the procedure. Non-ablative lasers and light sources, on the other hand, have demonstrated modest efficacy in the non-invasive treatment of mild facial rhytides and atrophic scarring with minimal side effects, but require multiple treatments with delayed and often inconsistent clinical results. Due to a need for more noticeable clinical improvement than these latter nonablative systems could provide, fractional photothermolysis was introduced into the skin resurfacing market to treat patients with rhytides, dyspigmentation, and atrophic scars.[103-107]

Techniques

Preoperative Management

- Adequate preoperative patient evaluation and education.

- Oral antiviral prophylaxis in patients with history of herpes labialis.

Adequate preoperative patient evaluation and education are essential. Sun exposure should be avoided prior to treatment in order to decrease risk of postoperative dyspigmentation. For patients with a strong history of herpes labialis, prophylactic oral antiviral medications should be considered when treating the perioral skin. Reactivation of prior herpes simplex infection can occur despite absence of an external wound due to the intense dermal heat produced by the laser.

Description of the Techniques

- Treatment is delivered concomitantly with forced air cooling. Energy setting of 25–40 mJ at densities of 125–250 MTZ/cm^2 are applied to treatment area in eight to ten passes, with total energies of 4–6 kJ delivered per session.

Fractional photothermolysis involves the use of a mid-infrared wavelength emitted by a 1,550 nm erbium-doped laser (Fraxel™, Reliant Technologies, MountainView, CA) to create microscopic non-contiguous columns of thermal injury in the dermis (referred to as microscopic thermal zones or MTZ) at depths of 200–500 µm surrounded by zones of viable tissue at 200–300 µm intervals.[102] The spatially precise columns of thermal injury produce localized epidermal necrosis and collagen denaturation at 125 or 250 MTZ/cm^2.[108] Because the tissue surrounding each MTZ is intact, residual epidermal and dermal cells contribute to rapid healing. Maintenance of the stratum corneum ensures continued epidermal barrier function. Histologic evaluation of the MTZ demonstrates homogenization of the dermal matrix and the presence of epidermal necrotic debris (MEND), representing the extrusion of damaged epidermal keratinocytes by viable keratinocytes at the lateral margin of the MTZ.[102] Microscopic epidermal necrotic debris exfoliates over the next several days, producing a bronzed appearance to the skin. The wound healing response differs from that after ablative laser techniques because the epidermal tissue that is spared between thermal zones contains viable transient amplifying cells capable of rapid re-epithelialization. Furthermore, because the stratum corneum has low water content, it remains intact immediately after treatment. Therefore, the wound created by fractional resurfacing is unique, not simply that of an ablative laser used to make "holes" in the skin. In addition, fractional resurfacing can provide an advantage over purely

Lasers for Resurfacing

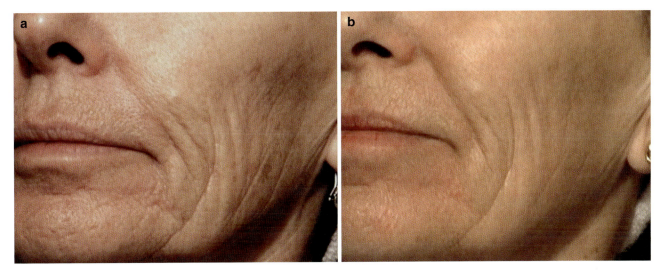

Fig. 5 Fractional photothermolysis (a) before and (b) after

non-ablative laser treatments due to the gradual exfoliation of the epidermis with resultant improvement in superficial dyspigmentation (Fig. 5a, b). Because only a fraction of the skin is treated during a single session, a series of fractional resurfacing treatments is required to achieve optimal clinical improvement.

The treatment areas should be cleansed of debris (including dirt, makeup, and powder) using a mild cleanser and 70% alcohol. A topical anesthetic cream is applied to the treatment sites for 60 min before treatment. The first generation fractional device required a water-soluble blue tinted tracking dye solution to be applied to the skin during treatment; however, current systems do not. Treatment is delivered concomitantly with forced air cooling using energy setting of 25–40 mJ and as high as 70 mJ. Total energies of 4–6 kJ are typically applied for full face treatment. Re-treatments with gradually higher fluences should be performed at 4 week intervals until patients are satisfied with clinical outcomes (typically three to five sessions are necessary to produce substantial clinical improvement).

Postoperative Management

- Mild cleanser, thermal spring water spray mist, and moisturizer several times daily for the first few postoperative days.

Patients are instructed to use a mild cleanser, thermal spring water spray mist, and moisturizer several times daily for the first few days after each treatment session (or as long as bronzing/xerosis is apparent).

Adverse Events

- Side Effects/Complications
  - Erythema, periocular edema, xerosis, and slight darkening of the skin (bronzing).
- Prevention and Treatment
  - Ice pack application for first 48 h.
  - Keep skin well-hydrated/moisturized for 48–72 h (or until xerosis/bronzing disappears).

Side effects of fractional resurfacing are typically mild and transient, including erythema, periocular edema, xerosis, and slight darkening of the skin (bronzing) during desquamation of the microscopic epidermal necrotic debris.[109] Erosions are uncommon and can be managed by liberal application of a healing ointment or plain petrolatum with cool wet compresses every 2–3 h. To date, permanent pigmentary alteration and scarring have not been reported. However, when an aggressive treatment protocol with a high density of microscopic thermal zones is used, the risk of visible epidermal ablation, along with the side effects associated with ablative laser procedures, is increased. Additional research is ongoing to determine optimal treatment parameters and the long-term benefits and sequelae of fractional resurfacing.

Conclusion

Ablative laser skin resurfacing has revolutionized the approach to photodamaged facial skin. Technology and techniques continue to evolve, further enhancing the ability to achieve substantial clinical improvement of rhytides, scars, and dyspigmentation with reduced postoperative morbidity. Utilizing proper technique and treatment parameters, excellent clinical results can be obtained with any one or combination of CO_2 and Er:YAG laser systems available. Therefore, the best choice of laser ultimately depends on the operator's expertise, clinical indication, and individual patient characteristics. Regardless of the type of ablative resurfacing laser used, the importance of careful postoperative follow-up cannot be overemphasized.

For those patients who desire a less aggressive approach to photorejuvenation than ablative laser skin resurfacing, non-ablative dermal remodeling or fractional laser photothermolysis represent viable alternatives for patients willing to accept modest clinical improvement in exchange for ease of treatment and a favorable side-effect profile. Treatments are typically delivered at monthly intervals with progressive clinical improvement observed after each session. Recent advances in fractional laser technology, in particular, have resulted in clinical effects approximating those of ablative laser treatment without its associated complications and risks.

References

1. Taylor CR, Stern RS, Leyden JJ, Gilchrest BA. Photoaging/photodamage and photoprotection. *J Am Acad Dermatol.* 1990;22: 1-15.
2. Lavker RM. Cutaneous aging: chronological versus photoaging. In: Gilchrest BA, ed. *Photodamage.* Cambridge: Blackwell Science; 1995:123-135.
3. Alster TS. Cutaneous resurfacing with CO_2 and erbium:YAG lasers: preoperative, intraoperative, and postoperative considerations. *Plast Reconstr Surg.* 1999;103:619-632.
4. Anderson RR, Parrish JA. Selective photothermolysis: precise microsurgery by selective absorption of pulsed radiation. *Science.* 1983;22:524-527.
5. Shapshay SM, Strong MS, Anastasi GW, Vaughan CW. Removal of rhinophyma with the CO_2 laser. A preliminary report. *Arch Otolaryngol.* 1980;106:257-259.
6. Dufresne RG, Garrett AB, Bailin PL, et al. CO_2 laser treatment of chronic actinic cheilitis. *J Am Acad Dermatol.* 1988;19:876-878.
7. Alster TS, Kauvar ANB, Geronemus RG. Histology of high-energy pulsed CO_2 laser resurfacing. *Semin Cutan Med Surg.* 1996;15:189-193.
8. Tanzi EL, Lupton JR, Alster TS. Review of lasers in dermatology: four decades of progress. *J Am Acad Dermatol.* 2003;49:1-31.
9. Lanzafame RJ, Naim JO, Rogers DW, Hinshaw JR. Comparisons of continuous-wave, chop wave, and super pulsed laser wounds. *Lasers Surg Med.* 1988;8:119-124.
10. Alster TS, Garg S. Treatment of facial rhytides with a high-energy pulsed CO_2 laser. *Plast Reconstr Surg.* 1996;98:791-794.
11. Alster TS. Preoperative preparation for CO_2 laser resurfacing. In: Coleman WP, Lawrence N, eds. *Skin Resurfacing.* Baltimore: Williams & Wilkins; 1998:171-179.
12. Hevia O, Nemeth AJ, Taylor JR. Tretinoin accelerates healing after trichloroacetic acid chemical peel. *Arch Dermatol.* 1991;127: 678-682.
13. West TB, Alster TS. Effect of pretreatment on the incidence of hyperpigmentation following cutaneous CO_2 laser resurfacing. *Dermatol Surg.* 1999;25:15-17.

14. Walia S, Alster TS. Cutaneous CO_2 laser resurfacing infection rate with and without prophylactic antibiotics. *Dermatol Surg.* 1999; 25:857-861.
15. Bernstein LJ, Kauvar ANB, Grossman MC, et al. The short- and long-term side effects of CO_2 laser resurfacing. *Dermatol Surg.* 1997;23:519-525.
16. Alster TS, West TB. Effect of topical vitamin C on postoperative CO_2 resurfacing erythema. *Dermatol Surg.* 1998;24:331-334.
17. Alster TS, Lupton JR. An overview of cutaneous laser resurfacing. *Clin Plast Surg.* 2001;28:37-52.
18. Alster TS, Nanni CA, Williams CM. Comparison of four CO_2 resurfacing lasers: a clinical and histopathologic evaluation. *Dermatol Surg.* 1999;25:153-159.
19. Walsh JT, Deutsch TF. Pulsed CO_2 laser tissue ablation: measurement of the ablation rate. *Lasers Surg Med.* 1988;8:264-275.
20. Fitzpatrick RE, Ruiz-Esparza J, Goldman MP. The depth of thermal necrosis using the CO_2 laser: a comparison of the superpulsed mode and conventional mode. *J Dermatol Surg Oncol.* 1991;17: 340-344.
21. Stuzin JM, Baker TJ, Baker TM, et al. Histologic effects of the high-energy pulsed CO_2 laser on photo-aged facial skin. *Plast Reconstr Surg.* 1997;99:2036-2050.
22. Walsh JT, Flotte TJ, Anderson RR, et al. Pulsed CO_2 laser tissue ablation: effect of tissue type and pulse duration on thermal damage. *Lasers Surg Med.* 1988;8:108-118.
23. Rubach BW, Schoenrock LD. Histological and clinical evaluation of facial resurfacing using a CO_2 laser with the computer pattern generator. *Arch Otolaryngol Head Neck Surg.* 1997;123:929-934.
24. Fitzpatrick RE, Smith SR, Sriprachya-anunt S. Depth of vaporization and the effect of pulse stacking with a high-energy, pulsed CO_2 laser. *J Am Acad Dermatol.* 1999;40:615-622.
25. Alster TS, Lupton JR. Prevention and treatment of side effects and complications of cutaneous laser resurfacing. *Plast Reconstr Surg.* 2002;109:308-316.
26. Lowe NJ, Lask G, Griffin ME, et al. Skin resurfacing with the ultrapulse CO_2 laser: observations on 100 patients. *Dermatol Surg.* 1995;21:1025-1029.
27. Alster TS. Comparison of two high-energy, pulsed CO_2 lasers in the treatment of periorbital rhytides. *Dermatol Surg.* 1996;22:541-545.
28. Apfelberg DB. Ultrapulse CO_2 laser with CPG scanner for full-face resurfacing of rhytides, photoaging, and acne scars. *Plast Reconstr Surg.* 1997;99:1817-1825.
29. Lask G, Keller G, Lowe NJ, et al. Laser skin resurfacing with the Silk Touch flash scanner for facial rhytides. *Dermatol Surg.* 1995;21:1021-1024.
30. Waldorf HA, Kauvar ANB, Geronemus RG. Skin resurfacing of fine to deep rhytides using a char-free CO_2 laser in 47 patients. *Dermatol Surg.* 1995;21:940-946.
31. Ratner D, Viron A, Puvion-Dutilleul F, et al. Pilot ultrastructural evaluation of human preauricular skin before and after high-energy pulsed CO_2 laser treatment. *Arch Dermatol.* 1998;134:582-587.
32. Ratner D, Tse Y, Marchell N, et al. Cutaneous laser resurfacing. *J Am Acad Dermatol.* 1999;41:365-389.
33. Fulton JE, Barnes T. Collagen shrinkage (selective dermoplasty) with the high-energy pulsed CO_2 laser. *Dermatol Surg.* 1998;24: 37-41.
34. Ross E, Naseef G, Skrobal M, et al. In vivo dermal collagen shrinkage and remodeling following CO_2 laser resurfacing. *Lasers Surg Med.* 1996;18:38.
35. Flor PJ, Spurr OK. Melting equilibrium for collagen fibers under stress: elasticity in the amorphous state. *J Am Chem Soc.* 1960; 83:1308.
36. Flor PJ, Weaver ES. Helix coil transition in dilute aqueous collagen solutions. *J Am Chem Soc.* 1989;82:4518.
37. Alster TS. Commentary on: increased smooth muscle actin, factor XIII a, and vimentin-positive cells in the papillary dermis of CO_2 laser-debrided porcine skin. *Dermatol Surg.* 1998;24:155.

38. West TB, Alster TS. Effect of botulinum toxin type A on movement-associated rhytides following CO_2 laser resurfacing. *Dermatol Surg*. 1999;25:259-261.

39. Katz BE, MacFarlane DF. Atypical facial scarring after isotretinoin therapy in a patient with a previous dermabrasion. *J Am Acad Dermatol*. 1994;30:852-853.

40. Roegnik HH, Pinski JB, Robinson K, et al. Acne, retinoids, and dermabrasion. *J Dermatol Surg Oncol*. 1985;11:396-398.

41. David L, Ruiz-Esparza J. Fast healing after laser skin resurfacing: the minimal mechanical trauma technique. *Dermatol Surg*. 1997;23:359-361.

42. Ruiz-Esparza J, Gomez JMB. Long-term effects of one general pass laser resurfacing: a look at dermal tightening and skin quality. *Dermatol Surg*. 1999;25:169-174.

43. Alster TS, Hirsch RJ. Single-pass CO_2 laser skin resurfacing of light and dark skin: extended experience with 52 patients. *J Cosmet Laser Ther*. 2003;5:39-42.

44. Tanzi EL, Alster TS. Single-pass CO_2 versus multiple-pass Er:YAG laser skin resurfacing: a comparison of postoperative wound healing and side-effect rates. *Dermatol Surg*. 2003;29:80-84.

45. Walsh JT, Flotte TJ, Deutsch TF. Er:YAG laser ablation of tissue: effect of pulse duration and tissue type on thermal damage. *Lasers Surg Med*. 1989;9:327-337.

46. Ross EV, Anderson RR. The erbium laser in skin resurfacing. In: Alster TS, Apfelberg DB, eds. *Cosmetic Laser Surgery*. 2nd ed. New York: Wiley; 1999:57-84.

47. Alster TS. Clinical and histologic evaluation of six erbium:YAG lasers for cutaneous resurfacing. *Lasers Surg Med*. 1999;24:87-92.

48. Hibst R, Kaufmann R. Effects of laser parameters on pulsed Er:YAG laser ablation. *Lasers Med Sci*. 1991;6:391-397.

49. Hohenleutner U, Hohenleutner S, Baumler W, et al. Fast and effective skin ablation with an Er:YAG laser: determination of ablation rates and thermal damage zones. *Lasers Surg Med*. 1997;20:242-247.

50. Alster TS, Lupton JR. Erbium:YAG cutaneous laser resurfacing. *Dermatol Clin*. 2001;19:453-466.

51. Khatri KA, Ross EV, Grevelink JM, et al. Comparison of erbium:YAG and CO_2 lasers in resurfacing of facial rhytides. *Arch Dermatol*. 1999;135:391-397.

52. Goldman MP, Marchell N, Fitzpatrick RE. Laser skin resurfacing of the face with a combined CO_2/Er:YAG laser. *Dermatol Surg*. 2000;26:102-104.

53. Sapijaszko MJA, Zachary CB. Er:YAG laser skin resurfacing. *Dermatol Clin*. 2002;20:87-96.

54. Pozner JM, Goldberg DJ. Histologic effect of a variable pulsed Er:YAG laser. *Dermatol Surg*. 2000;26:733-736.

55. Ross EV, McKinlay JR, Sajben FP, et al. Use of a novel erbium laser in a Yucatan minipig: a study of residual thermal damage (RTD), ablation, and wound healing as a function of pulse duration. *Lasers Surg Med*. 1999;15:17.

56. Newman JB, Lord JL, Ash K, et al. Variable pulse erbium:YAG laser skin resurfacing of perioral rhytides and side-by-side comparison with CO_2 laser. *Lasers Surg Med*. 1998;24:1303-1307.

57. Fitzpatrick RE, Rostan EF, Marchell N. Collagen tightening induced by CO_2 laser versus erbium:YAG laser. *Lasers Surg Med*. 2000;27:395-403.

58. Tanzi EL, Alster TS. Effect of a semiocclusive silicone-based dressing after ablative laser resurfacing of facial skin. *Cosmet Dermatol*. 2003;16:13-16.

59. Batra RS, Ort RJ, Jacob C, et al. Evaluation of a silicone occlusive dressing after laser skin resurfacing. *Arch Dermatol*. 2001;137:1317-1321.

60. Nanni CA, Alster TS. Complications of CO_2 laser resurfacing: an evaluation of 500 patients. *Dermatol Surg*. 1998;24:315-320.

61. Sriprachya-anunt S, Fitzpatrick RE, Goldman MP, et al. Infections complicating pulsed CO_2 laser resurfacing for photo-aged facial skin. *Dermatol Surg*. 1997;23:527-536.

62. McDaniel DH, Ash K, Lord J, et al. Accelerated laser resurfacing wound healing using a triad of topical antioxidants. *Dermatol Surg*. 1998;24:661-664.

63. Horton S, Alster TS. Preoperative and postoperative considerations for cutaneous laser resurfacing. *Cutis*. 1999;64:399-406.

64. Fisher AA. Lasers and allergic contact dermatitis to topical antibiotics, with particular reference to bacitracin. *Cutis*. 1996;58:252-254.

65. Alster TS, Nanni CA. Pulsed-dye laser treatment of hypertrophic burn scars. *Plast Reconstr Surg*. 1998;102:2190-2195.

66. Friedman PM, Geronemus RG. Use of the 308-nm excimer laser for postresurfacing leukoderma. *Arch Dermatol*. 2001;137:824-825.

67. Grimes PE, Bhawan J, Kim J, et al. Laser resurfacing-induced hypopigmentation: histologic alteration and repigmentation with topical photochemotherapy. *Dermatol Surg*. 2001;27:515-520.

68. Rohrer TE. Erbium:YAG laser resurfacing-experience of the first 200 cases. *Aesthet Dermatol Cosmet Surg*. 1999;1:19-30.

69. Tanzi EL, Alster TS. Side effects and complications of variable-pulsed erbium:yttrium–aluminum–garnet laser skin resurfacing: extended experience with 50 patients. *Plast Reconstr Surg*. 2003;111:1524-1529.

70. Rostan EF, Fitzpatrick RE, Goldman MP. Laser resurfacing with a long pulse erbium:YAG laser compared to the 950 ms pulsed CO_2 laser. *Lasers Surg Med*. 2001;29:136-141.

71. Ross VE, Miller C, Meehan K, et al. One-pass CO_2 versus multiple-pass Er:YAG laser resurfacing in the treatment of rhytides: a comparison side-by-side study of pulsed CO_2 and Er:YAG lasers. *Dermatol Surg*. 2001;27:709-715.

72. Zachary CB. Modulating the Er:YAG laser. *Lasers Surg Med*. 2002;26:223-226.

73. Alster TS, Lupton JR. Are all infrared lasers equally effective in skin rejuvenation. *Semin Cutan Med Surg*. 2002;21:274-279.

74. Zelickson B, Kilmer S, Bernstein E, et al. Pulsed dye laser therapy for sun damaged skin. *Lasers Surg Med*. 1999;25:229-236.

75. Zelickson B, Kist D. Effect of pulse dye laser and intense pulsed light source on the dermal extracellular matrix remodeling. *Lasers Surg Med*. 2000;12:68.

76. Bjerring P, Clement M, Heickendorff L, et al. Selective non-ablative wrinkle reduction by laser. *J Cutan Laser Ther*. 2000;2:9-15.

77. Goldberg DJ, Cutler KB. Non-ablative treatment of rhytides with intense pulsed light. *Lasers Surg Med*. 2000;26:196-200.

78. Bitter PH. Non-invasive rejuvenation of photodamaged skin using serial, full-face intense pulsed light treatments. *Dermatol Surg*. 2000;26:835-843.

79. Weiss RA, Weiss MA, Beasley KL. Rejuvenation of photoaged skin: 5 years results with intense pulsed light of the face, neck, and chest. *Dermatol Surg*. 2002;28:1115-1119.

80. Hardaway CA, Ross EV. Non-ablative laser skin remodeling. *Dermatol Clin*. 2002;20:97-111.

81. Goldberg DJ, Whitworth J. Laser skin resurfacing with the Q-switched Nd:YAG laser. *Dermatol Surg*. 1997;23:903-907.

82. Goldberg DJ, Metzler C. Skin resurfacing utilizing a low-fluence Nd:YAG laser. *J Cutan Laser Ther*. 1999;1:23-27.

83. Lee MW. Combination visible and infrared lasers for skin rejuvenation. *Semin Cutan Med Surg*. 2002;21:288-300.

84. Menaker GM, Wrone DA, Williams RM, et al. Treatment of facial rhytids with a non-ablative laser: a clinical and histologic study. *Dermatol Surg*. 1999;25:440-444.

85. Kelly KM, Nelson S, Lask GP, et al. Cryogen spray cooling in combination with non-ablative laser treatment of facial rhytides. *Arch Dermatol*. 1999;135:691-694.

86. Goldberg DJ. Non-ablative subsurface remodeling: clinical and histologic evaluation of a 1320 nm Nd:YAG laser. *J Cutan Laser Ther*. 1999;1:153-157.

87. Goldberg DJ. Full-face non-ablative dermal remodeling with a 1320 nm Nd:YAG laser. *Dermatol Surg*. 2000;26:915-918.

88. Trelles MA, Allones I, Luna R. Facial rejuvenation with a non-ablative 1320 nm Nd:YAG laser. A preliminary clinical and histologic evaluation. *Dermatol Surg*. 2001;27:111-116.

89. Fatemi A, Weiss MA, Weiss RA. Short-term histologic effects of non-ablative resurfacing: results with a dynamically cooled millisecond-domain 1320 nm Nd:YAG laser. *Dermatol Surg*. 2002;28:172-176.

90. Goldberg DJ, Rogachefsky AS, Silapunt S. Non-ablative laser treatment of facial rhytides: a comparison of 1450 nm diode laser treatment with dynamic cooling as opposed to treatment with dynamic cooling alone. *Lasers Surg Med*. 2002;30:79-81.

91. Hardaway CA, Ross EV, Paithankar DY. Non-ablative cutaneous remodeling with a 1.45 micron mid-infrared diode laser: phase II. *J Cosmet Laser Ther*. 2002;4:9-14.

92. Tanzi EL, Williams CM, Alster TS. Treatment of facial rhytides with a non-ablative 1450-nm diode laser: a controlled clinical and histologic study. *Dermatol Surg*. 2003;29:124-129.

93. Tanzi EL, Alster TS. The treatment of transverse neck lines with a 1450-nm diode laser. *Lasers Surg Med*. 2002;14(Suppl):33.

94. Tanzi EL, Alster TS. Comparison of a 1450-nm diode laser and a 1320-nm Nd:YAG laser in the treatment of atrophic facial scars: a prospective clinical and histologic study. *Dermatol Surg*. 2004;30:152-157.

95. Mordon S, Capon A, Creusy C. In vivo experimental evaluation of non-ablative skin remodeling using a 1.54 μm laser with surface cooling. *Lasers Surg Med*. 2000;27:1-9.

96. Ross EV, Sajben FP, Hsia J, et al. Non-ablative skin remodeling: selective dermal heating with a mid-infrared laser and contact cooling combination. *Lasers Surg Med*. 2000;26:186-195.

97. Lupton JR, Williams CM, Alster TS. Non-ablative laser skin resurfacing using a 1540 nm erbium:glass laser: a clinical and histologic analysis. *Dermatol Surg*. 2002;28:833-835.

98. Fournier N, Dahan S, Barneon G, et al. Non-ablative remodeling: a 14-month clinical ultrasound imaging and profilometric evaluation of a 1540 nm Er:glass laser. *Dermatol Surg*. 2002;28: 926-931.

99. Ruiz-Esparza J, Gomez JB. The medical face lift: a non-invasive, non-surgical approach to tissue tightening in facial skin using non-ablative radiofrequency. *Dermatol Surg*. 2003;29:325-332.

100. Alster TS, Tanzi EL. Improvement of neck and cheek laxity with a nonablative radiofrequency device: a lifting experience. *Dermatol Surg*. 2004;30:305-307.

101. Doshi SN, Alster TS. Combination radiofrequency and diode laser for treatment of facial rhytides and skin laxity. *J Cosmet Laser Ther*. 2005;7:11-15.

102. Manstein D, Herron GS, Sink RK, et al. Fractional photothermolysis: a new concept for cutaneous remodeling using microscopic patterns of thermal injury. *Lasers Surg Med*. 2004;34: 426-438.

103. Tannous ZS, Astner S. Utilizing fractional resurfacing in the treatment of therapy-resistant melasma. *J Cosmet Laser Ther*. 2005; 7:39-43.

104. Rokhsar CK, Fitzpatrick RE. The treatment of melasma with fractional photothermolysis: a pilot study. *Dermatol Surg*. 2005;31: 1645-1650.

105. Geronemus RG. Fractional photothermolysis: current and future applications. *Lasers Surg Med*. 2006;38:169-176.

106. Alster TS, Tanzi EL, Lazarus M. The use of fractional laser photothermolysis for the treatment of atrophic scars. *Dermatol Surg*. 2007;33:295-299.

107. Wanner M, Tanzi EL, Alster TS. Fractional photothermolysis: treatment of facial and nonfacial cutaneous photodamage with a 1,550-nm erbium-doped fiber laser. *Dermatol Surg*. 2007;33: 23-28.

108. Laubach HJ, Tannous Z, Anderson RR, Manstein D. Skin responses to fractional photothermolysis. *Lasers Surg Med*. 2006;38: 142-149.

109. Graber E, Tanzi EL, Alster TS. Side effects and complications of fractional laser photothermolysis: experience with 961 treatments. *Dermatol Surg*. 2008;34(3):301-305.

Fractional Photothermolysis

Dieter Manstein and Hans-Joachim Laubach

Abbreviations

FP	Fractional Photothermolysis
FR	Fractional Resurfacing
MEND	Microscopic-Epidermal-Necrotic-Debris
MTZ	Microthermal Treatment Zone
OPD	Optical Penetration Depth

Introduction and Background

- Traditional resurfacing techniques have their put period after drawbacks.

Traditional ablative resurfacing techniques and non-ablative laser and light procedures are well-established treatment modalities for modifying the appearance and characteristics of skin.[1-3] However, patients have become hesitant to accept the side effects and risks associated with traditional ablative techniques.[4] The main concerns of ablative resurfacing are prolonged procedural downtime, risk of scarring, and the incidence of delayed, long-lasting hypopigmentation, also known as 'alabaster skin'.[5,6] Further, traditional non-ablative techniques for collagen remodeling have shown inconsistent and often unpredictable results, frequently leading to unsatisfied patients and treating physicians.[7] For a detailed description of the advantages and disadvantages of traditional resurfacing techniques, see Chaps. 9, 12, and 13 of this volume.

- Fractional photothermolysis' (FP) is a relatively new concept introduced by Manstein et al. in 2004.
- FP is based on generating patterns of microscopically small lesions, also called 'microscopic treatment zones' (MTZs).
- FP has become an established treatment –technique in dermatological laser therapy.

To overcome the drawbacks of these traditional resurfacing approaches, fractional photothermolysis (FP) was developed by Manstein et al.[8] In contrast to traditional laser techniques, which provide laser exposure to the entire skin surface, FP creates a pattern of microscopically small, 3-dimensional treatment zones (microscopic treatment zones or MTZs) while leaving the skin surrounding each of these MTZs substantially undamaged (Fig. 1). The term "fractional photothermolysis" was selected to express that only a fraction (lat: frangere, to break into pieces) of the skin is exposed to light (photo) to thermally damage or destroy (thermolysis) small treatment zones. FP procedures have been demonstrated to successfully treat a wide variety of aesthetic and dermatological indications. There is a broad range of possible treatment settings that may be used to generate the resulting wound healing response. FP can be delivered in multiple treatments, each providing incremental improvement within the limits of individual patient's tolerance for downtime and side effects. Therefore FP gives the physician additional options to provide a customized treatment regime that is suited to fit their patient's needs and expectations. FP procedures have become increasingly popular over the past few years and have become an established concept in dermatological laser therapy. The rapid proliferation of publications in the dermatological literature related to FP is an indication of the significant impact that FP had on the field (Fig. 2). The success of FP is also documented by the wide variety of commercially available FP devices; virtually all dermatological laser device companies currently have at least one FP device in their product portfolio (Tables 1 and 2).

D. Manstein (✉)
Massachusetts General Hospital, Wellman Center for Photomedicine,
Harvard Medical School, Boston, MA, USA
e-mail: dmanstein@partners.org

K. Nouri (ed.), *Lasers in Dermatology and Medicine*,
DOI: 10.1007/978-0-85729-281-0_10, © Springer-Verlag London Limited 2011

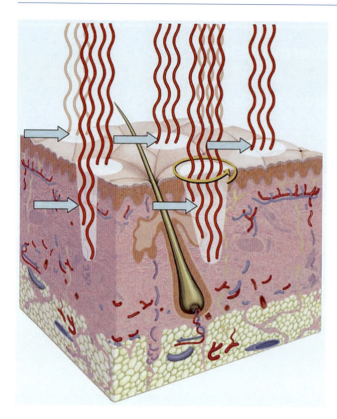

Fig. 1 Concept of fractional photothermolysis. An array of microscopically small zones of thermal injury, so called MTZs (microscopic treatment zones, gray arrows), is generated by multiple, focused laser pulses. Each of the MTZ is surrounded by undamaged skin (orange, circular arrow), allowing for fast repair (Laubach and Manstein[9])

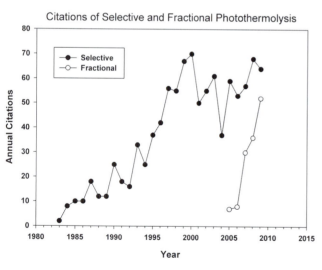

Fig. 2 Annual citations of the original article for fractional photothermolysis (FP) and selective photothermolysis (SP). Data obtained from 'ISI Web of Knowledge™', Thompson Reuters. The rapid proliferation of FP related publications indicates an increasing impact of this concept in the field of dermatology. The annual citations of FP have already reached a level comparable to that of SP. Further analysis reveals that recently SP citations are increasingly for non-dermatological indications, e.g., in ophthalmology or otorhinolaryngology. In contrast, FP citations are so far generally limited to dermatological indications (SP: Anderson and Parrish[10]; FP: Manstein et al.[8])

- Individual MTZs are typically so small that they induce neither extended inflammation nor fibrosis.
- MTZs heal quickly due to their small cross section and the presence of adjacent unharmed tissue.
- MTZs can extend down to the deep reticular dermis for certain laser parameters.

One of the key concepts of FP is that the individual damaged tissue regions (MTZs) are so small in at least one dimension that the damaged or destroyed tissue is rapidly repaired without any significant fibrosis. The close proximity of surrounding viable tissue facilitates the wound healing. Although the individual MTZs induce a guaranteed wound healing response, the extent of inflammation is limited and confined to their close proximity. The overall wound healing response is primarily determined by the shape of individual MTZs and their distribution (density) within the treatment area. This "fractional" approach contrasts with thermal wounds having larger dimensions and longer healing times, which are typically generated using conventional resurfacing procedures or the like. It remains a subject of further research to define the particular conditions favoring tissue repair over fibrosis. Another advantage of generating lesions on a microscopic scale is that the individual lesions are so small that typically they cannot be resolved with the naked eye under clinical conditions, thereby ensuring a homogenous appearance of the treated area. MTZs heal quickly due to their small cross section and the presence of unharmed tissue. They can extend down to the deep reticular dermis and still be well-tolerated in terms of rapid healing. Such deep tissue destruction has to be carefully avoided with traditional ablative resurfacing techniques, as confluent damage to such depth levels would impair the skin's ability to regenerate, and would most likely result in scarring similar to that seen in third-degree burns.[11]

- Two distinct types of FP exist: non-ablative FP (nFP) and ablative FP (aFP).
- Non-ablative FP (nFP) generates MTZs characterized by thermal coagulation.
- Ablative FP (aFP) generates MTZs exhibiting some degree of immediate tissue removal (vaporization) and a surrounding zone of coagulated tissue.
- A distinction between superficial, medium and deep FP procedures may facilitate description of the procedure, but is somewhat arbitrary.

Fractional Photothermolysis

Table 1 Characteristics of selected, commercially available non-ablative fractional photothermolysis (nFP) devices, including manufacturer, device name, laser type, emitted wavelength, nominal spot size and range of energy/MTZ. This table is not comprehensive, the pulse duration listed device parameters were obtained by manufacturer survey and are also subject to change.

Company	Device	Laser	Wavelength [nm]	Delivery	Spot size [µm/MTZ]	Energy [mJ/MTZ]	Pulse duration [ms]
Cynosure	Affirm	Nd:YAG	1320 / 1440	Stamping	100 – 150	up to 4.1	1, 1.5, 2
Lutronic	Mosaic	Er:Glass	1550	Scanned stamping		4 – 40	0.5 – 4.5
Palomar	Lux1540	Er:Glass	1540	Stamping		up to 100	5, 10
Quanta	Matisse	Er:Glass	1540	Stamping		up to 20	4 – 14
Sellas	1550	Er:Glass	1550	Scanned stamping	312 – 1000	1 – 30	0.5
Solta	Fraxel re:fine	Er:Glass	1410	Rolling		5 – 20	
Solta	Fraxel re:store DUAL	Er:Glass	1550 / 1927	Rolling	135 / up to 600	4 – 70, 5 – 20	0.015 – 3

Table 2 Characteristics of selected, commercially available ablative fractional photothermolysis (FP) devices, including manufacturer, device name, laser type, emitted wavelength, average optical emission power, nominal spot size and range of energy/MTZ. This table is not comprehensive, the pulse duration listed device parameters were obtained by manufacturer survey and are also subject to change.

Company	Device	Laser	Wavelength [nm]	Delivery	Power [W]	Spot size [µm/MTZ]	Energy [mJ/MTZ]	Pulse duration [ms]
Alma	Pixel CO_2	CO_2	10600	Scanned stamping	40, 70	250		50 – 300
AMT	Touch Cell	CO_2	10600	Scanned stamping	30	200		
Candela	QuadraLase	CO_2	10600	Scanned stamping	20			
Cutera	Pearl Fractional	YSGG	2790	Scanned stamping		300	60 – 320	0.6
Cynosure	Smart Skin	CO_2	10600	Scanned stamping				
Deka	SmartXide DOT HP	CO_2	10600	Scanned stamping	50	300		0.2 – 80
Ellipse	Juvia	CO_2	10600	Scanned stamping	10	500	5 – 15	5 – 7
Lasering	Mixto	CO_2	10600	Scanned stamping	20	180, 300		2.5 – 16
Lumenis	Active FX	CO_2	10600	Scanned stamping	60	1300	5 – 225	0.04 – 2
Lumenis	DeepFX	CO_2	10600	Scanned stamping	60	120	5 – 50	0.04 – 0.2
Lutronic	eCO2	CO_2	10600	Scanned stamping	30	120,180,300	4 – 120	
Palomar	Lux2940	Er:YAG	2940	Stamping		80 – 125	up to 25	
Quanta	youlaser CO_2	CO_2	10600	Scanned stamping	30			0.05 – 20
Quantel	BuraneFX	Er:YAG	2940	Scanned stamping		150	0.7 – 32	0.35 – 250
Quantel	ExelO$_2$	CO_2	10600	Scanned stamping	40	350	10 – 1000	1 – 100
Sciton	Profactional	Er:YAG	2940	Scanned stamping		250		
Solta	Fraxel re:pair	CO_2	10600	Scanned stamping	40	135, 600	5 – 70	0.15 – 3

At present, two distinct types of FP exist – non-ablative FP (nFP) and ablative FP (aFP) (Fig. 3). Non-ablative FP (nFP) generates MTZs having a small-diameter zone of thermally damaged epidermis and dermis extending down to a particular depth. The shape of such MTZs is either an inverted cone or a tapered column extending into the dermis. The degree of thermal damage within an MTZ is typically sufficient to cause cell necrosis and to coagulate collagen. The physical integrity of the skin remains intact, in spite of the marked localized thermal damage.[8] Ablative FP (aFP), on the other hand, creates MTZs by vaporizing microscopic zones of tissue up to a particular depth. This depth is primarily dependent on pulse energy and may extent into the deep reticular dermis. The resulting tapered cavity is lined by a thin layer of eschar and

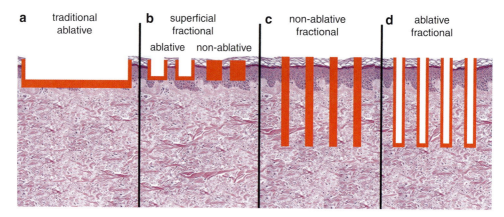

Fig. 3 Schematics of different resurfacing modalities. Traditional ablative procedures generate a confluent layer of tissue removal and with thermal coagulation to the adjacent remaining tissue (**a**). Mainly, two distinct types of FP procedures exist, ablative (aFP) and non-ablative (nFP) photothermolysis. nFP creates multiple microscopic treatment zones (MTZs) consisting of coagulated tissue. Despite of the thermal damage, the physical integrity of the skin remains intact (**c**). AFP vaporizes some tissue, creating multiple MTZs which consist of a cavity lined by a thin layer of eschar and surrounded by a cuff of coagulated tissue (**d**). Further differentiation of FP procedures according to the depth of individual MTZ is possible, e.g., superficial FP, but somehow arbitrary (**b**)

surrounded by a cuff of thermal denaturation, which is sufficient to destroy cells and coagulate collagen. Ablative FP results in immediate tissue loss due to the physical removal of portions of the skin by vaporization, and the physical integrity and barrier function of the skin is locally compromised.[12] As the depth of MTZ can vary greatly, it appears reasonable to further distinguish between FP procedures generating MTZs of different depths, e.g., superficial, medium and deep. While such a classification may serve to better describe a FP process, classification by damage depth is somewhat arbitrary. It remains to be determined how the depth of MTZs affects the clinical outcome for various FP protocols.

- The laser wavelength determines primarily if an FP procedure is ablative or non-ablative.
- Ablative FP procedures are performed with lasers emitting at wavelengths corresponding to strong absorption bands of water.
- The depth of an MTZ for nFP is limited by the optical penetration of the particular wavelength into skin tissue.

FP procedures generate a 3-dimensional pattern of MTZs in the skin and the wound healing response is primarily determined by the characteristics of individual MTZs and their spatial distribution. The laser tissue effects generated within individual MTZs depend primarily on applied wavelength, pulse energy, focused beam diameter and pulse duration.

The laser wavelength plays an important role in the characteristics and results of an FP procedure. The main chromophore absorbing the laser energy, either for nFP or aFP, is water. Wavelengths that are very strongly absorbed can result in local volumetric energy densities sufficient to vaporize tissue.[13] Therefore aFP procedures are performed with lasers emitting at wavelengths corresponding to strong absorption bands of water. The approximate optical penetration depth (OPD) in water for such lasers is minimal, e.g., 1 µm for the Er:YAG laser ($\lambda=2{,}940$ nm) and 10 µm for the CO_2 laser ($\lambda=10{,}600$ nm).[14] High volumetric energy densities are reached virtually instantaneously within the focus of the laser beam, and therefore such lasers can quickly advance a cavity deep into the tissue during the pulse. Due to this process it is possible that the resulting depth of an MTZ can greatly exceed the optical penetration depth of any particular laser wavelength. Once the local energy density exceeds the vaporization threshold, the depth of the laser created cavity is primarily related to the total energy delivered for a given spot size, and relatively independent of the applied wavelength. It should be noted, that the Er:YAG typically produces less thermal damage in the residual tissue as compared to the CO_2 laser due to the stronger absorption by water.

As nFP procedures do not physically remove tissue, the maximum depth of MTZs in nFP procedures is limited by the optical penetration depth of any particular laser wavelength. Variation of the applied laser energy allows some adjustment of the thermal injury depth within this physically imposed limit. However, several points should be considered when applying this concept to real procedures. The optical penetration depths provided are approximations of the penetration depth in water provided by Hall.[14] The water content of tissue can vary substantially and is approximately 30% for the epidermis and 70% for the dermis.[15] As the optical properties of water are also temperature dependent, it has been reported that the rapid change of tissue temperature during a laser pulse can dynamically alter the penetration depth substantially.[16] Also, other factors such as scattering, phase transitions (e.g., collagen denaturation), and non-linear phenomena should be taken into consideration for a more detailed analysis of the wavelength dependent effects on the shape of MTZs. The following are examples of lasers that can be used for nFP, together with their respective wavelengths (λ) and approximate optical penetration depth (OPD): Er:YAG ($\lambda = 1{,}440$ nm, OPD ≈ 300 μm) Er:Glass ($\lambda = 1{,}540$ and $1{,}550$ nm, OPD $\approx 1{,}000$ μm), and Thulium fiber laser ($\lambda = 1{,}927$ nm, OPD ≈ 100 μm). These differences in optical penetration lengths indicate why the Thulium laser, with a relatively shallow penetration depth, is often used to treat superficial lesions within the epidermis and papillary dermis, and why the Er:Glass laser with a relatively larger optical penetration depth can generate MTZs extending down into the mid to deep reticular dermis. Because these provided numbers are estimates that which can be affected by various factors, they should serve only as a general guideline, and not as a specific reference.

> - The pulse duration and temporal pulse profile can affect the amount of thermal damage in the surrounding tissue.

The pulse duration for FP systems is typically in the range of up to a few milliseconds, but varies with the preset energy applied per MTZ. The MTZ energy is controlled for most FP systems by adjustment of the pulse duration used to create individual MTZs. In a first approximation, such short pulse durations are within the thermal relaxation time of individual MTZs and minor variation of pulse duration should have limited effects on lesion shape. However, variation of pulse duration over an extended range of pulse profiles will affect the MTZ shape, e.g., ablation depth and/or extent of residual thermal damage. Tissue effects related to pulse duration and/or temporal pulse profile have not yet been characterized in detail, but these parameters are likely to be the focus of future studies for optimizing FP procedures. The available average power of an FP laser system is a critical factor that limits the maximum overall coverage rate. For example, a laser that delivers a higher average optical power can be capable of faster treatment of larger areas.

> - Coverage of a treatment area can be achieved by the 'stamping' or 'rolling' technique.
> - Typically, multiple passes are necessary to provide sufficient treatment coverage.
> - Variation of the number of passes and exposure settings in different areas can be used to adjust the clinical outcome in specific locations, e.g., 'feathering' at the edges of the treatment area.
> - Excessively high treatment densities should be avoided as they can result in undesirable side effects.

There are two general techniques currently available for generating the desired density of MTZs (number per unit area) within the treatment area: the 'stamping' technique and the 'rolling' technique. The 'stamping' technique is performed by forming a preset pattern of multiple MTZs on a skin region within a well-defined exposure area of the fixed handpiece, and then moving the handpiece to another skin region and repeating until the entire treatment area is covered. The density of MTZs at the end of a treatment session depends on the preset density within the exposure area of the handpiece and the number of passes performed over each skin region. A pass is defined as the coverage resulting from a single application of the handpiece to a particular area of the skin. The 'rolling' technique is performed by continuously rolling the handpiece across the entire treatment area. It is also referred as 'brushing' technique, because the movements of the operator are similar to using a paint brush. As the velocity of the handpiece relative to the skin varies during treatment, the delivery rate is adjusted automatically in order to maintain a defined, preset MTZ density per pass. The total density of MTZs at the end of a treatment session can be estimated as the density of MTZs per pass multiplied by the number of passes performed. However this presents only an estimate as with each pass the remaining undamaged skin surface decreases and therefore the effective amount of tissue that is newly damaged with each subsequent pass decreases. Some MTZs formed on subsequent passes may overlap or coincide with MTZs already formed during prior passes. A more detailed description of the determination of coverage in terms to number of passes is provided by Manstein et al.[17] There appears to be no single best technique for delivering the desired density of MTZs. The 'rolling' technique can facilitate treatment of larger areas, while the 'stamping' technique can facilitate the precise treatment of smaller areas, in particular areas having an irregular surface profile. It is the opinion of the authors that a reasonably well-defined MTZ density can be achieved with both techniques, and the choice between stamping and brushing ultimately comes down to a personal preference of the operator. FP systems generally allow the operator to adjust both MTZ density and MTZ characteristics independently within the treatment area. The MTZ density can be adjusted by varying the preset number of pulses per area and/or number of passes, while the dimensions of individual MTZs can be modified by adjustment of the MTZ energy, energy beam focal characteristics, etc. Such control allows, for example, formation of a decreased MTZ density at the periphery of a treatment area to avoid demarcation lines between treated and untreated areas (feathering), or an increased MTZ density or applied energy density within particular areas that can benefit from an enhanced treatment outcome. The overall extent of the wound healing response, and thus the extent of both clinical improvement and side-effects appear to be related to the total amount of thermal injury or total energy delivered per treatment area. Treatment densities that result in confluent thermal injury can result in blistering or even scarring.

- Bulk heating is the temperature rise of the tissue between individual MTZs by thermal conduction as each MTZ acts as a local heat source.
- Limited bulk heating may be desirable in FP procedures.
- Excessive bulk heating can result in confluent tissue damage and severe side effects including scarring.

- Excessive bulk heating can be avoided by limiting MTZ densities, extending the time interval between passes and application of cooling.
- Changes in tissue temperature effect the shape of individual MTZs.

While FP procedures are designed to deliver localized thermal injury within individual MTZs, it should be taken in consideration that energy deposited into the tissue may accumulate under certain conditions. The temperature gradient tends to be very high within a single MTZ, often resulting in a very sharp demarcation between coagulated and non coagulated collagen. However, each MTZ represents a small heat source within the surrounding tissue. This heating effect has two principal consequences.

First, although there is typically a very sharp demarcation at the perimeter of an individual MTZ, thermal effects on the tissue immediately surrounding an MTZ have been observed. For example, apoptotic cell death and induction of various heat shock proteins can be seen close to individual MTZs. Although the effects of such events on the clinical outcome have to be further investigated, it can be speculated, that up to a certain extent, these local heating effects around the MTZs may enhance wound healing and clinical outcome.

Second, as each of the MTZs acts as a local heat source, forming many MTZs within a short time period can lead to an increase in the average tissue temperature of the treated region due to heat conduction. Such tissue heating is described by the term 'bulk tissue heating.' Bulk tissue heating can become a significant problem when the local average tissue temperature rises above a critical temperature such that confluent areas of tissue are damaged or destroyed, rather than limiting such damage to discrete small microscopic zones. Such gross thermal injury mimics that of a third degree burn, which can lead to substantial side effects including scarring.

The following precautions should be taken into consideration in order to avoid excessive bulk heating during FP procedures:

(a) For higher individual MTZ formation energies, the spatial density of MTZs formed in the treatment region should be decreased.
(b) When multiple passes are performed on a treatment region, the time interval between passes should be long enough to allow the tissue to cool down between consecutive passes.
(c) External cooling, e.g., forced air cooling, can be used to remove some heat from the tissue region being treated.

Changes in tissue temperature have been shown to affect the geometry of individual lesions. Reduction of MTZ dimension due to decrease of tissue temperature have been shown to be more marked for nFP[18] as compared to aFP.[19] Skin cooling before, during and/or after FP treatments is often desirable because it can alleviate pain during treatment and also reduce the risk of bulk heating. Because skin cooling can also decrease the MTZ lesion size resulting from particular system settings during an nFP procedure, it is important to perform such procedures under standardized cooling conditions to control the thermal damage within individual MTZs. It should be noted that during aFP procedures, a substantial part of the laser energy is removed from the tissue with the hot laser plume. This is in contrast to nFP procedures, and therefore it is reasonable to conclude that for the same applied energy per MTZ energy and MTZ density, the overall (bulk) heating of tissue is greater for nFP as compared to aFP. Although, no studies have been carried out to either confirm or quantify this effect, the operator should be aware of such potential interrelated effects that are based on principles of laser tissue interaction.

- FP procedures are typically performed as multiple treatments.
- Treatment outcome is typically incrementally enhanced after additional FP treatments.
- Typically, a series of approximately 3–5 nFP or 1–3 aFP treatments are performed.
- There is some controversies regarding whether the clinical improvement of an aggressive treatment can be achieved by repetition of less aggressive treatments.
- FP treatments allow distribution of the thermal wounding resulting from individual MTZs at different densities and over distinct treatment sessions.

FP treatment of a particular skin region can be can be delivered in single or multiple treatment sessions. Typically 3–5 nFP or 1–3 aFP treatment sessions are performed, but the number of treatments can vary within a wider range depending on indications, treatment settings and patient response.

Each treatment is customized to a patient's individual condition to best manage side effects and downtime. The treatment is repeated until either the desired outcome is achieved or no further relevant improvement can be achieved. It should be remembered that some of the effects, e.g., collagen remodeling, can progress over a period of weeks or months after a treatment. Multiple treatments are generally performed at intervals of approximately 4–8 weeks. However there are no studies currently known that compare the outcomes achieved based on variation in treatment intervals. The current intervals of several weeks are generally preferred because they allow sufficient time for side effects to subside and also arguably because such intervals are convenient for the appointment scheduling of most offices and patients.

There is some controversy regarding the effect of multiple treatments sessions on enhancement of treatment outcomes. While it is generally accepted that multiple treatments sessions can improve the overall outcome, it is not clear exactly how the number of treatments sessions is related to the overall improvement. Also, it is still not known whether multiple treatments performed at well-tolerated settings can mimic the outcome of fewer or single treatments sessions performed with more aggressive settings that are associated with a marked wound healing response and prolonged downtime. FP treatments provide the possibility of obtaining particular degree of thermal wounding within individual MTZs and varying just the density of such MTZs and/or adjusting the number of sessions. In contrast, conventional treatments that cover the entire treatment area continuously do not allow for this freedom. These full-surface procedures only allow for adjustment of the treatment level by varying the fluence applied over the entire area.

- Several factors beyond the laser parameter settings can affect the thermal damage.
- Mechanical manipulation of the skin such as compression, stretching and contraction can affect the shape and density of MTZs.

A variety of factors beyond an FP system's preset MTZ exposure/energy and density settings can affect the thermal injury of the tissue. The operator should be aware of such factors, as they can impact the wound healing response, clinical outcome, and side effects experienced by the patient. For example, mechanical factors such as tissue stretching, contraction, or compression can affect MTZ lesion dimension and MTZ density. Stretching of the skin during exposure can lead to an increased actual density of MTZs. The density per pass is typically preset by the system for a fixed exposure area, but skin stretching during the exposure can actually

result in relatively higher MTZ density. This can occur because as the skin is able to retract after the stretching is relieved, any number of delivered pulses is located within a relatively smaller area. MTZs of smaller cross section can also result from stretching of the skin prior to treatment, as the MTZs that are formed in the stretched skin may shrink in size when the skin is allowed to retract. Point compression can distort the skin dimensions locally during exposure, and relatively deeper MTZs with smaller cross sections can result from such mechanical tissue manipulation. Also, because skin may contract as a result of localized thermal injury to the collagen, the dimensions of the skin can change during the delivery of a series of passes to generate individual MTZ patterns. Ablative FP procedures performed, particularly when performed with higher MTZ energies, tend to exhibit such shrinkage of the tissue during multiple FP passes over a particular treatment area.

- In addition to the shape and density of individual MTZs, the number of treatment sessions and intervals can be chosen by the operator.
- The broad variety of possible combinations allows tailoring patient treatment protocols to specific needs.
- The multivariate complexity of FP procedures represents a challenge to obtain comparative clinical data.
- Most FP treatments result in varying degrees of clinical improvement for appropriate indications.
- The three basic rules of any FP treatment are:
  A. Individual MTZs should induce wound healing but not fibrosis.
  B. Confluent damage and bulk heating should be avoided.
  C. The cumulative MTZ density should be sufficiently high to result in clinical improvement after the completion of a treatment course.

As discussed herein, many factors can affect thermal damage patterns generated in the skin and subsequent wound healing responses. Such factors include laser exposure parameters (e.g., energy per MTZ and focal spot size), the number of passes and time interval between them, mechanical tissue manipulation, use of skin cooling procedures, and others. The treatment interval between individual passes within a single treatment session and the number of sessions can also be varied. This virtually unlimited number of possible treatment combinations provides the possibility of tailoring patient treatment protocols to specific needs. However, this flexibility also leads to some complexity and uncertainty associated with the choice and control of all possible parameters and factors. The multivariate complexity of FP procedures explains in part the current lack of clinical studies comparing the effect of many specific FP parameters on patient outcomes. In spite of this complexity, it turns out that most FP treatment regimes result in some kind of clinical improvement for appropriate indications. Also, the fundamental principles of FP that guide the selection of treatment parameters are relatively simple and can be summarized by three basic rules. First, the dimensions of individual MTZs should not exceed certain dimensions, such that the induced wound healing results in tissue repair rather than inducing fibrosis. Second, the overall density of MTZs should not be excessively high to maintain sufficient undamaged tissue between the MTZs and facilitate tissue repair. In particular, thermal damage to confluent tissue via bulk heating should be avoided. Third, the cumulative density of MTZs should be sufficiently high to induce sufficient clinical improvement after a completed course of FP treatments.

When the concept of FP was first introduced, the laser was used as the energy source to generate fractional damage to the skin. The laser is still the most common energy source used in FP procedures. Its ability to quickly deliver energy in the form of focused optical radiation with high precision into small confined zones makes the laser a modality well suited for FP. Recently, other energy sources have emerged for generating fractional damage patterns. For example, radiofrequency (RF) and ultrasound devices are now commercially available that generate a pattern of small and confined thermal damage zones in skin tissue. The shape and anatomical location of MTZs generated using such modalities typically differ from those induced by focused optical radiation because of a different energy distribution within the tissue. As RF energy quickly diverges with increasing distance from the delivering electrode, it is possible to generate a spatially confined RF generated thermal injury only within the tissue directly adjacent to the tip of a needle electrode. Depending on the location of the tip of such RF electrode, damage can be generated either at the skin surface,[20] or virtually at any depth by inserting needle electrodes into the skin,[21] The use of stamping techniques with arrays or linear arrangements of multiple needle electrodes allows for coverage of a treatment area within a reasonable time. Focused ultrasound non-invasive generation of confined lesions,[22] in skin layers such as, e.g., the deep reticular dermis or even the superficial musculoaponeurotic system (SMAS) without causing any surface damage.[23] The MTZ cross section of RF or ultrasound generated MTZs is typically larger than that of laser generated MTZs because laser radiation can be more focused. However the ability to focus optical radiation decreases with increasing skin depth due to scattering and absorption of optical radiation. Further investigations are needed to investigate how the size and location of thermal lesions generated using RF and ultrasound sources affect the clinical outcome as compared to laser-generated MTZs.

- aFP and nFP can treat a wide variety of clinical conditions including some that have been traditionally the domain of selective photothermolysis (SP).
- The relative benefits and disadvantages of ablative and non-ablative FP approach are being investigated.

Both aFP and nFP target water-containing tissue and, unlike selective photothermolysis procedures,[10] there is no significant selectivity of specific components because virtually all cells of the skin are composed primarily of water. Nevertheless, FP can be used to treat certain conditions that traditionally have been a domain of selective photothermolysis, including treatment of pigmented and vascular lesions. FP targets aqueous tissue that contains such target lesions and therefore can affect a variety of lesions. Both, aFP and nFP have been applied successfully to a variety of clinical indications, including collagen remodeling and treatment of vascular and pigmented lesions. Further details of indications and the wound healing process are described in the following sections. The balance between improved clinical efficacy of aFP for selected indications as compared to nFP and the additional risks and side effects of aFP associated with a impaired epidermal barrier function and removal of entire columns of tissue in aFP is still being explored.

Non-ablative Fractional Photothermolysis (nFP)

- A variety of nFP devices are available in the marketplace.
- Principal treatment parameters for nFP are applied energy per MTZ and density of MTZs (number per square centimeter).
- To keep the areal fraction of damaged skin surface constant the MTZs density should be decreased when higher MTZ energies are applied.

An overview of certain systems currently available commercial systems for nFP procedures is presented in Table 1. These systems use various lasers emitting in the near IR range. Spot sizes in these systems are all in the sub-millimeter range, and the depth of the generated MTZs is mainly wavelength dependent, varies widely, and can extend into the deep reticular dermis for some systems. The depth and diameter of individual MTZs is positively correlated with energy.[24]

Variation of the focusing optics can also affect MTZ shape.[25] An example of the effects of different energies on the thermal damage and shape of MTZs is exhibited in Fig. 4. Primary treatment parameters for nFP include the energy applied per MTZ and the areal density of MTZs (e.g., the number per square centimeter). It is therefore necessary to decrease the MTZ areal density if higher energies are applied per MTZ to keep the areal fraction of damaged skin surface constant.

- Histologically, a column of necrotic, coagulated tissue is generally observed within the skin after formation of a MTZ via nFP.
- The skin barrier is preserved in nFP and the damaged epidermis is quickly replaced.
- Oval balls of microscopic epidermal necrotic debris (MEND) on the skin surface are often observed within 24 h of an nFP treatment.
- The 'MENDs shuttle' allows for controlled removal of epidermal and dermal content, e.g., melanin and elastin.
- nFP is well-suited for treatment of 'low contrast' superficial pigmented lesions.
- The remodeling of the damaged dermis can take several weeks and occurs without formation of fibrosis.

Histological analysis immediately after nFP treatment shows a column of thermally denatured dermis and epidermis that constitutes a microscopic treatment zone (MTZ) (Fig. 5a). In addition, subepidermal clefting may be observed in the area of the MTZ. This destruction of the dermal-epidermal (DE) junction corresponds to a microscopic blister, the size of which generally increases with the energy per MTZ. The tissue surrounding the MTZs appears microscopically undamaged. Further, the stratum corneum overlying the MTZ often appears unaltered, thus, preserving an intact skin barrier is preserved after nFP treatment. This is consistent with the early studies of Manstein et al.[8] who reported an absence of any significant change in trans-epidermal water loss after nFP. Due to the typically small (sub-millimeter) cross section of the MTZ, a rapid repair of the thermally damaged epidermis is generally observed. Within 24 h following an nFP procedure, necrotic cells in the epidermis are replaced by viable keratinocytes migrating to the damaged areas from the

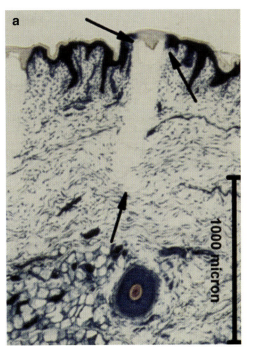

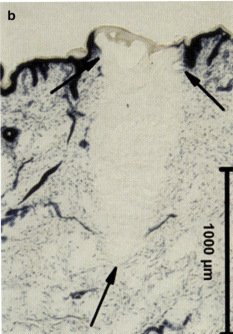

Fig. 4 Skin histology resulting from a nFP device at different energy levels. NitroBlueTetrazolium stain was used to monitor for thermal damage. Lack of blue staining indicates thermal cell injury. Lesions were produced with Fraxel re:store, Solta, $\lambda = 1,550$ nm within excised human skin. The depth and diameter of the MTZs vary with energy, 40 mJ (**a**) vs. 100 mJ (**b**). Note, the unstained part of the lesion consist of thermally damaged tissue rather than a cavity. Also, the commercial version of this laser is limited to a maximum energy of 70 mJ/MTZ (Thongsima et al.[25])

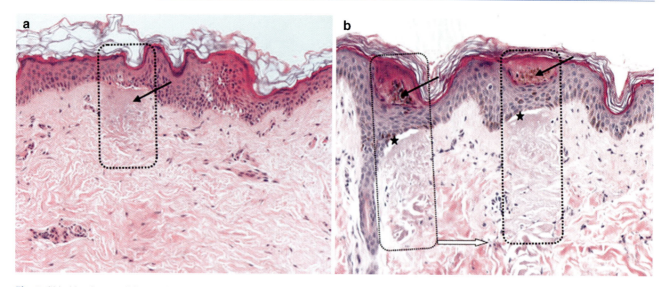

Fig. 5 Skin histology at different time points after nFP treatment. H&E stain, 200×. Lesions were produced with Solta prototype, λ = 1,500 nm, 5 mJ/MTZ. (**a**) 1 h after treatment a column of denatured collagen (*black arrow*) can be seen within the MTZ (*black outline*). The entire stratum corneum remains intact, even above the MTZ. There is no inflammatory infiltrate around the MTZ yet. (**b**) Day 1 after nFP. MTZs (*black outline*) contain microscopic epidermal necrotic debris (MENDs, *black arrows*), which represent the elimination of thermally damaged keratinocytes. MENDs are loaded with melanin. Subepidermal clefting is evident from 1 h after FP and lasts up to 5 days (*stars*). The dermal part of the MTZs appears the same as immediately post treatment and shows thermally altered collagen and a lack of nuclear staining. Subtle perivascular inflammatory infiltrate begins to form in the dermis (*white arrow*) (Laubach et al.[26])

unharmed tissue surrounding the MTZ (Fig. 5b) pushing the cellular debris of necrotic cells upwards towards the skin surface. Due to the excretion of the necrotic debris via the upper portion of the MTZs, oval balls of tissue may appear within about 24 h after nFP treatment. This tissue is referred to as microscopic epidermal necrotic debris (MEND).[8] Immuno-histochemical staining has revealed that MEND is mainly composed of necrotic epidermal tissue (including, e.g., melanin) but may also include portions originating from of dermal tissue (e.g., elastin).[27] In the days following an FP procedure, MEND migrates through the stratum corneum and can produce a small flaked shedding. The term 'MEND shuttle' describes the release of dermal and epidermal material through the MEND migration and shedding. During the migrational period of the MEND through the epidermis and stratum corneum, the number of dyskeratotic cells is reduced within the epidermis. About 1 week after the nFP treatment, the epidermis usually appears normal again. The MEND shuttle primarily facilitates controlled elimination of epidermal pigment, but it also allows for the removal of dermal content. The removal of pigment and dermal content by the MEND shuttle can be well-controlled by selection of the overall MTZ density formed during an nFP procedure. In contrast to laser procedures that utilize selective photothermolysis, the relative amount of pigment removed by the MEND shuttle is independent of the pigmentation of the treated tissue, because the wavelengths utilized to form the MTZs are primarily absorbed by water. This feature allows for a gradual removal of pigment of all skin colors by adjusting the density of MTZs. The pigment is also laterally re-distributed during the MEND shuttle process, so that a relative homogeneous removal of epidermal pigment can be achieved. As this process does not rely on the chromophore properties of melanin, all skin types can be effectively treated by the nFP process. Therefore nFP is a procedure of choice for removing pigment that presents as a 'low contrast lesion', i.e., where the difference in pigmentation levels between the lesion and the surrounding skin are relatively small. While the epidermal damage produced by nFP is quickly repaired, the dermal (deeper) portion of the MTZs is still well distinguishable for several weeks as a column of thermally coagulated collagen surrounded by minor perivascular, inflammatory infiltrate. Histological analyses performed 3 months after an nFP procedure indicate that the dermal portions of the MTZs are no longer distinguishable by standard H&E staining. However, overall dermal remodeling and restoration of a more undulated DE junction have been reported after nFP procedures.[8]

- nFP can also affect fine vessels, particularly for higher MTZ energies.

The effects of nFP are not limited to removal of epidermal pigment (Fig. 6a) and collagen remodeling (Fig. 6b). It has

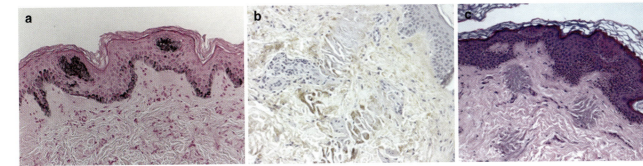

Fig. 6 Histological summary of the main effects of nFP procedures. (a) Pigment removal (*arrow*) by MENDs shuttle process (Fontana Masson stain). (b) Dermal remodeling as evidenced by positive collagen type III engulfing MTZs (*arrow*). (c) Coagulation of small blood vessels by statistical co-location of the MTZ and vessel (*arrow*)

been shown both histologically and clinically that nFP can also affect small vessels (Fig. 6c).[26] Although there is no significant selective absorption of energy by vascular targets in nFP procedures, it has been shown that small vessels having cross-section areas comparable to those of the MTZ lesions can be coagulated in a statistical manner, e.g., based on random intersection of the MTZs and vascular lesions. While selective photothermolysis remains the technique of choice for removal of vascular lesions, nFP can also have a beneficial effect on small vascular lesions. This vascular effect generally requires application of higher nFP energies to reach the tissue depth where the vascular targets are present. The clearance of vascular targets in the treatment region by using an nFP treatment with a high energy applied per MTZ was achieved (Fig. 7a, b), whereas a similar region of the same patient that was treated with the same total energy applied per unit area of the treatment region—but using a lower energy per MTZ formed—did not show any significant clearance of vascular lesions (Fig. 7c, d). The authors are not aware of any published clinical studies that have been performed to date on the treatment of vascular lesions with nFP, and further research is warranted in this area.

- The risk of bulk heating can be reduced by concurrent use of cooling.
- Cooling may alter the MTZ shape.

Forming relatively deep MTZs can be beneficial due to an increase in the local volume of thermally altered or destroyed tissue within the skin. However, increasing the diameter of the MTZs and/or the areal MTZ density ultimately results in unwanted side effects arising from increased damage to the dermo-epidermal junction (DEJ) and a stronger wound healing response. Although the optimal diameter and depth of MTZs formed during nFP to produce the greatest clinical efficacy and fewest side effects are yet to be determined, some limitations on these parameters have already been established. For example, it is well known that too much thermal damage per unit area of skin tissue (e.g., resulting from a large number of MTZs formed per unit area of tissue) can result in a loss of dermo-epidermal integrity and generation of severe unwanted side effects, such as blistering. Furthermore, creating too many MTZs within a region of skin in too short a time period can inhibit thermal relaxation of the tissue in-between passes and result in bulk heating of the entire treatment area. The thermal energy in such nFP procedures is no longer confined to the MTZs but instead diffuses into the surrounding tissue, leading to a thermal alteration of the entire tissue rather than limiting such thermal effects to the well-defined MTZ volumes. This spreading of the thermal energy ultimately may lead to unwanted side effects, including scarring of the treatment area. The combination of areal density of MTZs, energy used to form each MTZ, and the time interval in which they are created that can generate beneficial effects without introducing significant bulk heating to the treatment area remains an area in which more studies are needed. Several techniques for reducing the risk or extent of unwanted bulk tissue heating are described above. In particular, the use of skin cooling (e.g., forced-air cooling) and/or allowing sufficient time between consecutive nFP treatment passes can facilitate cooling of the treatment region. A decrease in skin temperature also tends to decrease the epidermal MTZ diameter for a particular set of applied energy parameters.[18] Therefore, tissue cooling effects should be considered when planning or comparing nFP treatments.

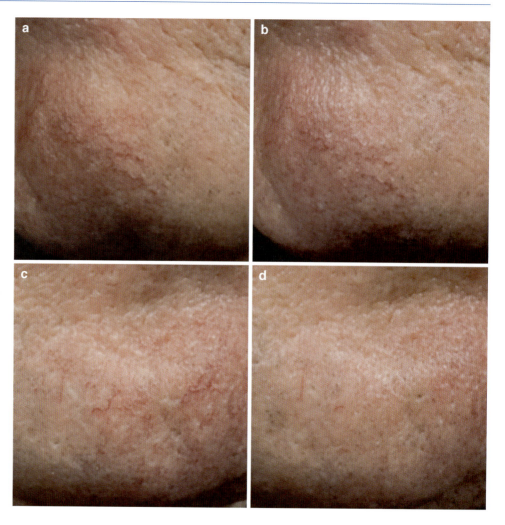

Fig. 7 Energy dependent response of telangiectasias to nFP treatment. A study patient with rosacea and acne scars had similar distribution of fine telangiectasias in contra-lateral areas of the face. 3 nFP treatments were performed at 1 month intervals with Fraxel re:store, λ=1,550 nm. A similar Fluence (average energy per area) was delivered at each side per treatment (approximately 13 J/cm^2) and outcome assessed 1 month after last treatment. The side treated with a lower MTZ energy (6 mJ/MTZ, ≈2,200 MTZ/cm^2) did not show any reduction of telangiectasias (**a**) and (**b**). The side treated with higher MTZ energy (70 mJ/MTZ, ≈200 MTZ/cm^2) showed significant reduction of telangiectasias (**c**) and (**d**)

- About 3–5 nFP treatment sessions are generally recommended; the exact number depends on the particular indication and desired end result.
- Other side effects associated with nFP treatment include a moderate erythema and/or edema developing immediately after the treatment and lasting up to 5 days; the severity of these side effects exhibit a positive correlation with MTZ energies and densities.

FP is based upon the concept of restricting thermal damage or alteration to well-defined microscopic zones within of the skin, whereby the surrounding healthy tissue can facilitate a rapid wound healing of the small damaged tissue volumes. Typically about 10–30% of the skin surface is thermally damaged or destroyed using focused laser beams in an nFP procedure. About 3–5 nFP sessions are generally recommended for treating a particular region of skin; the exact number of sessions can depend on the indication and desired end result. Although patient satisfaction (an indicator of treatment efficacy) generally improves with the number of treatment sessions, the improvement in satisfaction between the third and the fourth treatment appears to be only marginal.[28] The optimal number of nFP treatment sessions needed for greater patient satisfaction and clinical improvement is not generally known, and depend at least in part on the particular nFP parameters used and the condition being treated. The optimal time interval(s) between successive nFP treatment sessions for achieving optimal efficacy and a minimum of side effects also remains to be determined. In one particular example, it has been proposed that longer intervals between nFP treatment sessions, e.g., up to 2 months, are preferable when treating Fitzpatrick skin type IV–VI to reduce the risk of post inflammatory hyperpigmentation (PIH).[29]

- Discomfort during nFP treatment increases significantly with the energy applied per MTZ and the MTZ density per pass.
- Different approaches such as prior and/or simultaneous skin cooling, local application of a topical anesthetic, etc. can be used to reduce or eliminate perceived pain.

One of the side effects of nFP treatment is patient discomfort during the treatment itself. This discomfort increases mainly with the energy applied per MTZ, but also with the MTZ density per pass.[29] Several different approaches are currently used to decrease discomfort during treatment. Concomitant skin cooling during laser treatments not only reduces undesirable side effects such as bulk heating, but also reduces discomfort associated with nFP laser treatments.[30] Providers of various nFP systems often recommend either contact or air convection cooling. Some nFP laser system providers recommend the use of anesthetic cream prior to the nFP treatment, while others do not recommend the use of additional anesthetics. Because of a lack of comparative trials, it is currently not well investigated whether there is a significant difference in patient pain perception with different nFP systems.

> • Bronzing due to the MENDs formation and migration through the epidermis and stratum corneum can be observed 3–7 days after an nFP procedure.

Other side effects associated with nFP treatment include a moderate erythema and edema developing immediately after the treatment and typically lasting for up to about 1 week. The severity of these side effects show a positive correlation with MTZ energies; MTZ areal densities are not only associated with an increase in erythema and edema, but also correlate with observed post inflammatory hyperpigmentation (PIH).[29] Although a reduction in efficacy has been observed for nFP skin rejuvenation procedures with lower energy settings, lower applied energies are also correlated with a reduction in the duration and severity of side effects like erythema and edema.[29] A patient's downtime corresponds to the duration and the severity of the post-treatment erythema and edema, and is typically on the order of a few days. The authors' experience suggests that the consistent use of cooling pads during the first 24 h after nFP treatment further reduces the severity of erythema and edema. During the third to seventh days after an nFP procedure, the treated skin often shows a slight bronzing due to the MEND formation and migration through the epidermis and stratum corneum as noted above. This bronzing effect tends to be evenly distributed over the treated area, and most patients describe this effect as cosmetically not unpleasant and feeling slightly "suntanned." Such bronzing effect can contribute to the epidermal elimination of melanin. As this bronzing is related to transepidermal melanin elimination, it is generally more accentuated for darker skin types and within treatment areas of enhanced melanin density.

The 1,927 nm Thulium laser has been recently introduced in an nFP system and promoted among other indications the removal of superficial pigment, including for non-facial areas. Published details or studies of this system are not available as of the publication date of this volume. This system can produce a larger MTZ diameter of up to approximately 600 μm. Its wavelength is more superficially absorbed (OPD $\approx$ 100 μm) as compared, for example, to nFP systems based on the 1,540 nm or 1,550 nm lasers (OPD $\approx$ 1,000 μm) but less absorbed than aFP systems based on CO_2 lasers (OPD $\approx$ 10 μm). Thus it is designed to generate thermal injury in relatively superficially tissue without significant disruption of the epidermal barrier. A representative example of the clinical course after treatment with the Thulium laser is shown in Fig. 8.

For post-nFP aftercare, a hydrating, non-greasy moisturizer is generally recommended because patients commonly report a sensation of rough and dry skin, most likely due to the MEND shedding that commonly occurs several days after the procedure. Furthermore, there is an increased risk of the formation of acne-like lesions, especially with the use of higher treatment energies. Using a non-occlusive aftercare product may reduce this risk. Patients with a positive history of facial herpes simplex should take oral antiviral medication prior to nFP treatment to prevent or inhibit viral reactivation. The effectiveness of systemic or topical corticosteroids in reducing side effects such as edema and erythema without compromising treatment efficacy is yet to be determined.

> • The risk of post-inflammatory hyperpigmentation in patients having darker skin types can be decreased significantly by reducing the density of MTZs, and by simultaneous skin cooling.

Non-ablative FP procedures can be associated with minor petechial bleeding, especially if patients continue to traumatize the skin during the first few days after the treatment (e.g., by wearing tight wristbands, necklaces, etc.). Chan et al.[31] observed that a mild-to-moderate post-inflammatory hyperpigmentation (PIH) occurs in about 7.1–17.1% of Asians undergoing nFP treatment; the likelihood of this side effect depends on the laser settings and evaluation method. The risk of PIH, especially for darker skin type patients, can be reduced significantly by decreasing the extent (including the overall area) of dermo-epidermal junction destruction, e.g., by reducing total MTZ densities and using simultaneous skin cooling.[29,31,32] Furthermore, protection from sunlight during the weeks after nFP treatment should be emphasized to the patient to further reduce the likelihood of unwanted PIH. It remains to be determined whether lengthening the time intervals between successive nFP treatments can help to reduce the occurrence of PIH. Currently available data suggests that nFP treatments can be customized to the patients' desires to balance the aggressiveness of treatments to achieve a higher efficacy with the likelihood of causing undesirable side effects.

- The main indications for nFP are treatment of photoaging, various kinds of scars and treatment of dyschromia.
- Improvement of deep rhytides and skin tightening is limited.
- Melasma has a high risk of recurrence.

Non-ablative FP has been shown to be effective on a wide variety of conditions,[33-36] including but not limited to a variety of indications related to collagen remodeling, e.g., treatment of photoaging including fine and moderate rhytides (Fig. 9), treatment of traumatic (Fig. 10), surgical, burn (Fig. 11) and acne scarring, striae distensae, and treatment of dyschromia e.g., superficial pigmented lesions like solar lentigines. The authors would like to highlight the ability of nFP to improve various kinds of scars including textural skin

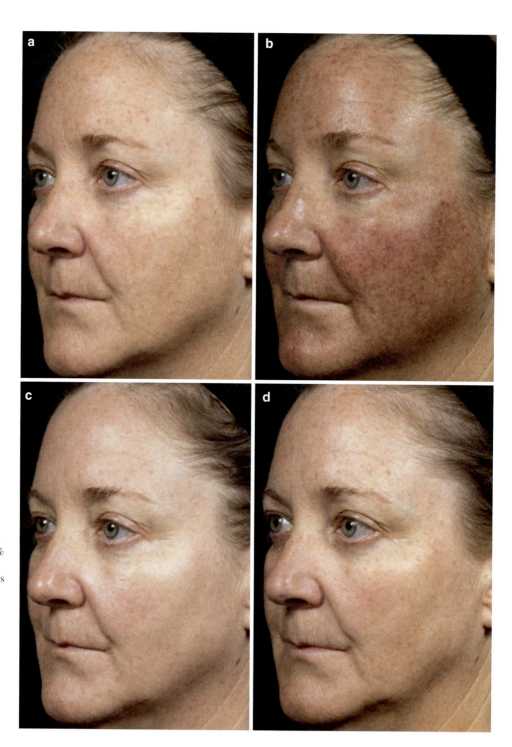

Fig. 8 Clinical course of after single treatment with Thulium laser. Treatment was performed with Fraxel Dual (Solta), $\lambda = 1,927$ nm, 10 mJ/MTZ, ≈ 800 MTZ/cm^2, treatment level 7, 50% density. Clinical appearance at baseline (**a**), 2 days (**b**), 6 months (**c**) and 10 months (**d**). After significant improvement of the dyschromia at 1 and 6 months, there is partial recurrence of dyschromia at the 10 months follow up. This is likely due to continued sun exposure as the patient participated in frequent outdoor sports without proper UV protection (Courtesy of Steven Struck, M.D.)

Fractional Photothermolysis 137

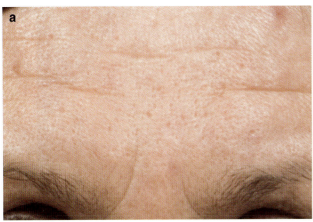
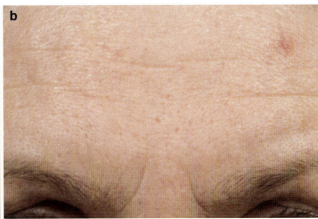

Fig. 9 Clinical improvement of fine and moderate (dynamic) rhytides. A series of 3 nFP treatments was performed with Fraxel re:store (Solta), λ = 1,550 nm, 70 mJ/MTZ, approx. 200 MTZ/cm^2. (**a**) Baseline. (**b**) 6 months after last treatment. *Note*: Treatment was performed as part of a clinical study, and the use of neurotoxins (not applied to this patient) would likely have provided similar results

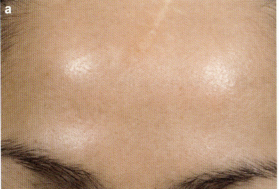
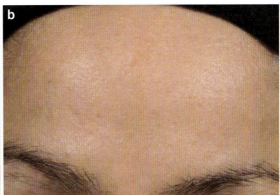

Fig. 10 Clinical improvement of a traumatic scar. A traumatic scar that was persistent for more than 10 years received a series of 3 nFP treatments with Fraxel re:store (Solta), λ = 1,550 nm, MTZ energy 70 mJ, ≈200MTZ/cm^2. The scar virtually disappeared after the completion of the series of treatments. (**a**) Baseline. (**b**) 6 months after last treatment

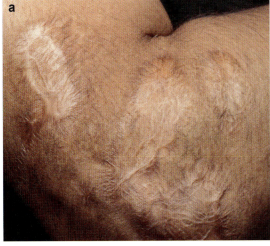
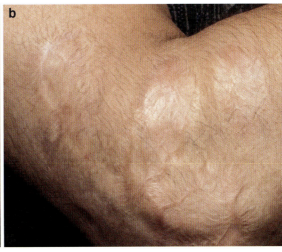
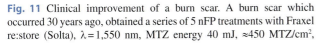

Fig. 11 Clinical improvement of a burn scar. A burn scar which occurred 30 years ago, obtained a series of 5 nFP treatments with Fraxel re:store (Solta), λ = 1,550 nm, MTZ energy 40 mJ, ≈450 MTZ/cm^2, 23% density, treatment level 8. Significant improvement of texture and pigmentation is observed. (**a**) Baseline. (**b**) 5 months after the last treatment (Courtesy of Steven Struck, M.D.)

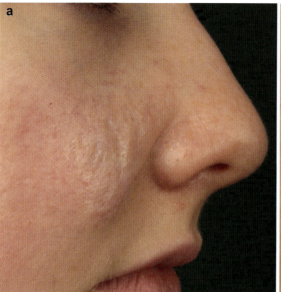 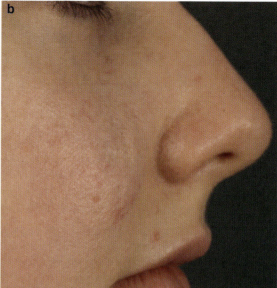

Fig. 12 Clinical improvement of scarring. Skin alterations mimicking dermal scarring had developed after the involution of an early childhood hemangioma and were stable for approximately 13 years prior to FP treatment. A series of 5 nFP treatments achieved a significant smoothening of skin surface (Solta, re:store, $\lambda = 1{,}550$ nm, ≈ 40 mJ/MTZ, treatment level 8). (**a**): Baseline. (**b**): 1 month after last treatment.

alterations after involution of hemangiomas (Fig. 12), as for these indications remarkable improvement was reported that was previously difficult to obtain. However, high efficacy of nFP procedures for improvement of deep rhytides and skin laxity has not yet been convincingly demonstrated. Treatment of melasma with nFP is an option but it should be used with caution, because of the relative high rate of repigmentation and sometimes even an increase in pigmentation after nFP treatments.[38]

- Many novel indications for nFP are emerging.
- Determination of optimal nFP parameters for particular indications is an area of ongoing study

Other indications that have shown some promise for treatment using nFP in small case studies are minocycline-induced hyperpigmentation,[39] granuloma anulare,[40] striae rubra,[41] Nevus of Ota,[42] alopecia areata,[43] and Poikiloderma of Civatte.[44] While results of these case reports suggest promising results, further clinical studies are needed before nFP can be established as a standard of care for such indications. Nevertheless, it is encouraging to see that nFP may be an option for treating such clinical problems.

Although a wide variety of nFP systems, treatment parameters, and regimens have been shown to provide measurable clinical improvement for various dermatological indications, determination of optimal parameters and conditions for particular indications remains an area of ongoing study.

Ablative Fractional Photothermolysis (aFP)

- A variety of different aFP laser systems are available, and most of them are based on CO_2 and Er:YAG lasers.

Ablative FP systems utilize wavelengths that are strongly absorbed within tissue as compared to wavelengths used in nFP systems. The resulting high energy densities lead to vaporization of tissue. An overview of selected aFP systems currently available commercially is provided in Table 2.

- Ablative Fractional Photothermolysis (aFP) is a procedure characterized by formation of microscopically small zones of removed (ablated) tissue surrounded by a small cuff of thermally damaged tissue embedded in viable tissue.

Vaporization of tissue within an MTZ generated in an aFP procedure forms a tapered cavity lined by a thin layer of eschar.[12] The thin layer of eschar is surrounded by an annular coagulation zone containing denatured collagen and cell necrosis. While the zones of denatured collagen and cell necrosis substantially overlap, the extent of the zone of cell necrosis is slightly larger due to the lower thermal damage threshold for cell necrosis as compared to that for collagen denaturation. A varying degree of thermal damage in the residual tissue immediately adjacent to the evaporated tissue of aFP procedures has been observed, similar to that resulting from conventional ablative resurfacing techniques. The thermal coagulation zone around the laser cavity typically varies with the type of laser and pulse duration used. For example, the CO_2 laser used in conventional resurfacing procedures produces typically more residual thermal damage as compared to the Er:YAG laser,[45] and thermal effects generated by a laser tend to increase with longer pulse duration.[46]

- The pulse duration and temporal pulse shape affect residual thermal damage.
- Mechanical factors applied during the post treatment regime might affect clinical skin tightening.

Analogous to traditional ablative procedures, the amount of residual thermal injury in aFP procedures may also be affected by the temporal profile of the laser pulse. Typical temporal profiles for energy delivery include continuous wave (CW), superpulsed,[47] and ultrapulsed[48] mode. Although such dependency of thermal injury on pulse profile appears reasonable, there is currently no investigational data available that specifically relates the extent of thermal damage for aFP procedures to the temporal pulse profiles. The amount of immediate skin shrinkage resulting from an aFP treatment (with CO_2 laser) is typically greater than that observed in nFP procedures. However, histological analysis indicates that nFP procedures may even exhibit a greater total volume of denatured collagen, as compared to an aFP process performed with similar energy per MTZ (comparison of data from Hantash et al.[12] and Thongsima et al.[25]). This seems to contradict the general observation that the extent of skin shrinkage is related to the total amount of denatured collagen. The authors hypothesize that as collagen denaturation and skin shrinkage occur at virtually the same time while the laser cavity is being formed, that part of the denatured collagen is removed during the cavity forming process. Histology reveals a static image of the amount of denatured collagen after the completion of the MTZ formation. Further research is indicated to investigate the dynamics of the various processes occurring within the short time of the formation of ablative MTZs.

In general, immediate tissue contraction during aFP due to collagen shrinkage is an indicator of anticipated skin tightening. However, the role of wound healing on the clinically relevant skin tightening should also taken into consideration. Animal studies have demonstrated that the skin tightening, including the direction of contraction can also be significantly affected by factors that were applied during the wound healing process after the completion of an aFP procedure. In particular, direction of mechanical forces (e.g., gravity or elastic wound dressings) applied during the initial several days have been shown to affect significantly the outcome.[49] These observations should stimulate further research before specific clinical recommendations on a modified post treatment regime can be made.

- Ablative FP impairs the epidermal barrier and can facilitate enhanced drug delivery but also bacterial infections.
- The use of antibiotic prophylaxis is typically indicated for aFP procedures of a larger areas.
- Impairment of epidermal barrier results in temporary serous oozing and punctuate bleeding.

The depth and diameter of MTZs formed using a particular aFP system is primarily dependent on the energy applied to the tissue to form each MTZ. Figure 13 illustrates the increase of depth and diameter of an ablated MTZ with increasing

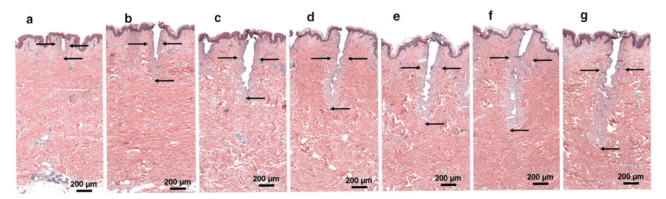

Fig. 13 Skin histology resulting from aFP at different energy levels. H&E staining. Lesions were produced within excised skin with Fraxel re:pair (Solta), $\lambda = 10{,}600$ nm. MTZ diameter and depth increases with energy. (**a**) 10 mJ, (**b**) 20 mJ, (**c**) 30 mJ, (**d**) 40 mJ, (**e**) 50 mJ, (**f**) 60 mJ, (**g**) 70 mJ (Courtesy of Solta Medical, Biomedical Research Team)

energy. Furthermore, because the stratum corneum is also evaporated in the core of MTZs formed during aFP, there is an actual disruption of the physical epidermal barrier that is proportional to the size and density of MTZs. Accordingly, aFP leads to more significant impairment of the protective and barrier function of the epidermis as compared with non-ablative techniques. This aspect presents opportunities for the concurrent delivery of drugs to the tissue but also imposes additional risks, such as an increased risk of bacterial infection following aFP procedures. Therefore, the use of antibiotic prophylaxis is typically indicated for aFP procedures of larger areas. The physical disruption of the epidermal barrier is also evidenced by serous oozing and punctuate bleeding following aFP. procedures. However, such side effects related to the disruption of the epidermal barrier resolve typically within about 12–24 h after the disruption occurs.[50] Although ablated MTZs can reach a depth in excess of 1 mm, they heal relatively fast. A representative time line of the histological wound healing for an aFP procedure is illustrated in Fig. 14. Analysis of in-vivo histology at different times after an aFP treatment revealed that re-epithelialization has taken place within 48 h of the treatment. The basement membrane was restored within 7 days, and a coagulation zone could be observed up to approximately 1 month after the procedure. A representative time line of the clinical course after an aFP procedure is presented in Fig. 15. The duration of wound healing from aFP is shorter as compared to traditional ablative CO_2 resurfacing procedures, but is considered longer than that observed in nFP procedures.

- Currently aFP is primarily used for dermatological indications that require collagen remodeling.
- The relative efficacy of aFP and nFP for various indications remains to be determined.

Almost all dermatological indications that have been treated by nFP procedures have also been treated by aFP procedures.[51-53] The authors are not aware of any extensive clinical studies performed to date that the authors are aware of comparing the outcomes of nFP and aFP procedures for the same conditions. It is important for the clinician to have more comparative data available to better assess whether the typically enhanced profile of side effects associated with aFP procedures is justified by improved clinical outcomes. Generally, aFP procedures are observed to provide enhanced collagen remodeling, e.g., for indications such as skin tightening,[54] treatment of skin laxity, and treatment of moderate to severe rhytides,[55] and overall produces satisfactory results for these collagen-sensitive responses with acceptable post-treatment patient downtime. Figures 16 and 17 illustrate cases of clinical improvement of photoaging with concurrent respectively moderate and severe rhytides. Although decreased patient downtime is desirable, traditional ablative resurfacing procedures—with generally long downtime periods—are still the gold standard of treatment for marked photodamage.

- Options for anesthesia are similar to conventional ablative resurfacing techniques.

Anesthesia for aFP treatments can be provided by topical agents, local infiltration, cooling, and/or nerve blocks. The level of patient pain tolerance, the laser parameters used (e.g., pulse energies and durations), and treatment location are all factors to be considered for individual pain management. The use of systemic agents, including narcotics, sedation or intravenous anesthesia, may be warranted for some patients, particularly when treatment of larger areas is performed on sensitive patients. Postoperative management is aimed to alleviate edema, exudates, and postoperative

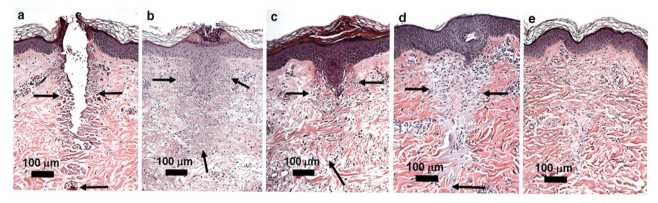

Fig. 14 Wound healing resulting from aFP at different time points. H&E staining. Skin lesions were produced with Fraxel re:pair (Solta), $\lambda = 10,600$ nm at 20 mJ/MTZ. Analysis of in-vivo histology at different times after an aFP treatment revealed that re-epithelialization has taken place within 48 h of the treatment. The basement membrane was restored within 7 days, and a dermal coagulation zone could be observed up to approximately 1 month after the procedure. At 3 months the lesions were resolved without evidence of fibrosis. (a) 0 day, (b) 2 days, (c) 7 days, (d) 30 days, (e) 90 days (Hantash et al.[50])

Fractional Photothermolysis

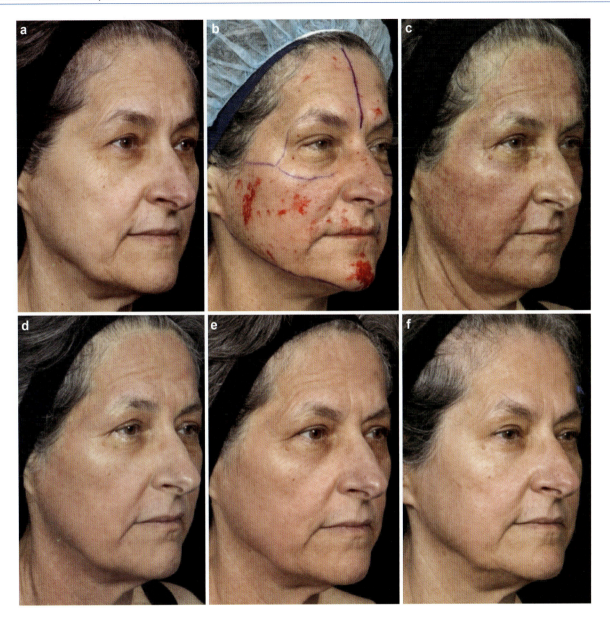

Fig. 15 Clinical course after aFP treatment. A single aFP treatment was performed with device Fraxel re:pair (Solta), 135 µm handpiece, $\lambda = 10{,}600$ nm, 70 mJ/MTZ, ≈300 MTZ/cm², treatment level 8, 30% nominal coverage. Photographs represent baseline (**a**), immediately after treatment (**b**), 3 days (**c**), 1 week (**d**), 1 month (**e**) and 6 months (**f**) (Courtesy of Steven Struck, M.D.)

discomfort. Elevation of the treatment area, cool compresses, and application of petrolatum ointment are typically used in postoperative care. When marked edema and/ or erythema occur following aFP treatment, a short term course of oral corticosteroids may be prescribed.

Adverse Events and Clinical Pitfalls of FP

- Excessive bulk heating (confluent thermal damage) must be avoided.
- Treatment of small areas can be particularly prone to bulk heating.
- In order to minimize the risk of bulk heating, the following strategies should be considered: skin cooling, lowering MTZ areal densities, and providing sufficient time between passes to allow cooling of the treated tissue.

Although fractional photothermolysis is generally considered to be safer than traditional ablative techniques that damage a confluent tissue layer, there are some clinical pitfalls that should be avoided. Following are several important considerations and cautions that should be recognized and addressed when performing FP procedures. One major concern for FP treatments is generation of bulk heating in the

Fig. 16 Clinical improvement of moderate rhytides. A single aFP treatment was performed with Active FX (80 mJ/MTZ, density 4) and Deep FX (15 mJ, 15% density) (Lumenis, $\lambda = 10{,}600$ nm). The images exhibit baseline (*left*) and 3 months after a single treatment (*right*) (Courtesy of Kevin Duplechain, M.D.)

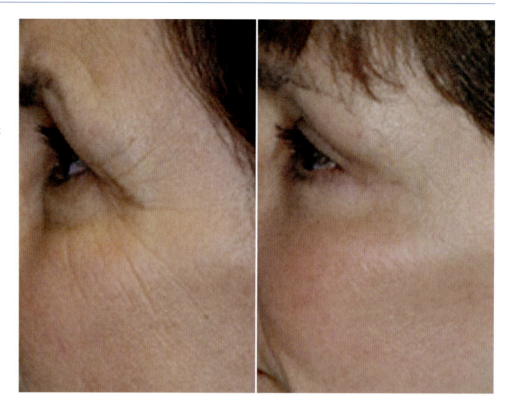

Fig. 17 Clinical improvement of severe rhytides. A single aFP treatment was performed with Active FX (80 mJ/MTZ, density 4) and Deep FX (15 mJ, 15% density) (Lumenis, $\lambda = 10{,}600$ nm). The images exhibit baseline (*left*) and 3 months after a single treatment (*right*) (Courtesy of Kevin Duplechain, M.D.)

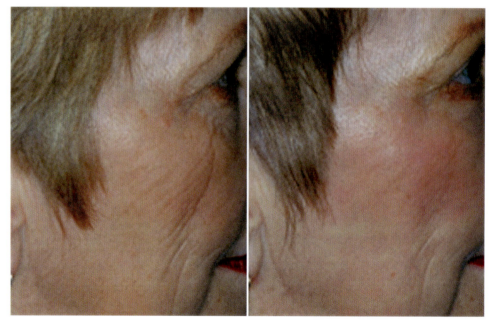

treated tissue. Bulk heating can facilitate undesirable effects such as post-inflammatory hyperpigmentation (which is more commonly observed in Asian patients) or even result in scarring (Fig. 18). To reduce the risk or extent of such side effects, proper evaluation of the condition being treated should be performed (e.g., acne scars, melasma, rhytides, etc.). An appropriate density of MTZ formation should also be selected based on the patient's skin type to produce effective results while minimizing the risk of side effects due to bulk heating. Furthermore, it is important to cool the tissue in the treatment region during FP procedures. For example, a dynamic air cooling device (such as the one produced by Zimmer, Inc.) has been used simultaneously with many FP treatments. It is also recommended to allow some time between successive treatment passes over a specific body area. However, treatment of small face or body areas may not

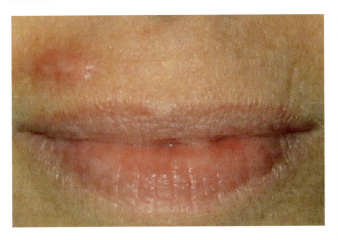

Fig. 18 Scar on the upper lip several months after nFP treatment delivered without adequate skin cooling. Bulk tissue heating has occurred due to delivery of multiple passes within small areas in relatively short time. *Note*: The lesion resolved over 6 months after intralesional steroid injections and the patient requested additional FP treatments because of otherwise excellent cosmetic improvement

allow sufficient time for skin cooling between passes, which can lead to bulk heating and scarring. Some observations of neck and periorbital area scarring, likely caused by local bulk heating, have been reported.[56]

- For highly-focused laser beams, a precise positioning of the handpiece is needed.
- Minor positional deviations from the focal plane could cause significant alteration of spot size and fill factor.

Operator technique is particularly important when using ablative FP (aFP) systems. The highly-focused laser beams generated by these ablative systems are configured to deliver a small spot size. Therefore, precise positioning of the handpiece is relative to the tissue being treated is extremely important. Any minor deviation of the laser beam focal point from the desired focal plane can cause significant alteration of the spot size and fill factor because of the convergent geometry of the focused beam. This can lead to bulk heating in specific areas, followed by potential scarring and pigmentation changes.

- Particular caution should be exercised at areas of thin skin and low density of skin appendages.

For patients seeking FP treatment of non-facial (e.g., poikiloderma of the neck, periorbital rhytides), the physician should also be aware of the lower density of appendageal units in such areas. This lower density may slow tissue healing and leave the treated area more susceptible to infection and scarring. Adequate selection of MTZ density becomes very important when treating such areas of the body to avoid unwanted side effects.

- The use of antiviral prophylaxis is not clearly established for FP; a history of herpes simplex virus (HSV), ablative treatments (aFP), and/or treatment of large areas are factors favoring antiviral prophylaxis.

Complications of FP treatment can be caused by local infections, particularly when performing aFP procedures that disrupt the stratum corneum. A universal prophylactic regimen has not yet been established for such procedures. Patients with a history of herpes simplex virus affecting the lips or any facial area are generally advised to undergo a 1- or 2-day course of oral antivirals concurrent with the FP procedure. A consensus for appropriate antibacterial antibiotic prophylaxis in conjunction with FP procedures is not clearly established, either. Antibiotic prophylaxis is typically indicated when treating large areas using ablative modalities.

- Pre-operative sun avoidance and discontinuation of retinoids are important factors for minimizing side effects.

Pre-operative and post-operative considerations must be discussed and addressed with the patient prior to initiating a course of FP treatments. During the pre-operative interview and physical examination, it is important to confirm the absence of sun burns and sun tanning, which should be strictly observed for at least 2–4 weeks prior to the procedure and, ideally, for the same length of time after the treatment. This is important in order to reduce the risk of post-inflammatory hyperpigmentation, and may be most relevant to patients living in the tropics and with a history of sun tanning. Similarly, patients with solar lentigos and melasma may be given a choice to first attempt chemical bleaching, followed by FP in order to remove remaining pigmentation and address textural and rhytides concerns. On the other hand, late-onset hypopigmentation is virtually never observed as resulting from FP treatments, in contrast to traditional resurfacing modalities. During the pre-operative period for FP, it is also important to address any prior use of retinoids, either alone or in combination with other topicals. The patient must be instructed to stop the use of topical retinoids for at least 1 week prior to each FP procedure. Use of oral retinoid therapy (isotretinoin) should preferably be discontinued for a period of a few months prior to performing an FP procedure.

- Post-operatively, sun avoidance, compliance with medication and proper recognition and management of complications are key.

Post-operatively, patients must be instructed on proper skin care and strict sun avoidance in order to prevent side effects and complications, including pigment alteration. Appropriate antiviral or antibiotic prophylaxis, if recommended, must be followed by the patient in order to avoid skin infection and/or potential scarring. Complications should be recognized early and without any delay appropriately managed.

Future Directions

- New indications treatable by FP will continue to be identified.

Fractional photothermolysis (FP) has been established as a treatment modality for various indications. To date, these indications are mostly aesthetic in nature. The beneficial effects of FP are not limited to collagen remodeling, pigment removal and closure of small vessels. Because FP can induce a strong wound healing reaction and induces HSP production, FP procedures may be developed to affect tissue regeneration, immune regulation, nerve fiber density, etc. Further investigation of these effects and others are warranted. FP appears to be an important tool that is capable of affecting many different biological pathways, and therefore it can be expected that more indications treatable using FP techniques, including a wide spectrum of dermatological diseases, will continue to emerge.

- Ablative FP can serve to facilitate drug and cell delivery into the skin.

Another important area of further development is the use of aFP for enhanced delivery of drugs and (stem) cells into different layers of the skin. It has been demonstrated that transcutaneous delivery of a photosensitizer can be enhanced

using a low-density aFP procedure.[57] The delivery of drugs or other substances that typically do not pass through the epidermis can thus be facilitated in a controlled manner over large areas using aFP treatment. aFP may make it possible to achieve topical delivery of a plethora of effective agents into the skin. For example, entire cell populations could be delivered through gateways formed by ablated MTZs and open up new strategies for controlled distribution of targeted (stem) cells into different layers of the skin. FP may potentially be used, not only for the delivery of (stem) cells, but also to simultaneously induce an appropriate and controlled wound healing response within the recipient tissue. Such wound healing response may create a microenvironment that facilitates growth and differentiation of delivered and/or resident stem cells.

- The channels created by aFP could be used for delivery of focused optical radiation of virtually any wavelength to deeper skin layers.

The microscopic ablated MTZ channels created by aFP could also be used as a gateway for delivery of focused optical radiation to deeper layers of the skin. The delivered optical energy could be virtually of any wavelength as the optical barriers of tissue absorption and scattering may be avoided when the radiation is directed through these small channels. Spatial and temporal alignment of ablative and delivered radiation sources is critical for forming such microscopic gateways and directing further radiation through the newly-formed gateways.

- FP has the potential to become soon a home-use product.

Home-use dermatology devices represent an area of growing interest and recent developments. The ability for the patient/consumer to perform a treatment conveniently at home and the huge commercial market potential are just two of the many factors driving the market for such devices. A primary concern when using a home-use device is guaranteed safety. This presents a challenge as the consumer, typically possesses only very limited skill with respect to medical device procedures. In particular, the ability to set the treatment parameters sufficiently high, to treat a wide range of skin types without jeopardizing without completely jeopardizing efficacy, is a prime challenge for home-use laser applications. FP offers three key characteristics that could facilitate the development of

FP-based home use products. First, the tissue effects of FP are not skin type dependent, as not melanin but water is the main chromophore. Second, although each individual MTZ induces a guaranteed wound healing response on a microscopic scale, the density needed to achieve a clinical improvement can be distributed over many treatments, e.g., using a daily application of low densities over a period of weeks. Such a treatment regime, which could be easily performed in an at home environment, could result in safe, minimal incremental effects but significant overall improvement after completion of a treatment course. And third, as relatively low energy is required to generate individual MTZs, the energy source (laser) could be produced relatively inexpensively and may even be battery operated. Although no FP home-use product is currently available, it would not be surprising if such an FP product will be marketed in the near future, considering the driving factors and the suitability of FP procedures for safe and effective applications in a home-use environment. (Note: Shortly after submission of this chapter the first FDA-approved home-use FP laser device was commercially released, the PaloVia device from Palomar Medical, MA.)

> • FP can potentially be applied to other organs besides skin.

Although the focus of FP procedures to date has been on treating skin tissue (skin is the most accessible organ of the body), the concepts and effects associated with FP treatment of skin tissue will likely be applicable to other biological organs and structures. For example, as we learn how to improve scars within the skin by FP, this could become a successful modality to improve fibrosis or degeneration in other organs. Virtually any organ system is plagued by diseases or conditions caused by such processes. FP procedures may become a novel treatment option to improve or restore the functionality of an affected organ. Potential examples of future non-dermatological indications treated with FP are scars (fibrosis) of the vocal cord or the heart. Obviously, the delivery systems for such FP procedures would have to be modified to be compatible with the specific anatomy, and further research has to be performed to investigate the effects of FP on different organ systems. Overall, it appears likely that in the future FP will also be utilized by specialties other than dermatology.

> • FP treatments show great future promise, but alternative concepts, such as conventional laser resurfacing and peeling techniques should still be considered.

Despite the efficacy and current popularity of FP procedures, the conventional resurfacing techniques including chemical peeling procedures should not be forgotten and will maintain a clinical role, in particularly when cost effectiveness is a consideration. Fractional treatments are not a universal solution to all types of dermatological conditions, but they certainly provide the clinician and patient additional options to achieve a desired clinical outcome. Further research is still needed to provide data that facilitates the selection of optimal parameters for FP treatment of various conditions.

Conclusion

Fractional Photothermolysis (FP) exploits the concept that 'size matters' with respect to laser-induced damage of biological tissue. Three-dimensional patterns of microscopic treatment zones (MTZs) promote tissue regeneration with fast wound healing in the absence of fibrosis. FP can be applied as a non-ablative (thermal damage) or ablative (tissue removal) modality. FP is currently used primarily to treat fine and moderate rhytides, scars of various types, pigmentary disorders, and to repair photodamaged skin. Novel indications treatable using FP continue to emerge. Due to the recognized efficacy of FP procedures, a proliferation of FP systems employing different wavelengths and exposure parameters have been introduced into the marketplace and FP procedures are offered by a large number of clinicians. Despite the significant progress in developing effective FP procedures to date, the search for ideal treatment parameters and conditions for the many indications is still ongoing. There is ample space for future developments of FP, including identification of additional treatable indications, adjuvant treatment modalities to modify the wound healing response, and improved delivery of drugs and/or (stem)cells in combination with aFP treatments. In the future, FP might not be limited to treatment of skin, but may become an effective technique for treating and regenerating different organ systems.

References

1. Hruza GJ, Dover JS. Laser skin resurfacing. *Arch Dermatol.* 1996;132(4):451-455.
2. Waldorf HA, Kauvar AN, Geronemus RG. Skin resurfacing of fine to deep rhytides using a char-free carbon dioxide laser in 47 patients. *Dermatol Surg.* 1995;21(11):940-946.
3. Williams EF III, Dahiya R. Review of nonablative laser resurfacing modalities. *Facial Plast Surg Clin North Am.* 2004;12(3):305-310. v.
4. Bernstein LJ, Kauvar AN, Grossman MC, Geronemus RG. The short- and long-term side effects of carbon dioxide laser resurfacing. *Dermatol Surg.* 1997;23(7):519-525.
5. Helm TN, Shatkin S Jr. Alabaster skin after CO_2 laser resurfacing: evidence for suppressed melanogenesis rather than just melanocyte destruction. *Cutis.* 2006;77(1):15-17.

6. Laws RA, Finley EM, McCollough ML, Grabski WJ. Alabaster skin after carbon dioxide laser resurfacing with histologic correlation. *Dermatol Surg*. 1998;24(6):633-636.

7. Hohenleutner S, Koellner K, Lorenz S, Landthaler M, Hohenleutner U. Results of nonablative wrinkle reduction with a 1,450-nm diode laser: difficulties in the assessment of "subtle changes". *Lasers Surg Med*. 2005;37(1):14-18.

8. Manstein D, Herron GS, Sink RK, Tanner H, Anderson RR. Fractional photothermolysis: a new concept for cutaneous remodeling using microscopic patterns of thermal injury. *Lasers Surg Med*. 2004;34(5):426-438.

9. Laubach HJ, Manstein D. Fractional photothermolysis. *Hautarzt*. 2007;58(3):216-218; 220–223.

10. Anderson RR, Parrish JA. Selective photothermolysis: precise microsurgery by selective absorption of pulsed radiation. *Science*. 1983;220(4596):524-527.

11. Grossman AR, Majidian AM, Grossman PH. Thermal injuries as a result of CO_2 laser resurfacing. *Plast Reconstr Surg*. 1998; 102(4):1247-1252.

12. Hantash BM, Bedi VP, Chan KF, Zachary CB. Ex vivo histological characterization of a novel ablative fractional resurfacing device. *Lasers Surg Med*. 2007;39(2):87-95.

13. Walsh JT Jr, Deutsch TF. Pulsed CO_2 laser tissue ablation: measurement of the ablation rate. *Lasers Surg Med*. 1988;8(3):264-275.

14. Hale GM, Querry MR. Optical constants of water in the 200-nm to 200-microm wavelength region. *Appl Opt*. 1973;12(3):555-563.

15. Warner DW, Morgan NE, Eby TA, Myers MC, Taylor DA. Water measurement in biological tissue. In: Romig AD, Chambers WF, eds. *Microbeam Analysis*, 21. San Francisco: San Francisco Press; 1987:238-240.

16. Walsh JT Jr, Cummings JP. Effect of the dynamic optical properties of water on midinfrared laser ablation. *Lasers Surg Med*. 1994;15(3):295-305.

17. Manstein D, Zurakowski D, Thongsima S, Laubach H, Chan HH. The effects of multiple passes on the epidermal thermal damage pattern in nonablative fractional resurfacing. *Lasers Surg Med*. 2009;41(2):149-153.

18. Laubach H, Chan HH, Rius F, Anderson RR, Manstein D. Effects of skin temperature on lesion size in fractional photothermolysis. *Lasers Surg Med*. 2007;39(1):14-18.

19. Kositratna G, Manstein D. Skin freezing during ablative fractional resurfacing: in-vitro effects on thermal lesion size. *Lasers Surg Med* 2009; Suppl.(21).

20. Brightman L, Goldman MP, Taub AF. Sublative rejuvenation: experience with a new fractional radiofrequency system for skin rejuvenation and repair. *J Drugs Dermatol*. 2009;8(11 Suppl):s9-s13.

21. Hantash BM, Ubeid AA, Chang H, Kafi R, Renton B. Bipolar fractional radiofrequency treatment induces neoelastogenesis and neocollagenesis. *Lasers Surg Med*. 2009;41(1):1-9.

22. Laubach HJ, Makin IR, Barthe PG, Slayton MH, Manstein D. Intense focused ultrasound: evaluation of a new treatment modality for precise microcoagulation within the skin. *Dermatol Surg*. 2008;34(5):727-734.

23. Gliklich RE, White WM, Slayton MH, Barthe PG, Makin IR. Clinical pilot study of intense ultrasound therapy to deep dermal facial skin and subcutaneous tissues. *Arch Facial Plast Surg*. 2007;9(2):88-95.

24. Bedi VP, Chan KF, Sink RK, et al. The effects of pulse energy variations on the dimensions of microscopic thermal treatment zones in nonablative fractional resurfacing. *Lasers Surg Med*. 2007;39(2): 145-155.

25. Thongsima S, Zurakowski D, Manstein D. Histological comparison of two different fractional photothermolysis devices operating at 1,550 nm. *Lasers Surg Med*. 2010;42(1):32-37.

26. Laubach HJ, Tannous Z, Anderson RR, Manstein D. Skin responses to fractional photothermolysis. *Lasers Surg Med*. 2006;38(2): 142-149.

27. Hantash BM, Bedi VP, Sudireddy V, Struck SK, Herron GS, Chan KF. Laser-induced transepidermal elimination of dermal content by fractional photothermolysis. *J Biomed Opt*. 2006; 11(4):041115.

28. Alster TS, Tanzi EL, Lazarus M. The use of fractional laser photothermolysis for the treatment of atrophic scars. *Dermatol Surg*. 2007;33(3):295-299.

29. Kono T, Chan HH, Groff WF, et al. Prospective direct comparison study of fractional resurfacing using different fluences and densities for skin rejuvenation in Asians. *Lasers Surg Med*. 2007;39(4): 311-314.

30. Fisher GH, Kim KH, Bernstein LJ, Geronemus RG. Concurrent use of a handheld forced cold air device minimizes patient discomfort during fractional photothermolysis. *Dermatol Surg*. 2005;31 (9 Pt 2):1242-1243; discussion 1244.

31. Chan HH, Manstein D, Yu CS, Shek S, Kono T, Wei WI. The prevalence and risk factors of post-inflammatory hyperpigmentation after fractional resurfacing in Asians. *Lasers Surg Med*. 2007;39(5): 381-385.

32. Lin JY, Chan HH. Pigmentary disorders in Asian skin: treatment with laser and intense pulsed light sources. *Skin Therapy Lett*. 2006;11(8):8-11.

33. Bak H, Kim BJ, Lee WJ, et al. Treatment of striae distensae with fractional photothermolysis. *Dermatol Surg*. 2009;35(8): 1215-1220.

34. Tierney EP, Kouba DJ, Hanke CW. Review of fractional photothermolysis: treatment indications and efficacy. *Dermatol Surg*. 2009;35(10):1445-1461.

35. Cohen SR, Henssler C, Johnston J. Fractional photothermolysis for skin rejuvenation. *Plast Reconstr Surg*. 2009;124(1):281-290.

36. Haedersdal M, Moreau KE, Beyer DM, Nymann P, Alsbjorn B. Fractional nonablative 1540 nm laser resurfacing for thermal burn scars: a randomized controlled trial. *Lasers Surg Med*. 2009; 41(3):189-195.

37. Laubach HJ, Anderson RR, Luger T, Manstein D. Fractional photothermolysis for involuted infantile hemangioma. *Arch Dermatol*. 2009;145(7):748-750.

38. Karsai S, Raulin C. Fractional photothermolysis: a new option for treating melasma? *Hautarzt*. 2008;59(2):92-100.

39. Izikson L, Anderson RR. Resolution of blue minocycline pigmentation of the face after fractional photothermolysis. *Lasers Surg Med*. 2008;40(6):399-401.

40. Karsai S, Hammes S, Rutten A, Raulin C. Fractional photothermolysis for the treatment of granuloma annulare: a case report. *Lasers Surg Med*. 2008;40(5):319-322.

41. Katz TM, Goldberg LH, Friedman PM. Nonablative fractional photothermolysis for the treatment of striae rubra. *Dermatol Surg*. 2009;35(9):1430-1433.

42. Kouba DJ, Fincher EF, Moy RL. Nevus of Ota successfully treated by fractional photothermolysis using a fractionated 1440-nm Nd:YAG laser. *Arch Dermatol*. 2008;144(2):156-158.

43. Yoo KH, Kim MN, Kim BJ, Kim CW. Treatment of alopecia areata with fractional photothermolysis laser. *Int J Dermatol*. 2010; 49(7):845-847.

44. Behroozan DS, Goldberg LH, Glaich AS, Dai T, Friedman PM. Fractional photothermolysis for treatment of poikiloderma of civatte. *Dermatol Surg*. 2006;32(2):298-301.

45. Khatri KA, Ross V, Grevelink JM, Magro CM, Anderson RR. Comparison of erbium:YAG and carbon dioxide lasers in resurfacing of facial rhytides. *Arch Dermatol*. 1999;135(4):391-397.

46. Walsh JT Jr, Flotte TJ, Anderson RR, Deutsch TF. Pulsed CO_2 laser tissue ablation: effect of tissue type and pulse duration on thermal damage. *Lasers Surg Med*. 1988;8(2):108-118.

47. Fitzpatrick RE, Ruiz-Esparza J, Goldman MP. The depth of thermal necrosis using the CO_2 laser: a comparison of the superpulsed mode and conventional mode. *J Dermatol Surg Oncol*. 1991;17(4): 340-344.

48. Fitzpatrick RE, Goldman MP, Satur NM, Tope WD. Pulsed carbon dioxide laser resurfacing of photo-aged facial skin. *Arch Dermatol.* 1996;132(4):395-402.
49. Wanner M, Farinelli W, Manstein D. Ablative fractional resurfacing – evaluation of different exposure parameters in a pig model. *Lasers Surg Med.* 2008;20(Suppl):28.
50. Hantash BM, Bedi VP, Kapadia B, et al. In vivo histological evaluation of a novel ablative fractional resurfacing device. *Lasers Surg Med.* 2007;39(2):96-107.
51. Hunzeker CM, Weiss ET, Geronemus RG. Fractionated CO_2 laser resurfacing: our experience with more than 2000 treatments. *Aesthet Surg J.* 2009;29(4):317-322.
52. Chapas AM, Brightman L, Sukal S, et al. Successful treatment of acneiform scarring with CO_2 ablative fractional resurfacing. *Lasers Surg Med.* 2008;40(6):381-386.
53. Waibel J, Beer K. Ablative fractional laser resurfacing for the treatment of a third-degree burn. *J Drugs Dermatol.* 2009;8(3): 294-297.
54. Rahman Z, MacFalls H, Jiang K, et al. Fractional deep dermal ablation induces tissue tightening. *Lasers Surg Med.* 2009;41(2): 78-86.
55. Dierickx CC, Khatri KA, Tannous ZS, et al. Micro-fractional ablative skin resurfacing with two novel erbium laser systems. *Lasers Surg Med.* 2008;40(2):113-123.
56. Avram MM, Tope WD, Yu T, Szachowicz E, Nelson JS. Hypertrophic scarring of the neck following ablative fractional carbon dioxide laser resurfacing. *Lasers Surg Med.* 2009;41(3):185-188.
57. Haedersdal M, Sakamoto FH, Farinelli WA, Doukas AG, Tam J, Anderson RR. Fractional CO(2) laser-assisted drug delivery. *Lasers Surg Med.* 2010;42(2):113-122.

Plasma Resurfacing

K. Wade Foster, Edgar F. Fincher, and Ronald L. Moy

- Plasma skin regeneration (PSR) is a novel method of skin resurfacing that uses plasma energy to create a thermal effect on the skin
- PSR is different from ablative lasers in that it is not chromophore dependent and does not vaporize tissue, but leaves a layer of intact, desiccated epidermis that acts as a biologic dressing and promotes rapid wound healing and faster recovery
- Histological studies performed on plasma resurfacing patients have characterized the changes that follow treatment and have confirmed continued collagen production, reduction of elastosis, and progressive skin rejuvenation beyond 1 year after treatment
- PSR has received FDA 510(k) clearance for treatment of rhytides of the body, superficial skin lesions, actinic keratoses, viral papillomata, and seborrheic keratoses. PSR has beneficial effects in the treatment of other conditions including dyschromias, photoaging, skin laxity, and acneiform scars.
- PSR has an excellent safety profile with no reports of hypopigmentation and only rare cases of scarring or prolonged erythema. There are no reports of demarcation lines in perioral, periorbital, or jawline areas, as can sometimes be observed following CO_2 resurfacing
- PSR is safe and effective in improving facial and periorbital rhytides and can be used on nonfacial sites including the hands, neck, and chest
- Numerous treatment protocols with variable energy settings allow for individualized treatments and provide the operator with fine control over the degree of injury and length of subsequent recovery time

K.W. Foster (✉)
Moy-Fincher Medical Group, 100 UCLA Medical Plaza, Suite 590, Los Angeles, CA 90024, USA
e-mail: wadefoster1@yahoo.com

Introduction

- PSR utilizes energy derived from nitrogen gas to create heat that is delivered onto the skin surface resulting in zones of thermal damage and thermal modification
- PSR is not chromophore dependent and does not result in vaporization of the epidermis, as is seen with ablative lasers, but leaves a layer of intact, desiccated epidermis that acts as a biologic dressing and promotes rapid healing
- The histological depth of cleavage is directly related to the pulse energy of the treatment. At settings of 1 J, the line of cleavage extends only to the superficial most portions of the epidermis and at 4 J, the line of cleavage is within the papillary dermis
- Seven treatment protocols are available to treat the full spectrum of patient conditions. These range from a low pulse energy (0.5 J) "lunch hour" procedure with effects and recovery times similar to those of fractional lasers to high energy (4 J) double pass procedures with more dramatic improvements and recovery times of 7–10 days. Protocols are comprised of either single or multiple treatments that can be matched to the patient's condition

Laser skin resurfacing remains the most effective modality for skin rejuvenation. Although numerous nonablative laser and light devices have been developed over the years, none of them is able to deliver results equivalent to ablative devices. The effectiveness of ablative lasers results from their ability to accomplish two major effects. First, complete vaporization of the epidermis removes unwanted pigment and solar damaged cells. Second, there is deeper penetration and diffusion of thermal energy that heats dermal tissues, causes tissue contraction, and stimulates new collagen production. These processes eventuate in a new, more uniform epidermis without unwanted pigmentation, removal of solar

K. Nouri (ed.), *Lasers in Dermatology and Medicine*,
DOI: 10.1007/978-0-85729-281-0_11, © Springer-Verlag London Limited 2011

elastosis from the superficial dermis yielding a brighter more lustrous skin tone, and immediate tissue contraction plus sustained neocollagenesis, leading to the reduction of wrinkles and laxity.

PSR employs the use of plasma, the fourth state of matter. Plasma results from heat-induced ionization of a gas. When energy is applied to a gas, electrons can escape their atom, resulting in positively charged atoms and negatively charged free electron particles. When the electron is "recaptured" by a positively charged atom, energy is emitted in the form of heat, and this thermal energy can be channeled onto a target (Fig. 1). The Portrait® PSR system (Rhytec Inc., Waltham, MA) creates a pulse of ultrahigh radiofrequency (UHF) energy from the device generator (Fig. 2a) that subsequently converts nitrogen gas into plasma within the handpiece. The plasma emerges from the distal end of the device handpiece (Fig. 2b) and is directed onto the skin area to be treated. Each pulse of plasma energy is released onto the target in a Gaussian distribution to provide even tissue heating and a uniform effect. The handpiece does not come in direct contact with the skin, and a turquoise blue non-contact targeting ring enables the user to maintain the plasma burst at an optimal angle and distance from the skin surface (Fig. 2c). The truly unique feature about plasma resurfacing that differentiates it from ablative lasers is the fact that it does not vaporize tissue, but leaves a layer of intact, desiccated epidermis that acts as a biologic dressing

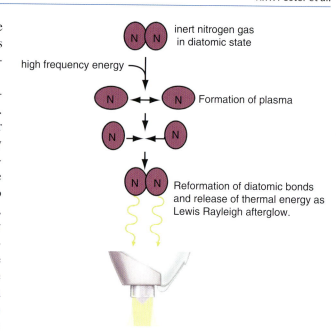

Fig. 1 Plasma generation by Portrait PSR®. An ultra-high-frequency radiofrequency generator excites a tuned resonator and imparts energy to nitrogen gas molecules flowing through the handpiece resulting in their ionization. The plasma is directed through a quartz nozzle out of the tip of the handpiece and onto the skin. Nitrogen is used for the gaseous source because it is able to purge oxygen from the surface of the skin, thus minimizing the risk of unpredictable hot spots, charring, and scar formation. The plasma appears as a characteristic lilac glow that transitions to a yellowish light called a Lewis–Raleigh afterglow[1]

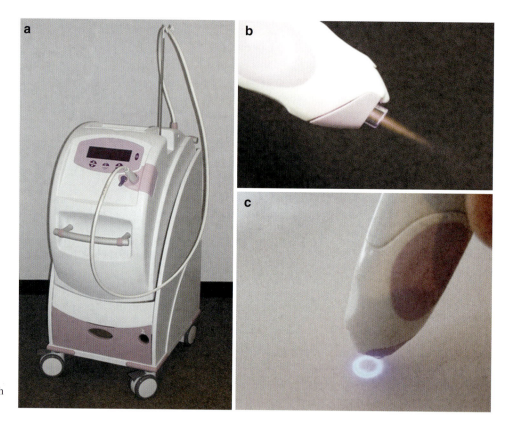

Fig. 2 Plasma skin resurfacing with Portrait® PSR. Plasma generating device (**a**) and handpiece (**b**) showing plasma energy emanating from tip are shown. Appearance of turquoise blue non-contact targeting ring used for gauging appropriate incident angle and distance from skin surface (**c**) (Reproduced with permission from Rhytec, Inc.)

Plasma Resurfacing

and promotes a more rapid recovery than would be observed with ablative treatments. The desiccated tissue sloughs over the ensuing 4–5 days leaving a new epidermis formed beneath. PSR is nonablative, not chromophore dependent, and rapid thermal penetration of the skin produces shallow zones of thermal damage and deeper zones of thermal modification with increased fibroblast activity. PSR can be used safely in Fitzpatrick skin types I–IV, and to date there have been no reports of hypopigmentation or demarcation lines in treated perioral, periorbital, or jawline areas, a major concern for both patients and physicians when contemplating CO_2 laser resurfacing.

The deep thermal effects of PSR share some similarity to that of CO_2 or erbium lasers. First, immediate tissue contraction is accomplished via thermal coagulation of dermal collagen. Second, thermal disruption of solar elastosis and activation of fibroblasts stimulate a wound healing cascade necessary for neocollagenesis. Histologically, immediately after a 3.5 J treatment an intact and nonablated epidermis with vacuolation of basal cell layer is noted (Fig. 3a). Four days after treatment, a line of cleavage can be noted which demarcates shedding epidermal and dermal remnants from newly formed stratum corneum and regenerated epidermis (Fig. 3b). The overlying epidermal and dermal remnants serve as a biologic dressing. Early changes in the superficial dermis, compatible with an evolving zone of thermal modification can also be seen. Ten days after treatment with 3.5 J, a fully regenerated epidermis is noted without basal cell layer vacuolation, and the zone of thermal modification, typified by an intense fibroplasia within the papillary and upper reticular dermis can be appreciated (Fig. 3c). Histological studies have also demonstrated that the depth of cleavage is directly related to the pulse energy of the treatment (Fig. 4), and confirmed continued collagen production up to 1 year after treatment (data not shown). Clinically visible improvements following PSR are a function of thermal penetration and dermal collagen denaturation, a process that requires temperatures of $\geq 60°C$.[2] Through finite element analysis, pulse energies of 4 J have been shown to result in thermal penetration well into the reticular dermis, such that temperatures of 60°C reach a depth of 600 μm in depth in normally hydrated skin (Fig. 5).

Seven treatment protocols are available to treat the full range of patient conditions and these can be categorized based on severity of rhytides, outcome expectations and recovery times (Table 1). The VLE (very low energy) protocol is a minimal recovery time procedure with 0.5 J pulse energy and is roughly equivalent to other "lunchtime" procedures, e.g., intense pulsed light or superficial chemical peel for facial skin rejuvenation. PSR NF (low energy) uses pulse energies ranging up to 1.8 and 2.5 J for dorsal and ventral surfaces, respectively, and improvements in chest, neck and dorsal hand skin have been recently demonstrated.[3, 4] PSR3

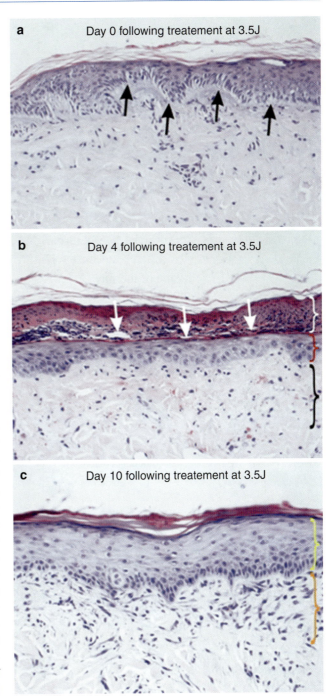

Fig. 3 Histological changes following treatment with PSR at 3.5 J. Immediately after treatment vacuolation of basal cell layer (*black arrows*) is noted near the dermoepidermal junction. This histological finding accompanies treatment with energy settings >2 J (**a**). Four days after treatment with 3.5 J, a developing line of cleavage (*white arrows*) between zones of thermal damage and thermal modification are noted. The zone of thermal damage (*white bracket*) containing epidermal and dermal remnants is being shed above the developing line of cleavage. Regenerated epidermis (*red bracket*) and the evolving zone of thermal modification (*black bracket*) are also visible (**b**). Ten days after treatment with 3.5 J, a regenerated normal appearing epidermis is noted (*yellow bracket*). The zone of thermal modification (*orange bracket*) is typified by an intense fibroplasia in the papillary and upper reticular dermis (**c**) (Reproduced with permission from Rhytec, Inc.)

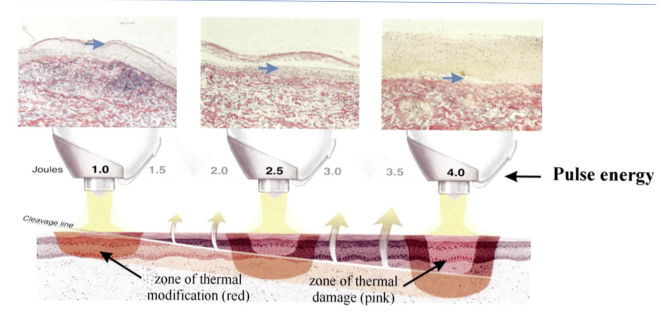

Fig. 4 The effects of pulse energy on depth of cleavage. Pulse energies of 1 J result in a very superficial cleavage line (*blue arrow*) just beneath the stratum corneum (*left*). The cleavage line (*blue arrow*) resulting from pulse energies of 2.5 J is localized within the basal cell layer (*middle*). Pulse energies of 4 J result in a cleavage line (*blue arrow*) within the papillary dermis (*right*) (Reproduced with permission from Rhytec, Inc.)

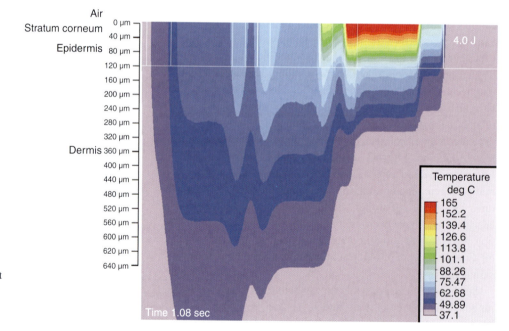

Fig. 5 Finite element analysis demonstrating the depth of thermal penetration resulting from three sequential 4 J pulses delivered over 1.08 s to adjacent areas of normally hydrated skin (Reproduced with permission from Rhytec, Inc.)

(high energy) utilizes 3–4 J pulse energies and can be used as a more aggressive treatment for facial skin resurfacing that produces a degree of injury similar to single pass CO_2 resurfacing laser, but is histologically different from CO_2 resurfacing in that the epidermis is not ablated and remains attached. Other protocols (e.g., PSR1, PSR2, PSR2/3) can be used to treat the full face or regional areas and are further detailed in Table 1.

Table 1 Characteristics of Portrait PSR® treatment protocols

Protocol	Energy (J/pulse)	Number of treatments/ passes required	Treated areas
VLE[a] (very low energy)	0.5	3–6/single	Full face ("no downtime" procedure)
PSR NF (low energy)	1–1.8[b]	1/single	Chest, hands, neck
Three-pass LE	1.5–1.8	1/triple pass	Full face or regional areas, periorbital skin-single treatment
PSR1 (low energy)	1–1.8	3/single	Full face or regional areas
PSR2 (high energy)	3–4	1/single	Full face or regional areas
PSR2/3 (high energy)	3–4	1/single pass for full face or regional areas with double pass on deep rhytides	Full face or regional areas
PSR3 (high energy)	3–4	1/double pass	Full face or regional areas

[a]Pending FDA clearance
[b]Alster and Konda (2007)[3]

- Plasma resurfacing is a relatively new technology that has been in clinical use for over 3 years, with 6 years of ongoing trials assessing its efficacy for facial and non-facial skin rejuvenation
- The Portrait PSR® system is currently the only commercially available plasma resurfacing system to date
- Published reports assessing high energy (3–4 J) single pass PSR for facial rejuvenation have demonstrated a mean 50% improvement in skin tone 30 days after treatment. Other reports have shown attenuated clinical improvement over time, e.g., a mean 39% reduction in depth of fine facial lines at 10 days after treatment that decreased to 23% 6 months after treatment.
- Published reports assessing PSR for acne scars showed a 23% reduction in scar depth at 6 months
- Published reports assessing PSR in the treatment of non-facial skin using low energy settings have demonstrated mean clinical improvements of 57%, 48%, and 41% in chest, hands, and neck sites, respectively, and significant reductions in wrinkle severity, dyschromia, and increased skin smoothness were achieved

The Portrait PSR® system is currently the only commercially available plasma resurfacing system to date. Previous clinical applications of plasma energy include a process known as coblation. Coblation remains in use as a therapeutic modality for tonsillectomy, for the treatment of sleep-related breathing disorders, and for the treatment of benign polyps or vocal cord nodules.[5] Coblation produces a low energy heating that enables only superficial ablation of the target lesions, and trials of coblation for skin resurfacing were examined but failed to produce any significant results, most likely due to the limited depth of energy penetration. In contrast to coblation, the Portrait PSR® system provides both higher energy, deeper thermal penetration, and superior outcomes.

With regard to skin rejuvenation, patient demands for treatment have been and continue to be affected by three major variables. These include the potential for improvement, risk of the procedure, and amount of recovery time. Historically, the potential for improvement has counterbalanced the risks and "downtime," and patient concerns over the long recovery times associated with ablative procedures have been the driving force behind the development of nonablative fractional lasers with reduced downtimes in spite of their more modest improvements. A broad range of treatment options is offered by the PSR system, and the relative improvement and recovery times of PSR protocols and other resurfacing modalities are represented diagrammatically (Fig. 6).

PSR is a relatively new technology with a handful of published reports documenting its efficacy in the treatment of facial and non-facial sites. In a pilot study evaluating the use of a single full-facial treatment at high energy (3–4 J), Kilmer et al.[6] demonstrated a mean improvement in overall facial rejuvenation of 50% by 1 month. Potter et al.[7] used silicone molding to demonstrate a 39% decrease in fine line depth 6 months after a single high-energy full-face treatment.

PSR has been also been evaluated in the treatment of non-facial skin including moderately photodamaged skin on the neck, chest, and dorsal hands.[3] The authors used three energy settings (1, 1.5, and 1.8 J) and clinical evaluations of skin texture, pigmentation, wrinkle severity, and side effects were conducted immediately and at 4, 7, 14, 30, and 90 days after treatment. Mean clinical improvements of 57%, 48%, and 41% were observed in chest, hands, and neck sites, respectively, and significant reductions in wrinkle severity, hyperpigmentation, and increased skin smoothness were achieved. Higher-energy settings were found to be of greater benefit but also had prolonged healing times. We performed a similar study using a series of

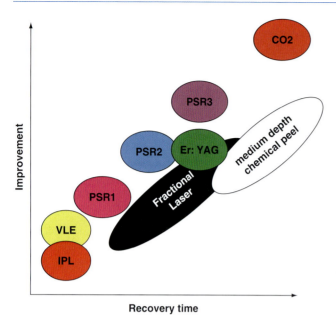

Fig. 6 Relative downtime versus improvement of different resurfacing modalities. *IPL* intense pulsed light, *VLE* very low energy plasma resurfacing with Portrait® PSR, *PSR1* single pass plasma resurfacing with Portrait® PSR at low energy (1–1.8 J), *PSR2* single plasma resurfacing with Portrait® PSR at high energy (3–4 J), *PSR3* double pass plasma resurfacing with Portrait® PSR at high energy (3–4 J), *Er:YAG* erbium yttrium-aluminum-garnet laser, CO_2 carbon dioxide laser

three low energy (1–2 J) PSR treatments on the neck and observed an overall improvement in skin tone, dyschromia and texture. Analysis of the degree of skin tightening showed patient-dependent results that ranged from minimal to excellent, and some patients had a 70–80% reduction in skin lines that was noted at 3-month follow up visits. The benefit of higher pulse energies was minimal and resulted in a more prolonged healing time.

A number of evolving applications for PSR were recently discussed at the 2007 American Society for Dermatologic Surgery Hot Topic Session in Chicago, IL entitled "Portrait Plasma Skin Rejuvenation Update: Treatment Protocols and Aesthetic Outcomes," and several of these will be mentioned below. VLE settings with pulse energies of 0.5 J have been used to provide "lunchhour" treatments to the face with minimal recovery times. With prototype PSR devices that were not originally designed to deliver such low energies, the low pulse energies could be approximated by increasing the distance of the handpiece from the skin surface from the normal distance of 5 mm to approximately 20 mm, and subsequent efforts by the manufacturer have resulted in production of a standardized 20 mm spacer device that can be used clinically for this purpose. In pilot and multicenter studies assessing the efficacy of VLE protocol, all subjects underwent three to six treatments separated by 3 weeks. Modest improvements in wrinkle severity and pigmentation were noted with minimal side effects.[8]

The effects of PSR on eyelid laxity and periorbital rhytides have also been evaluated.[9] Compared to a 91% improvement with blepharoplasty, treatment of upper eyelid skin with single or double pass high energy (3 J) resulted in a mean 22% and 35% improvement in upper eyelid tightening and periorbital wrinkles. With the high energies delivered in this protocol, double pass treatments resulted in mean 13.1 day recovery times, and mean 11.5 day recovery times were noted following single pass treatments. High energy treatments resulted in prolonged healing times and erythema, and these events were attributed to increased pulse count/density, high aggregate energies on relatively less tolerant eyelid skin, and post treatment care. In the second phase of the trial, energy and pulse density were subsequently decreased to 1.5 J double or triple pass with 25–30 pulses per pass. Peeling was noted between days 2–4, and no patients developed postoperative erythema. Results with low energy settings approximated those of high energy treatments, but were better tolerated with reduced healing times, and remained stable up to 4 months after treatment.

The effects of PSR on acne scars are also under investigation.[10] A recent trial included 30 patients who received one double pass high energy (3–4 J) treatment with follow up that extended to 180 days after treatment. EMLA cream under occlusion for 60 min was used before treatments, post-treatment care consisted of cool compresses and application of petrolatum, and photography and silicon molds of treatment areas were used to assess improvement. Mean improvement in acne scarring on the cheeks was 32%, 25% on the mouth and chin, and 13% on the forehead. Mean patient-rated improvement was 37% at 3 months and 35% at 6 months after treatment, and mean physician rated improvement was 29%. Mean recovery time was 4.6 days, and no hyper- or hypopigmentation was noted.

Indications and Contraindications

- PSR has received FDA 510(k) clearance for treatment of rhytides of the body, superficial skin lesions, actinic keratoses, viral papillomata, and seborrheic keratosis
- PSR has beneficial effects in the treatment of dyschromias and photoaged skin, and has been utilized for the treatment of acne scars, eyelid laxity, Hailey-Hailey disease, and linear porokeratosis
- Contraindications for PSR include patients with keloid prone skin, active infection, breaks in skin or any cutaneous inflammatory condition, patients who are pregnant or nursing, those who would be deemed ineligible for general surgery, patients with Fitzpatrick skin types V and VI, and those patients who have taken oral isotretinoin within the past 6 months[11]

As of September 2006, PSR is currently FDA 510(k) approved for the treatment of rhytides of the body, superficial skin lesions, actinic keratoses, viral papillomata, seborrheic keratoses, and benign skin lesions of the body. PSR has beneficial effects in the treatment of dyschromias and photoaged skin and has been used anecdotally for the treatment of acne scars, eyelid laxity, Hailey-Hailey disease, and linear porokeratosis. Contraindications to PSR include pregnancy, nursing mothers, predisposition to developing keloids, use of isotretinoin in the past 6 months, darker skin types (Fitzpatrick types V and VI), patients with skin defects, inflammatory skin conditions, active infections, and those deemed unfit for general surgery.[11]

helpful to minimize peri- and postoperative edema. Preoperative management should also include attempts to educate patients regarding wound care, including vinegar soaks and application of aquaphor or petrolatum.

Safety requirements for the procedure include eye protection for patients. Liberal application of petrolatum to eyelashes, eyebrows and the hairline reduces the chance of singeing. The surgeon should be aware of any flammable items (e.g., paper table coverings, oxygen, anesthetic inhalants), and when possible, these should be removed from the operative suite or covered with a moist towel. A fire extinguisher should be present for emergencies.

Techniques

Preoperative Management

- Patients being treated with high energy protocols should receive prophylactic antibacterial, antiviral, and antifungal medications (optional)
- Discomfort associated with PSR can be minimized through the use of topical anesthetic creams or nerve blocks
- Administration of opiate pain relievers, antihistamines, and oral anxiolytics may be necessary in some patients when high energy settings are used
- Prior to treatment, petrolatum should be applied liberally to eyelashes, eyebrows and the hairline to prevent singeing of facial and scalp hair
- All flammable substances should be removed from the area

While there are no consensus recommendations regarding preoperative management for plasma resurfacing patients, most surgeons adhere to the same precautions used for laser resurfacing. Bacterial prophylaxis should have *Staphylococcus* coverage, and we generally prescribe cephalexin 500 mg b.i.d. for 5 days, although levofloxaxin 500 mg q.d. for 7 days has also been advocated by some surgeons.[12] Antiviral (valacyclovir 500 mg t.i.d. for 7 days) and antifungal (fluconazole 200 mg once) prophylaxis may also be used. Topical anesthetic creams (lidocaine 2.5%/prilocaine 2.5% cream or specially compounded anesthetic creams consisting of 23% lidocaine/7% tetracaine) or nerve blocks are also useful to minimize discomfort, and oral anxiolytics (diazepam, alprazolam, lorazepam), opiate pain relievers (meperidine, hydrocodone/acetaminophen), and antihistamines (hydroxyzine) may also be useful in certain patients, especially with high energy treatments. Intramuscular dexamethasone may be

Description of the Technique

- Experienced users may prefer higher repetition rates (up to 2.5 Hz), whereas novice users may have better control with lower repetition rates (1–1.5 Hz)
- The non-contact target ring will be in sharp focus when the handpiece is at the correct angle (90°) and distance (5 mm) from the skin surface. Overhead lighting may need to be dimmed to better visualize the ring
- Spot overlap of 10–20% is generally preferred in single pass procedures
- In double pass procedures, spot staggering of the second pass ensures uniform treatment, and spot overlap is not necessary
- The operator should avoid skip areas and unintentional pulse stacking

Before beginning treatment, one must ensure that the skin surface is wiped clean of any residual anesthetic cream. After calibration is complete, the pulse energy (1–4 J) and repetition rate (1–2.5 Hz) are selected. Novice practitioners will have better control with pulse repetition settings of 1 Hz, but those with more experience may prefer higher pulse settings, up to 2.5 Hz. The hand piece is held 5 mm from the skin at a 90° angle such that the turquoise blue non-contact target ring is focused sharply around the area to be treated; visualization of the ring is best with dim overhead lighting. Although the presence of the target ring implies that all the thermal energy is delivered within the confines of the ring, some heat diffuses onto adjacent areas of skin that are outside of it. Single pass procedures are generally performed with 10–20% spot overlap, but double pass procedures do not require overlap since the spots of the second pass are staggered to ensure that the area is uniformly and completely treated. In contrast to CO_2 resurfacing, there is no wiping between the first and second passes. One drawback with the plasma system is lack of scanning technologies that define the exact size and shape of the treatment spot, a feature of most CO_2 lasers. For this reason, the operator must be exact with pulse placement to avoid skip areas or unintended pulse stacking.

Postoperative Management

- Following high energy treatment, patients should use open dressings with petrolatum ointment
- Strict sun avoidance is mandatory
- Desquamation generally begins on postoperative day 4–5 and is complete by postoperative day 7–8
- Postoperative erythema generally fades by postoperative day 14. Patients may generally apply makeup by day 7 (following a high energy treatment) or after desquamation is complete

Following each treatment at 1.5–2 J on the face, there is typically 4 days of erythema and some superficial exfoliation on days 3–4. The higher energy treatments at 3–4 J are performed as single treatments with an anticipated healing time of 7 days. The typical course following a high energy (4 J) double pass treatment is bronzing by day 2 followed by epidermal sloughing on days 4–5 and resolution of erythema between days 7–10 (Fig. 7). In contrast, low energy treatments have a much more rapid healing time with milder desquamation and full resolution of erythema by post-treatment day 4 (Fig. 8). The VLE protocol is accompanied by mild erythema following treatment, and desquamation does not usually occur. We have observed marked improvements in the appearance of periorbital and facial rhytides following treatment with high energy PSR protocols (Figs. 9 and 10), and treatment is generally accompanied with a high degree of patient satisfaction.

Postoperative wound care consists of an open dressing with petrolatum-based ointment with repeat applications three to four times daily along with gentle cleansing with a non-detergent based cleanser. Sunscreens and makeup are

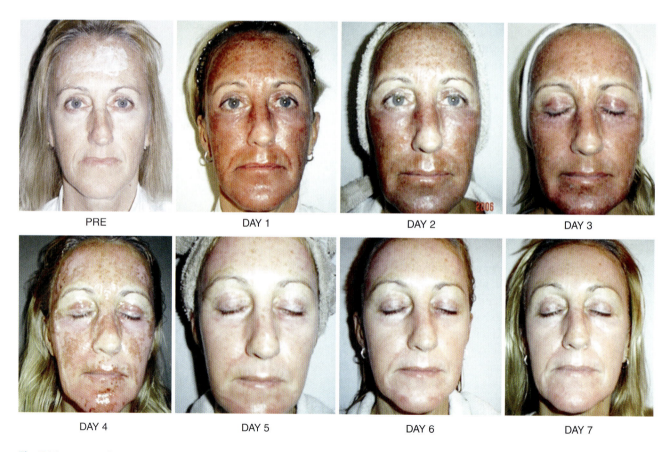

Fig. 7 Time course for healing following high energy treatment with PSR 2/3 for moderate to severe photodamage (Reproduced with permission from Rhytec, Inc. and J. David Holcomb, M.D.)

Plasma Resurfacing

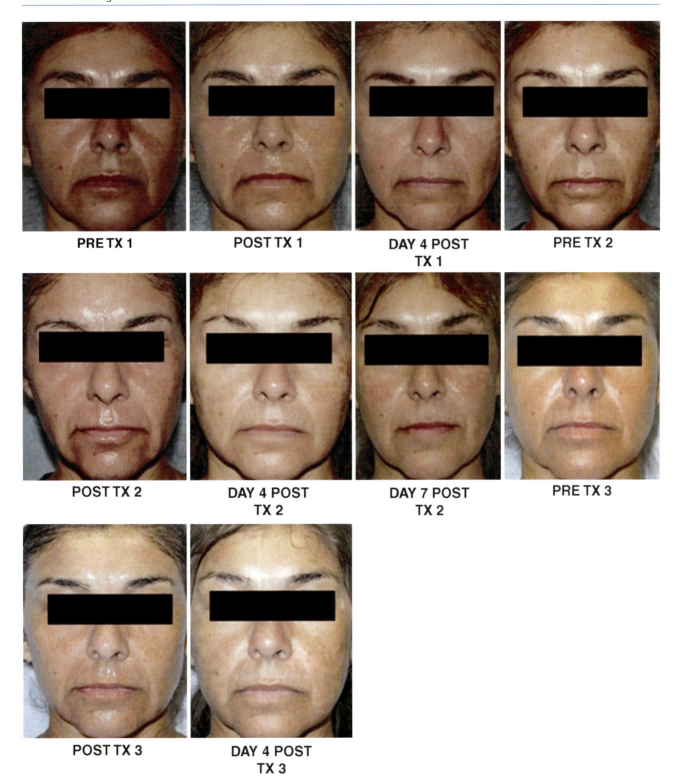

Fig. 8 Time course for healing following three low energy PSR1 treatments for mild to moderate photodamage (Reproduced with permission from Rhytec, Inc. and Richard Fitzpatrick, M.D.)

reduction in facial rhytides and 68% improvement in overall facial appearance. Low pulse energies in this trial resulted in decreased recovery times, manifest by complete reepithelialization and resolution of erythema by 4 and 6 days after treatment. Future directions in the field of plasma skin regeneration will focus on identifying treatment parameters to maximize patient outcomes and further expanding clinical indications.

Conclusion

PSR is a unique form of nonablative resurfacing that is not chromophore dependent and does not result in vaporization of the epidermis, but leaves a layer of intact desiccated epidermis that acts as a natural biologic dressing and promotes rapid healing. PSR improves fine lines and moderate to deep rhytides and the texture and tone of photoaged skin. The broad range of energy settings enables the operator to individualize treatments and control the degree of injury and length of subsequent recovery time. PSR is FDA approved for treatment of rhytides of the body, superficial skin lesions, actinic keratoses, viral papillomata, and seborrheic keratosis, can have beneficial effects in the treatment of dyschromias and photoaged skin, and has been utilized anecdotally for the treatment of acne scars (FDA clearance pending). PSR treatments have an excellent safety profile. Permanent hypopigmentation and demarcation lines have not been observed, and prolonged erythema and scarring are rare. These characteristics have validated PSR as an excellent and versatile modality that offers a wide range of treatment options, and as such it will undoubtedly command continued interest in the field of skin rejuvenation.

References

1. Bogle MA. Plasma skin regeneration technology. *Skin Ther Lett.* 2006;11:7-9.
2. Lin MG et al. Evaluation of dermal thermal damage by multiphoton autofluorescence and second-harmonic-generation microscopy. *J Biomed Opt.* 2006;11:064006.
3. Alster TS, Konda S. Plasma skin resurfacing for regeneration of neck, chest, and hands: investigation of a novel device. *Dermatol Surg.* 2007;33:1315-1321.
4. Moy RL, Fincher EF. Unpublished data; 2011.
5. Burton MJ, Doree C. Coblation versus other surgical techniques for tonsillectomy. *Cochrane Database Syst Rev.* 2007;CD004619.
6. Kilmer S, Semchyshyn N, Shah G, Fitzpatrick R. A pilot study on the use of a plasma skin regeneration device (Portrait PSR3) in full facial rejuvenation procedures. *Lasers Med Sci.* 2007;22:101-109.
7. Potter MJ et al. Facial acne and fine lines: transforming patient outcomes with plasma skin regeneration. *Ann Plast Surg.* 2007;58: 608-613.
8. Dover J, Arndt K. Very low energy plasma: portait study results. In: Portrait plasma skin regeneration: treatment protocols and aesthetic outcomes. In: American Society of Dermatologic Surgery Meeting; 2007; Chicago.
9. Biesman B. Portrait plasma blepharoplasty study and treatment results. In: Portrait plasma skin regeneration: treatment protocols and aesthetic outcomes. In: American Society of Dermatologic Surgery Meeting; 2007; Chicago.
10. Ueberhoer N. Portrait acne scar – study and treatment results In: Portrait plasma skin regeneration: treatment protocols and aesthetic outcomes. In: American Society of Dermatologic Surgery Meeting; 2007; Chicago.
11. Rhytec, Inc. Portrait® PSR3 System User Manual USA & Canada; 2006.
12. Fitzpatrick R. Plasma–CO_2 complication comparison, advanced treatment approach,latest portrait PSR3 research. In: Portrait plasma skin regeneration: treatment protocols and aesthetic outcomes. In: American Society of Dermatologic Surgery Meeting; 2007; Chicago.
13. Bogle MA, Arndt KA, Dover JS. Evaluation of plasma skin regeneration technology in low-energy full-facial rejuvenation. *Arch Dermatol.* 2007;143:168-174.

Sub-Surfacing Lasers

Michael H. Gold

Outline and Introduction

1. Sub-surfacing lasers consist of a variety of medical devices
   (a) KTP lasers
   (b) Pulsed dye lasers
   (c) 1,064 nm Q-Switched Nd: YAG lasers
   (d) 1,064 nm Long Pulsed Nd: YAG lasers
   (e) 1,319/1,320 nm Nd: YAG lasers
   (f) 1,450 nm Diode lasers
   (g) 1,540 Erbium Glass lasers
   (h) Intense Pulsed Light Sources
2. Developed to meet need of efficacy in rejuvenation without associated downtime
   (a) Erbium and CO_2 laser resurfacing standards
   (b) Adverse events, too much downtime
   (c) New devices to effect collagen in dermis, minimal downtime
   (d) Epidermal cooling required for treatment to be safe and effective
   (e) All have clinical studies showing effectiveness
   (f) All have a rejuvenation effect
   (g) All have potential for adverse events including blistering, burns, pigmentary concerns, scars

- Ablative laser resurfacing has been the gold standard throughout the 1980s and 1990s for improving skin texture by renovating photo damaged and aging skin.
- Although excellent results have been obtained with the use of ablative laser devices, the use of non-ablative laser systems have been increasingly popular as an alternative to obtaining the same results.
- The mechanism of ablative laser resurfacing involves the removal of the epidermis and the dermis, causing a wound to develop which may take up to several months to heal.
- The use of non-ablative laser systems have minimal side-effects by causing direct thermal damage to the dermis, while sparing the epidermis, and reducing the risks of post-treatment adverse effects and downtime.

Indications and Contraindications – *Clinical information regarding these devices with published evidence of safety and efficacy*

Introduction

The field of sub-surfacing lasers is also known commonly by the terms non-ablative laser resurfacing, photorejuvenation, and laser toning. A variety of lasers and light sources have been developed and utilized for sub-surfacing and will be the subject of this review.

Included in the overall category of sub-surfacing lasers are a diverse range of technologies which include the KTP lasers at 532 nm; the pulsed dye lasers at 585–595 nm; the Nd:YAG lasers which encompass the 1,064 nm long pulsed systems, the 1,064 nm Q-switched laser systems, and the 1,319/1,320 nm laser systems; the 1,450 nm diode laser systems; the erbium glass laser systems at 1,540 nm; as well as the spectrum of intense pulsed light (IPL) systems at a

M.H. Gold
Gold Skin Care Center, Tennessee Clinical Research Center,
The Laser Rejuvenation Center, Advanced Aesthetics Medi-Spa,
2000 Richard Jones Road, Suite 220,
Nashville, TN, USA and
Department of Dermatology,
Vanderbilt University School of Medicine, Vanderbilt University
School of Nursing, Nashville, TN, USA
e-mail: goldskin@goldskincare.com

K. Nouri (ed.), *Lasers in Dermatology and Medicine*,
DOI: 10.1007/978-0-85729-281-0_12, © Springer-Verlag London Limited 2011

wavelength range of 500–1,200 nm. All of these medical devices have proven successful for non-ablative laser/light source resurfacing, photorejuvenation, and the improvement of acne scars.[1,2]

These devices were developed, from a historical point of view, to rival the ablative laser resurfacing systems which enjoyed much popularity in the 1980s and 1990s. The ablative laser systems, predominantly identified by the erbium laser systems at 2,940 nm and the carbon dioxide resurfacing lasers with a wavelength of 10,600 nm, were and are the mainstays of the ablative laser resurfacing systems. The ablative laser resurfacing systems are the gold standard for skin resurfacing and still to this day are the standards to which all other laser or light sources for rejuvenation of the skin are judged as to their safety and efficacy. The ablative laser resurfacing systems work by removing the entire epidermis and portions of the dermis which results in a wound that, upon healing, gives a desired rejuvenation effect. These devices have been used for many years and have proven effective in improving skin roughness, fine lines and wrinkles, and skin dyschromias which are common manifestations associated with skin aging and photodamage. These ablative laser resurfacing devices can produce very nice and long-lasting results, as evidenced in Figs. 1 and 2. However, when performing these types of laser procedures, patients must understand that there will be significant downtime with these treatments, lasting upwards of 1 week or more before full reepithelization will occur, and then several more weeks where the skin is still pink until complete healing has occurred. As well, some patients have prolonged erythema, as seen in Fig. 3, which requires appropriate and thoughtful intervention from qualified clinicians to help minimize. And, as a long term sequelae to many of these procedures, a significant number (reported anywhere from 10–20%) may develop a post-treatment hypopigmentation, which may not be evident for several months to years following the initial procedure, as depicted in Fig. 4. However, these ablative laser resurfacing devices still remain the gold standard for skin resurfacing but other devices were developed in an attempt to reproduce these kinds of results, with minimal

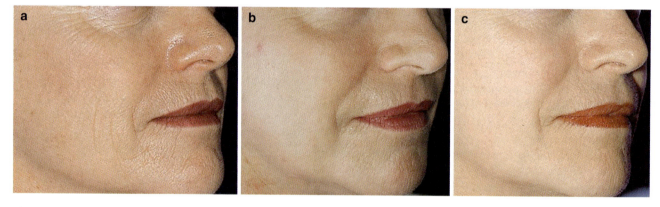

Fig. 1 (**a–c**) Clinical examples of ablative laser resurfacing with long-lasting results

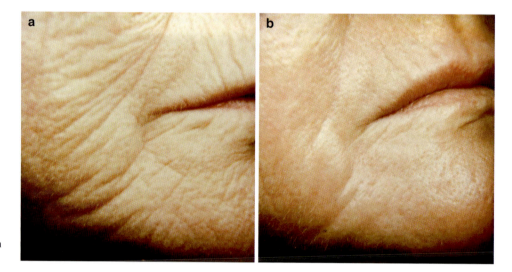

Fig. 2 (**a, b**) Clinical examples of ablative laser resurfacing with long-lasting results

Fig. 3 (a, b) Clinical example of prolonged erythema after ablative laser resurfacing

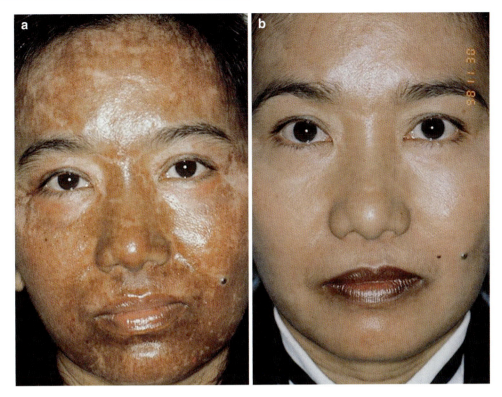

Fig. 4 Clinical example of long-term sequelae after ablative laser resurfacing

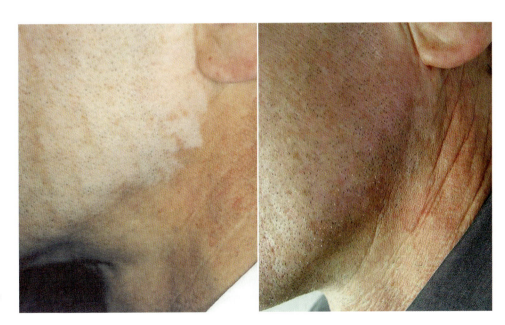

downtime, predictable results, and less chances for adverse or long term results.[3-5]

The purpose of the development of the non-ablative laser resurfacing is to affect changes in the skin similar to what the ablative laser resurfacing devices achieve. These devices were developed to improve the skin's texture, to improve facial lines and wrinkles and surface irregularities including facial scars. In addition, some of these devices also address pigmentary dyschromias and vascular changes in the skin associated with photodamage and actinically damaged skin. The non-ablative lasers and light sources work via thermal injury to the dermis, with epidermal sparing, thereby reducing the potential for any associated with these procedures. These medical devices have been demonstrated to work over a period of time and through a series of treatments, usually in the realm of 5–6 treatments given at 3–4 week intervals.[3]

Table 1 Sub-surfacing lasers

Device type	Device name	Manufacturer
(1) Vascular lasers		
KTP lasers	Aura (laserscope)	Iridex http://www.iridex.com/
	Viridis derma	Quantel medical http://www.quantelmedical.com/
Pulsed dye lasers	V-beam/	Candela http://www.candelalaser.com/
	Veam perfecta	Candela http://www.candelalaser.com/
	V-star	Cynosure http://www.cynosure.com/
	Cynergy	Cynosure http://www.cynosure.com/
	NLite	ICN Pharmaceuticals http://www.yestheyrefake.net/NLite.htm
(2) Mid-infrared lasers		
Q-switched 1,064 nm	Medlite C6/	Hoya ConBio http://www.conbio.com/
	RevLite	
Long-pulsed 1,064 nm	YAG 5	Palomar http://www.palomarmedical.com/
	Gentle YAG	Candela http://www.candelalaser.com/
	Apogee Elite	Cynosure http://www.cynosure.com/
1,319/1,320 nm	Profile 1,064 nm	Sciton http://www.sciton.com/
	CoolTouch® C3	CoolTouch® Corp http://www.cooltouch.com/
1,450 nm	Profile 1319	Sciton http://www.sciton.com/
1,540 nm	SmoothBeam	Candela http://www.candelalaser.com/
	Aramis	Quantel http://www.quantelmedical.com/
(3) Intense pulsed light sources	Lumenis one™	Lumenis http://www.lumenis.com/
	BBL	Sciton http://www.sciton.com/
	PhotoSilk	Cynosure http://www.cynosure.com/
	Harmony	Alma lasers http://www.almalasers.com/
	PPX/isolaz	Aesthera http://www.aesthera.com/
	Ellipse flex	DDD http://www.ellipse.org/

Maintenance therapy, although not addressed in many accounts of sub-surfacing lasers, is usually required at certain time intervals, as well as proper skin care to maintain the rejuvenation effect one is attempting to achieve. In contrast to the amount of literature which the ablative laser resurfacing devices have enjoyed in the medical literature, these sub-surfacing lasers have not had an overwhelming scientific base in the literature but have had descriptive coverage of the various devices and their effects.

Various classifications of these sub-surfacing lasers have been used over the past several years – we will classify them as shown in Table 1. Table 1 shows that these medical devices can be classified into (1) vascular lasers, (2) mid-infrared lasers and (3) intense pulsed light sources. The remainder of this chapter will review the literature of the vascular lasers, the mid-infrared lasers, and the IPLs.

- Studies have shown that KTP lasers have better collagen formation results when compared to 1,064 nm lasers in the treatment of skin photo-rejuvenation.
- Pulsed dye lasers (PDL) function best in the treatment of vascular lesions (i.e., port wine stains and hemangiomas) with significant production of procollagen type I and type III.
- Increased activity of dermal fibroblasts and mucin, as well as the thickening of the stratum spinosum in the dermis, has been noticed in the restoration of degenerated skin.
- The use of modern PDL systems for skin rejuvenation provides non-ablative results by minimizing side-effects and reducing purpura.

Vascular Lasers

KTP Lasers

The KTP lasers have traditionally been utilized to treat small caliber facial telangiectasias on the face and there is little in the medical literature which can be attributed to the use of the KTP lasers in rejuvenation of the skin. In a study by Lee,[6] 150 patients were treated with the KTP laser and the 1,064 nm laser separately and together for non-ablative facial rejuvenation. Patients in this series received 3–6 treatments of both the KTP laser alone, the 1,064 nm laser alone, and the combination of both devices. Skin biopsies looking at histologic effects in the skin were performed at 1, 2, 3, and 6 months following the last treatment. The results showed that the KTP laser was superior to the 1,064 nm laser in improving the parameters of photorejuvenation of the skin but that the combination of devices was superior to either one of the devices used alone. Post-therapy skin biopsies confirmed the presence of new collagen formation as well as a result of these lasers systems. Others, including Goldberg[7] found similar results in ten patients – again treated with a millisecond Nd: YAG laser and a millisecond KTP laser showed greater effects on tissue rejuvenation. Tan et al.[8] also demonstrated this synergistic effect of these two laser systems – 25% more improvement with the combined systems at 1 month for more than one third of the patients which increased to 40% at the end of 4 months.

Pulsed Dye Lasers

Pulsed dye lasers are also known commonly as flashlamp-pumped pulsed dye lasers are the prototype medical devices that were developed which adhere to the principle of selective photothermolysis.[9] Selective photothermolysis is a principle which stated that a specific wavelength of light can specifically destroy a chromophore within the skin, which in the case of the pulsed dye lasers is hemoglobin. The pulsed dye laser systems have improved in many facets over the years, especially in their methods of epidermal cooling and in that they have longer pulse durations than their predecessor devices, which reduces the incidences for purpura as a result of the therapy, considered one of the necessities of the early pulsed dye lasers but also one of the drawbacks from the treatment. These devices have been routinely used to treat vascular lesions (facial telangiectasia, diffuse erythema, and other superficial vascular lesions) and their successes in the treatment of port wine stains and hemangiomas have been reviewed in the medical literature.[10-12] Pulsed dye lasers have shown to be useful in reducing the erythema and improving

stretch marks[13] and these devices have also been used successfully to treat hypertrophic scars and keloidal lesions, especially being able to reduce the associated erythema sometimes associated with these lesions.[14,15] In the process, many of these scars have shown dermal remodeling and an associated shrinkage of the scar itself. The exact mechanism of pulsed dye induced collagen formation is not clear but it has been proposed that thermal induced damage to vascular endothelium may produce cytokines leading to dermal remodeling and thus the improvement of fine lines and wrinkles.[3]

Several clinical evaluations have been performed which support the use of the pulsed dye lasers for a non-ablative rejuvenation effect. Rostan et al.[16] utilized a long pulsed 595 nm laser in evaluating wrinkles of the cheeks. Fifteen patients received a series of four treatments at monthly intervals, either with the laser on or with cryogen only in the control group. The group performed skin biopsies prior to the pulsed dye laser treatments and at 4–6 weeks following the last laser treatment, as well as 3 months following the last laser treatment. They specifically looked at routine histology, procollagen I production and the activity of dermal fibroblasts. They found that the Grenz zone was moderately thicker in 50% of patients in both groups treated, but the degree of thickening was greater in the treatment groups than the controls. Similar findings were also seen at 3 months following the laser treatments, when an increase in dermal collagen was also observed in the treatment sites. A statistically significant improvement in the clinical grading scale for photodamage was also noted in the study.

Zelickson et al.[12] evaluated ten patients with mild to moderate facial lines and wrinkles and ten patients with moderate to severe facial lines and wrinkles that were treated with a single laser treatment with a 585 nm pulsed dye laser with a 450 um pulse duration. Clinically 9 out of 10 patients in the mild to moderate wrinkle group showed 50% or more improvement with 3/10 showing 75% or more improvement. All of the patients maintained their improvements for 6 months following their last laser treatment. In contrast, only 3/10 patients in the moderate to severe wrinkle group improved during the study. Skin biopsies from those patients in the mild to moderate group were performed at 6 and 12 weeks following the laser treatment. The biopsy specimens showed a thickened stratum spinosum and a thickened collagen layer in the superficial dermis as well as increased mucin in the superficial dermis. They also performed ultrastructural evaluations which demonstrated an increase in collagen fibers and an increase in the number of fibroblasts in the treated skin. They also noted that there was an increase in normal appearing elastic fibers and a decrease in the clumping of degenerated elastic fibers in the skin. Zelickson and Kist[17,18] have also reported results from skin biopsies performed after two periorbital 585 nm pulsed dye treatments or IPL treatments (6 week apart) in which in-situ hybridization mRNA probe studies were performed 6 weeks after the second treatment. These studies showed an 18% increase in type I collagen production after the IPL treatments compared to a 23% increase in type I collagen production after the pulsed dye therapy. Collagenase transcriptase activity was 32% for the IPL and 40% for the pulsed dye laser. The authors concluded that the observed increases in mRNA in fibroblasts indicated that through this non-ablative light, extracellular matrix protein production by dermal fibroblasts is increased, thus resulting in the effects seen.

Others have also looked at the pulsed dye lasers for its potential in rejuvenation of the skin. Bjerring et al.[19] utilized a 585 nm pulsed dye laser with a 350 um pulse duration and studied suction blisters which had been treated with the pulse dye laser. Using special markers for the production of type III procollagen they were able to demonstrate significant increases in type III procollagen levels after a single treatment with the pulsed dye laser, but also demonstrated a drop in type III procollagen levels after a retreatment. Goldberg et al.[20] also performed skin biopsies with a similar pulsed dye laser looking at facial lines and wrinkles. In this study, patients received two pulsed dye laser treatments. Pretreatment and 6 month post-treatment clinical evaluations and skin biopsies were analyzed. Forty percent of the individuals noted mild improvement in their wrinkle appearance. Ultrastructural analyses showed increases in type I and III collagen in those treated with the pulsed dye lasers. A second study by these authors[21] evaluated clinical, histologic, and ultrastructural changes after non-ablative treatments utilizing varying settings in the same subject. Ten patients were included in this clinical trial. The patients were randomly divided into two groups of five. All of the patients received 595 nm pulsed dye laser treatments to the periorbital areas. The first group was treated once, while the second group was treated twice at a 1 month interval. Each side of the face was treated with distinctly different laser settings. Seventy percent of the patients noted mild to moderate improvement clinically after treatment at 6 months following the last treatment. There was no difference between receiving one or two treatments in this study. Histologic and electron microscopy improvement was noted in all of the patients.

Examples of improvement in rejuvenation as a result of pulsed dye lasers are shown in Figs. 5 and 6.

The major side effect of pulsed dye lasers in the past was purpura, which has virtually been eliminated with today's more sophisticated machines, with longer pulse durations and improved epidermal cooling. However, purpura is a side effect still sometimes seen, and blister formation, pigmentary dyschromias, as well as scarring have been noted with the pulsed dye lasers.

- Q-switched 1,064 nm laser systems stimulate deep dermal collagen stimulation have shown to cause re-epithelization faster than carbon dioxide systems. Further studies have shown that Q-switched 1,064 nm laser devices significantly decrease solar elastosis and thicken upper papillary dermal zones of collagen.
- 1,064 nm Nd: YAG laser devices have useful skin tightening mechanisms for skin rejuvenation.
- With the use of epidermal cooling devices, such as cryogen, 1,319/1,320 nm laser devices have provided optimal results in the formation of new collagen, reduction of lines and wrinkles. These non-ablative laser systems leave the epidermis intact and provide great results in all skin rejuvenating procedures.
- 1,450 nm mid infrared diode laser systems have functioned successfully in the treatment of active inflammatory acne vulgaris, acne scars on the face, fine lines and wrinkles. This laser system targets dermal water, creates a wound in the dermis and triggers the regeneration process of collagen.
- 1,540 nm Erbium Glass laser devices have clinically proven dermal remodeling by treating fine lines and wrinkles, acne vulgaris and acne scars, and atrophic scars on the face. These lasers use a sapphire lens cooling device throughout the treatment process.

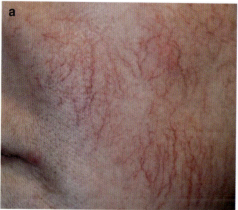
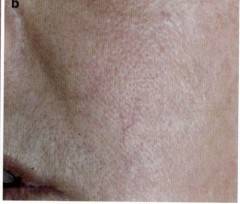

Fig. 5 (**a**, **b**) Clinical example of rejuvenation following pulsed dye laser treatment; 10 msec, 7 J/cm^2, Delay short, Nd:YAG 10 ms, 40 J/cm^2 (Photos courtesy of Cynosure/P. Boixeda M.D.)

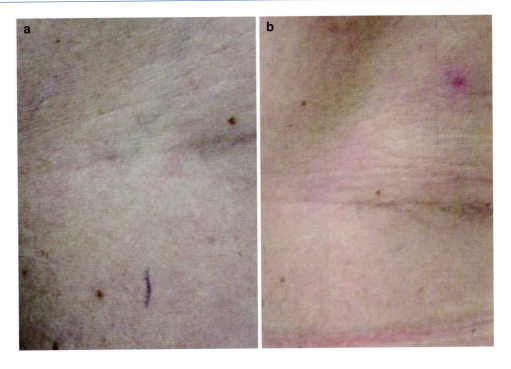

Fig. 6 (**a, b**) Clinical example of rejuvenation following pulsed dye laser treatment; Post 2 treatments, PDL 40 ms, 11 J/cm^2, Delay Medium, Nd:YAG 15 msec, 60 J/cm^2 (*Blue reticular vein.*) (Photos courtesy of Cynosure/R. Adrian M.D.)

Mid-Infrared Lasers

Q-Switched, 1,064 nm Nd: YAG Lasers

Several investigations have evaluated the effects of the Q-switched 1,064 nm laser system for the treatment of facial lines and wrinkles. These Q-switched laser systems were originally designed for the treatment of densely pigmented blue-black tattoos but have also been found to be potentially useful in the rejuvenation of the skin, due to its deep penetration into the skin and thereby stimulating dermal collagen. Goldberg and Whitworth[22] evaluated the Q-switched 1,064 nm laser in a comparative study to carbon dioxide laser systems. Eleven subjects were included in this evaluation. All of the patients treated with the carbon dioxide laser systems improved in this clinical study. Nine of the eleven patients improved with the Q-switched 1,064 nm laser. Complete reepithelization occurred faster (3–6 days earlier) in the patients treated with the Q-switched laser as compared to the carbon dioxide systems. The authors concluded that the Q-switched 1,064 nm laser may play a role in the treatment of rhytids. Goldberg and Metzler[23] utilized a 1,064 nm Q-switched laser and a topical carbon solution in an attempt to potentiate the laser effects. Two hundred forty two solar damaged sites were treated with three treatments on 61 patients. The investigators found that as a result of this adjuvant care, patients had improvements in skin texture and skin elasticity.

Goldberg and Silapunt[24] evaluated skin biopsies from infraauricular skin treated with two passes of the Q-switched laser before and after 3 months following the last treatment in eight patients. Clinically, 6 of the 8 patients in the trial showed improvement by an independent observer. Four of the six biopsy specimens evaluated showed decreases in solar elastosis and a mildly thickened upper papillary dermal zone of collagen. More organization of the collagen bundles was also seen in this clinical study. Cisneros et al.[25] evaluated 22 patients who were treated twice with the Q-switched laser system – all with improvement.

1,064 nm Nd:YAG Lasers

Very little literature exists as far as the efficacy of utilizing the 1,064 nm long pulsed Nd: YAG laser in the treatment of fine lines and wrinkles. In a recent study by Taylor,[26] a comparison was made to the skin tightening ability of the long pulsed 1,064 nm laser in comparison to the monopolar radiofrequency device. In this particular clinical trial the results showed that the 1,064 nm was as useful in skin tightening as the radiofrequency device. Clinical examples are shown in Figs. 7 and 8.

1,319/1,320 nm Laser Systems

These mid-infrared laser systems have had a lot of play in the non-ablative, sub-surfacing laser field of rejuvenation. The 1,320 nm laser system, known as CoolTouch®, from the CoolTouch® Corporation (Roseville, CA) was the original sub-surfacing device developed specifically for the treatment of facial lines and wrinkles utilizing the non-ablative technique.

Fig. 7 Clinical example of skin tightening using 1,064 nm

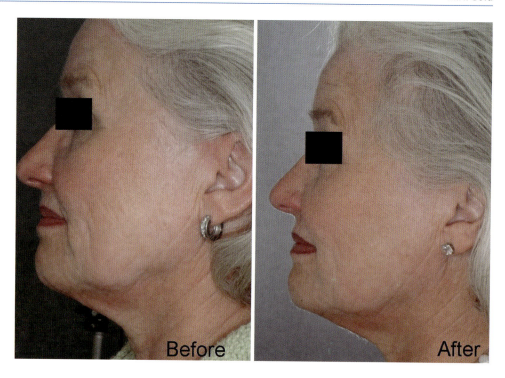

Fig. 8 Clinical example of skin tightening using 1,064 nm

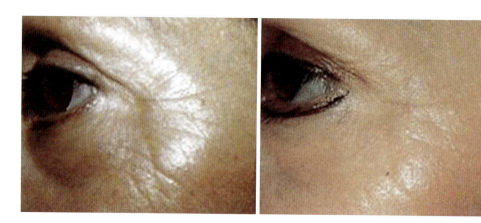

Subsequently, a 1,319 nm laser system from Sciton (Palo Alto) has also been introduced to this realm of sub-surfacing lasers.

The goal of these laser systems has always been to create a dermal wound resulting in the formation of new collagen, a reduction in lines and wrinkles, and to leave the epidermis intact. This has been achieved very well through the use of these devices and appropriate epidermal cooling. Clinical examples are shown in Figs. 9 and 10.

Utilizing unique delivery systems for cryogen spray delivery to the skin and with thermal sensors, the CoolTouch device was and is the prototype of the 1,319/1,320 nm laser systems on the market. It has had extensive clinical investigations performed using it over the years. Clinical assessment and skin biopsy clinical studies have been carried out by Goldberg,[27] Trelles et al.[28] and Levy et al.[29] In all of these clinical evaluations, skin biopsies performed at the end of the treatments showed evidence of new collagen formation. All of the patients had solar elastosis prior to treatment and demonstrated improvement clinically and histologically following the treatments. Goldberg[30] also evaluated ten patients with facial lines and wrinkles who received treatment five times with the CoolTouch device over 3–4 week intervals. At 6 months following the last treatment, all of the patients reported a subjective improvement in the quality of their skin; only 6 of the 10 were felt to be clinically improved by the investigator. All of the subjects showed evidence of new collagen formation at 6 months in skin biopsies.

Fatemi et al.[31] showed that with the 1,320 nm laser system that three passes from the device are better than a single pass in

Sub-Surfacing Lasers

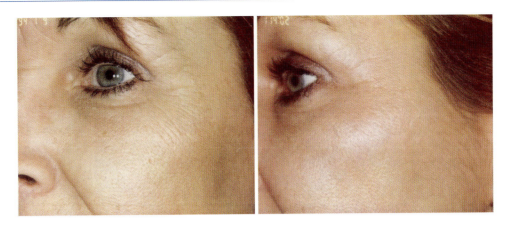

Fig. 9 Clinical example of 1,319/1,320 nm treatment

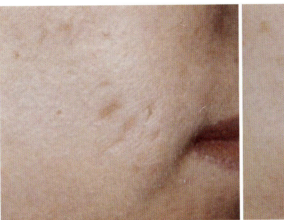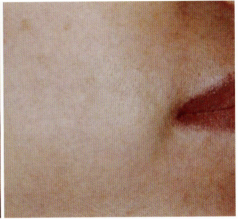

Fig. 10 Clinical example of 1,319/1,320 nm treatment

causing the early laser-induced histologic changes seen which noted included vascular damage, apoptosis, and edema – the beginning of the inflammatory mediator cascade required for collagen formation to occur.

1,450 nm Diode Lasers

The 1,450 nm mid infrared diode laser system, known as the SmoothBeam from Candela Corporation (Wayland, MA), has been used for the past several years as a treatment for active inflammatory acne vulgaris and for the treatment of acne scars on the face. It can also be used in a non-ablative fashion for the treatment of fine lines and wrinkles as well. This laser system works similarly to the 1,320 nm laser systems in that its wavelength targets dermal water, creates a wound in the dermis, and in the regeneration process forms new dermal collagen resulting in the desired effect.

In a study by Tanzi and Alster,[32] they compared the 1,450 nm diode laser to the 1,320 nm Nd:YAG laser in the treatment of atrophic facial scars. Twenty patients with mild to moderate atrophic facial acne scars received three monthly treatments with the 1,450 nm laser to one half of the face and the 1,320 nm laser to the other half of the face. Clinical evaluations and skin biopsy specimens were performed at various time intervals, including up to 1 year post the last treatment. Mild to moderate clinical improvement was observed clinically in the majority of patients studied. The 1,450 nm diode laser showed greater clinical scar response at the parameters studied (fluences from 9 to 14 J/cm^2). The same group also have investigated the 1,450 nm laser for the treatment of rhytids – periorbital rhytids improved more so than transverse neck lines.[33]

Acne vulgaris treatment with the 1,450 nm diode laser has received much attention. Paithankar et al.[34] treated patients with acne to their entire back area affected with acne and found that when treating four times at 3 week intervals, a statistical and clinical decrease in acne lesions was noted. Friedman et al.[35] also studied the effects of the 1,450 nm diode laser on sebaceous glands on the back and noted damage to the glands following therapy.

The SmoothBeam laser has shown quite a bit of efficacy over the years. Even with its sophisticated cryogen cooling, significant pain has been noted to occur in many patients, which has limited this machines ultimate further widespread use. A clinical example is shown in Fig. 11.

Fig. 11 Clinical example of 1,450 nm treatment

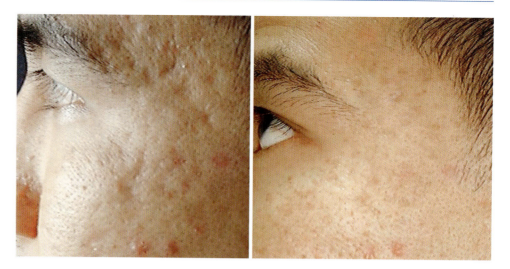

1,540 nm Erbium Glass Laser

The 1,540 nm erbium glass laser has seen extensive study in Europe for the treatment of fine lines and wrinkles, acne scars, and for the treatment of atrophic scars on the face. It has also been used successfully to treat active inflammatory acne vulgaris. Less clinical work appears to have been done on this device in the United States. This device utilizes a sapphire lens cooling device which delivers its contact cooling. Clinical evaluations with the device include Fournier et al.[36] in which patients treated with this device had a 40% reduction in wrinkles and a 17% increase in epidermal thickness at 6 weeks following the fourth treatment. The study evaluated 42 patients over a 14 month period of time. Lupton and Alster, looking at histologic effects from the erbium glass laser, demonstrated significant dermal remodeling and clinical satisfaction in 24 individuals 6 months after their final treatment (four treatments at 1 month intervals). In another study, Lupton et al.[37] evaluated the use of the 1,540 nm Er: Glass laser in 24 patients' facial wrinkles. Mild to moderate improvement in facial lines and wrinkles were seen in all of the study subjects; dermal fibroplasia was noted in the skin biopsy specimens.

All of the mid infrared devices have shown safety and efficacy. As noted with the 1,450 nm diode laser, pain is its most common adverse event. All of the mid infrared laser systems can cause significant discomfort without proper epidermal cooling. As well, most of these devices will result in some erythema and edema which, in the majority of cases, will resolve within 24–48 h. As with all laser systems, other adverse events can be seen with these devices, including pigmentary alterations and scarring of the skin.

A clinical example is shown in Fig. 12.

- Intense Pulsed Light (IPL) devices emit polychromatic light in broad ranges of wavelengths, selectively filtered to target specific chromophores, between 500 and 1,200 nm.
- IPLs treat vascular lesions, pigmentation, and have shown to have an effect in the production of collagen and elastic fibers in the dermis. Studies have shown that IPL photo-rejuvenation treatments using cooling apparatuses considerably increase epidermal thickness, and improve skin texture.
- The necessary cooling devices are required in all non-ablative devices to avoid the adverse effects relating to skin damaged. Blisters and pigmentary lesions can occur without the proper handling of cooling devices.

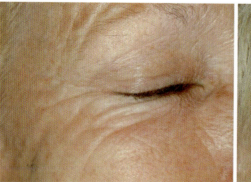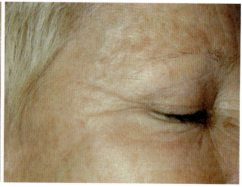

Fig. 12 Clinical example of 1,540 nm treatment

Intense Pulsed Light (IPL) Sources

IPLs have been around since the early 1990s and have withstood the test of time and criticism to become the most widely used medical devices in the world for photo-rejuvenation. The first of these light sources was a high-intensity flashlamp medical devices were initially developed for the treatment of vascular anomalies of the skin, specifically leg veins and telangectasias.[38] IPLs are pulsed light sources which emit polychromatic light in a broad wavelength of the light spectrum, usually between 500 and 1,200 nm. Many different variations on the IPL theme are now available, some with smaller absorption ranges, others with radiofrequency included to potentiate the effect of the broadband light, and still others with a vacuum apparatus included to bring the light in a colder relationship to the light itself. IPL devices of today are much more sophisticated than their predecessors but always are cautioned that not all IPLs are the same. In a recent well performed study by Town et al.[39] various IPLs were evaluated to determine their true pulse width (in an independent means) and to evaluate their true output in joules per centimeter squared over the time of the pulse. Differences were observed between devices and even based on some of the manufacturers' claims. These devices are very popular in today's culture; one must be aware of the company developing it and what clinical work rests behind it.

Although not true lasers, these devices also follows the principles of selective photothermolysis[9] in that with varying filters, or cut-off filters, one can use the IPL to selectively target a specific chromophore in the skin to cause a select affect upon that structure. It has been clearly demonstrated that the IPLs can treat vascular lesions, pigmentary concerns, and does have an effect on the collagen and elastic fibers in the dermal tissues.[40] These photorejuvenation effects of the IPL will now be reviewed.

The first major study in the field of photorejuvenation associated with a series of IPL treatments was published by Biter in 2000.[41] In this trial, 49 individuals received a series of treatments with an IPL device, with a minimum of four treatments given at 3 week intervals. In his study, he found that all of the parameters of photodamaged skin were improved in over 90% of those entered into this clinical trial. These included skin wrinkling, skin coarseness, irregular pigmentation, large pore size, and skin telangectasias. Skin biopsies taken from the forehead and 4 weeks after the last IPL treatment showed new collagen in both the papillary and reticular dermis as well as a resolution of any superficial dermal infiltrates.

Other studies utilizing an IPL demonstrating non-invasive resurfacing have also been performed. In his study, Hernandez-Perez et al.[42] evaluated five patients with five treatment sessions with an IPL. Moderate to very good improvement in the signs of photodamage were observed. Skin biopsy specimens were obtained at baseline and at 1 week following the final (5th) treatment. These biopsy specimens showed an increase in epidermal thickness, and an improvement in dermal concerns – specifically dermal elastosis, edema of the dermis, telangectasias present, as well as any dermal infiltrate. In another investigation, Negishi et al.[43] evaluated 73 individuals with an IPL. The patients in this clinical evaluation received at least five treatment sessions with the IPL. Clinical results noted a greater than 60% improvement in skin texture, in reduction of telangectasias, and in reducing pigmentary concerns in more than 80% of the patients who participated in the trial. Skin biopsies obtained at baseline and at 3 weeks following the final therapy showed an increase in types I and III collagen, as demonstrated by immunostaining. Goldberg, in several clinical trials, looked at rhytids following IPL therapy and clearly demonstrated an improvement in skin wrinkles which were also demonstrated histologically.[44,45] Prieto et al.[46] in their evaluation of IPL induced rejuvenation effects found similar collagen changes as compared to other authors but also found, through routine histology and electron microscope analyses, that after 1 week following therapy, there was no perifollicular infiltrate evident. Furthermore, at 3 and 12 months, demodex and an associated lymphoid infiltrate were observed. The authors postulated that because of the transient therapeutic effect of the coagulative necrosis of demodex organisms, a nonablative effect can occur. A long term evaluation by Weiss et al.[47] demonstrates that once the rejuvenation has had its effect, it can last for up to 5 years – 83% of patients followed continued improvement in skin texture; telangectasias improvement of 82%; and pigmentation remained improved in 79%.

Examples of photorejuvenation as a result of IPLs are shown in Figs. 13 and 14.

As noted, IPLs have much play in today's laser world. Because they are more sophisticated than ever before, most with exceptional cooling apparatus' to increase the safety of the devices, more and more physicians and others are utilizing them on a daily basis all over the world. Remember, these are medical devices that can damage the skin and cause horrific effects, as can all of the devices described in this report.

Techniques/Devices

Table 1 lists the names and manufacturers of the most commonly used lasers/light sources in each category along with the web address of those companies where further information to specifics may be obtained.

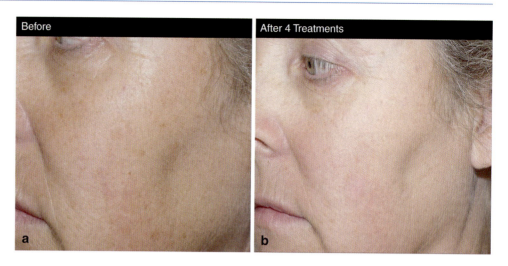

Fig. 13 (a, b) Clinical example of photorejuvenation with IPL

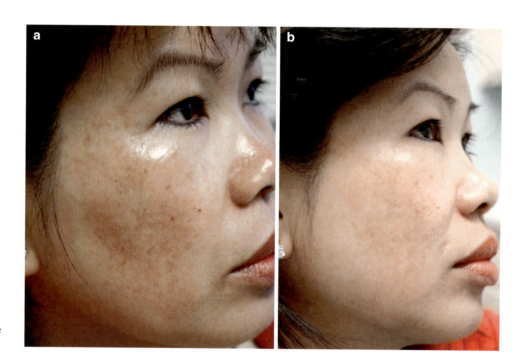

Fig. 14 (a, b) Clinical example of photorejuvenation with IPL

Adverse Events

All of the sub-surfacing devices have the potential to do harm. Because their mechanism of actions requires dermal injury with sparing of the epidermis, skin cooling becomes of paramount importance. Without proper epidermal cooling, which these machines do have, skin burning and blisters can occur. As a result, all of these devices have the potential to cause pigmentary changes and/or scars. These can be minimized by proper understanding and usage of the devices.

Future Directions

Personal opinion: The sub-surfacing devices have given us a good head start into the non-ablative laser world. I do believe other technology, more sophisticated and yielding even better results (safely) will be developed. I think that the IPLs have been an incredible addition to our rejuvenation efforts and I think they, in particular, will continue to be utilized, either alone or in combination, for the treatment of photodamage. I think that the newer fractional resurfacing devices offer increased efficacy over the sub-surfacing devices, and even in the fractionated realm it appears that the newer devices being developed are more ablative in nature than non-ablative. There will always be a role for the non-ablative resurfacing concept – positive results with none to minimal downtime. Hopefully, more devices of these kinds will be developed, benefiting physicians and patients alike.

Conclusions

Sub-surfacing, or non-invasive resurfacing, or photorejuvenation, have been a very popular part of the laser culture these past 10 years or so. Many of the devices described have shown a great deal of clinical efficacy, although at times, it has been difficult to document due to these changes being, at times, subtle. But our patients have been the ones who have benefited from these devices as they have always known the changes to be real, all with minimal to no downtime, one of the most important concepts of modern day lasers. Many of these procedures are now being replaced with the fractionated laser systems, which is covered elsewhere in this text. Sub-surfacing devices can provide you and your patients with much satisfaction.

References

1. Nelson JS, Majaron B, Kelly KM. What is nonablative photorejuvenation of human skin? *Semin Cutan Med Surg*. 2002;21:238-250.
2. Kelly KM, Kristen M, Majaron B, Nelson JS. Nonablative laser and light rejuvenation. The newest approach to photodamaged skin. *Arch Facial Plast Surg*. 2001;3:230-235.
3. Alam M, Hsu T-S, Dover JS, Wrone DA, Arndt KA. Nonablative laser and light treatments: histology and tissue effects – a review. *Lasers Surg Med*. 2003;33:30-39.
4. Papadavaid E, Katsambas A. Laser resurfacing review. *Int J Dermatol*. 2003;42:480-487.
5. Fitzpatrick RE. Laser resurfacing of rhytids. *Dermatol Clin*. 1997;15:431-447.
6. Lee MC. Combination aura 532 nm and lyra 1064 nm lasers for non-invasive skin rejuvenation and toning. *Lasers Surg Med*. 2002;30:32.
7. Goldberg DJ. Non-ablative dermal remodeling: comparing 3 different wavelengths: does it make a difference? *Lasers Surg Med*. 2002;30:31.
8. Tan MH, Dover JS, Hsu TS, Arndt KA, Stewart B. Clinical evaluation of enhanced nonablative skin rejuvenation using a combination of 532- and 1064-nm laser. *Lasers Surg Med*. 2004;34:439-445.
9. Anderson RR, Parrish RR. Selective photothermolysis: precise microsurgery by selective absorption of pulsed radiation. *Science*. 1983;220:524-527.
10. Alster TS, Kurban AK, Grove GL, Grove MJ, Tan OT. Alteration of argon laser induced scars by the pulsed dye laser. *Lasers Surg Med*. 1993;13:368-373.
11. Ashinoff R, Geronemus RG. Flashlamp-pumped pulsed dye laser for port wine stains in infancy: earlier versus later treatment. *J Am Acad Dermatol*. 1991;24:467-472.
12. Zelickson BD, Kilmer SK, Bernstein E, et al. Pulsed dye laser therapy for sun damaged skin. *Lasers Surg Med*. 1999;25:229-236.
13. McDaniel DH, Ash K, Zukowski M. Treatment of stretch marks with the 585 nm flashlamp-pumped pulsed dye laser. *Dermatol Surg*. 1996;22:332-337.
14. Alster TS. Improvement of erythematous and hypertrophic scars by the 585 nm flashlamp-pumped pulsed dye laser. *Ann Plast Surg*. 1994;32:186-190.
15. Alster TS, Williams CM. Treatment of keloid sternotomy scars with 585 nm flashlamp-pulsed dye laser. *Lancet*. 1995;345:1198-2000.
16. Rostan E, Bowes LE, Iyer S, Fitzpatrick RE. A double-blind, side by side comparison study of low fluence long pulse dye laser to coolant treatment for wrinkling of the cheeks. *J Cosmet Laser Ther*. 2001;3:129-136.
17. Zelickson BD, Kist DA. Pulsed dye laser and photoderm treatment stimulated production of type I collagen and collagenase transcriptase in papillary dermis fibroblasts. *Lasers Surg Med*. 2001;13:31.
18. Zelickson BD, Kist DA. Effect of pulsed dye laser and intense pulsed light source on the dermal extracellular matrix remodeling. *Lasers Surg Med*. 2000;12:17.
19. Bjerring P, Clement M, Heikendorff L. Selective non-ablative wrinkle reduction by laser. *J Cutan Laser Ther*. 2000;2:9-15.
20. Goldberg D, Tan M, Sarradet MD. Non-ablative dermal remodeling with a 585 nm, 350 um flashlamp pulsed dye laser: clinical and ultrastructural analysis. *Dermatol Surg*. 2003;29:162-164.
21. Goldberg DJ, Sarradet MD, Hussain M, Krishtul A, Phelps R. Clinical, histologic, and ultrastructural changes after nonablative treatment with a 595-nm flashlamp-pumped pulsed dye laser: comparison of varying settings. *Dermatol Surg*. 2004;30:979-982.
22. Goldberg DJ, Whitworth J. Laser skin resurfacing with the Q-switched Nd:YAG lasers. *Dermatol Surg*. 1997;23:903-906.
23. Goldberg DJ, Meltzer C. Skin resurfacing utilizing a low-fluence Nd:YAG laser. *J Cutan Laser Ther*. 1999;1:23-27.
24. Goldberg DJ, Silapunt S. Q-switched Nd: YAG laser: rhytid improvement by nonablative dermal remodeling. *J Cutan Laser Ther*. 2000;2:157-160.
25. Cisneros JL, Del Rio R, Palau M. The Q-switched neodymium (Nd) laser with quadruple frequency. *Dermatol Surg*. 1998;23:345-350.
26. Taylor MB, Prokopenko I. Split-face comparison of radiofrequency versus long-pulse Nd-YAG treatment of facial laxity. *J Cosmet Laser Ther*. 2006;8(1):17-22.
27. Goldberg DJ. Non-ablative subsurface remodeling: clinical and histologic evaluation of a 1, 320 nm Nd:YAG laser. *J Cutan Laser Ther*. 1999;1:153-157.
28. Trelles MA, Allones I, Luna R. Facial rejuvenation with a nonablative 1,320 nm Nd: YAG laser: a preliminary clinical and histologic evaluation. *Dermatol Surg*. 2001;27:111-116.
29. Levy JL, Trelles MA, Lagarde JM, Borrel MT, Mordon S. Treatment of wrinkles with the non-ablative 1,320 nm Nd: YAG laser. *Ann Plast Surg*. 2001;47:482-488.
30. Goldberg DJ. Full-face nonablative dermal remodeling with a 1320 nm Nd: YAG laser. *Dermatol Surg*. 2000;26:915-918.
31. Fatemi A, Weiss MA, Weiss RA. Short-term histological effects of nonablative resurfacing: results with a dynamically cooled millisecond-domain 1320 nm Nd: YAG laser. *Dermatol Surg*. 2002;28:172-176.
32. Tanzi EL, Alster TS. Comparison of a 1450-nm diode laser and a 1320-nm Nd: YAG laser in the treatment of atrophic facial scars: a prospective clinical and histologic study. *Dermatol Surg*. 2004;30: 152-157.

33. Alster TS, Tanzi EL. Treatment of transverse neck lines with a 1, 450 nm diode laser. *Lasers Surg Med.* 2002;14:33.

34. Paithankar DY, Ross EV, Saleh BA, Blair MA, Graham BS. Acne treatment with a 1, 450 nm wavelength laser and cryogen spray cooling. *Lasers Surg Med.* 2002;31:106-114.

35. Friedman PM, Jih MH, Kimyai-Asadi A, Goldberg LH. Treatment of inflammatory facial acne vulgaris with the 1450 nm diode laser: a pilot study. *Dermatol Surg.* 2004;30:147-151.

36. Fournier N, Dahan S, Barneon G, et al. Nonablative remodeling: a 14 month clinical ultrastructural imaging and profilometric evaluation of a 1540 nm ER: Glass laser. *Dermatol Surg.* 2002;28: 926-931.

37. Lupton JR, Williams CM, Alster TS. Nonablative laser skin resurfacing using a 1540 nm erbium glass laser: a clinical and histologic analysis. *Dermatol Surg.* 2002;28:833-835.

38. Goldman MP, Eckhouse S. Photothermal sclerosis of leg veins. *Dermatol Surg.* 1996;22:323-330.

39. Town G, Ash C, Eadie E, Moseley H. Measuring key parameters of intense pulsed light (IPL) devices. *J Cosmet Laser Ther.* 2007;9(3):148-160.

40. Raulin C, Greve B, Grema H. IPL technology: a review. *Lasers Surg Med.* 2003;32:78-87.

41. Bitter PH. Noninvasive rejuvenation of photodamaged skin using serial, full-face intense pulsed light treatments. *Dermatol Surg.* 2000;26:835-843.

42. Hernandez-Perez E, Ibiett EV. Gross and microscopic findings in patients submitted to nonablative full face resurfacing using intense pulsed light: a preliminary study. *Dermatol Surg.* 2002;28: 651-655.

43. Negishi K, Wakamatsu S, Kushikata N, Tezuka Y, Kotani Y, Shiba K. Full face photorejuvenation of photodamaged skin by intense pulsed light with integrated contact cooling: initial experiences in Asian skin. *Lasers Surg Med.* 2002;30:298-305.

44. Goldberg DJ, Cutler KB. Nonablative treatment of rhytids with intense pulsed light. *Lasers Surg Med.* 2000;26:196-200.

45. Goldberg DJ, Samady JA. Intense pulsed light and Nd: YAG laser. Nonablative treatment of facial rhytids. *Lasers Surg Med.* 2001;28:141-144.

46. Prieto VG, Sadick NS, Lloreta J, Nicholson J, Shea CR. Effects of intense pulsed light on sun-damaged human skin. Routine and ultrastructural analysis. *Lasers Surg Med.* 2002;30:82-85.

47. Weiss RA, Weiss MA, Beasley KI. Rejuvenation of photoaged skin: 5 year results with intense pulsed light of the face, neck, and chest. *Dermatol Surg.* 2002;28:1115-1119.

Non-invasive Rejuvenation/Skin Tightening: Light-Based Devices

Javier Ruiz-Esparza

Introduction

- The popularity of non-invasive cosmetic improvement of the skin has continued to grow amongst patients and practitioners alike.
- Cost and pain remain the principal limiting factors for patients.
- The safety of epidermal treatment in dark skin types has remained a challenge.
- Today, non-invasive treatment of photoaging can be achieved with light devices. A combination treatment which in my experience has proven to be safe and painless is described here.

A place in modern aesthetic procedures for non-invasive modalities is now well earned. The appeal of such procedures in the eyes of prospective patients is understandable. As for doctors, the possibility of improving someone's appearance without having to resort to drastic, painful and potentially risky procedures rapidly became the choice of many. It is to be understood that the changes induced are not as dramatic as those obtained by aggressive modalities, but they are not as drastic or irreversible either, thereby becoming a plus not a minus. Good candidates for these procedures are the ones who can live with the idea of gradual, subtle changes that, on the other hand, will not draw unnecessary stares, such as after an invasive Plastic Surgery correction. In addition, non-invasive procedures can now be directed at specific elements of photoaging, to specifically correct them. In such manner, the skin may be divided in three basic strata: Deep, being the reticular dermis; mid, being the papillary dermis and superficial being the epidermis. Each of these strata exhibit distinct changes attributable to premature

aging, namely: flaccidity, thinning or loss of substance, and brown (pigmentary) and red (vascular) dyschromias on the surface of the skin.

However, two are the limiting factors that need to be considered:

1. Cost: Being that multiple repeated procedures are needed to effect a change and
2. Pain: The interest of patients in these procedures is, in general, inversely proportional to the pain inflicted by them and therefore it is in the interest of the practitioner to be able to provide his patients with procedures that can be performed with as little pain as possible

The procedures described here can be carried out without pain and without anesthesia whatsoever. They are safe for all skin types and promote easy patient's acceptance because of lack of discomfort during and after treatment as well as carefree post operative time. As mentioned before, patients should understand that a series of treatments may be necessary to achieve the desired change. They are to understand as well, that the changes obtained after these procedures are subtle and may not be noticed after each individual session, but through completion of a series and or, upon photographic comparison of before and after pictures. Improvement however, can be seen after only one treatment session (Figs. 1–5) and improves after multiple or combined multiple sessions (Figs. 6–9). If the patient desires dramatic changes he or she is probably not a good candidate for these procedures.

On the other hand, we have gradually improved our understanding of how skin tightening takes place and how it can be induced painlessly and immediately using light. A long way has passed since we were trying to elicit a change using flash intense heating with radiofrequency. In a similar manner, when we use the Nd:YAG laser as later described, a change in skin quality is first noticeable after only a few days when treating the mid layer with laser, and there is even a change that is noticed immediately: pore size reduction. Dyschromias will also improve within a matter of days, again using light, intense pulsed light. So, all in all, these change account for an excellent acceptance level for the vast majority of patients who undergo these treatments, provided we have outlaid a

J. Ruiz-Esparza
Department of Dermatology, University of California,
San Diego, CA, USA
e-mail: thermalift@hotmail.com

K. Nouri (ed.), *Lasers in Dermatology and Medicine*,
DOI: 10.1007/978-0-85729-281-0_13, © Springer-Verlag London Limited 2011

Fig. 1 Six months post one Titan treatment

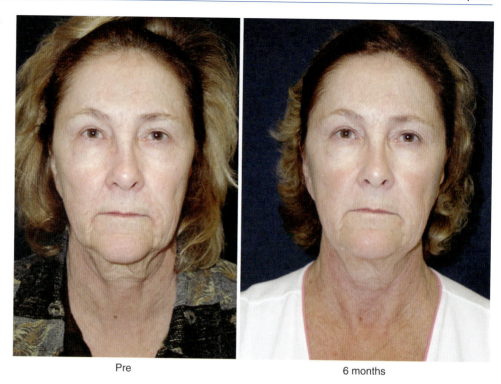

Fig. 2 Six months post one Titan treatment

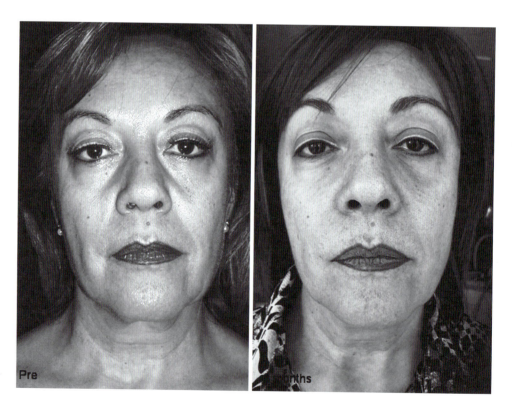

Non-invasive Rejuvenation/Skin Tightening: Light-Based Devices

Fig. 3 Eight months post one Titan treatment

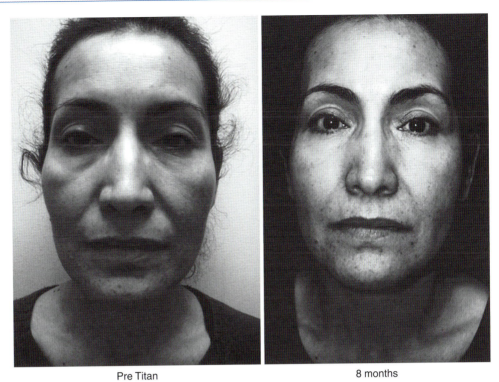

Pre Titan   8 months

Fig. 4 82 year old woman before and 1 month post a single Titan treatment

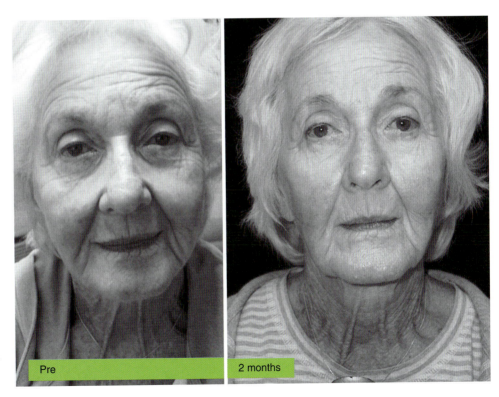

Pre   2 months

Fig. 5 One month post one Titan treatment

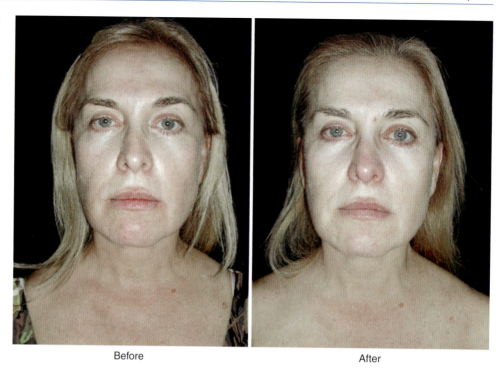

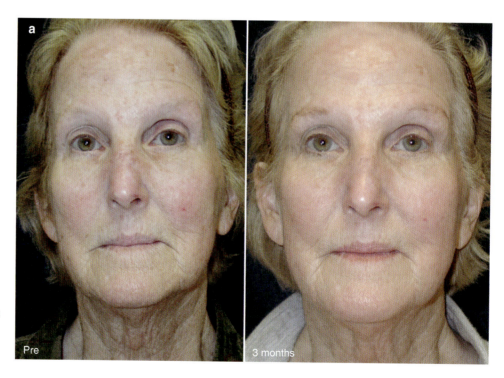

Fig. 6 (**a**) Three months post one Titan 3 Nd:YAG showing better skin quality and (**b**) in lateral view

Fig. 6 (continued)

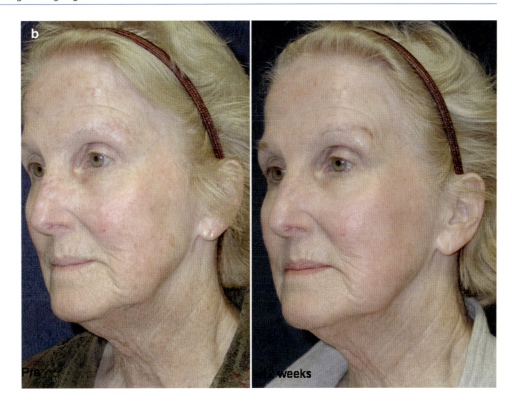

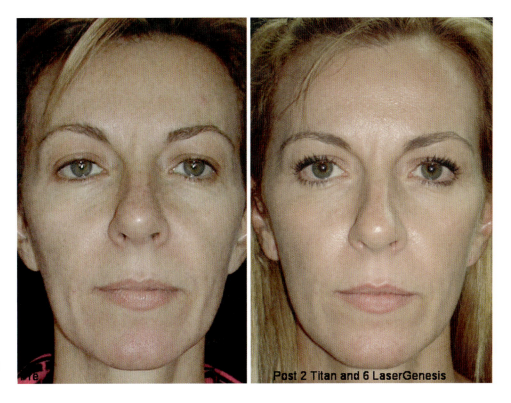

Fig. 7 Pre and 6 month post combination treatment Titan plus Nd:YAG

Fig. 8 Pre and post one Titan and 5 Nd:YAG

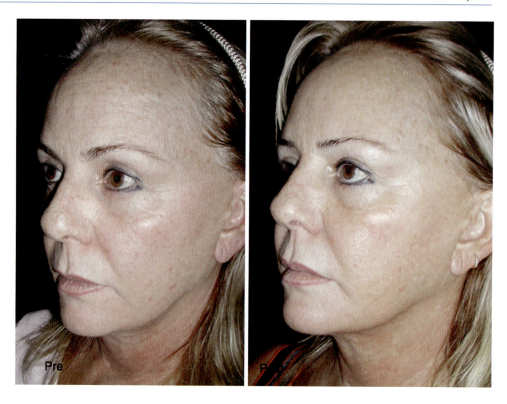

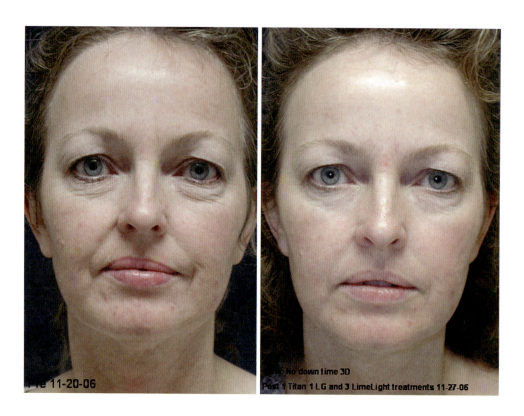

Fig. 9 Seven days after combination treatment of one Titan, 3 Nd:YAG and 5 IPL

plan of treatment and of expected level of improvement in all detail *prior* to starting the series and never *a posteriori*.

Photoaging in the Deep Stratum of the Skin Causing Skin Laxity Can Be Treated with Light

- Skin tightening can best be induced using long, gradual, sustained multi second pulses of heat
- If the tissue is heated in this manner, it can be done painlessly
- Immediate skin tightening is observed in nearly all patients regardless of age or skin type

For the purpose of this writing we will limit ourselves to the mid and lower thirds of the face and neck. Unwanted skin flaccidity starts at variable degrees for individual patients during the third decade of life. Jowls, loss of sharpness in the mandibular lines, laxity of cheeks and deepening of the nasal-labial fold individually or collectively may appear. The traditional approach years ago, was that of a rhytidectomy or face lift. The problem was that this procedure, alone, corrects by pulling the lax skin following one vector of movement, causing in some cases, distortion of landmarks of the face such as the corners of the mouth. Inducing skin contraction by delivering deep, sustained heat to the deep dermis, aims to cause a minute global shrinking, that will revert the skin to its original position to some degree. Achieving that with light, requires a source of heat that can be on for extended periods of time and that does not cause pain on contact with the skin. In other words, a long pulse of light, and cooling of the treatment surface of the device, the one that gets in contact with the surface of the skin while the light is on. The light must have a wavelength which allows for penetration to the level of the target, i.e.,: the deep reticular dermis. The closest to such a device is Titan® by Cutera, Inc.

Titan is an infrared light device emitting light at 1,100–1,800 nm in multi second cycles. At these wavelengths, there is a moderate level of water absorption and therefore it can thoroughly heat the dermis over a period of seconds. It differs from other infrared devices in that they usually have much smaller spot sizes and also have very short pulse durations (milliseconds) as well as a very high water absorption which results in shallow heating only. It has a spot area of 1 cm × 1.5 cm. Although it is an infrared lamp, it is not a

flashlamp. "Flashlamps" produce light at lower wavelengths (more visible light) and are usually pulsed at short (millisecond) durations. This is a broadband infrared lamp that emits longer wavelengths and is better suited for multi-second pulse durations. Heat penetration depth from this device is estimated to be about 1–2 mm, but some heating does occur down to about 5 mm. These calculations were done using dermal scattering coefficients and water penetration depths for near infrared wavelengths to estimate an "effective penetration depth" for a particular wavelength. The total intensity was then calculated by adding up the contribution from individual wavelengths. These models were then confirmed by actual thermal measurements of ex-vivo tissue samples and an appropriate filter design was selected based on the desired thermal profile obtained by the manufacturer.

Technique: Both, physician and patient should wear appropriate protection goggles. This author uses now a technique that differs from the traditional one for this device. It is a gliding technique, in which the treatment window is glided in vertical lines on the cheeks and neck. The machine is then set to emit the highest possible pulse which also has the longest possible pulse, lasting several seconds. The fluence is set at 65 J/cm². But since the device is engineered to emit a pre-cooling pulse of cold, as well as a trans-cooling and post cooling pulse, care is taken to avoid the pre and post-cooling because they are unnecessary in this particular technique. So, the device is made to begin contact with the skin surface immediately after the blue light indicator of cold emission is followed by the yellow light of infrared light emission. Then the handpiece is glided in a vertical fashion until the yellow light stops. When the blue light alone continues, at the end of each pulse, care should be taken to withdraw the handpiece from skin contact. This avoids unpleasant cold sensation for the patient. As mentioned above, I use the "S" handpiece at a setting of 65 J/cm², with pulses of 9.2 s duration. I find the "V" and "XL" handpieces less adequate for the glide technique due to their sharp edges.

At the beginning heat is almost imperceptible for the patient. The strokes are then repeated, over and over with some overlapping to produce the desired goal: incremental, sustained heating that because it is not sudden and intense, it is painless. Many strokes are necessary to elicit visible contraction, in my experience from 40 to 60 in each area, considering each cheek one area, and each side of the neck one area as well. Gliding is facilitated by the use of a hydrophilic gel such as K-Y Jelly® (Johnson and Johnson). Contraction can be seen with the patient lying down but it becomes more apparent when the patient sits up. The contrast with the untreated side demonstrates the contraction to the patient (Figs. 10–12) with the simple use of a mirror. As mentioned,

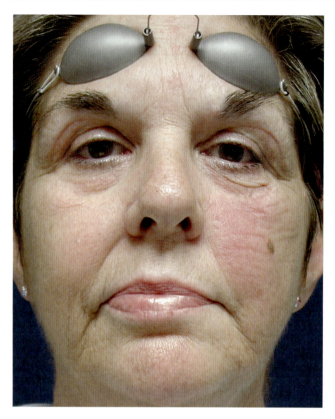

Fig. 10 Immediate skin contraction after Titan on left cheek

this technique, properly performed is painless even in the beard area in men, in which the traditional "stamping" technique usually hurts. The following principle must be understood: The skin will contract by applying heat slowly, steadily, progressively and sustainably. Overlapping strokes is permitted and desirable always guided by pain sensation. No pain is necessary to elicit contraction, with gentle heat applied for enough time, thus 40–60 gliding strokes of the handpiece are needed. Intense heat applied by the conventional "stamping technique" hurts and may not be the best for the patient. An animal hide will contract if put in a dryer with enough heat for enough time (Figs. 12 and 13). Sudden intense heat in brief pulses (such as that produced by a flame) will fail to contract the hide. Similar intense pulses in patients, whether originated by radiofrequency or light, will not offer the best contraction possible in clinical practice.

No post-operative care is required. Post-operative pain, swelling or bruising do not occur.

These treatment sessions can be repeated to improve results. Usually at monthly intervals until the desired level of improvement is achieved. I also recommend maintenance treatments every year for patients under 50 and every 6 months for patients over 50 years of age. Genetics, skin type, degree of sun protection and outdoor lifestyles will necessitate different maintenance schedules.

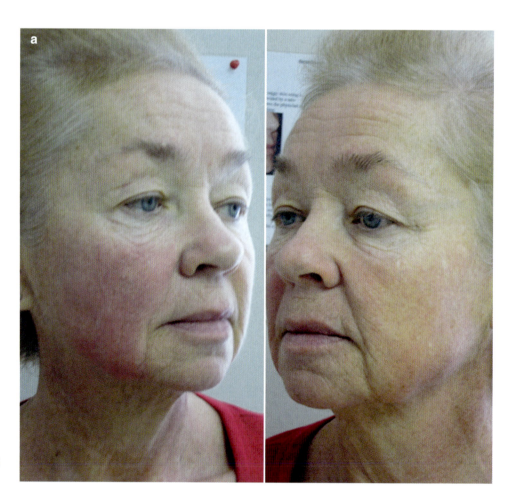

Fig. 11 (a) Immediate skin contraction on treated cheek and (b) in close up

Fig. 11 (continued)

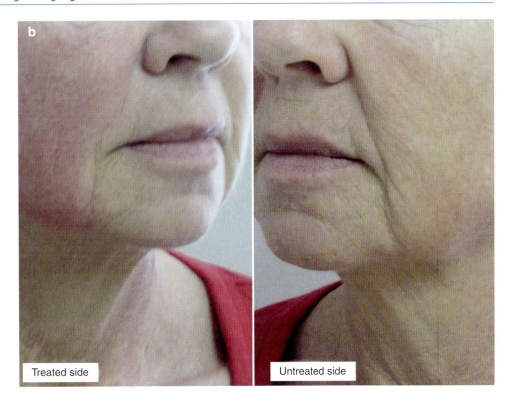

A Most Impressive Case of Tissue Contraction: Animal hide subjected to sustained slow heat for enough time

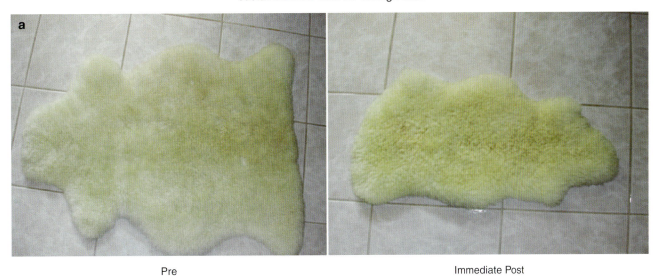

Fig. 12 (a, b) Animal hide contraction with slow sustained heat

A Most Impressive Case of Tissue
Contraction: Animal hide subjected to
sustained slow heat for enough time

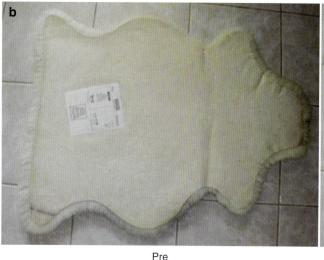
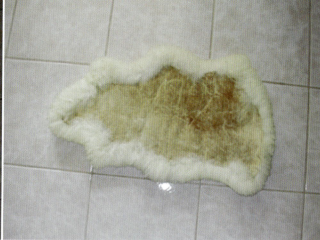

Pre

Immediate Post

Fig. 12 (continued)

Appropriate heating was applied to
elicit contraction

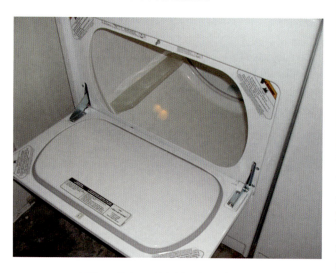

A Flame (intense brief heat) would have
burned the hide, not contracted it

Fig. 13 Slow and low heating can bring about appropriate contraction

A 1,064 Nm Nd:YAG Laser Is Used to Treat the Mid Stratum of the Skin

- The Nd:YAG laser can be used to improve skin quality.

- We use a repetition rate of 10 Hz at 15 J/cm², in 300 ms pulses.
- An airbrush technique about 1–2 cm from the skin surface is used.
- We use 5 sessions of 5,000 pulses each.
- Improvement can be observed within a month from each procedure.
- When adequately performed, the procedure is painless for most patients.

With this modality, an improvement in the quality of the skin is sought for. Improvement will start to be perceived by the patient usually after 1 week and will be at a peak after 1 month. An improvement in skin texture, softening of very fine static rhytids, a reduction of pore size, a diminution of actinic bronzing and an improvement in skin clarity and glow may result. Again, this technique is safe in all skin types.

Because of its wavelength, this laser can be used to reach the level of the papillary dermis. When engineered to deliver 15 J, in 300 ms pulses with a spot size of 5 mm, it can be delivered painlessly even at a repetition rate of 10 Hz.

Technique: Again, both, physician and patient should wear appropriate protection goggles.

First, we must understand the following principles:

1. The degree and speed of heating will be proportional to the speed of the hand of the operator as well as the distance between the handpiece and the skin.
2. Small areas heat up faster than larger ones. A repeated air brush movement is needed.

3. The face must be divided in relatively small areas rather than attempting to treat the entire face at the same time. In this manner, the forehead is considered one area, each cheek with the corresponding side of the nose will be another, and the perioral area and chin another area.
4. The operator will move to the next area in circles. Each will be treated generally with five consecutive passes. Pain or immediate redness are NOT treatment goals or endpoints.
5. The machine counts pulses automatically. The number of pulses will vary. Typically, 5,000 pulses for 5 monthly sessions. Lately, I have found that more pulses in a single session are more rewarding and safe. We now deliver 15,000–25,000 in a single treatment session.

Improvement of the Superficial Stratum of the Skin Using Light

- Intense pulsed light (IPL) can be used to improve some epidermal signs of photoaging.
- Pigmented or vascular dyschromias are exceedingly common and are ideal targets for this procedure.
- The procedure can be safely applied in dark skin types in the following manner: The procedure is done at daily intervals for 5 days.
- We use the "Limelight" device by Cutera, Inc.
- We start at 8 J/cm², "C" mode for skin types III–V and "B" for skin types I–II.
- We use increments of 2 J/cm² daily.
- Mild burning sensation during each pulse is expected. No pain afterwards.
- The cooled tip is kept in situ after each pulse long enough for the burning sensation to disappear.

Intense pulsed light (IPL) has been used for a number of years and an abundant body of literature has been published on the subject. We will deal in this chapter with the means to make this procedure safe for all skin types and to minimize discomfort and post-operative the undesirable treatment effects that we usually see when a conventional technique is used.

The device that we use ("Limelight" by Cutera, Inc.) emits light between 520 and 1,100 nm. It has a cooled sapphire handpiece. Three distinct factory-set programs are available labeled A, B and C. A delivers the shortest wavelength and pulse duration and is aimed to treat skin types I–II mainly with vascular dyschromias. B has a longer wavelength emission and correspondingly shorter cooling times. It is used in pigmented and vascular dyschromias in skin type I–III. The C program is the safest for darker skin types and emits in the longest wavelength range available for the machine. It also has the longest pulse duration. A so-called "Pigment mode" is available. This has a shorter cooling time and appears to be more effective in pigmentary targets. We use this mode carefully in darker types.

The initial fluence used for treatments will vary from 8 J/cm² for skin types II–IV to 12 J/cm² for skin type I–II. We do daily treatments for 1 week with increments in fluence of 2 J/cm² per day if tolerated. Two passes are the routine, per session. We take the time to cool the skin leaving the cool handpiece in situ for a few seconds or after the burning sensation from the light pulse disappears, after the emission of the light pulse. This aids significantly to decrease the level of the discomfort produced by these treatments, especially in dark skin types. We do not apply pre-or post-treatment cooling pads. Daily sessions will turn the chromophore in the skin darker by the day, augmenting the ultimate effect on pigmented lesions. On the other hand, gradual increments in fluence permit to reach higher levels safely. This is crucial in dark skin tones or suntanned skin.

Patients can expect darkening of the pigmented target lesions after 48 h and spontaneous sloughing of the lesions within 1 week. By doing daily treatments we curtail erythema post treatment and are able to deliver ultimately higher fluences, which, we feel aids in the final result. In this manner for example we are able to deliver up to 16 J/cm² in skin type IV by the fifth day.

Bibliography

Ruiz-Esparza J. Immediate skin contraction induced by near painless, low fluence irradiation by a new infrared device. A report of 25 patients treated with this novel non-invasive, non-ablative method. *Dermatol Surg.* 2006;32(5):601-610.

Negishi K, et al. An objective evaluation on the effects of non-ablative skin tightening with a broadband infrared light device. Presented at the 26th Annual Meeting of the American Society of Laser Medicine and Surgery; April 2006; Boston, MA.

Taub AF et al. Multicenter clinical perspectives on a broadband infrared light device for skin tightening. *J Drugs Dermatol.* 2006; 5(8):771-778.

Zelickson B, et al. Ultrastructural effects of titan infrared handpiece on forehead and abdominal skin. Presented and published in the meeting abstracts of the 25th Annual Meeting of the American Society for Laser Medicine and Surgery; April 2005;Orlando, FL.

Alexiades-Armenakas M. Assessment of the mobile delivery of infrared light (1100-1800 nm) for the treatment of facial and neck skin laxity. *J Drugs Dermatol.* 2009;8(3):221-226.

Sze-Hon C et al. Nonablative infrared skin tightening in type IV to V Asian skin: a prospective clinical study. *Dermatol Surg.* 2007;33: 146-151.

Schmults CD et al. Nonablative facial remodeling erythema reduction and histologic evidence of new collagen formation using a 300-microsecond 1064-nm Nd:YAG laser. *Arch Dermatol.* 2004;140:1373-1376.

Goldberg DJ. Non-ablative subsurface remodeling: clinical and histologic evaluation of a 1320-nm Nd:YAG laser. *J Cutan Laser Ther.* 1999;1(3):153-157.

Goldberg DJ, Silapunt S. Q-switched Nd:YAG laser: rhytid improvement by non-ablative dermal remodeling. *J Cutan Laser Ther.* 2000;2(3):157-160.

Goldberg DJ, Samady JA. Intense pulsed light and Nd:YAG laser non-ablative treatment of facial rhytids. *Lasers Surg Med.* 2001;28(2):141-144.

Tan MH, Dover JS, Hsu TS, Arndt KA, Stewart B. Clinical evaluation of enhanced nonablative skin rejuvenation using a combination of a 532 and a 1,064 nm laser. *Lasers Surg Med.* 2004;34(5):439-445.

Prieto VG, Diwan AH, Shea CR, Zhang P, Sadick NS. Effects of intense pulsed light and the 1,064 nm Nd:YAG laser on sun-damaged human skin: histologic and immunohistochemical analysis. *Dermatol Surg.* 2005;31(5):522-525.

Dang YY, Ren QS, Liu HX, Ma JB, Zhang JS. Comparison of histologic, biochemical, and mechanical properties of murine skin treated with the 1064-nm and 1320-nm Nd:YAG lasers. *Exp Dermatol.* 2005;14(12):876-882. Institute for Laser Medicine and Biophotonics, Shanghai Jiaotong University of Shanghai, China.

Dang Y, Ren Q, Hoecker S, Liu H, Ma J, Zhang J. Biophysical, histological and biochemical changes after non-ablative treatments with the 595 and 1320 nm lasers: a comparative study. *Photodermatol Photoimmunol Photomed.* 2005;21(4):204-209.

Trelles M, Allones I, Velez M, Mordon SJ. Nd:YAG laser combined with IPL treatment improves clinical results in non-ablative photo-rejuvenation. *J Cosmet Laser Ther.* 2004;6(2):69-78.

Min-Wei CL. Novel 3-in1 wavelength light source fpr photorejuvenation. *J Drugs Dermatol.* 2009;7(4):335-339.

Laser and Light Therapies for Acne

Voraphol Vejjabhinanta, Anita Singh, Rawat Charoensawad, and Keyvan Nouri

- Acne vulgaris is a very common cutaneous disorder which can cause permanent scarring and disfigurement.
- Acne is a multifactorial disorder of pilosebaceous units and affects the areas of skin with the greatest concentration of sebaceous follicles such as the face, neck, chest, and back.
- Common therapies for acne treatment include retinoids, keratolytic agents, antimicrobials, and anti-inflammatory agents.
- The need for an alternative treatment has led to the investigation of lasers and light sources as a new treatment.
- The laser and light based devices most commonly used are either the short wavelengths (400–700 nm) i.e., pulsed dye laser, red light or blue light; or longer wavelength lasers (near- and mid-infrared).
- The short wavelength lasers cause activation of protoporphyrin-IX resulting in a photodynamic reaction.
- The longer wavelength lasers target sebaceous glands resulting in reduction of sebum secretion and improvement of acne. They also induce collagen production resulting in improvement of acne scars.

Introduction

Acne vulgaris is the most common cutaneous disorder that affects approximately 80% of the population at some point during their lives.[1] Its prevalence has been estimated to be about 85–100% in boys aged 16–17 years, and 83–85% in girls of the same age.[2,3] In fact in the U.S., it is estimated that approximately 25 million adults and 40 million adolescents are affected by this condition.[4,5] However, even though it is common in teenagers and early adults, acne can occur in all age groups.[6,7]

This common cutaneous disorder can cause permanent scarring and disfigurement, which may lead to severe consequences in psychological and personality development. In fact, it is associated with a high prevalence of depression and is the second highest cause of skin disease related suicide. For these reasons effective management of acne can improve self esteem, body image and other life quality issues.[8,9]

Acne is a multifactorial disorder of pilosebaceous units and affects the areas of skin with the greatest concentration of sebaceous follicles. These areas include the face, neck, chest, and back. The main etiologic factors of acne are complex and multifactorial. There are four key components that contribute to the development of acne, these include (1) hypercornification of follicular epithelium at the infra-infundibulum with the development of a keratin plug blocking outflow of sebum to the skin surface; (2) hyperplasia of the sebaceous glands and hypersecretion of sebum with puberty or increased activity due to androgen hormone stimulation; (3) lipase-synthesizing bacteria (*Propionibacterium acnes*) colonizing the upper and midportion of the hair follicle, converting lipids within sebum to pro-inflammatory fatty acids; finally, (4) immune response and induction of inflammation in the follicle associated with release of cytotoxic and chemotactic factors.[10-13]

The severity of acne has been classified by the American Academy of Dermatology according to the following specifications: Mild acne is characterized by the presence of comedones, few papules and pustules (generally <10) but no nodules; Moderate acne has several to many papules and pustules (10–40) along with comedones (10–40); Moderately severe acne is characterized as the presence of <40 papules and pustules along with larger, deeper nodular inflamed lesions (up to 5); Severe acne is characterized by the presence of numerous or extensive papules and pustules, as well as many nodular lesions.[14] Although most patients will improve with time, some do not and have serious long term effects from acne. These include redness, hyperpigmentation, and permanent scars (atrophic, hypertrophic and keloids).[1]

V. Vejjabhinanta (✉)
Department of Dermatology and Cutaneous Surgery,
University of Miami, Leonard, M. Miller School of Medicine,
Miami, FL and
Department of Dermatology, Siriraj Hospital, Mahidol University,
Bangkok, Thailand
e-mail: vvoraphol@gmail.com

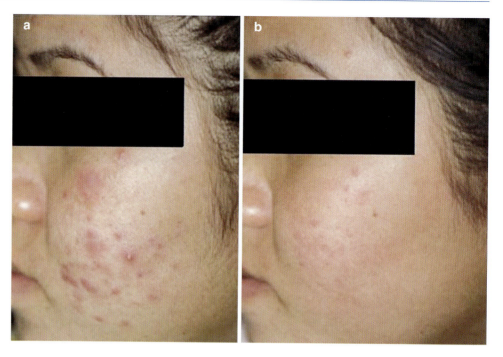

Fig. 1 Laser for acne (**a**) before treatment (**b**) result after four treatments with 1,064 nm Nd:YAG laser

Common therapies used for the treatment of acne vulgaris include keratolytic agents, antimicrobials, anti-inflammatories, retinoids, hormonal treatments, microdermabrasion, and chemical peels.[1,9] The need for an alternative treatment has led to the investigation of lasers and light sources as a new treatment. The mechanism of action relies upon the fact that lasers can emit wavelengths in the visible light spectrum (400–700 nm) which can cause self destruction of *P. acnes* because these bacteria have porphyrins with Q-band absorption peaks in the range of 500–700 nm.[15] In addition, long wavelength, near- and mid-infrared lasers, cause photothermal damage to the sebaceous glands because they can penetrate deeper into the skin (Fig. 1a, b).[16]

Laser Based Therapies

- The mechanisms of action are that lasers can emit wavelengths which are selectively absorbed by oxyhemoglobin of the dilated vasculature within inflamed acne, activate bacterial porphyrins resulting in self destruction of *P. acnes*, or decrease sebum production by photothermal damage to the sebaceous glands.

Pulsed Dye Lasers

The 585-nm and 595-nm pulsed-dye lasers (PDL) directly targets *P. acnes*. The PDL uses a yellow light which is mostly absorbed by oxyhemoglobin. For this reason it is especially useful for the treatment of vascular lesions as well as scars and fine wrinkles. However, the pulsed dye laser can also activate bacterial porphyrins and thereby produce selective photothermolysis of the dilated vasculature within inflamed acne.[17-19]

Orringer and co-workers conducted a randomized controlled split-face study with the 585-nm PDL, however their study did not find any significant improvement in treated versus non-treated skin.[20] In contrast, Seaton and co-workers found that this wavelength reduced inflammatory acne lesions by 49% at 12 weeks after one treatment.[21] No serious adverse affect to the treatment was noted in this study.

Potassium Titanyl Phosphate (KTP) Laser

The 532 nm potassium-titanyl-phosphate (KTP) laser uses a broad spectrum green light which is thought to photoactivate bacterial porphyrins and produce limited non-specific thermal injury to sebaceous glands.[22-24] Baugh and Kucaba conducted a study to evaluate the 532-nm KTP laser for the treatment of mild to moderate acne. This study was a randomized split-face study of 26 patients that showed a moderate reduction in acne score at 1 week and diminished reduction at 4 weeks post-treatment.[25]

Bowes and co-workers conducted another split-face study whereby they treated one-half of the face of 11 patients with mild to moderate acne with the KTP laser. After 1 month, the treated half had a 35.9% decrease in acne, while the control half had a 1.8% increase. They noted in this study that there was decreased sebum production but there was a minimal effect on *P. acnes*.[23]

1,450-nm Diode Laser

The 1,450 nm diode laser is a longer wavelength laser that penetrates to the level of the sebaceous gland within the mid-dermis.[26] This wavelength is primarily absorbed by water, so it does not greatly effect the epidermis but does thermally ablate sebocytes, along with *P. acnes*.[26,27] In a multicenter, blinded study, 61 patients were treated every month for 4 consecutive months using the 1,450 nm diode. There was a 26% drop out rate, but of the 45 patients remaining, 26 had 65% improvement 1 month following treatment, and at 6 months 5 patients required no additional acne therapy.[28]

Friedman and co-workers observed an 83% decrease in mean inflammatory facial acne lesions after three treatments using a 1,450 nm diode at 4–6-week intervals. Side effects were transient and local, including erythema, edema, and perioral pain. However, this study was limited in that there was no control and no long-term follow up.[27]

Alam and co-workers compared the 1,450 nm diode laser with the 595 nm PDL and determined that the 1,450 nm diode laser produced similar acne reduction with longer remissions (up to 3 months) when compared to the 595 nm PDL in a split-face trial of 25 patients after 4 monthly treatments.[29]

1,320 Neodymium: Yttrium Aluminum Garnet Laser (ND:YAG)

The 1,320 neodymium: yttrium aluminum garnet laser (Nd:YAG) is a deep-penetrating, long wavelength, mid-infrared laser that has been shown to have thermolytic effects upon sebaceous glands. In one study the 1,320 Nd: YAG laser was used to treat 50 moderate to severe acne patients with 6-weekly treatments. The patients were followed for 1 year thereafter. Eighty percent of patients felt they had 75–100% improvement after the fourth of these six treatments. However, 72% of the patients felt that the benefit seemed to fade beyond 3 months. Eighty two percent of the patients that had acne scarring had 'noticeable' improvement. The one major complication that was reported was one patient developed a pitted scar from the treatment.[30]

1,540 Erbium (ER): Glass Laser

The 1,540 erbium (Er): glass laser was initially used for non-ablative dermal remodeling and wrinkle reduction. However, this laser was shown to provide deep dermal penetration and subsequent alteration of sebaceous activity through thermal coagulation. Two studies that have looked at the effects of the 1,540 erbium (Er): glass laser have found very promising results. One study found that there was a 78% lesion reduction in 25 patients with facial and truncal acne after 4 monthly treatments with the 1,540 nm laser.[31] The other study found that there was a 70% reduction in 20 patients with facial acne who received four bi-weekly treatments.[32] Both studies had no reported adverse effects and had a reduction of oiliness in their patients.[31,32]

Light Based Therapies

- The three light based devices most commonly used are the blue light, red light, and intense pulsed light system.
- They can cause self destruction of *P. acnes* by activation of protoporphyrin IX to produce free radicals.

Blue Light

Light based therapies takes advantage of the photosensitivity of porphyrins produced by *P. acnes*. Activation of protoporphyrin IX, found in *P. acnes*, in the presence of oxygen produces a metastable intermediate that destroys the bacterium. Protoporphyrin IX absorption peaks occurs in wavelengths found in the visible light spectrum.[33-36]

In a study done by Elman and co-workers, 46 acne patients were treated with blue light. Of these 46 patients, 80% of them received approximately a 60% improvement of papulo-nodular acne lesions after 8 treatments. These patients had prolonged remission of their acne which was evident in the 8 weeks follow-up period. No adverse effects were noted in any of the patients.[37] In a split face study conducted by Tzung and co-workers, they found that the treated half when compared with the non-irradiated side, was markedly improved and concluded that blue light was effective in acne treatment.[38]

In a study by Tremblay and co-workers, 45 patients were treated with pure blue light (415 nm and 48 J/cm^2) for a period of 4–8 weeks. They found that the mean improvement score was 3.14 at 4 weeks and 2.90 at 8 weeks. In fact, nine patients experienced complete clearing at 8 weeks. The treatment was well tolerated, with 50% of patients highly satisfied with the treatment. There were no reported adverse effects in this study.[39]

In a study by Omi and colleagues, they investigated the use of high-intensity, narrow-band, blue light on acne. They recruited a total of 28 adult healthy volunteers with facial acne (mean age 28.1 years, range 16–56 years). These patients were treated with a total of eight serial biweekly 15-min treatment sessions. They found that overall there was a 64.7% improvement in acne lesions.[40]

Morton and co-workers tried to determine the effect of narrow-band blue light in the reduction of inflammatory and non-inflammatory lesions in patients with mild to moderate acne. They performed an open study utilizing a blue light source in 30 patients with mild to moderate facial acne. Over a 4 week period, patients received eight 10- or 20-min light treatments, peak wavelength 409–419 nm at 40 mW/cm^2. This study concluded that eight 10- or 20-min treatments over 4 weeks with a narrow-band blue light was found to be effective in reducing the number of inflamed lesions in subjects with mild to moderate acne. The onset of the effect was observable at week 5. However, the treatment was found to have little effect on the number of comedones.[41]

Blue/Red Light Combinations

Although by theory porphyrins should respond well to blue light, it is a shorter wavelength and therefore do not penetrate well into the skin.[42] Longer wavelengths with Q-bands, such as red light, has been combined with blue light in acne therapy. Red light (wavelength 600–650 nm) penetrates deeper into the skin than blue light. In fact, 635 nm light may penetrate through the skin up to 6 mm compared with 1–2 mm for light at 400–500 nm. Red light has also been shown to be effective in acne treatment by activating porphyrins in the Q band and decreases inflammation by controlling cytokine release from macrophages.[43-47]

In one study, Papageorgiou and co-workers randomized 107 patients with acne into four treatment groups: blue light, mixed blue and red light, cool white light, and 5% benzoyl peroxide cream. Treatment was given 15 min daily for 12 weeks. They concluded that there was a mean improvement was 76% for mixed blue and red light, with follow-up of 12 weeks.[43]

Intense Pulsed Light (IPL)

Intense pulsed light (IPL) uses a flashlamp to deliver wide spectrum, non-coherent visible light (green, yellow, and red) to near-infrared wavelengths. Treatment of acne with IPL has shown some very promising results (Fig. 2a, b). In a study by Gregory and co-workers, 50 patients with mild to severe acne were treated with IPL for 1 month. These patients showed a 60% lesion reduction at the 1-month follow-up, versus 32% increase in controls.[48] In a study done by Elman and co-workers of 19 patients with acne they showed that the IPL produced a 85% clearance of inflammatory lesions and 87% clearance of non-inflammatory lesions in 2 months.[49] He and co-workers also conducted a study to test the role of pulsed light and heat energy in acne clearance. A system with light pulses and heat was used in bi-weekly treatments for 4 weeks with wavelengths between 430 and 1,100 nm, this study showed approximately a 75% clearance of the inflammatory lesions 1 month after the last treatment.[50]

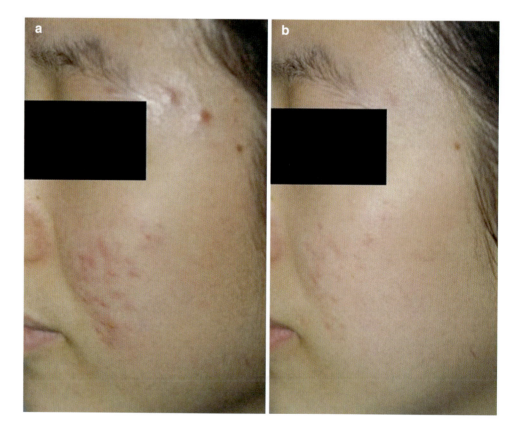

Fig. 2 Light based device for acne (**a**) before treatment (**b**) result after four treatments with an intense pulsed light

Conclusion

The treatment of acne is a difficult process due to its multifarious pathogenesis. For this reason more studies are needed to explore other possible treatments. For example, photodynamic therapy with δ-aminolevolunic acid or indocyanine green, IPL with suction (Photopneumatic therapy), combination therapies such as lasers/light based devices plus radiofrequency machines, etc. Using laser/ light based technology for the treatment of acne is rapidly evolving). The studies to date are promising; however, further investigation is necessary to determine safety, long-term efficacy, and optimal parameters of lasers and light sources. This comprehensive review of various lasers and light sources will hopefully provide a guide for physicians seeking to treat their acne patients utilizing technical innovations that are safe and effective.

References

1. Leyden JJ. Therapy for acne vulgaris. *N Engl J Med*. 1997;336: 1156-1162.
2. Kraning K, Odland GF. Prevalence, morbidity and cost of dermatologic diseases. *J Invest Dermatol*. 1979;73(Suppl):395-401.
3. Goodman G. Acne – natural history, facts and myths. *Aust Fam Physician*. 2006;35(8):613-616.
4. Del Rosso JQ. Acne in the adolescent patient: interrelationship of psychological impact and therapeutic options. *Today Ther Trends*. 2001;19:473-484.
5. Elman M, Lebzelter J. Light therapy in the treatment of acne vulgaris. *Dermatol Surg*. 2004;30:139-146.
6. Williams C, Layton AM. Persistent acne in women: implications for the patient and for therapy. *Am J Clin Dermatol*. 2006;7(5):281-290.
7. Harrington CI. Post-adolescent acne and marital break-up. *Br J Dermatol*. 1997;137(3):478-479.
8. Tan JK. Psychosocial impact of acne vulgaris: evaluating the evidence. *Skin Ther Lett*. 2004;9:1-3, 9.
9. Jappe U. Pathological mechanisms of acne with special emphasis on *Propionibacterium acnes* and related therapy. *Acta Derm Venereol*. 2003;83:241-248.
10. Leeming JP, Holland KT, Cunliffe WJ. The pathological and ecological significance of micro-organisms colonizing acne vulgaris comedones. *J Med Microbiol*. 1985;20:11-16.
11. Norris JFB, Cunliffe WJ. A historical and immunocytochemical study of early acne lesions. *Br J Dermatol*. 1988;118:651-659.
12. Cunliffe WJ et al. Comedogenesis: some new aetiological, clinical and therapeutic strategies. *Br J Dermatol*. 2000;142(6):1084-1091.
13. Zouboulis CC et al. What is the pathogenesis of acne? *Exp Dermatol*. 2005;14(2):143-152.
14. Pochi PE, Shalita AR, Strauss JS. Report of the Consensus Conference on Acne Classification. Washington, DC, March 24 and 25, 1990. *J Am Acad Dermatol*. 1991;24:495-500.
15. Cunliffe WB, Goulden V. Phototherapy and acne vulgaris. *Br J Dermatol*. 2000;142(5):855-856.
16. Lloyd JR, Mirkov M. Selective photothermolysis of the sebaceous glands for acne treatment. *Lasers Surg Med*. 2002;31(2): 115-120.
17. Bjerring P, Clement M, Heickendorff L, Lybecker H, Kiernan M. Dermal collagen production following irradiation by dye laser and broadband light source. *J Cosmet Laser Ther*. 2002;4:39-43.
18. Patel N, Clement M. Selective nonablative treatment of acne scarring with 585 nm flashlamp pulsed dye laser. *Dermatol Surg*. 2002;28:942-945.

19. Tan OT, Sherwood K, Gilchrest BA. Treatment of children with port-wine stains using the flashlamp pulsed tunable dye laser. *N Engl J Med*. 1989;320:416-421.
20. Orringer JS, Kang S, Hamilton T, et al. Treatment of acne vulgaris with a pulsed dye laser. A randomized controlled trial. *JAMA*. 2004; 291:2834-2839.
21. Seaton ED, Charakida A, Mouser PE, Grace I, Clement RM, Chu AC. Pulsed-dye laser treatment for inflammatory acne vulgaris: randomized controlled trial. *Lancet*. 2003;362:1347-1352.
22. Bowes LE. Clinical Case Report of Treatment of Acne Vulgaris with 532 nm KTP Laser Laserscope. White Paper 2003.
23. Bowes LE, Manstein D, Anderson RR. Effects of 532 nm KTP laser exposure on acne and sebaceous glands. *Lasers Surg Med*. 2003; 18:S6-S7.
24. Lee CMW. Aura 532 nm laser for acne vulgaris – a 3 year experience: Annual Combined Meeting of the American Society for Dermatolgic Surgery and the American Society for Mohs Micrographic Surgery and Cutaneous Oncology; October 2003; New Orleans.
25. Baugh W, Kucaba W. Nonablative phototherapy for acne vulgaris using the KTP 532 nm laser. *Dermatol Surg*. 2005;31:1290-1296.
26. Paithankar DY, Ross EV, Saleh BA, Blair MA, Graham BS. Acne treatment with a 1450 nm wavelength laser and cryogen spray cooling. *Lasers Surg Med*. 2002;31:106-114.
27. Friedman PM, Jih MH, Kimyai-Asadi A, Goldberg LH. Treatment of inflammatory facial acne vulgaris with the 1450-nm diode laser: a pilot study. *Dermatol Surg*. 2004;30:147-151.
28. Mazer JM. Treatment of facial acne with a 1450 nm diode laser: a comparative study. *Lasers Surg Med*. 2004;34:S67.
29. Alam M, Peterson SR, Silapunt S, Chopra K, Friedman PM, Goldberg LH. Comparison of the 1450 nm diode laser for the treatment of facial acne: a left–right randomized trial of the efficacy and adverse effects. *Lasers Surg Med*. 2003;32:S30.
30. Chernoff G. The Utilization of 1320 nm Nd:YAG Energy for the Treatment of Active Acne Vulgaris. Cooltouch Inc; White Paper 2004.
31. Boineau D, Angel S, Nicole A, Dahan S, Mordon S. Treatment of active acne with an Er:glass (1.54 um) laser. *Lasers Surg Med*. 2004;34:S55.
32. Kassir M, Newton D, Maris M, Euwer R, Servell P. Er:glass (1.54 mm) laser for the treatment of facial acne vulgaris. *Lasers Surg Med*. 2004;34:S65.
33. Lee W, Shalita A, Poh-Fitzpatrick M. Comparative studies of porphyrin production in *Propionibacterium acnes* and *Propionibacterium granulosum*. *J Bacteriol*. 1978;133:811-815.
34. Weishaupt K, Gomer C, Dougherty T. Identification of singlet oxygen as the cytotoxic agent in photoinactivation of a murine tumor. *Cancer Res*. 1976;36:2326-2329.
35. Niedre M, Yu C, Patterson M, et al. Singlet oxygen luminescence as an in vivo photodynamic therapy dose metric: validation in normal mouse skin with topical amino-levulinic acid. *Br J Cancer*. 2005;92: 298-304.
36. Taub AF. Photodynamic therapy in dermatology: history and horizons. *J Drugs Dermatol*. 2004;3(1 Suppl):S8-S25.
37. Elman M et al. The effective treatment of acne vulgaris by a high-intensity, narrow band 405–420 nm light source. *J Cosmet Laser Ther*. 2003;5(2):111-117.
38. Tzung TY et al. Blue light phototherapy in the treatment of acne. *Photodermatol Photoimmunol Photomed*. 2004;20(5):266-269.
39. Tremblay JF, Sire DJ, Lowe NJ, Moy RL. Light-emitting diode 415 nm in the treatment of inflammatory acne: an open-label, multicentric, pilot investigation. *J Cosmet Laser Ther*. 2006;8(1):31-33.
40. Omi T, Bjerring P, Sato S, et al. 420 nm intense continuous light therapy for acne. *J Cosmet Laser Ther*. 2004;6(3):156-162.
41. Morton CA, Scholefield RD, Whitehurst C, Birch J. An open study to determine the efficacy of blue light in the treatment of mild to moderate acne. *J Dermatol Treat*. 2005;16(4):219-223.
42. Kjelstad B, Johnson A. An action spectrum for blue and near ultraviolet inactivation of *Propionibacterium acnes*; with emphasis on a possible porphyrins photosensitization. *Photochem Photobiol*. 1986;43:67-70.

43. Papageorgiou P, Katsambas A, Chu A. Phototherapy with blue (415 nm) and red (660 nm) light in the treatment of acne vulgaris. *Br J Dermatol.* 2000;142:973-978. 22.
44. Cunliffe WJ, Goulden V. Phototherapy and acne vulgaris. *Br J Dermatol.* 2000;142:853-856.
45. Young S et al. Macrophage responsiveness to light therapy. *Lasers Surg Med.* 1989;9:497-505.
46. Lee SY et al. Blue and red light combination LED phototherapy for acne vulgaris in patients with skin phototype IV. *Lasers Surg Med.* 2007;39(2):180-188.
47. Goldberg DJ, Russell BA. Combination blue (415 nm) and red (633 nm) LED phototherapy in the treatment of mild to severe acne vulgaris. *J Cosmet Laser Ther.* 2006;8(2):71-75.
48. Gregory AN, Thornfeld CR, Leibowitz KR, Lane M. A study on the use of a novel light and heat energy system to treat acne vulgaris. *Cosmet Dermatol.* 2004;17:287-291.
49. Elman M, Lebzelter J. Evaluating Pulsed Light and Heat Energy in Acne Clearance Radiancy. White Paper, 2002.
50. Elman M, Lask G. The role of pulsed light and heat energy (LHE (TM)) in acne clearance. *J Cosmet Laser Ther.* 2004;6:91-95.

Lasers for Psoriasis and Hypopigmentation

Aaron M. Bruce and James M. Spencer

- Excimer Lasers
  - Psoriasis
  - Vitiligo
  - Other forms of Hypopigmentation
- Indications and Contraindications
  - Psoriasis
  - Vitiligo
- Techniques
  - Psoriasis
  - Vitiligo
- Adverse Events
- Future Directions
- Conclusion

References

Introduction

- Psoriasis and vitiligo have been found to benefit from light therapy in the UVB range (290–320 nm).
- The 308 nm xenon-chloride excimer laser is now utilized for select patients with psoriasis and vitiligo.
- The efficacy and safety of the excimer laser is well documented.
- Striae and post-resurfacing leucoderma have been found to respond to the 308 nm excimer laser.

One of the most recent advancements in phototherapy is the development of localized delivery systems. One such device is the excimer laser. The use of the excimer laser was first reported in dermatology by Bonis in 1997 for psoriasis

A.M. Bruce (✉)
Center for Surgical Dermatology, Westerville, OH, USA
e-mail: aaronmbruce@yahoo.com

treatment.[1] Psoriasis has been reported to respond best to light at a wavelength of 313 nm.[2] Since the excimer laser emits light at a wavelength of 308 nm, it was a logical choice for investigation. The excimer laser has been found to be efficacious for not only patients suffering from psoriasis but also several disorders of hypopigmentation including vitiligo. This chapter serves to discuss the use of the excimer laser for psoriasis and diseases of hypopigmentation.

Excimer lasers are a group of lasers utilized in a variety of medical specialties, most notably ophthalmology. There are several types of excimer lasers, all of which operate in the ultraviolet spectrum. Excimer refers to the formation of "excited dimers" via an inducible mixture of a halogen and noble gas. Electric current is delivered to the gas producing unstable, high-energy dimers that quickly dissociate giving off laser light.[3] The laser light is delivered to its target via a fiber optic cable. The mechanism of physiologic response is poorly understood, but does not appear to be a thermal mechanism. Thus, the excimer lasers do not operate under the theory of selective photothermolysis. Excimer lasers are capable of "cold ablation," which is precise tissue ablation with minimal surrounding thermal effects. This unique property enables the laser to be used in precision surgeries such as corneal reshaping. It is theorized that the energy of the photons from excimer lasers exceeds the energy of many chemical bonds which keep organic material together. This principle forms the theory termed "ablative decomposition," under which excimer lasers are thought to operate.

Excimer Lasers

Psoriasis

- Total cumulative dose is lower than traditional light therapy.
- Uninvolved skin is spared.
- Psoriatic plaques can tolerate several times the minimal erythema dose (MED).

K. Nouri (ed.), *Lasers in Dermatology and Medicine*,
DOI: 10.1007/978-0-85729-281-0_15, © Springer-Verlag London Limited 2011

The benefits of using the 308 nm excimer laser for psoriasis were fully elucidated in the late 1990s. Bonis showed that psoriatic lesions treated with the excimer laser cleared with fewer treatments than narrow band UVB therapy.[1] Utilization of the laser also spared the uninvolved skin from UV exposure, reducing the risk of carcinogenicity and photoaging. Kemeny also found that remissions for up to 2 years were seen in some patients.[4] Laser therapy demonstrated efficacy at lower cumulative doses when compared to conventional light therapy. It was also noted that psoriatic plaques can tolerate several times the minimal erythema dose (MED) of normal skin without burning. Exposure of three to four times the MED have demonstrated early clearance and long remissions. Doses greater than six times the MED, however, have shown to be complicated by blistering, pain and reduced compliance. In 2002, Feldman reported 80 patients treated with lower multipliers of the MED given twice weekly achieved 75% or greater clearance in 72% of subjects in an average of 6.2 treatments.[5]

The pulse dye laser (PDL) has also been studied for the treatment of psoriasis. The basis for using the PDL is selective photothermolysis of the exaggerated vascular network within psoriatic plaques. Small studies have revealed possible benefit.[6-8] Stronger data exists to support the use of the 308 nm excimer laser for the treatment of psoriasis.[5]

Vitiligo

- The excimer laser is as effective as oral PUVA, but with less associated risk.
- Over 25% of treated patients achieve 100% repigmentation.

The 308 nm excimer laser has also been shown to treat hypopigmentation of various etiologies. Vitiligo, which affects 1–2% of the population, is well known to be recalcitrant to most medical therapies. The disease has been treated with multiple forms of light therapy however, treatment requires many months of therapy exposing large areas of unaffected skin to ultraviolet radiation. Therapy is aimed at stimulating adjacent melanocytes to migrate and repopulate the affected skin. The use of the excimer laser for vitiligo was based on the finding that narrowband UVB therapy was as effective as oral PUVA with less associated risk. Hadi et al. demonstrated 50.6% of 221 vitiligo patients had 75%

or greater repigmentation after an average of 23 sessions. Also noteworthy is the fact that 25.5% of the patients achieved 100% repigmentation of the treated lesions. Two year follow-up did not reveal any loss of new pigmentation. Some patients even had continued repigmentation after treatment was completed.[9] These studies support the notion that the excimer laser works as well as NBUVB or PUVA for vitiligo, but in much less time. Kawalek et al. showed that the addition of tacrolimus 0.1% ointment in combination with the excimer laser induced faster and perhaps greater response to treatment.[10]

Other Forms of Hypopigmentation: Post-resurfacing Leucoderma and Striae

- Striae and post-resurfacing leucoderma can be safely treated with the excimer laser, although the results are not sustained.
- Striae associated atrophy remains unchanged after therapy.

Leucoderma is a generic term defined as, "deficiency of pigmentation of the skin."[11] Some authors have used this term more specifically to describe post-resurfacing hypopigmenation.[12] These hypopigmented macules and patches are known complications of carbon dioxide laser resurfacing. In 2001, Friedman and Geronemus reported using the 308 nm excimer laser for post carbon dioxide resurfacing leucoderma.[12] Two patients demonstrated 50–75% improvement with 8–10 treatments.

This therapy stimulates residual melanocytes while limiting cumulative UV-B exposure. Alexiades-Armenakas et al. in 2004 studied the response of hypopigmented scars, including striae alba, to the excimer laser. Thirty-one patients received up to ten treatments starting at 1 MED minus 50 mJ/cm². Visual analysis found 61% and 68% increase in pigmentation for leucoderma and striae, respectively, compared to control after nine treatments. However, the treated areas slowly depigmented back to baseline within 6 months of treatment cessation.[13]

In addition, Goldberg demonstrated 76% or greater darkening of striae after an average of eight treatments.[14] However, atrophy remained unchanged and the pigmentary improvements were not sustained. For patients with mature hypopigmented striae and hypopigmented scars, the 308 nm excimer laser presents a safe option for a common cosmetic concern with few other effective treatments.

Indications and Contraindications

Psoriasis

> Indications
>
> - Localized plaques that have not responded to medical therapy.
> - Mild to moderate psoriasis.
>
> Contraindications
>
> - Patients that report worsening of their lesions upon light exposure.

The excimer laser is indicated for mild to moderate psoriasis. Psoriatic lesions that occur in the groin and axilla (inverse psoriasis) respond well to the excimer laser. These areas are notoriously difficult to treat with traditional NBUVB. The excimer laser also works well for recalcitrant psoriatic lesions in areas such as the scalp. The most difficult areas to treat are the palms and soles. The excimer laser may also be used in conjunction with other systemic treatments for recalcitrant lesions. The excimer laser may be used in all skin types, however, skin types II, III, and IV appear to respond the best. Very fair skin may burn more easily and care must be taken when treating these patients. The only true contraindication is the rare psoriatic patient that reports worsening of lesions upon exposure to light.

A suitable patient is one who is able to commit to multiple treatments per week for potentially several weeks. Thus, compliance is usually the limiting factor for improvement. Increasing insurance copayments is also a substantial obstacle. Insurance coverage varies and documentation of prior treatment failure is usually required for approval. The ideal candidate lives or works near the unit location, has skin type II–IV, and has disease limited to the scalp or flexural areas. Most importantly, the patient must be committed to the course of treatment (Figs. 1a, b and 2).

Vitiligo

> Indications
>
> - Vitiligo with less than 20% involvement.
> - Locally distributed Lesions.
>
> Contraindications
>
> - Light sensitive patients.

The excimer laser is indicated for treatment of limited or localized lesions of vitiligo. Anatomic location is a major predictor of response rate when evaluating a vitiligo patient for possible excimer laser therapy. The most to least responsive areas are: face, scalp/neck, genitals, trunk, extremities, hands and feet, including bony prominences.[15] Skin type is also important, with Fitzpatrick III or higher skin types responding the best. Small lesions respond more quickly. Age, gender and duration of lesions do not appear to be a factor. It is not practical to treat large lesions due to the small spot size of the laser unit. The ideal candidate has Type III skin or darker with disease limited to the head, neck, or trunk. The only contraindication is a photosensitive patient. Patients taking medications that increase photosensitivity can be treated with caution. The inconvenience of multiple office visits and potential cost of therapy are significant hurdles when treating patients with psoriasis or vitiligo.

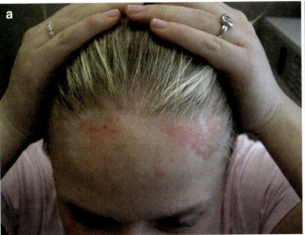 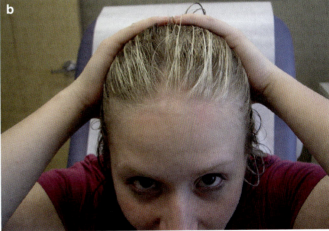

Fig. 1 (a) 21 y/o female with scalp psoriasis (b) after 12 treatments excimer laser

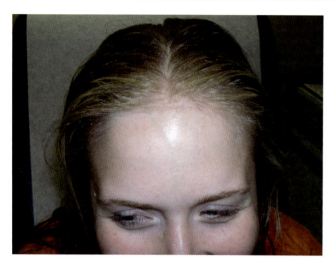

Fig. 2 One year follow up, still clear

Techniques

Psoriasis

- Preparation.
- Determine skin type and/or MED.
- Treat two to three times per week on non-consecutive days.
- Start at 3 MED and increase every other session unless burning occurs.

Initial evaluation of potential candidates should include extent, distribution, and past treatments of psoriatic lesions. The patient should be interviewed regarding any history of worsening psoriatic lesions upon light exposure. Risks and benefits should be discussed including the frequent and potentially long term visits for therapy. The cost of therapy including copayments should be addressed. Informed consent should be reviewed and obtained. Pretreatment photographs may also be useful. The skin should be free of any topical agents. Eye protection should be worn by all persons in the treatment room. It is also commonly recommended to apply a small amount of mineral oil to thick scaly plaques to help reduce light scatter.

Initial dosing can be chosen by skin type or determination of the MED. The MED is the minimal fluence required to induce pink erythema of unexposed skin. This is commonly tested on the lower back or gluteal area. A template is marked for orientation on a sun-protected area. Usually doses of 100 mJ/cm^2 through 350 mJ/cm^2 are used in 50 mJ/cm^2 increments. Therefore, six test doses are usually given. The patient avoids additional UV radiation to the area and returns for evaluation 24 h after test dosing. The lowest dose that induces detectable erythema is the MED.[16]

However, most manufacturers have treatment protocols for psoriasis based on plaque thickness and skin type. These guidelines avoid the inconvenience of determining the MED. Treatment guidelines usually consist of an initial dosing table followed by a protocol for subsequent treatments based on response. These guidelines are based on the following principles (see XTRAC Tables 1 and 2). Treatments should begin two to three times per week on non-consecutive days for up to a month or longer if needed. Treatment sessions may take longer than typical light therapy due to the small spot size, however it should be emphasized that less treatments are required (approximately 10 treatments versus 25 for conventional light therapy).

Treatment should start at 3 MED and increase every session, or every other session unless burning occurs. Dosage should be maintained to induce slight erythema within 24 h of treatment. The erythema should not last greater than 24 h and should not cause pain. If excessive erythema or pain occurs, decrease the subsequent dose by 25%. Most patients will continue topical therapy throughout the treatment.

Table 1 First dose determination for psoriasis Fitzpatrick skin type

Plaque thickness	Induration score	1–3 (mJ/cm^2)	4–6 (mJ/cm^2)
None	0		
Mild	1	300	400
Moderate	2	500	600
Severe	3	700	900

Adapted from Vitiligo Treatment Guidelines, 12-95362-01 Rev. A

Table 2 Subsequent dose determination for psoriasis

Clinical observation	No effect	Minimal effect	Good effect	Considerable improvement	Moderate/severe erythema
Typical dosing change	Increase dose by 25%	Increase dose by 15%	Maintain dose	Maintain dose, or reduce dose by 15%	Reduce dose by 25%

Adapted from Vitiligo Treatment Guidelines, 12-95362-01 Rev. A

Vitiligo

- Preparation and evaluation.
- Starting dose is 100–150 mJ/cm² on the head and neck.
- Dose is increased by 50 mJ/cm² per treatment until redness develops.
- Treatment is two to three times per week for up to 20 weeks.

Initial evaluation of potential candidates with vitiligo should include extent, distribution, and past treatments of hypopigmented lesions. A Wood's light may be used for examination of vitiligo lesions in patients with pale skin. This enhances any pigmentary changes not apparent under visible light. Risks and benefits should be discussed including the frequent and potentially long term visits for therapy. The cost of therapy including copayments should be addressed. Informed consent should be reviewed and obtained. Pretreatment photographs may also be useful. The skin should be free of any topical agents. Eye protection should be worn by all persons in the treatment room. The patient should be protected from natural light between treatments.

Determination of MED is not necessary for vitiligo patients as the calculated MED for the surrounding normal skin is not indicative for the skin affected by vitiligo. Other factors, such as, location, duration, and size are more important in determining response to laser therapy. The starting dose is 100–150 mJ/cm² on the head and neck. This dose is increased by 50 mJ/cm² per treatment until redness develops. If a severe burn occurs, reduce the dose by half or skip the following treatment. Avoid treatments on consecutive days. Much like psoriasis, a table and protocol for subsequent treatments is provided by the laser manufacturer (see XTRAC vitiligo Tables 3 and 4). Note the variability in initial dosing for various anatomical sites.

Recommended treatment is two to three times per week for up to 20 weeks. Most patients show response by 4 weeks, however, if there is no improvement by 20 weeks, then lesions may be deemed non-responsive to excimer laser therapy.

Adverse Events

- Erythema.
- Rarely bullae and pain.

Erythema is common and is the goal of treatment in vitiligo. Patients may perceive slight warmth upon laser application, however, most feel no sensation. Very few patients report transient stinging. Rare possible adverse events include sunburn reaction, corneal burn, freckling, irregular pigmentation, increase risk of skin cancer and accelerated aging. Eye protection and limiting treatment to the affected areas is recommended to minimize these risks.

Future Directions

- Psoriasis
  - Advances in medical therapy.
- Vitiligo
  - Advances in surgical and grafting techniques.

Table 3 First dose determination for vitiligo

Vitiligo location	Initial dose (mJ/cm²)
Periocular	100
Face, scalp, ear, neck, axilla, bikini	150
Arm, leg, trunk	200
Wrist	250
Elbow	300
Knee	350
Hands, feet	400
Finger, toes	600

Adapted from Vitiligo Treatment Guidelines, 12-95362-01 Rev. A

Table 4 Subsequent dose determination for vitiligo

Clinical observation	No effect	Good effect	Moderate erythema	Severe erythema
Typical dosing change	Increase dose by 50 mJ/cm²	Maintain dose	Decrease dose by 50 mJ/cm²	Postpone treatment or reduce by 100 mJ/cm²

Adapted from Vitiligo Treatment Guidelines, 12-95362-01 Rev. A

There has been great progress in understanding the nature of pigmentary and psoriatic disease. Advances in understanding the molecular pathogenesis of psoriasis has led to the development of the revolutionary class of medications known as the biologics. Currently there are 17 oral, topical, and injectable medications in phase II trials for psoriasis or psoriatic arthritis. Six oral and injectable medications are in phase III trials for psoriasis or psoriatic arthritis indications.[17] Despite the great advances in medical treatments for psoriasis, light therapy will likely continue to play a role for a large number of patients who may not be candidates for systemic therapy or may require systemic and localized light therapy for recalcitrant lesions. Other forms of treatment that are currently being researched include angiogenesis inhibitors, new retinoids, oral pimecrolimus, and photodynamic therapies.

Vitiligo patients that fail multiple medical therapies including topical and light therapy may be candidates for surgical techniques. Various grafting techniques such as mini-punch or blister grafts may be tried. Tattooing has also been used. The newest treatment includes the autologous melanocyte transplant. In this treatment, healthy skin is sampled, the melanocytes are grown in culture, and then they are transferred to the diseased skin. In addition to surgical therapy, research in gene therapy will shed more light on new and promising treatments.

Conclusion

Psoriasis and pigmentary disorders have a profound impact on the quality of life of affected patients. Despite multiple medical therapies for psoriasis, certain clinical scenarios present therapeutic dilemmas. The 308 nm xenon chloride laser provides another option that is both safe and effective for psoriatic and hypopigmented lesions such as vitiligo and post-resurfacing leucoderma. Combination therapy, including tacrolimus 0.1% and the 308 nm excimer laser, is likely the most effective and safest option for patients suffering from vitiligo.

References

1. Bónis B, Kemény L, Dobozy A, Bor Z, Szabó G, Ignácz F. 308 nm UVB excimer laser for psoriasis. *Lancet*. 1997;350:1522.
2. Parrish JA, Jaenicke KF. Action spectrum for phototherapy of psoriasis. *J Invest Dermatol*. 1981;76:359-362.
3. Spencer JM, Hadi SM. The excimer lasers. *J Drugs Dermatol*. 2004;3:522-525.
4. Kemény L, Bónis B, Dobozy A, Bor Z, Szabó G, Ignácz F. 308-nm excimer laser therapy for psoriasis. *Arch Dermatol*. 2001;137:95-96.
5. Feldman SR, Mellen BG, Housman TS, Fitzpatrick RE, Geronemus RG, et al. Efficacy of the 308 nm excimer laser for treatment of psoriasis: results of a multicenter study. *J Am Acad Dermatol*. 2002;46:900-906.
6. Erceg A, Bovenschen HJ, van de Kerkhof PC, Seyger MM. Efficacy of the pulsed dye laser in the treatment of localized recalcitrant plaque psoriasis: a comparative study. *Br J Dermatol*. 2006;155:110-114.
7. Ilknur T, Akarsu S, Aktan S, Ozkan S. Comparison of the effects of pulsed dye laser, pulsed dye laser + salicylic acid, and clobetasole propionate + salicylic acid on psoriatic plaques. *Dermatol Surg*. 2006;32:49-55.
8. Bovenschen HJ, Erceg A, Van Vlijmen-Willems I, Van De Kerkhof PC, Seyger MM. Pulsed dye laser versus treatment with calcipotriol/betamethasone dipropionate for localized refractory plaque psoriasis: effects on T-cell infiltration, epidermal proliferation and keratinization. *J Dermatol Treat*. 2007;18:32-39.
9. Hadi S, Tinio P, Al-Ghaithi K, et al. Treatment of vitiligo using the 308-nm excimer laser. *Photomed Laser Surg*. 2006;24:354-357.
10. Kawalek AZ, Spencer JM, Phelps RG. Combined excimer laser and topical tacrolimus for the treatment of vitiligo: a pilot study. *Dermatol Surg*. 2004;30:130-135.
11. Thomas C. *Taber's Cyclopedic Medical Dictionary*. 17th ed. Philadelphia: F.A. Davis Co; 1993:1102.
12. Friedman PM, Geronemus RG. Use of the 308-nm excimer laser for post resurfacing leukoderma. *Arch Dermatol*. 2001;137:824-825.
13. Alexiades-Armenakas MR, Bernstein LJ, Friedman PM, Geronemus RG. The safety and efficacy of the 308-nm excimer laser for pigment correction of hypopigmented scars and striae alba. *Arch Dermatol*. 2004;140:955-960.
14. Goldberg DJ, Sarradet D, Hussain M. 308-nm excimer laser treatment of mature hypopigmented striae. *Dermatol Surg*. 2003;29:596-599.
15. Ortonne JP, Passeron T. Melanin pigmentary disorders: treatment update. *Dermatol Clin*. 2005;23:209-226.
16. Asawananda P, Anderson RR, Chang Y, Taylor CR. 308 nm excimer laser for the treatment of psoriasis: a dose-response study. *Arch Dermatol*. 2000;136:619-624.
17. National Psoriasis Foundation, Research pipeline: drugs in development, www.psoriasis.org.

Lasers and Lights for Adipose Tissue and Cellulite

Molly Wanner and Mathew Avram

The use of lasers and light devices for the removal of adipose tissue and cellulite represents a new and exciting frontier in the laser field. To date, there are few non-invasive devices in the laser field all of which can only claim limited efficacy. This chapter will review the laser, light sources, as well as devices with radiofrequency and ultrasound devices that currently purport to treat cellulite or adipose tissue.

> - Non invasive options for adipose removal are few. The best studied non invasive treatment is focused ultrasound.
> - A significant barrier to non invasive treatments is the issue of fat localization after treatment. Adipose tissue stores triglycerides.
> - The Nd:YAG laser has been used alone or in combination with suction liposuction. SmartLipo™ (Cynosure, USA), a 300 um and 1,064 nm fiber encased in a micro-cannula, is an example of this type of device.

Devices for Removal of Adipose Tissue

While the demand for non-invasive removal is high, the effective means to do so is more limited. There are few laser or light based treatments for the removal of adipose tissue, and all currently available laser or light based options are invasive. The Nd:YAG laser has been used invasively, with or without liposuction, to remove adipose tissue. A low level 635 nm laser has also been combined with liposuction to remove adipose tissue. CO_2 laser has been used, in direct contact with adipose tissue to destroy it.[1] This section will review the light and laser based treatments for adipose tissue (Table 1). In addition, ultrasound approaches will be discussed as well.[13]

Non invasive options for adipose removal are few. The best studied non invasive treatment is focused ultrasound. Selective photothermolysis of adipose tissue has been reported at 1210 and 1720 nm wavelengths and may offer another non invasive option for treatment of adipose tissue, but a clinical device is not yet available.[14]

A significant barrier to non invasive treatments is the issue of fat localization after treatment. Adipose tissue stores triglycerides. Unlike cholesterol, which can be excreted, triglycerides are not excreted by the body; rather, they are metabolized for energy, stored, or used for such molecules as plasma lipoproteins.[15] Thus, the removal of large deposits of subcutaneous fat may yield redistribution to other sites in the body. Since increased visceral fat has been linked to increased cardiovascular disease, non invasive therapies should be approached cautiously, and their use may be limited to treatment of small deposits of fat.[16]

Focused Ultrasound

The Ultrashape™ System (Ultrashape Ltd, Israel), a focused ultrasound system, represents the only currently available non invasive device to destroy adipose tissue. This system delivers focused ultrasound waves at a precise depth to mechanically destroy adipose tissue and has been shown to decrease fat deposits with few side effects in one to three treatments.[17,18] Eighty-five percent of the fat reduction occurs in the first 14 days, so response to treatment can be assessed rapidly.[18] The procedure is quite lengthy, requiring topical anesthesia prior to treatment and a procedure time of 60–120 min.[18]

In a study of 30 patients, after three treatments, a statistically significant decrease of 2.3 cm in local deposits was found.[17] These patients maintained constant weight during the treatment period. In a larger prospective trial of 164 subjects

M. Wanner (✉)
Department of Dermatology, Massachusetts General Hospital,
Harvard Medical School, Boston, MA, USA
e-mail: mwanner@partners.org

K. Nouri (ed.), *Lasers in Dermatology and Medicine*,
DOI: 10.1007/978-0-85729-281-0_16, © Springer-Verlag London Limited 2011

Table 1 Laser and light treatment for adipose tissue

Technology	Example	Evidence in peer reviewed journal
1,064 nm Nd:YAG laser	SmartLipo™ (Cynosure® Inc.; Westford, MA)	Prospective, double blind, controlled trial of 25 patients and 110 treatments.[2] Patients served as their own control with suction lipoplasty on one half and laser-assisted lipoplasty on the other with a 2 mm and 1,064 nm Nd:YAG laser fiber follow by suction with a 3 mm cannula. Two blinded investigators evaluated photographs and found no difference between the groups. Postoperative pain was higher in the suction-assisted side versus the laser-assisted side at the first follow up visit only. Lipocrit (volume of red blood cells in the aspirated material) was lower on the laser-assisted side, a statistically significant difference. Histologic analysis showed more disruption of architecture on the laser-assisted side. Seventeen samples of infranatant were evaluated, and ten were found to have elevated triglycerides. These ten cases were laser-assisted cases. Statistical significance was not tested. It is unclear if the remaining seven cases were laser-assisted cases.
	FDA approved	Double blind study of 15 patients who received laser assisted liposuction on one side and standard liposuction on the other.[3] A 600 um Nd:YAG fiber in a 4 or 6 mm cannula at 40 W with a pulse duration of 0.2 s was used in combination with suction. In those patients who received both modalities, there was no difference in paresthesias or skin irregularities, and there was no scarring, infection, or hypopigmentation. Post operative pain seemed to be slightly less on the laser treated side. Lipocrit values did not show any trend. Laser assisted liposuction was not found to be more beneficial than standard liposuction.
		Review of 1,734 patients who received treatment with a 1,064 nm laser delivered through a 300 μm fiber in a 1 mm microcannula.[4] Fat was drained with negative pressure. Cosmetic results were similar to traditional liposuction.
		Randomized, controlled study of 30 female patients with focal areas of fat less than 100 cm^3 on the arm, submental area, thigh, and abdomen.[5] Ten received laser lipolysis with a 1,064 nm Nd:YAG laser with a 300 um fiber encased in a 1 mm microcannula. The procedure was not followed by suction. These patients had MRI pre and post procedure. Ten received and nine completed laser lipolysis followed by a biweekly treatment with the Tri-active system. Ten patients served as controls. Patients who received laser lipolysis reported an improvement of 37% at 3 months. An average 17% reduction in fat volume ($p<0.01$) was seen on MRI. Bruising and swelling were present in four and seven patients, respectively. Two patients had tingling that resolved, two had hyperpigmentation, four had tenderness, and one had a subcutaneous nodule that resolved.
		Report of 245 patients who received laser assisted liposuction with a 1,064 nm laser in a 1 mm cannula followed by aspiration with a 3 mm cannula.[6] Laser assisted liposuction was more time intensive, but less traumatic. There was no control group in this study, and statistical significance was not tested.
		Report of 82 patients who received laser assisted liposuction in the submental region with a 1,064 nm laser in a 1 mm cannula at 150 mJ with a 100 ms pulse.[7] Suction followed treatment in most cases. Biopsies were taken immediately following the procedure and 40 days following the procedure. On biopsy, coagulation of the blood vessels in the fat, adipocyte rupture, laser channels, "reorganization" of the reticular dermis, and coagulation of the collagen septa were seen. The author felt that the clinical result was similar to traditional liposuction. There was no control group in this study, and statistical significance did not appear to be tested.
		Report of one patient who received laser assisted liposuction with a 1,064 nm laser at 150 mJ followed by suction.[8] The purpose of this study was to understand histologic response to laser. The patient received conventional liposuction on one flank and laser assisted liposuction on the other flank. In the superior portion of the laser assisted side, she received a total energy of 3,000 J and 1,000 J in the inferior. Fat was sampled from all three areas. A control sample was obtained from an abdominoplasty obtained from the same patient. The average adipocyte diameter was found to be 73.48, 84.54, 95.69, and 82.63 from the control, conventional, 1,000 J site, and the 3,000 J site respectively. Standard deviations were reported. The standard deviation of the control site overlapped with the laser treated side. Statistical significance was not tested. The authors suggest that the laser treatment resulted in a larger adipocyte size due to alteration of the cell membrane that allows transport of extracellular material to the intracellular space. Ultimately, the treatment yielded adipocyte lysis or necrosis, explaining the larger diameter of the adipocyte at the 1,000 J rather than the 3,000 J site.
External 635 nm low level laser	Erchonia 3LT™ Lasers (Erchonia Medical, Inc.; McKinney, TX)	Study of 12 tissue samples.[9] Twelve tissue samples from 12 female subjects were exposed to the 635 nm laser for 0, 4, and 6 min with and without infusion of tumescent solution. After 4 min and tumescence or 6 min and no tumescence, adipocytes lost their round shape and fat spread to the intercellular space on scanning electron and transmission electron microscopy. After 6 min and tumescence, fat was completely removed from cells. A control portion of the sample, not exposed to laser or tumescence, was not noted to have changes in fat architecture.
	FDA approved	Report of 700 cases.[10] 635 nm diode laser applied to abdomen and thighs for 6 min and 10–12 min to back, sides, and axilla followed by liposuction. There was no control group and no statistical evaluation. Ninety-five percent of patients were satisfied with results. Asymmetry developed in 3% of procedures, hyperpigmentation in 0.1% of procedures, and fluid collections or seromas in 40% of patients. Two patients developed cellulitis.
		Placebo controlled, randomized, blinded study of low level laser followed by liposuction in 72 subjects.[11] 635 nm 14 mW dual diode laser used to treat 36 test subjects. A sham device was used to treat 36 subjects in the placebo group. One investigator was blinded. One investigator was not blinded. Subjects treated with laser were found to have less discomfort and swelling (both statistically significant) post operatively. Investigators found that fat extraction was easier after laser (statistically significant).
		Three human patients and two Yucatan pigs were treated with a 635 nm 10 mW laser.[12] Humans were treated with low level laser therapy. Biopsies were done to compare areas that were treated with and without low level laser. No adipocyte differences between irradiated and non irradiated sites were seen. Pigs were treated with ultrasound-assisted lipoplasty, suction lipoplasty, and low lever laser plus suction lipoplasty. Adipocytes were destroyed after ultrasound-assisted lipoplasty, but not suction lipoplasty or low level laser lipoplasty.

with 27 controls, subjects were treated once on the abdomen, thighs, or flanks.[18] At 3 month follow up, a statistically significant mean reduction of 1.9 cm was reported, in the setting of weight maintenance, compared to baseline, control group, and internal control for patients treated on the thigh. Liver ultrasound at 14–28 days and serial laboratory evaluations showed no "clinically significant" treatment associated changes, with no elevations in serum lipids or lipoproteins. No systemic adverse effects were noted, and cutaneous adverse effects were rare and included a tingling sensation, erythema, purpura, and blisters. Ninety-two percent of patients reported minimal to no discomfort after 90 min of topical anesthesia.

1,064 nm Laser with and without Liposuction

The Nd:YAG laser has been used alone or in combination with suction liposuction. SmartLipo™ (Cynosure, USA), a 300 um fiber encased in a micro-cannula, is an example of this type of device. The cannula is inserted subcutaneously to destroy lipid membranes and release lipids. Adipocytes appear to swell at lower energies and lyse at higher energies.[8] The laser heat also coagulates collagen fibers. This process is termed "laser lipolysis."[19] It is worth noting that the term "lipolysis" appears to be misused in this context. Strictly speaking, "lipolysis" is defined not as destruction of the adipocyte membrane, but rather as shrinkage of the fat cell due to the use of lipid for energy at the cellular level.

The Nd:YAG laser has been extensively studied, and these reports are described in Table 1.[2-8] There appears to be minimal cosmetic advantage to this procedure compared with traditional liposuction, although patients may have less post operative pain with laser-assisted lipoplasty. The procedure may be helpful for the surgeon, requiring less effort, particularly in difficult to treat areas,[4] but it can be more time consuming.[6]

An illustrative example is a prospective, double blind, controlled trial of 25 patients and 110 areas of treatment with patients serving as their own control with suction lipoplasty on one half and laser-assisted lipoplasty on the other with a 2 mm and 1,064 nm Nd:YAG laser fiber follow by suction with a 3 mm cannula.[2] No clinical difference in cosmetic result was found, although postoperative pain was higher in the suction-assisted side versus the laser-assisted side at the first follow up visit only.

Without liposuction, the Nd:YAG may have a role in the removal of local deposits of fat. The use of a 1,064 nm Nd:YAG laser with a 300 um fiber encased in a 1 mm micro-cannula, without combining it with liposuction was studied in a randomized study of 30 female patients with focal areas of fat less than 100 cm^3 on the arm, submental area, thigh, and abdomen.[5] An average 17% reduction in fat volume ($p < 0.01$)

was seen on MRI. Bruising, swelling, and tenderness were seen, and uncommonly, transient tingling, hyperpigmentation, and a subcutaneous nodule were reported. As with non invasive approaches, use of this device without liposuction may be best suited to small collections of fat.

635 nm Laser and Liposuction

Neira has combined low level 635 nm laser and liposuction in a technique labeled the "Neira 4 L technique".[10] Patients are irradiated with a low-level 635 nm laser after tumescent anesthesia. Following irradiation, removal of fat is accomplished with a cannula or other technique. Neira postulates that low level laser creates a pore in the adipocyte membrane, causing leakage of lipid into the interstitial space.[20] He studied 12 patients and found that after 6 min of low level laser, fat was completely removed from the cell.[9] He has reported a change in the consistency of fat with MRI evaluation.[21]

In contrast, another study did not find a histologic change in treated and untreated adipocytes, raising questions about the efficacy of the treatment.[12] Histologic analysis of the effects of low-level laser of adipose tissue in rats found enlargement and fusion of the brown, but not yellow fatty tissue.[22]

Neira reported a case series of 700 patients of whom 95% were satisfied with results.[10] A well designed randomized, controlled, blinded study found a statistically significant decrease in pain and swelling post operatively after treatment with low level laser.[11] Investigators reported a greater ease of fat extraction after low level laser therapy, also statistically significant. Based on these studies, low level therapy may influence healing, but the histologic effects and the effect on cosmesis remain unclear.

External Ultrasound and Liposuction

External ultrasound and liposuction have been combined to remove adipose tissue.[23-25] External ultrasound is theorized to relax the bonds between cells, affecting the septa, enhancing skin contraction after liposuction and allowing for the use of thin cannulas.[26] Fat cells can be used for grafting.[27] The typical procedure involves application of a 2–3 W/cm ultrasound device for 5–15 min.

Several studies have found external ultrasound to be beneficial,[27-30] although one double blind study casts doubt on the utility of this procedure.[31] In most of the studies, there appears to be a slight advantage of the ultrasound assisted approach in terms of physician fatigue (50–70% preferred the ultrasound treated side). Patients had less bruising (40–70% of patients), swelling (40–70% of patients), and discomfort

(50–80% of patients) on the ultrasound treated side.[28-30] The cosmetic result appears to be similar.[28-30] One of the studies reported increased skin retraction of 30% on the side treated with ultrasound.[29] These studies were randomized and controlled, but statistical significance was not tested. The surgeon was blinded in one of the trials.[28] The number of patients in these studies ranged from 10 to 30. Adverse effects including erythema, mild warmth, burns, blisters, and seroma were reported during the procedure.[24,26,27,30]

A larger study of 59 patients comparing external ultrasound assisted to standard liposuction also reported that patients had less bruising and discomfort.[27] A faster recovery time was reported, but patients receiving external ultrasound were given different instructions about reduction of physical activity, leading to a potential bias in recovery time. Skin shrinkage as evidenced by a smoothness of the skin was apparent on the ultrasound side at 30 days and on the standard liposuction side at 6 months; however, this smoothness was not quantitatively defined and no statistical evaluation was done.

These studies contrast with a double blinded study of 19 patients who served as their own control to evaluate external ultrasound-assisted liposuction.[31] The treatment side received ultrasound at 2–3 W/cm^2 for 10 min and the control side received 0.2–0.3 W/cm^2. Fat was sampled in two patients. There was no difference between resistance to removal and the rate of fat removal in 14 of 19 patients. Patients assessed the treatment as well, and only 4 of 19 reported a better operative and post operative course with external ultrasound. Statistical significance was tested for physician and patient assessments, and no benefit to using external ultrasound with liposuction was found. Histologic evaluation showed no difference between the experimental and control side. Although the study was limited by the small number of patients, the double blind, controlled framework provides strong support that the use of external ultrasound may not yield significant benefit.

Internal Ultrasound and Liposuction

Liposuction in combination with internal ultrasound was pioneered by Zocchi.[32] Several studies reported large series of patients treated with ultrasound assisted lipoplasty,[33-37] and the purported benefits of this technology include less blood loss, less surgeon fatigue, and improved skin retraction.[38,39] Ultrasound assisted liposuction has been found to be more selective for adipocyte removal; however, this selectivity may not yield superior results.[34] In studies that compare standard versus ultrasound-assisted lipoplasty, the ultrasound-assisted approach has not had better cosmetic outcome.[34,36,40] It may be that ultrasound-assisted lipoplasty is better for certain indications such as fibrous areas.[41]

A well designed study of 63 patients who received both traditional and ultrasound-assisted lipoplasty provides an example.[36] Patients were blinded to the procedure in this trial.

In addition to the evaluations by patient and surgeon, an independent panel evaluated ten randomly selective patients. Ultrasound-assisted lipoplasty was not found to be superior to traditional lipoplasty with no difference in sensory, pigment change, surface irregularity, skin contraction, bruising, or swelling. Similarly, a randomized, controlled study of ultrasound-assisted liposuction compared with traditional liposuction in 28 patients found no significant difference in cosmetic result and adverse effects.[40] Physicians reported less fatigue.

Skin necrosis, burn, fat necrosis and fibrosis, sensory alteration, infection, lower limb edema, and seromas have been reported.[33-35,40-43] Skin necrosis is a particularly concerning adverse effect. It is thought to be due to destruction of deep dermal vessels despite higher perfusion with ultrasound-assisted liposuction compared with suction liposuction.[44,45] Postoperative sensory changes occur in both traditional and ultrasound-assisted liposuction; immediately after surgery, these changes may be more prominent in those patients treated with ultrasound.[46,47] Surgeon experience and surgical technique may play a role in ultrasound assisted complications.[33]

With respect to invasive options for fat removal, internal or external ultrasound and laser assisted lipoplasty appear to offer minimal advantages over traditional lipoplasty. Nearly all blinded and controlled studies have failed to show improved cosmetic outcome with these devices. The Ultrashape™, an ultrasound based technology, is the only non invasive option currently available. Other non invasive options on the horizon may involve utilization of the 1,210 nm or 1,720 nm wavelength to destroy adipose tissue. However, it is clear that there is no panacea: non invasive removal of adipose tissue comes with an additional set of concerns and should be approached cautiously and systematically.

Devices for Removal of Cellulite

- Intense pulsed light (IPL) has been shown to stimulate collagen production, and it is used in the treatment of cellulite with the purpose of thickening the dermis to diminish the appearance of cellulite.
- Studies suggested that the light emitting diode had little effect.
- A few devices incorporate massage with light to treat cellulite. Massage is included in the treatments based on the idea that vascular and lymphatic alterations promote cellulite, although there is limited evidence to support this theory.
- Radiofrequency represents the best studied treatment for cellulite. The VelaSmooth™ is a bipolar radiofrequency, infrared heat, and suction device that is FDA.

Non invasive options for the removal of cellulite are more prevalent than those available for the removal of adipose tissue alone. There are several devices that have been used for treatment of cellulite including devices that incorporate laser or light sources. Most of these devices have temporary or limited efficacy or have been poorly studied, casting doubt on their efficacy. In this section, these devices will be reviewed as well as those that incorporate radiofrequency. Radiofrequency devices represent the best studied devices in the cellulite market.

Theoretically, those devices that best treat cellulite should be the devices that affect some aspect of the pathogenesis of cellulite. There are multiple theories to explain cellulite, but those with the most evidence suggest that cellulite is caused by sex specific differences in skin structure and hormonal milieu.[48-54] Cellulite is present in nearly 98% of women and rarely in men, except in cases of androgen deficiency.[48] Unlike in men, the subcutaneous tissue in women is loosely reinforced, and herniations of the superficial fat can be visualized more easily due to a thinner dermis. Therefore, therapies that remove the fat herniations, alter the septated connective tissue reinforcements in the subcutaneous fat, or thicken the dermis would be expected to improve cellulite.

Intense Pulsed Light

Intense pulsed light (IPL) has been shown to stimulate collagen production, and it is used in the treatment of cellulite with the purpose of thickening the dermis to diminish the appearance of cellulite.[55,56] A 12 week trial of 20 women of whom 8 received IPL alone and 12 received IPL in combination with retinyl based cream for a total of 9–12 treatments found that the majority of patients with improvement used the cream in combination with IPL.[57] Nine patients reported improvement greater than or equal to 50%, and seven maintained this improvement at 8 months. This study was limited as only 15 patients completed the study, and no statistical analysis was done. The use of IPL alone as a treatment for cellulite does not appear to be indicated.

Light Emitting Diode

A light emitting diode at 660–950 nm has been used in combination with a cellulite gel comprised of several active ingredients (*Bupleurum falcarum*, caffeine, coenzyme A, and phosphatidylcholine). A randomized, double blind controlled study evaluated nine patients who received an active gel on one thigh and placebo controlled gel on the control thigh in combination with light.[58] Cellulite was improved in eight of nine patients on the active thigh and no patients on the control side, suggesting that the light emitting diode had little effect.

Light Sources and Massage

A few devices incorporate massage with light to treat cellulite. Massage is included in the treatments based on the idea that vascular and lymphatic alterations promote cellulite, although there is limited evidence to support this theory.[59-61] Examples include TriActive™ (Cynosure™, USA), a low fluence 810 nm diode laser with vacuum massage; Synergie esthetic Massage System™ (Dynatronics, USA), a vacuum massage with or without a 660–880 nm probe or 880 nm light pad; and SmoothShapes® (Elemé Medical, USA), a 915 nm laser and 650 nm light source combined with vacuum and mechanical massage. All are FDA approved. The TriActive™ appears to yield a transient 21–25% improvement in cellulite after multiple treatments.

In an uncontrolled study of 16 patients who received twice weekly treatments of TriActive™ for 6 weeks, photographs evaluated by blinded investigators showed a 21% average improvement that was not present 1 month after the last treatment.[62] Significance was not tested. A comparison of 20 patients treated twice weekly for 6 weeks with the TriActive™ or VelaSmooth™, a radiofrequency device, found similar results.[63] In this study, photographs were evaluated by blinded investigators and significance was tested. The average improvement in cellulite was 7 and 25% for the VelaSmooth™ and the TriActive™, respectively. VelaSmooth™ and TriActive™ also yielded a 28–56% and a 30–37% improvement in the thigh circumference, respectively. The difference between the two devices was not significant. Adverse effects included bruising seen in 10 of 20 patients with VelaSmooth™ and 4 of 20 with TriActive™.

SmoothShapes is an FDA approved device with suction and mechanical massage combined with 650 nm and 915 nm laser light. A study of 65 subjects evaluated with MRI pre and post a mean of 14.3 treatments found that fat thickness decreased by 1.19 cm^2 in the leg treated with the device versus an increase of 3.82 cm^2 for the leg treated with massage alone.[70] There was no significant difference in thigh circumference. In another study of this device, 20 women were treated two times a week for 4 weeks.[71] Weight and BMI were similar throughout the study. Change in cellulite was evaluated using standard photography and VECTRA three-dimensional photographs, 76% of subjects improved with an average 2.3 mm elevation of cellulite dimples and 4.9 mm flattening of cellulite bulges six months after treatment.

Radiofrequency

Radiofrequency represents the best studied treatment for cellulite. The VelaSmooth™ is a bipolar radiofrequency, infrared heat, and suction device that is FDA approved for the treatment of cellulite. The Alma Accent RF System (Alma Lasers™, Israel) utilizes unipolar and bipolar radiofrequency and the ThermaCool® (Thermage®, USA) utilizes unipolar radiofrequency. Both of these devices are FDA approved for rhytides. Only the Alma System and the VelaSmooth™ have been studied in peer reviewed journals.

The VelaSmooth™ has been evaluated more extensively than any of the other devices for cellulite; however, many studies are flawed, without a control group or without statistical evaluation. Most studies report a decreased circumference of the treated area and an improvement in cellulite of 25–50% in most subjects.[64-68] The duration of benefit is unclear, and one investigator noted a diminution of effect at 6 months.[66] Bruising is a common side effect noted in up to 10–31%.[65-67] Crusting and burn have rarely been reported.[64,67]

One of the better and illustrative studies of the VelaSmooth™ is a controlled trial of 20 patients.[65] Of the 20 enrolled patients, 16 were treated twice weekly for 6 weeks on one leg, while the other leg served as control. A statistically significant decrease of thigh circumference (0.44–0.53 cm) was seen at 4 weeks, but not immediately or at 8 weeks. A greater than 51% improvement was seen in 25–31% of patients at 8 weeks after the last treatment. There was no histologic evidence of structural change, however. Lipid, hormone, and liver function tests were tested in five patients and showed no change. 31% of patients had bruising.

The Alma Accent RF System was evaluated in an uncontrolled study of 26 patients.[69] In this study, the patients received two treatments on the thigh and buttock. Patients were evaluated by ultrasound for a change in distance from the dermis to the first line of fibrous tissue (Camper's fascia) and the dermis to muscle. The majority of patients (64–72%) showed a 15.49–27.8% decrease in these measures. On average, there was a 6.8–11.55% decrease in the measurements among all patients, although some of the patients showed an increase in the distance. Findings were not uniformly significant, and this study is limited by the lack of a control group. The authors evaluated ultrasound for qualitative changes in the skin structure and found improvement in 50–57% of patients. Adverse effects were rare with small blisters developing in two patients and bruising in three patients.

Of the available devices on the market, those with radiofrequency seem to have the most effect, albeit marginal. These devices do not yield more than a 50% improvement in most subjects. Further, most do not employ clearly objective means of proving clinical efficacy, casting doubt on the true efficacy of these devices.

Conclusion

The currently available options for laser or light based removal of adipose tissue or cellulite are limited by evidence of efficacy. Although SmartLipo™ may have a role for removal of small collections of adipose tissue, it has not been shown to be cosmetically advantageous as compared with traditional lipoplasty. There are similar doubts about the use of the 635 nm laser as an adjunct to liposuction for fat removal. With respect to cellulite treatment, laser and light devices have either not been studied or have been proven to have modest, temporary effect.

In fact, the best studied devices, do not rely on light or laser. Yet even these alternatives have not been proven to be cosmetically superior to traditional methods (ultrasound-assisted lipoplasty), are new technologies and supported by few studies (focused ultrasound), or provide a limited benefit to the majority of patients (radiofrequency). However, the field is evolving and new developments on the horizon may prove to be more efficacious.

References

1. Prado A, Andrades P, Danilla S, et al. Nonresective shrinkage of the septum and fat compartments of the upper and lower eyelids: a comparative study with carbon dioxide laser and Colorado needle. *Plast Reconstr Surg*. 2006;117:1725-1735.
2. Prado A, Andrades P, Danilla S, et al. A prospective, randomized, double-blind, controlled clinical trial comparing laser-assisted lipoplasty with suction-assisted lipoplasty. *Plast Reconstr Surg*. 2006;118:1032-1045.
3. Apfelberg DB. Results of multicenter study of laser-assisted liposuction. *Clin Plast Surg*. 1996;23:713-719.
4. Goldman A, Schavelzon DE, Blugerman GS. Laserlipolysis: liposuction using Nd-YAG laser. *Rev Soc Bras Cir Plást*. 2002;17:17-26.
5. Kim KH, Geronemus RG. Laser lipolysis using a novel 1,064 nm Nd: YAG laser. *Dermatol Surg*. 2006;32:241-248.
6. Badin AZD, Moraes LM, Gondek L, et al. Laser lipolysis: flaccidity under control. *Aesthet Plast Surg*. 2002;26:335-339.
7. Goldman A. Submental Nd:YAG laser-assisted liposuction. *Lasers Surg Med*. 2006;38:181-184.
8. Badin AEZD, Gondek LBE, Garcia MJ, et al. Analysis of laser lipolysis effects on human tissue samples obtained from liposuction. *Aesthet Plast Surg*. 2005;29:281-286.
9. Neira R, Arroyave J, Ramirez H, et al. Fat liquefaction: effect of low-level laser energy on adipose tissue. *Plast Reconstr Surg*. 2002;110:912-922.
10. Neira R, Ortiz C. Low level laser assisted liposculpture: clinical report of 700 cases. *Aesthet Surg J*. 2002;22:451-455.
11. Jackson RF, Roche G, Butterwick KJ, Dedo DD, Slattery KT. Low lever laser-assisted liposuction: a 2004 clinical study of its effectiveness for enhancing ease of liposuction procedures and facilitating the recovery process for patients undergoing thigh, hip, and stomach contouring. *Am J Cosmet Surg*. 2004;21:191-198.
12. Brown SA, Rohrich RJ, Kenkel J, et al. Effect of low-level laser therapy on abdominal adipocytes before lipoplasty procedures. *Plast Reconstr Surg*. 2004;113:1796-1804.
13. Kuwahara K, Gladstone HB, Gupta V, et al. Rupture of fat cells using laser-generated ultra short stress waves. *Lasers Surg Med*. 2003;32:279-285.
14. Anderson RR, Farinelli W, Laubach H, et al. Selective photothermolysis of lipid-rich tissues: a free electron laser study. *Lasers Surg Med*. 2006;38(10):913-919.
15. Harvey RA, Champe PC. *Fatty Acid and Triacylglycerol Metabolism. Lippincott's Illustrated Reviews: Biochemistry*. 2nd ed. Philadelphia: JB Lippincott Company; 1994.

16. Grundy SM. Metabolic syndrome pandemic. *Arterioscler Thromb Vasc Biol.* 2008;4:629-636.
17. Moreno-Moraga J, Valero-Altes T, Martinez Riquelme A, et al. Body contouring by non-invasive transdermal focused ultrasound. *Lasers Surg Med.* 2007;4:315-323.
18. Teitelbaum SA, Burns JL, Kubota J, et al. Noninvasive body contouring by focused ultrasound: safety and efficacy of the contour I device in a multicenter, controlled, clinical trial. *Plast Reconstr Surg.* 2007;120:779-789.
19. Ichikawa K, Miyasaka M, Tanaka R, et al. Histologic evaluation of the pulsed Nd:YAG laser for laser lipolysis. *Lasers Surg Med.* 2005;36:43-46.
20. Neira R, Toledo L, Arroyave J, et al. Low-level laser-assisted liposuction: the Neira 4L technique. *Clin Plast Surg.* 2005:117-127.
21. Neira R, Jackson R, Dedo D, Ortiz CL, Arroyave JA. Low-level laser-assisted lipoplasty appearance of fat demonstrated by MRI on abdominal tissue. *Am J Cosmet Surg.* 2001;18:133-140.
22. Medrano AP, Trindade E, Reis SRA, et al. Action of the low-level laser therapy on living fatty tissue of rats. *Lasers Med Sci.* 2006;21:19-23.
23. Silberg B. The technique of external ultrasound-assisted lipoplasty. *Plast Reconstr Surg.* 1998;101:552.
24. Silberg B. The use of external ultrasound assist with liposuction. *Aesthet Surg J.* 1998;18:284-285.
25. Kinney B. Body contouring with external ultrasound. *Plast Reconstr Surg.* 1999;103:728-729.
26. Rosenberg GJ, Cabrera RC. External ultrasonic lipoplasty: an effective method of fat removal and skin shrinkage. *Plast Reconstr Surg.* 2000;105:785-791.
27. Wilkinson TS. External ultrasound-assisted lipoplasty. *Aesthet Surg J.* 1999;19:124-129.
28. Cook WR. Utilizing external ultrasonic energy to improve the results of tumescent liposculpture. *Dermatol Surg.* 1997;23:1207-1211.
29. Havoonjian HH, Luftman DB, Menaker GM, Moy RL. External ultrasonic tumescent liposuction. *Dermatol Surg.* 1997;23:1201-1206.
30. Mendes FH. External ultrasound-assisted lipoplasty from our own experience. *Aesthet Plast Surg.* 2000;24:270-274.
31. Lawrence N, Cox SE. The efficacy of external ultrasound-assisted liposuction: a randomized controlled trial. *Dermatol Surg.* 2000;26:329-332.
32. Zocchi M. Ultrasonic liposculpturing. *Aesthet Plast Surg.* 1992;16:287-298.
33. Tebbets JB. Minimizing complications of ultrasound-assisted lipoplasty: an initial experience with no related complications. *Plast Reconstr Surg.* 1998;102:1690-1697.
34. Scuderi N, Paolini G, Grippaudo FR, et al. Comparative evaluation of traditional, ultrasonic, and pneumatic assisted lipoplasty: analysis of local and systemic effects, efficacy, and costs of these methods. *Aesthet Plast Surg.* 2000;24:395-400.
35. Maxwell PG, Gingrass MK. Ultrasound-assisted lipoplasty: a clinical study of 250 consecutive patients. *Plast Reconstr Surg.* 1998;101:189-202.
36. Fodor PB, Watson J. Personal experience with ultrasound-assisted lipoplasty: a pilot study comparing ultrasound-assisted lipoplasty with traditional lipoplasty. *Plast Reconstr Surg.* 1998;101:1103-1116.
37. Kloehn RA. Liposuction with "Sonic Sculpture": six years experience with more than 600 patients. *Aesthet Surg Q.* 1996;16:123-128.
38. Adamo C, Mazzocchi M, Rossi A, et al. Ultrasonic liposculpturing: extrapolations from the analysis of in vivo sonicated adipose tissue. *Plast Reconstr Surg.* 1997;100:220-226.
39. Kenkel J, Robinson JB, Beran SJ, et al. The tissue effects of ultrasound-assisted lipoplasty. *Plast Reconstr Surg.* 1998;102:213-220.
40. Igra H, Satur NM. Tumescent liposuction versus internal ultrasonic-assisted tumescent liposuction. *Dermatol Surg.* 1997;23(12):1213-1218.
41. Rohrich RJ, Beran SJ, Kenkel JM, et al. Extending the role of liposuction in body contouring with ultrasound-assisted liposuction. *Plast Reconstr Surg.* 1998;101:1090-1102.

42. Cedidi CC, Berger A. Severe abdominal wall necrosis after ultrasound-assisted liposuction. *Aesthet Plast Surg.* 2002;26:20-22.
43. Scheflan M, Tazi H. Ultrasonically assisted body contouring. *Aesthet Surg Q.* 1996;16:117-122.
44. Gupta SC, Khiabani KT, Stephenson LL, et al. Effect of liposuction on skin perfusion. *Plast Reconstr Surg.* 2002;110:1748-1751.
45. Ablaza VJ, Gingrass MK, Perry LC, et al. Tissue temperatures during ultrasound-assisted lipoplasty. *Plast Reconstr Surg.* 1998;102:534-542.
46. Trott SA, Rohrich RJ, Beran SJ, et al. Sensory changes after traditional and ultrasound-assisted liposuction using computer-assisted analysis. *Plast Reconstr Surg.* 1999;103:2016-2025.
47. Howard BK, Beran SJ, Kenkel JM, et al. The effects of ultrasonic energy on peripheral nerves: implications for ultrasound-assisted liposuction. *Plast Reconstr Surg.* 1999;103:984-989.
48. Avram MM. Cellulite: a review of its physiology and treatment. *J Cosmet Laser Ther.* 2004;7:181-185.
49. Curri SB. Cellulite and fatty tissue microcirculation. *Cosmet Toiletries.* 1993;108:51-58.
50. van Vliet M, Ortiz A, Avram MM, et al. An assessment of traditional and novel therapies for cellulite. *J Cosmet Laser Ther.* 2005;7(1):7-10.
51. Draelos ZD. The disease of cellulite. *J Cosmet Dermatol.* 2005;4:221-222.
52. Nurnberger F, Muller G. So called cellulite: an invented disease. *J Dermatol Surg Oncol.* 1978;4:221-229.
53. Rossi ABR, Vergnanini AL. Cellulite: a review. *JEADV.* 2000;14:251-262.
54. Kligman AM. Cellulite: facts and fiction. *J Geriatr Dermatol.* 1997;5:136-139.
55. Iyer S, Carranza D, Kolodney M, et al. Evaluation of procollagen I deposition after intense pulsed light treatments at varying parameters in a porcine model. *J Cosmet Laser Ther.* 2007;9:75-78.
56. Goldberg DJ. New collagen formation after dermal remodeling with an intense pulsed light source. *J Cutan Laser Ther.* 2000;2:59-61.
57. Fink JS, Mermelstein H, Thomas A, et al. Use of intense pulsed light and a retinyl-based cream as a potential treatment for cellulite: a pilot study. *J Cosmet Dermatol.* 2006;5:254-262.
58. Sasaki GH, Oberg K, Tucker B, et al. The effectiveness and safety of topical PhotoActif phosphatidylcholine based anti-cellulite gel and LED (red and near-infrared) light on Grade II–III high cellulite: a randomized, double-blinded study. *J Cosmet Laser Ther.* 2007;9:87-96.
59. Rosenbaum M, Prieto V, Hellmer J, et al. An exploratory investigation of the morphology and biochemistry of cellulite. *Plast Reconstr Surg.* 1998;101:1934-1939.
60. Pierard G, Nizet JL, Pierard-Franchimont C. Cellulite: from standing fat herniation to hypodermal stretch marks. *Am J Dermatopathol.* 2000;22:34-37.
61. Curri SB, Bombardelli E. Proposed etiology and therapeutic management of local lipodystrophy and districtual microcirculation. *Cosmet Toiletries.* 1994;109:51-65.
62. Boyce S, Pabby A, Chuchaltkaren P, et al. Clinical evaluation of a device for the treatment of cellulite: triactive. *Am J Cosmet Surg.* 2005;22:233-237.
63. Nootheti PK, Magpantay A, Yosowitz G, et al. A single center, randomized, comparative, prospective clinical study to determine efficacy of the Velasmooth system versus the Triactive system for the treatment of cellulite. *Lasers Surg Med.* 2006;38:908-912.
64. Sadick NS, Mulholland RS. A prospective clinical study to evaluate the efficacy and safety of cellulite treatment using the combination of optical and RF energies for subcutaneous tissue heating. *J Cosmet Laser Ther.* 2004;6(4):187-190.
65. Sadick NS, Magro C. A study evaluating the safety and efficacy of the Velasmooth™ system in the treatment of cellulite. *J Cosmet Laser Ther.* 2007;9:15-20.

66. Alster TS, Tanzi EL. Cellulite treatment using a novel combination radiofrequency, infrared light, and mechanical tissue manipulation device. *J Cosmet Laser Ther*. 2005;7:81-85.

67. Kulick M. Evaluation of the combination of radio frequency, infrared energy and mechanical rollers with suction to improve skin surface irregularities (cellulite) in a limited treatment area. *J Cosmet Laser Ther*. 2006;8:185-190.

68. Waniphakdeedecha R, Manuskiatti W. Treatment of cellulite with a bipolar radiofrequency, infrared heat, and pulsatile suction device. *J Cosmet Dermatol*. 2006;5:284-288.

69. Pino ME, Rosado RH, Azuela A, et al. Effect of controlled volumetric tissue heating with radiofrequency on cellulite and the subcutaneous tissue of the buttocks and thighs. *J Drugs Dermatol*. 2006;5:714-722.

70. Lach E. Reduction of subcutaneous fat and improvement in cellulite appearance by dual-wavelength, low-level laser energy combined with vacuum and massage. *J Cosmet Laser Ther*. 2008;10: 202-209.

71. Kulick MI. Evaluation of a noninvasive, dual-wavelength laser-suction and massage device for the regional treatment of cellulite. *Plast Reconstr Surg*. 2010;125: 1788-1796.

Intense Pulse Light (IPL)

Robert A. Weiss, Girish S. Munavalli, Sonal Choudhary, Angel Leiva, and Keyvan Nouri

- Intense Pulsed Light (IPL) is a light-emitting system that is capable of emitting filtered polychromatic broad bandwidth wavelengths between 515 and 1,200 nm.
- The emission of wavelengths is controlled by both an internal filter that blocks undesired wavelengths from being emitted and a "heat-sink" effect that allows the controlled transfer of thermal energy from an object at high temperature to an object at lower temperature.

Introduction

Intense pulsed light (IPL) is a non-coherent filtered flash lamp capable of emitting a polychromatic broad bandwidth of light from 515 to 1,200 nm (approximately). It was first introduced in clinical studies in 1994 and cleared by the US FDA in late 1995, mainly for the treatment of leg veins. The device that first received approval was Photoderm™ (ESC/Sharplan, Norwood, MA-now, Lumenis, Santa Clara, CA). This technology is now marketed as the gold standard for treatment of signs of photoaging and its other recognized indications are treatment of virtually all skin vascular conditions, scarring, pigmentation, Poikiloderma of Civatte and hair removal.

IPL has the ability to minimize purpura which was a common drawback with Pulsed dye lasers (PDL) until the development of longer pulse durations.[1-8]

The IPL Device

The IPL device consists of a flashlamp housed in an optical treatment head with water cooled reflecting mirrors. An internal filter overlying the flashlamp prevents wavelengths less than 500 nm from being emitted. In certain devices, cut-off filters of various wavelengths (515, 550, 560,570, 590, 615, 645, 690, 755 nm) are available which are placed over the window of the optical treatment head to eliminate other wavelengths. Other devices required the changing of the IPL head to manipulate wavelengths. In some of the optical heads the water circulates around the flashlamp and helps reduce the recycling times. A water based gel is used for the purpose of allowing optimal light transmission to the skin by decreasing the index of refraction of light. Also, it creates a "heat-sink" effect. Heat sinks function by efficiently transferring thermal energy ("heat") from an object at a relatively high temperature to a second object at a lower temperature with a much greater heat capacity. This rapid transfer of thermal energy quickly brings the first object into thermal equilibrium with the second, lowering the temperature of the first object, fulfilling the heat sink's role as a cooling device.

Bio Physical Interactions

- Intense Pulse Light (IPL) systems function on the principle of selective photothermolysis by targeting specific ranges of wavelength.
- Small spot sizes used during treatment with IPL are associated with more scattering, yet heat distribution is better assimilated. In contrast, larger spot sizes have less scattering and are better targeted, but require greater thermal energy.
- A water-based gel filters out unnecessary wavelengths, such as near-infrared wavelengths that may be more damaging to the tissue.
- Tissue temperature is controlled by allowing thermal relaxation time (TRT) by a factor of $\varepsilon = 2.72$ between treatment sessions to prevent the elevation of epidermal temperatures above 70°C.

R.A. Weiss (✉)
Department of Dermatology, Johns Hopkins University School of Medicine, Hunt Valley, Baltimore, MD, USA
e-mail: rweiss@mdlsv.com

K. Nouri (ed.), *Lasers in Dermatology and Medicine*,
DOI: 10.1007/978-0-85729-281-0_17, © Springer-Verlag London Limited 2011

Wavelength

IPL, like lasers, works on the principle of selective photothermolysis, first described by Anderson and Parrish in 1983.[9] The target structures may have different absorption maxima such as hemoglobin absorbs at a wavelength of 580 nm while melanin has a spectral range of 400–750 nm. Longer wavelengths are absorbed lesser by the melanin and penetrate deep, thus reaching deeper blood vessels and avoiding epidermal damage. The bandwidth of IPL is modified by application of filters which exclude the lower wavelengths. In that spectrum, during a 10 ms pulse, relatively high doses of yellow light at 600 nm are emitted and other wavelengths are emitted much less.[4] This wavelength facilitates selective absorption by bright red superficial vessels.

Vascular lesion treatment filters require filters such as 515, 550, 560, 570 and 590 nm. Hair removal can be performed using longer filters such as 615, 645, 695 and 755 nm. These filters can also be used to cause fibroblast stimulation.

Spot Size

Spot size along with wavelength affects penetration depth. Smaller the spot size, more rapid the scatter and more rapid the decay of fluence by depth (Table 1). Thus larger spot size would result in greater amount of energy being delivered to the skin. The light emitting planar surface of the IPL device functions through a water-based interface between the crystal and the skin. This water based gel, as mentioned earlier has functions of enhancing optical coupling, minimizing reflections, acting as a "heat sink" and maintaining continuity of index of refraction of the skin/air interface. The gel also helps filter higher wavelengths, thus removing some of the ineffective or potentially tissue damaging near-infrared wavelengths before being absorbed by the target. In order to treat deeper or larger vessels, the fluence can be modified and increased and the gel can be chilled to protect the overlying epidermis. A 1–2 mm layer of chilling gel can be used between the crystal and the skin when working with a large footprint of IPL, as has been termed as "floating" the crystal. This is especially useful when an integrated chilled crystal is not being used.

Table 1 Spot size vs. wavelength

Spot size	1 mm	2 mm	5 mm
Light penetration depth (595 nm)	0.8 mm	1.1 mm	1.25 mm
Light penetration depth (800 nm)	1.5 mm	2.0 mm	2.5 mm

The penetration for the 800 nm appears to be approximately half the diameter of the spot size. This suggests that an 8 mm wide crystal should permit penetration down to 4 mm (Data on file, Lumenis, Santa Clara, CA)

Pulse Duration

Between two pulses, some amount of time is allowed for the epidermis to cool down and is referred to as thermal relaxation time (TRT). More accurately defined TRT is the amount of time taken for the temperature of a tissue to decrease by a factor of $\varepsilon = 2.72$ as a result of heat conductivity. TRT helps to prevent the elevation of epidermal temperatures above 70°C and prevents epidermal damage.

Epidermal thickness of 100 μ has a TRT of about 1 ms, a typical vessel of 100 μ has a TRT of approx. 4 ms. This can be used to predict that vessels greater than 300 μ would have a TRT of more than 10 ms and thus these vessels will cool more slowly than the epidermis, with a single pulse. For larger vessels, multiple pulses prove more advantageous with 10 ms or more delay times in between the pulses for epidermal cooling. The treatment of darker skin individuals (Fitzpatrick IV–VI), and/or patients with hyper-reactive melanocytes should be performed very carefully, best by using a 755 nm filter with a pulse delay of 50–100 ms, to allow sufficient cooling time for the epidermis. When treating leg veins, better results have been obtained with longer pulse duration (up to 50 ms).[10]

A study conducted to understand the principles of "double or multiple pulsing" using a 585 nm yellow dye laser on larger vessels of Port wine stains, showed that these vessels absorbed greater energy fluences before reaching purpura after double pulses spaced 3–10 ms apart.[11] After a pump pulse delivering 80% of the fluence necessary for causing purpura, the fluence of a second probe pulse necessary to cause purpura was determined and was found to increase the interval between the two pulses, in a manner consistent with the thermal diffusion theory. For a small vessel (0.3 mm), heat distribution was assumed to occur instantaneously. For a larger vessel, heat had to pass from the inside of the superficial vessel wall and through the vessel to the deeper wall. Larger vessels required longer cooling time periods for the accumulated heat inside the core. These principles are effective when using a double pulse 585 nm yellow dye laser in the treatment of larger vessels of PWS (larger than 0.1 mm). After double pulses spaced between 3 and 10 ms apart, larger vessels absorbed greater energy fluences upon reaching purpura.[11]

A study using pulsed laser irradiation at 585 nm with short pulse (0.45 ms) and long pulse (10 ms) durations showed that long-duration pulses caused coagulation of the larger diameter vessels. Small caliber vessels and capillaries demonstrated resistance to photothermolysis.[12] The use of IPL with extended pulse durations from 12–50 ms has caused larger vessels (0.5 mm or greater) to undergo more clinical photothermal coagulation while sparing the epidermis.[6]

Indications

- Leg vein treatment
- Hair removal
- Vascular skin conditions
- Scarring
- Pigmentation
- Poikiloderma of Civatte
- Photorejuvenation

- A two peak approach of dual short and long wavelengths is an effective method of treating the variably colored, multiple-diameter/depth array of vessels, which otherwise may be a challenge to treat.
- Each target chromophore, hemoglobin and its derivates, has a spectrum of light absorption. Proper administering of IPL devices can prevent damage to treated areas by selecting correct fluence levels, pulse type, wavelength, spot size, and delay periods for cooling of skin.
- Telangiectasias can be characterized as linear, arborizing, and punctiform, and can be treated with minimal side-effects using IPL systems, with cryogen cooling devices, at preferable wavelengths of 585 and 595 nm.

Treatment of Benign Vascular Lesions

Reticular Leg Veins with Associated Telangiectasias

Leg telangiectasias are visible, ectatic dermal arterioles, capillaries, or veins with a diameter of 0.1–1 or 2 mm. The chromophores for vascular lesions are represented by the hemoglobin and its derivates: oxyhemoglobin, deoxyhemoglobin, and methemoglobin.[13] Each target chromophore has a variable spectrum of light absorption. Oxyhemoglobin has a very high coefficient of absorption up to 630 nm, although the absorption is poor at longer wavelengths and increases again in the near infra-red range of 800–900 nm. Deoxyhemoglobin absorbs in the range of 600–750 nm, and unlike oxyhemoglobin, does not drop as much as 600–750 nm. Blue leg telangiectasias are slightly more deoxygenated compared to red telangiectasias.[14] Additionally, when a vessel is treated with multiple closely spaced pulsing (up to 20 ms), oxygenated hemoglobin is converted to deoxygenated hemoglobin during the first portion of sequential pulsing, leading to predict that 600–750 nm range is preferable for treating relatively deoxygenated blue leg telangiectasias. Shorter wavelengths have been found to be effective in treating superficial red vessels, but are refractory in terms of treating deeper blue venulectases and reticular veins. These findings can be attributed to the following reasons:

- Lower extremity vein have shown to vary in size depth and diameter.[15]
- Tyndall effect may play a role in giving a bluish hue to the blood vessels deep in the reticular dermis and the degree of oxygenation of the blood in the vessels contribute in determining the reddish or bluish hue of blood vessels. The red telangiectasias have an increased concentration of oxygenated hemoglobin while the blue venulectases and reticular veins have been shown to have an increased concentration of deoxygenated hemoglobin.[13,16]
- Hemoglobin saturation/wavelength-chromophore factors indicate that deoxygenated hemoglobin is a favored chromophore for longer wavelength.
- Background variations may contribute to redness or bluishness of background structures.[17]

Use of multiple devices in combination may be necessary for lower extremity vessels. For example, red vessels <1 mm in diameter can be treated with 578 nm KTP laser, 585–600 nm PDL, 532 nm Copper bromide laser and 500–1,200 nm IPL source, and blue vessels 1–4 mm in diameter can be treated with 755 nm Alexandrite laser, 800 nm Diode laser and 1,064 nm Nd:YAG laser.[18] Longer wavelengths may be used to treat larger diameter blue venulectasia and small reticular veins.

A great advantage of IPL devices is that the parameters are adjustable in a way that the risk of epidermal injury is minimized. This can be done by proper selection of fluence levels, pulse type, wavelength, delay periods and always cooling of the skin immediately after treatment. The bigger the spot size is also important; the bigger the spot size, the more area is covered and more light penetration is assured.[19]

The lasers currently available to eradicate leg veins emit green light (532 nm), yellow light (578–600 nm), red light (755–810 nm), near infrared light (1,064 nm), and a broad spectrum IPL (515–1,200 nm).[20] With appropriate wavelength matching for specific vessel color, luminal diameter and depth, improved results have been achieved. Extended pulse durations, higher fluences and improved contact and dynamic cooling technologies; contributed to more reliable clinical as more energy can be delivered while sparing the epidermis.

In a review of literature conducted by Fodor et al., data collected from 28 patients with small vascular lesions on face, neck, chest and hands, it was shown that the satisfaction level and grade of improvement was reported to vary from 45% to 100%.[21] They suggested that the type of vascular lesion and the number of treatment parameters can influence the success rate. Amongst all the types of vascular lesions, cherry angiomas and reticular and telangiectatic veins had the best response to IPL. Immediate posttreatment reactions, such as urticaria or bruising, were the most commonly seen adverse reactions. These were actually considered as signs of effectiveness.[22] Erythema and pigmentary alterations were noted to be the most encountered complications; the latter being attributed to vessel breakage and hemosiderin deposits. A combined IPL and Nd:Yag laser (1,064 nm) or Nd:Yag laser alone gave better results for larger lower extremity veins, blue, and deeper veins.[18,22]

The parameters for IPL devices can be adjusted according to the response at the previous treatment. Therefore, when a side-effect is encountered, the fluence can be reduced or pulse delay increased. This is a possible benefit of IPL devices avoiding damage to the epidermis by proper selection of fluence levels, pulse type, wavelength, spot size, delay periods, and always cooling of the skin immediately after treatment. The spot size is important because the bigger the spot, the more area is covered, and more uniform light penetration is assured.[23] The most frequently used intervals between treatments reported in the literature vary between 3 and 8 weeks. IPL is not the treatment of choice for leg veins, but may be employed.

- Although the Q-switched laser system remains the method of choice, studies have shown that intense pulsed light (IPL) devices have obtained the desired results with minimal adverse effects in the removal of pigmented lesions.
- Ultraviolet light damaged collagen and elastic fibers of skin may be treated with non-ablative photorejuvenation of IPL used to reduce mottled pigmentation, telangiectasias and skin texture.
- The mechanism of IPL may be relating to maintain the balance of oxidation and anti-oxidation, restoring oxidase activity and regulating the death of skin cells by increasing Bcl-2 expression.
- IPL wavelengths of 1,064, 1,320 and 1,450 nm enhance dermal collagen formation.
- Photodynamic Therapy (PDT) uses an IPL light source along with a photosensitizer, 5-aminolevulinic acid (ALA), for the treatment of photodamaged skin, actinic keratoses, skin cancers, and cystic acne.

Telangiectasias

Clinically, telangiectasias can be classified as linear, arborizing, spider and punctiform.[24] The reason for the development of facial telangiectasias in most cases is unknown, but sun exposure, topical or systemic steroids and hormonal replacement therapy play a role. Facial telangiectasias on nose and cheeks are a cosmetic blemish for many a patient. IPL and lasers have been very effective in improving these telangiectasias.[25] PDL with 0.5 ms pulses are the most preferred way of treatment but intracutaneous hematomas have frequently been encountered.[25,26] (Fig. 1a, b) On the other hand, IPL systems have less of these side-effects and have become increasingly popular for telangiectasia treatment.[7,27] Clearance rates of 75–100% have been achieved in treating patients with essential telangiectasias, as demonstrated on 153 such patients by Angermeier.[28] In another study by Schroeter et al. achieved 90–95% clearance in one session with PhotoDerm VL in 45 patients with telangiectasias and spider nevi.[29] Clementoni et al. demonstrated a 75–100% clearance but did not find any correlation with lesion size, age, skin type but was related to operator's experience.[30]

Erythematotelangiectatic (ET) rosacea clinically manifests as facial telangiectasias, persistant erythema and flushing involving the central face. PDL at wavelengths of 585 and 595 nm, have been used and considered to be an effective modality for their treatment.[31,32] But, purpura was frequently a less tolerated side-effect of PDL treatment, which was quite a lot improved with the modifications that were introduced such as the use of higher fluences and incorporation of cooling devices. Besides, cryogen cooling sprays also aided much in protecting the epidermis while still delivering the heat sufficiently to target the deeper vessels.[33] On the other hand, the main advantage with the IPL device is the absence of postoperative purpura when treating vascular lesions. In fact, in a study with 29 patients, a comparison was made between the nonpurpuragenic PDL and IPL treatment in the ability to reduce erythema, telangiectasia and symptoms in patients with moderate facial ET rosacea. With split face treatments with IPL/PDL, PDL/no treatment and IPL/no treatment combinations in three groups of patients, it was observed that both IPL and PDL had similar efficacy and safety and both modalities were reasonable choices for treating ET rosacea.

Schroeter et al. in a study to test the effect of IPL on 60 patients, observed that an average of four treatments, 77.8% clearance of facial telangiectasias occurred. The forehead showed the best (87%) clearance.[34] Of the different, sites treated, the nose needed the maximum number of treatments (five) for the lesions to disappear. They also observed and suggested that IPL has the following advantages in treating facial telangiectasias over other lasers:

- The PDL, argon laser and CO_2 lasers are coherent light sources while IPL is a non-coherent broad spectrum of light. Deeper penetration into the skin can be achieved

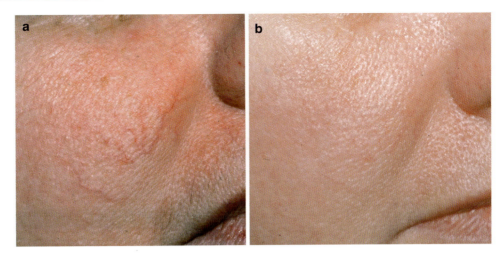

Fig. 1 (**a**) Patient with facial telangiectasias before treatment. (**b**) Patient with facial telangiectasias after treatment with IPL

using the longer wavelengths. The shorter pulse time of microseconds as with PDL is not sufficient to close the vessels. Also, a higher selection of a broad range of vessel colors of the vascular system.

- With one shot of IPL, a surface of 2.8 cm^2 can be treated, whereas with the PDL, it is a surface of 19.6 mm^2 for a diameter of 5 mm and for Argon laser it is only 3 mm^2. Thus the large surface area of IPL offers more time efficient treatment with less patient discomfort.
- By splitting the energy into two or three pulses with different pulse delays, the skin can be allowed to cool between pulses.

A case of hereditary benign telangiectasia treated with 12 treatments of IPL in 18 months and the condition showed vast improvement.[35]

- Hemangiomas are characterized as spontaneous proliferated growth of abnormal atrophic blood vessels that form ulceration. Several lasers, such as the preferred flashlamp-pulsed dye laser, have proven to be effective in the treatment of hemangiomas.
- Erythematous, pigmented and finely wrinkled appearance of the skin are common manifestations of Poikiloderma of Civatte (POC) and can be efficiently treated with an intense pulsed light (IPL) laser system at wavelengths from 515 to 590 nm.
- Nodular hypertrophic port-wine stains (PWS) have been effectively treated using IPL.
- Improved results can be attained when treating leg telangiectasias by using the appropriate wavelength matching the specific vessel color, luminal diameter and depth.

Hemangiomas

Hemangiomas are characterized by a proliferation growth phase followed by slow, inevitable regression (involution phase) between 1 and 10 years of age. Although hemangiomas resolve, lesions persist in 35–50% of children who begin school.[36] Even after spontaneous involution of the lesions, 15% of children have residual skin changes, including depigmentation or hyperpigmentation, telangiectasia, atrophy and wrinkling of the skin, and cutaneous depression. If skin changes occur, remaining changes of the skin may correspond to the largest size of the hemangioma.[37] However, spontaneous regression is no guarantee of a satisfactory cosmetic result, as is often presumed.

Various lasers, particularly the flashlamp-pulsed dye laser, have been proven to be effective in the treatment of hemangiomas.[38-42] (Fig. 2a, b) Nevertheless, the post-treatment side effects, such as pronounced purpura and changes in pigmentation, have been a matter of concern until longer pulse durations became available.

Ulceration is the most common complication of infantile hemangiomas and poses a therapeutic challenge due to associated pain, infection, hemorrhage and subsequent scarring. In a report on the use of an IPL system in the treatment of ulcerated hemangiomas in a 4-month-old girl, with hemangioma affecting the entire cutaneous surface of the left limb and development of four ulcerations on the inner aspect of this extremity.[43] Two sessions with an IPL system using a triple pulse mode; (a 570-nm lower cut-off filter and a fluence of 38 J/cm^2) were performed. Good results were rapidly obtained after two and four sessions of IPL treatment, respectively. Pain was soon relieved and complete epithelization was obtained by between 1 and 2 months in both patients. Yet, due to the pain being a very commonly associated complaint and more complications occur while treating hemangiomas with IPL, pulsed dye laser is still the preferred method of treatment for initial superficial hemangiomas.[44]

Poikiloderma of Civatte

Poikiloderma of Civatte (POC) is a common manifestation of photoaging and presents as erythematous, pigmented and

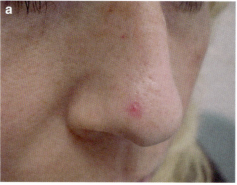
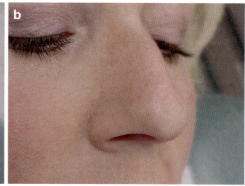

Fig. 2 (**a**) Patient with hemangioma of the nose before treatment. (**b**) Patient with hemangioma of the nose after treatment with IPL

finely wrinkled appearance of the skin in sun exposed areas mainly on the neck, forehead and upper chest, with sparing of submental area.

Because of their ability to target vascular and pigment abnormalities simultaneously, IPL is an ideal device to treat POC. The use of 515 nm filter allows absorption, both by melanin and hemoglobin simultaneously. In patients with more dyspigmentation, initial use of higher filters (550 and 560 nm) prevents too much epidermal absorption and thus avoids crusting and swelling. Additional treatments with IPL using 550, 560 or 570 nm filter to treat the vascular component of POC may be required. Patients with severe form of POC may need initial treatments to begin with 590 nm filter followed by the use of lower filters. In different studies, a clearance of more than 75% of telangiectasias and hyperpigmentation was observed. An incidence of 5% of side effects including pigment changes has been seen.[45]

Port Wine Stains

Although PDL has been proven to be the preferred treatment for port-wine stains (PWS) in children and adults, lesions with nodular parts and hypertrophic and extended PWS may not achieve great outcomes, thus making it necessary to look out for more options.[46-48] The reason for the resistance to treatment with PDL is probably the large size and the greater depth of the vessels in PWS.[11,49] (Fig. 3a, b)

In a certain multi-center study, it was shown that PhotoDerm VL yielded good results in both therapy resistant and hypertrophic PWS (Table 2).[4]

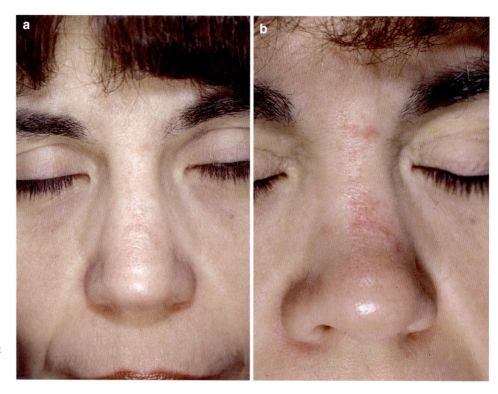

Fig. 3 (**a**) Patient with port-wine stain before treatment. (**b**) Patient after port-wine stain after treatment with IPL

Intense Pulse Light (IPL)

Table 2 Suggested parameters for photorejuvenation for various commercially available systems

Device	Filters (nm)	Fluence (J/cm^2)	Delay time (ms)	First pulse (ms)	Second pulse (ms)	Number of sequential pulses
Lumenis M 22 (Fig. 4)	560	20–35	5–150	4–10	4–10	1, 2 or 3
Lumenis One/Quantum	560	22–28	5–150	2.4–3.0	3.0–4.0	1, 2 or 3
Cutera (Limelight)	560–1,100 Setting B	16–26	12–30	N/A	N/A	N/A
Starlux	Lux G 500–670, 870–1,200	30–40	10–100	N/A	N/A	N/A

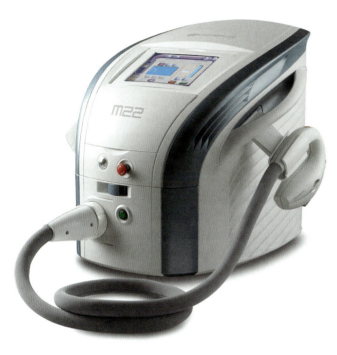

Fig. 4 M 22, a new generation pulsed light device

Pigmented Lesions

Pigmented lesions have a spectrum ranging from epidermal lentigines and café-au-lait macules to acquired Ota's/Ito's nevus, Becker's nevus and congenital nevi to post-inflammatory hyperpigmentation, melasma and decorative and traumatic tattoos. IPL systems have pulse durations in millisecond range, they do not appear to be optimally suited for treating pigmented lesions still have been reports of successful use and Q-switched laser system remains the method of choice for treating benign pigmented lesion. In a study by Bjerring et al. on 96 patients with solar lentigines and melanocytic nevi were treated.[50] The IPL device used for treatment was characterized by the fact that the emitted light is conditioned by two types of optical filters: a hot mirror filter and a water chamber which work together to create the desired spectral range of light. A single session of this treatment led to a 96% reduction in pigment, 74.2% clearance for lentigo solaris and 66.3% for melanocytic nevi.

In another study, treatment of solar lentigines and ephelides was performed in three to five sessions. A total of 48% of patients showed 50% improvement in pigmentation.[51]

With the objective of studying the efficacy and safety of a new IPL device in the treatment of melasma in Chinese patients, Li et al. treated 89 women with melasma with a total of four IPL treatments at 3-week intervals.[52] Among all the results obtained, noticeable was that 77.5% of the patients obtained 51–100% improvement. Patients with epidermal-type melasma responded better to treatment than the mixed type. The patients younger than 35 years or older than 45 years responded significantly better to the treatment, especially after one session. Minimal adverse effects were observed.

Non-ablative Photorejuvenation

IPL is very commonly used for changes of photoaging as IPL has the potential to treat multiple components simultaneously including pigmentation, telangiectasias and degraded collagen. The quantitative effects of sun exposure with resultant UV damage of structural components such as collagen and elastic fibers impact the overall appearance of aging skin. Besides, genetic factors, intrinsic factors, disease processes (rosacea) and overall loss of cutaneous elasticity associated with age also have a role to play. Photorejuvenation "photofacial" has been described a dynamic non-ablative process involving the use of the IPL to reduce mottled pigmentation, telangiectasias and smoothen the textural surface of skin.[2] The treatment is in the form of three to six procedures in 3–4 week intervals where the entire face is treated and the patient may return to all activities immediately (Fig. 5).

In a study, Zelickson demonstrated that IPL treatment results in an 81% increase in collagentype-1 transcripts while PDL treatment results in a 23% increase in Collagen type-1 transcripts improving the fine wrinkles.[53,54] Another investigation demonstrated collagen I, III, elastin and collagenase to be increased in 85–100% of patients and procollagen increased in 50–70% of patients.

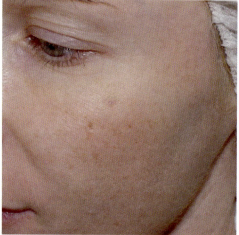 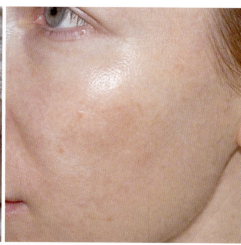

Fig. 5 Before and after pictures of a patient after 3 treatments with IPL for photorejuvenation

The histologic effects of five IPL treatments with 570–645 nm (2.4–6.0 ms, 25–42 J/cm²) showed epidermal thickening of 100–300 μm, better cellular polarity, a decrease in horny plugs, new rete ridge formation, decreased elastosis and dermal neo-collagen formation.[55] In a study by Wong et al. to examine the effects of IPL irradiation on normal human dermal fibroblasts grown in contracted collagen lattices, a dose-dependent increase in viable cells was demonstrated after the IPL irradiation. No significant change in mRNA levels of collagen I and fibronectin occurred, but expression of collagen III and TGF-beta 1 in dermal fibroblast was upregulated.[56]

In a study in the murine model to understand the effect and mechanism of IPL on skin aging, it was found that Superoxide dismutase (SOD) activity and Hydroxyproline (Hyp) content in the IPL treatment groups was lower than that in the control group.[57] IPL irradiation increased Bcl-2 protein content in rat skin cells but had no effect on Bax protein expression. Therefore, it was concluded that the mechanism of IPL may be relating to maintain the balance of oxidation and anti-oxidation, restoring oxidase activity and regulating the death of skin cells by increasing Bcl-2 expression.

With the original IPL, Negishi et al. conducted a study in 97 Japanese patients using 550 nm filter for the pigment and 570 nm cut-off filter for telangiectasia. Patients were treated three to six times at 2–3 week intervals with IPL 28–32 J/cm², 2.5–4.0/4.0–5.0 ms, 20–40 ms delay without topical anesthesia. It was seen that 49% of patients had greater than 75% improvement in pigmentation with 33% having greater than 75% improvement in telangiectasia and 13% having a greater than 75% improvement in skin texture. There were no reports of hyperpigmentation, even in four patients with melasma. Also, histologic evidence of collagen and elastic fiber proliferation in papillary and subpapillary layer was present in biopsies, performed at the end of the study.[58] In a different study by this group, 73 Japanese patients were treated with Quantum IPL every 3–4 weeks. Quantum IPL has an integrated skin cooling crystal that cools the epidermis to 40°C during IPL versus 65°C without cooling. They demonstrated a greater than 60% improvement in pigmentation and erythema along with smooth skin; in 80% of the patients.

Another sign of photoaging that improved with IPL treatment is freckling. Huang et al. used 550–590 nm filters (25–35 J/cm², 4 ms single or double pulse, 20–40 ms delay time), one to three treatments at 4 week intervals. Their endpoint consisted of graying or perilesional erythema with 91.7% of the patients extremely satisfied with the results.[59] Kawada et al. also treated freckling and lentigos in Asian skin with Quantum IPL (560 nm, 20–24 J/cm², 2.6–5.0 ms, 20 ms delay) for three to five treatments at 2–3 week intervals.[51] Patients reported that small patches and ephelides responded best and no adverse effects were reported.

Weiss et al. used IPL to treat vascular lesions but evaluated 80 of their initial patients for possible "photorejuvenation".[60] This was performed using photographic images from three subsequent visits including one follow-up at 4 years. An 80% improvement in pigmentation, telangiectasia and skin texture was seen. Some adverse events such as hypopigmentation lasting for 1 year occurred in 2.5%, temporary mild crusting occurred in 19%, erythema for more than 4 h in 15%, hypo- or hyperpigmentation in 5%, and rectangular foot-printing in 5% (Fig. 6).

In 49 subjects (except in males, who elected to avoid treatment of beard area to prevent any potential hair loss) with varying degrees of photodamage including wrinkling, skin coarseness, irregular pigmentation, pore size and telangiectasias was improved in more than 90% of the patients when they were treated with a series of four or more full-face treatments at 3-week intervals using IPL.[2] In this study 72% of subjects reported a 50% or greater improvement in skin smoothness; 44% reported a 75% or greater improvement. Side effects reported were temporary discoloration consisting of a darkening of lentigines which resolved completely within 7 days.

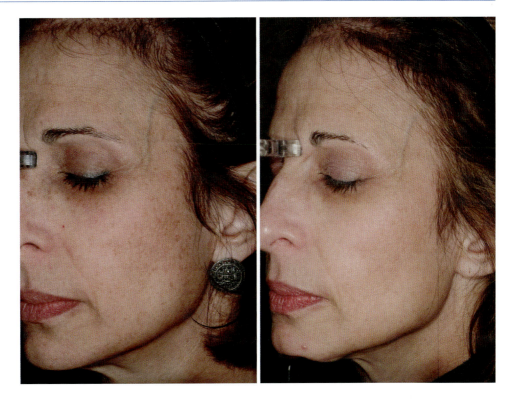

Fig. 6 Before and after pictures of a patient after IPL photorejuvenation with Lumenis one

It has been suggested that enhanced photorejuvenation may be achieved with combination procedures, such as the use of Intense Pulsed Light with 1,064 and 1,320 nm Nd:YAG laser treatments,[61,62] microdermabrasion[63] and the use of botulinum toxin A (Botox.®, Allergan, Irvine, CA)[64]. The use of 1,064, 1,320 and 1,450 nm wavelengths can cause significant structural change in the dermis which can enhance new collagen formation further reducing wrinkling. Muscle relaxation with botulinum A allows for parallel collagen formation over a static dermis.

Photodynamic Therapy (PDT) for Photorejuvenation

This advanced technique has also been termed as Photodynamic Skin Rejuvenation (PSR). PDT using IPL as the light source and sensitizers such as 5-aminolevulinic acid (ALA) can be used in the treatment of severely photodamaged skin.[65] Besides offering treatment for conditions such as actinic keratoses,[66] early skin cancers,[67] and cystic acne[68] it can provide a significant cosmetic benefit. This technique involves activation of a specific photosensitizing agent, 5-ALA (a precursor in the heme biosynthesis pathway of protoporphyrin-9), activated by the conventional IPL as provided by VascuLight or Quantum system. This leads to the production of activated oxygen species within cells, resulting in their elimination or their destruction. FDA cleared the use of ALA with 410 nm continuous blue light for the treatment of AKs although in clinical practice, variety of light sources with different wavelengths have shown efficacy in treatment of AKs.[69] However, a broader wavelength such as that found with the IPL should be even more efficacious in activating ALA. IPL treatments are under study for such enhanced benefits of photodynamic therapy.[70]

IPL for Scars

IPL applied following suture removal was found in a pilot study to be effective on surgically induced scars and on various types of scars on another study.[71,72] The mechanism of IPL is not fully understood, but it probably targets the vascular proliferation essential to the collagen overgrowth and its effect on the pigmentation (both melanin and artificial pigments) that results in scar development (hyperpigmented, erythematous, and proliferative scars).[73]

In a study by Erol et al., with the aim of assessing the safety and efficacy of IPL on scars originating from burns, trauma, surgery and acne, an overall clinical improvement in the appearance of scars and reductions in height, erythema and hardness were seen in the majority of the patients (92.5%) and over half of the patients had good or excellent improvement.[74] It was concluded by the investigators that IPL is effective not only in improving the appearance of hypertrophic scars and keloids regardless of their origin, but also in reducing the height, redness and hardness of scars.

Bellew et al. in a prospective study aimed to compare the safety and efficacy of LPDL and IPL on surgically induced scars (breast reduction scars and abdominoplasty scars).[71] Two treatments were done 2 months apart. It was found that LPDL and IPL are equally effective in improving the appearance of hypertrophic surgical scars but the differences in improvement between the LPDL and IPL sides were not statistically significant. Patients rated IPL as more painful than LPDL.

Another kind of scars, striae distensae, are common cutaneous lesions characterized terminally by linear bands of atrophic skin, commonly seen in adolescents and young adults especially pregnant women.[75-77] There is no widely accepted treatment for improving the appearance of stretch marks. Lasers, microdermabrasion, topical tretinoin etc. have been tried with limited success. With the aim of establishing that IPL can provoke clinical and microscopical improvement in the stretch marks, Hernandez-Perez et al. studied on 15 women on their striae distensae of the abdomen.[78] All the patients showed clinical and microscopical improvement in each one the parameters assessed and statistically significant difference was observed in the post-treatment dermal thickness.

- Intense pulse light (IPL) has shown to improve the appearance of hypertrophic scars and keloids, as well as reducing the height, redness and hardness of scars.
- IPL hair removal must be used at different wavelengths to treat the various depths of hair follicles. Increasing Fitzpatrick skin types may have adverse effects such as redness, crusts, and other pigmentary alterations.

IPL for Hair Removal

In addition to the treatment of vascular malformations, the treatment of unwanted hair is one of the most important indications for the use of high-intensity pulsed light sources, even though the exact mechanism of action has not been decisively determined. A number of studies have demonstrated good results using IPL systems.[79-83]

One of the theories suggests that lasers may induce damage to the isthmus and upper stem and interfere with the interaction between dermal and epidermal germinative cell, thus inhibiting or altering the normal hair cycle.[84] Another theory postulated says that the damage to the hair follicle and the hair shaft in the anagen phase cause a long-term interruption in the hair growth cycle.[85,86]

Gold et al. and Weiss et al. included 31 and 71 patients, respectively, with hypertrichosis of different parts of the body. After one treatment session and a 3-month follow-upperiod, Gold et al. reported that an average of 60% of the hair had been removed.[79] Similarly, Sadick et al. treated a total of 34 patients with excessive body hair using a filtered IPL system which was an early prototype. The mean hair removal efficiency (HRE) achieved was 76% after a mean of 3.7 treatments. In a subgroup of 14 patients followed-up for more than 12 months (mean 20 months), a final HRE of 83% was achieved after a mean of 3.9 treatments.[87]

The clearance rate and satisfaction level after IPL hair removal varies greatly. The results depend on hair type, skin type, number of treatments, and treatment parameters. A larger spot size offers faster treatment and better light distribution. Black hairs show the best clearance.[23,88] (Fig.7a, b) IPL hair removal seems to be effective for most patients, although some may experience side-effects. According to Raulin et al., IPL hair removal has more complications than other IPL applications.[89] With increasing skin type (Fitzpatrick classification), more complications occur. Redness, crusts, and pigmentary alterations are the most frequent side-effects.[88,90] They represent the response of perifollicular erythema and edema.

Yellow discoloration of the terminal hairs was reported by Radmanesh[91] and is caused by the destruction of melanocytes within the hair follicles without the destruction of germinative cells. Leukotrichia and "paradoxical effect" seem to be the most unpleasant side-effects and have a 0–10% chance of appearance.[88,90,92] This can be explained by the difference in thermal relaxation times of melanocytes and germinative cells.

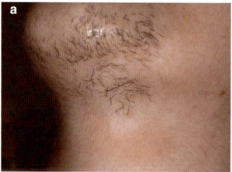 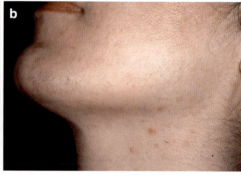

Fig. 7 (**a**) Before hair removal. (**b**) After hair removal with IPL

Adverse Reactions

Moreno-Arias et al. assessed all possible side-effects after IPL hair removal in a series of 49 females with facial hirsutism during a total 390 treatment sessions of IPL photodepilation. Evaluations were performed clinically, photographically, and using a 2 month post-treatment questionnaire. The side effects observed were transient erythema, late evanescent erythema, mild pain, moderate pain, crust formation, superficial burning, isolated vesicles, transient hyperpigmentation, transient hypopigmentation, paradoxical effect, persistent local heat sensation and minimal scar. The most interesting of these was the "paradoxical effect" which was seen as the growth of new, fine, dark terminal hair in untreated areas in the proximity of treated areas. Although the cause of this is unknown, it is believed to be due to the sublethal doses of IPL that may have induced activation of dormant follicles (Table 3).

The risk of side effects can be reduced with some safety measures such as skin lightening/sun avoidance prior to treatment, cooling devices or cold gel to diminish skin temperature during treatment, sun avoidance/blockers after treatment.[93]

Conclusions

IPL is a non-coherent source of light with a broad bandwidth approximately ranging from 515 to 1,200 nm which, based on the principle of photothermolysis, has been utilized for several indications such as leg vein treatment, hair removal, vascular lesions, scarring, pigmentary disorders, poikiloderma of civatte and photorejuvenation. By varying parameters such as wavelength, spot size and pulse duration IPL can be made suitable for a specific treating each of these indications. IPL has been used as the light source in photodynamic therapy for the treatment of range of conditions. The choice of patients and expertise in using the device are essential to achieve successful results and minimize complications.

Table 3 Recommended parameters for IPL

Fitzpatrick skin type	Filter (nm)	Fluence (J/cm²)	Pulse durations	Delay between pulses (ms)
II	615	39–42	3.3–5 ms 2 pulses	30
III	645	34–36	3.0 ms 3 pulses	30
IV	695	34–40	3.0 ms 3 pulses	40
V	695, 755	38–40	5–7 ms 2 pulses	50–60

References

1. Weiss RA, Goldman MP, Weiss MA. Treatment of poikiloderma of Civatte with an intense pulsed light source. *Dermatol Surg.* 2000;26(9):823-827; discussion 828.
2. Bitter PH. Noninvasive rejuvenation of photodamaged skin using serial, full-face intense pulsed light treatments. *Dermatol Surg.* 2000;26(9):835-842; discussion 843.
3. Goldberg DJ, Cutler KB. Nonablative treatment of rhytids with intense pulsed light. *Lasers Surg Med.* 2000;26(2):196-200.
4. Raulin C, Schroeter CA, Weiss RA, Keiner M, Werner S. Treatment of port-wine stains with a noncoherent pulsed light source: a retrospective study. *Arch Dermatol.* 1999;135(6):679-683.
5. Jay H, Borek C. Treatment of a venous-lake angioma with intense pulsed light. *Lancet.* 1998;351(9096):112.
6. Weiss RA, Weiss MA, Marwaha S, Harrington AC. Hair removal with a non-coherent filtered flashlamp intense pulsed light source. *Lasers Surg Med.* 1999;24(2):128-132.
7. Raulin C, Schroeter C, Maushagen-Schnaas E. Treatment possibilities with a high-energy pulsed light source (PhotoDerm VL). *Hautarzt.* 1997;48(12):886-893.
8. Raulin C, Weiss RA, Schönermark MP. Treatment of essential telangiectasias with an intense pulsed light source (PhotoDerm VL). *Dermatol Surg.* 1997;23(10):941-945; discussion 945-946.
9. Parrish JA, Anderson RR, Harrist T, Paul B, Murphy GF. Selective thermal effects with pulsed irradiation from lasers: from organ to organelle. *J Invest Dermatol.* 1983;80(Suppl):75s-80s.
10. Adrian RM. Treatment of leg telangiectasias using a long-pulse frequency-doubled neodymium:YAG laser at 532 nm. *Dermatol Surg.* 1998;24(1):19-23.
11. Dierickx CC, Casparian JM, Venugopalan V, Farinelli WA, Anderson RR. Thermal relaxation of port-wine stain vessels probed in vivo: the need for 1-10-millisecond laser pulse treatment. *J Invest Dermatol.* 1995;105(5):709-714.
12. Kimel S, Svaasand LO, Hammer-Wilson M, et al. Differential vascular response to laser photothermolysis. *J Invest Dermatol.* 1994;103(5):693-700.
13. Goldman MP, Bennett RG. Treatment of telangiectasia: a review. *J Am Acad Dermatol.* 1987;17:167-182.
14. Sommer A, Van Mierlo PL, Neumann HA, Kessels AG. Red and blue telangiectasias. Differences in oxygenation? *Dermatol Surg.* 1997;23(1):55-59.
15. Sadick NS. A histologic bimodal approach to lower extremity veins. *Cosmet Dermatol.* 2000;June:17-30.
16. Goldman MP, Eckhouse S. Photothermal sclerosis of leg veins. *Dermatol Surg.* 1996;22:323-330.
17. Reisfeld PL. Blue in the skin. *J Am Acad Dermatol.* 2000;42:597-605.
18. Sadick NS. A dual wavelength approach for laser/intense pulsed light source treatment of lower extremity veins. *J Am Acad Dermatol.* 2002;46(1):66-72.
19. Lask G, Eckhouse S, Slatkine M, Waldman A, Kreindel M, Gottfried V. The role of laser and intense light sources in photo-epilation: a comparative evaluation. *J Cutan Laser Ther.* 1999;1(1):3-13.
20. Dover JS, Sadick NS, Goldman MP. The role of lasers and light sources in the treatment of leg veins. *Dermatol Surg.* 1999;25(4):328-335; discussion 335-336.
21. Fodor L, Carmi N, Fodor A, Ramon Y, Ullmann Y. Intense pulsed light for skin rejuvenation, hair removal, and vascular lesions: a patient satisfaction study and review of the literature. *Ann Plast Surg.* 2009;62(4):345-349.
22. Fodor L, Ramon Y, Fodor A, et al. A side-by-side prospective study of intense pulsed light and Nd:YAG laser treatment for vascular lesions. *Ann Plast Surg.* 2006;56:164-170.
23. Lask G, Eckhouse S, Slatkine M, et al. The role of laser and intense light sources in photo-epilation: a comparative evaluation. *J Cutan Laser Ther.* 1999;1:3-13.

24. Redisch W, Pelzer RH. Localized vascular dilatations of the human skin, capillary microscopy and related studies. *Am Heart J.* 1949;37(1):106-113.
25. Raulin C, Greeve B, eds. *Laser und IOL-Technologie in der Dermatologie and Aesthetischen Medizin.* 1st ed. New York: Schattauer Stuttgart; 2001.
26. Ruiz-Esparza J, Goldman MP, Fitzpatrick RE, Lowe NJ, Behr KL. Flash lamp-pumped dye laser treatment of telangiectasia. *J Dermatol Surg Oncol.* 1993;19(11):1000-1003.
27. Podmore P. Treatment of widespread generalized congenital aberrant telangiectasia with a flashlight source. *J Cutan Laser Ther.* 2000;2(2):79-80.
28. Angermeier MC. Treatment of facial vascular lesions with intense pulsed light. *J Cutan Laser Ther.* 1999;1:95-100.
29. Schroeter CA, Neumann M. An intense light source. The PhotoDerm VL-flashlamp as a new treatment possibility for vascular skin lesions. *Dermatol Surg.* 1998;24:743-748.
30. Clementoni MT, Gilardino P, Muti GF, et al. Facial teleangectasias: our experience in treatment with IPL. *Lasers Surg Med.* 2005;37(1):9-13.
31. Clark SM, Lanigan SW, Marks R. Laser treatment of erythema and telangiectasia associated with rosacea. *Lasers Med Sci.* 2002;17(1):26-33.
32. Tan SR, Tope WD. Pulsed dye laser treatment of rosacea improves erythema, symptomatology, and quality of life. *J Am Acad Dermatol.* 2004;51(4):592-599.
33. Chang CJ, Nelson JS. Cryogen spray cooling and higher fluence pulsed dye laser treatment improve port-wine stain clearance while minimizing epidermal damage. *Dermatol Surg.* 1999;25(10): 767-772.
34. Schroeter CA, Haaf-von Below S, Neumann HA. Effective treatment of rosacea using intense pulsed light systems. *Dermatol Surg.* 2005;31(10):1285-1289.
35. Purcell E, Condon C. Intense pulsed light therapy in the management of hereditary benign telangiectasia. *Br J Plast Surg.* 2004; 57(5):453-455.
36. Poetke M, Philipp C, Berlien HP. Flashlamp-pumped pulsed dye laser for hemangiomas in infancy: treatment of superficial vs mixed hemangiomas. *Arch Dermatol.* 2000;136(5):628-632.
37. Poetke M, Philipp C, Berlien HP. Clinical features and classification of congenital vascular disorders. In: Berlien HP, Schmittenbecher PP, eds. *Laser surgery in children.* Berlin: Springer; 1997:72-81.
38. Ashinoff R, Geronemus RG. Flashlamp-pumped pulsed dye laser for port-wine stains in infancy: earlier versus later treatment. *J Am Acad Dermatol.* 1991;24:467-472.
39. Geronemus RG. Pulsed dye laser treatment of vascular lesions in children. *J Dermatol Surg Oncol.* 1993;19:303-310.
40. Goldman MP, Fitzpatrick RE, Ruiz-Esparaza J. Treatment of port-wine stains (capillary malformation) with the flashlamp-pumped pulsed dye laser. *J Pediatr.* 1993;122:71-77.
41. Reyes BA, Geronemus RG. Treatment of port-wine stains during childhood with the flashlamp-pumped pulsed dye laser. *J Am Acad Dermatol.* 1990;23:1142-1148.
42. Tan OT, Sherwood K, Gilchrest BA. Treatment of children with port-wine stains using the flashlamp-pulsed tunable dye laser. *N Engl J Med.* 1989;320:416-421.
43. Jorge BF, Del Pozo J, Castiñeiras I, Mazaira M, Fernández-Torres R, Fonseca E. Treatment of ulcerated haemangiomas with a non-coherent pulsed light source: brief initial clinical report. *J Cosmet Laser Ther.* 2008;10(1):48-51.
44. Raulin C, Greeve B, eds. *Laser und IPL-Technologie in der Dermatologie und Ästhetischen Medizin.* 1st ed. New York: Schattauer Stuttgart; 2001.
45. Weiss RA, Goldmann MP, Weiss MA. Treatment of poikiloderma of Civatte with an intense pulsed light source. *Dermatol Surg.* 2000;26:283-828.

46. Alster TS, Wilson F. Treatment of port-wine stains with the flashlamp pumped dye laser: extended clinical experience in children and adults. *Ann Plast Surg.* 1994;32:478-484.
47. Ashinoff R, Geronemus RG. Flashlamp-pumped dye laser for port-wine stains in infancy: early versus later treatments. *J Am Acad Dermatol.* 1990;24:467-472.
48. Fitzpatrick RE, Lowe NJ, Goldman MP, Borden H, Behr KL, Ruiz-Esparza J. Flashlamp-pumped dye laser treatment of port wine stains. *J Dermatol Surg Oncol.* 1994;20:743-748.
49. Fiskerstrand EJ, Svaasand LA, Kopstad G, Ryggen K, Aase S. Photothermally induced vessel-wall necrosis after pulsed dye laser treatment: lack of response in port-wine stains with small sized or deeply located vessels. *J Invest Dermatol.* 1996;107:671-675.
50. Bjerring P, Christiansen K, Troilius A. Intense pulsed light source for the treatment of dye laser resistant port-wine stains. *J Cosmet Laser Ther.* 2003;5(1):7-13.
51. Kawada A, Shiraishi H, Asai M, et al. Clinical improvement of solar lentigines and ephelides with an intense pulsed light source. *Dermatol Surg.* 2002;28(6):504-508.
52. Li YH, Chen JZ, Wei HC, et al. Efficacy and safety of intense pulsed light in treatment of melasma in Chinese patients. *Dermatol Surg.* 2008;34(5):693-700; discussion 700-701. Epub 2008 Mar 3.
53. Zelickson B, Kist D. Pulsed dye laser and photoderm treatment stimulates production of type-1 collagen and collagenase transcripts in papillary dermis fibroblasts. *Lasers Surg Med Abstr Suppl.* 2001;13:33.
54. Zelickson B, Kist D. Effect of pulse dye laser and intense pulsed light source on the dermal extracellular matrix remodeling [abstract]. *Lasers Surg Med.* 2000(Suppl 12):17.
55. Hernandez-Perez E, Ibiett EV. Gross and microscopic findings in patients undergoing microdermabrasion for facial rejuvenation. *Dermatol Surg.* 2001;27(7):637-640.
56. Wong WR, Shyu WL, Tsai JW, Hsu KH, Pang JH. Intense pulsed light effects on the expression of extracellular matrix proteins and transforming growth factor beta-1 in skin dermal fibroblasts cultured within contracted collagen lattices. *Dermatol Surg.* 2009;35(5):816-825. Epub 2009 Mar 30.
57. Yaping X, Wang B, Lu J, et al. Effect and mechanism of intense pulsed laser on skin aging in rats. *Zhong Nan Da Xue Xue Bao Yi Xue Ban.* 2009;34(5):375-381.
58. Negishi K, Tezuka Y, Kushikata N, Wakamatsu S. Photorejuvenation for Asian skin by intense pulsed light. *Dermatol Surg.* 2001;27(7):627-631; discussion 632.
59. Huang YL, Liao YL, Lee SH, Hong HS. Intense pulsed light for the treatment of facial freckles in Asian skin. *Dermatol Surg.* 2002;28:1007.
60. Weiss RA, Weiss MA, Beasley KL. Rejuvenation of photoaged skin: 5 years results with intense pulsed light of the face, neck, and chest. *Dermatol Surg.* 2002;28(12):1115-1119.
61. Goldberg DJ, Whitworth J. Laser skin resurfacing with the Q-switched Nd:YAG laser. *Dermatol Surg.* 1997;23(10):903-906; discussion 906-907.
62. Fatemi A, Weiss MA, Weiss RA. Short-term histologic effects of nonablative resurfacing: results with a dynamically cooled millisecond-domain 1320 nm Nd:YAG laser. *Dermatol Surg.* 2002;28(2): 172-176.
63. Tan MH, Spencer JM, Pires LM, Ajmeri J, Skover G. The evaluation of aluminum oxide crystal microdermabrasion for photodamage. *Dermatol Surg.* 2001;27(11):943-949.
64. Fagien S, Brandt FS. Primary and adjunctive use of botulinum toxin type A (Botox) in facial aesthetic surgery: beyond the glabella. *Clin Plast Surg.* 2001;28(1):127-148.
65. Ruiz-Rodriguez R, San-Sanchez T, Cordoba S. Photodynamic photorejuvenation. *Dermatol Surg.* 2002;28:742-744.
66. Fritsch C, Goerz G, Ruzicka T. Photodynamic therapy in dermatology. *Arch Dermatol.* 1998;134:207-214.

67. Kalla K, Merk H, Mukhtar H. Photodynamic therapy in dermatology. *J Am Acad Dermatol*. 2000;42:389-413.
68. Hongcharu W, Taylor CR, Chang Y, Aghassi D, Suthamjariya K, Anderson RR. Topical ALA-photodynamic therapy for the treatment of acne vulgaris. *J Invest Dermatol*. 2000;115(2):183-192. PMID: 10951234.
69. Fowler JF, Zax RH. Aminolevulinic acid hydrochloride with photodynamic therapy: efficacy outcomes and recurrence 4 years after treatment. *Cutis*. 2002;69(6S):2-7.
70. Gold MH. The evolving role of aminolevulinic acid hydrochloride with photodynamic therapy in photoaging. *Cutis*. 2002;69(Suppl 6):8-13.
71. Bellew SG, Weiss MA, Weiss RA. Comparison of intense pulsed light to 595-nm long-pulsed pulsed dye laser for treatment of hypertrophic surgical scars: a pilot study. *J Drugs Dermatol*. 2005;4:448-452.
72. Kontoes PP, Marayiannis KV, Vlachos SP. The use of intense pulsed light in the treatment of scars. *Eur J Plast Surg*. 2003;25:374-377.
73. Hedelund L, Due E, Bjerring P, Wulf HC, Haedersdal M. Skin rejuvenation using intense pulsed light: a randomized controlled split-face trial with blinded response evaluation. *Arch Dermatol*. 2006; 142:985-990.
74. Erol OO, Gurlek A, Agaoglu G, Topcuoglu E, Oz H. Treatment of hypertrophic scars and keloids using intense pulsed light (IPL). *Aesthet Plast Surg*. 2008;32(6):902-909. Epub 2008 Jun 17.
75. Requena L, Sánchez-Yus E. Striae distensae. *Dermatopathol Pract Concept*. 1997;3:197-202.
76. McDaniel D, Ash K, Zukowski M. Treatment of stretch marks with the 585-mm flash lamp-pumped pulsed dye laser. *Dermatol Surg*. 1996;22:332-337.
77. Elson ML. Treatment of striae distense with topical tretinoin. *J Dermatol Surg Oncol*. 1990;16:267-270.
78. Hernández-Pérez E, Colombo-Charrier E, Valencia-Ibiett E. Intense pulsed light in the treatment of striae distensae. *Dermatol Surg*. 2002;28(12):1124-1130.
79. Gold MH, Bell MW, Foster TD, Street S. Long-term epilation using the EpiLight™ broad band, intense pulsed light hair removal system. *Dermatol Surg*. 1997;23:909-913.
80. Dierickx CC. Hair removal by lasers and intense pulsed light sources. *Semin Cutan Med Surg*. 2000;19:267-275.
81. Dierickx CC. Hair removal by lasers and intense pulsed light sources. *Dermatol Clin*. 2002;20:135-146.
82. Bjerring P, Cramers M, Egevist H, Christiansen K, Troilius A. Hair reduction using a new intense pulsed light irradiator and a normal mode ruby laser. *J Cutan Laser Ther*. 2000;2:63-71.
83. Moreno-Arias GA, Vilalta-Solsona A, Serra-Renom JM, Benito-Ruiz J, Ferrando J. Intense pulsed light for hairy grafts and flaps. *Dermatol Surg*. 2002;28:402-404.
84. McCoy S, Evans A, James C. Histological study of hair follicles treated with a 3-msec pulsed ruby laser. *Lasers Surg Med*. 1999;24:142-150.
85. Schroeter CA, Raulin C, Thuerlimann W, Reineke T, de Potter C, Neumann M. Hair removal in 40 hirsute women with an intense laser-like light source. *Eur J Dermatol*. 1999;9:374-379.
86. Sadick NS, Shea CR, Buchette JL Jr, Prieto VG. High-intensity flashlamp photoepilation. *Arch Dermatol*. 1999;135:668-676.
87. Sadick NS, Weiss RA, Shea CR, Nagel H, Nicholson J, Prieto VG. Long-term photoepilation using a broad-spectrum intense pulsed light source. *Arch Dermatol*. 2000;136:1336-1340.
88. Fodor L, Menachem M, Ramon Y, et al. Hair removal using intense pulsed light (EpiLight): patient satisfaction, our experience, and literature review. *Ann Plast Surg*. 2005;54:8-14.
89. Raulin C, Greve B, Grema H. IPL technology: a review. *Lasers Surg Med*. 2003;32:78-87.
90. Moreno-Arias GA, Castelo-Branco C, Ferrando J. Side-effects after IPL photodepilation. *Dermatol Surg*. 2002;28:1131-1134.
91. Radmanesh M. Temporary hair color change from black to blond after intense pulsed light hair removal therapy. *Dermatol Surg*. 2004;30:1521.
92. MorenoArias G, CasteloBranco C, Ferrando J. Paradoxical effect after IPL photoepilation. *Dermatol Surg*. 2002;28:1013-1016; discussion 1016.
93. Liew SH. Laser hair removal: guidelines for management. *Am J Clin Dermatol*. 2002;2:107-115.

Photodynamic Therapy

Robert Bissonnette

- Photodynamic therapy with ALA or MAL is an excellent treatment for multiple actinic keratoses
- Large field photodynamic therapy can eradicate multiple actinic keratoses with a shorter downtime than 5-fluorouracil or imiquimod
- Multiple large field photodynamic therapy sessions can delay the appearance of actinic keratoses
- Photodynamic therapy with MAL is approved in several countries for the treatment of superficial basal cell carcinoma and Bowen's disease
- Photodynamic therapy with ALA or MAL has been successfully used off-label for the treatment of acne vulgaris and to improve photoaging.
- Intense pulsed light and pulsed dye lasers can be used to activate porphyrins after ALA or MAL application

Introduction

- Photodynamic therapy was officially discovered at the turn of the twentieth century
- The use of photodynamic therapy with ALA to treat actinic keratoses and basal cell carcinoma was pioneered in Canada by Kennedy and Pottier
- Both ALA and MAL are transformed into porphyrins which can be activated by blue or red light

Photodynamic therapy (PDT) combines the administration of a photosensitizer or photosensitizer precursor with its activation by light of the appropriate wavelengths. In the presence of oxygen, this leads to generation of reactive oxygen species and free radicals. Treatment with plants containing photosensitizers followed by sunlight exposure was practiced by several civilizations since antiquity, but PDT was officially discovered at the turn of the twentieth century by Oscar Raab, a medical study working in Germany in the laboratory of Von Tappeiner.[1] The discovery that pre-malignant and malignant skin lesions can be treated with topical aminolevulinic acid (ALA) application followed by light exposure was made in Canada by Kennedy and Pottier in the late 1980s.[2]

Aminolevulinic acid (ALA) can enter the heme biosynthetic pathway which leads to production of porphyrins and ultimately of heme, as protoporphyrin IX is transformed into heme by the enzyme ferrochelatase. Heme has a negative feedback on ALA synthesis. The addition of exogenous ALA bypasses this negative feedback leading to accumulation of porphyrins which can be activated with visible light (Fig. 1). Blue light is the most efficient waveband for porphyrin activation but red light is also often used as it penetrates deeper than blue light. Following this discovery, researchers experimented with several ALA derivatives including methylaminolevulinate (MAL)[3]. This ester of ALA also enters the heme biosynthetic pathway where it is transformed into porphyrins.

With the approval of ALA and MAL in several countries, photodynamic therapy is now a well established procedure in

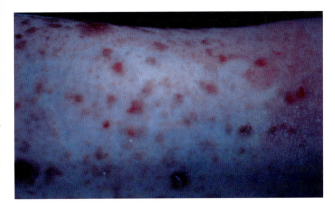

Fig. 1 Accumulation of porphyrins (*pink-red*) in basal cell carcinomas of a patient with Gorlin's syndrome 3 h after application of ALA. Photograph taken under Wood's lamp

R. Bissonnette
Innovaderm Research Inc., Montreal, Quebec, Canada
e-mail: rbissonnette@innovaderm.ca

Dermatology. Both drugs are approved to treat actinic keratoses (AK). In addition, MAL is approved in several countries, but not in the US, for the treatment of various types of non-melanoma skin cancers. Since the approval of MAL and ALA, physicians have successfully used these two photosensitizer precursors for the treatment of several other skin diseases and have combined them with different lasers, intense pulsed light and other non-coherent light sources for porphyrin activation.

Indications and Contraindications

Indications
Aminolevulinic acid: minimally to moderately thick actinic keratoses of the face and scalp
Methylaminolevulinate: non hypertrophic actinic keratoses of the face and scalp
PDT with MAL is approved in several countries, but not in the US, for the treatment of superficial basal cell carcinoma and Bowen's disease

Contraindications
Porphyria and sensitivity to visible light
Presence of invasive squamous cell carcinoma in the treatment field
Morpheiform basal cell carcinoma
Topical or systemic medications inducing visible light sensitivity
Allergy to MAL
Warning: MAL contains peanut oil

Indications

Aminolevulinic acid is approved in the US, Canada and Brazil for the treatment of minimally to moderately thick actinic keratosis of the face and scalp in combination with the Blu-U unit (Fig. 2). The original approval was for non-hypertrophic actinic keratoses. This has recently been changed to minimally to moderately thick AK at the FDA's request. In practice, this wording is similar and refers to the fact that PDT is not approved for thick and hypertrophic AKs. There are two issues related to treatment of hypertrophic AKs with PDT. The first is inadequate penetration of ALA through the hyperkeratotic portion of the lesion and the second is the possibility that some of the more hypertrophic

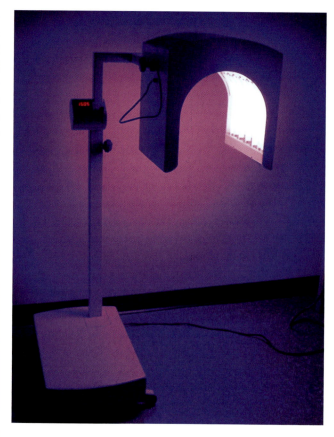

Fig. 2 Blu-U device. This non-coherent light source is approved for the treatment of actinic keratoses with ALA

lesions might be micro-invasive SCCs. The current approval is based on phase III studies where ALA was applied on visible lesions for 14–18 h followed by 10 J/cm^2 of blue light from a Blu-U unit.[4] However, in practice very few physicians use ALA-PDT with a 14–18 h incubation. Most will use a shorter incubation of 45 min to 2 h. This off label use is supported by a small pilot study which showed that incubation of 1–3 h in patients with extensive sun exposure leads to AK lesion cure rates that are similar to what has been reported with longer incubations in phase III studies.[5] Complete responses on BCC have been reported following ALA-PDT,[6] however the efficacy of ALA-PDT for the treatment of BCC has never been studied in multicenter phase III trials and the long term recurrence rates have not been well studied.

MAL is currently FDA-approved for the treatment of non hypertrophic actinic keratoses of the face and scalp in immunocompetent patients when used in conjunction with lesion preparation and when other therapies are considered medically less appropriate. AK cure rates following either a single MAL-PDT session repeated at 3 months if necessary or 2 MAL-PDT sessions performed 7 days apart have been reported to be around 90%.[7,8] Studies presented at meetings suggest that multiple large surface ALA or MAL PDT sessions can delay the appearance of new actinic keratoses in organ transplant patients. This suggests that large surface PDT may be able to prevent skin cancer.

Several countries have also granted approval of MAL-PDT for the treatment of various non-melanoma skin cancers. The indications vary from one country to another but in general most countries approved MAL-PDT for the treatment of Bowen's disease and superficial BCC when other therapies such as surgery are considered inappropriate.[9-11] The complete response rate of superficial BCC following MAL-PDT has been shown to be 97% and the 48-month long-term recurrence rate 22%.[12,13] The main advantage of PDT for the treatment of sBCC and Bowen's disease is the excellent cosmetic outcome as compared to surgery, cryotherapy or electrodessication and curettage.[6,9] Some countries have also approved MAL-PDT for thin nodular BCC, but because the cure rate is lower than with sBCC many countries have restricted their approval to sBCC. Recurrences for superficial BCCs, nodular BCCs and Bowen's disease usually occur during the first 2–3 years after therapy with no increase in recurrence between the third and the fifth year.

At the time this text was written, MAL was not yet commercially available in the US because the FDA approved MAL only in combination with the Curelight device, an earlier LED light source that is rather cumbersome. In most countries MAL is approved with the Aktilite (Fig. 3), a smaller and more convenient device. Studies comparing the efficacy of Curelight and Aktilite in the treatment of AK are currently being completed in the US. These studies should lead to FDA approval of MAL-PDT performed with the Aktilite device.

Initial studies conducted with PDT for skin diseases often used lasers. However, the current off-label trend with ALA-PDT is to use broad area application ALA or MAL in order to treat non-visible lesions, improve photoaging and eventually prevent the appearance of new lesions. This trend combined with the cost and limited availability of lasers in the 400–450 nm and 630–640 nm ranges has limited the use of lasers for PDT in Dermatology. When physicians are using ALA with a non-approved light source, they tend to favor LEDs or intense pulsed light. However, the pulsed dye laser at 595 nm has also been used for the treatment of actinic keratoses and acne.[14]

ALA and MAL have been reported to successfully treat various non oncologic skin conditions in small pilot studies or in single case reports. These include acne, sebaceous hyperplasia, hidradenitis suppurativa and photoaging.[14-19] MAL and ALA are both in phase II for the treatment of acne. A number of small controlled studies have shown that MAL and ALA can improve acne.[14,15,20,21] This is related in part to the intense accumulation of porphyrin in sebaceous glands following topical application of ALA and MAL (Fig. 4). Light exposure could induce partial necrosis of sebaceous glands and reduce sebum excretion thus reducing acne lesions. Preliminary findings with ALA suggest that this is one of the mechanisms of ALA-PDT when used for the treatment of acne.[22] Studies performed with PDT in acne are complicated by the fact that blue or red light alone can improve acne by elimination of propionibacterium acnes as these bacteria naturally accumulate porphyrins.[23] The best treatment parameters for acne are currently unknown. Most controlled studies which have shown good efficacy report a strong post PDT phototoxic reaction. Clinical photographs published in some of the articles which used MAL under occlusion for 3 h show moderate to severe erythema with crusting 1 day post-PDT. These publications report severe pain in many patients during light exposure.[15,21] Such a strong phototoxic reaction is probably not needed to see improvement in acne. However, it is possible that prolonged remission requires a certain degree of phototoxic reaction as necrosis of sebaceous gland tissue might be necessary. The current literature suggests that PDT for acne is more efficacious for patients with moderate to severe inflammatory acne.

Touma and colleagues have demonstrated that the use of ALA-PDT with a 1–3 h incubation followed by blue light exposure in patients with multiple actinic keratoses can improve photoaging.[5] Small wrinkles, pigmentation and

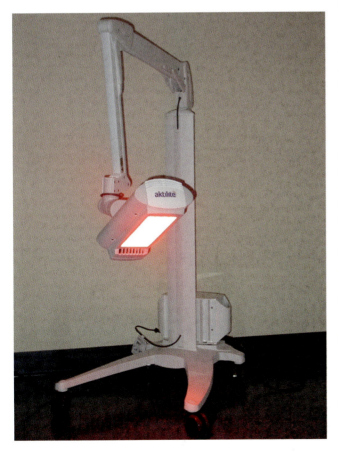

Fig. 3 Aktilite device. This LED light source is approved in several countries for the treatment of AK and/or Bowen's disease and/or superficial basal cell carcinoma with MAL

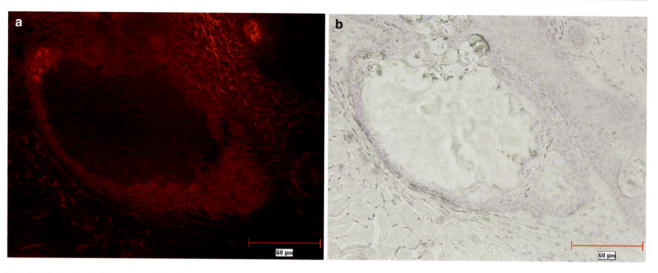

Fig. 4 (**a**) Porphyrin fluorescence in sebaceous glands 3 h after application of MAL. (**b**) Same section stained with hematoxylin

sallowness were the parameters best improved with ALA-PDT. ALA-PDT performed with IPL has also been shown to improve photoaging.[18,24] Small studies have also shown complete response in AKs treated with ALA and IPL.[24,25] There are currently a very wide variety of devices approved and used for the treatment of photoaging. Most physicians using ALA or MAL-PDT for photoaging either combine PDT with other devices and treatments or favor ALA or MAL-PDT for patients with actinic keratoses who would also like to have improvement in photoaging.

Contraindications

ALA and MAL are contraindicated in patients sensitive to visible light corresponding to the spectral output of the light source used (400–450 nm for Blu-U and 630–640 nm for Aktilite). Patients with porphyria and some patients with solar urticaria are also sensitive to visible light. ALA and MAL-PDT performed on patients using concomitant photosensitizing drugs such as phenothiazines, tetracyclines, thiazides and sulphonamide have not been thoroughly studied and could theoretically increase the phototoxic reaction seen after PDT. Current use of topical or systemic retinoids such as tretinoin, adapalene, acitretin or isotretinoin could also increase the phototoxic reaction. MAL contains peanut oil. It should not contain the protein allergen present in peanuts, but many physicians refrain from using MAL-PDT in patients allergic to peanuts.

Histological variants of BCCs that are at high risk of recurrence such as morpheiform BCC are a contraindication to PDT with MAL. Pigmented basal cell carcinoma is usually considered a contraindication to PDT as pigment limits light penetration. However several physicians have reported complete responses of pigmented BCCs with PDT.

Techniques

Pre-operative management

- Informed consent with emphasis on difficulty to predict phototoxic response
- Thorough examination of skin areas to be exposed to detect malignant lesions
- Consider herpes simplex prophylaxis

Description of the technique

- Skin preparation to enhance penetration (mandatory for MAL)
- Photosensitizer application
- Interval to allow porphyrin build-up
- Light exposure

Post operative management

- Sun avoidance
- Ferrous oxide containing sunscreen
- Moisturizer

Pre-operative Management

A complete skin examination of the areas to be treated is necessary. This is of the utmost importance when performing large surface PDT. This examination should focus on the identification of malignancies such as basal cell carcinoma, squamous cell carcinoma and melanoma. Sub-optimal treatment of these malignant lesions could lead to later, deeper recurrences. Any suspicious lesion should be biopsied. If PDT is performed to treat a malignant lesion such as BCC or Bowen's disease, a pre-treatment biopsy is recommended. A complete medical history including the existence of visible light sensitivity diseases such as porphyria or solar urticaria should be recorded. Patients should be asked about current use of any topical product on the areas to be treated. Products that can alter the stratum corneum such as topical retinoids can increase ALA and MAL penetration and create a more severe phototoxic reaction following PDT. The use of systemic treatments that increase visible light sensitivity such as St-John's wort should be avoided.

Patients should be well informed about the procedure including difficulty in predicting the phototoxic reaction generated by PDT. If only a few AKs or a single BCC are treated, the phototoxic reaction is usually not a problem. However a full face treatment can lead to erythema associated with tenderness and sometimes with focal areas of crusting. It is suggested to obtain a written informed consent which should mention this information as well as potential complications such as hyperpigmentation, hypopigmentation, scarring (mostly when treating basal cell carcinoma), sun and visible light sensitivity and prolonged erythema. Patients should be advised to bring a hat (when treating the face) or other pieces of clothing to cover the area to be treated.

The risks of triggering light sensitive recurrences of herpes labialis following PDT are currently unknown. For patients who experience recurrences following sun exposure, antiviral prophylaxis should be discussed.

Light exposure during PDT sometimes leads to an urticarial reaction immediately after PDT. This is more intense when red light is used and when large surfaces are exposed. This phenomenon has recently been attributed to histamine release by mastocytes and could be prevented by pre-treatment with antihistamines such as cetirizine.[26]

Description of the Technique

Treatment of Actinic Keratoses with ALA

A gentle curettage of keratotic AKs should be performed prior to ALA application. This is not included in the current product monograph but the author finds that this increases the clinical response of individual lesions, probably by increasing drug penetration. Skin preparation is suggested when performing short ALA incubations. The face can be washed vigorously with acetone or treated with microdermabrasion. Theses techniques are believed to increase ALA penetration through degreasing and/or partial removal of the stratum corneum.

Microdermabrasion can significantly reduce ALA incubation time.[27] Care should be taken to use the same technique with the same pre-treatment method and performed by the same person when treating a patient at different sessions as differences in skin preparation can have a dramatic impact on porphyrin buildup and therefore on the extent of the post-PDT phototoxic reaction.

ALA (Levulan) is available in the form of two glass vials inserted in a plastic tube that is covered by cardboard (Fig. 5). The two vials should be crushed with fingers and the stick shaken for about 3 min to ensure proper mixing of ALA powder and hydroalcoholic vehicle. ALA should be applied on all AKs present in the treatment area. Most physicians will also apply ALA on the entire face in order to treat non visible lesions and prevent new AKs. Broad area ALA application also has the advantage of improving signs of photoaging.[5] Care should be taken to avoid applying ALA too close to the eyes as inadvertently gets the hydroalcoholic solution will sting if it inadvertently gets into the eyes. Facial zones with more sebaceous glands, such as the nose and chin, often display a more important phototoxic reaction than the rest of the face when performing PDT. This is probably due to more intense accumulation of porphyrins in sebaceous glands. If ALA or MAL is applied on these zones during a full face treatment, patients should be told to expect a strong phototoxic reaction the day following light exposure. A delay of 45 min to 2 h is suggested between ALA application and light exposure when ALA-PDT is used on large skin surfaces for the treatment of AK. The intensity of the phototoxic reaction generated by ALA-PDT varies greatly from one patient to another and is highly dependent on the type of pre-treatment used. For patients with extensive photodamage and numerous ill defined AKs, a 45–60 min incubation is usually enough and will even sometimes lead to a severe phototoxic reaction post PDT. Some physicians prefer to perform the first treatment with a 30–45 min incubation time in these patients. The incubation time can be adjusted at subsequent treatments based on the phototoxic reaction and the clinical response observed.

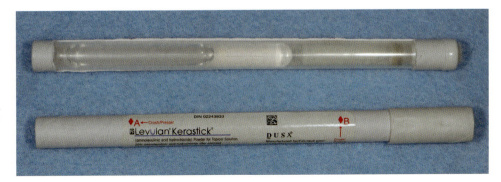

Fig. 5 ALA (Levulan Kerastick). The cardboard has been removed to show the 2 glass vials. Areas where pressure needs to be applied to crush the two glass vials are identified in *red*

After a proper incubation time, patients are placed inside the Blue-U device with their eyes protected with appropriate eyeshields as the blue light is very intense. As the U-shaped unit rotates, treatments can be performed with the patients sitting or lying down. The current product monograph recommends a light dose of 10 J/cm^2 of blue light which corresponds to an incubation time of 16 min 40 s. This was the fluence used in phase III, but a lower fluence is probably enough in most patients to completely photobleach porphyrins present in lesions. Many physicians use a shorter incubation time, but the efficacy of shorter incubation times has not been thoroughly studied in clinical trials.

Blue light exposure after ALA application generates a burning sensation that gradually increases to reach a plateau around 3–8 min and is followed by a gradual decrease. This decrease in burning sensation intensity corresponds to photoinactivation of porphyrins present in skin lesions. Blue light exposure is usually well tolerated by most patients if they have been properly warned about the sensation to expect during light exposure. An assistant should be present in the room during PDT, especially for the first PDT session, to reassure patients and to monitor the burning sensation. The assistant can use cool air, spray cool water or even temporarily interrupt light exposure if pain is too intense.

Treatment of BCC with MAL

A biopsy is suggested before treating a BCC with MAL-PDT. The purpose of the biopsy is to confirm the diagnosis and exclude histological subtypes, such as morpheiform BCCs, for which PDT is contraindicated. Gentle curettage of the lesion is mandatory before MAL application as 5 year cure rates for MAL-PDT have been established with pre-treatment curettage. Figure 6 shows a patient with multiple BCCs before and immediately after lesion preparation. MAL is provided in 2g tubes. Once opened the cream must be used within 7 days. This allows for treatment of more than one patient with the same tube or treatment of the same patient 7 days later with the same tube. MAL should be applied on the entire lesion to be treated plus a margin of 1 cm and should be occluded (with Opsite). Three hours later the occlusion is removed, the cream wiped out of the treatment field and the device (Aktilite) positioned at 5–8 cm from the skin. There is a risk of under treatment if the device is positioned beyond 8 cm as the head is flat and the irradiance varies according to the distance between skin and light source. The area where MAL has been applied should be exposed to 37 J/cm^2 (Aktilite device) of red light which corresponds to approximately 7 min and 30 s.

Post-operative Management

Excess ALA and MAL should be removed by thorough washing with tap water to prevent further porphyrin synthesis which would make the patient more sensitive to visible light. This is especially important when ALA or MAL has been applied to large areas such as the entire face. As patients are mostly sensitive to the visible part of the electromagnetic spectrum, the use of high SPF sunscreens does not provide adequate sun protection in the days following PDT. Patients can use a sunscreen containing inorganic sunscreening agents such as Avene 50 Compact which provides some (but not complete) protection.[28] Patients should avoid sun exposure or exposure to intense visible light such as surgical lighting or a high power dentist lamp for 2 days after PDT. Patients should avoid driving or walking under the sun on the day PDT is performed. They should also be reminded that there is significant visible light exposure even on cloudy days and through window glass. There is no visible light sensitivity beyond 2 days after PDT with ALA or MAL. However, patients should

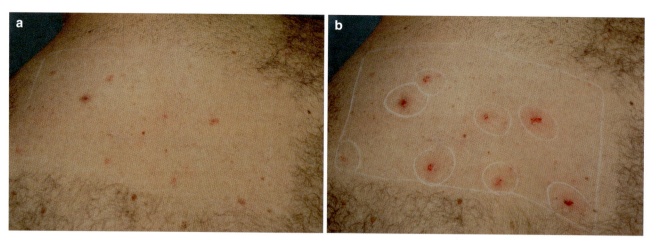

Fig. 6 Patient with multiple BCCs (Gorlin's syndrome) on the back before lesion preparation (**a**) and immediately after lesion preparation but before MAL application (**b**)

use a high SPF sunscreen providing adequate UVA protection to prevent hyperpigmentation. The use of Avene thermal water, a low mineral content water, after PDT has been shown to be superior to a higher mineral content water comparatively for decreasing post treatment pruritus.[29]

Crusting and erosions over AK and BCC is expected and desirable when treating malignant or pre-malignant lesions with PDT. Simple occlusion combined with the use of petrolatum jelly or an antibiotic ointment is usually all that is required to promote healing and to decrease pain. Regular use of a bland moisturizer is recommended. Patients should avoid any topical products containing urea, retinoic acid or other alpha hydroxyl acids, alcohol or propylene glycol in the days and weeks following PDT. Patients should be advised to call if the reaction increases beyond 2 days as this may be suggestive of bacterial infection or reactivation of extensive herpes simplex.

Adverse Events

Expected

- Erythema
- Burning sensation during light exposure
- Crusting on AKs and BCCs

Possible

- Pain after light exposure
- Hyperpigmentation
- Hypopigmentation
- Scarring by loss of substance (e.g., nodular basal cell carcinoma)
- Urticarial reaction on exposed area
- Prolonged erythema
- Cellulitis, impetigo
- Reactivation of herpes simplex

Side Effects/Complications

Most patients will report a burning sensation, pain or pruritus during light exposure. This is usually well tolerated. When large surfaces are treated with MAL or ALA, the use of water spray, fan or cold air (such as from a Zimmer device) can alleviate this sensation. Temporary interruption of light exposure is another alternative as the burning sensation subsides rapidly when the light device is turned off.

All patients should expect a phototoxic reaction after PDT. The absence of a phototoxic reaction on pre-malignant

or malignant lesions following PDT is usually a sign that the treatment will not be efficacious. The phototoxic reaction manifests itself primarily by erythema on exposed sites that can vary from mild to severe. This is usually associated with crusting on areas were AKs were present and sometimes associated with vesicles, pustules and/or erosions. Erythema and edema are often more severe when the lesion to be treated is located on the nose. This is probably related to the abundance of sebaceous glands on the nose. Tenderness is usually present for a few days after PDT. Whole face treatments are often associated with pain and tenderness that are exacerbated with pressure (contact with pillow when sleeping for example) and followed by desquamation.

Bacterial infections such as impetigo and/or cellulitis or reactivation of herpes simplex are possible but very rarely seen with ALA and MAL-PDT. PDT can induce hyperpigmentation on treated areas. This is rarely seen in patients with phototype I or II. Hypopigmentation is possible but rare. Scarring by loss of substance can be seen after treatment of lesions that invade the dermis such as nodular basal cell carcinoma.

A few cases of prolonged erythema have been reported following PDT on the face.[30] This phenomenon can sometimes last many months. In the author's experience, this is more frequent in patients with rosacea and usually fades over time.

Allergy to MAL has been reported and documented by patch testing.[31] Clinicians should think about this possibility in patients who have undergone several MAL-PDT treatments and present with a dermatitis type of reaction that was not present at previous treatments.

Prevention and Treatment of Side Effects/Complications

As discussed in the post operative management section, application of petrolatum jelly, a bland moisturizer or an antibiotic ointment will make the phototoxic reaction more tolerable.

Removal of MAL and ALA after PDT is important in order to reduce the continuous synthesis of porphyrin which increases post-treatment sensitivity to visible light. Patients should thoroughly wash their face with soap and water after light exposure. In a small pilot study where MAL was applied for 3 h under occlusion, porphyrin fluorescence was maximum at 1 h after cream removal but there was enough porphyrin present in the skin at 24 h after MAL application to induce a phototoxic reaction following light exposure in 6 out of 16 subjects.[32]

Patients must be warned to avoid sun exposure for 2 days after PDT. The use of a sunscreen containing the physical sunscreening agent iron oxide such as Avene Compact 50 is recommended during the first 2 days. Sun protection with a high SPF sunscreen with good UVA protection is also important during the weeks following PDT in order to prevent hyperpigmentation.

Future Directions

- Treatment of acne
- Treatment of sebaceous hyperplasia
- Treatment of hidradenitis suppurativa
- Prevention of skin cancer with larger surface PDT
- Development of new photosensitizers

PDT with ALA and/or MAL is now a well established treatment modality for actinic keratoses, basal cell carcinoma and/or Bowen's disease. Some studies have suggested that large surface ALA or MAL PDT could prevent AK and maybe even SCC. Further prevention studies are needed in patients with multiple AKs, SCCs and BCCs. There is evidence that PDT performed with these photosensitizers has good efficacy in the treatment of acne vulgaris and both are currently in phase II for this indication. Future studies should determine the best treatment parameters to obtain improvement in acne vulgaris while limiting the phototoxic reaction. Other areas where MAL and/or ALA PDT has shown promising efficacy include sebaceous hyperplasia and hidradenitis suppurativa.

New photosensitizers are also currently being studied in phase I/II for various skin diseases including acne and hair removal. This should lead to more dermatological applications for PDT in the coming years.

Conclusion

Photodynamic therapy with ALA and MAL is currently widely used for the treatment of actinic keratoses, superficial basal cell carcinoma and Bowen's disease. One of the main advantages of PDT for sBCC and Bowen's disease as compared to surgical interventions is the superior cosmetic outcome observed with PDT. For most indications, the use of a non-coherent light source is more convenient. For multiple AKs, a full face or large surface PDT treatment is associated with less downtime than topical 5-fluorouracil or imiquimod. Preliminary studies also suggest that large surface PDT can prevent actinic keratoses. Preventive treatments and treatment of non neoplastic skin diseases probably represents the future of PDT in Dermatology.

References

1. Taub AF. Photodynamic therapy for the treatment of acne: a pilot study. *J Drugs Dermatol*. 2004;3(6 Suppl):S10-S14.
2. Kennedy JC, Pottier RH, Pross DC. Photodynamic therapy with endogenous protoporphyrin IX: basic principles and present clinical experience. *J Photochem Photobiol B*. 1990;6(1–2):143-148.
3. Kloek J, Akkermans W, van Beijersbergen Henegouwen GM. Derivatives of 5-aminolevulinic acid for photodynamic therapy: enzymatic conversion into protoporphyrin. *Photochem Photobiol*. 1998;67(1):150-154.
4. Piacquadio DJ, Chen DM, Farber HF, et al. Photodynamic therapy with aminolevulinic acid topical solution and visible blue light in the treatment of multiple actinic keratoses of the face and scalp: investigator-blinded, phase 3, multicenter trials. *Arch Dermatol*. 2004;140(1):41-46.
5. Touma D, Yaar M, Whitehead S, et al. A trial of short incubation, broad-area photodynamic therapy for facial actinic keratoses and diffuse photodamage. *Arch Dermatol*. 2004;140(1):33-40.
6. Wang I, Bendsoe N, Klinteberg CA, et al. Photodynamic therapy vs. cryosurgery of basal cell carcinomas: results of a phase III clinical trial. *Br J Dermatol*. 2001;144(4):832-840.
7. Pariser DM, Lowe NJ, Stewart DM, et al. Photodynamic therapy with topical methyl aminolevulinate for actinic keratosis: results of a prospective randomized multicenter trial. *J Am Acad Dermatol*. 2003;48(2):227-232.
8. Tarstedt M, Rosdahl I, Berne B, et al. A randomized multicenter study to compare two treatment regimes of topical methyl aminolevulinate (Metvix)-PDT in actinic keratosis of the face and scalp. *Acta Derm Venereol*. 2005;85:424-428.
9. Horn M, Wolf P, Wulf HC, et al. Topical methyl aminolaevulinate photodynamic therapy in patients with basal cell carcinoma prone to complications and poor cosmetic outcome with conventional treatment. *Br J Dermatol*. 2003;149(6):1242-1249.
10. Rhodes LE, de Rie M, Enstrom Y, et al. Photodynamic therapy using topical methyl aminolevulinate vs surgery for nodular basal cell carcinoma: results of a multicenter randomized prospective trial. *Arch Dermatol*. 2004;140(1):17-23.
11. Vinciullo C, Elliott T, Francis D, et al. Photodynamic therapy with topical methyl aminolaevulinate for 'difficult-to-treat' basal cell carcinoma. *Br J Dermatol*. 2005;152(4):765-772.
12. Basset-Seguin N, Ibbotson SH, Emtestam L, et al. MAL-PDT versus cryotherapy in primary sBCC: results of 48-month follow up. *J Eur Acad Dermatol Venereol*. 2005;19(Suppl 2):237.
13. Basset-Seguin N, Ibbotson SH, Emtestam L, et al. MAL-PDT versus cryotherapy in primary sBCC: results of 36 months follow-up. *J Eur Acad Dermatol Venereol*. 2004;18(Suppl 2):412.
14. Alexiades-Armenakas M. Long-pulsed dye laser-mediated photodynamic therapy combined with topical therapy for mild to severe comedonal, inflammatory, or cystic acne. *J Drugs Dermatol*. 2006;5(1):45-55.
15. Wiegell SR, Wulf HC. Photodynamic therapy of acne vulgaris using methyl aminolaevulinate: a blinded, randomized, controlled trial. *Br J Dermatol*. 2006;154(5):969-976.
16. Gold M, Bridges TM, Bradshaw VL, et al. ALA-PDT and blue light therapy for hidradenitis suppurativa. *J Drugs Dermatol*. 2004;3 (1 Suppl):S32-S35.
17. Dover JS, Bhatia AC, Stewart B, et al. Topical 5-aminolevulinic acid combined with intense pulsed light in the treatment of photoaging. *Arch Dermatol*. 2005;141(10):1247-1252.
18. Alster TS, Tanzi EL, Welsh EC. Photorejuvenation of facial skin with topical 20% 5-aminolevulinic acid and intense pulsed light treatment: a split-face comparison study. *J Drugs Dermatol*. 2005;4(1):35-38.
19. Alster TS, Tanzi EL. Photodynamic therapy with topical aminolevulinic acid and pulsed dye laser irradiation for sebaceous hyperplasia. *J Drugs Dermatol*. 2003;2(5):501-504.

20. Horfelt C, Funk J, Frohm-Nilsson M, et al. Topical methyl aminolaevulinate photodynamic therapy for treatment of facial acne vulgaris: results of a randomized, controlled study. *Br J Dermatol.* 2006;155(3):608-613.

21. Wiegell SR, Wulf HC. Photodynamic therapy of acne vulgaris using 5-aminolevulinic acid versus methyl aminolevulinate. *J Am Acad Dermatol.* 2006;54(4):647-651.

22. Hongcharu W, Taylor CR, Chang Y, et al. Topical ALA-photodynamic therapy for the treatment of acne vulgaris. *J Investig Dermatol.* 2000;115(2):183-192.

23. Borelli C, Merk K, Schaller M, et al. In vivo porphyrin production by P. acnes in untreated acne patients and its modulation by acne treatment. *Acta Derm Venereol.* 2006;86(4):316-319.

24. Avram DK, Goldman MP. Effectiveness and safety of ALA-IPL in treating actinic keratoses and photodamage. *J Drugs Dermatol.* 2004;3(1 Suppl):S36-S39.

25. Gold MH, Bradshaw VL, Boring MM, et al. Split-face comparison of photodynamic therapy with 5-aminolevulinic acid and intense pulsed light versus intense pulsed light alone for photodamage. *Dermatol Surg.* 2006;32(6):795-801. Discussion 801-803.

26. Brooke RC, Sinha A, Sidhu MK, et al. Histamine is released following aminolevulinic acid-photodynamic therapy of human skin and mediates an aminolevulinic acid dose-related immediate inflammatory response. *J Invest Dermatol.* 2006;126(10):2296-2301.

27. Katz BE, Truong S, Maiwald DC, et al. Efficacy of microdermabrasion preceding ALA application in reducing the incubation time of ALA in laser PDT. *J Drugs Dermatol.* 2007;6(2):140-142.

28. Bissonnette R, Nigen S, Bolduc C, et al. Protection afforded by sunscreens containing inorganic sunscreening agents against blue light sensitivity induced by aminolevulinic acid. *Dermatol Surg.* 2008; 34(11):1469-1476.

29. Goldman MP, Merial-Kieny C, Nocera T, et al. Comparative benefit of two thermal spring waters after photodynamic therapy procedure. *J Cosmet Dermatol.* 2007;6(1):31-35.

30. Misra A, Maybury K, Eltigani TA. Late erythema after photodynamic therapy to the face. *Plast Reconstr Surg.* 2006;117(7):2522-2523.

31. Harries MJ, Street G, Gilmour E, et al. Allergic contact dermatitis to methyl aminolevulinate (Metvix) cream used in photodynamic therapy. *Photodermatol Photoimmunol Photomed.* 2007;23(1):35-36.

32. Angell-Petersen E, Christensen C, Muller CR, et al. Phototoxic reaction and porphyrin fluorescence in skin after topical application of methyl aminolaevulinate. *Br J Dermatol.* 2007;156(2):301-307.

.

Light-Emitting Diode Phototherapy in Dermatological Practice

R. Glen Calderhead

Introduction

- Phototherapy is not new! It was being used more than 4,000 years ago
- Light-emitting diodes have attracted interest as a phototherapeutic source
- LEDs are solid state and robust
- LEDs are comparatively inexpensive

History of Phototherapy

Phototherapy in its broadest sense means any kind of treatment (from the Greek *therapeia* 'curing, healing,' from *therapeuein* 'to cure, treat.') with any kind of light (from the Greek *phos, photos* 'light'). The modern accepted definition of phototherapy, however, has become accepted as: "the use of low incident levels of light energy to achieve an athermal and atraumatic, but clinically useful, effect in tissue". Under its basic original definition, phototherapy is an ancient art because the oldest light source in the world is the sun, and therapy with sunlight, or heliotherapy, has been in use for over 4,000 years with the earliest recorded use being by the Ancient Egyptians.[1] They would treat what was probably vitiligo by rubbing the affected area with a crushed herb similar to parsley, then expose the treated area to sunlight. The photosensitizing properties of the parsley caused an intense photoreaction in the skin leading to a very nasty sunburn, which in turn hopefully led to the appearance of postinflammatory secondary hyperpigmentation, or 'suntan' thereby repigmenting the depigmented area. In their turn the Ancient Greeks and Romans used the healing power of the sun, and it

was still being actively used in Europe in the eighteenth, nineteenth and early twentieth century, particularly red light therapy carried out with the patient placed in a room with red-tinted windows. One famous patient was King George III of Great Britain and Northern Ireland who ruled from 1760 to 1801, popularly though erroneously known as 'Mad King George'. We now strongly suspect that he was actually suffering from the blood disease porphyria, so being shut in a room with red-draped walls and red tinted windows to treat his depression probably only served to make him even more mad, since porphyria is often associated with severe photosensitivity! Entities treated this way included the eruptive skin lesions of rubella and rubeola, and even 'melancholia', as was the case with King George III, now recognised as clinical depression. Hippocrates, the Father of Medicine, certainly concurred with the latter application some two millennia before King George: Hippocrates prescribed sunlight for depressive patients and believed that the Greeks were more naturally cheerier than their northern neighbors because of the greater exposure to the sun.

In the field of wavelength-specific phototherapy research, red light therapy was examined at a cellular level under the newly-invented microscope by Fubini and colleagues in the late eighteenth century,[2] who were able to show that visible red light, provided *via* lenses and filters from sunlight, selectively activated the respiratory component of cellular mitochondria. There is nothing new under the sun. However, the sun is a fickle medical tool, particularly in northern Europe, and modern phototherapy as we know it started around the turn of the last century with Finsen's electric arc lamp-based system, giving phototherapy at the turn of a switch, independent of the sun.[3] However, apart from the use of blue light therapy for neonatal bilirubinemia which continues to the present day, phototherapy was, in the majority of its applications, overtaken in the first part of the twentieth century by better medication or improved treatment techniques.

The development of the first laser systems, a race which was narrowly won by Theodore Maiman in 1960 with his flashlamp-pumped ruby-based laser, next gave clinicians and researchers a completely different and unique light source to play with. In the 4 years between 1960 and 1964, the ruby laser

R.G. Calderhead
Japan Phototherapy Laboratory, Tsugamachi, Tochigi-ken, Japan
e-mail: docrgc@cc9.ne.jp

K. Nouri (ed.), *Lasers in Dermatology and Medicine*,
DOI: 10.1007/978-0-85729-281-0_19, © Springer-Verlag London Limited 2011

was followed by the argon, helium-neon (HeNe), neodymium: yttrium-aluminum-garnet (Nd:YAG) and carbon dioxide (CO_2) lasers all of which have remained as workhorses in the medical field, and the HeNe laser (632.8 nm) has in fact provided a large bulk of the phototherapy literature over the last three decades. As for light-emitting diodes (LEDs), the first light from a semiconductor was produced in 1907 by the British experimenter H. J. Round. Independently in the mid 1920s, noncoherent infrared light was produced from a semiconductor (diode) by O-V Losev in Russia. These studies were published in Russia, Germany and the UK, but their work was completely ignored in the USA.[4] It was not till 1962 that the first practical and commercially-available visible-spectrum (633 nm, red) LED was developed in the USA by Holonyak, regarded as the 'Father of the LED' while working with the General Electric Company. In the next few years, LEDs delivering other visible wavelengths were produced, with powers ten times or more that of Holonyak's original LED. For reasons which will be discussed later, these LEDs were really inappropriate as therapeutic sources, although they were extremely bright and very cheap compared with laser diodes, and it was not till the late 1990s that a new generation of extremely powerful, quasimonochromatic LEDs was developed by Whelan and colleagues as a spin-off from the National Aeronautic and Space Administration (NASA) Space Medicine Program.[5] Unlike their cheap and cheerful predecessors, the so-called 'NASA LEDs' finally offered clinicians and researchers a new and truly practical therapeutic tool.[6]

The What and Why of LEDs

What Is an LED?

Light-emitting diodes belong to the solid state device family known as semiconductors. These are devices which fall somewhere between an electrical conductor and an insulator, although when no electrical current is applied to a semiconductor, it has almost the same properties as an insulator. Simply explained, light-emitting semiconductors or diodes consist of negative (N-type) and positive (P-type) materials, which are 'doped' with specific impurities to produce the desired wavelength. The n-area contains electrons in their ground or resting state, and the p-area contains positively charged 'holes', both of which remain more or less stationary (Fig. 1a–c). When a direct current electric potential with the correct polarity is applied to an LED, the electrons in the N-area are boosted to a higher energy state, and they and the holes in the P-area start to move towards each other (Fig. 1d), meeting at the N/P junction where the negatively-charged electrons are attracted into the positively-charged holes. The electrons then return to their resting energy state and, in doing

so, emit their stored energy in the form of a photon, a particle of light energy (Fig. 1e). The wavelength emitted is noncoherent, ideally very narrow-band, and depends on both the materials from which the LED is constructed, the substrates, and the p-n junction gap. Table 1 shows a list of the main substrates and associated colors. Figure 2 shows the anatomy of a typical dome-type LED. These can be mounted on circuit boards at regular and precise distances from each other to provide an LED array, part of which is shown in Fig. 3. However, the latest generation of LEDs actually form part of the board (so-called 'on-board' chips) which are much more compact than the dome-type LED and more efficient.

What Is the Difference Between LEDs and Lasers or IPLs?

The laser is a unique form of light energy, possessing the three qualities of monochromaticity, collimation and phase which make up the overall property of 'coherence'. Monochromaticity means all the photons are of exactly the same wavelength or color; collimation means the built-in parallel quality of the beam superimposed by the conditions of the laser resonator; and phase means that all of the photons march along together exactly equidistant from each other in time and in space. Laser diodes do not have inherent collimation, but because they are still true lasers, and therefore a so-called point source, the light can be gathered and optically collimated: the humble but ubiquitous laser pointer works on this principle. Intense pulsed light is, on the other hand, totally noncoherent, with a very large range of polychromatic (multicolored) light from near infrared all the way down to blue; has no possibility of collimation with extreme divergence; and has its vast variety of photons totally out of phase. The new generation of LEDs, on the other hand, has an output plus or minus a few nanometers of the rated wavelength, and so are classed as quasimonochromatic; some form of optical collimation can be imposed on the photons which are divergent but do have some directionality; but they are not in phase. Laser energy can easily produce high photon intensity per unit area, IPLs much less so, but provided LEDs are correctly arrayed, they are capable of almost laser-like incident intensities. Figure 4 schematically illustrates the differences between lasers, IPLs and LEDs. In short, LEDs for therapeutic applications must be quasimonochromatic, be capable of targeting wavelength-specific cells or materials, have stable output, and be able to deliver clinically useful photon intensities.

Why Use LEDs?

There are many excellent laser and intense pulsed light (IPL) systems available to the dermatologist. Why should LEDs be

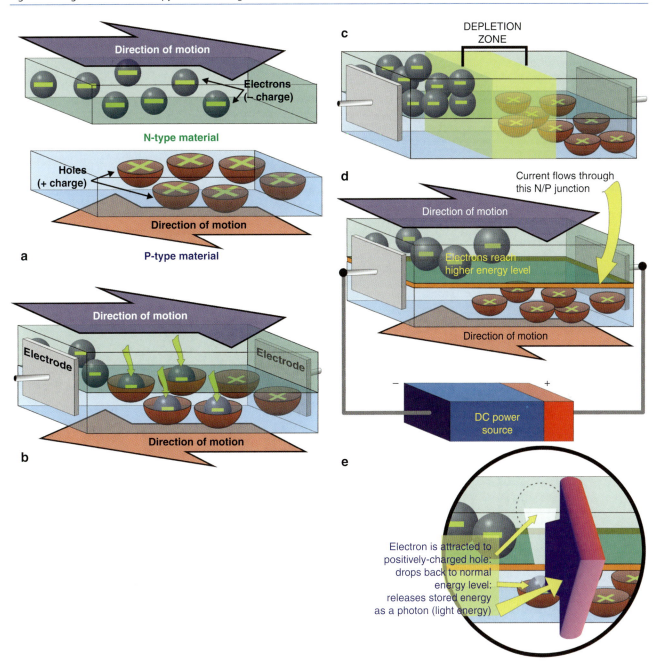

Fig. 1 What is an LED and how can it produce light? (**a**) An LED is basically composed of two materials, the N-type or negative material and the P-type or positive material. The N-material contains negatively charged electrons which move as shown, and the P-material contains positively charged holes, which move in the opposite direction. When the materials are apart and not connected to any power source, movement continues, so both materials are conductors. (**b**) When the materials are sandwiched together, however, without any power applied to the electrodes attached to opposite ends, the negatively charged electrons in the center of the chip are attracted to the holes, and form an area called the depletion layer as seen in (**c**) and all movement ceases in both the N- and P-materials: the chip is now an insulator. (**d**) Power is applied to the electrodes, with the positive electrode or anode at the origin of movement of the holes and the negative electrode or cathode at the origin of movement of the electrons. Observing the polarity when connecting a direct current (DC) power source is extremely important. Power flows through the junction between the materials, called the N/P junction, and movement of both electrons and holes starts again, but with power applied the electrons move to a higher energy level from their ground or resting state. (**e**) As in 1b above, the N-electrons are attracted to the P-holes, but in moving down through the N/P junction they must return to their ground energy level, and lose their extra stored energy in the form of a photon, the smallest packet of light energy. Unlike the situation in 1b, however, when power is applied this action continues endlessly and no depletion layer is formed. The N- and P-materials are 'doped' with other materials which determine the distance of the 'fall' between electrons and holes: the greater the distance the electrons have to fall, the higher is the energy level of the photons emitted. Photons with high energy levels have shorter wavelengths than those with lower energy levels, thus the wavelengths of the emitted light are determined by the materials and their doping. High quality N- and P-materials and pure doping substances will give photons of very nearly the same wavelength, i.e., quasimonochromatic light

Table 1 Most common substrate combinations and the colors they are capable of producing

Substrates	Formula	Colors produced
Aluminum gallium arsenide	(AlGaAs)	Red, infrared
Aluminum gallium phosphide	(AlGaP)	Green
Aluminum gallium indium phosphide	(AlGaInP)	Green, yellow, orange, orange-red(all high-intensity)
Gallium arsenide phosphide	(GaAsP)	Yellow, orange, orange-red, red
Gallium phosphide	(GaP)	Green, yellow, red
Gallium nitride	(GaN)	Blue, green, pure green (emerald green): also white (if it has an AlGaN Quantum Barrier, so-called 'white light' LED)
Indium gallium nitride	(InGaN)	Near ultraviolet, blue, bluish-green

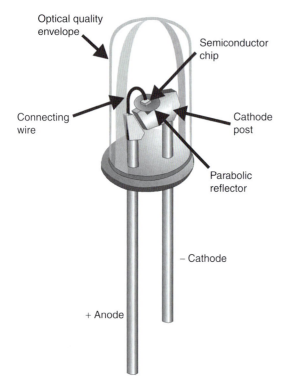

Fig. 2 Anatomy of a typical high-quality dome-type LED. The cathode is always shorter than the anode and there is a flat surface in the base of the LED by the cathode so polarity is clearly determined when connecting to a DC power source. On top of the cathode post and forming part of the negative electrode of the LED chip is a parabolic reflector in which the chip itself is mounted thus ensuring as much light as possible is directed forwards, with a consistent angle of divergence, typically 60° steradian or less depending on the specifications of the LED. A fine wire connects the positive electrode of the chip to the anode post, thus completing the circuit. The entire assembly is encapsulated in an optical quality clear plastic envelope, giving the final assembly its robust nature

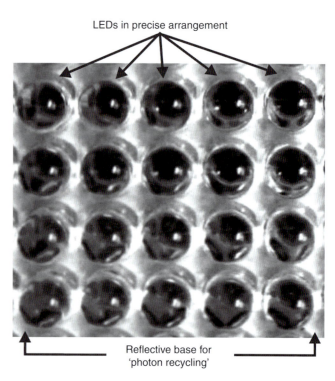

Fig. 3 Close-up view of dome-type LEDs mounted in an actual array from a therapeutic system. Note the precise x-y spacing of the LEDs, (cf Fig. 6 and associated text), and the reflective backing into which they are mounted. When light is incident on living skin, a certain amount will be reflected from the outer layer of skin, the stratum corneum. The longer the wavelength, the greater this reflection will be. In addition, some light is always back-scattered out of skin. The purpose of the reflective backing of the array is to capture these photons and reflect them back into the skin, known as 'photon recycling'

considered as a viable alternative phototherapy source? The main reasons are efficiency and price. The electricity-light conversion ratio of a typical laser is very low, requiring 100 or even 1,000 of watts in to give an output of a few watts. The same applies to IPL systems, where the flashlamp has to be pumped with enormous amounts of energy to provide polychromatic light, which may however be filtered (cut-on or cut-off). Even when filtered, IPL energy is delivered over a waveband rather than at a specific wavelength. In the case of LEDs, which are quasimonochromatic and require no filtering, the conversion efficiency is very high so that very few watts at a low voltage are required to produce a clinically useful output. LEDs are much less expensive than even laser diodes. Depending on quality and wavelength, anywhere from 300 new-generation LEDs can be purchased for the cost of a single laser diode. The cost of laser and IPL systems

Light-Emitting Diode Phototherapy in Dermatological Practice

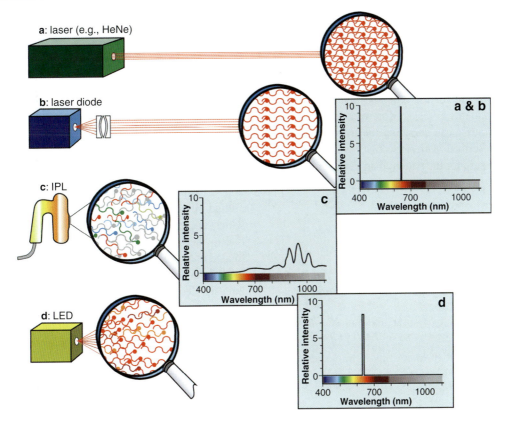

Fig. 4 Comparison among the output characteristics of a laser, laser diode, intense pulsed light system and a new generation LED. (**a**) A laser emits all of its energy at one precise wavelength, in a coherent beam, i.e., monochromatic, collimated and with the photons all in phase both temporally and spatially. If a 'special magnifying glass' could view the beam, it would show the picture as seen in the figure. All of the energy is delivered at a precise wavelength, as illustrated in the spectrogram, so the relative intensity of the beam is extremely high. (**b**) A laser diode has all the characteristics of a laser, except that the beam is divergent, without collimation. However, because it is a point source the beam can be collimated with condensing optics. The magnified view of the beam shows a lower photon intensity than the laser, but the relative intensity is still very high. (**c**) An IPL system emits a pulse of broad-band polychromatic noncoherent light, so the 'magnifying glass' would show a plethora of widely divergent photons of many different wavelengths, but with the majority in the near infrared as seen from the spectrogram. Because of the very broad waveband, the relative intensity at any given wavelength is low to very low. (**d**) The LED is somewhat similar to the laser diode, but the light is noncoherent, highly divergent and quasi-monochromatic. The 'magnifying glass' shows plenty of photons, mostly the same color, with some degree of directionality but without the true collimation and phase associated with the laser diode. The relative intensity is still very high, however, because the vast majority of the photons are being delivered at the nominal wavelength with a very narrow waveband of plus or minus a very few nanometers

is very high, so a much cheaper LED-based system offers the possibility to halt the ever-upward spiralling costs of health care for both the clinicians and their patients. A further advantage is the solid state nature of LEDs. There are no filaments to be heated up, and no flashlamps are required to produce light or to pump the laser medium: LEDs thus run much cooler than their extremely higher-powered cousins, so less is required in the way of dedicated cooling systems, again helping to reduce the cost. However, some cooling of LEDs is still required, especially when LEDs are mounted in multiple arrays, because as the temperature of an LED increases, its output will move away from the rated wavelength. When wavelength cell- or target-specificity is required, this could be a major problem. The solid state nature of LEDs also makes them much more robust than either lasers or IPL systems, so they tend to be able to take the sometimes not-so-gentle handling which is part of a busy clinical practice without causing either output power loss or alignment problems. Finally, LEDs can be mounted in flat panel arrays, which may in turn be joined together in a treatment head which can be adjustable to fit the contour of the large area of tissue being treated, whether it is the face, an arm, the chest or back, or a leg. Compare this potentially very large treatment area of some 100 of square centimeters with that of a laser, usually a very few millimeters in diameter, or that of an IPL treatment head, typically 1 cm × 3 cm, and the clinician-intensive nature of the latter two is quickly evident when large areas are to be treated such as the entire face. Multiple shots are required, and the handpiece has to be manually applied and controlled by the user. The LED-based treatment head can be attached to an articulated arm to make individual adjustment even easier. Heads with different wavelengths can be designed to be easily interchangeable, controlled by the same base unit. With 'set-it-and-forget-it' microprocessor-controlled technology, the clinician simply sets the head up over the area to be treated, following the manufacturer's recommendations, turns the system on, and he or she can then leave the patient for the requisite treatment time and attend to other patients or tasks. Moreover, in many cases a suitably trained nurse can carry out the treatment once the clinician has prescribed it, because LED systems are much more inherently safe for the patient than lasers or IPLs.

Basics of Light-Tissue Interaction

- Light-emitting diodes provide athermal and atraumatic photoactivation
- LEDs are a viable and valuable phototherapeutic tool
- LEDs are capable of interesting light-tissue interactions, provided certain criteria are met. The most important criteria are:
  - Wavelength.
    Determines both the target and the depth at which the target can be reached
    Quasimonochromaticity is essential
    Wavelengths should be applied separately and sequentially, and not combined at the same time
  - Photon density.
    Gives suitably high intensity at all levels of target cells or materials
    Ensures sufficient athermal energy transfer to raise targets' action potentials
  - Dosimetry.
    Provided the wavelength and intensity are appropriate, correct dosage obtains the optimum effect with the shortest irradiation time
  - Temporal beam profile.
    Continuous wave would appear to be more efficient for most cell types *in vivo*, compared with 'pulsed' (frequency modulated) light

The main purpose of using phototherapy is to achieve some kind of clinical reaction in the target tissue through the use of light energy. If the incident power is high, heat will be the end product as with the surgical laser. If a too-low photon intensity is delivered, there will be very little or no reaction. The trick in LED phototherapy is to deliver just the right amount of photon intensity to achieve the desired clinical effect but in an athermal and atraumatic manner.

Photothermal and Athermal Reactions

Despite their very different output powers, lasers, IPLs and LEDs all depend on the 'L' which is found in all their names, standing for 'light'. It could be said that they are all different facets of the same coin, but even in photosurgery, phototherapy plays a very important role. If we consider the typical beam pattern of a surgical CO_2 laser in tissue, we see the range of temperature-dependent bioeffects as illustrated schematically in Fig. 5, ranging from carbonization above 200°C, vaporization above 100°C, through coagulation around 60–85°C, all the way down to photobiomodulation, which occurs atraumatically when there is no appreciable rise in the tissue temperature at the very perimeter of the treated area. These effects occur virtually simultaneously as the light energy propagates into the target tissue with photon intensity decreasing with depth, and can be divided as shown into varying degrees of photosurgical destruction and reversible photodamage, and athermal, atraumatic photobiomodulation. The zones are also shown in a typical CO_2 laser specimen stained with hematoxylin and eosin (Fig. 5).

Laser surgery involves all zones, but the importance of the photobiomodulative zone cannot be stressed enough. It is the existence of this zone which sets laser surgery apart from any other thermally-dependent treatment, such as electrosurgery, or even athermal incision with the conventional scalpel, and it is the photoactivated cells in this zone which provided the results that interested the early adopters of the surgical laser compared with the cold scalpel or electrosurgery, namely better healing with less inflammation and much less postoperative pain. IPL systems, and so-called nonablative lasers, produce areas of deliberate but controlled coagulative damage beneath a cooled and intact epidermis (Fig. 6), however they also produce the photobiomodulative zone to help achieve the desired effect of neocollagenesis and neoelastinogenesis through the wound healing process in the dermal extracellular matrix (ECM). LED-based phototherapy systems, on the other hand, deliver only athermal and atraumatic effects, but are still capable of inducing the wound healing process almost as efficiently as IPLs and nonablative lasers, as will be shown in detail in a later section.

Wavelength and Its Importance

The first law of photobiology, the Grotthus-Draper Law, states that only energy which is absorbed in a target can produce a photochemical or photophysical reaction. However, any such reaction is not an automatic consequence of energy absorption. It may be simply converted into heat, as in the surgical and non-ablative lasers or IPL systems, or re-emitted at a different wavelength (fluorescence). The prime arbitrator of this

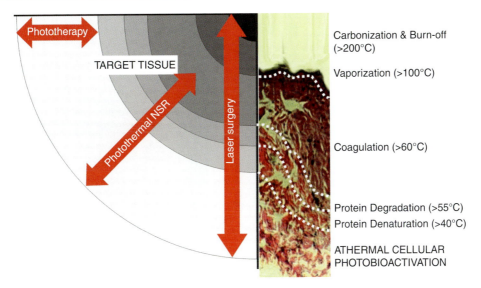

Fig. 5 Range of photothermal and athermal photobioreactions in tissue following a typical surgical laser impact, e.g., a CO_2 laser. A hematoxylin and eosin stained specimen of actual CO_2 laser treated skin is also included to show the typical histopathological changes for each of the bioreactions: the epidermis has been totally vaporized leaving a layer of carbon char above the coagulated dermis. The outermost layer, the photobioactivation layer, shows normal tissue architecture, even though some photons will have reached this layer and transferred their energy to the cells in an athermal and atraumatic manner. Laser surgery involves all levels of bioreactions. Photothermal nonablative skin rejuvenation (NSR) delivers controlled coagulative photothermal damage, with all the subsequent layers, whereas phototherapy only delivers athermal and atraumatic photobioactivation

'no absorption-no reaction' precept is not the output power of the incident photons, but their *wavelength*, and this comprises two important considerations: wavelength specificity of the target, or the target chromophore; and the depth of the target. Based on these two considerations, the wavelength must not only be appropriate for the chosen chromophore, but it must also penetrate deeply enough to reach enough of the target chromophores with a high enough photon density to induce the desired reaction. In theory, a single photon can activate a cell, but in actual practice multiple photon absorption is required to achieve the desired degree of reaction.

Phototherapy is athermal and atraumatic, hence achieving selective photothermolysis is of no concern as it would be for surgical or other photothermal applications. On the contrary, penetration of light into living tissue is, however, extremely important in phototherapy, and very frequently displays characteristics which are often in discord with results produced by mathematical models, a point often totally ignored by some researchers. A favorite, but photobiologically false, axiom beloved of phototherapy opponents, is that 'all light is absorbed within the first millimeter of tissue'. Anyone who has shone a red laser pointer through their finger, transilluminating the entire fingertip and completely visible on the other side, has already disproved that statement. A totally different finding is seen with green or yellow laser pointers, however. Figure 7 is based on a transmission photospectrogram of a human hand captured *in vivo* over the waveband from 500 nm (visible blue/green) to 1,100 nm in the near infrared.[7] The photospectrometer generator was positioned above the hand, delivering a 'flat spectrum' of 'white light', and the recorder placed beneath it. The wavelength is shown along the *x*-axis, and the calculated optical density (OD) is on the *y*-axis, from lower ODs to higher. The higher the OD, the greater is the absorption of incident light, and hence the lower the transmission, or penetration depth into the tissue. It must also be remembered that the OD is not an arithmetic but a logarithmic progression, so that the difference between an OD of 4 and one of 6 is not simply 2, but 2 *orders of magnitude*, i.e. a factor of 100.

From 500 to 595 nm (blue-green to yellow), the OD was from 8.2 to approximately 7.6, respectively, resulting in poor penetration. At 633 nm, the approximate wavelength of the HeNe laser, the photobiological efficacy of which is well recorded, the OD was approximately 4.5. In other words, red light at 633 nm penetrated living human tissue by 3 orders of magnitude better than yellow at 595 nm, because of the pigment-specific absorption characteristics of the two wavelengths. Visible yellow at 595 nm is at the peak of the oxyhemoglobin absorption curve, and is also much higher absorbed in epidermal melanin than 633 nm, which is why the yellow light in the spectrogram did not penetrate at all well into the tissue due to competing chromophores of epidermal melanin and superficial dermal blood. Accordingly, cellular and other targets in the mid to deep reticular dermis are inaccessible to yellow light with sufficient photon intensities to achieve multiple photon absorption in the target cells. The deepest penetration was achieved at 820–840 nm

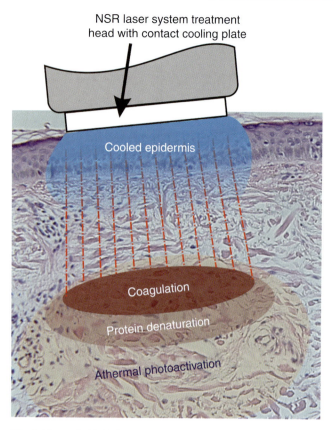

Fig. 6 Theory behind photothermal nonablative skin rejuvenation: the laser energy passes through the cooled epidermis without harming it, and delivers a controlled area of coagulation in the typically elastotic dermis associated with photoaged skin. However, the photons do not stop there, and there are zones of protein denaturation and, most importantly for the good result, athermal and atraumatic photoactivation around and beyond the controlled thermal damage. The photoactivated cells in the last of these three zones will assist with the wound healing process

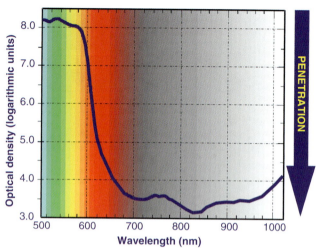

Fig. 7 Photospectrogram of a human hand *in vivo*. The generator, delivering uniform 'white light' at the waveband shown on the x-axis, was placed above the hand and the sensor below the hand. Optical density on the y-axis is shown in logarithmic units. Penetration is shown on the right-hand axis. The further down the curve reaches, the better the penetration at that wavelength into living human tissue (Adapted from Smith[7])

in the near infrared. At this waveband, pigment is not a primary chromophore with proteinous targets as the major chromophore, and this 820–830 nm waveband coincides with the bottom of the water absorption curve. The most successful of the laser diode systems used in laser therapy as distinct to laser surgery, or low level laser therapy (LLLT) as it was also known, delivered a wavelength of 830 nm for this very reason,[8] and was shown to penetrate living hands, and even bone, very successfully.[9] After around 1,000 nm, water absorption once again starts to play a significant role, and in the curve in Fig. 2 the OD was seen to increase thereafter. In general, shorter visible wavelengths penetrate less than longer visible and near IR wavelengths, up to a given waveband, depending on the absorbing chromophore.

Following these findings, it made a great deal of sense to source LEDs for LED systems at wavelengths already tried, tested and proven in the more than three decades of laser therapy application and research, so LED systems delivering 633 nm or thereabout in the visible red and 830 nm in the near infrared, and at high enough photon densities, have been reported as having significant effects on their target tissues at a good range of depths well into the mid and even the deep reticular dermis. The usefulness of visible red and near IR LED phototherapy has already been reported in a wide range of medical specialties, including dermatology. Yellow light at 590–595 nm has also attracted attention, but the penetration properties of yellow light must be carefully considered, as illustrated *in vivo* in Fig. 7. From the standpoint of photobiological theory, yellow light has very good potential specificity in a number of subcellular and haematological targets, such as cytochrome-c oxidase, however its poor penetration into the intermediate and deeper dermis, where cellular targets such as fibroblasts lie, limits the practical efficacy of yellow light in living tissue. Blue light at around 415 nm has very interesting properties regarding the eradication of the bacterium *Propionibacterium acnes* (*P. acnes*) although the photoreaction is different and will be discussed later in the chapter. LED systems with many other wavelengths have been produced, but basically they have very little or no published work to back up the claims of the manufacturers. 'Any old LED will not do' is an axiom which must be borne in mind by the dermatologist wishing to incorporate LED phototherapy into his or her practice.

Finally, the different wavebands, visible light and invisible infrared light, have different primary mechanisms. Absorption of visible light photons at appropriate levels induces a photochemical reaction, and a primary photochemical cascade occurs within the cell, usually instigated by specific components in the respiratory chain of the mitochondria, the adenosine triphosphate-producing power-houses of the cell.[10] Infrared photons, on the other hand, are primarily involved in photophysical reactions which occur in the cell membrane, changing the rotational and vibrational characteristics of the membrane molecules. Through subsequent activation of the various membrane-located transport mechanisms, such as the Na^{++}/Ca^{++} and Na^{++}/K^{++} pumps and changes in the cell permeability, changes occur in the chemical and osmotic balance in the cytosol, finally resulting in the induction of a secondary chemical cascade which gives more or less the same endpoint as the visible light photons, namely cellular activation or proliferation.[11] These photoreactions are illustrated schematically in Fig. 8.

To sum up, the wavelength of a therapeutic source therefore has a double importance, namely to ensure absorption of the incident photons in the target chromophores, and to be able to do so at the depths at which these chromophores exist. The waveband in which the wavelength of the incident photons is located determines not only which part of the cell is the target, but also the primary photoaction. Wavelength is thus probably the single most important consideration in LED phototherapy, because without absorption, there can be no reaction.

Photon Density

Light energy travels in the form of photons. It is obvious that the more photons are incident per unit area of tissue, the greater will be the bioeffect. This incident photon intensity is called the power density, or irradiance, of a beam of light. The power density (PD) is an extremely important factor, following wavelength, and is calculated using the following formula:

$$PD = \frac{OP}{TA} \ (W/cm^2)$$

where OP is the output power incident on the target in watts (W) and TA is the irradiated area in square centimeters (cm^2). PD is usually expressed in watts per square centimeter (W/cm^2) or milliwatts (mW)/cm^2. It is the power density of a beam that will determine more than anything else (apart from wavelength) the magnitude of the bioeffect in the target tissue. Consider Table 2, where a laser with a constant incident output power of

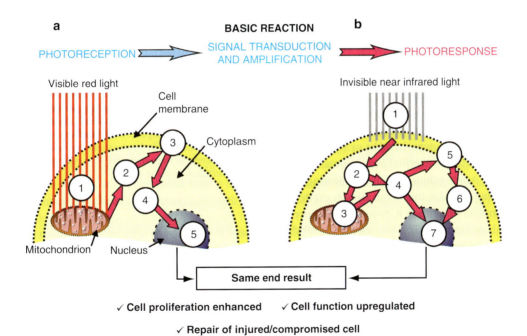

Fig. 8 Schematic depicting photoreception (absorption) of light in a cell, and the subsequent wavelength-specific response. The basic reaction as defined by Karu is absorption, which is followed by signal transduction and amplification within the cytosol, and leads to the photoresponse. (**a**) (1): Visible red light induces a primary photochemical cascade initiated in the mitochondrion, the energy factory and cell power house, which results in increased levels of nicotinamide adenine dinucleotide (NAD) extremely important in a wide range of redox (reduction-oxidation) reactions, one of the results of which is the generation of adenosine triphosphate (ATP) which is the 'gasoline' for the cell. (2): The increased levels of cytoplasmic ATP fuel the membrane transport pumps, the $Na^{++}K^{++}$ and $Ca^{++}K^{++}$ pumps (3) which induce extra- and intracellulation of messenger Ca^{++} ions and protons (H^+) which are elementary particles carrying a positive electric charge, the flow of which is used to generate energy from ATP via ATPase. Cytoplasmic levels of Ca^{++} ions and H^+ dramatically increase. (4) This in turn upregulates intracellular signaling including mRNA production from ribosomes on the rough endoplasmic reticulum, and finally (5) nuclear activity is also up regulated. (**b**) In the case of near infrared light, the primary mechanism of absorption is completely different (1) resulting in a photophysical reaction which changes the energy levels of the cell membrane, in which near IR energy is absorbed. This kick-starts the $Na^{++}K^{++}$ and $Ca^{++}K^{++}$ pumps so that cytoplasmic levels of Ca^{++} and H^+ dramatically increase (2) and (4), prompting the mitochondrion to manufacture more ATP to fuel the increased energy requirement (3), thereby raising cytoplasmic levels of ATP (4) which again impacts on the transport mechanisms of the membrane not affected by the near IR light. Despite the totally different pathways, the end result is however the same as in the case of visible light, namely further cyclic increased energy levels in the cytoplasm (6) and upregulation of nuclear activity (7)

The most interesting point in both studies was that the improvement obtained after the final treatment session, which ranged from 50% to 60% clearance of inflammatory lesions, continued to improve up to 12 weeks after the final treatment with no other therapeutic intervention, reaching from 83% to 90% clearance, and if extrapolated beyond the trial period would have in many patients reached 100%, which from personal communication with the authors of both papers, it in fact did. Figure 16 is a graphic representation of the inflammation reduction curves of the two referenced papers.

No secondary hyperpigmentation was seen in any patients in both studies, which is of particular interest in the Asian skin type. In addition, overall skin condition was subjectively assessed to have improved, and in the case of the Asian population, skin lightening was objectively shown across the population with an instrumental assay. Figure 17 shows examples of the treatment efficacy courtesy of the authors of the papers. At 6 months after the final session, recurrences in both trial centers were extremely few and mild, easily treated with another regimen of the blue/red LED therapy (David Goldberg and Celine SY Lee, personal communication).

As with all approaches not involving excisional surgery, there will always be a small percentage of patients in whom light-only LED phototherapy for acne vulgaris will have disappointing results, but from the above studies the overall efficacy is high enough to warrant applying this approach as the primary treatment of choice. Sequential combination LED phototherapy for acne can be combined with other approaches with even better results and improved maintenance, provided none of these involves any kind of photosensitizing agents, any of which have the potential to create painful and possibly severe side effects. The validity of the addition of a third LED wavelength to the current protocol, namely near infrared at 830 nm with its own unique cellular and tissue targets, is currently being assessed in ongoing clinical studies.

Skin Rejuvenation

Skin rejuvenation and antiageing have become very 'hot' topics. Excessive skin exposure to solar UVA and UVB brings about damaging morphological and metabolic changes in the epidermis and dermal extracellular matrix (ECM), combining with and accelerating the effects of chronological ageing and resulting in the lax, dull and wrinkled appearance of 'old' skin. Oxidative stressors such as singlet oxygen are photochemically generated following absorption of UV radiation in the ECM and damage the matrix integrity with elevated levels of the matrix metalloproteinases (MMPs) 1 and 2, formerly known as collagenase and gelatinase; elastotic damage to the underlying connective tissue occurs, with interstitial spaces appearing in a poorly-organized matrix; the viscosity and quality of the ECM ground substance glycosaminoglycans is reduced; and an inflammatory infiltrate can be identified. As this damage is cause by light, an elegant concept to use the power of light to reverse the damage led to the application of lasers, usually the CO_2 or/and the Er:YAG, in what became known as ablative laser resurfacing. Although still regarded as the 'gold standard' in the rejuvenation of

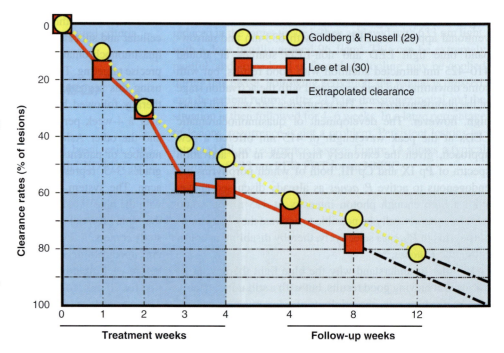

Fig. 16 Inflammatory lesion clearance rates following the blue/red combination LED phototherapy for acne adapted from the studies by Goldberg and Russell[29] and Lee et al.[30] The Goldberg study had a 12-week follow-up after the final treatment, i.e. 16 weeks from baseline, whereas the Lee study had an 8-week follow-up (12 weeks from baseline). However, by extrapolating the clearance rates in both studies, which were clearly linear in nature, the continued improvement is evident. No other therapy was used in either study. The system used was the Omnilux® fitted with the blue™ and revive™ heads

Fig. 17 Representative examples from the Goldberg and Lee studies on light-only combination blue/red LED phototherapy for inflammatory acne. (**a**) Cystic acne at baseline in a 21-year-old female, skin phototype II, from the Goldberg and Russel series. (**b**) Six weeks after the final treatment session (10 weeks from baseline). Excellent clearance and very good cosmesis. Photographs courtesy of Bruce Russell MD. (**c**) Inflammatory acne on the cheek and jaw line of a 19-year-old Korean male patient from the Lee series, skin type IV. (**d**) Eight weeks after the final treatment session (12 weeks from baseline). Good clearance with no secondary hyperpigmentation, a major problem in the Asian skin. The remaining small areas of redness will fade with time (Photographs courtesy of SY Celine Lee MD. Same system used in both trials as in Fig. 16)

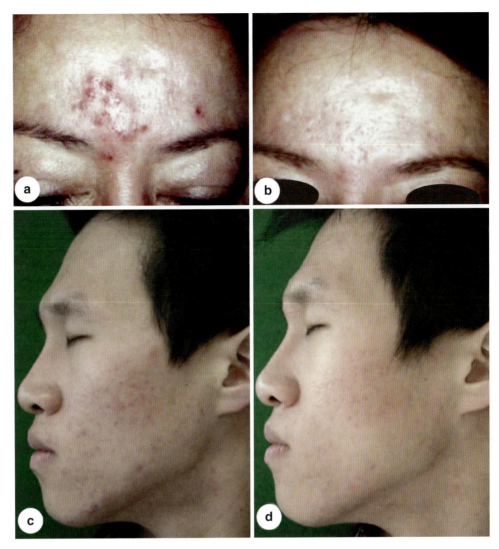

severely photoaged skin in general and wrinkles in particular, the possibly severe side effects and a prolonged patient downtime of up to several months associated with this approach drastically reduced its popularity.

To attempt to overcome these problems, so-called nonablative resurfacing was developed using specially adapted laser or intense pulse light sources. The theory was to deliver a controlled zone of deliberate photothermal damage beneath an intact epidermis, so that the wound-healing processes, including collagenesis and remodeling, could occur under the undamaged epidermis, thereby obtaining rejuvenation of the skin without any patient downtime and was popularized as the 'lunch-break rejuvenation'. The theory was good, but in clinical practice patient satisfaction was very low,[31,32] because the good dermal neocollagenesis seen in post-treatment histological analysis was not reflected in a 'younger' epidermis.[33] In an attempt to bridge this gap between ablative and pure nonablative rejuvenation, so-called fractionated or fractional technology was developed whereby many spots of almost grossly invisible epidermal and dermal 'microdamage' were delivered via a scanner or 'stamp-type' head, all surrounded by normal epidermis and dermis to obtain swift reepithelialization and dermal wound healing.[34] Unfortunately, once again the clinical results were not satisfactory to the majority of patients, with good dermal neocollagenesis not being echoed in the epidermis. In both the nonablative laser/IPL and the first generation of fractional technologies, the big problem was that what the patient first sees when looking in a mirror is the *epidermis*, not the dermis. It does not matter to the patient (or her friends) that her dermis is wonderfully better organized if her epidermis remains unchanged, what the author refers to as the SOE syndrome – 'same old epidermis'. Recognizing this, manufacturers of the more recent second generation of fractional systems have returned to the orginal ablative wavelengths, the CO_2 and the Er:YAG, in addition to newer media such as Er-doped fiber, to deliver fractionated microbeams that visibly damage the skin, with a recognizable amount of erythema and some edema post-treatment.

This in some way takes us back towards our gold standard of ablative resurfacing, as once again heat deposition, combined with controlled epidermal damage, becomes a pivotal consideration to achieve the ideal rejuvenation results on a patient-by-patient basis.[35] This approach has been much more successful from the patient satisfaction criterion, although at the cost of a little downtime, because it is involving the epidermis more than the previous nonablative and fractional approaches.

In the meantime, other clinical researchers were wondering if there was a role for LED phototherapy in skin rejuvenation, and the first approach was to use a lower strength of topically-applied 5-ALA activated with 633 nm LED in LED PDT.[36] The results were good, but begged the question as to why more damage, and indeed some pain, should be inflicted to treat what was essentially comparatively mild skin damage. One approach has been to deliver the 5-ALA at very low concentrations (<2%) via liposomes and activate the target tissue using intense pulsed light, achieving complete quenching of the porphyrins and thus avoiding the side effect of residual photosensitivity.[37,38] Because of its totally noninvasive, athermal and atraumatic nature, light-only LED phototherapy for skin rejuvenation has also attracted attention first with a single wavelength system in the visible yellow,[39] but once again a sequential combination technique proved more effective than the single wavelength just as was the case with LED phototherapy for acne.[40,41] The wavelengths used for LED skin rejuvenation have been near IR at 830 nm applied first, followed by 633 nm 72 h later, repeated over 4 weeks. The reasons for these wavelengths and the order in which they are applied are photobiologically based on the precepts of the wound healing cycle, and will be covered in some detail in the next subsection dedicated to wound healing. Both of these wavelengths involve the mother keratinocytes in the basal layer of the epidermis, however, in addition to the target dermal cells, with beneficial effects to both the cellularity and organization of the epidermis, but with no heat and no damage.

Lee and colleagues, in the first and only really detailed controlled study in the peer-reviewed literature, which was published in the very prestigious *Journal of Photochemistry and Photobiology (B)*,[42] compared LED skin rejuvenation in a total of 76 patients randomly assigned to four groups: 830 nm LED therapy on its own, 633 nm LED therapy on its own, the combination therapy with 830 nm and 633 nm and a sham irradiated group. All patients were treated hemifacially, so there was intrapatient as well as intergroup controls. In addition to clinical photography and subjective patient assessment, Dr Lee tested the results with profilometry and instrumental measurement of skin melanin and elasticity. She also carried out histological, immunohistochemical and biochemical assays. She found that wrinkles and skin elasticity were best improved in the 830 nm-treated groups,

skin lightening was best in the 633 nm group, so the combination of the two wavelengths was able to achieve the best overall efficacy and high patient satisfaction with the results, with statistical significance seen between all treated groups and the sham-irradiated controls, and a statistically significant improvement between the treated and occluded sides in all of the experimental groups, but not in the sham irradiated group. The clinical photography was backed up by the histological findings for both collagenesis and elastinogenesis, which was proved to take place in all dermal layers down to the deep reticular dermis. No MMP activity was noted, and on the contrary the levels of tissue inhibitors of MMPs (TIMPs) one and two were significantly elevated in all treatment groups, suggesting a photoprotective effect against degradation of the newly-formed extracellular matrix. This was an excellent and thorough study, and the author recommends the reader to get hold of it and read it, all 17 pages of it. It will go a long way to convincing even the most skeptical of the real efficacy of combination LED skin rejuvenation, backed up with real science. An even more recent discussion on the 830 nm/633 nm LED combination has appeared in Viewpoint 3 (Trelles, Mordon and Calderhead) and Comment three (Goldberg) in an article on redressing UV-mediated skin damage in Volume 17 of *Experimental Dermatology*.[43] The wavelengths and systems that have been reported in the five studies cited above are 595 nm (Gentlewaves®, Light Bioscience, VA, USA)[39] and the 830 nm/633 nm combination (Omnilux® plus™ and revive™, respectively: Photo Therapeutics, Fazeley, UK, and Carlsbad, CA, USA).[40-43] Figure 18 shows examples of the efficacy of light-only combination LED skin rejuvenation, including histological findings from the Lee study demonstrating photorejuvenation of both the dermis and epidermis at only 2 weeks after the final treatment session: as remodeling progresses, these histological results will become even better. The important point is the epidermis also shows improved morphology and not just the dermis, thus avoiding the SOE (same old epidermis) syndrome which was the major problem with photothermal nonablative skin rejuvenation. As with LED phototherapy for acne, adjunctive complementary treatment and maintenance techniques will certainly improve the good results consistently shown for light-only LED skin rejuvenation in these studies.

Wound Healing

Wound healing underpins all applications of LED phototherapy involving photon absorption therapy (PAT), and plays a major role in obtaining good cosmetic results in combination LED PDT/PAT for the treatment of acne, and in LED skin rejuvenation, in addition to the treatment of traumatic

Light-Emitting Diode Phototherapy in Dermatological Practice 251

Fig. 18 Representative examples of combination near IR/red light-only LED skin rejuvenation. (**a**) A 29-year-old female, skin type II, at baseline: note the mild rosacea on her cheek. (**b**) The result at 6 weeks after the final treatment session (10 weeks from baseline). Smoothing of the periocular wrinkles can be seen, with overall better skin tone. The rosacea has almost gone. Photographs courtesy of Bruce Russell MD.[40] **c:** Baseline findings in a 26-year-old Korean female, skin type IV. (**d**) Result 12 weeks after the final treatment session. Excellent removal of the fine 'crow's feet' wrinkles and overall improvement and lightening of the skin tone. (**e**) Histological findings at baseline, showing a typical elastotic dermis under a thinned epidermis with a highly disorganized stratum corneum. (**f**) Histology at only 2 weeks after the final treatment session. Note the much better-organized dermal collagen, extending down into the deeper reticular dermis, and the highly visible Grenz layer running under and attached to the basement membrane at the dermoepidermal junction. The epidermis is much thicker with good cellularity and a very well-delineated stratum corneum. (Hematoxylin and eosin, original magnification ×200) (Photographs and photomicrographs courtesy of SY Celine Lee MD.[42] The system used in both studies was the Omnilux® with the plus™ (830 nm) and revive™ (633 nm) heads)

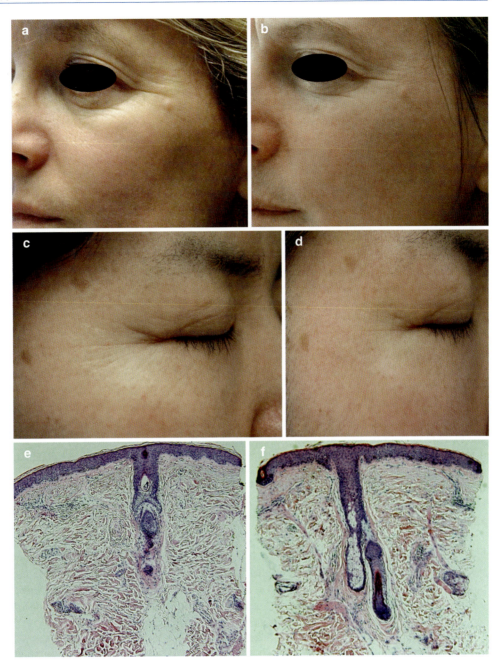

or post-surgical wounds themselves. A brief overview of the wound healing process is therefore warranted. Three distinct phases make up the wound healing process, namely inflammation, proliferation and remodeling, and although they are distinguished by their timing and cellular components, there is always some degree of overlap between them.

The Three Stages of Wound Healing

Inflammation is often regarded as a major problem, but in the wound healing process it is absolutely essential that inflammation occurs before proceeding into the proliferative phase. Inflammation only becomes a problem when it is out of control, such as the end product of the vicious circle instigated by *P. acnes* and rogue t-cells in acne vulgaris.

In the inflammatory phase, from wounding until about day 3–5, mast cells (already present or recruited through chemotaxis), macrophages (already present, recruited or differentiated from monocytes or pericytes) and neutrophils (recruited or differentiated from hematopoietic stem cells) peak in the wound and surrounding tissue. The macrophages ensure that all debris and detritus from the wound are removed through engulfment and internalization, and the leukocytes are the first line of defence of the autoimmune system against invading pathogens. When they are at work, the macrophages release an important trophic factor, fibroblast growth factor (FGF), and leukocytes are associated with TGFα and β (transformational growth factor). Connective tissue mast cells are granule-filled cells differentiated from CD34-expressing bone marrow precursors which circulate in the ECM till they mature *in situ*, found normally around capillaries and arterioles. Their part in the wound healing process is to release their granules into the ECM. Although the majority of the granules are proinflammatory, which are amongst the first to be released, the later granules contain antiinflammatory chemokines and cytokines, chemotactic factors to recruit more wound-healing cells to the area, and the most powerful antioxidant endogenous to our bodies, superoxide dismutase (SOD). In fact, the mast cell was first described and named by the German physiologist Paul Ehrilch in the latter part of the 1800s. Mistakenly believing that the purpose of the granules was to nourish the ECM, he called the cells '*mastzellen*', (German for 'feeding cells'), giving us our Anglicized version. The combined efforts of the inflammatory stage cells thus leave the ECM in an ideal and favorable condition for the proliferative stage cells.

In the proliferative stage, from around day 4 to day 21, as the inflammatory stage cells decrease in number, fibroblasts and endotheliocytes peak. Fibroblasts, (already in the area or differentiated from pericytes), are an extremely important multifunctional cell. They are not only responsible for synthesizing collagen to replace damaged ECM collagen fibers, but they also produce new elastin to form elastic fibers and additionally manufacture the ground substance, the glycosaminoglycans and glycoproteinous viscous gel-like liquid which lubricates and hydrates the ECM, and which also facilitates intercellular signalling. It is also their task to maintain ECM morphological integrity through constantly monitoring the state of the collagen and elastic fibers, lying along which they can often be seen. In this respect, the quality of both proliferative wound repair and the final wound appearance rests firmly on the back of the fibroblast. Endotheliocytes, (already present in the wound or differentiated from endothelial progenitor cells) clump together to start the neovasculogenesis process, culminating in the repair of damaged blood vessels and production of new blood vessels to oxygenate the newly-forming ECM and provide essential nutrients. From a peak at around day 12–18, the increased number of fibroblasts and endotheliocytes gradually returns by day 20–22 to the pre-wound baseline, leaving the ECM in a regenerated state with newly formed clumps of collagen and elastin fibers, a fresh supply of glycosaminoglycans and well-vascularized.

In the final and much longer stage of the wound healing process, remodeling, which starts around day 19–23, these new fibers and structures gradually mature and are slowly reorganized into better alignment to give a strong, flexible and resilient ECM under an epidermis firmed and tightened by the Grenz layer of collagen fibers running under and attached to the dermoepidermal junction basement membrane. One of the transformational cells of great importance in this phase is the myofibroblast, fibroblasts with smooth muscles at each end of their longitudinal axis. These cells lie along the newly-formed collagen fibres and exert force on them to bring them into good linear alignment. The remodeling process can take up to 6 months, or even longer, to complete, and this is important when thinking of patient education regarding when they can anticipate the final optimal appearance of their treated tissue. Once they have completed their task, the myofibroblasts enter apoptosis and die off, whereas the excess fibroblasts differentiate into quiescent fibrocytes. Figure 19 illustrates in schematic form the time course of the wound healing process, showing the peaks and lows of the cells associated with each of the three phases.

The Influence of Different Wavelengths of Light on the Wound Healing Cells

When we consider LED phototherapy, it is very tempting to go ahead and invent 'new' wavelengths for 'new' photoprocesses. It must never be forgotten that LLLT, laser therapy, has a rich and well-documented history which extends back over the last three decades, so by examining this wealth of published literature it should be possible not to have to reinvent the wheel all over again. Sadly, because the US Food and Drug Administration did not grant 510k approval to a laser therapy system in the process erroneously called 'biostimulation' until 2002, there is not a lot to be found in the US literature until more recently. However, those early US papers which are there, have been quietly forgotten, probably on the principle that if one doesn't understand it, one simply ignores it.

A great deal of literature exists on red light-cell reactions, because the mainstay light source of the early pre-LED investigators was the HeNe laser, delivering 632.8 nm, basically the same as the 633 nm of current array-based LED systems, also in continuous wave (C/W) rather than frequency modulated as discussed already. As mentioned in the Introduction, the effect of red light specifically on subcellular organelles was first published by Fubini and colleagues in the late eighteenth century! The last three decades, however, have added tremendously to the knowledge regarding red light and skin cells. It was reported that 633 nm red light from the HeNe laser induces fibroblast monosheet formation *in vitro* faster and with much better alignment, almost double the speed of the unirradiated controls.[44] Furthermore, a 'wound' created in the monosheet was repaired much faster in the HeNe-irradiated groups. More recent *in vivo* work

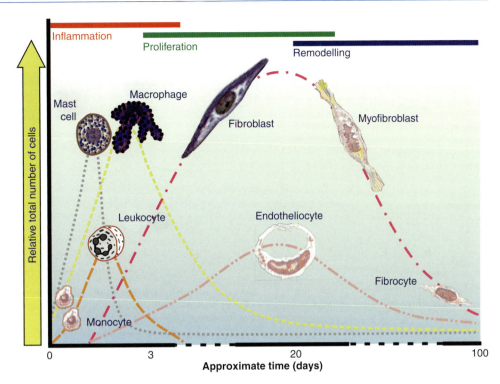

Fig. 19 Schematic illustration of the cell cycles and numbers during the 3 phases of wound healing. During inflammation, which occurs from day zero to day 3–5, the inflammatory cells (leukocytes, mast cells and macrophages) increase in number, peak and then return to baseline levels. During proliferation, the collagen-producing cells, fibroblasts, and neovascularization cells, endotheliocytes, increase in number, and then as remodeling starts, gradually decrease. In the case of fibroblasts, some remain as active fibroblasts, but some transform into myofibroblasts, literally fibroblasts with muscles, whose task is to ensure good linear alignment of the new collagen fibres. It should be noted that the phases overlap, with no clear border between each

with 633 nm LED energy in human subjects demonstrated dramatic fibroplasic changes in specimens from irradiated subjects compared with unirradiated controls.[45] Tiina Karu, probably the most well-known living photobiologist, has produced an enormous amount of work in her lifetime on the effects of low incident levels of light on cells and their organelles. She confirmed the much earlier work by Fubini and further identified the specific target for 633 nm light as the cytochrome-c oxidase resident at the end of the mitochondrial respiratory chain.[46] She also showed that coherent light was not essential to achieve effects *in vivo*, provided the photon intensity at the target was high enough. Mast cells have been stimulated *in vitro* and *in vivo* to degranulate when irradiated with 633 nm light, and much faster than when unirradiated: stimulation with 830 nm speeds up degranulation even more.[47,48] The author has very recently shown that, 48 h after a single irradiation with 830 nm LED energy, mast cells in the forearms of healthy human subjects had almost 50–70% degranulated compared with specimens from unirradiated controls, where no degranulation was seen at all (Unpublished data). Near IR energy at 830 nm stimulates macrophages to perform their chemotactic, phagocytic and internalizing functions better and faster, while releasing almost 30-fold the amount of fibroblast growth factor (FGF) compared with unirradiated controls,[49] and the same is true for neutrophils.[50,51] The epidermal basal layer keratinocyte is too often forgotten in LED phototherapy, but research has shown that both 633 and 830 nm noncoherent light both *in vitro* and *in vivo* can activate the keratinocytes to release a large amount of cytokines which drop down into the dermis to assist with the dermal wound healing processes, so much so that keratinocytes have been nicknamed 'cytocytes'.[52] Additionally, the photoactivated keratinocytes can improve the cellularity and organization of the epidermal strata, with a better organized stratum corneum.[42]

If the wound healing cells, including epidermal keratinocytes, are examined for increased wavelength-specific action potential based on the last 30 years of both LLLT and non-laser light source literature, the results could be presented as in Table 4. The wavelengths which have the most verified and published results at a cellular and subcellular level are 633 and 830 nm in the near IR, but very importantly they do not have the same efficacy in the same cell types. Near IR at 830 has excellent results in activating the activity levels of the inflammatory stage cells, mast cells, macrophages and neutrophils, in addition to epidermal keratinocytes. On the other hand, red at 633 nm is best for photoactivating fibroblasts *in vivo*, due to its superior penetrating powers compared with 595 nm yellow, and epidermal keratinocytes. This is why the skin rejuvenation protocol was set to start always with 830 nm and then, 48–72 h later, 633 nm, because of the specific cellular targets and their temporal appearance in the wound healing process, because with LED therapy at these wavelengths, although there is no wound, exactly the same response is achieved as seen after any examples of the nonablative photothermal damage approach.

The data displayed in this table can also help to explain why the 830 nm/633 nm combination is effective for skin

Table 4 Phototherapeutic wavelength-specific actions in raising the action potentials of dermal and epidermal cells specifically associated with wound healing and skin rejuvenation. All results are for low incident power densities (15 mW/cm² to 1.0 W/cm²) and a range of doses (2–60 J/cm²) delivered in continuous wave with the exception of the yellow waveband which is a frequency modulated (so-called 'pulsed') beam and 904 nm which is from a true pulsed diode laser. Many of these studies in the 633 and 830 nm rows have also been replicated *in vivo* with LED energy

Nominal wavelength (nm)	Wound healing phase/cell types and action level					
	Inflammation			Proliferation	Remodeling	All
	Mast	Neutro	Macro	Fibro	Fibro-Myo	Keratino
590–595	?	?	?	+++[a]	?	?
633	++[a,b]	+[a]	++[a]	+++[a,b]	±	+++[a,b]
670	?	?	++[a]	++[a]	?	?
790	++[a]	?	?	++[a]	?	?
830	+++[a,b]	+++[a]	+++[a]	+[a]	+++[b]	+++[a,b]
904	–	?	±[a]	–	–	?
1,064	?	?	?	+[b]	?	?
10,600	?	?	?	++[b]	?	?

[a] *in vitro* studies;
[b] *in vivo* studies; *Mast* mast cells, *Neutro* neutrophils, *Macro* macrophages, *Fibro* fibroblasts, *Fibro-Myo* fibroblast to myofibroblast transformation, *Keratino* keratinocytes. Degree of action potential: +++, very high; ++, high; +, some; ± little or none; –, retardation; ?, unknown

rejuvenation, even though it is not wound healing *per se*. The 830 nm energy first degranulates the mast cells, dumping a load of proinflammatory substances into normal tissue, such as heparin, trypsin, histamine and bradykinin. This gives the tissue the impression that it has been 'wounded', even though there is actually no wound because of the athermal and atraumatic action of LED phototherapy. Macrophages are also photoactivated, helping to give a clean ECM 'seeded' with FGF, with some TGF released from neutrophils recruited into the area by the degranulating mast cells. Because the inflammatory stage has been established especially by this mast cell-mediated 'quasi-wounding', the tissue has no option but to proceed into the next stages of the wound repair process, starting with proliferation in which 633 nm has its best effect on fibroblasts. When this 830 nm/633 nm sequence of irradiation is repeated over 4 weeks, separated each week by 2–3 days, the dermal cells (and epidermal keratinocytes) are upregulated in a step-wise manner and maintained in the inflammatory/proliferative stages. After the final treatment session the remodeling is allowed to start, and this explains why the best results are not seen at this immediately post-treatment stage, but later on at 4, 8 and 12 weeks or more after the final treatment, as was the case in the acne and skin rejuvenation studies already mentioned.[29,30,42]

The same sequential wavelength principle applies to frank wound healing, whether it is accidental or iatrogenic trauma. Burns, for example, are an ideal injury for LED phototherapy, because of the noncontact and hands-free application, and the large area of the treatment heads. In a recent study, the 830 nm/633 nm combination produced excellent results in large area burns, as illustrated in Fig. 20.[53] As mentioned already above, ablative laser resurfacing lost popularity due to the potential of serious side effects, especially edema and prolonged erythema, leading to prolonged patient downtime.

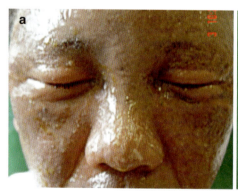 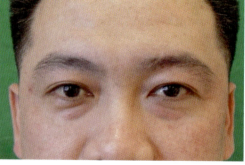

Fig. 20 A 39-year-old male patient with severe full facial electric spark burn injury before (**a**) and 3 months after the final treatment with combination 830 nm/633 nm LED phototherapy. One full 4 week session was performed with the wavelengths being sequentially applied as usual, a resting period of 4 weeks, and then another 4-week regimen (Photographs courtesy of Prof Jin-wang Kim MD PhD, Burns Center, Haelym University School of Medicine, Seoul, Korea. System used: Omnilux® with the plus™ (830 nm) and revive™ (633 nm) heads)

The wound left following laser ablative resurfacing is simply a full facial burn. In a recent publication Trelles and co-workers used the 830 nm/633 nm combination LED therapy following laser ablation of the face with a combined Er:YAG/CO_2 laser system.[54] There were two groups of patients, 30 in each group. The experimental group received the LED therapy following laser ablative treatment, and the control group received sham treatment from the standby setting of the 633 nm head only. The average healing times (full reepithelization and resolution of erythema) for the control and experimental groups were 13 weeks and 6 weeks respectively. The extent of post-procedure pain, bruising and erythema was significantly less for the LED-treated group (60.1%, 72.3% and 59.7%, respectively), whereas improvement in the skin condition was much more clearly seen in the LED-treated group, with a satisfaction index (SI) of 89% compared with 51% for the control group. The SI was calculated by adding only the number of 'excellent' and 'very good' scores from a standardized 5-element scoring system, and expressing the result as a percentage of the total population. Healing following upper blepharoplasty and periocular laser resurfacing in a hemifacial study was reported to be cut by one-half to one-third following LED therapy at 633 nm, and the improvement was subjectively rated as 2–4-fold better compared with the unirradiated side.[55] LED treatment (830 nm/633 nm) following Er:YAG laser ablation of deep and extensive plantar warts roughly halved the healing time, cut the postoperative pain by at least one-tenth and gave less than 6% recurrence rate in 121 cases.[56] Long-term nonhealing ulcers which healed following low incident levels of red light (HeNe laser, 633 nm) was the first subject to appear in the literature from the Godfather of phototherapy, the late Prof. Endre Mester of Semmelweis University, Budapest, Hungary, and started all the controversy surrounding LLLT in the early 70s.[57] Very interestingly, Mester reported that ulcers on the limb contralateral to the one treated also eventually healed, although more slowly than the irradiated wounds. This was the first report on the systemic theory in phototherapy, whereby photoproducts created in the irradiated tissue were carried systemically through the body to have an effect wherever they were required. More recent studies with 830 nm showed even quicker healing of recalcitrant crural ulcers.[58] Near IR 830 nm does not only work in soft tissue wounds, but also in bone where it accelerates the union of fractures, even in the case of delayed union healing, replacing the usual poorly-organized callus with better-quality bone so that the remodeling stage is much shorter.[59,60]

Some of the mechanisms behind the efficacy of LED phototherapy-accelerated wound healing at the appropriate wavelength have already been at least partly elucidated, such as the wavelength-specific activation of the dermal and epidermal cells associated with the three phases of wound healing. Karu has suggested that the latency effect of phototherapy in cells actually continues in subsequent generations of the irradiated cells in a chapter of her latest book (*Ten Lectures on Basic Science of Laser Phototherapy*, 2007, Prima Books AB, Grängesberg, Sweden), which is an important consideration in skin rejuvenation.[61] Another important mechanism involves improvement of blood flow following irradiation with 830 nm, and this has been shown to positively impact on flap survival in the rat model.[62] Improved blood flow not only brings in oxygen and nutrients, but establishes a higher oxygen tension in the treated area which can establish gradients between the wound at the surrounding tissue, used as 'super-highways' by the reparative cells.[63] In the case of bony tissues, 830 nm has been shown to increase the metabolism of osteoblasts,[64] and to upregulate some of the genetic pathways leading to better differentiation of new, active osteoblasts from mesenchymal cells.[65]

In conclusion, the sequential application of 830 and 633 nm LED energy, and even of each of these wavelengths used on its own, has been shown to enhance all aspects of wound healing, always provided the incident irradiance (power density, photon intensity) is sufficiently high and an appropriate dose is given. In addition to the excellent and growing reputation of LED phototherapy as a stand-alone light-only therapy, this means that LED therapy has proved to be an ideal adjunctive therapy to any of the conventional approaches seen in dermatological practice and this is perhaps the most exciting aspect of LED phototherapy in the future. No matter how the dermatologist alters the epidermal or dermal morphology of his or her patient, be it through microdermabrasion, ablative and nonablative skin rejuvenation, fractional technology or conventional surgery, the addition of an appropriate LED phototherapy regimen will help to improve already good results but at a very reasonable cost, thus improving the satisfaction rates of both the clinician and the patient.

Other Clinical Indications

The indications already discussed have been well-researched, and are being reported in the literature. Some other applications exist which are very much at the experimental stage, but which should be mentioned to prepare the reader for what's coming in the not-too-distant future and for which LED phototherapy is proving very interesting. At this stage the author cannot go into details, because of the early stage of the clinical and related basic science experiments, but the reader should watch for articles on LED therapy and eczema, psoriasis, stretch marks, vitiligo and even cellulite reduction, although in the last-mentioned LED therapy is being used adjunctive to other approaches. Particularly in psoriasis, several multinational pilot studies have produced very interesting results, and this may well be the first of the list to appear in print in a peer-reviewed article. Yet another exciting field is the potential use of LED phototherapy in combination with platelet-rich plasma (PRP) for wound healing and for skin rejuvenation. PRP is well-established as a valid method in wound healing to speed up the process and give good cosmesis or in recalcitrant healing situations. Knowing how cell-specific certain LED wavelengths are, the obvious step is to combine the two approaches to achieve even better results, even faster. Some preliminary studies are currently underway in Tokyo, and the early results indicate that this will be a field to watch closely.

Safety with LEDs

- LED phototherapy is intrinsically safe
- Eye protection sometimes required against potential optical hazards
- LED phototherapy is essentially side effect free
- Few contraindications exist, but sensible precautions should be taken
  - Patient history must be checked for any photosensitivity-related diseases or conditions.
  - Drugs, ointments and even cosmetics being used by the patient must be checked for photosensitizing elements.

Surgical lasers and even intense pulsed light systems are by their very nature designed to create thermal damage and are thus subject to stringent safety codes to prevent accidental irradiation of tissue, other than the planned target tissues. Because LEDs are incapable of creating photothermal damage in tissues, the same stringent codes regarding accidental irradiation of tissue do not apply. However, as all of the LED systems discussed above operate in the visible and near infrared waveband, there is a potential for optical damage, as the eye is capable of gathering this waveband and focusing the light onto the retina at the back of the eye, particularly the macula and fovea, the area responsible for visual acuity. This will be looked at in a little more detail below.

Most LED phototherapy systems are run from conventional mains electricity, and so present potential hazards in common with any other such mains-driven equipment as, for example, DVD players and television sets. Common sense dictates the safe handling of this group of equipment, leading to the following guidelines:

DO NOT connect or disconnect the mains plug with wet or damp hands

DO NOT pull the plug from the mains socket using the power cable

DO NOT place any containers with liquid in them on top of the unit (e.g., coffee mugs) to prevent damage from accidental spillage. If such spillage should occur immediately turn off the system and have it serviced before using it again.

DO NOT attempt to perform and unauthorized servicing of the system which involves opening up the case and/or defeating any interlocks.

DO connect the mains cable to the system before plugging the mains plug into the socket

DO check that the power to the wall socket is off before inserting the mains cable plug

DO switch off the wall socket before removing the mains plug

Apart from these rather obvious points, common sense should prevent any electrical-related damage to therapist or patient.

Optical Hazards with LED Phototherapy

As already mentioned above, any LED system operating in the visible to near-infrared waveband emits light which the human eye can gather, and focus onto the back of the retina as illustrated in Fig. 21. If the incident power density is great enough,

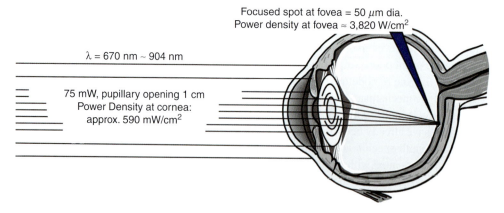

Fig. 21 Schematic illustration of how a low incident power of 75 mW is capable of being focused by the unaccommodated eye into a very small spot, with damaging power densities, right in the center of the fovea. The importance of appropriate protective eyewear is quite clear

permanent damage to the fovea could occur leading to uncorrectable loss of visual acuity. For example, an incident power density of as low as 75 mW focused to a 50 μm spot produces a power density of over 3,800 W/cm^2, perfectly capable of severely damaging target biological tissue. However, a set of values has been established for the maximum permissible exposure, or MPE, to light at a range of wavelengths. If an LED phototherapy system has been independently tested to deliver light below the MPE for its nominal wavelength, then even prolonged direct viewing of the beam is theoretically safe. In clinical practice, however, visible light LED arrays are extremely bright, even when below the MPE for their wavelength, so some form of eye protection is usually a good idea if only for patient comfort. Small, opaque eye cups held in place with an elasticated cord are popular, which will still allow the light to reach the periocular region in the case of LED phototherapy for skin rejuvenation. However, if the system delivers light which is over the MPE, then protective eyewear becomes mandatory for the patient, and also for any ancillary staff spending any length of time in the treatment room to help protect their eyes against diffuse reflection from the target tissue. For shorter visible wavelengths such as the blue waveband, the inherent photon energy of the light is approximately one-third as high again as visible red light even though the incident power density is the same, as discussed above, and so has greater potential for optical damage. Appropriate eyewear is necessary in this case.

The 'blink reflex' is nature's way of helping us protect our own eyes against an over-bright visible light source, but near-IR light cannot be 'seen' by the human eye and so the blink reflex is not triggered by energy in this invisible waveband. Near-IR is still gathered and focused by the unaccommodated eye just as visible light is, however, so suitable protective eyewear is thus mandatory for LED systems delivering energy in the near-IR waveband.

If the goggles or glasses are not opaque, then they have to be specifically sourced with an appropriate optical density for the wavelength of the system. Eyewear designed for red light will not protect adequately against IR or visible blue light, for example. The eyes of the patient, and indeed anyone with the patient in the treatment room during LED therapy, must be assiduously protected even though LEDs are often discounted as inherently 'safe', compared with a surgical laser or IPL. It is better to err on the side of caution!

Finally, national and federal regulatory agencies, such as the US Food and Drug Administration (FDA), issue approvals of systems for specific applications for which they have been proved '**safe and effective**'. Although some manufacturers have received such approvals, they are few and far between. Some less than truthful manufactures will claim FDA approval, when in fact all they hold is a letter from FDA recognizing that their LED system is a **nonsignificant risk device**, or NSRD. This is NOT the same as a system's having gone through the due regulatory process to obtain what is known as a **510(k) approval**, based on which, and only on which, can that device be legally sold in the USA for clinical use. 510(k) approvals for existing LED systems can be searched for on the FDA website (www.fda.gov/cdrh/510khome.html).

Side Effects

Once again, the inherently 'safe' output of LED systems helps to keep unwanted side effects to a minimum, but with any kind of phototherapy there is always the outside chance of triggering such a side effect. These are almost 100% photosensitivity-related, so a careful history of the patient must always be taken to identify the existence of pre-existing photosensitivity issues. For example, if a patient reports that he or she regularly comes out in an itchy rash when exposed to terrestrial sunlight, LED phototherapy should not be given. Some skin types, such as the Asian skin, are incredibly sensitive to other wavelengths despite being very resilient to UV skin damage. Particularly in the Asian skin, secondary hyperpigmentation can occur without any apparent physical insult, and a carefully-taken history will show if the patient is predisposed to this very upsetting side effect. A very small proportion of patients treated with LED therapy have reported post-treatment headaches of varying magnitudes, all of which have resolved spontaneously. No reason has been elucidated for this, and treatment with mild analgesics has been found to speed up the resolution of the headache. Almost all of those so afflicted have been undergoing LED phototherapy for facial skin rejuvenation, but interestingly only a very few have actually stopped turning up for their treatments. The main point is to take a very careful and thorough patient history to identify the potential of any LED therapy-related problems, but they are very much extremely few and far between. For longer sessions of LED phototherapy, for example in facial skin rejuvenation, the main side effect is that the patients tend to fall asleep during the treatment and 'wake up' feeling great!

Contraindications

Leading on from the previous subsection, any kind of endogenous or exogenous photosensitivity is a contraindication to LED phototherapy. Patients with any form of porphyria, for example, should never be treated with LEDs. Those whose history includes solar-mediated eruptions are likewise not good subjects. The careful dermatologist should also ascertain what the patients are putting on their skins prior to an LED therapy session. Ointments or creams containing known photosensitizers such as coumarins or porphyrins must be discontinued at least 2 weeks before any LED treatment.

from the chip with a series of condensing optics, as is currently the case with laser diode-based pointers, so that an almost parallel beam would emerge: this would obviously instantly increase the incident photon intensity of the beam. Alternatively, a lens could be incorporated in the capsule, to deliver a beam with a fixed focal length, i.e., coming to a focused point at a predetermined distance from the LED. This would increase the incident photon intensity even more. An array of convergent and individually focused LEDs would therefore offer a real alternative to a laser diode, probably still at less cost than a laser diode-based system, once the problem of the cost of the optics has been resolved. Again, this is an area which deserves watching carefully.

The final area is the home market, which is tied into the previous subsections as far as appropriately selected LEDs are concerned. There are already a large number of very pretty colored, happily twinkling LED-based systems being touted as suitable for home use, however the vast majority of them are mere toys, especially the ones with multicolored LEDs, and the poor user might as well stand in front of their christmas tree lights as use these systems. This does not mean that responsible manufacturers have not been researching correct combinations of appropriate wavelengths and intensities in ergonomically-designed hand-held self-contained units which will be safe and effective for home use: some indeed have. It is anticipated that these units will be available in a number of ways: for prescription by a dermatologist or other specialist as a maintenance program for their in-office LED treatment regimen; as an over-the-counter product from chemists or pharmacists with product-related training; or from reputable self-health mail-order companies. The author is aware of one company who has two such self-contained hand-held products, one blue/red for treatment of acne, and one infrared/red for skin rejuvenation, which are in the final stages of FDA approval process. Despite their size, they have the same high quality LEDs delivering the same intensity in mW/cm^2 as the medical versions of the systems based on LED arrays. When used for the recommended time they will thus deliver exactly the same dose as their much larger cousins. Naturally they cover a very much smaller area than the full-sized planar arrays, but because of their lightweight nature, it is anticipated that the user will be able to watch TV or listen to music while irradiating the target area one bit at a time, and they will be absolutely ideal for a maintenance program following office or clinic treatment with the full-sized systems. Yet another area to be watched with great interest.

Applications: Combination Is Key

The applications for light-only LED phototherapy continue to grow in a pan-speciality manner, so that a large range of

clinicians are finding useful applications for LED phototherapy of appropriate wavelength and incident photon intensity. However, as with lasers, a saturation point will be reached. This can be postponed by combining the effects of different LED wavelengths, such as the blue/red combination for acne, and the near-infrared/red combination for wound healing and skin rejuvenation. I firmly believe that we should go beyond that, as in fact is already happening, and use LED phototherapy in combination with the existing more conventional approaches to achieve even better results. A perfect example where this is happening is full face laser ablative resurfacing. Initially hailed as a superb approach to rejuvenating severely photoaged skin, in recent years it has declined dramatically in popularity because of potential side effects such as scarring, unpleasant-looking sequelae and a very long downtime before the patient can once again return to work or to society. However, everyone agrees it is still the 'gold standard', particularly for deep wrinkles and severe photodamage. Some reports have now appeared on the use of near infrared/red combination LED phototherapy together with ablative laser resurfacing. The controlled study already discussed above by Trelles et al. is an excellent example which compared two groups of full-face ablative resurfacing patients[54]: one group was also treated with combination LED phototherapy, and the control group was not, but otherwise the resurfacing and wound care regimens were exactly the same. The healing time in the LED-treated group was cut by more than one-half, postoperative pain was cut by more than 70% and the erythema cleared in less than 7 weeks compared with 4–6 months.

LED phototherapy can and does offer even better results in any case where the dermatologist has in some way altered the epidermal and dermal architecture of his or her patient, whether it is as mild as an epidermal powder peel, through chemical peels to nonablative resurfacing with lasers or IPL systems, and full-face ablative resurfacing. The adjunctive application of LED phototherapy will, I believe, drive its acceptance even more strongly than its use as a stand-alone modality, and the major advantage of LED-based systems is their very competitive pricing in addition to their portability and versatility. Combination therapy is the key.

Conclusions (and Questions You Should Ask)

- LED phototherapy is here to stay!
- 'Any old LED' will NOT fit the bill!
- When considering buying an LED system, ask the right questions!
- Combination treatment is the key!

LED phototherapy is certainly here to stay, but unfortunately the medicoscientific waters are being muddied by a number of manufacturers who have jumped on the LED bandwagon, making extravagant claims and barefacedly using the data amassed by those companies who have been responsible enough to go through regulatory approvals, such as FDA 510k clearances, as if the data were their own. Statements such as '.... uses NASA technology ....' are common, but totally misleading. The current generation of LEDs actually exceeds the 1990s NASA technology as far as output power and quasimonochromaticity are concerned, and in fact have absolutely nothing to do with NASA! Even worse than these manufacturers are the companies which import 'lookalikes' from countries such as China and Korea. They may be cheap, but they are certainly not cheerful, and the heart of an LED system is the quality and pedigree of the LEDs used in its arrays: you get what you pay for. To make sure you get what you actually want, i.e., an LED phototherapy system that will actually do something that you want it to do, and make you and your patients happy, please see the following, which will not only summarize the main points of the chapter but will also reinforce my favorite maxim which is; 'Any old LED will NOT do'.

Caveat Emptor (Let the Buyer Beware!)

When considering purchasing an LED-based phototherapy system for his or her practice, the wise dermatologist should always ask the manufacturer or salesperson the following questions (and take a written note of verified or verifiable answers!).

What Regulatory Approvals Does the System Have?

This means appropriate FDA 510k approvals in the USA (no LED system has yet got full premarketing approval, PMA), Health Canada in Canada, TGA in Australia, Ministry of Health, Labour and Welfare (*Kohseishou*) in Japan, appropriate CE marking for medical devices in Europe, and so on. It does not mean having 'NASA technology LED's' or 'Approved by the FDA', the latter of which usually simply means a letter from FDA recognizing that the system is a nonsignificant risk device (NSR) or minimal risk device (MSR). This is not an approval to market, but is simply a guide based on which the institutional review board (IRB) of a research center can classify the system when it does take part in a properly structured study.

What Is (Are) the Wavelength(s)?

As has been said many times, wavelength is the most important single factor when attempting to achieve a photoreaction: no absorption, no reaction. Some targets require a fairly broad waveband of 30 nm or so, but most of the targets in LED phototherapy are much more specific. Ask what the nominal wavelength of the system is, and what is the deviation either side. For example, the Omnilux® revive™ mentioned elsewhere in this chapter has a nominal wavelength of 633 nm, and the spread is ±3 nm. That means that the vast majority of the light is at the nominal wavelength of 633 nm, and will therefore optimally target wavelength-specific chromophores at that wavelength such as cytochrome c oxidase, and the porphyrins Cp III and Pp IX. Visible red at 670 nm, for example, will still have some effect on cytochrome c oxidase, but that wavelength just misses the boat as far as porphyrin activation is concerned.

While on the subject of wavelength, some manufacturers offer all the colors of the rainbow in the one system, in one particular system mounted in a semicircular bar which scans over the face with the claim that 'blue is for serenity, green is for inner peace, yellow is for well-being, and red is for relaxation'. In fact, this manufacturer is not offering phototherapy, but 'chromotherapy' also known as 'colorology' which is an alternative medical approach based on 'chakras' and their associated colors to achieve balance in an unbalanced system.[68] As with reflexology, the origin of the approach is Russian, as is a great deal of the literature, but chromotherapy has a large following. The methods and English language studies used to prove that it works, however, have been severely criticized.[69] In addition, as Karu and colleagues have well-demonstrated, the intermingling of wavelengths way well include some which cancel each other out thus having no effect, or indeed downregulate cellular activity compared to the wavelengths applied individually.[10] The fact that the light is scanned over the face should sound another warning bell, since this dramatically lowers the dose, even if the photon intensity were high enough (which it is not). The answer? Keep to well-proven wavelengths, applied singly. This does not mean to say they cannot be applied in combination, but sequentially .... indeed they should, but a suitable period (48–72 h) must be allowed between applications to allow the first wavelength to do what it is supposed to do at a cellular and tissue level before the second wavelength involves its specific targets.

What Is the Intensity?

You are looking for answer here in mW/cm^2 (milliwatts per square centimeter) of the entire array, not the 'lumens' of an individual LED or indeed the whole head. If in doubt about this parameter and its paramount importance, next to wavelength, please re-review subsection 2.3 above on photon density, another way of saying 'intensity'. A good range, depending on wavelength, would be anywhere from 40 mW/cm^2 up to 150 mW/cm^2, although the higher the intensity, the more problems will exists in keeping the head cool enough to avoid discomfort to the patient and a drift away from the LED nominal wavelength. If this range seems low compared with a diode laser therapy system, for example, always bear in mind that the better LED systems cover a large area of tissue, for example some offer an active array area of 220 cm^2, unlike the laser therapy system which usually irradiates a spot of only a few mm in diameter per 'shot'.

If you get an answer in joules, ignore it ... better still, laugh loudly. If you get an answer in joules per square centimeter (J/cm^2), that's better, but it is actually the answer to the next question! The incident intensity or power density is extremely important, because a higher power density enables a shorter irradiation time, and it has been reported for a continuous wave system that shorter irradiation times with a higher intensity got significantly better results in first passage human gingival fibroblast proliferation *in vitro* compared with longer irradiation times at a lower intensity, even though the dose (in J/cm^2) was the same.[70] Of course, the Arndt-Schultz curve must always be remembered (subsection 2.3 above), and the upper limit of photoactivation must never be exceeded or a photothermal reaction will occur.

What Is the Recommended Dose?

This is where the J/cm^2 unit should be the correct answer, but NOT the dreaded joule. If you see a joule running around an LED system, kill it. As discussed above, the joule is simply a unit of energy and has no significance whatever on the clinical effect in a prescribed area of target tissue. Correlate the dose with the recommended irradiation time. As a matter of interest, if you cannot find out the intensity from the manufacturer, by dividing the dose (J/cm^2) by the irradiation time (in seconds), you will end up with the intensity in W/cm^2.

For this category, here is no 'correct' dose, although it should certainly be higher than 40 J/cm^2 depending on the wavelength. If the intensity or power density is correct, then it is almost impossible to overdose. Overdosing is not recommended, however, simply because it wastes time and will not often produce dramatically better results than the recommended dose, which the responsible manufacturer will have arrived at by conducting dose-ranging response-related studies. If the recommended dose is, for example, 120 J/cm^2 over 20 min, increasing the irradiation time by 10–30 min will not get a 50% better effect, but on the other hand, cutting the time down by half to 10 min may well give a result well below 50% of that achieved at the recommended time. If the system supports heads with different wavelength, the manufacturer may well have standardized the treatment time to the same for each of the heads, but the dose will almost always be different for each wavelength, simply because of a combination of LED characteristics, wavelength/tissue interactions and the individual photon energy associated with each wavelength.

How Is the LED Energy Delivered?

The answer here will be 'in continuous wave (or CW)', which is good; or 'frequency modulated (also known as photomodulated)' which is not so good; or 'pulsed', which is actually the incorrect way of saying the second answer and is totally wrong! Light at a given wavelength already contains its own frequency, as discussed in subsection 2.5 above, and light represents 'information' to cellular targets. Imposing a secondary frequency on that primary frequency cannot only disrupt the flow of information, it also cuts down on the dose since there is no light incident on the target cells when the source is switched off. It is true that cells have a 'dark reaction' time as shown by Karu,[71] but it occurs well after irradiation, and not in the short off-duty interval in a frequency modulated beam cycle (cf Fig. 10b). Figure 22 is by the same independent research group, Almeida-Lopes and colleagues at the University of Sao Paulo, Brazil, as the data on power density in reference 70, and shows the growth pattern of first

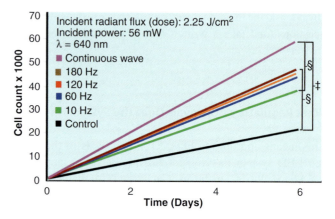

Fig. 22 An *in vitro* experiment to assess the effects of various frequencies in frequency modulated beams compared with a continuous wave beam and an unirradiated control on the cell proliferation of first passage pooled human gingival fibroblasts. The dose was kept constant at 2.25 J/cm^2. All of the frequencies were statistically significantly better at increasing proliferation (§, $p < 0.01$ for all). The CW beam, however, was significantly more efficient than both the control and the frequency modulated beams (‡, $p < 0.001$ and §, $p < 0.01$, respectively). The results represent the averaged data from 10 repeated experiments (Used with the permission of Pra. Luciana Almeida-Lopes, personal communication, data as yet unpublished)

passage human gingival fibroblasts exposed *in vitro* to 640 nm at several frequencies and continuous wave (CW), with constant incident power density and dose as ascertained in earlier studies. There was a significant difference seen between the group of frequencies and the unirradiated controls ($p > 0.01$ for all), with the higher frequencies inducing better cell proliferation, but the continuous wave beam induced greatest and most significant proliferation compared with both the unirradiated controls ($p < 0.001$) and the frequency modulated beams ($p < 0.01$). The experiment was repeated 10 times and the results averaged. (Data and graph reproduced with the permission of Pra. Luciana Almeida-Lopes, as yet unpublished data). Cells, especially fibroblasts, seem to prefer CW to frequency modulated energy.

What Has Been Published on the System/Technology?

What you are looking for here are papers by reputable authors published in the indexed and peer-reviewed literature, or at least in well-established and peer-reviewed journals (15 or more volumes) which have not yet been indexed by MedLine and/or PubMed but which do none-the-less have scientific credence. An example of the latter is *Laser Therapy* (Editor-in-Chief, Toshio Ohshiro, published by JMLL, Tokyo, Japan, now entering its 17th edition). An alternative source is appropriate chapters in books from reputable publishers. What you are NOT looking for are so-called 'white papers' which any manufacturer can produce to look like a genuine publication, or articles from the commercially-oriented medical press unless they are also in turn backed up by 'real' papers. All of the referenced works in this chapter fall under this latter category. Also, make very sure that the articles offered by the manufacturer/salesperson are on their specific system and wavelength(s). Very often articles on approved systems will be cited as 'proof' that their (unapproved) system works, even though sometimes the intensity, dose or even wavelength is not the same as in the published articles.

Finally...

Despite the moaning of the sceptics, LED phototherapy has definitely arrived, has been proven to work in many areas, and is finding a steadily increasing number of applications both within and outside dermatology. It is comparatively inexpensive, robust, easy to administer, safe, effective, pain free (in fact it can be used to treat pain), side-effect free and minimally contraindicated. It offers the possibility of a stand-alone noninvasive phototherapy method, but when used together with any of the methods currently used by the dermatologist to alter his or her patient's skin, already good

results can be expected to become even better. LED phototherapy will not turn a poor dermatologist into a good one, but it will help the good dermatologist to become even better, with happier patients. And finally, please remember, above all, not any old LED will do the job!

References

1. Giese AC. *Living with Our Sun's Ultraviolet Rays*. New York: Springer; 1976.
2. Fubini S. Influenza della luce sulla respirazione del tessuto nervoso. *Annali Universali di Medicina e Chirurgia*. 1897; Serie 1, 250: Fascicolo 7.
3. Finsen NR. Om de kemiske Straales skadelige Virkning paa den dyriske Organisme. In: *Behandlung af Kopper Med Udestaengning af de kemiske Straaler*. Copenhagen: Hospitalstidende; 1893.
4. Zheludev N. The life and times of the LED – a 100-year history. *Nat Photonics*. 2007;1:189-192.
5. Whelan HT, Houle JM, Whelan NT, et al. The NASA light-emitting diode medical program- progress in space flight and terrestrial applications. *Space Technol Appl Int Forum*. 2000;504:37-43.
6. Whelan HT, Smits RL, Buchmann EV, et al. Effect of NASA light-emitting diode (LED) irradiation on wound healing. *J Clin Laser Med Surg*. 2001;19:305-314.
7. Smith KC. *The Science of Photobiology*. New York: Plenum Press; 1977.
8. Ohshiro T, Calderhead RG. *Low Level Laser Therapy: A Practical Introduction*. Chichester: Wiley; 1988.
9. Asagai Y, Ueno R, Miura Y, Ohshiro T. Application of low reactive-level laser therapy (LLLT) in patients with cerebral palsy of the adult tension athetosis type. *Laser Ther*. 1995;7:113-118.
10. Karu T. Primary and secondary mechanisms of action of visible to near-IR radiation on cells. *J Photochem Photobiol B*. 1999;49:1-17.
11. Smith KC. The photobiological basis of low level laser radiation therapy. *Laser Ther*. 1991;3:19-24.
12. Kudo C, Inomata K, Okajima K, Motegi M, Ohshiro T. Low level laser therapy pain attenuation mechanisms, 1: histochemical and biochemical effects of 830 nm gallium aluminium arsenide laser radiation on rat saphenous nerve Na-K-atpase activity. *Laser Ther*. 1988;Pilot Issue: 3-6.
13. Dougherty TJ. Photodynamic therapy (PDT) of malignant tumors. *Crit Rev Oncol Hematol*. 1984;2:83-116.
14. Garcia-Zuazaga J, Cooper KD, Baron ED. Photodynamic therapy in dermatology: current concepts in the treatment of skin cancer. *Expert Rev Anticancer Ther*. 2005;5:791-800.
15. Gold MH, Goldman MP. 5-aminolevulinic acid photodynamic therapy: where we have been and where we are going. *Dermatol Surg*. 2004;30:1077-1083.
16. Charakida A, Seaton ED, Charakida M, Mouser P, et al. Phototherapy in the treatment of acne vulgaris: what is its role? *Am J Clin Dermatol*. 2004;5:211-216.
17. Kjeldstad B, Johnsson A. An action spectrum for blue and near ultraviolet inactivation of Propionibacterium acnes; with emphasis on a possible porphyrin photosensitization. *Photochem Photobiol*. 1986;43:67-70.
18. Sigurdsson V, Knulst AC, van Weelden H. Phototherapy of acne vulgaris with visible light. *Dermatology*. 1997;194:256-260.
19. Arakane K, Ryu A, Hayashi C, Masunaga T, et al. Singlet oxygen (1 delta g) generation from coproporphyrin in *Propionibacterium acnes* on irradiation. *Biochem Biophys Res Commun*. 1996;223:578-582.
20. Lavi R, Shainberg A, Friedmann H, Shneyvays V, et al. Low energy visible light induces reactive oxygen species generation and stimulates

an increase of intracellular calcium concentration in cardiac cells. *J Biol Chem.* 2003;278:40917-40922. Epub July 7, 2003.

21. Morton CA, Whitehurst C, Moseley H, et al. Development of an alternative light source to lasers for photodynamic therapy. Clinical evaluation in the treatment of pre-malignant non-melanoma skin cancer. *Lasers Med Sci.* 1995;10:165-171.

22. Babilas P, Kohl E, Maisch T, Backer B, et al. *In vitro* and *in vivo* comparison of two different light sources for topical photodynamic therapy. *Br J Dermatol.* 2006;154:712-718.

23. Pollock B, Turner D, Stringer M, Bojar RA, et al. Topical aminolae-vulinic acid-photodynamic therapy for the treatment of acne vulgaris: a study of clinical efficacy and mechanism of action. *Br J Dermatol.* 2004;151:616-622.

24. Hong SB, Lee MH. Topical aminolevulinic acid-photodynamic therapy for the treatment of acne vulgaris. *Photodermatol Photoimmunol Photomed.* 2005;21:322-325.

25. Omi T, Bjerring P, Sato S, Kawada S, et al. 420 nm intense continuous light therapy for acne. *J Cosmet Laser Ther.* 2004;6:156-162.

26. Webber J, Luo Y, Crilly R, Fromm D, Kessel D. An apoptotic response to photodynamic therapy with endogenous protoporphyrin *in vivo. J Photochem Photobiol B.* 1996;35:209-211.

27. Nitzan Y, Kauffman M. Endogenous porphyrin production in bacteria by δ-aminolevulinic acid and subsequent bacterial photoeradication. *Lasers Med Sci.* 1999;14:269-277.

28. Papageorgiou P, Katsambas A, Chu A. Phototherapy with blue (415 nm) and red (660 nm) light in the treatment of acne vulgaris. *Br J Dermatol.* 2000;142:973-978.

29. Goldberg DG, Russell B. Combination blue (415 nm) and red (633 nm) LED phototherapy in the treatment of mild to severe acne vulgaris. *J Cosmet Laser Ther.* 2004;8:71-75.

30. Lee SY, You CE, Park MY. Blue and red light combination LED phototherapy for acne vulgaris in patients with skin phototype IV. *Lasers Surg Med.* 2007;39:180-188.

31. Trelles MA, Allones I, Luna R. Facial rejuvenation with a nonablative 1320 nm Nd:YAG laser: a preliminary clinical and histologic evaluation. *Dermatol Surg.* 2001;27:111-116.

32. Nikolaou VA, Stratigos AJ, Dover JS. Nonablative skin rejuvenation. *J Cosmet Dermatol.* 2005;4:301-307.

33. Orringer JS, Voorhees JJ, Hamilton T, Hammerberg C, et al. Dermal matrix remodeling after nonablative laser therapy. *J Am Acad Dermatol.* 2005;53:775-782.

34. Rahman Z, Alam M, Dover JS. Fractional laser treatment for pigmentation and texture improvement. *Skin Ther Lett.* 2006;11:7-11.

35. Wanner M, Tanzi EL, Alster TS. Fractional photothermolysis of facial and nonfacial cutaneous photodamage with a 1,550-nm erbium-doped fiber laser. *Dermatol Surg.* 2007;33:23-28.

36. Lowe NJ, Lowe P. Pilot study to determine the efficacy of ALA-PDT photo-rejuvenation for the treatment of facial ageing. *J Cosmet Laser Ther.* 2005;7:159-162.

37. Alster TS, Surin-Lord SS. Photodynamic therapy: practical cosmetic applications. *J Drugs Dermatol.* 2006;5:764-768.

38. Christiansen K, Peter Bjerring P, Troilius A. 5-ALA for photodynamic photorejuvenation - optimization of treatment regime based on normal-skin fluorescence measurements. *Lasers Surg Med.* 2007;39:302-310.

39. Weiss RA, Weiss MA, Geronemus RG, McDaniel DH. A novel non-thermal non-ablative full panel LED photomodulation device for reversal of photoaging: digital microscopic and clinical results in various skin types. *J Drugs Dermatol.* 2004;3:605-610.

40. Russell BA, Kellett N, Reilly LR. A study to determine the efficacy of combination LED light therapy (633 nm and 830 nm) in facial skin rejuvenation. *J Cosmet Laser Ther.* 2005;7:196-200.

41. Goldberg DJ, Amin S, Russell BA, Phelps R, et al. Combined 633-nm and 830-nm led treatment of photoaging skin. *J Drugs Dermatol.* 2006;5:748-753.

42. Lee SY, Park KH, Choi JW, Kwon JK, et al. A prospective, randomized, placebo-controlled, double-blinded, and split-face clinical study

on LED phototherapy for skin rejuvenation: clinical, profilometric, histologic, ultrastructural, and biochemical evaluations and comparison of three different treatment settings. *J Photochem Photobiol B.* 2007;88:51-67. Available online as Epub ahead of print.

43. Trelles M, Mordon S, Calderhead RG, Goldberg D. (Viewpoint 3 and comment 3) How best to halt and/or revert UV-induced skin ageing: strategies, facts and fiction. *Exp Dermatol.* 2008;17:228-240.

44. Rigau J, Trelles MA, Calderhead RG, Mayayo E. Changes in fibroblast proliferation and metabolism following *in vitro* helium-neon laser irradiation. *Laser Ther.* 1991;3:25-34.

45. Takezaki S, Omi T, Sato S, Kawana S. Ultrastructural observations of human skin following irradiation with visible red light-emitting diodes (LEDs): a preliminary *in vivo* report. *Laser Ther.* 2005; 14:153-160.

46. Karu T. Identification of the photoreceptors. In: *Ten Lectures on Basic Science of Laser Phototherapy.* Grangesberg: Prima Books AB; 2007.

47. Trelles MA, Rigau J, Velez M. LLLT *in vivo* effects on mast cells. In: Simunovic Z, ed. *Lasers in Medicine and Dentistry (Part 1).* Switzerland: LaserMedico; 2002:169-186.

48. Trelles MA. Phototherapy in anti-aging and its photobiologic basics: a new approach to skin rejuvenation. *J Cosmet Dermatol.* 2006;5:87-91.

49. Young S, Bolton P, Dyson M, Harvey W, Diamantopoulos C. Macrophage responsiveness to light therapy. *Lasers Surg Med.* 1989;9:497-505.

50. Osanai T, Shiroto C, Mikami Y, Kudou E, et al. Measurement of GaAlAs diode laser action on phagocytic activity of human neutrophils as a possible therapeutic dosimetry determinant. *Laser Ther.* 1990;2:123-134.

51. Dima VF, Suzuki K, Liu Q, Koie T, et al. Laser and neutrophil serum opsonic activity. *Roum Arch Microbiol Immunol.* 1996;55(4): 277-283.

52. Samoilova KA, Bogacheva ON, Obolenskaya KD, Blinova MI, et al. Enhancement of the blood growth promoting activity after exposure of volunteers to visible and infrared polarized light. Part I: stimulation of human keratinocyte proliferation *in vitro. Photochem Photobiol Sci.* 2004;3(1):96-101. Epub September 1, 2003.

53. Kim JW, Lee JO. Low level laser therapy and phototherapy assisted hydrogel dressing in burn wound healing: light guided epithelial stem cell biomodulation. In: Eisenmann-Klein M, Neuhann-Lorenz C, eds. *Innovations in Plastic and Aesthetic Surgery.* Berlin: Springer; 2007:36-42.

54. Trelles MA, Allones I, Mayo E. Combined visible light and infrared light-emitting diode (LED) therapy enhances wound healing after laser ablative resurfacing of photodamaged facial skin. *Med Laser Appl.* 2006;21:165-175.

55. Trelles MA, Allones I. Red light-emitting diode (LED) therapy accelerates wound healing post-blepharoplasty and periocular laser ablative resurfacing. *J Cosmet Laser Ther.* 2006;8:39-42.

56. Trelles MA, Allones I, Mayo E. Er:YAG laser ablation of plantar verrucae with red LED therapy-assisted healing. *Photomed Laser Surg.* 2006;24:494-498.

57. Mester E, Szende B, Spiry T, Scher A. Stimulation of wound healing by laser rays. *Acta Chir Acad Sci Hung.* 1972;13:315-324.

58. Kubota J. Defocused diode laser therapy (830 nm) in the treatment of unresponsive skin ulcers: a preliminary trial. *J Cosmet Laser Ther.* 2004;6:96-102.

59. Glinkowski W. Delayed union healing with diode laser therapy (LLLT); case report and review of literature. *Laser Ther.* 1990;2:107-110.

60. Pretel H, Lizarelli RF, Ramalho LT. Effect of low-level laser therapy on bone repair: histological study in rats. *Lasers Surg Med.* 2007;39(10):788-796.

61. Karu T. Irradiation effects are detectable in the cells of subsequent generations. In: *Ten Lectures on Basic Science of Laser Phototherapy.* Grangesberg: Prima Books AB; 2007.

62. Kubota J. Effects of diode laser therapy on blood flow in axial pattern flaps in the rat model. *Lasers Med Sci.* 2002;17:146-153.
63. Niinikoski J. Current concepts of the role of oxygen in wound healing. *Ann Chir Gynaecol.* 2001;90(Suppl 215):9-11.
64. Kim YD, Kim SS, Hwang DS, Kim SG, et al. Effect of low-level laser treatment after installation of dental titanium implant-immunohistochemical study of RANKL, RANK, OPG: an experimental study in rats. *Lasers Surg Med.* 2007;39:441-450.
65. Nagasawa A, Kato K, Negishi A. Bone regeneration effect of low level lasers. *Laser Ther.* 1991;3:59-62.
66. Dima VF, Ionescu MD. Ultrastructural changes induced in walker carcinosarcoma by treatment with dihematoporphyrin ester and light in animals with diabetes mellitus. *Roum Arch Microbiol Immunol.* 2000;59:119-130.
67. Skobelkin OK, Michailov VA, Zakharov SD. Preoperative activation of the immune system by low reactive level laser therapy (LLLT) in oncologic patients: a preliminary report. *Laser Ther.* 1991;3:169-176.
68. Simpson S. *Chakras for Starters.* 2nd ed. Nevada City: Crystal Clarity Publishers; 2002.
69. Carey SC. *A Beginner's Guide to Scientific Method.* 2nd ed. Belmont: Wadsworth Publishing Inc; 2004.
70. Almeida-Lopes L, Rigau J, Zângaro RA, Guidugli-Neto J, Jaeger MM. Comparison of the low level laser therapy effects on cultured human gingival fibroblasts proliferation using different irradiance and same fluence. *Lasers Surg Med.* 2001;29:179-184.
71. Karu T. *Ten Lectures on Basic Science of Laser Phototherapy.* Grangesberg: Prima Books AB; 2007.

Laser and Light for Wound Healing Stimulation

Navid Bouzari, Mohamed L. Elsaie, and Keyvan Nouri

Introduction

Understanding wound healing is critical for health care professionals mainly because of the enormous burden of chronic wounds on society. In addition, in many medical specialties, creating wounds for diagnostic and therapeutic purposes is part of a physician's daily practice.

Acute wounds are usually closed using sutures, staples, or other methods of wound closure. Conventional modalities include maintenance of a moist wound bed, and prevention of infection. Although acute wounds are not challenging in most settings, they may influence the hospital stay or expenses related to medical procedures. Chronic wounds however, are more challenging. The incidence of chronic wounds in the United States is approximately five to seven million per year[1] and the annual costs for management of these wounds is greater than \$20 billion.[2,3] Accurate diagnosis is the key, and can be clinically made in less than 75% of cases.[4] Treatment usually consists of debridement of necrotic tissue, maintenance of a moist wound bed, and control of infection. Unfortunately, despite much progress, treating chronic wounds is still challenging.

Laser and light based technologies have recently emerged as alternative therapies for wound healing. A variety of lasers and light sources have been introduced as a non-invasive tool for chronic wound healing as well as an alternative method of closure of surgical wounds. This chapter will discuss the role of this new technology in wound healing.

N. Bouzari (✉)
Department of Dermatology, University of Miami,
Miller School of Medicine, NW. 10th Ave. 1600, Miami,
FL 33136, USA
e-mail: nbouzari2@med.miami.edu

Wound Healing

- Cutaneous wound healing is divided into three phases: the inflammatory phase, the proliferative phase, and the remodeling phase
- Inflammatory phase starts with tissue injury which causes extravasation of platelets, neutrophils, and monocytes to the site of injury. These cells release a variety of cytokines, inducing epithelial cell migration and proliferation
- In the proliferative phase, keratinocytes and fibroblasts proliferate and migrate to the wound bed in order to close the defect
- In the remodeling phase, remodeling of the collagen into a more organized structure occurs in order to increase the wound's tensile strength
- The wound healing process can be applied to both acute and chronic wounds. Acute wounds are generally less than 8 weeks, and usually result in a sustained restoration of anatomic and functional integrity. Chronic wounds are defined as wounds that have failed to proceed through the usual stepwise fashion. Lasers are used for healing of both acute and chronic wounds

Understanding the processes involved in wound repair is a prerequisite to maximize our knowledge regarding the use of lasers for wound healing. Cutaneous wound healing involves the complex interaction of several types of cells, their cytokines or mediators, and the extracellular matrix. After cutaneous injury, a cascade of events is observed, which mediates tissue repair and eventually the reestablishment of the barrier function of the skin. Tissue repair is divided into three phases: the inflammatory phase, the proliferative phase, and the remodeling phase (Fig. 1).[5]

K. Nouri (ed.), *Lasers in Dermatology and Medicine*,
DOI: 10.1007/978-0-85729-281-0_20, © Springer-Verlag London Limited 2011

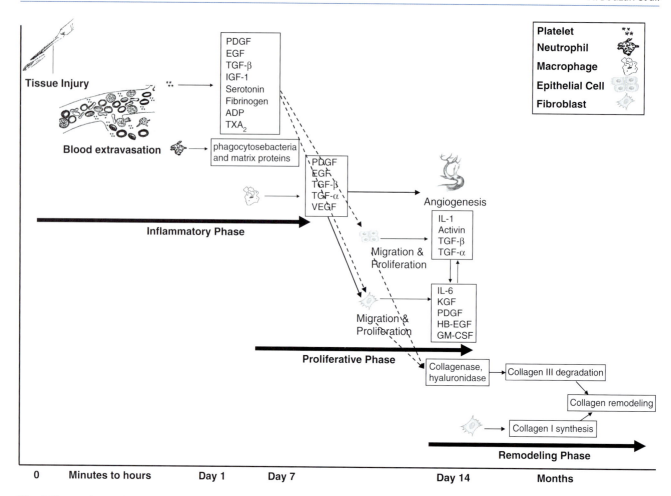

Fig. 1 Phases of wound healing. The inflammatory phase starts within minutes after tissue injury with extravasation of blood followed by activation of platelets, monocytes and macrophages, release of mediators and cytokines. These cytokines induce the proliferative phase by activating keratinocyte and fibroblast proliferation and migration, as well as release of a variety of growth factors involve in angiogenesis and granulation tissue formation. The last phase of wound healing is remodeling via replacing collagen III by collagen I. *IL* interleukin, *KGF* keratinocyte growth factor, *FGF* fibroblast growth factor, *VEGF* vascular endothelial growth factor, *PDGF* platelet-derived growth factor, *EGF* epidermal growth factor, *HB-EGF* heparin binding EGF, *TGF-α* transforming growth factor-alfa, *TGF-β* transforming growth factor-beta, *IGF-1* insulin-like growth factor-1, *GM-CSF* granulocyte-macrophage colony stimulating factor, *ADP* adenosine diphosphate, *TXA2* thromboxane A2

Inflammatory Phase

The initial event in tissue injury is the damage to endothelial cells and blood vessels. This causes extravasation of blood into the wound and collagen exposure which leads to blood clotting, platelet aggregation and activation, as well as migration of neutrophils and monocytes (and subsequently macrophages) to the site of injury. Activated platelets release a variety of mediators (Fig. 1) which initiate the wound healing cascade by attracting and activating fibroblasts, endothelial cells and macrophages. Neutrophils, once in the wound environment, phagocytose bacteria and matrix proteins. Later in the inflammatory phase, monocytes and macrophages become the dominant figures, and release a variety of cytokines, inducing epithelial cell migration and proliferation as well as matrix production.[5-7]

Proliferative Phase

This phase involves the creation of a permeability barrier as well as the establishment of an appropriate blood supply and reinforcement of the injured tissue. Keratinocytes and fibroblasts proliferate and migrate to the wound bed. Fibroblast proliferation and migration are modulated by PDGF, EGF, TGF-α, TGF-β and FGF. Macrophages play a key role in initiating fibroblast proliferation and migration. When the number of macrophages begins to diminish, fibroblasts and keratinocytes are the main source of the growth factors. The interplay of keratinocytes with fibroblasts gradually shifts the microenvironment away from an inflammatory to a synthesis-driven granulation tissue.

In the granulation tissue, mesenchymal cells become maximally activated, proliferate, and synthesize huge amounts of extracellular matrix which supports the developing capillary loops. Keratinocytes proliferate and migrate over the provisional matrix of the underlying granulation tissue, eventually closing the defect.[5,8,9]

Remodeling Phase

In this phase, remodeling of the collagen into a more organized structure occurs in order to increase the wound's tensile strength. The type III collagen of the granulation tissue is replaced by type I collagen through a tightly controlled synthesis of new collagen and lysis of old until the normal skin ratio of 4:1 for type I collagen to type III collagen is present. In addition, the composition of other matrix material such as water, fibronectin, hyaluronic acid, and proteoglycans changes over the period of a year or more.[5,10]

Acute Versus Chronic Ulcers

The wound healing process can be applied to both acute and chronic wounds. Acute wounds are generally less than 8 weeks, and usually result in a sustained restoration of anatomic and functional integrity. Chronic wounds are defined as wounds that have failed to proceed through the usual stepwise fashion. As a result, the healing process is prolonged and incomplete, with lack of restoration of integrity.[11] A large number of factors can impede wound healing and may predispose a patient to the development of a chronic wound. These include both local factors (wound infection, tissue hypoxia, repeated trauma, the presence of debris and necrotic tissue) and systemic causes (diabetes mellitus, malnutrition, immunodeficiency, and the use of certain medications).[12,13]

Lasers for Wound Healing

The use of lasers for wound healing has been focused in two fields: lasers to augment the healing of acute wounds (e.g., tissue welding, tissue soldering), and lasers for chronic wounds (e.g., low intensity laser devices)

The use of laser energy for wound healing was proposed more than 35 years ago.[14] It was first suggested for bonding skin incisions, and termed "laser welding." Interest in the efficacy of lasers as a noninvasive tool for treatment of all types of wounds soon grew among researchers in both animal

models[15] and clinical studies.[16] The concept that surgeons can replace their scalpels and tedious suturing techniques with a simple, non–operator-dependent, safe, and rapid technique, has inspired many investigators to experiment on different laser systems.[17] The areas of research can be divided in two major groups: lasers to augment the healing of acute wounds (tissue welding, tissue soldering, etc. *see below*), and lasers for chronic wound (e.g., low intensity laser devices, *see below*). Although these two groups of lasers share many similarities, there are differences in their mechanism of action, laser systems, laser parameters, etc. These factors will be discussed in this chapter.

Lasers for Acute Wounds

- The main techniques of laser-assisted wound closure of acute wounds are: simple tissue welding, tissue soldering, dye-enhanced tissue welding, and addition of growth factors
- The potential advantages of laser-assisted tissue bonding over conventional methods include increased immediate wound strength, fluid-tight closure, decreased operative repair time, reduced probability of infection and bleeding, and improved cosmetic results. However, lasers have disadvantages such as their high cost, risk of dehiscence, risk of thermal damage, and inconsistency of results
- The exact mechanism involved in laser-assisted wound closure is not completely understood. The heat produced by laser energy in the tissue causes collagen fibers to lose their triple helix structure and become fused, intertwined, swollen, and dissolved

Interest for tissue welding for closure of acute wounds first came out of early experiences with the use of electrocautery energy.[18] Later, laser energy was introduced for vascular anastomosis and then for other types of acute wounds. After the introduction of laser-assisted wound closure, it was rapidly evident that welding of skin was difficult. In fact, the initial tensile strength of the wound was weak compared with conventional sutures in the first few days post incision.[15,19,20] However, the wound healing process was generally accelerated, and the cosmetic aspect of the scar was improved. In order to enhance the tensile strength and minimize the thermal damage, various improvements have been suggested. The main techniques are simple tissue welding, tissue soldering, dye-enhanced tissue welding, and addition of growth factors (Table 1).

Tissue welding: The first method introduced for laser-assisted wound closure was "tissue welding." The principle

Table 1 Lasers commonly used in acute wound healing

Technique	Laser system + solder/dye
Tissue welding	CO_2
	Argon
	Nd:YAG
	Diode
Tissue soldering	Diode + albumin-genipin
	Diode + methylene blue
	Diode + albumin
	Diode + fibrinogen
	CO_2 + albumin
	Nd:YAG + albumin
	Argon + fibrinogen
Dye-enhanced	Alexandrite + indocyanine green
	Argon + fluorescein isothiocyanate
	Diode + indocyanine green
	Diode + gold nanoshells

of laser-assisted tissue welding is based on the heat produced by the laser irradiation. The increased temperature in the skin causes collagen denaturation and the crosslinking of fibrils.[21] It is crucial to estimate the optimal photonic energy that is to be delivered to tissue. In this respect, major determining factors are laser wavelength, power, exposure time, and mode of operations (continuous wave or pulsed). For this reason, various types of laser systems were investigated (Table 1).[15,22-24] The first successful use of a laser in tissue welding was in 1979 when ND:YAG was used to repair incisions made in blood vessels of a rat.[25] Later, tissue welding was successfully performed for skin closure as well as for anastomosis of other tissues.[15] Despite progresses made in tissue welding, surgeons still do not embrace this new laser technology. The main reasons can be summarized in three main drawbacks of laser welding: (1) low tensile strength during the first few days, (2) noticeable thermal damage, (3) inconsistency of results.[26]

Tissue soldering: Laser-assisted tissue soldering uses an additional component known as a "solder" for better wound closure. The solder (bovine albumin, human albumin, blood, etc.) absorbs the laser energy, coagulates, and as a result, enhances the tensile strength while minimizing the thermal damage of the surrounding tissue.[17,27] Laser-assisted tissue soldering has been carried out using two types of lasers: lasers such as Nd:YAG and GaAs, whose radiation penetrates deep into tissue[28]; and lasers such as CO_2, whose radiation is highly absorbed by surface tissue.[19] A variety of solders have also been studied (Table 1). Albumin as a solder, was introduced in 1988, and showed to be promising in studies with CO_2, diode and Nd:YAG lasers.[15,29-31] Other solders such as fibrinogen,[32] Albumin-genipin,[33] and methylene blue[34] have also been suggested. Again, the major drawback of this technique was the weak tensile strength of the repairs due to the decreased solubility of the partially denatured solder. To

overcome this problem, "2-layer" soldering was developed. In "2-layer" soldering, the layer in contact with tissue absorbs the laser and bonds to tissue while the second layer provides cohesive strength and flexibility. The main limitation of this method is lack of flexibility of bonded tissue.[35]

Dye-enhanced tissue welding: The concept of using a topical tissue-staining dye to facilitate selective delivery of laser energy by the target tissue has been postulated to improve tissue welding. A nontoxic dye that is strongly absorbed by a specific laser wavelength can serve to confine photon absorption and the resultant thermal energy to the weld site. A variety of combinations of dyes and lasers have been studied with variable success rates.[16,32,36,37] It seems that combination of indocyanine green with either pulsed alexandrite or pulsed diode laser is superior to other dye-enhanced tissue welding techniques. Nonetheless, it is worth noting that very limited clinical data have been available yet that confirm the clinical value of dye-enhanced tissue welding.

Nanoshells are a new class of nanoparticles consisting of a dielectric core surrounded by a thin metal shell. Use of gold nanoshells in conjunction with near infrared light has recently been suggested as a means of dye-enhanced tissue welding. Application of lasers at wavelengths within the near infrared, between approximately 650 and 900 nm, where tissue components have minimal absorption, decreases the chance of widespread thermal damage and improves penetration depth.[38] The use of nanoshells has several advantages over indocyanine green. For example, the small size of nanoshells reduces diffusion from the site of treatment and concentrates heating at the interface to be welded. Also, they are less photosensitive hydrolytically sensitive and susceptible to photobleaching in the presence of light compared to indocyanine green.

Addition of growth factors: Attempts have been made to use recombinant growth factors, as an adjunct to laser-assisted tissue soldering to accelerate wound healing. A variety of growth factors such as HB-EGF, FGF, TGF-β, etc. have been studied. The result of an animal study by Poppas and colleagues showed that addition of TGF-β to the solder (albumin in their study) increases the tensile strength of the wound by more than 50%. Using this technique, it is imperative to maintain a predetermined tissue temperature in order to prevent thermal degradation of growth factors.[39]

Lasers Versus Conventional Methods of Acute Wound Closure

Conventional techniques for tissue bonding (sutures, staples, and adhesives) are highly reliable procedures that have proven themselves over the years to be good clinical practice.

Table 2 Advantages and disadvantages of different methods of wound closure

	Advantage	Disadvantage
Suture	Reliable	Cause trauma to the tissue
	Flexible	Time consuming
	Inexpensive	Operator dependant
	Available	Introduce foreign body
		No immediate watertight closure
		Risk of needle-stick
		Risk of infection (due to lack of sealing)
		Need suture removal
Staple	Reliable	Cause trauma to the tissue
	Available	Inflexible (predetermined size)
	Relatively quick	Introduce foreign body
	Not operator dependant	No immediate watertight closure
		Risk of needle-stick
		Risk of infection (due to lack of sealing)
		Need staple removal
Adhesive	Immediate watertight closure	Expensive (controversial)
	Painless	Does not provide hemostasis
	No trauma to tissue	Introduce foreign body
	"No needle" procedure	(Possible) need for subcutaneous sutures
	Less risk of infection	Risk of tissue reactivity
	No need for removal	Not flexible (comparing to sutures)
	Fast	
Laser	Immediate watertight closure	Expensive
	better scar	Not readily available
	"No needle" procedure	Foreign body (Soldering, dye-enhanced)
	Less risk of infection	Risk of dehiscence
	No need for removal	Complicated (many parameters to consider)
	Fast	Risk of thermal damage
	Dynamic effects (may increase growth factors)	Inconsistent results

Sutures have been successfully used for centuries. They are inexpensive, flexible, reliable, and readily available.[15] However, they are not the perfect technique due to several reasons (Table 2). Since sutures cause trauma to the skin, and introduce a foreign body, they can result in inflammation, granuloma formation, and scarring. Many technical factors such as position of the needle in the holder, the slope of the tissue at needle entrance, suture spacing, knot tension, and choice of suture material can affect wound healing.[23,40] Staples are another mean of wound closure which share many common characteristics with sutures. However, they are faster and more uniform than sutures. Their main disadvantage is that they come in predetermined size which precludes their use in some anatomical sites. Adhesives are a clean, fast, non-operator-dependant, painless method of wound closure. They are an excellent "no needle" alternative in pediatric patients. However, for most applications, they have not been able to provide adequate strength.[15,41,42]

As shown in detail in this chapter, laser-assisted tissue bonding can transcend the limitations of conventional methods in many aspects. Their potential advantages over conventional methods include increased immediate wound strength, fluid-tight closure, decreased operative repair time, reduced probability of infection and bleeding, and improved cosmetic results. However, there have been several obstacles which prevented physicians from using laser welding clinically. These included collateral thermal injuries, inconsistency of results, and a lack of understanding of the exact mechanism by which laser irradiation induces tissue bonding. In addition, there are many parameters that need to be optimized in the welding process. These parameters include wavelength, fluence, pulse duration, repetition rate, irradiation time, spot size, and solder selection. Indeed, the parameter window for optimum tissue bonding is very small. All parameters should be chosen appropriately to provide enough heat for denaturation and crosslinking of collagen fibers, but not to the level of tissue necrosis and sloughing of wound edges. What makes the use of laser even more complicated is the fact that energy levels and exposure times that may work very well with certain tissues may not be the best for other situations.[15,17] As we discuss later in this chapter, several thermal feedback systems have been suggested to overcome the above limitations.

Mechanism of Laser-Assisted Wound Bonding

The exact mechanism involved in laser-assisted wound closure is not completely understood. Nonetheless, what is commonly believed is that tissue bonding occurs mainly due to the thermal effect of laser. The heat produced by laser energy in the tissue causes collagen fibers to lose their triple helix structure and become fused, intertwined, swollen, and dissolved. This generates a coagulum that serves both as a coating for sealing the wound and as a sophisticated scaffold for re-colonization of cells, as in the case of re-epithelialization.[24,43,44] Other theories have been postulated, as Helmsworth and colleagues believe that welding effect is the result of reorganization of intramolecular disulfide bonds of laminin, type IV collagen, and entactin rather than covalent bonds of type I collagen.[45] Despite the controversies, it seems that collagen plays a major role although bonding is most likely dependant on extracellular proteins rather than collagen alone.

Laser Systems and Parameters for Optimal Wound Bonding

In order to achieve a reliable tensile strength, it is crucial to estimate the optimal photonic energy that is to be delivered to tissue. In this respect, major determining factors are laser wavelength, power, exposure time, and mode of operations (continuous wave or pulsed). For this reason, various types of laser systems were investigated.[15,23] CO_2 was one of the first lasers employed for wound bonding because of its availability. However, it is a poor choice of wavelength and unlikely to yield a reliable high strength bonds. Due to the high absorption at the surface, the outermost tissue layers are "overcooked," whereas the deeper layers are hardly affected at all. Therefore, the temperature in the dermis is not high enough for collagen alteration and fusion. If the energy is increased to achieve the suitable temperature in the dermis, the surface will burn. Increasing the pulse duration will also result in producing a large zone of thermal damage. Like CO_2 laser, holmium:YAG (Ho:YAG) has a high absorption by water, hence it causes thermal injury at the surface. To overcome this problem, these lasers need to be used under a temperature-controlled system. Near Infrared lasers (650–900 nm) such as diode lasers are also becoming more popular in welding studies. While the wavelengths between 780 and 850 nm have the advantage of less absorption by water, their relatively high absorption by melanin prevents their deeper penetration.[46,47] Recently, 980 nm diode was suggested as a better wavelength for wound closure due to its better absorption by water and less absorption by melanin compared to other infrared lasers.[47] In general, although near infrared lasers would allow deeper penetration of the light, their absorption by tissue components is minimal; hence, they may need to be used in conjunction with exogenous absorbers to induce welding. Due to its water and melanin absorption coefficient values,[46] Nd:YAG (1,064 nm) is another infrared laser used in tissue welding. Like many of the near infrared lasers, Nd:YAG laser needs to be used with solders for optimal welding. It should be noted that most of our knowledge about lasers used for wound bonding is on either in vitro or animal studies. Therefore, the optimal laser systems and parameters for human wound closure is yet to be determined.

Lasers for Chronic Wounds

- Different lasers for treating chronic wounds include helium-neon, gallium-arsenide (GaAs), gallium-aluminum-arsenide (GaAlAs), Nd:YAG, carbon dioxide, ruby, krypton, and argon dye lasers

- The exact mechanism of action of low intensity laser therapy is not known. Current hypotheses are: stimulation of Ca influx and mitosis rate, increased expression of Heat-Shock-Proteins (e.g., HSP70), increased expression of growth factors such as TGF-β, alteration of mitochondrial activity and increased ATP synthesis, augmented formation of mRNA and protein secretion, enhancement of fibroblast and keratinocyte proliferation and migration, angiogenesis, improvement of phagocytosis, and increased rate of transformation of fibroblasts into myofibroblasts

Laser irradiation was introduced as a noninvasive therapeutic modality for acceleration of wound healing in the late 1960s, and has since been used for the treatment of a variety of chronic ulcers.[48] Different laser systems such as helium-neon, gallium-arsenide (GaAs), gallium-aluminum-arsenide (GaAlAs), Nd:YAG, carbon dioxide, ruby, krypton, and argon dye lasers have been studied.[49,50] Despite differences in wavelengths, the common characteristic of all these lasers is that they all employ low energy for wound healing. This method of therapy has been known as low-intensity, low-power, or low-level laser therapy. It has been suggested to increase the speed, quality and tensile strength of tissue repair, resolve inflammation and provide pain relief. The use of low intensity laser therapy is not limited to wound healing; and it has been used in odontological, rehabilitative, and other medical specialties. The basic principle of laser therapy is that low intensity laser radiation has the capability to alter cellular behavior in the absence of significant heating. Previous works have been focused on three areas: in vitro studies on molecular and cellular function, animal studies, and human trials. Unfortunately, the clinical data is mostly anecdotal, poorly controlled, and more variable than might be desired. The in vitro and animal studies are less arguable, and provide most of the scientific rationale of laser therapy.

Lasers have been used for healing of a variety of chronic wounds such as pressure ulcers, venous ulcers, and diabetic ulcers (Table 3). The first implication of lasers for pressure ulcers was to use them as a surgical tool for debridement. Controlled trials on CO_2 laser versus conventional debridement showed less bleeding, less infection, and shorter hospital stays with the use of CO_2 laser.[51,52] Later, low intensity lasers such as diode and GaAs were attempted. While some reports found impressive wound healing outcomes, some others showed no advantages.[53-55] There is insufficient evidence to suggest a benefit of treating venous ulcers with low-intensity laser therapy. Most of the data is anecdotal, and there is only one small randomized controlled trial suggesting the therapeutic benefit of laser therapy for venous ulcers.[56]

Table 3 Commonly used lasers for different types of chronic ulcers

Type of chronic ulcer	Laser type and wavelength	Energy	Result[a]
Venous	810 nm GaAlAs	4.0 J/cm²	Not effective
	660–950 nm GaAlAs	12.0 J/cm²	Effective
	904 nm GaAs	1.0 J/cm²	Effective
	632.8 nm HeNe	4.0 J/cm²	Effective
	810 nm diode	4.0 J/cm²	Effective
Pressure	904 nm GaAs	1.0 J/cm²	Effective
	830 nm diode	5.0 J/cm²	Effective
Diabetic	670 nm diode	18 and 36 J/cm²	Not effective with 36 J/cm²
	632.8 nm HeNe	1.0, 4.0, 4.8, 5.0, 10.0, and 16.0 J/cm²	Effective with all except 16 J/cm²
	904 nm GaAs	1.0 J/cm²	Effective
	830 nm diode	5.0 J/cm²	Effective

[a]The results given are based on authors' conclusion. Not all the studies are well controlled randomized trials

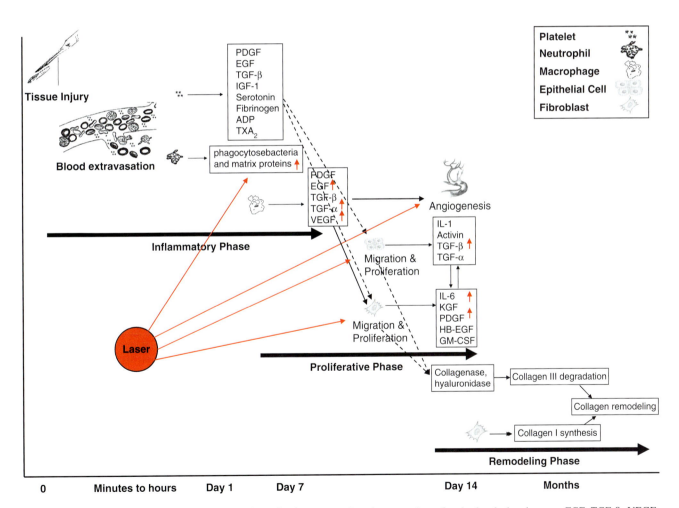

Fig. 2 The molecular and cellular effects of low intensity lasers on chronic wounds: Lasers mainly affect inflammatory and proliferative phases of wound healing. At cellular level, lasers improve phagocytosis, enhance angiogenesis, and increase proliferation of fibroblasts and keratinocytes. At molecular level, they increase FGF, TGF-β, VEGF, IL-6, and PDGF. *IL* interleukin, *FGF* fibroblast growth factor, *VEGF* vascular endothelial growth factor, *PDGF* platelet-derived growth factor, *TGF-β* transforming growth factor-beta

Low intensity laser therapy has been shown by various studies to be effective in the treatment of diabetic wound healing. Some of the suggested advantages of this method are increased microcirculation, increased speed of healing, improved wound epithelialization, increased granulation tissue formation, and increased collagen deposition.[57-59] However, some authors emphasize that depending on the applied dose, wavelength, irradiation time, and also the conditions of the treated tissue, different positive and negative biological answers can be achieved.

Mechanism of Laser-Assisted Wound Healing

The exact mechanism of action of low intensity laser therapy is not completely understood. Currently there is no accepted theory to explain the mechanism of low-intensity lasers, and this lack of knowledge complicates the evaluation of conflicting reports in the literature. Another limitation is the lack of ideal models of chronic wounds. Most of the studies have been conducted on surgically excised skin. These wound models excluded common problems associated with delayed healing, such as ischemia, infection, and necrotic debris. What makes the data even more confusing is that a variety of laser parameters such as wavelength, fluence, and time of treatment onset can influence the biologic effects of low intensity lasers.

The suggested mechanisms at the molecular level are stimulation of Ca influx and mitosis rate, increased expression of Heat-Shock-Proteins (e.g., HSP70), increased expression of growth factors such as TGF-β, alteration of mitochondrial activity and increased ATP synthesis, augmented formation of mRNA and protein secretion. On the cellular level, laser-induced changes are enhancement of fibroblast and keratinocyte proliferation and migration, angiogenesis, improvement of phagocytosis, and increased rate of transformation of fibroblasts into myofibroblasts (Fig. 2).[60-66] Some of the animal studies on laser-assisted wound healing are in accordance with molecular and cellular studies, showing decreased inflammatory period, increased collagen and granulation tissue in the wound bed, increased tensile strength, and faster epithelialization.[54,67,68] However, repeated experiments on many of the above in-vitro and animal models have failed to verify these benefits. These conflicting reports may partly be explained by considering discordance among the laser types used, the parameters selected, and the wound models chosen. In summary, to better understand the role of low intensity lasers in healing of chronic wounds, well-controlled studies that correlate cellular effects and biologic processes are needed. In the absence of such studies, the literature does not appear to support widespread use of lasers in wound healing at this time.

References

1. Petrie NC, Yao F, Eriksson E. Gene therapy in wound healing. *Surg Clin N Am*. 2003;83(3):194-199.
2. Harding KG, Morris HL, Patel GK. Science, medicine and the future: healing chronic wounds. *BMJ*. 2002;324:160-163.
3. Frykberg RG, Armstrong DG, Giurini J, et al. Diabetic foot disorders: a clinical practice guideline. American College of Foot and Ankle Surgeons. *J Foot Ankle Surg*. 2000;39(5 Suppl):S1-S60.
4. de Araujo T, Valencia I, Federman DG, et al. Managing the patient with venous ulcers. *Ann Intern Med*. 2003;138:326-334.
5. Kirsner R. Wound healing. In: Bolognia JL, Jorizzo JL, Rapini RP, et al., eds. *Dermatology*. Edinburgh: Mosby; 2003:2207-2215.
6. Clark RAF. Wound repair: overview and general considerations. In: Clark RAF, ed. *The Molecular and Cellular Biology of Wound Repair*. London: Plenum Press; 1996:3-50.
7. Clark RA, Ghosh K, Tonnesen MG. Tissue engineering for cutaneous wounds. *J Invest Dermatol*. 2007;127(5):1018-1029.
8. Werner S, Krieg T, Smola H. Keratinocyte-fibroblast interactions in wound healing. *J Invest Dermatol*. 2007;127(5):998-1008.
9. Mast BA, Schultz GS. Interactions of cytokines, growth factors, and proteases in acute and chronic wounds. *Wound Repair Regen*. 1996;4:411-420.
10. Booth BA, Polak KL, Uitto J. Collagen biosynthesis by human skin fibroblasts. *Biochim Biophys Acta*. 1980;607:145-160.
11. Lazarus GS, Cooper DM, Knighton DR, et al. Definitions and guidelines for assessment of wounds and evaluation of healing. *Arch Dermatol*. 1994;130(4):489-493.
12. Steed DL. Wound-healing trajectories. *Surg Clin N Am*. 2003;83(3):206-208.
13. Williams JZ, Barbul A. Nutrition and wound healing. *Surg Clin N Am*. 2003;83(3):193-197.
14. Mester E, Spiry T, Szende B, et al. Effect of laser rays on wound healing. *Am J Surg*. 1971;122(4):532-535.
15. Bass LS, Treat MR. Laser tissue welding: a comprehensive review of current and future clinical applications. *Lasers Surg Med*. 1995;7:315-349.
16. Kirsch AJ, Cooper CS, Gatti J, et al. Laser tissue soldering for hypospadias repair: results of a controlled prospective clinical trial. *J Urol*. 2001;65:574-577.
17. Simhon D, Halpern M, Brosh T, et al. Immediate tight sealing of skin incisions using an innovative temperature-controlled laser soldering device: in vivo study in porcine skin. *Ann Surg*. 2007; 245(2):206-213.
18. Sigel B, Acevedo FJ. Vein anastomosis by electrocoaptive union. *Surg Forum*. 1962;13:291.
19. Garden JM, Robinson JK, Taute PM, et al. The low-output carbon dioxide laser for cutaneous wound closure of scalpel incisions: comparative tensile strength studies of the laser to the suture and staple for wound closure. *Lasers Surg Med*. 1986;6(1):67-71.
20. Abergel RP, Lyons RF, White RA, et al. Skin closure by Nd:YAG laser welding. *J Am Acad Dermatol*. 1986;14(5):810-814.
21. Wang S, Grubbs PE Jr, Basu S, et al. Effect of blood bonding on bursting strength of laser-assisted microvascular anastomoses. *Microsurgery*. 1988;9(1):10-13.
22. McKennan KX. "Tissue welding" with the argon laser in middle ear surgery. *Laryngoscope*. 1990;100(11):1143-1145.
23. Talmor M, Bleustein CB, Poppas DP. Laser tissue welding: a biotechnological advance for the future. *Arch Facial Plast Surg*. 2001;3:207-213.
24. Tang J, Godlewski G, Rouy S, et al. Morphologic changes in collagen fibers after 830 nm diode laser welding. *Lasers Surg Med*. 1997;21(5):438-443.
25. Jain KK, Gorisch W. Repair of small blood vessels with the neodymium-YAG laser: a preliminary report. *Surgery*. 1979,85(6):684-688.

26. Simhon D, Ravid A, Halpern M, et al. Laser soldering of rat skin, using fiberoptic temperature controlled system. *Lasers Surg Med.* 2001;29(3):265-273.

27. Capon A, Mordon S. Can thermal lasers promote skin wound healing. *Am J Clin Dermatol.* 2003;4(1):1-12.

28. Abergel RP, Lyons R, Dwyer R, et al. Use of lasers for closure of cutaneous wounds: experience with Nd:YAG, argon and CO_2 lasers. *J Dermatol Surg Oncol.* 1986;12:1181-1185.

29. Massicotte JM, Stewart RB, Poppas DP. Effects of endogenous absorption in human albumin solder for acute laser wound closure. *Lasers Surg Med.* 1998;23:18-24.

30. Lauto A. Repair strength dependence on solder protein concentration: a study in laser tissue-welding. *Lasers Surg Med.* 1998;22:120-125.

31. Levanon D, Katzir A, Ravid A. A scanning electron microscopy study of CO_2 laser-albumin soldering in the rabbit model. *Photomed Laser Surg.* 2004;22(6):461-469.

32. Wider TM, Libutti SK, Greenwald DP, et al. Skin closure with dye-enhanced laser welding and fibrinogen. *Plast Reconstr Surg.* 1991;88:1018-1025.

33. Lauto A, Foster LJ, Ferris L, et al. Albumin-genipin solder for laser tissue repair. *Lasers Surg Med.* 2004;35(2):140-145.

34. Birch JF, Mandley DJ, Williams SL, et al. Methylene blue based protein solder for vascular anastomoses: an in vitro burst pressure study. *Lasers Surg Med.* 2000;26(3):323-329.

35. Lauto A, Kerman I, Felsen D, Poppas D. Two-layer film as a laser soldering biomaterial. *Lasers Surg Med.* 1999;25:250-256.

36. DeCoste SD, Farinelli W, Flotte T, et al. Dye-enhanced laser welding for skin closure. *Lasers Surg Med.* 1992;12(1):25-32.

37. Small W 4th, Heredia NJ, Maitland DJ, et al. Dye-enhanced protein solders and patches in laser-assisted tissue welding. *J Clin Laser Med Surg.* 1997;15(5):205-208.

38. Gobin AM, O'Neal DP, Watkins DM, et al. Near infrared laser-tissue welding using nanoshells as an exogenous absorber. *Lasers Surg Med.* 2005;37(2):123-129.

39. Poppas DP, Massicotte JM, Stewart RB, et al. Human albumin solder supplemented with TGF-beta 1 accelerates healing following laser welded wound closure. *Lasers Surg Med.* 1996;19(3):360-368.

40. Seki S. Techniques for better suturing. *Br J Surg.* 1988;75: 1181-1184.

41. Gennari R, Rotmensz N, Ballardini B, et al. A prospective, randomized, controlled clinical trial of tissue adhesive (2-octylcyanoacrylate) versus standard wound closure in breast surgery. *Surgery.* 2004;136(3):593-599.

42. Ong CC, Jacobsen AS, Joseph VT. Comparing wound closure using tissue glue versus subcuticular suture for pediatric surgical incisions: a prospective, randomised trial. *Pediatr Surg Int.* 2002;18:553-555.

43. Schober R, Ulrich F, Sander T, et al. Laser-induced alteration of collagen substructure allows microsurgical tissue welding. *Science.* 1986;232:1421-1422.

44. Simhon D, Brosh T, Halpern M, et al. Closure of skin incisions in rabbits by laser soldering: I: wound healing pattern. *Lasers Surg Med.* 2004;35:1-11.

45. Helmsworth TF, Wright CB, Scheffter SM, et al. Molecular surgery of the basement membrane by the argon laser. *Lasers Surg Med.* 1990;10:576-583.

46. Peavy GM. Lasers and laser-tissue interaction. *Vet Clin North Am Small Anim Pract.* 2002;32(3):517-534.

47. Gulsoy M, Dereli Z, Tabakoglu HO, et al. Closure of skin incisions by 980-nm diode laser welding. *Lasers Med Sci.* 2006;21:5-10.

48. Mester E, Mester AF, Mester A. The biomedical effects of laser application. *Lasers Surg Med.* 1988;5:607-614.

49. Wheeland RG. Lasers for stimulation or inhibition of wound healing. *J Dermatol Surg Oncol.* 1993;19:747-752.

50. Kawalec JS, Hetherington VJ, Pfennigwerth TC, et al. Effect of a diode laser on wound healing by using diabetic and nondiabetic mice. *J Foot Ankle Surg.* 2004;43(4):214-220.

51. Dixon JA. Current laser applications in general surgery. *Ann Surg.* 1988;207(4):355-372.

52. Juri H, Obeide A, Young S. CO_2 laser in decubitus ulcers. *Lasers Med Surg.* 1985;5:143-144.

53. Schindl A, Schindl M, Schindl L. Successful treatment of persistent radiation ulcer by low power laser therapy. *J Am Acad Dermatol.* 1997;37:646-648.

54. Allendorf JD, Bessler M, Huang J, et al. Helium-neon laser irradiation at fluences of 1, 2, and 4 J/cm^2 failed to accelerate wound healing as assessed by wound contracture rate and tensile strength. *Lasers Surg Med.* 1997;20:340-345.

55. Basford JR. Low-energy laser therapy: controversies and new research findings. *Lasers Surg Med.* 1989;9:1-5.

56. Bilhari I, Mester AR. The biostimulative effect of low level laser therapy of long-standing crural ulcers using helium neon laser, helium neon plus infrared lasers, and noncoherent light: preliminary report of a randomized double-blind comparative study. *Laser Ther.* 1989;1(Pt 2):97-98.

57. Schindl A, Heinze G, Schindl M, et al. Systemic effects of low-intensity laser irradiation on skin microcirculation in patients with diabetic microangiopathy. *Microvasc Res.* 2002;64(2):240-246.

58. Reddy GK, Stehno-Bittel L, Enwemeka CS. Laser photostimulation accelerates wound healing in diabetic rats. *Wound Repair Regen.* 2001;9(3):248-255.

59. Yu W, Naim JO, Lanzafame RJ. Effects of photostimulation on wound healing in diabetic mice. *Lasers Surg Med.* 1997;20(1):56-63.

60. Abergel RP, Meeker CA, Lam TS, Dwyer RM, Lesavoy MA, Uitto J. Control of connective tissue metabolism by lasers: recent developments and future prospects. *J Am Acad Dermatol.* 1984;11: 1142-1150.

61. Pourreau-Schneider N, Ahmed A, Soudry M, et al. Helium-neon laser treatment transforms fibroblasts into myofibroblasts. *Am J Pathol.* 1990;137:171-178.

62. Boulton M, Marshall J. He-Ne laser stimulation of human fibroblast proliferation and attachment in vitro. *Lasers Life Sci.* 1986;1: 125-134.

63. Posten W, Wrone DA, Dover JS, et al. Low-level laser therapy for wound healing: mechanism and efficacy. *Dermatol Surg.* 2005; 31(3):334-340.

64. Pereira AN, EduardoCde P, Matson E, Marques MM. Effect of low-power laser irradiation on cell growth and procollagen synthesis of cultured fibroblasts. *Lasers Surg Med.* 2002;31:263-267.

65. Medrado AR, Pugliese LS, Reis SR, Andrade ZA. Influence of low level laser therapy on wound healing and its biological action upon myofibroblasts. *Lasers Surg Med.* 2003;32:239-244. 12605432.

66. Schindl A, Merwald H, Schindl L, et al. Direct stimulatory effect of low-intensity 670 nm laser irradiation on human endothelial cell proliferation. *Br J Dermatol.* 2003;148:334-336.

67. Lyons RF, Abergel RP, White RA, et al. Biostimulation of wound healing in vivo by a helium-neon laser. *Ann Plast Surg.* 1987;18: 47-50.

68. Stadler I, Lanzafame RJ, Evans R, et al. 830-nm irradiation increases the wound tensile strength in a diabetic murine model. *Lasers Surg Med.* 2001;28:220-226.

Lasers in Hair Growth and Hair Transplantation

Nicole E. Rogers, Joseph Stuto, and Marc R. Avram

Introduction

- Results from hair transplantation are consistently natural
- Demand for the procedure has increased significantly
- Lasers have been implemented in the field of hair transplantation to create recipient sites and enhance hair growth

The field of hair transplantation has undergone a significant transformation during the last 10–15 years. With the advent of follicular unit transplantation, patients achieve far better results than they could with the original unnatural punch grafts (Figs. 1–4). This cosmetic revolution has resulted in an

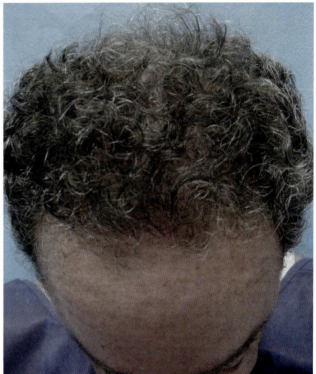

Fig. 2 Patient 1: after 1,000 grafts

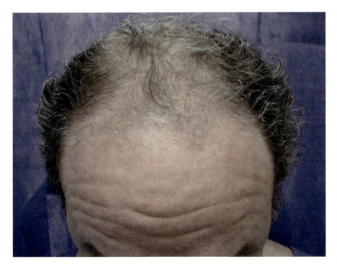

Fig. 1 Patient 1: before hair transplantation

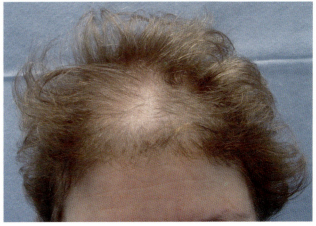

Fig. 3 Patient 2: before hair tansplantation

N.E. Rogers (✉)
Department of Dermatology, Tulane Medical Center,
New Orleans, LA 70112, USA
e-mail: nicolerogers11@yahoo.com

K. Nouri (ed.), *Lasers in Dermatology and Medicine*,
DOI: 10.1007/978-0-85729-281-0_21, © Springer-Verlag London Limited 2011

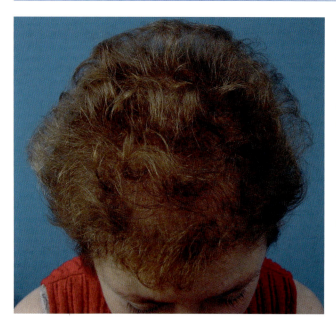

Fig. 4 Patient 2: after 900 grafts

ever increasing demand for the procedure. According to the International Society of Hair Restoration Surgery, practice census results from 2006 demonstrated that over 100,000 hair restoration procedures were performed in the United States, up from 88,000 in 2004. Worldwide, over 225,000 people underwent hair transplant surgery in 2006. This translates to a market size of over 1.2 billion dollars in the U.S. alone.[1]

In the last decade, there has been an equally important revolution in the field of laser surgery. The theory of selective photothermolysis introduced in 1983 by Anderson and Parrish served as the intellectual foundation for the laser revolution.[2] This chapter will focus on the two major laser applications affecting the hair: (1) laser-assisted creation of recipient sites in hair transplantation, and (2) the use of low-level-laser therapy to increase hair growth. Both applications have faced considerable controversy within the laser and hair transplant community. We attempt to provide a balanced perspective of each so that their roles may be fairly assessed and possibly even implemented.

Lasers in Hair Transplantation

- Recipient sites for hair transplantation are usually made with needles
- Difficulties with hemostasis called for the use of CO_2 lasers for recipient site creation
- In 1996, the FDA approved lasers for use in hair transplantation

Most physicians performing hair transplant surgery use traditional steel blade trephines or needles to create their recipient sites. In doing so, they face several challenges. The foremost among these is hemostasis. As each new recipient site is created, bleeding makes graft placement difficult and time-consuming. Heavy drinkers or patients on aspirin or blood-thinning supplements may present even more of a challenge. Grafts may pop out and require re-placement. This challenge prevents many interested dermatologic surgeons from entering the field.

Carbon dioxide lasers were introduced in the mid-1960s. They were popularized in the 1970s in dermatologic surgery because of their ability to vaporize tissue and seal blood vessels. The problem with *continuous* wave carbon dioxide lasers was the peripheral non-specific spread of heat, resulting in widespread scarring of the skin. In the 1990s, the concept of selective photothermolysis was applied to carbon dioxide lasers. By limiting the exposure time of the laser to less than one-half of the thermal relaxation time of the surrounding tissue, there was a significant reduction in lateral thermal damage. This allowed CO_2 lasers to vaporize tissue with excellent hemostasis and no scarring. Pulsed CO_2 lasers were introduced to treat dermatoheliosis and acne scarring with dramatic results.

At that same time this laser revolution in CO_2 lasers was occurring, the field of hair transplantation underwent a similar revolution. The traditional large "pluggy" grafts were abandoned in favor of natural 1–3 hair follicular unit grafts. The problems of bleeding and popping of grafts at recipient sites remained. The investigation of handpieces for creating recipient sites in pulsed CO_2 lasers was begun in the mid-1990s to overcome this problem. High energy pulsed CO_2 lasers would vaporize tissue and seal dermal vessels with excellent hemostasis.

Initial studies found that average graft hair counts were greater in laser-created sites in four of the ten patients, and looked more natural.[3] They also found that there was less bleeding in the laser-created sites, and that the associated grafts required less handling. One pitfall from the excellent hemostasis was that a few of the grafts fell out. By adjusting the laser's energy down slightly, there was an increase in "biological glue" that kept future grafts from falling out.

Subsequent studies confirmed the ability to make recipient sites with excellent hemostasis and growth of transplanted hair (Figs. 5 and 6).[4,5] These studies led to FDA approval of lasers for hair transplantation in 1996.[6-8] FDA approval resulted in a worldwide interest and use of lasers to create recipient sites. Yet, today very few hair surgeons use laser to make recipient sites. What happened?

- Lasers have a minor role in hair transplantation
- Steel needles can provide closer site creation, with less lateral damage, resulting in greater density and less post-surgical hemorrhagic crusting

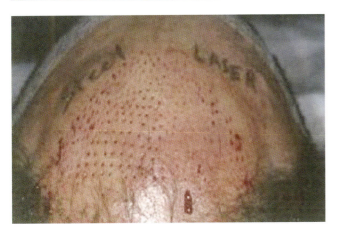

Fig. 5 Laser recipient sites versus steel created sites

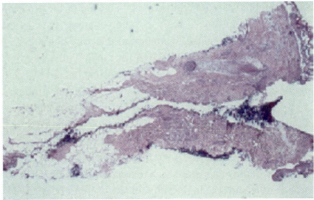

Fig. 7 Pathology showing CO_2 laser assisted recipient sites for hair transplantation

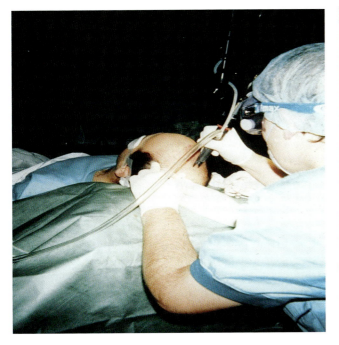

Fig. 6 Physician making CO_2 laser assisted recipient sites

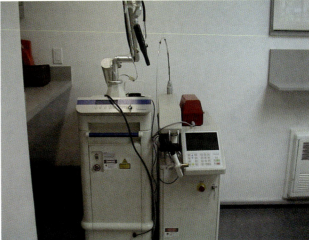

Fig. 8 CO_2 laser and Erbium laser

Some clinicians and investigators reported superficial de-epithelialization surrounding the sites. This led to greater and longer-lasting crusts post-operatively. Delayed hair growth of 2–6 weeks was also observed.[4] The chief obstacle over time was density. Histologic studies of laser-created site showed a minimum of 20–50 μm of lateral thermal damage through the dermis (Fig. 7).[9-11] This was enough to create excellent hemostasis and growth of transplanted hair, but it did not allow for close placement of recipient sites among existing hair follicles. Nineteen gauge needles could more safely create closely spaced sites than pulsed CO_2 lasers. Physicians who tried placing recipient sites too close together often had a massive telogen of existing hair, poor growth, and in some cases necrosis of the skin.

To overcome the lateral tissue necrosis associated with CO_2 lasers, clinicians have tried to use holmium:YAG or erbium:YAG lasers instead of traditional CO_2 lasers for recipient site creation. Histologic studies of the Ho:YAG (λ = 2,120 nm) demonstrated no advantage over traditional CO_2.[12] It created jagged, irregular-shaped channels with even larger zones of thermal injury. The Er:YAG (λ = 2,940 nm) has shown promising results in creating recipient sites for both androgenetic alopecia[13] and cicatricial alopecia.[14] Its use in a 2-year clinical trial produced greater than 95% yield of 1–4-hair follicular units with no reported side effects.[15] However, its use has been limited by the lack of hemostasis and the inability to create sites deep enough with single pulse (Fig. 8).

Risks Inherent in CO_2 Laser Usage

- Damage to water-containing organs, such as the cornea
- Formation of smoke plume containing possibly infectious disease
- Potential for igniting a fire with concomitant oxygen use with sedation

Besides the disadvantages stated above, there are risks inherent in the CO_2 laser because it targets water as its primary chromophore. Laser operators must be aware of the possibility of damaging organs high in water content, such as the cornea. There is also the formation of a smoke plume which could contain bacteria, viral DNA, or viable cells. The high voltage of a CO_2 laser may pose an electrical hazard by igniting tissue, oxygen, or volatile solvents used in hair products.

As seen in (Table 1), there are as many advantages as there are disadvantages to using lasers for hair transplantation. The technique can be helpful for novices to the field, in controlling bleeding and reducing time to place the grafts. However, it may take more time to create sites with an appropriate angle and spacing. Recipient sites cannot be made too close together due to the dermal necrosis. If they are too closely made, widespread necrosis of the scalp may occur. It is unclear whether the vaporization of tissue by laser creates enough density to outweigh this requirement. Ultimately, one must consider factors like the cost of the laser and

whether this technique is superior to current standard of practice. It may be hard for an expensive, complex laser to beat the ease and economy of using needles or steel blades, especially when bleeding is not a significant problem for the experienced hair transplant surgeon.

Perhaps novel fractional ablative devices will be able to create recipient sites as close as #19 and #20 gauge needles without the increased risk of necrosis. Creating a fractional ablative handpiece with a scanner would allow recipient sites to be created quicker, with better hemostasis leading to reduced operating time for patient and physician.

- CO_2 ablative lasers have FDA approval for hair transplantation.
- Not used in hair transplants due to density.
- If laser transplant is performed, spacing too close will result in telogen effluvium.
- Fractional ablative lasers may allow greater density in the future.

Table 1 Pros and Cons of Lasers in Hair Transplantation

Pros of lasers in hair transplantation

1. Improved hemostasis because blood vessels are sealed by laser
2. Reduced time to plant grafts
3. May be easier for beginner hair transplant doctors, as well as their assistants
4. Nerve endings, like blood vessels, are sealed with theoretical reduction in pain[3]
5. May achieve higher density because tissue is vaporized, not just pushed apart[12]
6. Less graft compression, again because alopecic skin measuring 1–2 mm wide is vaporized[3]
7. Less handling of the graft itself, because the laser-prepared sites are wider (1–2 mm) than scalpel created sites.
8. Don't have to constantly sharpen 1–2 mm trephines[3]
9. Less risk of cobblestoning (from graft elevation) or pitting (from graft depression) because there is a constant depth of laser-created site[3]
10. Use of less epinephrine[9]
11. Shorter operative time, which translates to less patient discomfort and less staff frustration[16]
12. Lower risk of cyst formation as a result of tissue left behind[17]

Cons of lasers in hair transplantation

1. Expense of laser, required office space, and maintenance[18,19]
2. May fray epithelial edges and cause superficial de-epithelialization[4]
3. Greater postoperative crusting[12,20]
4. Delayed (2–6 weeks) regrowth of transplanted follicles[4]
5. Risk of telogen effluvium from heat of laser – may thin sites with existing hair
6. Increased risk of secondary infection[4]
7. Risk of injury to adjacent hair follicles in recipient area[4]
8. May achieve lower density because cannot place so close as to risk necrosis[18,19]
9. Longer operating time, because of difficulty creating site at the appropriate angle[4]
10. Persistent erythema[20]
11. Learning curve associated with using laser[4]
12. Plume may contain noxious and carcinogenic chemicals

Lasers in Hair Growth

- LLLT (Low Level Light Therapy) is a relatively new modality
- Few studies have so far demonstrated its efficacy in treating hair loss
- Devices are sold without a prescription, through direct-to-consumer marketing

Given that lasers have historically been used to *remove* unwanted hair, many physicians are debating whether the low-level-light lasers can really enhance hair growth. Numerous products are being marketed directly to consumers that employ low-level-light-therapy (LLLT) to theoretically thicken and promote the growth of existing follicles. However, these products have so far undergone few double-blind, placebo-controlled trials. It would seem that the manufacturers, in their eagerness to make the products available to the public at large, have forgotten to first convince the scientific community.

Nonetheless, there does seem to be fairly good evidence that these products may work. The earliest study was done by Hungarian researcher Endre Mester in 1967, when he was trying to find out if laser radiation could cause cancer in mice.[21] He shaved off their dorsal hair and divided the mice into control and treatment groups, the latter receiving a low-powered ruby laser therapy (694 nm). He found no evidence of cancer in the mice, but did observe that the laser-treated group had faster hair regrowth. This was the origin of "biostimulation" using "cold laser" or "soft laser" therapy administered at lower powers of 1–500 mW. Higher powered lasers, emitting 1–10 W, are used to clear blood vessels or hyperpigmentation.

Several other parameters are involved in administering LLLT. Wavelengths of 600–700 nm are used to treat superficial tissues, while 780–950 nm wavelengths are used for deeper tissues. There is a biphasic dose response curve, in which the central distribution, 700–770 nm is not considered to have as much activity. The dose of energy is comparable to regular laser use, between 1 and 20 J, but it is delivered in a much slower way (Power = J/s = watts).

Basic Science of LLLT

- Stimulates the mitochondrial transport chain
- Enhances ATP production
- Stimulates wound healing
- Reduces inflammation
- Improves neurologic damage, such as with stroke
- Improves musculoskeletal and joint pain

The use of LLLT is based on several scientific papers showing that it can increase ATP levels in tissues by stimulating the mitochondrial transport system.[22-24] To fully understand this we must briefly review the structure and mechanisms of ATP synthesis in mitochondria. These intracellular organelles are considered to be the powerhouses of the cell. They have an outer membrane and an inner membrane, which has numerous infoldings or cristae. Between these two membranes there is an intramembranous space. The very center of the mitochondria is called the matrix (Fig. 9).

The respiratory chain has five major complexes that shuttle electrons from the intramembranous space into the matrix. These include NADH dehydrogenase (Complex I), ATP succinate dehydrogenase (Complex II), cytochrome c reductase (Complex III), cytochrome c oxidase (Complex IV), ATP synthase (Complex V) and two freely diffusible molecules ubiquinone and cytochrome c that shuttle electrons from one complex to the next.[25] By transferring electrons centrally, a proton gradient is built up in the intermembranous space. These protons enter back into the mitochondrial matrix through channels in the ATP synthase enzyme complex. This entry is coupled to ATP synthesis from ADP and phosphate (P_i) (Fig. 10).

LLLT has been found to increase the activity of Complex II and Complex IV in particular.[26] This was demonstrated in a controlled study of wounds treated with AsGa (gallium arsenate, 904 nm) low level laser. This study also showed a clinical improvement in the rate of wound healing after LLLT. Another study using the same laser but at a slightly different wavelength (808 nm) showed enhancement of ATP production in human neuronal cells in culture.[22] This supports the observation that LLLT can help in the setting of neurologic damage following strokes.[27,28] Its ability to repair neurologically damaged tissue may be a function of inhibiting

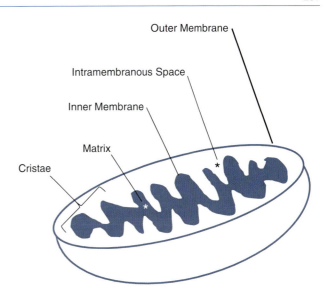

Fig. 9 Structure of mitochondria

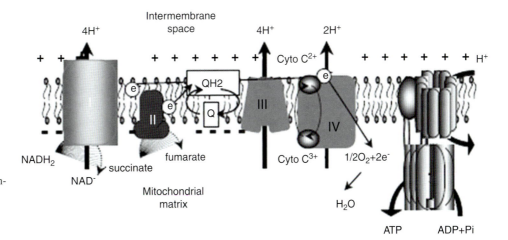

Fig. 10 Structure of the mitochondrial transport chain (Reprinted from Hamblin and Demidova[25] with permission from the SPIE)

nitric oxide synthase and up-regulating the expression of transforming growth factor-beta 1.[29]

It appears that low-level-lasers can help not only with neurologic damage but also with neurogenic pain and musculoskeletal complaints. Peer-reviewed studies found it helpful in treating low back pain,[30] temporomandibular joint disorders,[31] and rheumatoid arthritis patients with carpal tunnel syndrome.[32] In fact, the MicroLight 830 is a low-level-laser which received 510K medical device clearance by the FDA in 2002 for the treatment of carpal tunnel syndrome. Some chiropractors and practitioners of holistic medicine attest to its usefulness in treating patients with other chronic disorders like fibromyalgia.[33,34] They liken it to acupuncture, in providing a noninvasive treatment where other options have failed.

As mentioned above, LLLT can improve wound healing. One study showed that the helium neon laser, at a wavelength of 633 nm, was effective in stimulating the cellular responses of wounded fibroblasts and promoting cell migration.[35] Another study looking at LLLT for wound healing in diabetic rats found faster healing in the treatment group, again with an optimum wavelength of 633 nm.[36]

Perhaps most important is the evidence that LLLT can reduce levels of inflammation in the tissues. It was found to reduce the levels of TNF-alpha in rats treated with a 650 nm Ga-Al-As laser.[37] It has also been found to reduce levels of serum prostaglandin E2 in rats with zymosan-induced arthritis that underwent illumination with 810 nm laser.[38] The authors also observed a reduction in joint swelling that was comparable to treatment with dexamethasone. Finally, levels of COX-2 mRNA expression are also reduced in patients treated with LLLT.[39]

These results suggest that LLLT may be useful in treating autoimmune and other disorders based on inflammation, where primary treatments have failed. Hair disorders such as lichen planopilaris and alopecia areata may even benefit. Androgenetic alopecia, which is not an inflammatory process, may improve more from increased energy and ATP created by the laser. Studies are lacking to directly link the production of ATP with the enhancement of hair growth. However, there are many drugs whose mechanism of action is still unclear. It would be a shame to omit a helpful treatment from our armamentarium simply because we do not yet understand it. Hopefully more studies will soon bring this to light.

- Intellectual basis for potential use for hair including paradoxical growth from laser hair removal and PUVA
- Few clinical trials to date
- FDA 510K approval for male pattern hair loss in 2007

LLLT Products

- Hairmax Lasercomb™
- Sunetics® Laser Hair Brush and Clinical unit
- Revage® 670 Laser (Chair unit)
- Spencer Forrest X5 (Handheld) Hair Laser™

The Hairmax Lasercomb™ has been one of the most publicized products on the market today. It was developed and patented by Lexington International in 2000. Although the exact wavelength and other parameters are kept confidential, the manufacturers do reveal that it uses a diode laser operating in the red portion of the visible color spectrum.[40] It gives off a monochromatic, collimated laser energy. It is indicated to promote hair growth in males with androgenetic alopecia who have Norwood Hamilton Classifications of Ia to V and Fitzpatrick skin types I to IV. Reports of the data they submitted to the FDA are positive, showing increased hair counts among almost all patients in their four-site study. However, they have chosen to keep the specifics of this data proprietary. And although the trials were done only in men, they market the product to women as well. The FDA approved it in January 2007 after the company filed a 510(k) notice, requesting that it be registered as a medical device.

One caveat is that FDA approval of medical devices is far less rigorous than it is for standard pharmaceutical drugs. This labeling indicates that the FDA has reviewed the product and found it to be safe and 'substantially equivalent' to predicate devices already on the market. The most similar predicate device is the TerraQuant, a handheld LLLT device emitting 60–90 W within the 600–900 nm wavelength for treatment of musculoskeletal pain.[41] Other such devices include the Violet Ray device, which was manufactured in the 1950s as a treatment for nearly everything but later its makers were charged with libel and misbranding.[42]

So far, just three studies have been published to investigate the efficacy of low-level-lasers in the treatment of hair loss. The first, by Satino and Markou[43] enrolled 35 patients with androgenetic alopecia (28 males, 7 females) and gave them a Lasercomb to use at home for 6 full months, combing for 5-10 minutes daily. They found that overall, for men and women, there was a 93.5% increase in hair counts in both temporal and vertex sites. Tensile strength of individual hairs also increased by 78.9%. A second study was performed by the authors, which demonstrated a decrease in the number of vellus hairs, and increase in the number of terminal hairs, and an increase in shaft diameter, but the results were not statistically significant[44]. A third study was published in 2009 by the manufacturers of HairMax LaserComb. It did demonstrate statistically significant improvements in hair growth in men over a sham device[45]. More independent studies will be helpful in establishing the role of LLLT in treating hair loss.

Some other names in the industry of LLLT for hair growth are Sunetics® International, located in Las Vegas, NV[46] and the Revage 670® laser.[47] The Sunetics product comes either as a brush ($200–400) or as a free-standing machine for total scalp treatments ($39,900). It uses a 650 nm wavelength at a fluence of 5 mW. It is marketed especially among hair transplant offices to increase the quality/quantity of the donor area, to reduce the pain and to speed wound healing after transplant, and to prevent or reduce hair loss from post-transplant shock. It also is sold as an option for men and women who do not want to undergo a hair transplant procedure and haven't improved with minoxidil or finasteride. The Revage 670® is a chair-based laser that uses rotational phototherapy containing 30 diodes that rotate 180° around the scalp. It is given as in-office treatments 2×/week for 6 weeks then once weekly for 16 weeks. Each treatment session is 30 min each.

Conclusion

- The use of lasers in hair growth and transplantation remains controversial
- Needles remain the standard of treatment for transplant site creation, due to efficiency, economy, and improved density
- FDA approval of lasers for hair growth suggests that they are safe
- More well-designed clinical trials are needed to assess their efficacy

There is a great deal of debate about the use of lasers to enhance hair growth. While seemingly safe, the paucity of peer-reviewed studies validating LLLT for hair loss makes it hard to convince physicians of its efficacy.[19] It is unclear why so few studies exist, given the positive anecdotal reports described above. In contrast, many studies have been done on lasers for creating hair transplantation sites. The difficulty with their implementation is weighted more by technical and economic factors. Can we identify the best laser settings, and use them to create graft sites that are better than those created manually? And if so, will the improvement in the quality and quantity justify the costs of the laser, and risks of thermal damage to surrounding skin?

No matter how we implement lasers to treat patients with hair loss, we must first identify the etiology. Frequently conditions such as lichen planopilaris or alopecia areata may present in a way that mimics androgenetic alopecia. We should be sure that the patients undergo medical evaluation and biopsy where necessary. This crucial step may be left out when treatments such as LLLT are available directly to the public without a prescription. Consumers should be protected from buying expensive items that may not be applicable or aggressive enough for their type of hair loss. Likewise, physicians should be open to the use of such devices where other options have failed, so long as reproducible studies can demonstrate their safety and efficacy.

Terms	Definitions	Units
Energy	Fundamental unit of work	Joule
Power	Rate at which energy is delivered	Watt = J/s
Fluence	Amount of energy delivered per unit area	J/cm^2
Irradiance	Power delivered per unit area	$Watt/cm^2$

References

1. http://www.ishrs.org/PDF/ISHRS_Practice_Census_Survey_Report_2007.pdf
2. Anderson RR, Parrish JA. Selective photothermolysis: precise microsurgery by selective absorption of pulsed radiation. *Science*. 1983;220:524-527.
3. Unger WP, David LM. Laser hair transplantation. *J Dermatol Surg Oncol*. 1994;20:515-521.
4. Unger WP. Laser hair transplantation II. *Dermatol Surg*. 1995;21:759-765.
5. Unger WP. Laser hair transplantation III. *Dermatol Surg*. 1995;21:1047-1055.
6. Grevelink JM, Brennick JB. Hair transplantation facilitated by flashscanner-enhanced carbon dioxide laser. *Otolaryngol Head Neck Surg*. 1994;5:278-280.
7. Grevelink JM. Laser hair transplantation. *Dermatol Clin*. 1997;15:479-486.
8. Villnow M. 2300 grafts/laser session. *Hair Transplant Forum*. 1994;4:6-7.
9. Grevelink JM, Farinelli W, Bua D, et al. Hair transplantation aided by CO_2 lasers. *Lasers Surg Med*. 1995;7:47.
10. Smithdeal CD. Carbon dioxide laser-assisted hair transplantation: the effects of laser parameters on scalp tissue – a histologic study. *Dermatol Surg*. 1997;23:835-840.
11. Kauvar AN, Waldorf HA, Geronemus RG. A histopathological comparison of "char-free" carbon dioxide lasers. *Dermatol Surg*. 1996;22:343-348.
12. Chu EA, Rabinov CR, Wong BJF, Krugman ME. Laser-assisted hair transplantation: histologic comparison between CO_2 and Ho: YAG lasers. *Dermatol Surg*. 2001;27:335-342.
13. Neidel FG, Fuchs M, Krahl D. Laser-assisted autologous hair transplantation with the Er: YAG laser. *J Cutan Laser Ther*. 1999;1: 229-231.
14. Podda M, Spieth K, Kaufmann R. Er:YAG laser-assisted hair transplantation in cicatricial alopecia. *Dermatol Surg*. 2000;26:1010-1014.

15. Uebel C. The use of erbium:YAG laser in hair micro-transplant surgery. *Clin Appl Notes*. 1999;7:1.
16. Ho C, Nguyen Q, Lask G, Lowe N. Mini-slit hair transplantation using the Ultrapulse carbon dioxide laser handpiece. *Dermatol Surg*. 1995;21:1056-1059.
17. Unger WP. What's new in hair replacement surgery. *Dermatol Clin*. 1996;14:783-802.
18. Avram MR. Laser-assisted hair transplantation – a status report in the 21st century. *J Cosmet Dermatol*. 2005;4:135-139.
19. Avram MR, Leonard RT Jr, Epstein ES, Williams JL, Bauman AJ. The current role of laser/light sources in the treatment of male and female pattern hair loss. *J Cosmet Laser Ther*. 2007;9:27-28.
20. Fitzpatrick RE. Laser hair transplantation. Tissue effects of laser parameters. *Dermatol Surg*. 1995;21:1042-1046.
21. Mester E, Szende B, Gartner P. The effect of laser beams on the growth of hair in mice. *Radiobiol Radiother (Berl)*. 1968;9:621-626.
22. Oron U, Ilic S, De Taboada L, Streeter J. Ga-As (808 nm) laser irradiation enhances ATP production in human neuronal cells in culture. *Photomed Laser Surg*. 2007;25:180-182.
23. Gavish L, Asher Y, Becker Y, Kleinman Y. Low level laser irradiation stimulates mitochondrial membrane potential and disperses subnuclear promyelocytic leukemia protein. *Lasers Surg Med*. 2004;35:369-376.
24. Yu W, Naim JO, McGowan M, Ippolito K, Lanzafame RJ. Photomodulation of oxidative metabolism and electron chain enzymes in rat liver mitochondria. *Photochem Photobiol*. 1997;66:866-871.
25. Hamblin MR, Demidova TN. Mechanisms of low level light therapy. *Proc SPIE*. 2006;6140:614001.
26. Silveira PC, Streck EL, Pinho RA. Evaluation of mitochondrial respiratory chain activity in wound healing by low-level laser therapy. *J Photochem Photobiol B*. 2007;86:279-282.
27. Oron A, Oron U, Chen J, et al. Low-level laser therapy applied transcranially to rats after induction of stroke significantly reduces long-term neurological deficits. *Stroke*. 2006;37:2620-2624.
28. Lampl Y, Zivin JA, Fisher M, et al. Infrared laser therapy for ischemic stroke: a new treatment strategy: results of the NeuroThera Effectiveness and Safety Trial-1 (NEST-1). *Stroke*. 2007;38:1843-1849.
29. Leung MC, Lo SC, Siu FK, So KF. Treatment of experimentally induced transient cerebral ischemia with low energy laser inhibits nitric oxide synthase activity and up-regulates the expression of transforming growth factor-beta 1. *Lasers Surg Med*. 2002;31:283-288.
30. Djavid GE, Mahrdad R, Ghasemi M, Hasan-Zadeh H, Sotoodeh-Manesh A, Pouryaghoub G. In chronic low back pain, low level laser therapy combined with exercise is more beneficial than exercise along in the long term: a randomized trial. *Aust J Physiother*. 2007;53:155-160.
31. Fikackova H, Dostalova T, Navratil L, Klaschka J. Effectiveness of low-level laser therapy in temporomandibular joint disorders: a placebo-controlled study. *Photomed Laser Surg*. 2007;25:297-303.
32. Ekim A, Armagan O, Tascioglu F, Oner C, Colak M. Effect of low level laser therapy in rheumatoid arthritis patients with carpal tunnel syndrome. *Swiss Med Wkly*. 2007;137:347-352.
33. www.laser-therapeutics.net/articles.htm
34. www.healing.org/only-7.html
35. Hawkins D, Abrahamse H. Effect of multiple exposures of low-level laser therapy on the cellular responses of wounded human skin fibroblasts. *Photomed Laser Surg*. 2006;24:705-714.
36. Al-Watban FA, Zhang XY, Andres BL. Low-level laser therapy enhances wound healing in diabetic rats: a comparison of different lasers. *Photomed Laser Surg*. 2007;25:72-77.
37. Aimbire F, Albertini R, Pacheco MT, et al. Low-level laser therapy induces dose-dependent reduction of TNF-alpha levels in acute inflammation. *Photomed Laser Surg*. 2006;24:33-37.
38. Castano AP, Dai T, Yaroslavsky I, et al. Low-level laser therapy for zymosan-induced arthritis in rats: importance of illumination time. *Lasers Surg Med*. 2007;39:543-550.
39. Albertini R, Aimbire F, Villaverde AB, Silva JA Jr, Costa MS. COX-2 mRNA expression decreases in the subplantar muscle of rat paw subjected to carrageenan-induced inflammation after low-level laser therapy. *Inflamm Res*. 2007;56:228-229.
40. www.hairmax.com
41. www.coldlasertherapies.com.
42. www.museumofquackery.com/devices/ut.htm
43. Satino JL, Markou M. Hair regrowth and increased hair tensile strength using the HairMax LaserComb for low-level laser therapy. *Int J Cosmet Surg Aesthet Dermatol*. 2003;5:113-117.
44. Avram MR, Rogers NE. The use of low-level light for hair growth: part I. *J Cosmet Laser Ther*. 2009;11:110-117.
45. Leavitt M, Charles G, Heyman E, Michaels D. HairMax LaserComb Laser Phototherapy device in the treatment of male androgenetic alopecia. *Clin Drug Invest*. 2009;29:283-292.
46. www.sunetics.com.
47. www.laserhaircare.com

Reflectance-Mode Confocal Microscopy in Dermatological Oncology

Juan Luis Santiago Sánchez-Mateos, Carmen Moreno García del Real, Pedro Jaén Olasolo, and Salvador González

- Imaging techniques capable of non-invasive, high-resolution, skin imaging *in vivo* have been the focus of recent attention in the dermatology field. These efforts are directed to improve the diagnostic accuracy of skin cancer, especially cutaneous melanoma.
- Reflectance-mode confocal microscopy (RCM) allows real time non-invasive histological imaging with cytological detail comparable to conventional histology of the skin when exploring cutaneous structures between the stratum corneum and the upper reticular dermis.
- Reflectance-mode confocal microscopes consist of a light source for illumination of a small spot within translucent tissue; and a point detector that detects back-scattered and reflected light though a pinhole. The pinhole prevents out-of-focus light from reaching the detector; as a result, only the optical plane in focus (confocal) is detected.
- Similar to dermoscopy images, real time images obtained by RCM are oriented horizontal to skin surface (optical transversal sections).
- Melanin provides strong contrast because of its high refractive index (1.7) relative to the surrounding epidermis; the melanosome size, similar to the near-infrared wavelengths (800–1,064 nm), produces strong back scattering of the beam. Thus, cells containing melanin, such as pigmented keratinocytes, melanocytes, or melanophages, appear very bright when illuminated in this manner.

- Similarly, other organelles or cytoplasmic granules provide good contrast (albeit less intense than melanin), resulting in good imaging of cells containing them, such as Langerhans cells, lymphocytes, or cytoplasmic granules in keratinocytes at the stratum granulosum.
- Major confocal imaging criteria of pigmented lesions such as benign and malignant melanocytic tumors have been established. RCM imaging criteria of other skin cancers such as basal cell carcinoma, squamous cell carcinoma, oral cavity neoplasm, and mycosis fungoides have also been evaluated.
- Reflectance-mode confocal microscopy shows promise for: (1) guidance during biopsy collection; (2) monitoring histological architectural changes or dynamic process such as inflammatory response or capillary flow; (3) histological correlation with dermoscopic features; (4) monitoring of the response of a given lesion to treatment; and (5) demarcation of the extension of a lesion before proceeding to invasive treatments such as surgical excisions.
- The main limitation of RCM is its relatively low penetration through the dermis; currently, a maximum depth of 250–300 μm can be achieved, preventing imaging of structures located in deep dermis and hypodermis.
- The main challenge is the interpretation of images. Specific photographic atlas, courses and development of teledermatology may solve this problem.

S. González (✉)
Dermatology Service, Memorial Sloan-Kettering Cancer Center, New York, NY, USA and
Ramón y Cajal Hospital, Alcalá University,
Madrid, Spain
e-mail: gonzals6@mskcc.org

Introduction

- A wide variety of non-invasive imaging techniques provides the potential for high-resolution skin imaging *in vivo* including dermoscopy, optical coherence tomography, high-frequency ultrasound, magnetic resonance imaging, fluorescence-mode confocal microscopy, and reflectance-mode confocal microscopy.
- Reflectance-mode confocal microscopy is a technique with many possible applications, offering real time non-invasive microscopic images between stratum corneum and reticular dermis.

Dermatology is an area of medical specialization in which diagnosis is frequently based exclusively on bare eyed clinical examination. Recent advances in imaging techniques provide the potential for non-invasive high-resolution skin imaging *in vivo*. These can overcome some of the disadvantages of the conventional biopsy and histologic analysis. Such advances include dermoscopy,[1] optical coherence tomography,[2] high-frequency ultrasound,[3] magnetic resonance imaging (MRI),[4] fluorescence-mode confocal microscopy,[5] and reflectance-mode confocal microscopy (RCM). Of these, RCM is the technique with more potential applications, offering real time non-invasive microscopic images with the highest resolution comparable to routine histology when exploring cutaneous structures between stratum corneum and reticular dermis.[6-8]

History

- Marvin Minsky invented confocal scanning microscopy in 1955.
- Development of light sources and computerization since the 1980s have significantly improved the hardware and software of confocal microscopy.
- Since the 1980s, several studies have demonstrated potential applications *of in vivo* RCM imaging in dermatology.
- The first paper using confocal scanning laser microscopy for imaging human skin *in vivo* was reported in 1995 by Rajadhyaksha et al.[8]

Marvin Minsky invented the confocal scanning microscope while working as a postdoctoral fellow at Harvard in 1955.[9] However, its employment to image tissue *in vivo* required extensive development of light sources and computerization technologies. Since the 1980s, several research groups have employed tandem scanning confocal microscopy to image human and animal tissue *in vivo*.[10-13] The first reported use of confocal scanning laser microscopy to image human skin *in vivo* dates back to 1995.[8] Since then, many reports have suggested its possible applications in dermatology, particularly in the diagnosis of skin tumors.

Advantages of *In Vivo* Imaging in Dermatology

- *In vivo* RCM imaging offers several important advantages over conventional histology: it is painless, causes no tissue damage and minimizes disruption of the native structure in the skin.
- The same region of the skin can be repeatedly imaged over time in order to evaluate tissue growth, wound healing, lesion progression or response to therapy.
- This technique collects data in real time and may be useful to study dynamic processes such as capillary flow or leukocyte trafficking.

In vivo RCM offers several important advantages over conventional histology. Imaging is painless and non-invasive, causing no tissue damage. The skin is not altered by post-collection processing (fixation, sectioning, and mounting) or staining, minimizing artifacts or disruption of the native structure of the tissue. Real-time data collection is faster than routine histology, and the same location of the skin can be repeatedly imaged over time to evaluate dynamic changes such as tissue growth, wound healing, lesion progression or response to therapy.[14-18] This is one of the main advantages of the technique compared to conventional histology, which can only reveal information about the tissue at the time of collection of the sample.

Principles of Reflectance-Mode Confocal Microscopy

- Reflectance-mode confocal microscopy uses a point source of laser light (800–1,064 nm) that illuminates a small spot within translucent tissue such as skin or mucosa.

- The reflected light (reflectance) is imaged onto a detector after passing through a small pinhole. Backscattering of light occurs due to local variations of the refractive index within the tissue.
- The pinhole prevents out-of-focus light from reaching the detector in order to create a bidimensional image of a plane that is in focus (confocal) within tissue.
- The resolution depends on the pinhole size, the numerical aperture of the objective lens, and the wavelength used. Usually, RCM provides images with a lateral resolution of 1 μm and an axial resolution of 3–5 μm.
- The current depth that can be reached in the dermis with RCM varies among different microscopes (wavelengths), but averages 200–250 μm across.
- Water immersion lenses are used since the refractive index of water (1.33) is close to that of epidermis (1.34), minimizing spherical aberrations caused when the light passes through the tissue-air interface.
- A skin contact device is used to reduce motion artifacts and contain the water or gel interface during imaging.
- Melanin provides endogenous contrast because of its high refractive index relative to the surrounding epidermis and size of the melanosomes, similar to that of the illuminating wavelength. This means that cells containing melanin (pigmented keratinocytes, melanocytes, and melanophages) are bright under these conditions.
- By moving the lens along the "z" (vertical) axis with respect to the skin surface, it is possible to image different horizontal layers within the tissue.
- Images can be converted into static pictures of horizontal skin sections as well as recorded to produce movies of dynamics events, such as blood flow or trafficking leukocytes.

Reflectance confocal microscopy is based on the use of a point source of light that illuminates a small spot within translucent tissue, such as skin or mucosa. The reflected light (reflectance) is imaged onto a detector after passing through a small pinhole. This pinhole prevents out-of-focus light from reaching the detector, so that only light from the exact in-focus plane (confocal) is detected. An entire image of the whole plane of the sample under study is generated using line scanning of the point source beam. This enables a virtual sectioning of a thin horizontal tissue plane *in vivo*, such as computerized tomography or MRI. Such optical sectioning of the tissue allows intact tissue to be studied without physical sectioning, as in conventional histology, preserving the physical structure and physiology of the tissue.

The resolution depends on the pinhole size, the numerical aperture of the objective lens, and the wavelength used. Although lasers of different wavelengths may be used as the light source for RCM, only longer wavelengths penetrate deep enough into the skin. Therefore, confocal microscopes use sources of illumination near the infrared wavelength (800–1,064 nm). Backscattering of light occurs due to local variations of the refractive index within the tissue as well as when the scattering structure has a size similar to the illuminating wavelength. For example, near-infrared wavelengths produce strong backscattering from melanosomes (despite melanin absorption at this wavelength) because they contain material with a high refractive index relative to the surrounding skin structures and have a size similar to the illuminating wavelength.[14] This can be used in order to detect cells containing melanin, such as basal keratinocytes, melanocytes, and melanophages, which appear very bright upon imaging. Other microstructures similar in size to the illuminating wavelength, such as organelles or granules in the cytoplasm also act like reflectance surfaces and may determine other endogenous sources of contrast in Langerhans cells and lymphocytes.

New microscopes use a single optical fibre that is common to both the illumination optical path and the detection optical path. This single-moded optical fibre acts as a spatial filter that discards out-of-focus information collected by the objective lens. This system simplifies the opto-mechanical complexity by eliminating the bulky optical components and confocal apertures (pinholes) associated with conventional confocal implementations. This fiber-optic approach has enabled miniaturization of the confocal scanner into a handheld device that provides the flexibility and mobility necessary for actual clinical use.

The currently commercially available RCM has a wavelength of 830 nm and 30× objective lens of NA 0.9, which provides a lateral resolution of approximately 1 μm and an axial resolution (section thickness) of 3–5 μm.[14] It is possible to image normal skin from the stratum corneum to a depth of 200–250 μm, at the level of upper reticular dermis.[14] Imaging deeper layers within the skin may also be achieved by using greater laser power, but the laser power used in the commercially available device is less than 30 mW because it causes no tissue damage or eye injury. Water immersion lenses are used since the refractive index of water (1.33) is close to that of the epidermis (1.34), which minimizes spherical aberrations caused when the light passes through the tissue-air interface.[14] Other immersion media, such as water-based gels, are useful when imaging a scaly or hyperkeratotic lesion since the gel settles between disrupted corneocytes, reducing refractive irregularities. Such gels are also useful when imaging irregular skin sites, since the gel does not run off of the skin the way water or other aqueous solutions would do.

Skin movement is an important limitation when imaging *in vivo*. To reduce motion artefacts and contain the water or the gel interface when imaging, a skin contact device is used. This device consists of a metal ring that is fixed to the skin with adhesive, and is coupled to the microscope housing with a magnet during imaging. It has a concave shape to hold the immersion medium over a round window, which allows passing of light on to the sample as well as reflected light from the tissue.

Images are obtained after sequential illumination of multiple pixels according to the density of the reflected light from focal plane. This plane is scanned in two dimensions in order to create a mosaic image; architectural patterns can be evaluated this way. By moving the objective lens in the "z" stage (vertical) with respect to the skin surface, it is possible to image at different horizontal levels within the tissue since the focal plane is progressively moved deeper or closer to the surface. We can select each imaged square to compose a mosaic image and study cytological or architectural details. Images can be captured to produce static pictures of horizontal skin sections as well as recorded on videotape (20–30 frames per second) to produce movies that reveal dynamics events such as blood flow.[8,14-18]

Findings of Normal Skin

- Confocal images obtained are horizontal or *en face* compared to vertical sections as normally obtained from routine histology. These images are grayscale (bright-scale) similar to radiographs or echographic examinations.
- The level of the skin under study can be ascertained by the morphologic appearance of tissue at a given depth or by measuring the depth of section, using a micrometer attached to the "z" stage of the objective lens.
- Starting from the surface and progressing deeper we elucidate the following tissue structures:

Epidermis

1. *Stratum corneum.* It appears as bright images of anucleated polygonal corneocytes 10–30 μm in size, and grouped in "islands" separated by skin folds, which appear very dark.

2. *Stratum granulosum.* It has 2–4 layers of cells measuring 25–35 μm. The nuclei of these cells appear as dark central ovals, surrounded by bright grainy cytoplasms.
3. *Stratum spinosum.* It has the aspect of a tight honeycomb pattern of smaller cells, measuring 15–25 μm in size, with well-demarcated cell borders.
4. *Basal layer.* It consists of bright clusters of cells measuring 7–10 μm. The suprapapillary epidermal plate at the dermo-epidermal junction is apparent as rings of bright basal cells surrounding dark dermal papillae (bright dermal papillary rings).

Dermis

5. *Papillary dermis.* It consists of a network of reticulated gray fibers, with central capillary vessels surrounded by bright cellular rings correlated with basal keratinocytes.
6. *Reticular dermis.* It shows a reticulated pattern, correlated with collagen bundles and elastic fibers.
7. *Skin appendages.*
   - Eccrine ducts appear as bright hollow structures that spiral through epidermis and dermis.
   - Pilo-sebaceous units appear as whorled centrally hollow structures with elliptical elongated cells at the circumference and a central refractile long hair shaft.
- Although these are the classical features of normal skin, other variables such as anatomical site, sun-exposure, skin color, age, and physiological condition need to be analyzed.

Real-time reflectance-mode confocal microscopy offers a novel view of the skin in terms of the orientation and image content. Compared to routine histology, it offers two main differences. First, the image obtained is horizontal or *en face* rather compared to the vertical sections typical in histology. Second, images are greyscale (bright scale), similar to radiographs or echographic examinations. The field of view provided by RCM varies with different microscopes, but is generally 250–500 μm across.[14] The layer of the skin under study can be ascertained by the morphologic appearance of tissue at a given depth or by measuring the depth of section, using a micrometer attached to the "z" stage of the objective lens.

When imaging the skin, the most superficial images obtained are of the stratum corneum. The morphologic appearance of that section includes anucleated polygonal corneocytes 10–30 µm in size grouped in "islands" separated by skin folds, which appear very dark (Fig. 1a). Images are very bright because the refractive difference at the interface between the immersion medium and stratum corneum results in a large amount of back-scattered light. The next layer is the stratum granulosum, which consists of two to four layers of cells measuring 25–35 µm. The nuclei appear as dark central ovals within the cell surrounded by a bright grainy cytoplasm (Fig. 1b). The next layer is the stratum spinosum, which consists of a tight honeycomb pattern of smaller cells 15–25 µm in size with well-demarcated cell borders (Fig. 1c). The deepest layer of the epidermis is the basal layer, visualized as bright clusters of cells due to their content in melanin, 7–10 µm in size. The suprapapillary epidermal plate at the dermo-epidermal junction appears as rings of bright basal cells surrounding dark dermal papillae, which often show a central area of blood flow consistent with papillary dermal vascular loops (Fig. 1d). The papillary dermis images consist of a network of reticulated fibres with central capillary vessels (Fig. 1e). In the reticular dermis, confocal images show a thick reticulated pattern consisted of collagen bundles and elastic fibres (Fig. 1f). We can also observe eccrine ducts, which appear as bright, centrally hollow structures that spiral through epidermis and dermis, and hair shafts with pilo-sebaceous units. These appear as whorled, centrally hollow structures with elliptical, elongated cells at the circumference and a central, refractile long hair shaft.

The appearance of normal skin varies according to the anatomical site, sun-exposure, skin color, age, and physiological condition being imaged.[19] Skin from sun-exposed or darkly pigmented sites, for example, appears generally brighter because of what appears to be more pigment at the basal layer.

Non-Pigmented Lesions

- *Basal Cell Carcinoma (BCC)*
  - Confocal features of BCC have been defined retrospectively so that the presence of two of five criteria has a sensitivity of 100%, with a specificity of 95.7% when the number of criteria is four.[21]
  - Diagnostic criteria:
    1. Islands of monomorphic, elongated, tumor cells.
    2. Polarization of elongated, monomorphic nuclei along the same axis of orientation.

- Streaming: polarization of nuclei in an entire aggregate of tumor cells.
- Peripheral palisading of nuclei: peripheral monolayer of tumor cells oriented parallel to each other and perpendicular to the stroma.
    3. Variable epidermal disarray (nucleated corneocytes, loss of the honeycombed pattern, and keratinocytic nuclear pleomorphism).
    4. Prominent inflammatory cell infiltrate.
    5. Increase of capillary vessels, which are dilated and may show leukocytes rolling and their adhesion on endothelium.
- *Actinic keratoses (AK)*
    1. Irregular hyperkeratosis.
    2. Architectural disarray at the epidermal level: epidermal cell nuclear enlargement with pleomorphism and nucleated corneocytes (parakeratosis).
    3. Pattern of architectural disarray that does not involve the full thickness of the epidermis.
  - The lack of depth of the illuminating wavelength restricts the potential of RCM to accurately differentiate between hypertrophic AK and SCC.
- *Squamous cell carcinoma (SCC)*
    1. Irregular hyperkeratosis.
    2. Architectural disarray at the epidermal level: epidermal cell nuclear enlargement with pleomorphism and nucleated corneocytes (parakeratosis).
    3. Pattern of architectural disarray involving the full thickness of epidermis.
    4. Vascular patterns and keratin pearls are not well characterized yet.
  - The lack of depth of the illuminating wavelength restricts the potential of RCM to accurate distinguish AK from SCC, or between superficially invasive SCC and SCC *in situ* (Bowen's disease).
- *Oral cavity neoplasm*
    1. Densely packed, pleomorphic tumor nuclei.
    2. Architectural disarray at the level of the epithelium with parakeratotic areas.
    3. Areas of inflammation.
- *Mycosis fungoides (MF)*
    1. Weakly refractile, round to oval point cells at epidermal levels (epidermotropic lymphocytes).
    2. Vesicle-like dark spaces filled with weakly refractile, round to oval point cells (Pautrier's microabscesses).

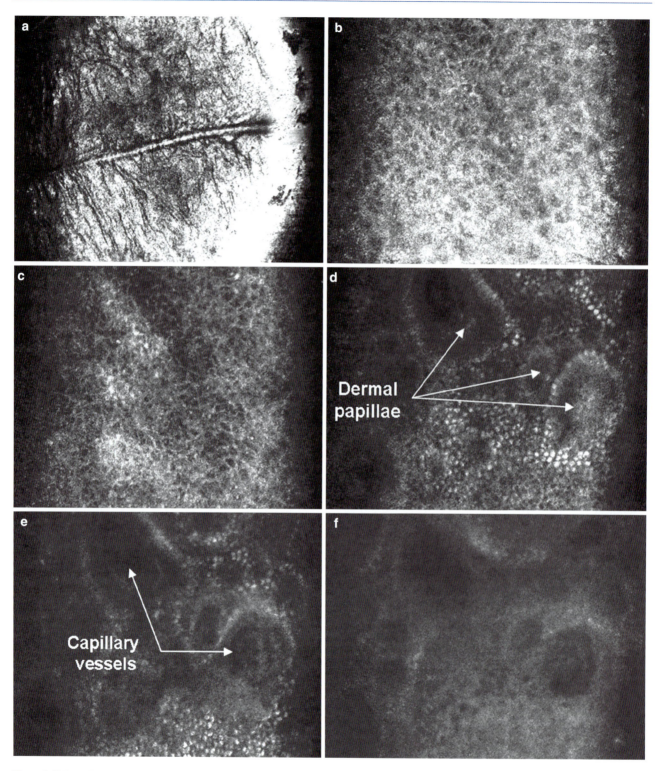

Fig. 1 RCM parallel images of normal skin obtained moving the objective lens in the "z" stage (vertical) with respect to the skin surface. Stratum corneum appears as a bright surface, with dark skin folds (**a**). The stratum granulosum has a regular honeycomb web pattern, where granular cells have dark oval areas (nuclei) within bright grainy cytoplasms (**b**). The stratum spinosum has a honeycombed pattern too, but spinous keratinocytes are smaller, with polygonal and well demarcated cell borders (**c**), The basal layer consists of small bright cells usually without nuclei visualized. They are located around of apertures of dermal papillae, which are delimited with uniform bright rings of basal cells (**d–e**). Dermal papillae have a thin network of reticulated grey fibres around dark spaces (capillary vessels), where blood flow can be visualized during real time imaging (**e–f**)

3. Increase of the intercellular space at epidermal levels; visualization of interkeratinocytic junctions (spongiosis).
4. Tagging of the dermo-epidermal junction by weakly bright, round to oval point cells (lymphocytic infiltration).
5. Hyporefractility of the basal cells surrounding the dermal papillae.

These confocal features are not specific since they have also been observed in lichenoid dermatitides and acute contact dermatitis.

The characterization of skin neoplasm using RCM is an important area of clinical research with potential for non-invasive diagnosis and management of a variety of skin cancers. The advent of newer, less invasive topical therapies such as topical imiquimod or photodynamic therapy demands the development of non-invasive diagnostic tools to identify tumor subtypes and tumor margins accurately, and to monitor the response to treatment.

Basal Cell Carcinoma

Basal Cell Carcinomas (BCCs) are the most common skin tumors in humans (Fig. 2a, b); RCM features of BCC have been defined.[20] They include the presence of islands of monomorphic tumor cells (Fig. 2c, d), elongated in shape and with nuclei oriented along the same axis, producing a polarized appearance (basaloid nuclei). This polarized cell pattern persists through the thickness of the epidermis (Fig. 2e), with loss of the normal progressive size difference of differentiating epidermal cells, loss of the normal honeycomb pattern, and loss of dermal papillae architecture. The presence of keratinocyte disarray and architectural disorder of the overlying epidermis is indicative of actinic damage or consequence of reactivity to the tumor. Reactive fibrosis is featured by thick, bright bundles near tumor islands (Fig. 2c, d). In addition, pronounced superficial blood vessels, dilation, tortuosity, and rolling of leukocytes along the endothelial wall have been frequently observed. It is also possible to visualize inflammatory cell infiltrates among the tumor cells (Fig. 2e).

A retrospective, multicentric study from 152 lesions[21] has determined that the presence of at least two of these criteria has a sensitivity of 100% for the diagnosis of BCC. As the number of criteria is higher, the specificity increased, so that when at least four criteria are present the specificity was 95.7%, showing the best correlation between high sensitivity

and specificity. The most sensitive and specific criterion was the presence of polarized nuclei (91.6% and 97% respectively). These results showed little variability across BCC locations and subtypes. RCM may be also useful to noninvasively monitor the response to cryotherapy or new therapies such as topical imiquimod or photodynamic therapy.

Actinic Keratoses

Actinic keratoses (AKs) are keratinocytic dysplasias (Fig. 3a–c) that can develop into squamous cell carcinomas (SCC). Confocal features of AK include irregular hyperkeratosis with parakeratosis (Fig. 3d), architectural disarray, and epidermal cell nuclear enlargement with pleomorphism (Fig. 3e). The pattern of architectural disarray does not involve the full thickness of the epidermis.[22] As BCCs, RCM images of AKs shows thick refractile bundles in dermis correlating with solar elastosis (Fig. 3f). The most important limiting factor of RCM is the shallow depth of the illuminating wavelength, which prevents accurate visualization of the dermo-epidermal junction, particularly in hyperkeratotic lesions. This restricts the potential of this tool to distinguish accurately between hypertrophic AK *vs.* SCC. On the other hand, recent evidence suggests the presence of multilocular preneoplastic changes in the areas surrounding the affected skin sites, thus RCM may be useful to detect subclinical AKs.[23] The same report evaluated the sensitivity of RCM in the diagnosis of AKs. Sensitivity was an estimated 97.7% (44 AKs cases were included in this study). Thus, RCM may be a useful diagnostic tool in the management and follow-up of patients with low skin phototypes and a history of intense sun-exposure to permit an early diagnosis of AKs or BCCs.

Squamous Cell Carcinoma

Confocal features consistent with SCC are full thickness architectural disarray and nuclear enlargement with pleomorphism in the stratum granulosum and stratum spinosum[22] (Fig. 4a–e). Other changes consistent with SCC, such as vascular patterns and keratin pearls, need further investigation. Leukocyte rolling along the endothelial wall has been observed as well (Fig. 4f). Lack of depth of the RCM illumination wavelengths makes differential diagnosis between hyperkeratotic AKs and SCC difficult due to lack of adequate visual assessment at the dermo-epidermal junction. This also makes differential diagnosis between superficially invasive SCC and SCC *in situ* (Bowen's disease) impossible as of today.

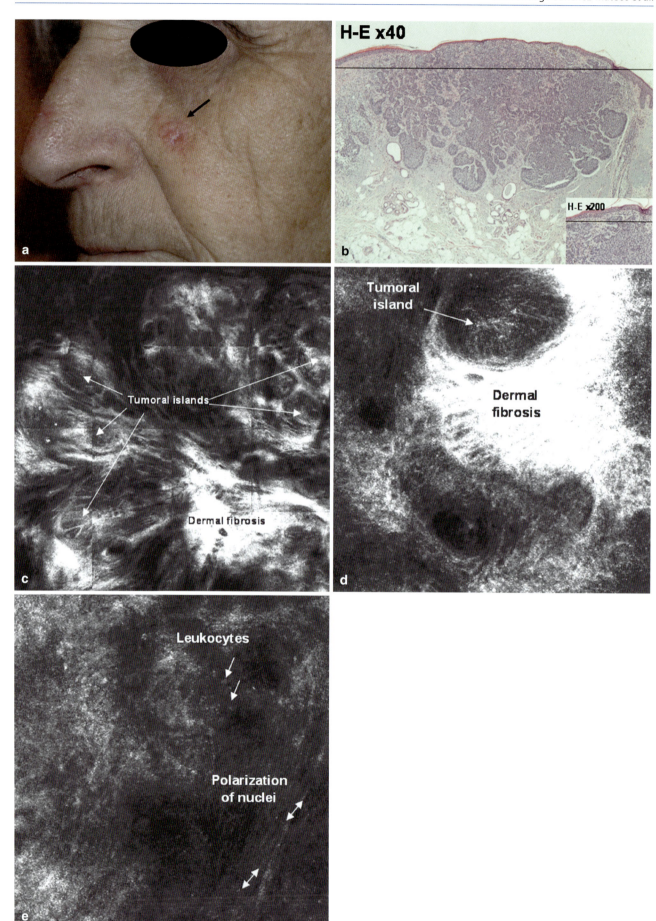

Oral Cavity Neoplasm

Reflectance-mode confocal microscopy-based *ex vivo* examination allows imaging the oral mucosa with resolution comparable to conventional histology without tissue preparation and staining.[24] In SCCs, densely packed, pleomorphic tumor nuclei, and architectural disarray at the level of epithelium could be visualized. Others features that could be identified included areas of inflammation. *In vivo*, imaging was possible up to 490 and 250 μm in the lip and tongue, respectively.[25] Reflectance-mode confocal microscopy provides details of normal human oral mucosa at the cellular level; it has the potential for use in clinical practice as a diagnostic tool for the early detection of oral cancer and precancer.

Mycosis Fungoides

Reflectance-mode confocal microscopy is able to image epidermotropic lymphocytes, Pautrier's microabscesses, spongiosis, and tagging of the dermo-epidermal junction by lymphocytes.[26] Confocal features were hyporefractility of the basal cells surrounding the dermal papillae, corresponding to basal layer infiltration by atypical lymphocytes, and vesicle-like dark spaces filled with small, weakly refractile, round to oval cells, corresponding with Pautrier's microabscesses. The latter was typically limited to plaque-type mycosis fungoides (MF). Hyporefractility of the basal cells surrounding the dermal papillae is a result of the presence of less refractile lymphocytes within and around the basal layer of the epidermis. Unfortunately, this hyporefractility has also been observed in lichenoid dermatitides and the vesicular structures may be difficult to distinguish from other vesicles filled with inflammatory cells, such as those seen in allergic contact dermatitis. Other limiting factor is the lack of depth, which is a key factor in tumoral-type MF. Reflectance-mode confocal microscopy may be a real-time guide for optimal biopsy site selection in patients with multiple lesions consistent with MF.

Pigmented Lesions

Pigmented Non-Melanocytic Lesions

- *Seborrheic keratosis*
  1. Epidermal thickening without keratinocytic disarray.
  2. Long, parallel, dermal papillae.
  3. Homogeneous bright rings surrounding dermal papillae (*edged papillae*).
  4. Epidermal lesion with cerebriform architecture.
- *Dermatofibroma (DF)*
  1. Honeycomb pattern or cobblestone pattern at epidermal levels.
  2. Homogeneous bright rings surrounding dermal papillae (*edged papillae*).
  3. Papillary rings have poor demarcation.
  4. Increase of papillary density at dermo-epidermal junction.
  5. Absence of bright nucleated cells at dermo-epidermal junction.
  6. Highly refractile, thick collagen bundles at papillary and reticular dermis.
- *Pigmented BCC*
  1. Similar features to non-pigmented BCC.
  2. Melanin is not uniformly distributed throughout the tumor cords.
  3. Melanin contrast is due to benign pigmented keratinocytes, pigmented tumor cords, melanocytes, and dermal melanophages.
  4. Presence of melanophages in papillary dermis.
- *Pigmented mammary Paget disease*
  1. Large atypical bright cells arranged in pagetoid fashion.
  2. Keratinocytic disarray.
  3. Irregular dermal papillae without homogeneous bright rings surrounding them (*non-edged papillae*).
  4. Confocal images similar to melanoma *in situ*.

Fig. 2 (**a**) Clinical photograph of a BCC located on the left cheek of a 65 year old male showing superficial telangiectases and bright pearly borders. (**b**) H&E original magnification 40×, the corresponding histologic section shows tumor islands consisting of basaloid cells on a sun exposed (solar elastosis) skin. H&E original magnification 200×, corresponding histologic detail shows well-circumscribed tumor islands and their typical peripheral palisading. (**c**) RCM mosaic image taken at dermal level shows several tumor islands surrounded by thick gray collagen bundles. There are areas with brightly, dense, dermal fibrosis.

(**d**) RCM image reveals loss of dermal papillae architecture and intense bright area, correlated with reactive dermal fibrosis, surrounding tumor islands (RCM image 500×500 μm). (**e**) RCM image shows a detail with long dark nuclei oriented along the same axis (polarized cell pattern) in a tumor island. Red arrows point to weakly bright cells among the tumor cells near the capillary vessels, which has been correlated with trafficking leukocytes and inflammatory cell infiltrate (RCM image 500×500 μm)

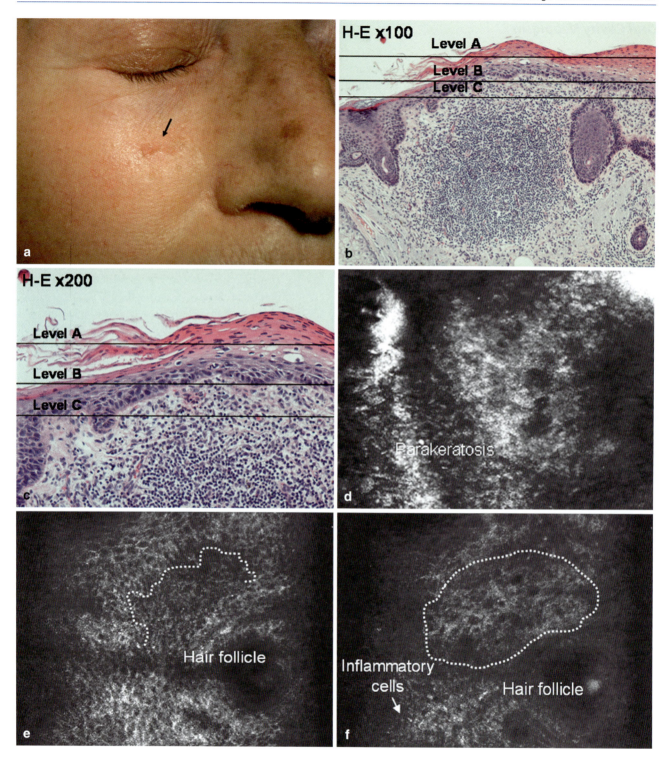

Fig. 3 (**a**) Clinical photograph of an actinic keratosis located on the right cheek of a 55 year old female. (**b**) H&E original magnification 100×, corresponding histologic section reveals parakeratosis and epidermal dysplasia involving interadnexal epidermis on sun exposed skin. These features support the diagnosis of actinic keratosis. (**c**) H&E original magnification 200×, corresponding histologic detail shows epidermal dysplasia affecting typically the basal layers, with parakeratosis and inflammatory infiltrates in dermis. (**d–f**) RCM images 500×500 μm at different levels of depth. *Level A* shows areas with bright polygonal and nucleated cells (parakeratosis) at the stratum corneum (RCM image 500×500 μm). *Level B* exhibits keratinocytic disarray and loss of honeycombed pattern. Dermal papilla (*dotted line*) is not well delimited showing the loss of uniform bright rings and distortion of DEJ limits (RCM 500×500 μm). *Level C* shows weakly bright point cells (inflammatory cells) and a thick gray network at the superficial dermis (*dotted limited area*) which has been related with actinic damage and correlated with solar elastosis (RCM image 500×500 μm)

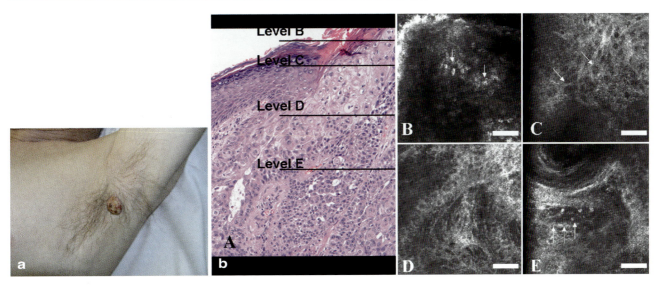

Fig. 4 (a) Clinical photograph of SCC located at the left axilla of a 57 year old male. (b) H&E original magnification 200×, corresponding skin biopsy exhibiting neoplastic cells with squamous differentiation grouped in tumoral nests within skin. (c–f) RCM images 500×500 μm at different levels of depth. *Level B* demonstrates nucleated corneocytes corresponding with parakeratotic cells (*arrows*). *Level C* shows keratinocytic disarray and the loss of honeycombed pattern at stratum spinosum. *Level D* exhibits several tumor islands and disruption of dermal papillae at DEJ level. *Level E* shows a RCM image taken at dermal level with dilated capillaries and weakly bright, point cells along the internal capillary surface (*arrows*) which have been correlated with rolling and trafficking leukocytes

Seborrheic Keratosis

Seborrheic keratosis is a common benign epidermal proliferation (Fig. 5a–c). Sometimes this tumor can be pigmented; it is then important to distinguish it from melanocytic lesions such as melanoma. On confocal microscopy, epidermal thickening without keratinocytic disarray is observed, including long, parallel, dermal papillae (Fig. 5d), which are well delimited by bright rings of basal keratinocytes (*edged papillae*). This pattern, together with cerebriform morphology (Fig. 5e), is usually interpreted as benign.

Dermatofibroma

Dermatofibroma (DF) is a common benign dermal proliferation of histiocytes with an even distribution in males and females regardless of age; however, it is more typically seen in young adult women. Darkly pigmented lesions can simulate dysplastic nevi or melanoma. Reflectance confocal microscopic examination of DF reveals a normal epidermis with homogeneously bright papillary rings and refractile keratinocytes above the dermo-epidermal junction, corresponding histologically to the pigmentation of the basal layer. Moreover, the dermis shows highly refractile, thick collagen bundles corresponding to the sclerotic stroma of the tumor. Specific images of the primary features of DF by RCM have been hard to collect because spindle fibroblast-like cells, histiocytes and sclerotic stroma are too deep in the reticular dermis. However, this technique may still be useful in differential diagnosis with other cutaneous tumors, particularly when DF is darkly pigmented, simulating melanocytic lesions.

Pigmented Basal Cell Carcinoma

Pigmented BCC is a clinical and histologic variant of BCC that may be difficult to distinguish clinically from benign pigmented lesions and melanoma. Agero et al.[27] have characterized pigmented BCC with RCM. The features include similar features to those described previously for BCC. Melanin was not uniformly distributed throughout the tumor cords. The variable amounts of melanin present, together with the melanin distribution within the tumor nests, determined the variability in brightness of tumor nest visualized on RCM. Melanin from benign epidermal keratinocytes, from melanocytes interspersed among the tumor cells, and from melanophages in papillary dermis all contribute to the pigmentation of the BCC tumor. Melanin and melanosomes provide strong contrast compared to the surrounding edematous or mucinous dermal stroma of BCCs under RCM.

Pigmented Mammary Paget Disease

Pigmented mammary Paget disease represents a rare variant of mammary Paget disease that is often clinically and histologically similar to melanoma. On RCM, the presence of

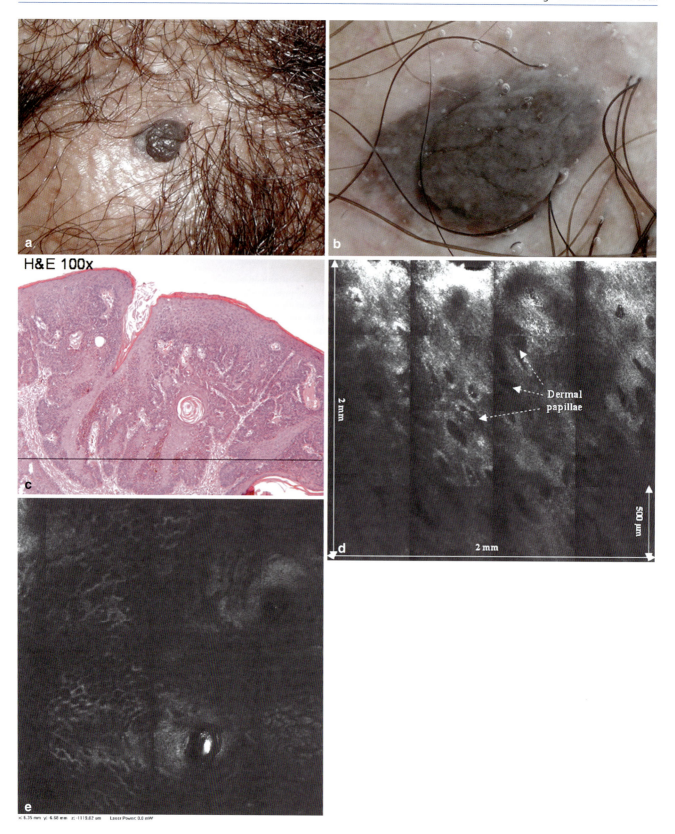

large atypical cells arranged in pagetoid fashion (resembling pagetoid melanocytosis observed in malignant melanocytic lesions), as well as the epidermal disarrangement and papillae without distinct edges suggested a superficial spreading melanoma.[28] Immunohistochemical analysis provided conclusive evidence because most of the Paget cells stained positively for *c-erb-b2* expression.

Melanocytic Lesions

- *Lentigo simplex*
  1. Normal architecture of the epidermis: spinous and granular layer show no alteration.
  2. Cobblestone pattern: normal epidermal pattern consisting of homogenous, bright, and well demarcated cells (pigmented keratinocytes).
  3. Small monomorphous, round or oval bright cells with central nuclei (nevomelanocytes) at the dermo-epidermal junction, near dermal papillae.
  4. Dermal papillae well circumscribed by a ring of bright monomorphous cells (*edged papillae*).
  5. Regular distribution and morphology of dermal papillae.
  6. Absence of bright nucleated cell clusters.
- *Melanocytic nevi*
  1. Normal architecture of the epidermis: spinous and granular layers show no alteration.
  2. Cobblestone pattern: normal epidermal pattern consisting of homogenous, bright, and well demarcated cells (pigmented keratinocytes).
  3. Uniform population of small monomorphous, round or oval bright cells with central nuclei (nevomelanocytes) at the dermo-epidermal junction.
  4. Dermal papillae circumscribed by a ring of refractive monomorphous cells (*edged papillae*).
  5. Regular distribution and morphology of dermal papillae.
  6. In compound nevi, melanocytes are observed at the dermo-epidermal junction but also in superficial dermis, where they are grouped in rounded clusters (nests), often near capillary vessels.

- *Dysplastic nevi*
  1. Focal loss of cell demarcation at epidermal levels associated with bright, fine dendrites and granular structures (melanin dust).
  2. Heterogeneous population of bright nucleated cells in terms of shape, size, and brightness (atypical melanocytes) at the dermo-epidermal junction.
  3. Bright nucleated cells (melanocytes) tend to be round or oval as in common nevi, rather than dendritic as in melanoma.
  4. Atypical nevi may show focal disruption at the dermo-epidermal junction, especially on the face.
  5. Dermal papillae without uniform bright contours (*non-edged papillae*).
  6. Cell clusters (melanocytic nests) may be less demarcated.
- *Malignant melanoma*

Superficial Spreading Melanoma

  1. Bright nucleated cells at epidermal levels, some of them ascending within the epidermis (pagetoid infiltration). Variable cellular morphology in pagetoid cells (round, polygonal, fusiform or dendritic).
  2. Coarse branching dendrites.
  3. Disarray of keratinocytes. Focal/total loss of the normal epidermal pattern.
  4. Bright grainy particles distributed within the epidermis (melanin dust).
  5. Irregular dermal papillae without uniform bright contours (*non-edged papillae*).
  6. Atypical nucleated cells with irregular morphology and brightness at dermo-epidermal junction.
  7. Bright nucleated cells (melanocytes) within the papilla.

Facial Lentigo Maligna Melanoma

  - An important criterion for malignant melanoma is the appearance of asymmetrical bright contour surrounding follicular apertures with bright dendrites or atypical nucleated bright cells on the face.

Fig. 5 (**a**) Clinical image of pigmented lesions located on the penis of a 41 year old man. (**b**) Dermoscopic image reveals a nodular area on a flat pigmented lesion, without other specific data of melanocytic lesion. Based on this evidence, it was removed to make a definitive diagnosis. (**c**) H&E original magnification 100× revealed an epidermal tumor with a benign pattern. This tumor was characterized by proliferation of basaloid cells, some of them pigmented, with squamoid differentiation, suggesting the diagnosis of pigmented seborrheic keratosis. Black line corresponds with confocal optical section in RCM image. (**d**) RCM mosaic image 2×2 mm taken before the excision corresponds with an oblique optical section due to the exophytic surface of the lesion. This shows a non-malignant pattern consisting of several elongated, digitiform dermal apertures oriented along the same axis within a background of cobblestone pattern. Note the presence of edged papillae as well as the architectural pattern, compatible with seborrheic keratosis. (**e**) RCM mosaic image 2×2 mm exhibits an epidermal cerebriform pattern, which is characteristic of seborrheic keratosis

Nodular Areas in Superficial Spreading Melanoma

1. Papillary apertures are not visible in nodular areas.
2. Below epidermal layers, pleomorphic cells with bright cytoplasm and dark nuclei (atypical melanocytes) are present in the basal layer, sometimes with a distribution in sheet-like structures.
3. Dermal cell clusters with irregular morphology and brightness:
   - Sparse cell nests are irregularly bright nucleated cell aggregates, which contain dark spaces and grey fibrous tracts.
   - Cerebriform nests are irregularly bright cell aggregates with non-visualized nuclei and poly-lobular architectural contours, correlated with nodular areas.
4. Plump cells at dermal levels (melanophages).
5. Weakly bright, point cellular infiltration at papillary and reticular dermis (inflammatory infiltration).
6. Enlarged and tortuous vessels near atypical cell nests (angiogenesis).

Pure Nodular Melanoma

1. Absence of characteristic melanoma features, such as epidermal disarrangement or pagetoid melanocytosis within the epidermis.
2. Pure nodular melanoma and nodular areas in superficial spreading melanoma exhibit similar features at dermo-epidermal and dermal levels.

Lentigo Simplex

On reflectance-mode confocal microscopy, lentigo simplex (Fig. 6a, b) shows homogenous, bright, well demarcated keratinocytes at the level of epidermal layers (cobblestone pattern). This characteristic epidermal image represents the negative of honeycomb pattern, revealing bright cells (pigmented keratinocytes) in pigmented lesions. Cobblestone pattern is particularly pronounced at the level of the basal layer in these lesions. Dermal papillae are surrounded by a ring with a single layer of bright monomorphic cells (Fig. 6c, d), some of them with a dark central nucleus and bright dendrites (melanocytes). Sometimes, lentigo simplex may be confused with other pigmented lesions clinically. RCM may be useful in the diagnosis of these lesions. So, the presence of bright nucleated cells grouped in cell clusters (melanocytic nests) on RCM image suggests the diagnosis of lentiginous nevus or small dysplastic nevus. On the other hand, the absence of bright nucleated cells (melanocytes) on RCM is compatible with solar lentigo.

Melanocytic Nevi

Confocal microscopy is particularly well suited to image melanocytic lesions, since the large amount of melanin they possess provides very good contrast. Accurate characterization of the features of benign and malignant melanocytic lesions has important implications for the diagnosis and/or screening of pigmented lesions. Confocal features of common melanocytic nevi have recently been identified. They include the presence of a homogeneous population of small monomorphous, round or oval bright cells with central nuclei (nevomelanocytes).[29,30] In benign nevi both spinous and granular layers show no alteration; their normal pattern consists of homogenous, bright, well demarcated keratinocytes (cobblestone pattern). Dermal papillae are uniformly distributed and circumscribed by a ring of refractive monomorphous cells that are small melanocytes and basal keratinocytes (*edged papillae*), without any cytologic atypia. In junctional nevi, nevomelanocytes are observed within the epidermis at the dermo-epidermal junction, typically surrounding dermal papillae.[29] In compound nevi (Fig. 7a), cells consistent with nevomelanocytes may be observed at the dermo-epidermal junction but also in the superficial dermis. These are often grouped in rounded clusters or "nests" containing several cells (Fig. 7b, c), often near blood vessels. In both these nevus types, melanocytes arranged in small nests or as a single cell may also be seen higher in the epidermis, but the architecture of the stratum corneum, granulosum, spinosum, and basal cell layer remains otherwise unchanged (normal epidermis).

Dysplastic Nevi

Confocal features of dysplastic nevi are different from other melanocytic nevi. Common melanocytic nevi maintain the epidermal architecture and feature a symmetrical architectural pattern and homogeneous cytological characteristics. On the other hand, dysplastic nevi (Fig. 8a) exhibit features similar to common nevi and melanoma.[29] These nevi have irregular shape in dermal papillae, including homogenously bright keratinocytic rings (Fig. 8b, c). Dysplastic nevi also show a great variety in nevomelanocyte refractivity, size and shape (nevomelanocytic population more heterogeneous). However, nevomelanocytic cells tend to be round or oval as in common nevi, rather than dendritic as in melanomas.[29,30] Atypia is seen with melanocytes weakly bright, with isolated big epithelioid cells with a peripheral nucleus.[31] Cell nests

Reflectance-Mode Confocal Microscopy in Dermatological Oncology 299

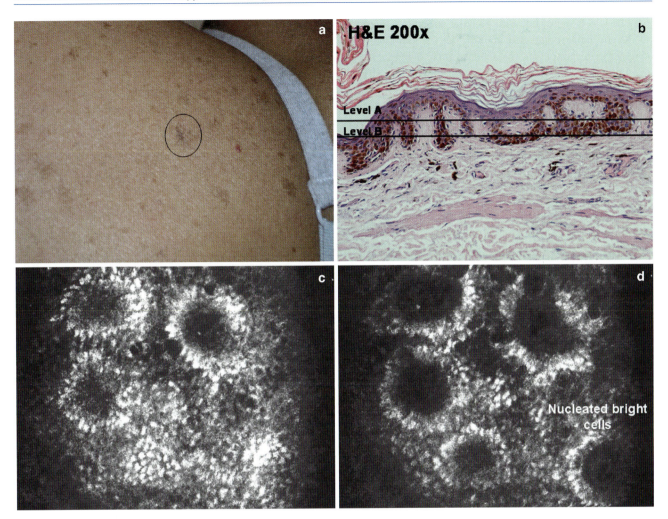

Fig. 6 (a) Clinical photograph of a melanocytic lentigo on the back of a 26 year old woman. (b) H&E original magnification 100× and 200×, respectively, corresponding skin biopsy demonstrates melanocytic cells grouped in epidermal crests, without form nests, and pigmented keratinocytes. (c, d) RCM parallel optical sections (500×500 μm) corresponding with levels A and B. They show dermal apertures surrounded by uniformly bright rings, which consist of nucleated bright cells (melanocytes) and small bright cells (pigmented keratinocytes) at the level of DEJ

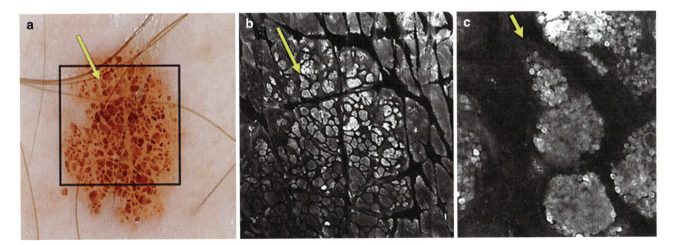

Fig. 7 (a) Dermoscopic image reveals a melanocytic nevus with typical cobblestone pattern. (b) RCM mosaic image shows bright cell clusters at the dermo-epidermal junction. (c) detail of one melanocytic nest (*arrow*), which corresponds exactly with dermoscopic image (Source: Scope et al.[39] Reprinted with permission of Archives of Dermatology)

may be less demarcated, with globular structures composed of bright cells connected to the dermal papillae rings (Fig. 8d). Keratinocytes focally lose their demarcations at the spinous layer associated with dendrites and occasionally "melanin dust" (high refractive granular particles that probably represent melanin bodies). On the face, atypical nevi frequently exhibit focal disruption at the dermo-epidermal junction (focal loss of the cell-cell keratinocytic borders), with low homogeneous dermal papillae and absence of demarcation by refractive cells.

Malignant Melanoma

Pigmented melanomas (Fig. 9a, b) imaged with RCM show the presence of enlarged atypical nucleated cells with pleomorphic morphology, variable refractivity and angulus nuclei, which may be found in several layers of the epidermis (pagetoid dissemination) and in the dermis (Fig. 9c–e). These cells may be oval (Fig. 9c–e), stellate, or fusiform (Fig. 9d) in shape and posses coarse branching dendritic processes and eccentrically placed large, dark nuclei. There is also disruption of the regular architectural pattern of the stratum spinosum, with indistinct cell borders and bright, grainy particles, probably melanin ("melanin dust"), distributed within the epidermis.[31] Linear dendrites are thickened and bright more than in healthy skin. These alterations in suprabasal layers are defined as keratinocytic disarray, typically, with atypical cobblestone pattern (Fig. 9d). In basal layers, cells may be grouped, simulating a dysplastic nevus, or isolated. Dermal papillae are smaller, more irregular and with worse ill-defined borders (*non-edged papillae*) than in common nevi (Fig. 9e). Their architectural pattern is very asymmetric both in size and refractivity. In the dermis, we may find cerebriform clusters (nodular areas) or sparse cell nests consisting of irregularly bright cell aggregates, with non-demarcated cell borders and pleomorphism, surrounded by "melanin dust". This "melanin dust" may be thicker (1–3 μm) than in atypical nevi, and can be visualized along the epidermis. On the face (Fig. 10a–d), an atypical cobblestone pattern with asymmetrical bright contour is usually observed (Fig. 10e) surrounding follicular apertures with bright dendrites or atypical nucleated bright cells (Fig. 10f). This is considered an important criterion for malignant melanoma. The architecture of dermal papillae is similarly disrupted in lentigo maligna melanoma (Fig. 10g), with bright non nucleated cells (melanophages) within the dermis (Fig. 10h).

Criteria to distinguish accurately between benign and malignant pigmented lesions need to be further defined, developed, and tested in large blinded studies; however, it is feasible to distinguish between benign nevi vs. atypical or malignant melanocytic lesions. Interestingly, some features typical of melanomas can also be identified in amelanotic

melanomas using RCM.[32] It appears that it is possible to detect melanocytes in a clinically amelanotic melanoma, presumably because of the presence of some melanin in premelanosomes and also, as previously indicated, by their size, similar to the illuminating wavelength. Images from patients diagnosed with cutaneous amelanotic melanoma showed the presence of bright round, oval or fusiform cells, sometimes with dendritic processes. These cells were present either isolated around dermo-epidermal junction and spinous layer, or in confluent, ill-defined groups. As with pigmented melanomas, there was architectural disruption and loss of distinct cell borders at epidermal levels. These RCM features correlated well with conventional histology.

Gerger et al.[33] have addressed the application of RCM to the diagnostic classification of benign and melanocytic skin tumors. That study found the images derived from dermo-epidermal junction to be more useful for diagnosis. Melanocytic cytomorphology and architecture, as well as keratinocyte cell borders assessment were the most useful markers, reporting high interobserver and intraobserver agreement. On the other hand, evaluation of melanocytic cell brightness and dendrite-like structures had close to none diagnostic importance. The fact that observers without specific dermatopathology experience performed better than trained dermatopathologists may indicate that micromorphologic features relevant in paraffin histology cannot be compared directly to RCM images. This study concludes that an unprejudiced approach is more successful with respect to diagnostic accuracy. Recently, a diagnostic semi-quantitative algorithm for RCM evaluation of clinically and dermoscopically equivocal melanocytic lesions has been proposed by Pellacani et al.,[34] showing a total score ranging from 0 to 8. This algorithm has two major and four minor RCM criteria associated to malignancy. Major criteria (scored two points in the diagnostic algorithm) are the presence of *non-edged papillae* and cytological atypia (Fig. 9e), whereas the minor criteria (scored one point) are the presence of round, bright, and nucleated cells within the epidermis (Fig. 9c, d), pagetoid cells widespread throughout the lesion (Fig. 10f), and cerebriform clusters and bright nucleated cells within the dermal papilla (Fig. 10g). Lesions with a score equal to or greater than three were quantified for final scores of 97.3% sensitivity and 72.3% specificity.[34]

Infiltration of the epidermis by melanocytes (pagetoid melanocytosis) is considered a relevant criterion for melanoma by pathologists, although sporadically observable in benign melanocytic lesions.[35] RCM enables the visualization of superficial layers at cellular-level resolution; pagetoid melanocytosis may be exposed by this technique indicating that melanoma diagnosis should be considered, whereas it can not be excluded in the absence of pagetoid cells, which are absent in at least 10% of malignant lesions.[35] Similar results could be obtained in eczematous lesions, where bright

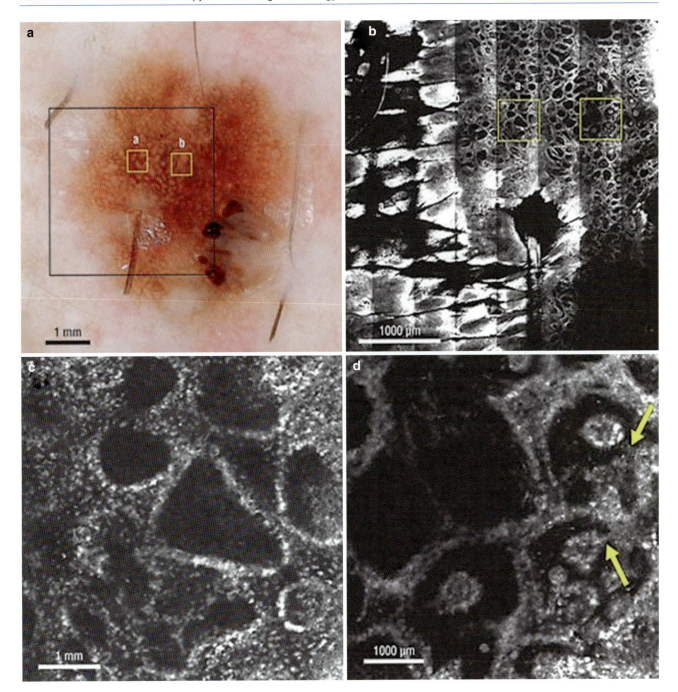

Fig. 8 (a, b) Dermoscopic and RCM mosaic images at dermo-epidermal level in dysplastic nevus. *Squares a* and *b* on dermoscopic image correspond with *figures 8c* and *d*, respectively. (c) irregular shape of dermal papillae, neatly surrounded by bright rings within a background of pigmented cells (keratinocytes). (d) globular structures of bright cells (melanocytic nests) conected to the dermal papillae rings (*arrows*) (Source: Scope et al.[39] Reprinted with permission of Archives of Dermatology

dendritic cells located at the epidermis correspond to Langerhans cells.[36] Thus, although the presence of pagetoid dissemination is relevant, observation of round pagetoid cells is more specific and it can be considered a further criterion for melanoma (Fig. 9c).

Whereas superficial areas of malignant melanoma have been imaged and their RCM features have been defined, nodular areas in melanoma or pure nodular melanomas have not been studied as thoroughly as the former. Nodular areas exhibited differential features when imaged by RCM compared to superficial spreading ones. Pure nodular melanomas lacked characteristic epidermal features of superficial spreading melanomas, such as epidermal disarray and pagetoid melanocytosis. Nodular areas of superficial spreading

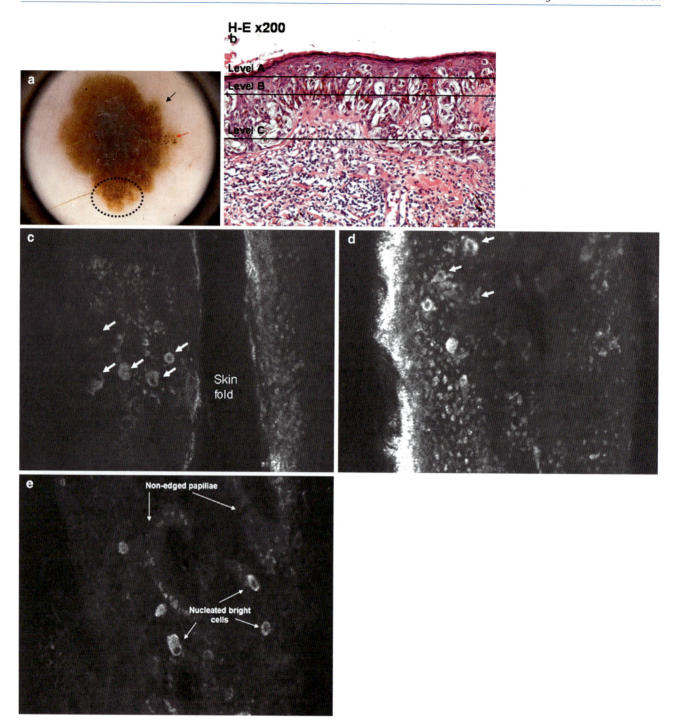

Fig. 9 (**a**) Dermoscopic image of superficial spreading melanoma with multicomponent pattern: peripheral streaks (*black arrow*), atypical network (*dotted circle*), irregular pigmented globules (*red arrow*), and heterogeneous coloration. (**b**) H&E original magnification 200×, histologic section shows pagetoid dissemination of atypical melanocytes within epidermis corresponding with superficial spreading melanoma. (**c–e**) RCM image at *level A* demonstrates several nucleated, bright and round cells within epidermis (*arrows*) which are correlated with pagetoid dissemination. Pagetoid dissemination is an important and evident RCM feature in superficial spreading melanoma (RCM image 500×500 μm). (**d**) RCM image at *level B* shows an atypical cobblestone pattern consisting of atypical nucleated bright cells within epidermis (*arrows*) and bright keratinocytes (RCM image 500×500 μm). (**e**) At the dermoepidermal junction (*level C*), RCM image demonstrates atypical nucleated bright cells and dermal apertures without uniform bright rings surrounding them (non-edged papillae) which are the two more important confocal criteria in the diagnosis of cutaneous melanoma (RCM image 500×500 μm)

melanomas usually show a disarranged pattern and pagetoid cells within the epidermis. At the dermoepidermal junction, both nodular areas (pure nodular and superficial spreading melanomas) have similar RCM features. Papillary apertures are surrounded by bright rings of cells not visible in nodular areas. In these areas, RCM shows pleomorphic cells with bright cytoplasms and dark nuclei (atypical melanocytes) distributed in sheet-like structures between the basal layer and upper dermis, sometimes aggregated in heterogeneous clusters. At the reticular dermis, RCM visualizes aggregates of hyporefractive and nucleated cells with lobular architectural pattern called cerebriform nests, which have been correlated with deep melanoma infiltration. Plump cells, corresponding to dermal melanophages, and various inflammatory reactions have two common features in nodular components in melanoma: enlarged and tortuous vessels are

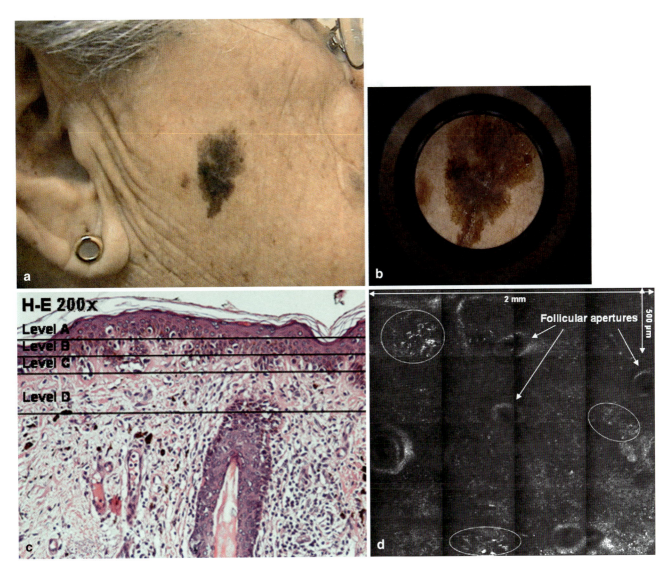

Fig. 10 (a) Clinical photograph corresponding to lentigo maligna in an 82 year old woman. (b) Dermoscopic image with irregular pigmented network and rhomboidal pigmented structures corresponding with dermoscopic features of lentigo maligna. (c) H&E original magnification 200×, histologic section presents pagetoid dissemination of atypical melanocytes within epidermis, especially near follicular structures. Histologic image shows numerous melanophages and solar elastosis in superficial dermis. (d) RCM mosaic image shows bright cells and dendrites (*dotted circles*) within epidermis and surrounding follicular apertures at the level of spinosum stratum (RCM mosaic image 2×2 mm). (e–h) RCM image at *level A* exhibits an atypical cobblestone pattern consisting of bright dendrites and nucleated bright cells (*red arrows*). Background is very heterogeneous regarding both, morphological and bright structures (RCM image 500×500 μm). RCM image at *level B* demonstrates atypical nucleated bright cells surrounding a follicular aperture, within a background of keratinocytic disarray marked with an asterisks (RCM image 500×500 μm). RCM image at *level C* shows irregular dermal apertures with atypical nucleated bright cells inside at DEJ (RCM image 500×500 μm). RCM image at dermis (*level D*) exhibits non nucleated bright cells with not well delimited borders (*red arrows*) corresponding with melanophages, within a background of heterogeneous gray bundles correlated with dermal actinic damage (RCM image 500×500 μm)

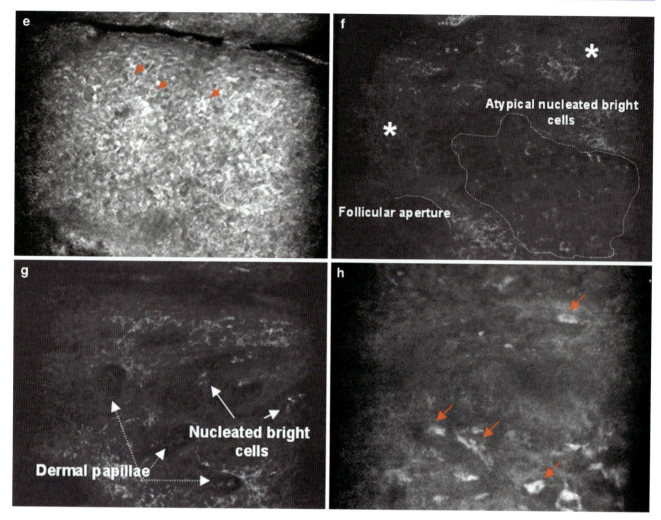

Fig. 10 (continued)

situated below nodular areas, corresponding to angiogenesis-phase in thicker malignant lesions. Since the presence of this nodular component has been correlated to deep melanoma infiltration, these RCM features require further investigation in order to discover a possible prognostic use in RCM analysis.

Besides its potential diagnostic capability, RCM has shown promise as a guide for biopsy collection in the most relevant lesion area[37]; to monitor the response to treatment[38]; and to delineate the extension of a lesion before proceeding to surgical excision.[32,38] It may also serve to study possible prognostic features depending on the correlation of specific RCM features with superficial spreading or nodular areas in malignant melanoma.

One of the main drawbacks of RCM is a certain inability to reach deep tissue in the dermis, reaching a maximum depth of 250 μm.[14] This limiting factor prevents imaging of structures located deep in the dermis, especially in cases of hyperpigmented lesions. In these cases, there is strong attenuation of the contrast due to massive absorption and light scattering going through those structures. The presence of inflammatory cells and collagen bundles may also diminish contrast and difficult melanocyte visualization.

Other Applications in Dermatological Oncology

- *Dermoscopy-RCM correlation.*
  1. Study and classification of the specific dermoscopic structures.
  2. Increase accuracy of differential diagnosis of pigmented lesions where clinical and dermoscopic examinations are equivocal.
  3. Dermoscopy-RCM correlations:

- *Pigment network*: bright rings of pigmented keratinocytes surrounding dermal papillae (*edged papillae*) and bright thickenings consist of melanocytic cells located at basal at dermo-epidermal junction (junctional thickenings).
- *Atypical pigment network*: architectural disarray of the basal layer around papillary dermis. The presence of atypical melanocytes is revealed in melanomas.
- *Dermoscopic globules*: clusters of nucleated, bright cells with morphology similar to melanocytes located at the dermo-epidermal junction level or in the upper dermis.
- *Peripheral streaks*: aggregates of elongated cells, well delineated from the bordering dermis and contiguous to the central mesh of the lesion. Some aggregates appeared to be round, curving around existing dermal papillae (pseudopods). Other aggregates produced an arrow-like arrangement (linear streaks).
- *Blue whitish veil*: focal disruption of the arrangement of the basal cells, and suprabasal epidermal architecture with bright, plump cells corresponding to melanophages and of some melanocytes in the superficial dermis.
4. The level of dermo-epidermal junction is the most useful for the correlation of dermoscopic global pattern with the RCM mosaic image.
- *Guide to perform a biopsy on a focused area.*
- *Margin assessment and adjunct to surgery.*
  1. Tumors with radial growth phases:
     - lentigo maligna melanomas.
     - melanomas *in situ*.
     - basal cell carcinomas.
  2. Tumors that are difficult to see clinically:
     - amelanotic melanomas.
     - sclerosing infiltrative basal cell carcinomas.
  3. Adjunct to Mohs micrographic surgery:
     - margin assessment *in vivo*.
     - may be useful *ex vivo* to evaluate presence or absence of margin involvement by non-melanoma skin cancer.
- *Use of RCM to evaluate the response to treatment.*
  - Monitoring therapies:
  - surgical treatment.
  - cryotherapy.
  - non-invasive treatments such as topical imiquimod or photodynamic therapy.

Dermoscopy-RCM Correlation

The precise correlation between dermoscopy and RCM of melanocytic lesions (Figs. 7a–c, 8a–d) has several potential applications. First, it enables the study of specific dermoscopic structures.[31,39] Confocal microscopy may have an added value in refining the classification of dermoscopic structures.[40] On the other hand, RCM may be useful to distinguish between benign lesions and those suggestive of malignancy in areas of equivocal dermoscopic findings because RCM evaluates tissue architecture and cytomorphological features, such as pagetoid spread, that may evade dermoscopic resolution.[31,39,40] Due to the close relationship between early diagnosis and life prognosis of the patient, RCM may be particularly useful to increase clinical and dermoscopic sensitivity.

The precise layer within the dermo-epidermal junction is the most useful piece of information for the correlation of dermoscopic global pattern with the RCM mosaic image.[31,39] The dermoscopic appearance of a network has been correlated to pigmented keratinocytes of the basal layer surrounding dermal papillae (*edged papillae*) and bright thickenings consisting of melanocytic cells located at basal at the dermo-epidermal junction (junctional thickenings). Atypical pigment networks can result from an architectural disarray of the basal layer around the papillary dermis. Atypical melanocytes could be seen in melanomas. Dermoscopic globules were correlated with nests of melanocytes at the dermo-epidermal junction or the papillary dermis. Each globule on dermoscopy could be identified as a cluster of bright cells on RCM. Peripheral streaks were correlated with aggregates of elongated cells, well delineated from the bordering dermis and contiguous with the central mesh of the lesion. Some aggregates appeared to be round, curving around existing dermal papillae and producing a pseudopod-like appearance. Other aggregates produced an arrow-like arrangement, representing more linear streaks.[31,40]

Reflectance-mode confocal microscopy presents limitations in identifying compact orthokeratosis and the corresponding pigmented structures in deeper dermis reported in the histopathological correlation of the dermoscopic blue whitish veil. However, RCM can provide a complementary horizontal overview of the architectural arrangement at the dermo-epidermal junction level; such application clearly showed focal disruption of the arrangement of the basal cells, with bright, plump cells, consistent with melanophages and of some melanocytes in the superficial dermis.[31]

Guide to Perform a Biopsy

Reflectance-mode confocal microscopy can be useful for clinicians prior to performing a biopsy on a focused area that shows concerning confocal findings.[20-23,25,26,37]

Margin Assessment and Adjunct to Surgery

Reflectance-mode confocal microscopy has the potential to define lesion margins before surgical or non-surgical therapy. This can prove particularly helpful in margin assessment of tumors with radial growth phases, including lentigo maligna melanomas,[38] some basal cell carcinomas,[41] or tumors that are difficult to visualize clinically, such as amelanotic melanomas[32] or sclerosing infiltrative basal cell carcinomas.[20] Again, the main limiting factor is the limited depth that can be reached with this technique, which prevents accurate imaging at depths below the superficial dermis. Lack of contrast can also pose a problem, which might be solved by the future development of exogenous contrast agents.[42] Despite the present limitations, RCM can help identify areas that are atypical and need a biopsy to provide histologic confirmation.

Confocal microscopy may also aid in the rapid establishment of tumor margins by examining excised specimens during procedures such as Mohs micrographic surgery.[41,43] Mohs micrographic surgery is a histologically guided method of removing skin cancers that maximally preserves normal tissue. Thin layers of tissues are removed, and the margins are examined histologically to determine if cancerous cells remain. Selective removal of residual tumor tissue is performed until tumor-free margins are obtained. This procedure can be time-consuming since each excised specimen must be processed by frozen histopathology requiring embedding, sectioning, and staining. With RCM of *ex vivo* unprocessed tissue, it is possible to detect neoplastic cells by using 5% acetic acid and cross-polarized illumination. This technique enhances the brightness of the neoplastic nuclei and darkens the surrounding dermis. Recently, it has been demonstrated that RCM may be useful in examining non-melanoma skin cancers in *ex vivo* tissue during Mohs micrographic surgery without frozen sections.[41,43] This novel application of RCM offers the advantage of rapid visualization of margins compared to permanent sectioning and the ability to do specific or permanent staining in areas that are equivocal. RCM has also been used in vivo during Mohs surgery to help locate tumors and rapidly visualize the margins of BCCs and melanoma. However, poor visualization of non-flat wounds, wound fluid interference, and limited depth reach make it impractical to use *in vivo* RCM for Mohs surgery at present.

Use of RCM for Evaluating Response to Treatment

To assess histological changes that occur after new treatments, a biopsy is often required. If a treated lesion is small, this may be possible only once. It is possible to repeat RCM on the same skin lesion or site repeatedly, unlike biopsy collection. This permits evaluation of dynamic processes such as epidermal architectural changes or inflammatory infiltration. There are ongoing RCM studies evaluating the histopathological responses of actinic keratoses treated with imiquimod or 5-aminolevulinic acid and photodynamic therapy, as well as BCCs treated with imiquimod. To date, RCM has proven to be accurate in establishing the presence of BCCs before treatment and responsiveness of BCCs to the treatment regimen with imiquimod.[44] These studies may also be useful in order to understand the physio-pathological mechanisms (inflammatory response, microvascular changes, tissue restitution, etc.) involving these novel non-invasive therapies.

Limitations and Potential Solutions

- Instrumentation:
  1. Confocal microscopes are available in only a minority of dermatology departments.
     Solution: Diffusion.
  2. Size and versatility of the equipment (i.e., microscopes).
     Solutions: development of more versatile and smaller instruments.
- Interpretation of RCM findings:
  1. Interpretation depends on the observer and on his cumulative experience.
     Solutions: development of teledermatology, consensus glossary, courses, and specific atlas.
  2. Pathological knowledge.
     Specific formation.
- Problems related to imaging:
  1. Lack of deep reach of the light source limits its application to the superficial dermis.
     Solutions: additional signal filtering techniques (coherence gating) or different immersion media (glucose or glycerol).
  2. Decrease in contrast.
     Solution: development of exogenous contrast agents.
  3. Difficulty to use the current contact device on non-flat surfaces (ears or noses).
- Problems related to visual quality of images:
  1. Uneven brightness within an image.
  2. Lack of contrast (limited subset of gray levels).
  3. Considerable degree of noise.
     Solution: digital enhancement.
- Future:
  1. Three-dimensional sections.
  2. Vertical sections.

Although RCM may be considered as a useful new technology for the diagnosis and study of skin cancer, especially cutaneous melanoma, a number of limitations need to be considered at present. Reflectance-mode confocal microscopes themselves are available in only a minority of dermatology departments and require a learning curve to operate them and interpret the images. Interpretation of RCM findings depends on the observer and, as such, relies on cumulative experience. This observer dependence is not dissimilar to histopathological or radiological interpretations. In the future, development of teledermatology may solve this problem; RCM specialists may be contacted and images sent in real-time for their evaluation.

Problems related to imaging include the lack of reach of the light source, which limits its practical range to the superficial dermis or even less if the lesion is particularly hyperkeratotic or hyperpigmented. Thickness of the melanoma lesion is an important prognostic factor, thus improvements in the technique will be necessary in order to increase RCM potency and imaging depth. Some solutions can be provided by the use of different immersion media and illumination sources. The use of additional signal filtering techniques such as coherence gating[45] to better isolate backscattered light from the focal plane, as well as chemical agents such as glucose and glycerol[46] to improve index matching at the surface could improve penetration depth. Decrease in contrast may be solved through development of exogenous contrast agents.[47] Current contact devices are also cumbersome and difficult to use on a non-flat surface such as ears, noses or genitalia.

Regarding the visual quality of RCM images, there are three main problems: uneven brightness within an image, mostly caused by reflection from the skin surface or from poorly reflecting structures of the superficial dermis; lack of contrast, where details of certain structures are displayed with a limited subset of grey levels; and a considerable degree of noise. This last feature is implicit to the scanning process and the *in vivo* situation in which images are taken. Digital image enhancement can address all these problems, at least to a certain extent.[48]

Finally, work is in progress to facilitate the creation of vertical sections and three-dimensional sections,[49] which would vastly increase the potential of RCM. Also a portable prototype using fiber optics is under development and testing. This would make it much more practical and would facilitate the diffusion of this new technology for the *in vivo* diagnosis in dermatology.

Conclusions

Reflectance-mode confocal microscopy bears the potential to represent a new era for skin oncology, making a large contribution to the advancement of dermatological research and clinical care. In research, RCM offers benefits both *ex vivo* and *in vivo*. *Ex vivo*, it allows to sample tissue and noninvasively evaluate it to determine what further testing may be required on the same tissue. *In vivo*, RCM can be used to study normal processes or physiopathologic processes noninvasively over time. It can also be used to establish the presence or absence of a reactive immunologic event and guide tissue sampling such as fine needle aspiration for cells or molecular analysis (DNA, RNA or proteins) of a specific immunological response against neoplastic cells. RCM can also be used to establish timing and dosing responses to non-invasive therapies such as cryotherapy, imiquimod, and photodynamic therapy.

Clinically, RCM has value both *ex vivo* and *in vivo*. *Ex vivo*, tissue can first be evaluated by RCM, and specific findings can be confirmed on the same exact tissue using appropriate markers or staining techniques. *In vivo*, RCM may be useful for *in vivo* diagnosis, accurate assessment of lesion margins, for monitoring response to non-invasive therapies. Although RCM is a promising technique, it seems clear it is taking its first baby steps, and further investigations are necessary to determine its real potential in the future management of skin cancer.

Acknowledgement This work has been partially supported by a grant from the Spanish Ministry of Health (FISS, PI060499).

References

1. Carli P, De Georgi V, Soyer HP, Stante M, Mannone F, Giannotti B. Dermatoscopy in the diagnosis of pigmented skin lesions: a new semiology for the dermatologist. *J Eur Acad Dermatol Venereol.* 2000;14:353-369.
2. Tearney GT, Brezinski ME, Southern JF, et al. Determination of the refractive index of highly scattering human tissue by optical coherence tomography. *Opt Lett.* 1995;20:2258-2260.
3. Mansotti L. Basic principles and advanced technical aspects of ultrasound imaging. In: Guzzardi R, ed. *Physics and Engineering of Medical Imaging.* Boston: Martinus Nijhoff; 1987:263-317.
4. Markitz JA, Aquilia MG. *Technical Magnetic Resonance Imaging.* Stamford: Appleton & Lange; 1996.
5. Suihko C, Swindle LD, Thomas SG, Serup J. Fluorescence fibre-optic confocal microscopy of skin in vivo: microscope and fluorophores. *Skin Res Technol.* 2005;11:254-267.
6. New KC, Petroll WM, Boyde A, et al. In vivo imaging of human teeth and skin using real-time confocal microscopy. *Scanning.* 1991;13:369-372.
7. Corcuff P, Leveque JL. In vivo vision of the human skin with the tandem scanning microscope. *Dermatology.* 1993;186:50-54.
8. Rajadhyaksha M, Grossman M, Esterowitz D, et al. In vivo confocal scanning laser microscopy of human skin: melanin provides strong contrast. *J Invest Dermatol.* 1995;104:946-952.
9. Minsky M. Microscopy apparatus. US patent 3 013 467. November 7, 1957.
10. Cavanagh HD, Jester JV, Essepian J, et al. Confocal microscopy of the living eye. *CLAO J.* 1990;16:65-73.
11. Jester JV, Andrews PM, Petroll WM, et al. In vivo, real-time confocal imaging. *J Electron Microsc Tech.* 1991;18(1):50-60.

12. Andrews PM, Petroll WM, Cavanagh HD, et al. Tandem scanning confocal microscopy (TSCM) of normal and ischemic living kidneys. *Am J Anat*. 1991;191:95-102.
13. Masters BR, Thaer AA. In vivo human corneal confocal microscopy of identical fields of subepithelial nerve plexus, basal epithelial, and wing cells at different times. *Microsc Res Tech*. 1994;29:350-356.
14. Rajadhyaksha M, González S, Zavislan J, et al. In vivo confocal scanning laser microscopy of human skin II: advances in instrumentation and comparison to histology. *J Invest Dermatol*. 1999;113: 293-303.
15. González S, White WM, Rajadhyaksha M, et al. Confocal imaging of sebaceous gland hyperplasia in vivo to assess efficacy and mechanism of pulsed dye laser treatment. *Lasers Surg Med*. 1999;25: 8-12.
16. González S, Sackstein R, Anderson RR, et al. Real-time evidence of in vivo leukocyte trafficking in human skin by reflectance confocal microscopy. *J Invest Dermatol*. 2001;117:384-386.
17. Agasshi D, Anderson RR, González S. Time-sequence histologic imaging of laser-treated cherry angiomas using in vivo confocal microscopy. *J Am Acad Dermatol*. 2000;43:37-41.
18. Agasshi D, González E, Anderson RR, et al. Elucidating the pulsed dye laser treatment of sebaceous hyperplasia in vivo using real-time confocal scanning laser microscopy. *J Am Acad Dermatol*. 2000;43:49-53.
19. Huzaira M, Rius F, Rajadhyaksha M, et al. Topographic variations in normal skin histology, as viewed by in vivo confocal microscopy. *J Invest Dermatol*. 2001;116:846-852.
20. González S, Tannous Z. Real-time in vivo confocal reflectance microscopy of basal cell carcinoma. *J Am Acad Dermatol*. 2002;47: 869-874.
21. Nori S, Rius-Diaz F, Cuevas J, et al. Sensivity and specifity of reflectance.mode confocal microscopy for in vivo diagnosis of basal cell carcinoma: a multicenter study. *J Am Acad Dermatol*. 2004;51: 923-930.
22. Agasshi D, Anderson RR, González S. Confocal laser microscopy imaging of actinic keratoses in vivo: a preliminary report. *J Am Acad Dermatol*. 2000;43:42-48.
23. Ulrich M, Maltusch A, Rowert J, et al. Actinic keratoses: non-invasive diagnosis for field cancerisation. *Br J Dermatol*. 2007; 156(Suppl 3):47-52.
24. Clark AL, Gillenwater AM, Collier TG, Alizadeh-Naderi R, El-Naggar AK, Richards-Kortum RR. Confocal microscopy for real-time detection of oral cavity neoplasia. *Clin Cancer Res*. 2003;9:4714-4721.
25. White WM, Rajadhyaksha M, González S, Fabian RL, Anderson RR. Noninvasive imaging of human oral mucosa in vivo by confocal reflectance microscopy. *Laryngoscope*. 1999;109:1709-1717.
26. Agero AL, Gill M, Ardigo M, Myskowski P, Halpern AC, González S. In vivo reflectance confocal microscopy of mycosis fungoides: a preliminary study. *J Am Acad Dermatol*. 2007;57(3):435-441.
27. Agero ALC, Busam KJ, Rajadhyaksha M, et al. Reflectance confocal microscopy for imaging pigmented basal cell cancers in vivo. *J Am Acad Dermatol*. 2006;54(4):638-643.
28. Longo C, Fantini F, Cesinaro AM, Bassoli S, Seidenari S, Pellacani G. Pigmented mammary Paget disease. dermoscopic, in vivo reflectance-mode confocal microscopic, and inmmunohistochemical study of a case. *Arch Dermatol*. 2007;143:752-754.
29. Langley RGB, Rajadhyaksha M, Dwyer PJ, Sober AJ, Flotte TJ, Anderson RR. Confocal scanning laser microscopy of benign and malignant melanocytic skin lesion in vivo. *J Am Acad Dermatol*. 2001;45:365-376.
30. Busam KJ, Charles C, Lee G, Halpern AC. Morphologic features of melanocytes, pigmented keratinocytes, and melanophages by in vivo confocal scanning laser microscopy. *Mod Pathol*. 2001;14: 862-868.

31. Pellacani G, Cesinaro AM, Longo C, et al. Microscopic in vivo description of cellular architecture of dermoscopic pigment network in nevi and melanomas. *Arch Dermatol*. 2005;141:147-154.
32. Busam KJ, Hester K, Charles C, et al. Detection of clinically amelanotic malignant melanoma and assessment of its margins by in vivo confocal scanning laser microscopy. *Arch Dermatol*. 2001;137:923-929.
33. Gerger A, Koller S, Weger W, et al. Sensitivity and specificity of confocal laser-scanning microscopy for in vivo diagnosis of malignant skin tumors. *Cancer*. 2006;107(1):193-200.
34. Pellacani G, Cesinaro AM, Seidenari S. Reflectance-mode confocal microscopy of pigmented skin lesions-improvement in melanoma diagnostic specificity. *J Am Acad Dermatol*. 2005;53:979-985.
35. Pellacani G, Cesinaro AM, Seidenari S. Reflectance-mode confocal microscopy for the in vivo characterization of pagetoid melanocytosis in melanomas and nevi. *J Invest Dermatol*. 2005;125:532-537.
36. Gonzalez S, Gonzalez E, White M, Rajadhyaksha M, Anderson RR. Allergic contact dermatitis: correlation of in vivo confocal imaging to routine histology. *J Am Acad Dermatol*. 1999;40:708-713.
37. Tannous ZS, Mihm MC, Flotte TJ, Gonzalez S. In vivo examination of lentigo maligna and malignant melanoma in situ, lentigo maligna type by near-infrared reflectance confocal microscopy: comparison of in vivo confocal images with histologic sections. *J Am Acad Dermatol*. 2002;46:260-263.
38. Curiel-Lewandrowski C, Williams CM, Swindells KJ, et al. Use of in vivo confocal microscopy in malignant melanoma: an aid in diagnosis and assessment of surgical and nonsurgical therapeutic approaches. *Arch Dermatol*. 2004;140:1127-1132.
39. Scope A, Gill M, Benvenuto-Andrade C, Halpern AC, Gonzalez S, Marghoob AA. Correlation of dermoscopic structures of melanocytic lesions to reflectance confocal microscopy. *Arch Dermatol*. 2007;143:176-185.
40. Scope A, Gill M, Benvenuto-Andrade C, Halpern AC, Gonzalez S, Marghoob AA. Correlation of dermoscopy with in vivo reflectance confocal microscopy of streaks in melanocytic lesions. *Arch Dermatol*. 2007;143:727-734.
41. Rajadhyaksha M, Menaker G, Flotte T, Dwyer PJ, González S. Confocal examination of nonmelanoma cancers in thick skin excisions to potentially guide Mohs micrographic surgery without frozen histopathology. *J Invest Dermatol*. 2001;17:1137-1143.
42. Tannous Z, Torres A, González S. In vivo real-time confocal reflectance microscopy: a noninvasive guide for Mohs micrographic surgery facilitated by aluminum chloride, an excellent contrast enhancer. *Dermatol Surg*. 2003;29:839-846.
43. Chung VQ, Dwyer PJ, Nehal KS, et al. Use of ex vivo confocal scanning laser microscopy during Mohs surgery for nonmelanoma skin cancers. *Dermatol Surg*. 2004;30:1470-1478.
44. Goldgeier M, Fox CA, Zavislan JM, Harris D, Gonzalez S. Noninvasive imaging, treatment, and microscopic confirmation of clearance of basal cell carcinoma. *Dermatol Surg*. 2003;29(3):205-210.
45. Izatt JA, Kulkarni MD, Wang HW, Kobayashi K, Savak MV. Optical coherence tomography and microscopy in gastrointestinal tissues. *IEEE J Sel Top Quantum Electron*. 1996;2:1017-1028.
46. Vargas G, Chan KF, Thomsen SL, Welch AJ. Use of osmotically active agents to alter optical properties of tissue: effects on the detected fluorescence signal measured through skin. *Lasers Surg Med*. 2001;29:213-220.
47. Rajadhyaksha M, González S, Zavislan JM. Detectability of contrast agents for confocal reflectance imaging of skin and microcirculation. *J Biomed Opt*. 2004;9(2):323-331.
48. Gruber MJ, Wackernagel A, Richtig E, Koller S, Kerl H, Smolle J. Digital image enhancement for in vivo laser scanning microscopy. *Skin Res Technol*. 2005;11:248-253.
49. Oho I, Sakemoto A, Ogino J, Kamiya T, Yamashita T, Jimbow K. The real-time, three-dimensional analyses of benign and malignant skin tumors by confocal laser scanning microscopy. *J Dermatol Sci*. 2006;43:135-141.

Laser Clinical and Practice Pearls

Lori A. Brightman and Roy Geronemus

Safety Measures

- All laser operators should be up to date on associated laser risks and standard safety measures for each laser that they use.
- Different wavelengths of light are responsible for different ocular damage and therefore appropriate eyewear should be used with each laser treatment.
- Corneal eyeshield placement is a safe and effective method of eye protection.
- Surgical lubricant can be applied to protect hair, eyelashes and eyebrows from laser treatment
- Diligence must be of utmost importance in avoidance of combustible products in the laser treatment field

Safety is of utmost importance in laser treatments for the patient as well as treating physician. All laser operators should be up to date on the associated laser risks and standard safety measures for each machine that they use.

Here we discuss additional safety measures. See Chaps. "Laser-Tissue Interactions" and "Laser Safety: Regulations, Standards and Practice Guidelines" for complete laser safety discussion.

Eye Safety

Unprotected eyes are at great risk for injury during laser treatment from direct or indirect laser beams. Different wavelengths of laser light are responsible for various ocular damage, which can be permanent. As the injury may be painless and the laser beam invisible to the eye, damage can occur inconspicuously. Hence, appropriate eye protection should be consistently used during any laser treatment.

There are different types of eyewear available for protection. For the practitioner, there are optically coated goggles, spectacles and wraps. One must make certain whichever eyewear is used must fit tightly on face and cover entire eye or any additional vision-correction lens. The chosen eyewear should also be of appropriate wavelength and optical density for the laser being employed. The parameters are most often written on the frame of the eyewear. For the patient, when treating non-facial areas, one can use plastic or metal eye shield goggles that completely cover the orbit as well as partial periorbital area. When treating in the facial area, one should use metal corneal eye shields.[1,2]

Corneal eye shield placement begins with a thorough tray set up (Fig. 1). Choose the appropriate size shield for the patient; sizes range from infant to adult (Fig. 2). Use topical ophthalmic anesthetic (i.e. tetracaine hydrochloride 0.5% ophthalmic solution) for corneal anesthesia followed by lower lid retraction, placement of shield with slight pressure inferiorly. This will allow the upper lid to be placed over shield

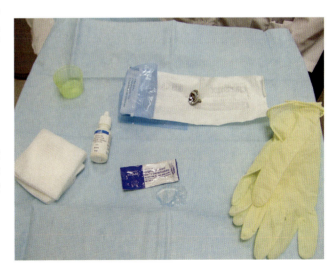

Fig. 1 Tray set up for corneal eye shield placement

R. Geronemus (✉)
Laser and Skin Surgery Center of NY,
New York, NY, USA
e-mail: rgeronemus@laserskinsurgery.com

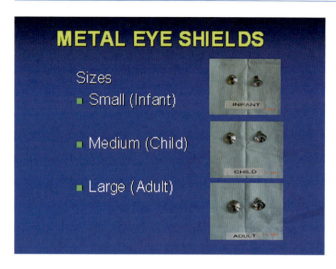

Fig. 2 Various sizes of corneal eye shields

simultaneously with ease (Figs. 3 and 4). The reverse approach can also be used beginning with upper lid retraction.

Hair Protection

During periorbital laser treatment, one must be certain to protect the eyelashes and eyebrows, as the laser beam can inadvertently singe these hairs. Surgical lubricant acts as a semi-hydrated coating medium that does not allow laser penetration.

After eye shield placement, use a cotton tip applicator or tongue depressor to apply surgical lubricant to the eyebrows and eyelashes prior to commencement of laser treatment (Figs. 5 and 6). One can also use a tongue depressor to cover the eyebrows in lieu of surgical lubricant for hair protection (Fig. 7).

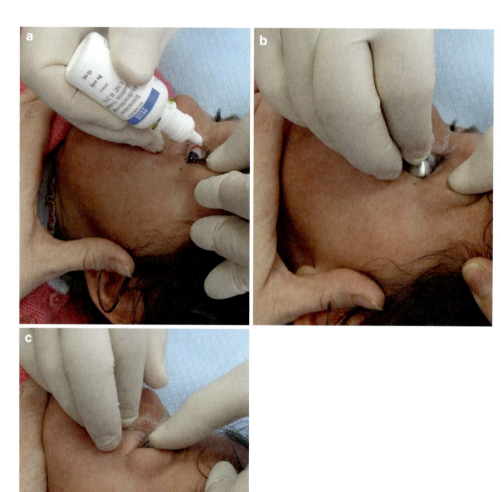

Fig. 3 Placement of child corneal eye shield. (**a**) With upper lid retraction, place ophthalmic drops for mucosal anesthesia; (**b**) retract upper lid, place shield with slight pressure superiorly; (**c**) retract lower lid slightly, allowing the lower lid to then slide over the eyeshield. Eyeshield is now in place

Laser Clinical and Practice Pearls

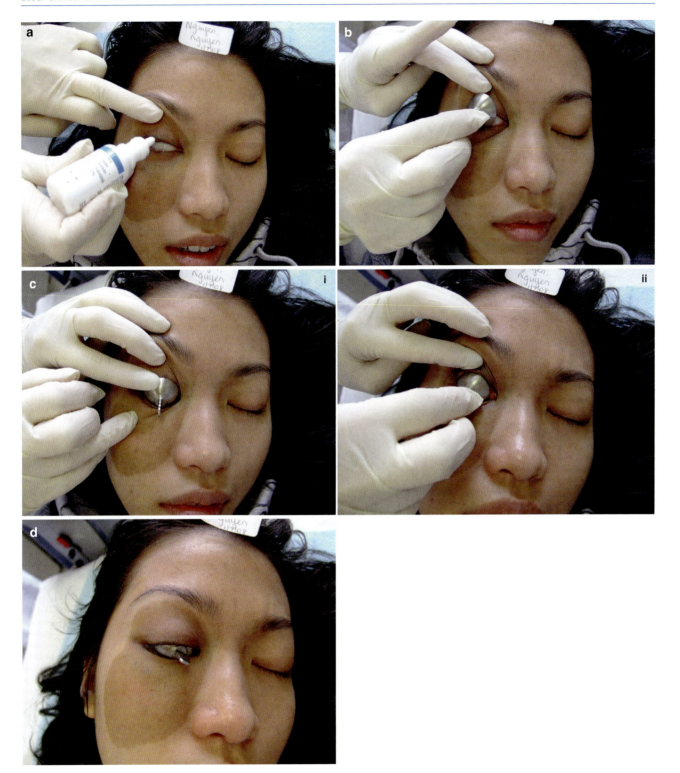

Fig. 4 Placement of adult corneal eye shield. (**a**) Ophthalmic anesthesia is placed; (**b**) retract upper lid. With slight pressure inferiorly, place adult-sized eyeshield; (**c**) retract upper lid (**i**), allowing eyeshield to glide into superior sclera space (**ii**); (**d**) adult eyeshield in place

Anesthesia Safety

When the laser beam of the pulsed dye laser strikes a combustible object such as oxygen and or nitrous oxide in an endotracheal tube, there is a risk of spontaneous fire eruption. This risk is not only applicable to laser use but also has been reported during electrosurgical coagulation. Regulatory groups as well as laser manufacturers have well documented the items that are at risk for igniting and advise these items be kept out of the laser field; these items include oxygen, nitrous oxide,

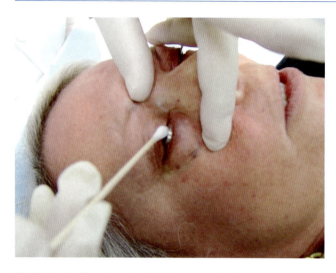

Fig. 5 Application of surgical lubricant on eyelashes

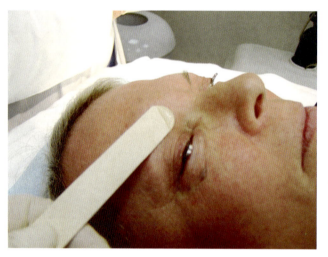

Fig. 6 Application of surgical lubricant on eyebrows

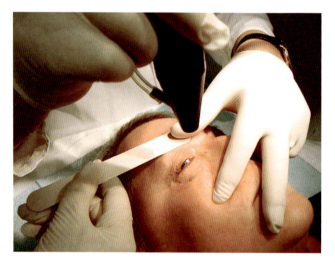

Fig. 7 Tongue depressor to protect eyebrows

hair, gauze, paper drapes, clothing, masks, cannulas, airway materials and even flame retardant paper drapes. Therefore, all of these potential ignitable materials must be diligently kept away from the laser field. Those that must remain in the field must be kept wet with saline or water- based lubricant.

Most cases of pulse dye laser treated port wine stains are in office procedures without sedation and its accompanying oxygen supplementation and monitoring equipment. In these cases, one must be cognosent of the aforementioned ignitable materials. When the oxygen supplementation and monitoring equipment is needed in cases of sedation, it is important to choose an airway with lower risk of igniting. Nasal cannulas are an open system and can ignite quite easily. Face masks are not considered a tight seal and therefore can also leak oxygen. Endotracheal tubes are a consideration however, in the pediatric population, there is a greater risk of oxygen leak if the cuff is not tight and during positive pressure ventilation. Colored airways and or masks should not be used, especially green, as they are likely to ignite.

Laryngeal mask airway (LMA) is a device that can be inserted into the patient's pharynx. With spontaneous ventilation, the LMA prevents oxygen and nitrous oxide leakage by approximately 95%. Leakage is more likely to occur with positive pressure ventilation. In all types of ventilation, one can employ an oxygen analyzer or capnograph to detect oxygen level at airway. Whichever airway is used, one should drape wet gauze around the airway, use a non-flammable petrolatum over hair bearing areas and use ocular shields. When not using the laser it should be placed in standby mode.

Even with all precautions taken, there is still a risk that exists and it is prudent for all staff involved in the patient's care to be up to date on American National Standard for the Safe Use of Lasers. During all operative room laser procedures, there should always be readily available a basin of water and a fire extinguisher.[3]

Tattoos

- Cosmetic tattoos have higher likelihood of containing ferric oxide or titanium dioxide pigments which darken with Q switch laser treatment.
- Ablative or fractional ablative laser treatment allow for cosmetic tattoo removal without risk of tattoo pigment darkening.
- Fractional erbium doped 1,550 nm and fractional CO_2 lasers can be employed when treating dark skin patients with known contact allergen to tattoo pigment to minimize risk of anaphylaxis
- Hypopigmentation seconvdary to laser treatment for tattoo removal can be treated with fractional erbium doped 1,550 nm and fractional CO_2 lasers.

Laser Clinical and Practice Pearls

Tattoos come in many forms including amateur, professional, cosmetic, medicinal and traumatic. Laser treatment is a method of tattoo removal with minimal risk of scarring particularly when compared with alternative tattoo removal methods such as dermabrasion or surgical excision. Amateur tattoos are generally easier to treat than professional tattoos as the ink is usually more superficial and of less dense particles. Multicolor tattoos will require different lasers in order to treat the various colors. Double treated, densely pigmented and multi-colored tattoos are more likely to be recalcitrant to laser therapy. See Chap. "Laser Treatment of Tattoos" for complete discussion of laser tattoo removal.

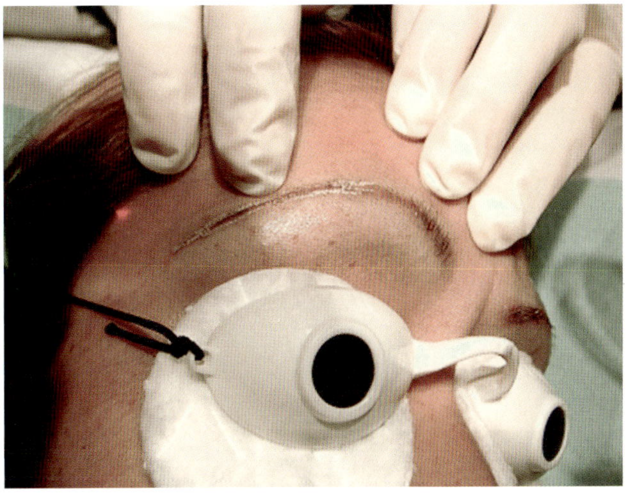

Cosmetic Tattoo Removal

Cosmetic tattoos are generally composed of pigments in the beige, white and red families of which most contain ferric oxide or titanium dioxide pigment. When exposed to Q switch lasers, oxidation of the pigment to ferrous oxide occurs, resulting in an immediate pigment darkening.[4,5]

As there is no standardization of tattoo ink, all tattoo pigments are different. It can be very difficult to predetermine which cosmetic tattoos will be able to undergo laser tattoo removal without darkening. One may preemptively treat cosmetic tattoos with ablation or fractional ablation to avoid this oxidation risk. The superficial fractional ablation will allow pigment removal in the sloughing of skin. There is minimal risk of scarring or pigmentary changes as the zones of untreated skin in between ablative zones act as a resource for epithelial repair (Figs. 8–11). In this patient, a fractional CO_2 laser was used for eyebrow tattoo removal. One can appreciate immediate lessening of tattoo pigment after two passes of fractional ablative laser treatment (Figs. 11–13).

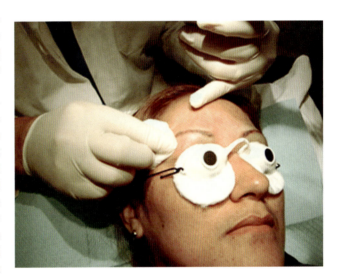

Fig. 9 Fractional CO_2 treatment of cosmetic eyebrow tattoo

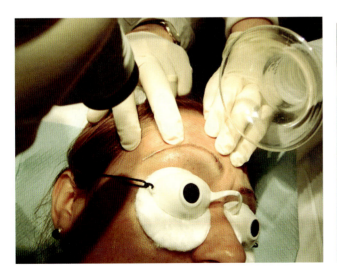

Fig. 8 Fractional CO_2 treatment of cosmetic eyebrow tattoo

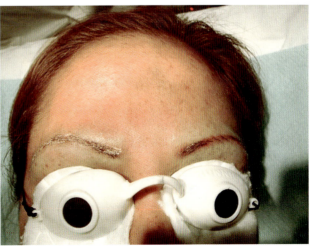

Fig. 10 Remove sloughed skin in between laser passes with wet gauze

Fig. 11 Right eyebrow after second laser pass

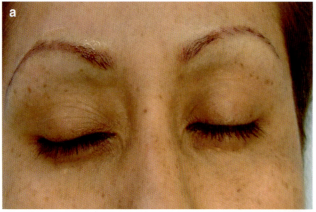

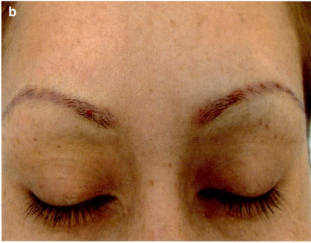

Fig. 12 (**a**) Before treatment. (**b**) After treatment

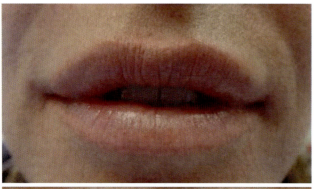

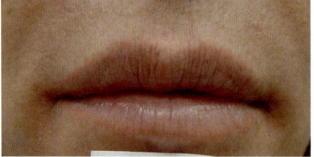

Fig. 13 Removal of cosmetic lip tattoo

Tattoo Removal in Dark Skin Types

The principal of tattoo removal is destruction of unwanted pigment with minimal collateral damage. This concept is particularly challenging when treating darker skin types as the melanosomes act as competing targets with the potential to cause epidermal damage. The 1,064-nm wavelength has the least absorption by melanocytes and is therefore the best choice for laser tattoo removal in darker skin types. There is less risk for hypopigmentation, scarring or textural change. However, the 1,064-nm wavelength will not treat all tattoo colors. Therefore, one must employ alternate methods for multicolored or densely colored tattoos in dark skin types.[4,5]

Fractional ablation of tattoos in dark skin types will allow extraction of tattoo pigment particles with minimal risk of scarring or pigmentary change. This concept is particularly useful in dark skin types with in a patient that has demonstrated allergic reaction to the tattoo pigment. For instance, red pigment is the most common known tattoo allergen and can result in a granulomatous reaction. If targeted with a 532-nm wavelength for removal, the pigment can shatter into many smaller particles followed by uptake systemically with the potential for anaphylaxis. To avoid this issue, fractional CO_2 laser can be used for sloughing of the pigment through epidermal loss with limited systemic elimination. Non-fractional CO_2 laser has limited use in this circumstance as it has significant potential to permanently depigment or scar the skin. This was the case in the patient in Figs. 14 and 15.[5-8]

Complications in Laser Tattoo Removal

Even in the most experienced hands, lasers can induce scarring, textural changes and hypopigmentation. When hypopigmentation does occur, the majority of time it is transient and will resolve over the course of months with appropriate care. There are a small percentage of cases in which the hypopigmentation is permanent. This is cosmetically unappealing and in the view of the patient sometimes worse than the original tattoo. Again, the fractional CO_2 laser can be employed to stimulate repigmentation. This is accomplished via melanocyte stimulation in the zones of untreated skin, adjacent to ablated zones, acting as a pigment resource.[6-10] (Figs. 16–18).

Laser Clinical and Practice Pearls 315

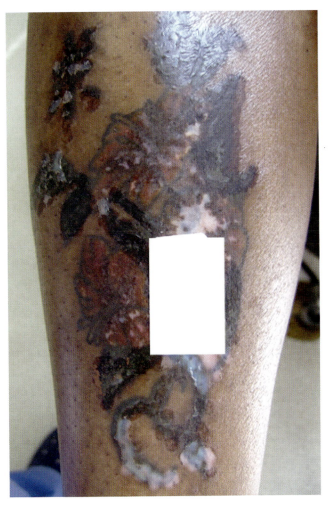

Fig. 14 Noted depigmentation after CO_2 laser treatment for tattoo removal

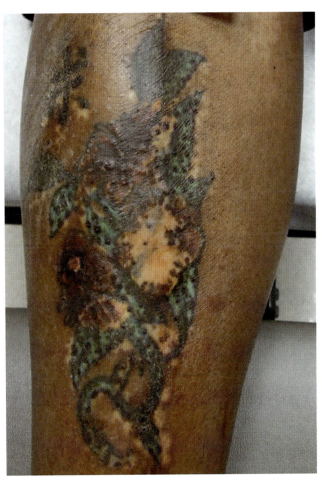

Fig. 15 Noted repigmentation of prior treated area, accomplished with fractional CO_2 laser treatment

Scars

- Hypertrophic, keloid and atrophic scars, whether traumatic, surgical or acne etiology, can be significantly improved with fractional erbium doped 1,550 nm and fractional CO_2 laser treatments.
- Hypopigmented scars can be repigmented with fractional erbium doped 1,550 nm and fractional CO_2 laser treatments.

Any injury to the skin that goes beyond the epidermis, will result in scarring. Scars come in many varieties. They can be categorized according to etiology, such as traumatic scar, surgical scar or acne scar. They can also be grouped by wound healing response, such as hypertrophic or keloid scars, resulting from excessive wound healing. Regardless of etiology, there are limited resources for significant cosmetic improvement with limited down time or risk. See Chap. "Laser for Scars" for complete discussion of scar treated with lasers.

Hypertrophic, Keloid and Atrophic Scars

Past studies have demonstrated mild to moderate reduction in scar erythema, thickness and pruritus with PDL treatment. This is theorized to be secondary to reduction in vasculature of the scar. Ablative lasers (erbium or CO_2) can be used to reduce the excess tissue however there is great risk of further scarring or dyspigmentation from the laser treatment itself. More recent technology, such as fractional photothermolysis, can result in significant cosmetic improvement of scars via collagen

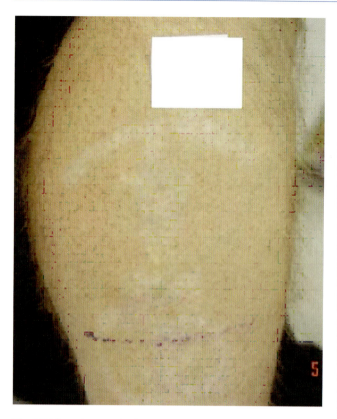

Fig. 16 Hypopigmentation in skin type II after ruby laser used in black tattoo removal

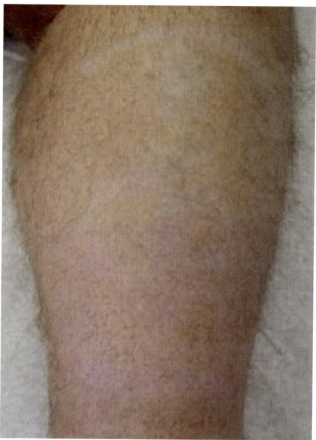

Fig. 17 Repigmentation of skin accomplished with fractional CO_2 laser

remodeling with limited risk of side effects. Ablative fractional photothermolysis allows for reduction of excess tissue in a controlled capacity within the thermal microzones. This leaves the normal adjacent tissue to act as the resource for repair minimizing risk of dyspigmentation and scarring. The deep coagulation allows for scar contraction and smoothing of texture resulting in a remodeling of scar tissue to clinically appear closer to normal tissue. Non-ablative fractional photothermolysis is also effective in treating scars. The collagen remodeling allows for improvement in overall texture as well as repigmentation of hypopigmented scars. The scars continue to improve in pliability, texture and pigmentation with each successive treatment. Both non-ablative and ablative fractional resurfacing allow for scar improvement in all skin types in contrast to standard ablative lasers (Figs. 18–21).[8-13]

Acne Scars

Facial acne scarring plagues many patients, of all skin types. There are multiple options for treatment however, not all have significant improvement and not all can be used in darker skin types. Non-ablative lasers such as Nd:Yag have been used for dermal collagen stimulation with a low risk profile and convenient treatment course but limited results. More recently, fractional photothermolysis has demonstrated consistent efficacy in scar improvement with limited risk of side effects and importantly can be used in all skin types with appropriate parameter selection (Figs. 22–24).[11-16]

Laser Clinical and Practice Pearls

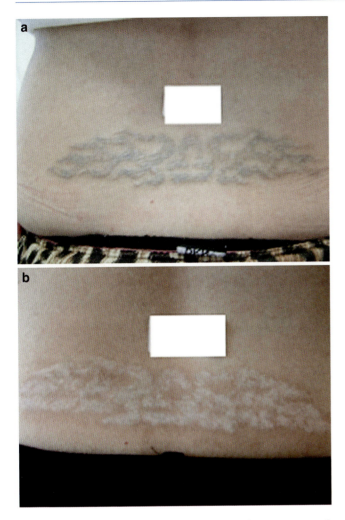

Fig. 18 (**a**) After multiple ruby laser treatments for tattoo removal, slight tattoo pigment remains as well as mild hyperpigmentation of normal surrounding skin; (**b**) after four treatments of non-ablative fractional erbium treatments, no appreciable tattoo pigment remains. Normalizing of normal surrounding skin tissue

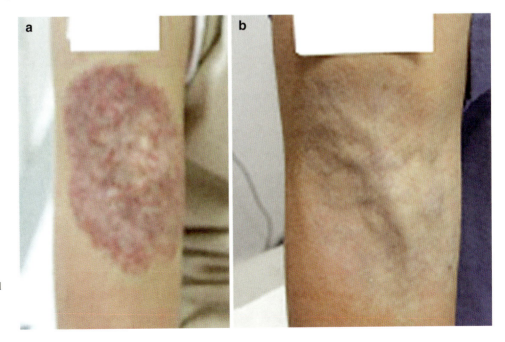

Fig. 19 (**a**) Involuted hemangioma with resulting atrophy, hypopigmentation and textural changes; (**b**) significant improvement after five fractional non-ablative 1,550 nm erbium-doped laser and pulse dye laser treatments

Fig. 20 (**a**) Atrophic scars with hypopigmentation and textural changes in skin type III; (**b**) Significant improvement after five fractional non-ablative 1,550 nm erbium-doped laser treatments

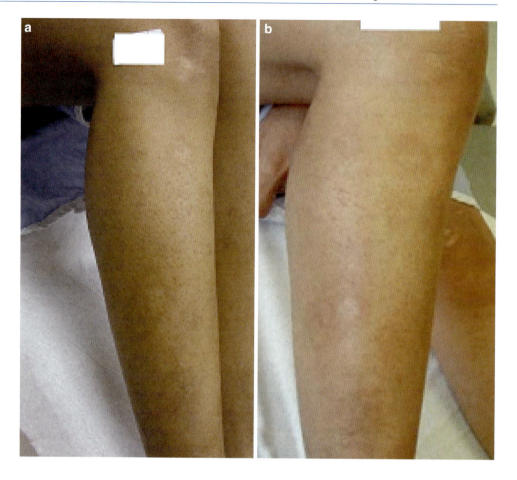

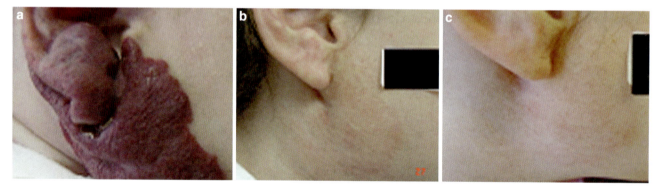

Fig. 21 (**a**) Infantile hemangioma; (**b**) Involution of hemangioma with resulting textural and pigmentary changes; (**c**) Significant improvement after three erbium-doped 1,550 nm laser treatment

Laser Clinical and Practice Pearls

Fig. 22 (a) Linear atrophic scar, traumatic injury 18 years prior; (b) Near complete resolution of atrophic scar status post fractional CO_2 laser treatment (1 month post treatment #1)

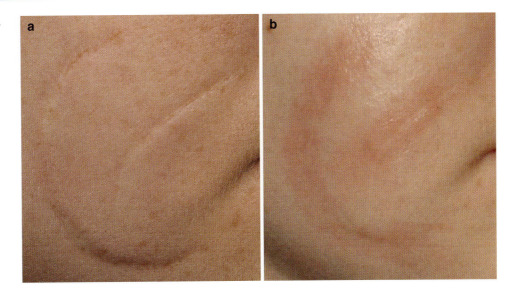

Fig. 23 (a) Skin type II, with moderate acne scarring; (b) After a series of five treatments with fractional 1,550 nm erbium-doped fiber laser and significant reduction of scar appearance

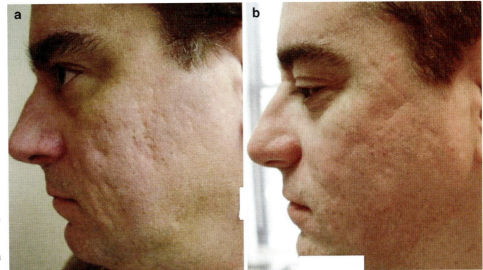

Fig. 24 (**a**) Baseline with moderate acne scarring and melasma; (**b**) After five fraxel 750 nm laser treatments and one fractional CO_2 laser treatment with notable resolution of acne scars as well as melasma

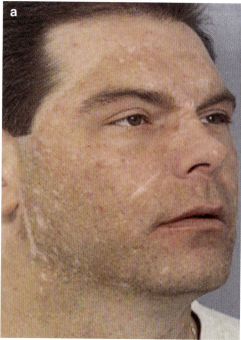 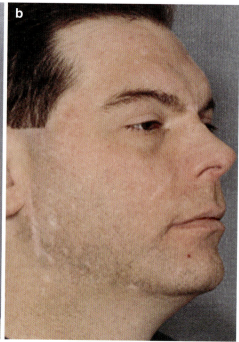

References

1. Halkiadakis I, Skouriotis S, Stefanki C, et al. Iris atrophy and posterior synechiae as a complication of eyebrow epilation. *J Am Acad Dermatol*. 2007;57(suppl 2):S4-S5.
2. Bader O, Lui H. *Laser Safety and the Eye: Hidden Hazards and Practical Pearls*. Washington, DC: American Academy of Dermatology Annual Meeting; 1996.
3. Waldorf H, Kauvar A, Geronemus R, Leffell D. Remote fire with the pulsed dye laser: risk and prevention. *J Am Acad Dermatol*. 1996;34:503-506.
4. Lapidoth M, Aharonowitz G. Tattoo removal among Ethiopian Jews in Israel: tradition faces technology. *J Am Acad Dermatol*. 2004;51(6):906-909.
5. Kuperman-Beade M, Levine VJ, Ashinoff R. Laser removal of tattoos. *Am J Clin Dermatol*. 2001;2(1):21-25.
6. Manstein D, Herron G, Sink R, et al. Fractional photothermolysis: a new concept for cutaneous remodeling using microscopic patterns of thermal injury. *Lasers Surg Med*. 2004;34:426-38.
7. Geronemus R. Fractional photothermolysis: current and future applications. *Lasers Surg Med*. 2006;38:169-76.
8. Hantash B, Mahmood M. Fractional photothermolysis: a novel aesthetic laser surgery modality. *Dermatol Surg*. 2007;33:525-34.
9. Laubach H, Tannous Z, Anderson R, Manstein D. Skin responses to fractional photothermolysis. *Lasers Surg Med*. 2006;38(2):142-149.
10. Rahman Z, Alam M, Dover J. Fractional laser treatment for pigmentation and texture improvement. *Skin Ther Lett*. 2006;32:298-301.
11. Alster T, Tanzi E, Lazarus M. The use of fractional photothermolysis for the treatment of atrophic scars. *Dermatol Surg*. 2007;33:295-299.
12. Glaich A, Zakia R, Goldberg L, Friedman P. Fractional resurfacing for the treatment of hypopigmented scars: a pilot study. *Derm Surg* March 2007;33(3): 289-294.
13. Behroozan D, Goldberg L, Dai T, et al. Fractional photothermolysis for the treatment of surgical scars: a case report. *J Cosmet Laser Ther*. 2006;8:35-38.
14. Friedman P, Jih M, Skover G, Payonk G, Kimyai-Asadi A, Geronemus R. Treatment of atrophic facial acne scars with the 1064-nm Q-switched Nd: YAG laser: six-month follow-up study. *Arch Derm*. 2004;140(11):1337-41.
15. Tanzi E, Alster T. Comparison of a 1450-nm diode laser and a 1320-nm Nd:YAG laser in the treatment of atrophic facial scars: a prospective clinical and histological study. *Dermatol Surg*. 2004;30(2 pt1):152-7.
16. Hasegawa T, Matsukura T, Mizuno Y, Suga Y, Ogawa H, Ikeda S. Clinical trial of a laser device called fractional photothermolysis system acne scars. *J Dermatol*. 2006;33(9):623-7.

The Selection and Education of Laser Patients

Murad Alam and Natalie Kim

- Basic Considerations in Patient Selection
- Procedure Delegation to Non-Physician Caregivers
- Initial Consultation and Patient Education
- Exclusion Criteria for Laser Treatments
- Patient Education Regarding Undesired Effects

Introduction

Several measures can affect the likelihood of optimal treatment results and patient satisfaction. First, a suitable candidate must be selected. As with many cosmetic procedures, unreasonable expectations, body dysmorphic disorder, relevant psychiatric illness, and chronic dissatisfaction with prior physicians are concerning factors. Additionally, patient dissatisfaction is frequent following treatment of minor complaints or those for which reliable, efficacious treatments are not available. Tanned patients or patients of color are at risk for dyschromia, and treatment may need to be delayed or modified accordingly.

Following patient selection for laser procedures, there is a detailed pretreatment consultation during which patient education occurs. When counseling patients, physicians may first listen to patient concerns, then ask salient questions for clarification, and finally suggest a range of appropriate options. To further ensure redundancy and clarity, physicians may involve multiple caregivers in the education process and utilize photographs and brochures. Patients should be informed of the approximate number of laser treatments that may be necessary, expected downtime after treatment, and potential alternatives or combination therapies. Physicians may also preemptively disclose that some patients do not respond with the same success as others to certain procedures.

M. Alam (✉)
Department of Dermatology, Otolaryngology – Head and Neck Surgery, Northwestern University, Chicago, IL, USA
e-mail: m-alam@northwestern.edu

Lastly, patients should be told of common undesired effects before treatment, and be given contact information to encourage prompt reporting of unexpected adverse events after treatment. In the event of procedure-related adverse events, calm and honest discussion is the guiding principle. Physicians should explain corrective options and assure their commitment to the patient. Careful patient selection and education will prove beneficial for both patient and physician.

Selecting the Laser Patient

Potential Contraindications in Patient Selection

1. Unreasonable expectations
2. Body dysmorphic disorder
3. Unmanaged psychiatric illness
4. Complaints regarding prior physicians and treatments
5. Hard to see, hard to treat problems
6. Selection of procedures with highly variable efficacy

Finding the Reasonable Patient

In discourses on patient selection in cosmetic and laser surgery, there is an emphasis on ensuring that the patient has so-called "reasonable expectations." The difficulty lies in defining this phrase and in ascertaining whether a particular patient meets the test. Among the useful cues are facial expressions and the patient's responses to the physician's discourse.[1] A patient who nods in response and asks appropriate questions in a modulated voice of moderate volume is reassuring for the physician. The implication is that the patient is a partner in the discussion and is both understanding what the physician is saying and agreeing with the physician's plan. An excessively emotional, or alternatively stone-face and hostile, patient is cause for concern.

K. Nouri (ed.), *Lasers in Dermatology and Medicine*,
DOI: 10.1007/978-0-85729-281-0_24, © Springer-Verlag London Limited 2011

Body Dysmorphic Disorder

Much has also been written about the unsuitability for cosmetic procedures of patients with body dysmorphic disorder. The full-blown disorder is probably uncommon among patients seeking laser treatment. But less extreme variants are seen often. In brief, the problem is that some patients perceive their own bodies in an unrealistic manner.[2] Minor flaws are seen as major disfigurement, and some normal features are viewed as problems needing correction. Such patients are chronically dissatisfied with their appearance, and there may be no limit to the number of complaints they have. Correcting a given complaint with a perfectly executed laser procedure will be of no value: either the patient will immediately generate another complaint, or they will deny that the first was adequately treated despite objective evidence to the contrary.[3]

Identifying the patient with body dysmorphic disorder or a lesser subtype is not always simple. Patients may be expert at concealing their pathology. They may appear eminently reasonable. Evidence in support of a diagnosis of body dysmorphic disorder is a large number of prior surgeries or procedures to address the same problem.[4] These may be invasive surgeries like rhinoplasty or rytidectomy that are seldom repeated multiple times, and they may have been performed by a number of different physicians.

A surgeon who is convinced that a patient has body dysmorphic disorder should refer the patient for appropriate counseling with a mental health professional. If there is some doubt about the diagnosis, it may be appropriate to consult with or refer the patient to another cosmetic surgeon for a second opinion. If the diagnosis is far from certain and the physician thinks the patient is anxious but not mentally ill, it may still be preferable to avoid any major procedures until the patient has undergone some minor nonablative procedures and evinced a satisfactory post-treatment course.

Patients with Psychiatric Illness and Factitial Dermatoses

Patients with depression and anxiety disorders, schizophrenia, and other psychiatric disorders may present for laser surgery. Importantly, these conditions are not absolute contraindications for treatment. Patients who understand their illness, are appropriately medicated, and are under the care of a physician who is both managing their mental illness and supportive of their desire for laser surgery may in fact be appropriate laser patients. Needless to say, patients with mental illness who lack insight and whose underlying disease is not managed are not suitable candidates for laser procedures.

One problem in the post-operative period is picking and self-mutilation.[5] Picking behaviors are often exacerbated by the appearance of what is perceived as "damaged" skin, such as the re-epithelializing skin after ablative resurfacing. Since picking can lead to prolonged healing and scarring, picking should be treated before ablative or partially ablative laser treatments are commenced.

Patients Who Have Been Dissatisfied with Prior Physicians

Not uncommonly, laser physicians see patients who are unhappy with doctors who have treated them previously. On initial presentation, such patients may convey delight at having finally found the perfect, best qualified physician for their needs. They may relate the horrors of prior experiences with different physicians, who were in their estimation incompetent and dangerous quacks. These patients may be effusive and smiling, and convey their relief at finally being under the care of a master and magician, the physician in question.

While this level of approbation can be intoxicating for the physician toward whom it is directed, caution should be exercised in treating patients who present thus. Often, dissatisfaction with prior physicians is founded not on the incompetence of these professionals but rather on unrealistic patient expectations that could not have been, and hence were not, met.[6] Patients who hated their other doctors, may soon come to hate their current doctor. In such patients, there is a pervasive tendency to view physicians as either all good, or all bad. Oversimplification of this type is incompatible with the more shades-of-grey medical model, in which good care often results in partial resolution of ill-defined problems.

In working with a patient of this type, it may be wise for the physician to communicate forcefully early in the consultation that he or she is quite certainly unable to help the patient in the manner they seek. Additional referrals may be provided to other physicians who may or may not be able to assist the patient. Disappointing the patient early in the process may, for the physician, be preferable to managing an unhappy patient after treatment.

Identifying Problems That Are Difficult to Treat

Some patients have very high standards. They may ask to have removed minute lentigines that are difficult to see. Or they may request a further scar revision for an accident-induced scar that was previously expertly revised and is now a faint flat line.

In considering the needs of such patients, it is important to maintain a realistic appraisal of what is possible. One approach is for the physician to communicate that he or she definitely understands the patient's concern, but is unsure that he or she has the means to resolve it. The physician may wish to share that given the subtlety of the defect, it is difficult to say whether it would be improved, unchanged, or even exacerbated after a laser procedure. Since no physician is omniscient, it is reasonable to concede that some other laser surgeon may offer a superior treatment strategy associated with a greater likelihood of success; it may thus be appropriate for the physician to suggest a second opinion be obtained from another laser expert in the area. If the initial physician chooses to treat the minor defect perceived by the patient as a major one, the physician should be prepared for a dissatisfied patient after treatment. To avoid this, the physician should be clear about the weak prospects for improvement, and the likely need for many treatments; a comprehensive oral and written consent may be obtained.

Performing Procedures to Which Some Patients Do Not Respond

Some energy procedures, such as nonablative skin tightening, do not provide all patients with similar benefits. Perhaps a fourth of patients obtain excellent results, another half have modest improvement, and a quarter may have no discernible change from baseline. If there is a reasonable likelihood that a laser procedure will be unsuccessful for a particular patient, it is important to communicate this before the procedure is performed. It is more credible for the physician to predict lack of response than to justify it after it has happened. Prediction implies superior knowledge and honesty; justification after the fact suggests lack of competence and the possibility that a mistake is being rationalized. Of course, any laser procedure, and any medical procedure in general, can be ineffective in a specific case without any physician fault. But when such an outcome is probable, it behooves the physician to clearly communicate this in a pre-emptive manner. In general, it is better to lose a patient than to regret having performed a procedure on a now unhappy patient, who feels mislead and whose needs have not been met.

Delegating Procedures to Non-physician Caregivers

Smaller laser procedures are frequently delegated to nurses, physician assistants, and other non-physician providers. After a consultation with the physician, who may recommend a series of laser treatments, the patient may follow up on a monthly basis with a trained non-physician provider who performs these treatments under physician supervision. Medical practices vary with regard to the degree of delegation: on-site versus off-site delegation; the types of laser procedures that are delegated; and the level of training and education of the providers performing the delegated functions.

Another variable is patient acceptance of delegation. Some patients insist upon treatment by the attending physician. Others may be more flexible, but may want the attending physician to be in-house or to perform at least part of the procedure. Still others may be indifferent as to who provides the service as long as the physician is in charge and responsible for the outcome. Before delegating a procedure, the physician must make sure that the patient is accepting of this. If the patient insists on the physician performing the procedure, it is appropriate to charge a higher fee, which accounts for the additional physician time required. When procedures are delegated, if the patient is dissatisfied with the non-physician provider, this should be conveyed forthwith to the physician by the provider; the physician can then see the patient, address the concerns, and repair the patient-physician relationship.

Educating Laser Patients Presenting for Consultation

Presenting Complaints in Laser and Cosmetic Patients

Patients who present for laser procedures either have a specific complaint they wish addressed, or have a general interest in laser therapy. In the latter case, they are typically unsure what laser might be able to do for them, but are attracted to laser therapy, which they consider precise and definitive.

Counseling Patients Who Know What They Want Treated

Listen to Patient Concerns

If patients present with a specific concern, say excess hair on the upper lip or telangiectasia on the nose, the first step is for the physician to assess the problem. It is best to let the patient speak for several minutes, as this will help the physician understand the exact concerns as well as the degree of emotional overlay. For instance, if the patient has telangiectasia over much of her face but is only bothered by a large spider angioma on her nasal tip, this is useful information. Similarly, it is useful to understand whether the patient is only mildly disturbed by a concern or whether this subjectively a life-altering problem for which she is willing to consider most any treatment option. As the patient is describing her presenting complaint, it is helpful to offer her a handheld mirror, so that she can point to the relevant areas, and the physician can see these clearly.

Ask Questions to Clarify the Extent of the Concern, and Prior Treatment History

Once the patient has had an opportunity to describe the problem, the physician should ask salient questions. If the physician believes that the patient may have omitted some concerns or not have provided adequate history, questions may be asked to elicit this information. For example, the physician may ask, "I know the red spot on your nose bothers you, but what about the blood vessels on your cheek, and the redness elsewhere on your head and neck?" The purpose here is not to induce insecurity in the patient, but rather to obtain complete information. If the patient comments that other areas of redness are not too noticeable and looks to the physician for confirmation, it behooves the physician to say something reassuring, like "I see what you mean, it's really only the nose that is a problem at this time." With regard to history, it is important to know the genesis of a problem and what prior treatments may have been undertaken. A red, indented scar caused by a motor vehicle accident 2 days ago may be treated with conservative wound therapy, a waiting period, and then laser for redness and scar; conversely, a long-standing red scar may be treated immediately with laser. In the same vein, an angioma previously treated unsuccessfully three times with pulsed-dye laser may require either higher fluence therapy with bruising or possibly a more aggressive vascular laser, such as an Nd:YAG; a so-called "virgin" angioma may only require gentle pulsing from a KTP or pulsed-dye laser. While laser procedures are often elective, and not reimbursed by insurance, it is imperative that the physician retain the vigilance usually required when confronted with serious medical problems. For instance, if there is a scar adjacent to the presenting complaint that the patient has not explained, the doctor should ask about it. If the patient has complicating medical illnesses, like lupus or scleroderma, that may inhibit healing, the physician should glean this information from the chart or ask the patient directly.

Communicate to the Patient that You Are Carefully Considering Options

Having had the patient describe the problem and having asked additional questions for clarification, the physician

should take a moment to think. It is best to be sitting down for this, as studies have shown that patients prefer this, and view a physician who sits as one who spends more time with them.[7] Patients are used to being interrupted hurried by their physicians, so some quiet thinking time may give them the correct impression that their concerns are being evaluated. A furrowed brow, leaning back in a chair, or even saying aloud, "let me consider what you have said," will communicate that the physician is hard at work solving the problem. Of course, this phase should not last too long to avoid creating the impression that the physician is confused or unsure.

Suggest a Range of Appropriate Treatment Options

Based on the information provided, the physician should provide treatment options to the patient. In some cases a specific treatment may be suggested. In other cases, a range of options, from the less costly and minimally invasive to the more expensive and more downtime-intensive, can be presented. Whether one or several options are presented will depend on: (1) the medical issue being addressed, and whether multiple therapies exist for its management; (2) patient preference, with some patients wanting the doctor to decide and others wanting to select from a series of well-described options themselves. Patients vary in the degree of risk they wish to assume. Should the physician have a sense of their set point for risk, this can be taken into account. To wit, a patient who wants something very gentle, like a topical cream, for facial rejuvenation, may be amenable to microdermabrasion, superficial chemical peels, and nonablative laser; another equally photodamaged person who has previously had a two face-lifts and a blepharoplasty may not be satisfied with anything less than maximal therapy with full face laser resurfacing or fractional carbon dioxide laser treatment.

Involve Other Caregivers, Photographs, and Written Materials to Ensure Redundancy and Enhance Clarity

In providing information about therapeutic options, it is useful to include other educators and visual aids. Due to the inordinate time commitment associated with initial patient consultations, mid-level professionals may be asked to participate. Nurses, clinical nurse practitioners, physician assistants, and residents or fellows in training may join the attending physician in the patient room, and they may stay after the physician exits to answer additional questions. Alternatively, a similar professional may be the first to see the patient, elicit a history, and prepare a possible list of therapeutic options before the attending enters the room. From the patient perspective, meeting with several caregivers sequentially may allow patients to refine their thoughts and to have all their questions answered. From the perspective of the attending physician, this serial approach reduces the amount of attending time to be spent with each patient while ensuring that nothing salient is missed by the treating team and that routine elements of the consultation, such as description of adverse events, prices, and preoperative instructions, are conveyed clearly. While some practitioners do not like to provide representative before and after photographs, these can be very helpful. A nurse or other caregiver may review a book of such photographs with a prospective patient, thus creating reasonable expectations, affording the patient a further opportunity to ask questions, and providing the patient with information that she may need before deciding to proceed with the laser therapy. Brochures about procedures and a carefully customized menu of recommended services with prices are also beneficial for patient information.[8] Patients often forget what they have heard. Written materials can be used to refresh memories, and perused at home with a spouse or significant other. For major procedures requiring some downtime ad risk, phone numbers of willing patients who have previously been satisfied with similar procedures may allay patient worries. A designated cosmetic coordinator or cosmetic consultant from the physician practice may contact the patient at home or provide a contact number in case the patient has further queries. Some practices will permit a free or low-cost reconsultation with the physician to address lingering issues before a procedure.

Counseling Patients Who Offer No Specific Complaints but Want to Look Better

The patient who is unsure about precisely what she wants but desires to look better overall is slightly more challenging in initial consultation. Usually, even such relatively unsophisticated or indecisive patients do have some internal view of their flaws. Gentle questioning can often lead them to reveal these self-assessments. If adequate information is thus obtained, management of these concerns can proceed as if the patient initially presented with them. If, on the other hand, the patient is not providing much guidance even after some pointed queries, the physician may prompt pursue a systematic approach: Starting on the face, the physician can assess color and textural irregularities. The physician can verbally list the apparent problems and visible signs of aging, and then suggest the modalities that may be suitable for improving each. The physician may also allude to the approximate degree of invasiveness, downtime, and cost associated with various treatment options. Finally, the physician may suggest a step-by-step program for proceeding. High on the list should be procedures that are simple, inexpensive, and highly likely to produce an appreciable improvement; the successful outcome of these may help diminish patient anxiety and increase patient willingness to undergo more invasive or complex procedures in the future.

Explaining the Laser Treatment in the Context of a Larger Treatment Plan

One laser treatment will seldom completely correct a patient complaint. The exception may be full-face laser resurfacing or aggressive fractional resurfacing with carbon dioxide laser. In most cases, 3–6 or more laser treatments may be needed to mostly treat a problem; for instance, a series of nonablative treatments with various lasers will improve telangiectasia, diffuse facial erythema, lentigines, acne scars, and excess hair. Tattoo removal may require 10–20, or more, treatments.

Treatments That Can Be Combined with Lasers

- Injectable fillers
- Surgical excision
- Neurotoxins
- Other energy devices (radiofrequency, ultrasound)

Further, laser is not the only treatment type that may be appropriate. Other methods, like injectable fillers, surgical excision, neurotoxins, and other energy devices, may be used in combination. Such multimodality treatments can maximize the efficacy and persistence of results while maintaining an excellent safety profile. If appropriate, patients should be counseled during the consultation phase about the utility of other treatments to enhance the effect of laser. Considerations of cost and time may intrude, but patients should be offered the choice. Also, in raising this issue, the physician will clarify that complete resolution of the target complaint is not possible by laser alone.

When Laser Treatments Should Be Deferred or Modified

In certain cases, laser treatment may be inappropriate or at least need to be postponed. Different lasers may have specific exclusion criteria. For example, if a Caucasian patient has plucked their chin hair recently, they would not be a candidate for laser hair removal until several weeks later since the presence of hair roots at the target site is essential for the efficacy of this procedure. Some cautions are more general, applying to all cutaneous laser devices.

Tanned Patients

Caucasian patients who are intensely tan due to tanning beds, prolonged outdoor exposure, or a recent sunny vacation should not receive laser treatment as they are at risk for brownish discoloration. While dyschromia of this type will eventually resolve, it can be disfiguring and take months to remit. Patients about to embark on a vacation where they will be sun-exposed should also defer laser treatment. Athletes pending a major outdoor sporting event, such as a triathlon, or tennis or golf tournament, may wish to be treated a few weeks after this is over. In general, laser treatments should be avoided a few weeks before and a few weeks after significant sun exposure. Tanning booths are considered sun exposure, but artificial tanning solutions are not; even so, artificial tanners should be discontinued 4–5 days prior to laser procedures.

Patients of Color

Darker skinned patients, especially those of Fitzpatrick skin types IV-VI, are at greater risk of post-inflammatory hyperpigmentation after laser procedures. Ablative and partially ablative lasers are much more likely to induce pigmentary change in susceptible patients, but all lasers are a potential risk. Bruising after pulsed-dye laser procedures can also culminate in brownish discoloration. In darker skinned patients, including those of Indian, Middle Eastern, Far Eastern, and Latino origin, post-inflammatory hyperpigmentation may be slow to resolve, and may last many months or even years. Higher energy treatments are commonly avoided in patients with ethnic skin. More numerous lower-energy treatments may be substituted in lieu of fewer more aggressive treatments.

Educating Patient About Common Undesired Effects

Common Undesired Effects

Before treatment

- Redness
- Swelling
- Bruising
- Erosions
- Downtime

After treatment

- Hives
- Blisters

Redness and Swelling

Patients should be told that a certain degree of redness and swelling are inevitable after most laser procedures. Such sequelae can be covered with makeup and will remit in hours, or at most 1–2 days. In describing these results, it is preferable to avoid using the technical terms "erythema" and "edema," as these are not understood by most patients. It may be helpful to also explain that there is individual variation, and some patients may become redder or swell more than most. When the upper cheeks and lower forehead area are treated, periorbital swelling is extremely common. In such cases, patients should be apprised that their eyes may almost swell shut for a day or two, and that this can occur a day or two after treatment. Eyelid swelling is a common stimulus for a worried phone call from patients; proper pretreatment counseling can avert this needless anxiety, and inconvenience to both patient and physician.

Bruising

Bruising (ecchymoses) can occur after some laser treatments, including pulsed-dye laser and some ablative resurfacing lasers. Bruising can persist for a week or longer, with more protracted course periorbitally. In the initial consultation, it is important to ascertain the degree to which patients can tolerate bruising. Some patients in the public eye may not want even the smallest, faintest bruise; for them, laser treatment parameters should be adjusted to ensure that bruising is entirely avoided. Pretreatment or postreatment with oral arnica montana supplementation can also reduce the degree and duration of bruising. Many patients have great faith in vitamins, herbals, and dietary supplements, and the recommendation to acquire a supply of arnica may be well-received.

Erosions

Even nonablative laser treatments may result in a few pinpoint or small erosions. These reddish, crusted areas are best treated with bland emollients. Hard crust should not be allowed to form. Since patients are often reluctant to disturb crust or scabs, they should be told something like, "greasy wounds without crust heal better." For many patients, this is a revelation, and they can be useful allies in facilitating wound healing once they know what to do.

Hives and Blisters

Urticaria and blisters occur infrequently after laser treatment, but can be very striking and worrisome when they manifest.

It is probably not necessary to educate patients preemptively about these unusual outcomes. However, if urticaria and transient micro-blisters occur, antihistamines and topical steroids can be commenced immediately. Concurrently, the patient should be reassured that these problems look very bad but are not serious and easily treated.

Downtime

After every laser procedure, there is a recovery period. For nonablative lasers like Q-switched lasers, pulsed-dye lasers, hair removal lasers, and nonablative tightening devices, this may be brief. No time off from work or social engagements is usually necessary after these "lunchtime" procedures. However, some partially ablative and fully ablative modalities may be followed by more substantial downtime. Fractionated laser treatments may have 3–4 days of post-procedure downtime, and higher energy treatments with fractionated carbon dioxide devices may be associated with downtime of 7–10 days. Notably, even though traditional full-face laser resurfacing with carbon dioxide laser has approximately equivalent downtime in days, the character of downtime after fractionated carbon dioxide is better. Patients in the latter case do not have extreme crusting and scabbing for the duration, and they are not as uncomfortable; they still look unpresentable for many days, but the degree of disfigurement is less and the associated discomfort largely lacking. When counseling patients, it is important to understand their limits for downtime. Some patients are relatively more relaxed, and older patients who are no longer working may be able to remain at home for a longer period. Other patients may know exactly how many days of work they can miss, and the intensity of partially ablative procedures may need to be titrated to fit these bounds. That being said, there is a balance between providing adequate information about downtime, and needlessly scaring patients to the point where they decline an otherwise effective, indicated procedure.

Encouraging Patients to Promptly Report Unexpected Adverse Events

Apart from common adverse events, unusual or rare undesired events can occur after laser treatments. Providing patients with contact information to report such outcomes increases the likelihood that problems can be corrected without permanent sequelae. Sometimes, patients will forget instructions, and be unable to manage even an expected adverse event. If they feel their physician is approachable, they will be motivated to contact the office for help. In this manner, patients will not only protect their health but also allow the physician to avoid the risk that an untreated minor problem devolves into a serious treatment-associated complication.

Discussing Procedure-Related Problems with Patients

Not every laser procedure is entirely successful. Problems can occur preoperatively, intraoperatively, or postoperatively. Preoperative problems may pertain to anesthesia adverse events, device malfunctions, and patient anxiety. Intraoperative problems may be excessive pain, inappropriate laser parameters, cooling failures, incorrect use of protective eyewear, and the like. Post-operative adverse events are discussed elsewhere in this book, but may commonly include dyspigmentation, bruising, infection or inflammation, delayed healing, and scar.

In discussing procedure-associated issues with patients, the guiding principles are clarity, calmness, honesty, and reassurance. Full information should be provided in a timely manner. The physician should be empathetic, clearly showing his or her commitment ensuring the best possible outcome for the patient. Explanations should be accurate and concise, not colored by excessive emotion or rationalization. The physician should explain what needs to be done now, if anything, to correct residual problems. Corrective action should be compatible with the patient's schedule; efforts should be made to respect the patient's time and finances. Finally, the physician should state clearly that he or she will do everything in his or her power to resolve the situation, and will continue to work closely with the patient for the duration.

One excellent strategy is to bring the patient back weekly to assess the problem, and the extent to which it is responding to treatment. Not only does this communicate to the patient that the doctor cares, it also allows the physician to provide timely interventions when necessary and to detect any new problems as they arise. Regular follow-up also protects the physician from any subsequent charges of abandoning a patient in need.

References

1. Mast MS. On the importance of nonverbal communication in the physician-patient interaction. *Patient Educ Couns*. 2007;67: 315-318.
2. Phillips KA. Body dysmorphic disorder: the distress of imagine ugliness. *Am J Psychiatry*. 1991;148:1138-1149.
3. Veale D, Boocock A, Gournay K, et al. Body dysmorphic disorder: a survey of fifty cases. *Br J Psychiatry*. 1996;169:196-201.

4. Phillips KA, Grant J, Siniscalchi J, Albertini RS. Surgical and non-psychiatric medical treatment of patients with body dysmorphic disorder. *Psychosomatics*. 2001;42:504-510.

5. Stein DJ, Hollander E. Dermatology and conditions related to obsessive-compulsive disorder. *J Am Acad Dermatol*. 1992;26:237-242.

6. Ward CM. Consenting and consulting for cosmetic surgery. *Br J Plast Surg*. 1998;51:547-550.

7. Renzi C, Abeni D, Picardi A, et al. Factors associated with patient satisfaction with care among dermatological outpatients. *Br J Dermatol*. 2001;145:617-623.

8. Ellis DA, Hopkin JM, Leitch AG, Crofton J. 'Doctors Orders': controlled trial of supplementary, written information for patients. *Br Med J*. 1979;1:456.

Anesthesia for Laser Surgery

Voraphol Vejjabhinanta, Angela Martins, Ran Huo, and Keyvan Nouri

- A number of laser procedures such as laser resurfacing or tattoo removal are associated with some discomfort.
- Anesthesias provide a reversible loss of sensation and alleviate most of the discomfort.
- The techniques most commonly used are topical anesthesia and regional anesthesia with or without systemic analgesics and/or anxiolytics.
- Concomitant cooling, vibration or pinching of the area can be use to minimize the pain perception.

Introduction

Local anesthesia has been one of the most notable advancements in surgery for the past century. Prior to the advent of local anesthetics, patients had few options for dealing with pain. Inebriation was a common, albeit ineffective, practice.

In the early nineteenth century, it was reported that the Peruvian Indians experienced numbness around the lips after chewing leaves of the coca plant, *Erythroxylon coca*. In 1859, Albert Niemann, a German chemist, first extracted and isolated cocaine from the coca plant in a purified form.

Local anesthetics were first introduced into medical practice in 1884 when ophthalmologist Carl Kollar used purified cocaine as a topical agent by applying it to the cornea of animal models. In its first clinical application, cocaine was used in an operation for glaucoma. In the same year, Halsted and Hall infused cocaine into the brachial vein of a patient to achieve regional anesthesia.

Dentists used to dissolve cocaine hydrochloride pills in water and performed nerve infiltrations and blocks after drawing the mixture into a syringe. Although it provided profound local anesthesia that revolutionized dentistry and medical practice, the extreme vasoconstrictive action of cocaine often lead to tissue necrosis.

By the 1900s, cocaine's narcotic effects had become well recognized, including its mood-altering effects and cardiac and central nervous system stimulation. In addition, due to cocaine's severe physical and psychological dependence, its use for local anesthesia was discontinued.

In 1904, Alfred Einhoin synthesized procaine (Novacaine), an ester anesthetic, in search for a safer and less toxic local anesthetic. Novacaine was the gold standard for topical anesthetics for the following 40 years, until Nils Lofgren synthesized lidocaine. Lidocaine was the first of the amide group of local anesthetics, which exhibited greater potency, fewer allergic reactions, and a more rapid onset of action.

Proper local anesthesia is vital in laser surgery, as most laser procedures are associated with some discomfort, ranging from mild warmth to sever burning pain. An understanding of various local anesthesia indications, techniques, and side effects will provide a basis for the selection of the most appropriate anesthetic agent for the given procedure.

Classification and Mechanism of Action

- Local anesthetics share a similar chemical structure: a hydrophilic amine portion, an intermediate chain, and a lipophilic aromatic ring.
- They are divided into amide or ester groups due to the intermediate chain.
- Anesthetics act by disrupting sodium channel activity and blocking electrical impulse transmission at nerve endings.
- Most local anesthetics except cocaine have vasodilatory effects.
- Epinephrine is often added as a vasoconstrictive agent and has the added benefit of minimizing systemic effects and increasing the length of anesthetic effect.

V. Vejjabhinanta (✉)
Department of Dermatology and Cutaneous Surgery,
University of Miami, Leonard M. Miller School of Medicine,
Miami, FL and
Department of Dermatology, Siriraj Hospital, Mahidol University,
Bangkok, Thailand
e-mail: vvoraphol@gmail.com

K. Nouri (ed.), *Lasers in Dermatology and Medicine*,
DOI: 10.1007/978-0-85729-281-0_25, © Springer-Verlag London Limited 2011

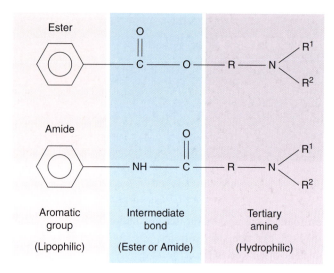

Fig. 1 Chemical structure of local anesthetic agents

Topical Anesthesia

- Topical anesthetics are used for superficial laser surgery and minor dermatological procedures.
- Quick procedures that require only a few seconds of anesthesia can utilize cooling agent.
- Lidocaine is the most widely used topical anesthetics.
- Occlusion with a plastic wrap is a way of enhancing anesthetic penetration and delivery to the dermis.
- Methemoglobinemia is a major concern regarding the use of EMLA, particularly in neonates.

Local anesthetic agents are functionally divided into the amino amide and amino ester groups (Fig. 1). Both groups share a similar chemical structure that contains three components: a hydrophilic amine portion, an intermediate chain, and a lypophilic aromatic ring. The intermediate chain contains either an ester or amide linkage which categorizes the agent.

Pain sensation is carried via C fiber (unmyelinated nerve, 0.5–1 μm) and A-delta fiber (2–5 μm). These fibers are more sensitive to the actions of local anesthetics as compared to large nerve fibers. Consequently, patients may be able to feel sensations such as pressure and vibration while being insensitive to pain.

The effectiveness of a local anesthetic depends on its ability to diffuse across the nerve cell's membrane (lipophilic properties) and then convert to a cationic form that results in better protein binding (hydrophilic properties). Higher lipid solubility of an agent increases its diffusion through a cell's membrane, leading to higher potency and lower concentrations needed to produce the desired result. However, greater protein-binding ability leads to a longer duration of action due to a higher affinity for intracellular receptors.

Most local anesthetics except cocaine have vasodilatory effects, which increases chances of excessive bleeding during the course of the procedure. To counteract this, epinephrine is often added as a vasoconstrictive agent, which has the added benefit of increasing the local sequestration of the anesthetic, minimizing systemic effects and increasing the length of anesthetic effect.

Topically-applied anesthetic agents are suitable for use in superficial laser surgery and minor dermatological procedures. Topical anesthetics act by disrupting sodium channel activity and blocking electrical impulse transmission at nerve endings. They can also be used to permit painless needle insertion when infiltrative anesthesia is required. These agents are usually encountered in an oil-in-water base or similar cream compound. For quick procedures, cooling sprays such as dichlorotetrafluoroethane or ethylchloride may be used.

The skin's stratum corneum serves as a mechanical barrier slowing down topical anesthesia penetration. Thus, the vehicle is very important in helping the anesthetic traverse the epidermis. The thickness of the stratum corneum varies with anatomical locations, altering the time to achieve adequate anesthesia. Occlusion with a plastic wrap is one way of enhancing product penetration and delivery to the dermis. This method also hydrates the skin, which may help explain the lower incidence of side effects seen after its use in carbon dioxide resurfacing laser procedures.

The most widely used topical anesthetic is EMLA cream, a 5% eutectic mixture of lidocaine 2.5% and prilocaine 2.5% in an oil-in-water emulsion. It must be applied under an occlusive dermal dressing for 60 min for adequate dermal anesthesia. EMLA has been shown to provide adequate anesthesia for pulsed dye laser treatments of Port Wine Stains (PWSs) without affecting the laser treatment's efficacy. It is also used in ablative laser resurfacing. The major concern regarding the use of EMLA relates to the potential risk of methemoglobinemia, also a known side effect of prilocaine. It is more likely in neonates, especially in pre-term infant.

LMX-4 (formerly called ELA-Max) is a 4% lidocaine cream in a liposomal vehicle that only requires 15–45 min of application time without the need of an occlusive dressing following its application. LMX-5 is the 5% concentration and although it is marketed for anorectal use, it can also be applied as a topical anesthetic agent.

Betacaine-LA ointment contains lidocaine, prilocaine and a vasoconstrictor in a liquid paraffin ointment. It has a recommended application time of 30–45 min without the requirement of an occlusive dressing.

Tetracaine gel is a long-acting ester anesthetic composed of 4% tetracaine in a lecithin gel. Its time application is 30 min under an occlusive dressing.

The 7% lidocaine and 7% tetracaine (LT) peel is a self occlusive topical anesthetic, presenting as a 1:1 eutectic mixture that is applied as a cream and air-dries to form a flexible membrane that can be peeled from the skin. The recommended application time is 30 min. LT peel has been successfully used in a variety of dermatological procedures such as PDL therapy, laser-assisted hair removal, non-ablative facial laser resurfacing, laser therapy for leg veins, cutaneous laser resurfacing and laser-assisted tattoo removal. It has shown to have a superior anesthetic efficacy in adult patients undergoing a variety of cutaneous procedures when compared to EMLA cream.

Quick procedures that require only a few seconds of anesthesia can utilize cooling refrigerant sprays, such as dichlorotetrafluoroethane or ethyl chloride. Ice cubes can also be used, especially to give painless injections in children.

Infiltrative Anesthesia

- Local infiltration can be performed for procedures associated with more pain such as ablative laser resurfacing.
- The ester-linked anesthetics have a much greater allergenic potential than the amide-linked anesthetics.
- Cross reactivity exists among ester-linked anesthetics, PABA, paraphenylenediamine, and sulfonamides.

Infiltrative anesthesia is the most commonly performed form of skin anesthesia. The concentration and selection of infiltrative anesthetics depend on the procedure to be performed, the speed of onset desired, and duration of action required. For quick and simple procedures, a short-acting anesthetic with rapid onset can be chosen. As for larger procedures, longer-acting agents will be needed.

When an extensive area of the skin is to be anesthetized, the anesthetic should be diluted in order to limit the total amount applied to the tissue and to reduce possible systemic adverse reactions. Conversely, higher concentrations can be used in smaller quantities for specific nerve blocks.

The ester-linked anesthetics (i.e. procaine, cocaine, tetracaine) have decreased in popularity due to allergic and cross-reactions with benzocaine, para-aminobenzoic acid (PABA), paraphenylenediamine, and sulfonamides.

Most procedures are performed using 1% or 2% lidocaine providing quick onset, long duration (45 min to 3 h without epinephrine), and low allergic reaction potential. When combined with epinephrine, an even longer anesthetic response can be achieved.

Bupivacaine and etidocaine are first-line agents used to achieve longer anesthetic periods, such as in the cases for nerve blocks. Etidocaine has a short onset of action, a long duration, and high potency without excessive increase in toxicity, and is ideal when a long procedure is planned and epinephrine is contraindicated. A summary of the most commonly used anesthetics, their onset, and duration of action are displayed on Table 1.

Injections may be placed subcutaneously or intradermally. Intradermal injection has a faster onset and longer duration of action, although it is much more painful than subcutaneous injection. Distortion of the skin by injection can be compensated for in procedures by marking the skin before injection and massaging it afterwards.

If amide and ester anesthetics cannot be used for a patient, a 1% solution of diphenhydramine (an antihistamine) can be used, with an anesthetic effect equivalent to that of 1% lidocaine. However, the duration of action is shorter and the pain upon injection is greater than that of lidocaine.

Procedures and Anesthesia of Choice

The specific laser procedure to be performed impacts the choice of anesthesia. The dermatologist has to consider factors such as onset of action, potency, potential vasoactivity, depth and length of anesthesia required, and potential adverse events and host sensitivity.

Laser Treatment for Tattoos, Pigmented Lesions, and Hair Removal

LMX 4–5% is the most practical choice in laser treatment of tattoos, pigmented lesions, and hair removal. It can be prescribed ahead of time with instructions to the patient to apply

Table 1 Common anesthetic agents

Anesthetic agents	Onset plain (min)	Duration plain (min)	Duration with epinephrine (min)	Max dose plain (mg/kg)	Max dose with epinephrine (mg/kg)
Amides					
Lidocaine	<2	30–120	60–400	4.5	7
Prilocaine	<2	30–120	60–400	5.5	8.5
Bupivacaine	3–5	120–240	240–480	2.5	3
Esters					
Procaine	<2	15–30	30–90	7	8.5
Tetracaine	<15	120–40	240–480	1.4	–

it prior to the clinic visit. Since the laser targets in these procedures are pigment chromophores, the vasoactivity of the anesthetic agent does not influence the outcome of the procedure.

Non-ablative Rejuvenation

Vasoactive agents such as anesthetics will diminish the target chromophore, hemoglobin, in non-ablative rejuvenation, thus interfering with the clinical outcome. For that reason, it is recommended the use of a non-vasoactive or vasodilating agent.

Some non-ablative treatments do not require anesthesia. In order to assess patient's discomfort level, the practitioner can perform a spot test prior to the application of the anesthetic; the patient may be able to tolerate the treatment without anesthetics. If anesthesia is needed, the use of LMX 4–5% cream may be applied.

Tumescent Anesthesia

Jefferey Klein introduced low-concentration lidocaine anesthesia (tumescent technique) for cutaneous surgery in the late 1980s. It is defined as direct infiltration of dilute lidocaine (<1 mg/L), epinephrine (<1 mg/L), and sodium bicarbonate (10 mEq/L), and provides excellent pain control with minimal adverse effects. Initially used for liposuction, this method has been successfully applied to many other dermatologic procedures such as hair transplantation, removal of skin tumors, localized phlebectomy, laser surgery, and dermabrasion. This approach has the advantage of achieving anesthesia in a very large area of skin. The safest maximum dose for the tumescent technique with lidocaine with epinephrine (1:100,000) in concentrations of 0.05% and 0.1% is between 45 and 50 mg/kg. The solution preparation and concentration of the solutions is displayed on Table 2.

Table 2 Tumescent local anesthesia mixture

0.1% solution (0.1% lidocaine, epinephrine 1:1,000,000, pH 7.4)	
0.9% normal saline	1 l
2% lidocaine	50 ml
Epinephrine 1:10,000	1 ml
8.45% sodium bicarbonate	12.5 ml
0.05% solution (0.05% lidocaine, epinephrine 1:1,000,000, pH 7.4)	
0.9% normal saline	1 l
2% lidocaine	50 ml
Epinephrine 1:10,000	1 ml
8.45% sodium bicarbonate	12.5 ml

The use of the tumescent anesthesia technique reduces blood loss, bruising, and postoperative soreness. It has been reported that this type of local anesthesia has contributed to pain relief for up to 18 h after procedure, therefore minimizing the need for post operative narcotics.

Nerve Blocks

A detailed knowledge of the head and face neuroanatomy allows the cosmetic surgeon to perform facial surgical procedures with minimal pain in the patient. Skillful administration of the chosen anesthesia can also minimize the potential risks involved, including nerve laceration, hematoma, and paralysis.

A specific nerve block provides pain relief without the local distortion sometimes seen with local infiltration. The central face allows the use of field block anesthesia due to multiple foramina and their respective nerve roots accessibility. With the knowledge of anatomical nerve landmarks, the surgeon can perform nerve blocks according to the area that needs to be anesthetized by injecting anesthetic solution in adequate concentration throughout the nerve foramen either by a percutaneous or intraoral approach. Due to the complexity of nerve ramifications, an infiltrative anesthesia may be added to the nerve block.

Peripheral nerve blocks commonly used in dermatologic practice include digital blocks, supraorbital and supratrochlear/infratrochlear blocks (forehead and vertex of the scalp), infraorbital blocks (nose except the tip, medial cheek, lower eyelids and upper lip), anterior ethmoidal nerve block (tip of the nose), mental blocks (chin, lower cheek and lips) and inferior alveolar blocks (tongue and lower lip).

Many of the facial nerves can be easily approached either percutaneously or intraorally. The supraorbital nerve exits the orbit through the supraorbital foramen which is palpable in most patients. The supratrochlear nerve exits the orbit through a foramen approximately 17 mm from the glabellar midline. The infratrochlear nerve exits the orbit trough a foramen bellow the trochlea. The infraorbital nerve exits the orbit through the infraorbital foramen 4–7 mm below the orbital rim. The mental nerve exits the mental foramen on the hemimandible at the base of the root of the second premolar (Fig. 2). Injection of 2–4 cc's of local anesthetic solution, about 10 mm inferior to the gum line or 15 mm inferior to the top of the crown of the second premolar tooth, usually leads to a successful nerve block. Alternatively, the mental nerve may be blocked with a facial approach aiming for the same target. After the procedure, the numbed area will extend from the unilateral lip down to the mentolabial fold. The anesthesia may also reach other areas like the anterior chin and cheek, depending on the patient's anatomy and nerve ramification.

Nerve damage is a possible complication of nerve blocks, and care should be employed to avoid direct injection of anesthesia into a nerve or foramen.

Digital nerve blocks of fingers can effectively provide anesthesia by injecting the anesthetic solution (usually 2 ml of 2% plain lidocaine) on the side of the finger just distal to the metacarpophalangeal joint. By directing the needle

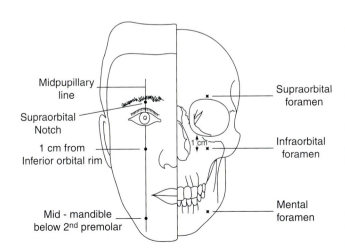

Fig. 2 Landmarks for facial nerve blocks

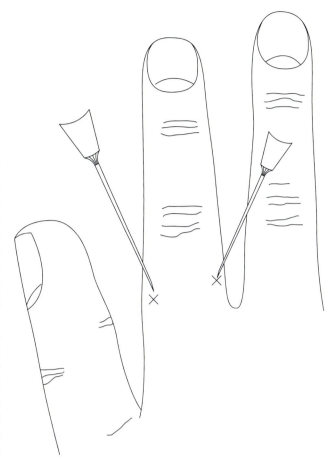

Fig. 3 Digital nerve block

inferiorly and then superiorly, both inferior and superior digital nerves can be anesthetized (Fig. 3).

Adverse Effects of Local Anesthetics

Local anesthesia adverse events can be divided into two groups – those involving the needle insertion and those attributable to the anesthetic solution itself. Possible consequences of needle insertion include fainting, pain, ecchymosis, edema, infection, hematoma, hyperalgesia, nerve damage, and muscle trismus. Psychogenic reactions may occur due to pain of the injection or to the patient's fear of pain or needles, and a vasovagal response involving skin pallor, diaphoresis, bradycardia, and hypotension may result. For this reason, the patient should always be lying down during injections. Commonly used needles are between 25 and 30 gauge, with smaller needles preferred to minimize injection pain.

Adverse events of anesthetic solutions include local and systemic toxicity, allergy and anaphylaxis, and idiosyncratic responses. Local reactions may occur secondary to improper injection of the anesthetic solution and the consequences may be lethal if the targeted area is a large vessel.

Allergic responses can be immediate or delayed. Type I immediate response occurs more often with ester group anesthetics, when the compounds are metabolized to PABA. Preservative-free lidocaine should be used for allergic patients; these formulations do not contain preservatives that may cause type I reactions. Type IV delayed hypersensitivity reactions are characterized angioedema, tachycardia, urticaria, and anaphylaxis. If a patient is reactive to one group of anesthetics (amide or ester), the other group can be used since the groups do not cross-react.

Systemic reactions to anesthetics occur most often when the agent is used over the maximum recommended dose or when the agent is accidentally injected intravenously. Aspirating before injection can help reduce instances of intravenous injection. Central nervous system toxicity of local anesthetics can lead to tinnitus, blurred vision, light-headedness, nausea, hallucinations, slurred speech, and ultimatedly, tonic-clonic seizures and respiratory arrest. Cardiovascular effects can lead to mild tachycardia, tremors, palpitations, and at higher doses, hypotension and arrhythmias. Amide group anesthetics are more dependent on the liver for metabolism; for patients with liver problems, ester-linked anesthetics are recommended.

Patients with have coagulation disorders or those using anticoagulants are more prone to develop ecchymosis and hematomas. Patients taking beta blockers should not be given epinephrine, due to paradoxical hypertension followed by reflex bradycardia that can lead to cardiac arrest or hypertensive stroke. A detailed medical history is essential to prevent and manage these aforementioned complications. Direct injection of anesthesia into a nerve or foramen should be avoided, as it can lead to nerve damage.

Local Anesthesia in Special Patients

Anesthesia and Pregnancy

Due of concerns about potential harm to the mother or fetus, dermatologic surgeons are frequently hesitant to perform cutaneous surgery on pregnant patients.

Low doses of most local anesthetics with epinephrine as well as nitrous oxide less than 50% are safe to use during pregnancy. However, use of epinephrine should be avoided during labor. Sedatives and opioids are potential teratogens and should be avoided.

Anesthesia in Pediatric Patients

Local anesthetic toxicity is rarely seen in infants and children. Lidocaine has been widely used in infants and children

for topical, regional, plexus, epidural, and spinal anesthesia. Prilocaine has been linked to methemoglobinemia, and thus may not be suitable for use in infants and children.

Systemic Sedation for Outpatient Clinic

Conscious sedation is typically used in conjunction with local anesthesia and may be preferable over general anesthesia in dermatologic surgery in many cases. Conscious sedation utilizes a combination of sedatives, analgesics, and tranquilizers to induce a state of amnesia, anxiolysis, and analgesia.

Some of the advantages of conscious sedation as compared to general anesthesia include

1. Reduced risk of drug-related side effects since fewer drugs and smaller doses are used
2. Faster recovery and less postoperative nausea and vomiting
3. Absence of complications from airway manipulation since there is no need for intubation
4. Less expensive because general anesthesia equipment is not needed

However, some disadvantages of conscious sedation include

1. Measures to control the airway must be prepared in case of oversedation
2. Patients who suffer from extreme anxiety may benefit more from general anesthesia

Conclusion

The advent of local anesthesia has dramatically improved patient experience in dermatologic surgery. Physician experience and attention to patient history are two of the most important factors in choosing the right anesthetic. When used correctly and with mindfulness of potential adverse effects, local anesthesia can be extremely safe and effective.

Suggested Reading

Amin SP, Goldberg DJ. Topical anesthetics for cosmetic and laser dermatology. *J Drugs Dermatol.* 2005;4(4):455-461.

Cunningham BB, Gigler V, Wang K, et al. General anesthesia for pediatric dermatologic procedures: risks and complications. *Arch Dermatol.* 2005;141(5):573-576.

Eaton JS, Grekin RC. Regional anesthesia of the face. *Dermatol Surg.* 2001;27(12):1006-1009. J Am Acad Dermatol. 2000 Aug;43 (2 Pt 1):286-298.

Friedman PM, Mafong EA, Friedman ES, Geronemus RG. Topical anesthetics update: EMLA and beyond. *Dermatol Surg.* 2001;27(12): 1019-1026.

Huang W, Vidimos A. Topical anesthetics in dermatology. *J Am Acad Dermatol.* 2002;47(1):158-159.

Isago T, Kono T, Nozaki M, et al. Ambulatory anesthesia for children undergoing laser treatment. *Surg Today.* 2006;36(9):765-768.

Kilmer SL, Chotzen V, Zelickson BD, et al. Full-face laser resurfacing using a supplemented topical anesthesia protocol. *Arch Dermatol.* 2003;139(10):1279-1283.

Koay J, Orengo I. Application of local anesthetics in dermatologic surgery. *Dermatol Surg.* 2002;28(2):143-148.

Niamtu J III. Local anesthetic blocks of the head and neck for cosmetic facial surgery, I: a review of basic sensory neuroanatomy. *Cosmet Dermatol.* 2004a;17(8):515-522.

Niamtu J III. Local anesthetic blocks of the head and neck for cosmetic facial surgery, II: techniques for the upper and mid face. *Cosmet Dermatol.* 2004b;17(9):583-587.

Niamtu J III. Local anesthetic blocks of the head and neck for cosmetic facial surgery, III: techniques for the maxillary nerve. *Cosmet Dermatol.* 2004c;17(10):645-647.

Niamtu J III. Local anesthetic blocks of the head and neck for cosmetic facial surgery, III: techniques for the lower face. *Cosmet Dermatol.* 2004d;17(11):714-720.

Ramos-Zabala A, Pérez-Mencía MT, Fernández-García R, Cascales-Núñez MR. Anesthesia technique for outpatient facial laser resurfacing. *Lasers Surg Med.* 2004;34(3):269-272.

Laser Application for Ethnic Skin

Heather Woolery-Lloyd and Mohamed L. Elsaie

- The use of lasers on skin of color has been limited due to the risks involved with hyperpigmentation and scarring.
- Fractional resurfacing is a safe method for skin rejuvenation in ethnic skin since melanin is not selected for targeted destruction. It has been proven that patients with skin types IV-V have been successfully treated with minimal side effects, such as transient erythema.

Acne Scars

Ablative Devices

CO_2 laser has been used for the treatment of acne scars in skin of color. The laser's usefulness has been limited due to the risk associated with hyperpigmentation and scarring. For that reason other modalities have been investigated for optimum acne scar treatment in ethnic skin.[1]

Fractional Devices

Fractional photothermolysis (Fraxel SR, Reliant Lasers, Palo Alto, CA, USA) is a novel nonablative erbium:glass (1,500 nm) laser treatment for facial rejuvenation.[2] It is also used for the treatment of melasma and acneiform scarring. Fractional photothermolysis is performed with a midinfrared laser, which creates microscopic columns of thermal injury. These zones of thermal injury, called microthermal zones (MTZs), have a diameter that is energy dependent and ranges from 100 to 160 µm. At the energies commonly used for facial rejuvenation (8–12 mJ/MTZ), the depth of penetration ranges from 300 to 700 µm.[3] Relative epidermal and follicular structure sparing account for rapid recovery without prolonged downtime. Melanin is not at risk of selective, targeted destruction; therefore, fractional resurfacing has been used successfully in patients with skin of color.

Studies have demonstrated the effectiveness of fractional photothermolysis in the treatment of acne scars. Alster et al examined the use of fractional photothermolysis in the treatment of atrophic scars. Fifty-three patients (skin phototypes I –V) with mild to moderate atrophic facial acne scars received monthly treatment with a 1,550-nm erbium-doped fiber laser (Fraxel, Reliant Technologies Inc., San Diego, CA). Clinical response to treatment was determined at each treatment visit and 6 months after the final treatment session by two independent investigators. 91% of patients had at least 25–50% improvement after a single treatment. 87% of patients receiving three treatments demonstrated at least 51–75% improvement in the appearance of their scars. Skin phototype also did not significantly affect the clinical responses observed. It was concluded that Fraxel procedures were effective in acne scar treatment for all skin types.[4]

One study specifically examined Fraxel in skin of color. This study included Asian patients with acne scars and skin types IV and V. One treatment consisted of four passes of the device to attain a final microscopic treatment zone of thermal injury with a density of $1,000–1,500/cm^2$. The fluence was set to 6 mJ per microscopic treatment zone. The treatment was repeated up to three times at 2–3-week intervals. Clinical improvement was achieved in all the patients. Rare adverse events included mild transient erythema. No patients showed scarring or hyperpigmentation as a result of treatment.[5]

Non Ablative Devices

One study comparing the 1,320 nm Nd:YAG and the 1,450 nm diode laser in the treatment of atrophic scars included skin types I-V. In this study both devices offered clinical improvement without significant side effects.[6]

H. Woolery-Lloyd (✉)
Department of Dermatology and Cutaneous Surgery,
University of Miami, Miller School of Medicine, Miami, FL, USA
e-mail: woolerylloyd@yahoo.com

K. Nouri (ed.), *Lasers in Dermatology and Medicine*,
DOI: 10.1007/978-0-85729-281-0_26, © Springer-Verlag London Limited 2011

- It has been observed that fractional laser devices used at higher densities are more likely to produce swelling, redness, and hyperpigmentation than when used at high fluences.
- Although the 532 nm laser is not the preferred device for treatment on ethnic skin, it has been reported that pigmented and telangiectatic areas can be successfully treated.
- Applications have been prudent and results are better secured when test spots are done prior to application.
- Thickening of the upper papillary collagen and improvement of collagen fibrils have been observed using long-pulsed and Q-switched 1,064 nm lasers.
- At a wavelength of 1,064 nm, heating of dermal tissue is likely and may cause adverse effects on darker skin patients.
- Intense Pulsed Light (IPL) devices use cutoff filters which eliminate wavelengths that target melanin absorption. By selecting wavelengths and pulse widths, the appropriate parameters can be set to prevent hypopigmentation in ethic skin.
- Light Emitting Diodes (LEDs) use monochromatic light therapy for the treatment of photoaged skin by causing the up-regulation of procollagen and down-regulation of matrix metalloproteinase I.

Photorejuvenation

In general, all races are susceptible to photoaging. However, it is clear that in patients with Fitzpatrick's skin phototypes IV to VI photoaging is delayed and less severe due to the photoprotective role of melanin. Published studies on photoaging in blacks have been limited to African Americans. In African Americans, photoaging is more prominent in lighter-complexioned individuals. In addition photoaging may not be apparent until the late fifth or sixth decade of life. Clinically, the features of photoaging in African Americans can include fine wrinkling, mottled pigmentation, and dermatosis papulosa nigra. In Asian and Hispanic patients photoaging is most prominently manifested by solar lentigos and other pigmentary changes.[7]

Fractional Devices

Kono et al.,[8] has described the use of the Fraxel in 35 type IV and V Asian skin patients for photorejuvenation. It was

noted that increased density was more likely to produce swelling, redness, and hyperpigmentation when compared to increased energy. In this study, the authors concluded that patient satisfaction is significantly higher when their skin is treated with high fluences, but not when treated with high densities. Overall they concluded that fractional photorejuvenation can be safe and effective in darker ethnic skin types.[8]

532 nm Laser

Although not a prominent feature in ethnic skin, treatment of the pigmented and telengectatic component of photoaging has been reported in ethnic skin.[9,10] Rashid and colleagues reported on the use of a quasicontinuous wave 532 nm laser in the treatment of lentigines in type IV skin patients. They showed 50% improvement in lesion clearance, with a 10% incidence of hyperpigmentation and 25% incidence of hypopigmentation after multiple treatments. These side effects abated after 2–6 months.[10]

Lee reported 150 patients with skin types ranging from I to V who were treated in multiple sessions with 532 nm laser (4 mm spot, 6–15 J/cm^2, 30- to 50-ms pulse duration), 1,064 nm laser (10 mm spot, 24–30 J/cm^2, 30- to 65-ms pulse duration), or a combination of both. Sapphire-tipped contact cooling was utilized. Improvement in erythema, texture, pigmentation, and rhytides was reported in both study arms but was highest in the combination group. An incidence of 5% postinflammatory hyperpigmentation was reported in patients with type III and IV skin treated with the 532 nm laser alone, which resolved after 4–6 weeks.[9]

Safety data on the use of the 532 nm laser in ethnic skin is limited. For this reason, the use of conservative settings to achieve the desired results is prudent. Test spots are essential to assess the initial patient response and to decrease the risk of hypopigmentation which can be challenging to treat.

1,064 nm Laser

Long-pulsed and Q-switched 1,064 nm lasers target melanin as well as hemoglobin and water. Although safer for darker skin, there is a diffuse heating of dermal tissue due to the deep penetrating nature of 1,064 nm laser. The typical depth of penetration ranges from 5 to 10 mm.[11]

One study has shown evidence of improvement with a Q-switched 1,064 nm laser for nonablative treatment in type IV skin.[12] Sun-damaged 4 cm × 4 cm areas of infra-auricular skin were exposed to a 1,064 nm Q-switched Nd:YAG laser at fluence of 7 J/cm^2 and a 3 mm spot size. Two laser passes with a 10–20% overlap, were used on all subjects in an attempt to promote petechiae as the visible end point. Petrolatum dressings were applied for 1 week after treatment. Three millimeter punch biopsy specimens were taken from each subject before treatment and 3 months after the last treatment. Histologic specimens were evaluated blindly by a board certified dermatopathologist. Four of six skin biopsy specimens obtained 3 months after the last laser treatment showed mild fibrosis with histologic improvement in pretreatment solar elastosis. There was a mildly thickened upper papillary collagen zone, with an improvement in the organization of collagen fibrils. The remaining two specimens showed no changes. Clinically, none of the treated, nonbiopsied areas showed any evidence of pigmentary changes or scarring.[12]

Another study utilized the 1,064 nm Nd:YAG (Laser genesis, Cutera, Inc., Brisbane, California)for rejuvenation of facial skin in skin types I-V. Patients and masked physician assessment demonstrated overall improvement. Specific improvement was also seen in coarse wrinkles and skin laxity. No adverse events were noted in this study.[13] The Nd:YAG may offer greater safety in treatment of skin rejuvenation in sklin of color.

Intense Pulsed Light

Another device for photorejuvenation is Intense Pulsed Light (IPL). IPL is produced by a noncoherent flashlamp pumped light source that is capable of emitting light from 500 to 1,200 nm.[11] The use of cutoff filters allows the elimination of some of the shorter wavelengths of the visible light spectrum to limit melanin absorption. Different pulse widths can be chosen so that appropriate parameters match the thermal relaxation time of the targets. Cooling of the epidermis is achieved with contact cooling in the device head or external cooling devices.

Negishi and colleagues were among the first to investigate the use of IPL in types IV and V Japanese patients. They applied a thin-layer of ice-cold gel and they utilized a 550 nm cutoff filter. Settings were 28–32 J/cm^2 and 2.5- to 4.0 and 4.0- to 5.0-ms pulse durations. Excellent results were reported in 73 out of 97 patients.[14] No evidence of dyspigmentation was reported in either series. Negishi and colleagues have also employed UV photography to identify and treat subclinical epidermal hyperpigmentation with IPL in skin of color.[15]

Although IPL has been utilized with success in skin of color, when treating these patients conservative settings are prudent to achieve a favorable result with the least unwanted side effects. Moreover the use of IPL should be limited in skin types V and VI skin due to the significant risk of hyperpigmentation.

Light Emitting Diode (LED)

Light Emitting Diodes (LEDs) offers advancement in visible spectrum, monochromatic light therapy for photoaged skin. Typically, LEDs in devices are arrayed in panels. Each LED emits visible light in a ± 10 to 20 nm band around the dominant emitted wavelength. Energy output is less than 25 W, representing a fluence of about 0.1 J/cm^2.[16] The mechanism of this device is thought to act by targeting stimulation of fibroblast mitochondrial metabolic activity. In addition concomitant up-regulation of procollagen and down-regulation of matrix metalloproteinase I has been demonstrated.[17,18] Although there are no studies on LED in ethnic skin, based on the mechanism of action, these devices should be and are generally considered safe in skin of color.

Skin Tightening

Radiofrequency (RF)

- Radio Frequency (RF) energy ranges from 3 kHz to 300 GHz and does not target specific chromophores or epidermal melanin making RF a safe choice for treating all skin types by inducing dermal heating and collagen.
- Infrared tightening heats the dermis and thermally induces collagen synthesis, while protecting the epidermis with the use of pre and post operative cooling devices.

Radio frequency (RF) is electromagnetic radiation in the frequency range of 3 kHz–300 GHz. These devices induce dermal heating, denature collagen and induce collagen remodeling. Wound healing mechanisms promote wound contraction, which ultimately clinically enhances the appearance of mild to moderate skin laxity. One device (Thermacool, Thermage Inc, Hayward, CA, USA) has reported efficacy in the treatment of laxity involving the periorbital area and jowls.[19] Because RF energy is not dependent on a specific chromophore interaction, epidermal melanin is not targeted and treatment of all skin types is possible.

Kushikata et al.[20] reported the use of RF in a series of 85 Asian patients of skin types IV and V and concluded that RF treatment was effective for skin tightening in Asian facial skin. Although there is a small risk of hyperpigmentation with RF treatments in ethnic skin, RF does offer safe and effective treatment of skin laxity in ethnic skin.

Infrared Tightening

Titan, (Cutera, Inc., Brisbane, California) uses infrared light to volumetrically heat the dermis. It is designed to thermally induce collagen contraction, with subsequent collagen remodeling and neocollagen synthesis. The epidermis is protected via pre-, parallel, and post-treatment cooling. With this device, improvements in skin laxity and facial and neck contours have been achieved. Response rates are variable and can be influenced by patient selection. [21]

Chua et al investigated the use of infrared light on 21 patients of Fitzpatrick skin types IV and V. At 6 month follow up 86% of patients had improvement as measured by the physician assessment. They concluded that Titan was effective to achieve mild to moderate gradual clinical improvement of facial and neck skin laxity. The procedure is associated with minimal downtime and is safe for use in darker skin, including skin types V and VI. [22]

- The Ruby (694 nm) laser was the first laser used for hair removal, which targets the pigment in the hair follicle and epidermal melanin. The Alexandrite (755 nm) and the Diode (800–1,000 nm) have longer wavelengths that serve to better target hair follicles.
- The Diode laser has been used at higher fluences to safely treat darker skinned people with fewer complications.
- Studies have shown that the Nd:YAG (1,064 nm) laser has been most successful for hair removal in patients with skin types V and VI.

Laser Assisted Hair Reduction

Laser assisted hair reduction also targets pigment but this pigment is in the hair follicles. The Ruby (694 nm) was the first laser introduced for laser assisted hair removal and is highly absorbed by all melanin in the skin. This melanin absorption includes not only the targeted melanin in the hair follicle but also epidermal melanin. The Alexandrite (755 nm) and the Diode (800–1,000 nm) were later introduced for laser hair removal. These lasers have longer wavelengths allowing for a larger variety of patients to be treated.

The Alexandrite laser has been studied in Fitzpatrick skin types IV to VI. In one study, a long pulsed 755 nm laser with a 40 ms pulse width was used to treat 150 patients with skin types IV to VI. A test site with a fluence of 16 J/cm^2 was first performed and energy fluence was selected according to response. The authors reported an overall complication rate of 2.7%, however, only two patients with skin type VI were included in the study and both developed blistering. [23]

A smaller study of the Alexandrite (755 nm, 3 ms pulse width) included four women with Fitzpatrick skin type VI. In this study, lower fluences were used (8–14 J/cm^2) and no side effects were noted. [24] Although treatment of skin types IV to VI is possible with the Alexandrite, the associated risk is still great in these patients.

The Diode laser has been studied with greater success in the treatment of darker skinned patients. The 800 nm diode laser was studied with pulse widths of 30 ms and 100 ms. Adrian et al. reported that although both settings could be used safely, longer pulse widths (100 ms) allowed higher fluences to be utilized with less complications. [25] Another study utilized the 810 nm Diode laser to treat eight patients with skin types V and VI. These patients were treated with low fluence of 10 mj/cm^2 and a pulse width of 30 ms. Transient blistering and pigment alterations were noted in some patients despite the lower fluence utilized. [26] Overall, the diode laser offers increased safety over the Alexandrite laser in African-American patients, however, complications remain an issue.

The Nd:YAG (1,064 nm) laser was introduced which provides safe laser hair removal in all skin types including skin types V and VI. In one study, 20 patients with skin types IV through VI were treated with a series of three laser sessions. The pulse width utilized was 50 ms, the fluence ranged from 40 to 50 J/cm^2, and a contact sapphire tip cooling device was used. Adverse events from all 60 treatments included transient pigment alteration (5%) and rare vesiculation (1.5%). [27] In another study 37 patients with psuedofolliculitis barbae were successfully treated with the long-pulsed Nd:YAG with few side effects. [28]

The long-pulsed Nd:YAG laser is the laser of choice for laser-assisted hair removal in skin phototypes IV to VI because of its high safety profile. [29]

- Pulsed Dye laser has proven to be successful in the treatment of vascular lesions on skin type V patients.
- No improvement has been noticed on patients treated for port wine stains using a 585 nm flashlamp-pump dye laser.
- Darker skinned patients may encounter side effects when treated with lasers at an absorption range of 577 nm due to the presence of oxyhemoglobin.

Vascular Lesions

The treatment of vascular lesions with lasers in patients with darker skin types poses an especially great challenge since a major peak absorption of oxyhemoglobin (577 nm), is also in the range of the peak absorption of melanin. This makes targeting vascular lesions while sparing epidermal pigment difficult. Reported success rates of laser treatment of vascular lesions in skin types V and VI vary.[30–32] In one series of three patients the 585 nm flashlamp-pumped dye (FLPD) was used to treat vascular malformations. In this series, the FLPD was effective but transient color and textural changes occurred at treated sites.[30] Another report of a single patient treated with the 585 nm FLPD found no improvement in a port wine stain and persistent hyperpigmentation in treated sites.[31] One of the largest reviews involved 13 patients with skin type V who received a total of 97 pulsed dye laser treatments. Transient pigmentary changes occurred in 7 of the 13 patients. Two patients developed limited atrophic scarring. Out of 97 total laser treatments, 85 were not associated with significant problems. Overall six patients (46%) achieved good or excellent results. The authors concluded that if treatment expectations and risks are discussed appropriately, pulsed dye laser treatment of port wine stains is a viable treatment option in patients with skin type V.[32]

Epidermal cooling may improve unwanted side effects when treating vascular lesions, however this has not been specifically studied in patients skin type IV-VI. One study compared pulsed dye laser (PDL) in conjunction with cryogen spray cooling (CSC) to PDL alone in Chinese patients. In this study half of the port wine stain was treated with PDL and the contralateral half was treated with PDL-CSC. There was no difference in long term adverse efects between the two sides, however, acute blistering and pain was diminished on the PDL-CSC treated sites.[33]

A computer model has been developed to examine epidermal and port wine stain thermal damage induced by pulsed dye laser in skin types V and VI. This model demonstrated that a single cryogen spurt followed by a single pulsed dye laser exposure did not provide enough epidermal protection for skin types V and VI. Interestingly, this model did show that multiple intermittent cryogen spurts and laser pulses provided adequate epidermal protection while still permitting port wine stain photocoagulation.[34] To achieve a favorable outcome with the least unwanted side effects. In patients of skin of color, a test spot is needed to assess the patient's initial response and limit complications.

> • Mild hyperpigmentation and no scarring for tattoo removal have been observed in darker skinned patients, skin types V and VI, using the Q-switched Nd:YAG laser.

Tattoos

Laser treatment of tattoos has always presented a challenge in patients with darker skin types. As with other laser treatments in dark skin, the epidermal melanin absorption of laser energy is the main limiting factor in treating tattoos. Interestingly, there are several reports of tattoos treated successfully in skin types V and VI. The Q-switched Nd:YAG has been used to treat amateur tattoos in darkly pigmented patients. In a series of 13 patients, only two developed mild hypopigmentation at treated sites.[35] In another small series the Q-switched Nd:YAG laser effectively removed tattoos in darkly pigmented patients without permanent pigment alterations of normal skin.[36] The procedure is often risky and can carry a risk of side effects unless a test spot is carried out to limit complications and asses the patients initial response.

A large study conducted by Lapidoth et al consisted of 401 women and 3 men of Ethiopian origin with Fitzpatrick skin type V or VI. Ages ranged from 15 to 53 years. In most cases (n=380, 94%),the Q-switched Nd:YAG laser (Continuum Biomedical, Livermore, Calif) at 1,064 nm was used. The parameters used were a pulse width of 10 nsec, spot size of 3 mm, and fluences ranging from 4.2 to 7.0 J/cm2. The other patients (n=24) were treated with the Q-switched ruby laser, (Wavelight Laser Technologie AG, Erlangen, Germany) at 694 nm, The parameters used were a pulse width of 20 nsec, spot size of 4 mm, and fluences ranging from 5.0 to 7.0 J/cm2. Good clearance (90–100% was achieved in 92% of the patients after the last laser treatment. In the remaining 32 patients, 75–90% clearance was documented. Most of the patients showed no changes in skin pigment or texture after treatment. Transient (2–4 months) mild hyperpigmentation was noted in 177 (44%) patients, and mild textural changes in two, both treated with the Q-switched Nd:YAG laser. There were no cases of scarring or permanent pigmentary changes.[37] Although these results are encouraging, treatment of tattoos in darkly pigmented skin can be unpredictable. A test spot is essential before treating large areas.

Conclusion

In conclusion, laser procedures in darker skinned patients are challenging but can be successfully achieved if certain treatment guidelines are followed. Appropriate discussion of risks and patient expectations are essential in treating this patient population. Pre and post laser cooling can be helpful to minimize side effects and improve patient comfort. This is especially true with laser hair removal.

Photorejuvenation can be successfully achieved with low risk when the appropriate settings are used. Fractional technology has increased treatment options for rhytides and atrophic scars. Although there are no studies on LED treatments in skin of color, it can be used as either a primary or adjunctive treatment modality with low risk. The 532 nm laser proved to be risky in skin of color and conservative guidelines should apply when using it. The 1,064 nm lasers may offer greater safety when treating rhytides and acne scars ethnic skin. The IPL is an option for treating skin of color, though limited use for skin types V and VI is advisable. Encouraging data and large studies suggesting that treatment of tattoos can be successful in the ethnic skin patients, however, test spots remain essential in these patients. Finally newer tightening technologies are safe modalities to treat skin laxity in ethnic skin.

Test spots are no longer necessary in laser hair removal with the long pulsed Nd:YAG since safety with these lasers in darker skin types is very well established. In conclusion, when treating darker skinned patients the use of conservative settings to achieve the desired results is prudent. Following these guidelines, the clinician is most likely to achieve a favorable result with the least unwanted side effects.

References

1. Kim JW, Lee JO. Skin resurfacing with laser in Asians. *Aesthetic Plast Surg.* 1997;21(2):115-117.
2. Manstein D, Herron GS, Sink RK, et al. Fractional photothermolysis: a new concept for cutaneous remodeling using microscopic patterns of thermal injury. *Lasers Surg Med.* 2004;34:426-438.
3. Fisher GH, Geronemus RG. Short-term side effects of fractional photothermolysis. *Dermatol Surg.* 2005;31:1245-1249.
4. Alster TS, Tanzi EL, Lazarus M. The use of fractional laser photothermolysis for the treatment of atrophic scars. *Dermatol Surg.* 2007;33(3):295-299.
5. Hasegawa T, Matsuka T, Mizuno Y, et al. Clinical trial of laser device called fractional photothermolysis system for acne scars. *J Dermatol.* 2006;33(9):623-627.
6. Tanzi EL, Alster TS. Comparison of a 1,450 nm diode laser and a 1320nmNdYAG laser in the treatment of atrophic facial scars: a prospective clinical and histological study. *Dermatol Surg.* 2004;30(2pt1):152-157.
7. Kligman AM. Solar elastosis in relation to pigmentation. In: fitzpatrick TB, Pathak MA, eds. *Sunlight and Man.* Tokyo: University of Tokyo Press; 1974:157-163.
8. Kono T, Chan HH, Groff WF, et al. Prospective direct comparison study of fractional resurfacing using different fluences and densities for skin rejuvenation in Asians. *Lasers Surg Med.* 2007;39(4):311-314.
9. Lee MW. Combination 532-nm and 1064-nm lasers for noninvasive skin rejuvenation and toning. *Arch Dermatol.* 2003;139:1265-1276, 14568830.
10. Rashid T, Hussain I, Haider M, Haroon TS. Laser therapy of freckles and lentigines with quasi-continuous, frequency-doubled, Nd:YAG (532 nm) laser in Fitzpatrick type IV: a 24-month follow-up. *J Cosmet Laser Ther.* 2002;04:81-85.
11. Weiss RA, McDaniel DH, Geronemus RG. Review of nonablative photorejuvenation: reversal of the aging effects of the sun and environmental damage using laser and light sources. *Semin Cutan Med Surg.* 2003;22:93-106.
12. Goldberg DJ, Silapunt S. Histologic evaluation of a Q-switched Nd:YAG laser in the nonablative treatment of wrinkles. *Dermatol Surg.* 2001;27:744-746.
13. Dyan SH, Vartanian AJ, Menaker G, Mobley SR, Dayan AN. Nonablative laser resurfacing using the long-pulse (1064-nm) Nd:YAG laser. *Arch Facial Plast Surg.* 2003;5(4):310-315.

14. Negishi K, Tezuka Y, Kushikata N, Wakamatsu S. Photorejuvenation for Asian by intense pulsed light. *Dermatol Surg.* 2001;27:627-631.
15. Negishi K, Wakamtsu D, Kushikata N, et al. Full face photorejuvenation of damaged skin by intense pulsed light with integrated contact cooling: initial experiences in Asian patients. *Lasers Surg Med.* 2002;30:298-305.
16. Gentlewave approval FDA Gentlewave FDA approval. Cosmetic surgery–news. Available at: http://www.cosmeticsurgery-news.com/article2357.html. 2005.
17. Weiss RA, Weiss MA, Geronemus RG, McDaniel DH. A novel non-thermal non-ablative full panel led photomodulation device for reversal of photoaging: digital microscopic and clinical results in various types. *J Drugs Dermatol.* 2004;03:605-610.
18. Weiss RA, McDaniel DH, Geronemus RG, Weiss MA. Clinical trial of a novel non-thermal LED array for reversal of photoaging: clinical, histologic, and surface profilometric results. *Lasers Surg Med.* 2005;36:85-91.
19. Hsu TS, Kaminer MS. The use of nonablative radiofrequency technology to tighten the lower face and neck. *Semin Cutan Med Surg.* 2003;22:115-123, 12877230.
20. Kushikata N, Negishi K, Tezuka Y, Takeuchi K, Wakamatsu S. Non-ablative skin tightening with radiofrequency in Asian skin. *Lasers Surg Med.* 2005;36(2):92-97.
21. Bunin LS, Carniol BJ. Cervical facial skin tightening with an infra-red device. *Facial Plast Surg Clin North Am.* 2007;15(2):179-184.
22. Chua SH, Ang P, Khoo LS, Goh CL. Nonablative infrared skin tightening in Type IV to V Asian skin: a prospective clinical study. *Dermatol Surg.* 2007;33(2):146-151.
23. Breadon JY, Barnes CA. Comparison of adverse events of laser and light-assisted hair removal systems in skin types IV-VI. *J Drugs Dermatol.* 2007;6:40-46.
24. Nouri K, Jimenez G, Trent J. Laser hair removal in patients with Fitzpatrick Skin type VI. *Cosmet Dermat.* 2002;15(3):15-16.
25. Adrian RM, Shay KP. 800 nanometer diode laser hair removal in African American patients: a clinical and histologic study. *J Cutan Laser Ther.* 2000;2(4):183-190.
26. Greppi I. Diode laser hair removal of the black patient. *Lasers Surg Med.* 2001;28(2):150-155.
27. Alster TS, Bryan H, Williams CM. Long-pulsed Nd:YAG laser-assisted hair removal in pigmented skin: a clinical and histological evaluation. *Arch Dermatol.* 2001;137(7):885-889.
28. Ross EV, Cooke LM, Timko AL, Overstreet KA, et al. Treatment of pseudofolliculitis barbae in skin types IV, V, and VI with a long-pulsed neodymium:yttrium aluminum garnet laser. *J Am Acad Dermatol.* 2002;47(2):263-270.
29. Aldraibi MS, Touma DJ, Khachemoune A. Hair removal with the 3-msec alexandrite laser in patients with skin types IV-VI: efficacy, safety, and the role of topical corticosteroids in preventing side effects. *J Drugs Dermatol.* 2007;6(1):60-66.
30. Garrett AB, Shieh S. Treatment of vascular lesions in pigmented skin with the pulsed dye laser. *J Cutan Med Surg.* 2000;4(1):36-39.
31. Ashinoff R, Geronemus RG. Treatment of a port-wine stain in a black patient with the pulsed dye laser. *J Dermatol Surg Onc.* 1992;18(2):147-148.
32. Sommer S, Sheehan-Dare RA. Pulsed dye laser treatment of port-wine stains in pigmented skin. *J Am Acad Dermatol.* 2000;42(4):667-671.
33. Chiu CH, Chan HH, Ho WS, Yeung CK, Nelson JS. Prospective study of pulsed dye laser in conjunction with cryogen spray cooling for treatment of port wine stains in Chinese patients. *Dermatol Surg.* 2003;29(9):909-915, discussion 915.
34. Aguilar G, Diaz SH, Lavernia EJ, Nelson JS. Cryogen spray cooling efficiency: improvement of port wine stain laser therapy through

multiple intermitent cryogen spurts and laser pulses. *Lasers Surg Med.* 2002;31(1):27-35.

35. Jones A, Roddey P, Orengo I, Rosen T. The Q-switched Nd:YAG laser effectively treats tattoos in darkly pigmented skin. *Dermatol Surg.* 1996;22(12):999-1001.

36. Grevelink JM, Duke D, van Leeuwen RL, Gonzalez E, DeCoste SD, Anderson RR. Laser treatment of tattoos in darkly pigmented patients: efficacy and side effects. *J Am Acad Dermatol.* 1996;34(4):653-656.

37. Moshe L, Aharonowitz G. Tattoo removal among ethipian jews in Israel: tradition faces technology. *J Am Acad Dermatol.* 2004;51: 906-909.

Laser Applications in Children

Mercedes E. Gonzalez, Michael Shelling, and Elizabeth Alvarez Connelly

Introduction

Lasers can be used to treat a wide variety of dermatological disorders in children. This chapter outlines the conditions amenable to laser surgery in children (Table 1) and discusses the special issues surrounding parental counseling, heightened anxiety and safety precautions when performing laser surgery in children.

Lasers for Vascular Lesions

- The flashlamp- pulsed dye laser (PDL) has revolutionized the treatment of vascular lesions in children.
- The PDL's well-established safety profile makes it the treatment of choice for vascular lesions in the pediatric population.
- It uses 577–600 nm wavelengths to target the last oxyhemoglobin peak within the blood vessels.
- PDL has been used successfully to treat vascular lesions such as port-wine stains, superficial hemangiomas, telangiectasias, angiofibromas and pyogenic granulomas; and non-vascular conditions in children such as viral warts, molluscum contagiosum, hypertrophic scars and others.
- Adverse effects although rare include dyspigmentation, scarring, infection and pain.

Oxyhemoglobin, the target chromophore in blood vessels, has absorption peaks at 418, 542 and 577 nm and thus the best suited lasers for treatment of vascular lesions emit light in this range (See Table 2). The earliest lasers used to treat vascular lesions in children were the quasi-continuous lasers such as the Argon pumped tunable dye, copper bromide and copper vapor lasers but these have since fallen out of favor due to the high risk of hypertrophic scarring and textural changes.[1] In 1989, the flashlamp-pumped PDL revolutionized the treatment of vascular lesions, and today it is the treatment of choice for some hemangiomas, port-wine stains, and telangiectasias in children.[2] It uses a flashlamp to energize rhodamine dye and generates a pulse of yellow light. Today's most commonly used PDL systems emit wavelengths of 585 or 595 nm and are used not only for vascular lesions but also to target blood vessels in non-vascular lesions in children. More recently developed PDLs have longer wavelengths (595 and 600 nm), larger spot sizes (10–12 mm), and higher peak fluence potential, allowing for better treatment of deeper vessels in hemangiomas and port-wine stains. They also have longer pulse durations (1.5–40 ms), which allows for the targeting of larger vessels in more complicated lesions. As long as the pulse duration is shorter than or equal to the thermal relaxation time of target vessels, the laser can achieve selective destruction of target vessels without damage to the surrounding normal tissue. Larger blood vessels have longer thermal relaxation times (TRT) and thus longer pulse durations can be used. In addition, certain PDL systems have excellent dynamic cooling devices which reduce epidermal damage and intraoperative pain.[3]

Other lasers such as the 532 nm KTP, 755 nm alexandrite, 1,064 Nd:Yag or Intense Pulsed light (IPL) are used less frequently, for PDL resistant lesions and have less favorable outcomes.

E.A. Connelly (✉)
Department of Dermatology and Cutaneous Surgery,
University of Miami, Miller School of Medicine,
Miami, FL, USA
e-mail: econnelly@med.miami.edu

K. Nouri (ed.), *Lasers in Dermatology and Medicine*,
DOI: 10.1007/978-0-85729-281-0_27, © Springer-Verlag London Limited 2011

Table 1 Dermatologic conditions in the pediatric population amenable to laser therapy

Vascular lesions
Port-wine stains
Superficial hemangiomas
Telangiectasias
Spider angiomas
Pyogenic granulomas
Facial angiofibromas
Lymphangiomas
Pigmented lesions
Café Au Lait
Small congenital nevi
Nevus of ota
Nevus of ito
Lentigines
Becker's nevus
Other conditions
Viral warts
Molluscum contagiosum
Hypertrophic scars
Morphea
Hypertrichosis
Vitiligo
Acne and acne scarring

Table 2 Vascular lesions

Lasers used to treat vascular lesions in children	
Quasi continuous lasers	
Argon pumped tunable dye	577–585 nm/yellow
Copper bromide	578 nm/yellow
Copper vapor	578 nm/yellow
Krypton	568 nm/yellow
Pulsed lasers	
Flashlamp-pumped pulsed dye laser (PDL)	585 nm/yellow
Long pulsed dye laser (LPDL)	595 nm/yellow
Potassium titanyl phosphate (KTP)	532 nm/green

Indications and Contraindications

- Indications
- Port-wine stains
  - Superficial hemangiomas of infancy in the proliferative or involution phase, those encroaching upon vital structures or those that are cosmetically disfiguring
  - Ulcerated hemangiomas of infancy
  - Telangiectasias
  - Pyogenic granulomas
  - Facial angiofibromas
  - Verrucae vulgaris
  - Molluscum contagiosum
- Contraindications
  - Patients with unrealistic expectations
  - Patients who form scars will be at a greater risk for this post-operative complication
  - Deep or mixed hemangiomas of infancy
  - Pyogenic granulomas wider or higher than 5 mm

Port Wine Stains

Port-wine stains (PWS) are benign vascular malformations composed of ectatic capillary-sized blood vessels in the papillary dermis that are usually present at birth.[4] They occur in 0.3–0.5% of newborns. Early in life, PWS are pink and macular (See Fig. 1). After puberty some become darker, resembling the color of "port wine," and hypertrophy. They are usually unilateral and are commonly found on the face. The flashlamp-pumped PDL is the established treatment of choice for PWS in children. One older study used Candela® flashlamp-pumped PDL with a 585 nm wavelength in 89 patients ages 0–31 years of age and compared lightening among the different ages. Using a colorimeter, they measured lightening after five treatments in four different age groups. Good lightening was seen in all age groups and the authors concluded that PDL treatment can be effective at any age.[5] However, data from more recent studies using the Candela® V-Beam 595 nm PDL have shown that early treatment of PWS can leads to improvement of the lesion with minimal side effects. The earlier the treatment, the lesion size is proportionately smaller and the thickness of skin is lesser, allowing deeper penetration of the light.[6] Starting the treatment early may also require fewer treatments[7-9] and may help to increase the chances of complete resolution of the lesion.[10] One study reported that treating PWS in children younger than 1 year old seem to have the most effective lightening.[11] In addition, aging PWS become thicken and develop nodularity, which can lead to asymmetrical deformity of the face. Once hypertrophy and nodularity occur, the lesion then become very difficult to treat and might not response to PDL.

Many clinicians have recommended that the decision of when to initiate PWS treatment should be based on patient's psychosocial benefit, discomfort and anxiety from the procedure. When they are on the face or other cosmetically significant location, PWS can have a profound effect on a child's social and psychosocial adjustment. For this reason, many physicians have suggested that treatment of PWS is

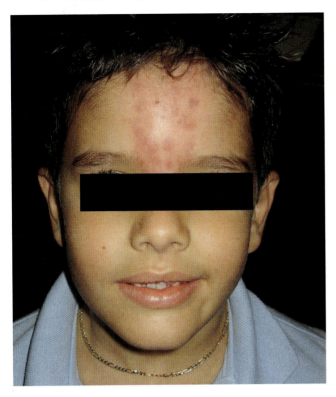 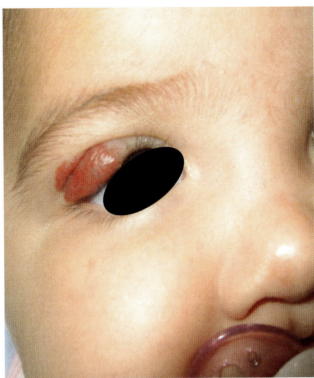

Fig. 1 Post-treatment purpura secondary to blood vessel destruction typically resolves within several days

Fig. 2 Hemangioma of infancy involving upper eyelid may threaten function and therefore require treatment

a medical necessity.[12,13] According to a psychology study, children develop their body self-awareness around the latter half of the second year of age.[14] The development of body self-awareness in toddlers is the foundation of ego development and self-esteem later in life.[15] Many families choose to begin treatment before children start school to reduce their psychosocial impact. Studies have shown that adult patients with PWS have lower self confidence,[16] which is increase after a significant improvement of PWS has achieved with PDL treatment.[17]

So far, there is no recommended setting of PDL due to the lack of controlled studies with a single parameter difference. In general, the ranges of parameters are: 585–600 nm wavelength, 4–12 J/cm^2 fluence, 0.45–10 ms pulse duration and a minimum of 7 mm spot size.[1] Longer wavelengths and larger spot sizes may allow the laser beam to penetrate deeper into the lesion.[18] Pulse durations should be chosen according to the presumed size of the blood vessels within the lesion. Do keep in mind that capillaries have a TRT in the tens of microseconds and PWS venules have a TRT of tens of milliseconds.[1] Post-treatment purpura secondary to blood vessel destruction, is a desired result, and typically resolve within several days (See Fig. 2).[19] Many clinicians choose the initial fluence based on their personal experience and adjust the fluence based on the PWS appearance immediately after the laser pulse.[20] Some physicians prefer to perform a test spot and gauge PDL settings based on the patient's response. Using a PDL system that has a cooling device can help reduce epidermal damage and intraoperative pain. PDL with a cryogen cooling spray device was found to enhance clinical efficacy because higher fluences could be used without an increased risk of permanent scarring or dyspigmentation.[21]

When treating PWS, it is recommended to target the smaller blood vessels and the edges of the lesion first and leave the larger blood vessels for later treatments.[4] Multiple treatment sessions are necessity and should be scheduled at 4–8 week intervals. There is no agreement on how many treatment sessions required to achieve complete clearance of the lesion. For facial PWS, the average number of sessions is between 9 and 12 in order to achieve ~80% clearance.[13] The most drastic improvement is noted after the first five treatments. Predictive factors for improvement have been examined by several studies. A study of 91 children with an average age of 4.5 years found that the maximal improvement is noted in the first five treatments in all patients regardless of age, location or size of the lesion. The best result of treatment was observe when treating lesions over bony prominences of the face such as the central forehead, size less than 20 cm^2 and those in children less than 1 year of age.[11] Lesions of the head and neck require fewer treatments than those on the trunk and extremities and those in the V2 dermatomal distribution of the trigeminal nerve lightened significantly less with the same number of treatments than those in the V1, V3 and C2/C3 regions.[22] One study in 16 children recommended that using higher fluences (11–12 J/cm^2) and longer pulse durations (1.5 ms) can achieve faster lightening; >75% clearance was attained in four treatment sessions.[23] The number of treatments is often determined by when the patient and/or family are cosmetically pleased with the result, or decide not to continue the treatment.

Challenging PWS with larger and deeper blood vessels tend to require more treatment sessions. Repetitive treatments, even when greater than 20 does not increase the risk of side effects and can offer additional lightening.[24] Very resistant PWS not responded to repetitive treatments with PDL may require longer wavelength lasers such as 595–600 nm LPDL, 755 nm Alexandrite, 1064 Nd:Yag, KTP and IPL. A recent study demonstrated that KTP laser can help to further lighten PDL treatment-resistant PWS. Of 30 adult and pediatric patients in the study all who have had at least five PDL treatments, 16 patients (53%) experienced some lightening (>25%).[25]

It is important to note that redarkening can occur after treatment. In a 10 year follow up study of 51 patients who received PDL for PWS, 35% reported redarkening of their stains.[26] The further out from last treatment, the more likely the patient is to report recurrence.[27]

Hemangiomas of Infancy

While PDL treatment for PWS is well established, the role of PDL in the treatment of hemangiomas of infancy (HOI) is less clear. Hemangiomas are the most common benign tumor of infancy and are composed of capillary-sized blood vessels.[1] HOI are estimated to affect 1.1–2.6% of newborns. Their natural history is characterized by three stages: rapid proliferation (usually the first 6–8 months of life), plateau and involution. The duration of each stage in a particular lesion is difficult to predict, however the onset of involution is indicated by a color change from bright red to gray or purple. The vast majority of hemangiomas undergo spontaneous involution without residual defect. On the other hand, about 5–13% of hemagiomas will ulcerate in the proliferative phase and some leave a yellowish discoloration, atrophic scarring, redundant skin, fibrofatty tissue or residual telangiectasias. Treatment of HOI includes active nonintervention, topical, intralesional and oral corticosteroids, vincristine, recombinant interferon alpha 2a and 2b, imiquimod, cryotherapy, and surgery. More recently, vascular lasers such as the PDL have been added to the armamentarium. Due to their unpredictive growth of the lesion and spontaneous resolution of hemangiomas, the indication to treat is controversial. Most experts agree that hemangiomas in locations that is functionally disabling or life threatening (See Fig. 3), that will permanently scar, located on the face and ulcerated should required treatment. Most pediatric dermatologists prefer a wait and see approach with uncomplicated HOI that do not have the aforementioned characteristics.

Batta et al. compared PDL treatment of uncomplicated HOI to active nonintervention and concluded that there was no useful benefit of early treatment with PDL in uncomplicated hemangiomas. Furthermore, lesions that were treated with PDL experienced an increased risk of skin atrophy and hypopigmentation compared to untreated hemangiomas.[28] This study, however, was criticized for not using a cooling device[29] which not only allow the use of higher fluences but also prevented post treatment pigment alteration.

PDL treatment is currently used for thin, superficial lesions, ulcerated hemangiomas and the residual redness and telangiectasias left after HOI involute.[30,31] LPDL versus traditional PDL may help to limit the average time period of maximum hemangioma proliferation with less adverse effects.[32]

Clear beneficial results have been seen when PDL is used to treat an early pink macular lesion. One study showed that treating early hemangiomas with 595 nm PDL at fluences of 6–7 J/cm^2 can induce involution and prevent the development of the deep components.[33] Unfortunately, most HOI do not present to a dermatologist until they are in the proliferative phase.

Clear benefits of PDL are also seen with superficial hemangiomas. In one study, lesions less than 3 mm thick achieved resolved quicker than thicker lesions (>3 mm). However, these are also the ones more likely to involute spontaneously with a good cosmetic outcome. The authors recommended that only superficial hemangiomas impinging on vital structures should be treated with the PDL.[33] Furthermore,

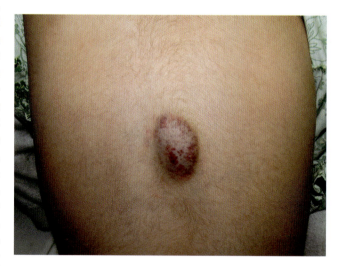

Fig. 3 Deeper hemangiomas may be less amenable to treatment with lasers

superficial hemangiomas in proliferative and involution phases both respond well to PDL therapy.[34]

In addition, PDL treatment in ulcerating hemangiomas can effectively decrease pain and improve healing of the affected area.[35] In a study of 78 patients with ulcerated hemangiomas, 91% of patients experienced epithelialization of the ulceration after an average of two laser treatments. No significant complications were noted in this study.[36]

When treating hemangiomas, it is important to recognize how HOI differ from PWS. As opposed to PWS, hemangiomas are high flow tumors, and composed of smaller blood vessels that close to skin surface.[37] Lower fluences and shorter pulse durations should be used in PDL treatment. The average parameter used in PDL treatment for hemangioma studies are: 585–595 nm wavelength, 5–10 J/cm^2 fluence, 0.3–0.5 ms pulse duration and a 3–7 mm spot size. Treatment sessions are usually repeated every 1–4 weeks. Kono et al. studied superficial hemangiomas in preproliferative or early proliferative stages in patients 1–3 months of age and compared treatment with a 585 nm PDL (7 mm spot size, 6–7 J/cm^2, 0.45 ms pulse duration, no epidermal cooling device) with a 595 nm LPDL (7 mm spot size, 9–15 J/cm^2, 10–20 ms pulse duration with an epidermal cooling device). Both groups were treated at 4 week intervals until the lesion cleared. Although the number of children whose lesions showed complete clearance or minimal residual signs at 1 year of age was similar in both groups, the PDL-treated group had more dyspigmentation and more textural changes than the LPDL-treated group. The average time of maximal proliferation in the LPDL group was significantly shorter than in the PDL group. The authors concluded that LPDL is safer and more effective than PDL in the treatment of early hemangiomas.[32] However, it is difficult to know which factor confers superiority of the result in LPDL group; the longer pulse duration, the higher fluence, or the use of the cryogen cooling spray.

While the efficacy of PDL is limited to treat deeper hemangiomas (See Fig. 4), 1,064 nm Nd:YAG laser has been used successfully to treat PDL-failed lesions.[38] Several studies have used both percutaneous and intralesional applications of the laser with positive results. Nd:YAG laser should only be used by experienced laser surgeons. More recently a dual –wavelength laser system (595 and 1,064 nm) (Cynergy with Multiplex®, Cyanosure, Westford, MA) has been found to be superior than PDL or Nd:YAG alone in clearing facial telangiectasias.[39] Combining the 595 nm PDL and the 1,064 nm Nd:YAG wavelengths results in a synergistic effect and would theoretically be beneficial for deeper vascular malformations in children. Studies with this laser in children are ongoing.

KTP laser is a modified Nd:YAG that emits 532 nm through a KTP crystal. Pulse durations range from 1 to 100 ms. The laser is administered to tissue via a fiberoptic hand piece. Advantages

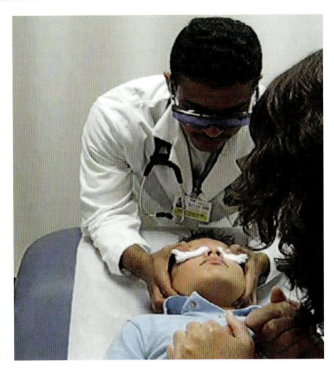

Fig. 4 Overlapping 2×2-in. gauzes may be held in place over the child's eyes and may be an alternative to standard safety goggles

of using 532 nm wavelength in treatment of hemangiomas include selective absorption by hemoglobin with minimal purpura. Disadvantage includes the limited penetration depth and the higher risk of post treatment dyschromias.[1] Achauer et al. demonstrated successful use of the KTP bare fiber at 15 J and 0.6 mm spot size in treating bulkier hemangiomas.[40]

Although successful treatment of superficial hemangiomas is evident, there are some controversies about an optimal laser treatment and treatment indication. Clinical treatment criteria include rapid enlargement of the lesion, involvement of large surface area, actual or potential functional impairment, ulceration, cosmetic disfigurement, and recurrent bleeding or trauma to the area.[41] Laser treatment should be considered when the lesion failed conventional medical therapy.[42] Superficial hemangiomas respond quite easily and effectively to the PDL, while a more variable response is noted in deeper hemangiomas, early proliferative lesions, and ulcerated hemangiomas.[33,43]

Other Lesions Amenable to Vascular Laser Therapy

In addition to PWS and hemangiomas, other vascular lesions in children can be effectively treated with vascular laser. Telangiectasias are small dilated capillaries, most commonly seen as spider telangiectasias in children.[4,44] Telangiectasias, especially on the face, are highly responsive to laser therapy. Complete resolution of the lesion can be achieve with a single treatment in some cases.[45] Pyogenic granulomas are solitary vascular proliferations that can be seen in childhood, typically present as rapidly growing, bright red papules. PDL has been found to be more effective for smaller, flatter lesions and should be used to treat the lesion smaller than 5 mm.[46] When pyogenic granuloma is not responding to PDL treatment, alternative diagnoses such as spitz nevi should be considered.

There are a growing number of other conditions in children that can be successfully treated with PDL. For example, angiofibromas may be treated effectively when they are first developed and small. The lesions may require follow-up treatments at 6- or 12-month intervals.[47] Several studies on the use of PDL in verrucae vulgaris (VV)[48] and in molluscum contagiosum[49] have shown it to be a useful treatment. VV, or common wart, is estimated to occur in 10–22% of children and young adults with a peak incidence between 12 and 16 years of age.[50] Nearly two-thirds of warts resolve spontaneously within 2 years. There are many treatment options for VV including topical salicylic acid, cryotherapy and PDL, which recently been added as a third line treatment of choice for recalcitrant warts.[51] The mechanism of PDL is still unknown, but thought to be either selective photothermolysis, targeting oxyhemoglobin in dilated capillaries within the lesions, or by destroying the heat sensitive-human papilloma virus ladden cells.[48] The efficacy of PDL in VV has been examined by many studies, and has been shown to be as high as 92–95% clearance rate.[52,53] A few studies showed less favorable outcomes.[54] Only some of these studies included children. In one study of 56 children less than 12 years of age, warts were pre-treated with EMLA, then pared down with a razor, and treated with the 585-nm flashlamp-pumped PDL (5-mm spot size, 7–10 J/cm^2, double pulsed with a 1 mm overlap, 2–3 week intervals). The overall clearance rate was 48.1% with an average of three visits needed to achieve complete remission.[55] The most effective fluences for eradication is between 8.5 and 9.5 J/cm^2. The authors concluded that PDL is safe, tolerable and relatively effective to treat VV in children and can be considered a therapy for recalcitrant warts, but not as the first line therapy. PDL is also a safe, quick and effective treatment for molluscum contagiosum.[56] Using a 585 nm PDL with pulse duration of 0.450 ms, a 7-mm spot size and fluence of 6–7 J/cm^2, nearly 84% of children had complete remission with one treatment and the remainder responded by the third treatment session. All patients tolerated the treatment well.[49] Using pulse duration of 0.25–0.45 ms, fluences of 2–10 J/cm^2 for 1–3 sessions can also give a successful treatment of the lesion.[57,58]

PDL has been effective in the early treatment of hypertrophic scars, with scars on the face being most responsive.[59] Other pediatric conditions that have been successfully treated by using PDL include inflammatory linear verrucous epidermal nevus,[60] morphea,[61] angiofibromas,[62] granuloma annulare[63] and lymphangiomas.[64]

Potassium Titanyl Phosphate (KTP)

At this time, KTP seems to have a significant therapeutic role in the treatment of several different conditions commonly seen in the pediatric population. First, KTP laser has demonstrated significant clinical efficacy for lightening PDL treatment-resistant PWS. Over 50% of the patients showed >25% improvement and 17% showed >50% response, with the best results achieved at fluences ranging from 18 to 24 J/cm^2 with pulse width 9–14 ms.[25] Interestingly, patients described less discomfort during treatment and less post-treatment purpura with KTP, as compared to PDL. In another similar study that included children, this laser was proven safe and effective treatment for common superficial cutaneous vascular lesions, specifically in patients with Fitzpatrick skin types I–III.[65] Because of its shorter wavelength, KTP laser may only be able to effectively treat these superficial lesions.[66] Also, the shallow penetration of the laser results in an increase targeting of epidermal melanin and thus a greater risk for non-specific tissue injury in darker skin types.[67] In addition, KTP appears to be successful for the treatment of facial angiofibromas early in life, secondary to its photothermal destruction.[68] Lastly, KTP laser has been used for recalcitrant viral warts. In one study, 80% of patients responded to therapy with 532-nm KTP continuous wave laser, with complete clearance observed in nearly 50% of the group.[48] While there are a growing number of conditions treatable with the KTP laser, more research needed to be done to evaluate its safety and efficacy in the pediatric population.

Quasi Continuous Lasers

The argon pumped tunable dye (577–585 nm/yellow), Copper bromide (578 nm/yellow) Copper Vapor (578 nm/yellow), and Krypton (568 nm/yellow) lasers were used in the past for the treatment of vascular skin lesions. There use has fallen out of favor due to the success of the PDL.

Adverse Events

Fortunately, the safety and efficacy of PDL has made it an ideal laser system for treatment of pediatric conditions. However, no laser treatment is risk free and there exists a very small chance of hypertrophic scarring and atrophic scarring when treating pediatric PWS.[7,69] Purpura is a desired adverse event but occasionally prolonged purpura lasting up to 14 days can occur and is distressing.[70] The risk of post inflammatory hyperpigmentation is higher in darker-skinned and tanned patient because of a possible competitive absorption of melanin. To treat this subset of patients, longer interval between 3 to 6 months is recommended.[71]

Pain is common during and immediately after the procedure. Its intensity is less when using a cooling device with PDL. An ice pack to the treated area can help lessen pain. Infection can also occur as a consequence of a diminished skin barrier following epidermal damage. This risk may be higher in patients with coexisting atopic dermatitis.[72]

Another concern in children is psychological sequelae from the treatment. The pain, restraint and darkness associated with the procedure can be psychologically scarring and can lead to fear and stress in future doctor's visits. Special considerations particular to children such as techniques on allaying heightened anxiety in children and the use of analgesic and sedative agents for laser treatments will be discussed in more detail later in the chapter.

Pigmented Lesions

Lasers Used to Treat Pigmented Lesions in Children

Potassium-titanyl-phosphate (KTP) laser	532 nm
Q-Switched alexandrite	755 nm
Q-Switched ruby	694 nm
Q-Switched Nd:YAG, frequency-doubled	532 nm
Q-Switched Nd:YAG	1,064 nm

- The main chromophore of pigmented lesions, melanin, is the target of laser treatments.
- While PDL has become the standard of care for many lesions in this population, KTP and the Q-switched lasers have proven to be a safe and effective alternative in certain cases.
- KTP may be a better alternative than PDL for treatment of resistant hypertrophic PWS and some superficial facial telangiectasias.

Pigmented lesions can be effectively treated by selecting a specific laser therapy with a target wavelength and depth of penetration that match the target lesion. Melanin is the major target chromophore for the treatment of pigmented lesions.[4] It has wide absorption spectrum ranging from 300 to 1,000 nm, and slowly decreasing from the ultraviolet to the near infrared. Because of its wide range of light absorption, there are a large number of different lasers that can selectively treat a large number of benign pigmented lesions in this population. In general, pigment-specific lasers tend to have very short pulse durations, which minimize heat spread from the melanosome to surrounding tissue, allowing for single pigment cell destruction.[4] Based upon the depth of lesion being treated (epidermal, dermal or mixed), individual laser systems can be optimally selected to maximize the treatment of the target lesions. While treatment efficacy decreases as the wavelength of light increases, longer wavelength laser systems may be required for improved penetration and treatment of deeper lesions.[73]

Indications and Contraindications

- Indications
  - Epidermal Lesions
    - Lentigines
    - Café Au Lait Macules
    - Nevus Spilus
  - Dermal Lesions
    - Nevus of Ota or Ito
    - Tattoos
  - Mixed Lesions
    - Congenital Melanocytic Nevi (Still Controversial at this Time)
- Contraindications
  - Patients with unrealistic expectations.
  - Patients who tend to scar will be at a greater risk for this post-operative complication.
  - Patients with clinically atypical melanocytic nevus.

Lentigines are small, flat darkly-pigmented lesions that can involve any cutaneous surface in a spotty distribution, and can be seen on the lips in children.[74,75] They result from an increase in the number of melanocytes at the dermo-epidermal junction without the formation of nests. Histologically, they consist of enlarged melanosomes throughout the epidermis. Lentigines can be effectively treated by pigment-specific lasers. Taylor and Anderson have demonstrated that, by using 694-nm Q-switched ruby laser, nearly all lentigines were cleared after a single treatment. The laser parameter used in this study is 4.5–7.5 J/cm^2 and pulse duration of 40 ns.[76] Similarly, using the frequency-doubled Q-switched Nd:YAG laser can leads to >75% clearance after a single treatment using 2.0-mm spot size, 10 ns pulse duration, and fluences of 2–5 J/cm². [77] Another report showed 595-nm LPDL delivered with the compression method was effective in the treatment of facial lentigines in adult Asian patients. Using settings of 9–13 J/cm² and 1.5 ms pulse duration, this traditional "vascular" LPDL can be used for treating pigmented lesions. [78] Currently, there is no consensus on the best laser system and settings in the treatment of lentigines, since these lesions tend to be quite responsive to treatments.

Café-au-lait macules are flat, sharply-demarcated lesions of uniformly light tan to brown, with uniform melanin pigmentation. The lesions can range from a few millimeters to 20 cm in diameter. Solitary café-au-lait macule is not uncommon and can be founded in 10–28% of normal individuals, with the prevalence increasing during infancy and decreasing in adult life. [74] The response to laser treatment is vary, not only among different lasers treatments but also among café-au-lait macules treated with the same laser. [4] The macules may darken, lighten, or recur after laser treatment. [79] Given the benign nature of these lesions, there are not so many documented reports of clinical trial in the pediatric population. Most of the studies have been done in adolescence and adult population. Taylor and Anderson demonstrated substantial clearing with the 694-nm Q-switched ruby laser using fluences of 4.5 and/or 7.5 J/cm² and a pulse duration of 40 ns. [76] A comparative study of the Q-switched ruby laser and Q-switched Nd:YAG laser showed the results from both treatment groups to be quite similar in efficacy, with the ruby laser having slightly better treatment response. [80] Grossman attempted to identify clinicopathologic correlations between café-au-lait macules and laser therapy used in treatment. Using a fluence of 6.0 J/cm² for the frequency-doubled Q-switched Nd:YAG laser (532 nm, 2 mm beam diameter) and the Q-switched ruby laser (994 nm, 5 mm diameter), they concluded that both lasers yielded variable response and that patients should be aware of recurrences or darkening of the lesions. [79]

Nevus spilus is a well-defined patch of hyperpigmentation with scattered smaller, darker pigmented macules or papules, frequently found on trunk or extremities. Size can be varied from 1 to 20 cm in diameter and the prevalence of nevus spilus is <1% in newborns. [74] Normally, the lesion consists of café-au-lait and nevocellular melanocytic components. The melanocytic component can range from lentigines to melanoma, [81] therefore, any suspicious lesions should be biopsied and followed-up. [82] The Q-switched ruby, Q-switched alexandrite, Q-switched frequency-doubled Nd:YAG lasers, as well as normal ruby and alexandrite lasers, have all been used to treat nevus spilus. [4] The treatment outcome is unpredictable, similar to those for café-au-lait macules. Given their response to multiple lasers and the heterogeneity of such responses, there is no agreement upon standard laser therapy for this condition. Several laser settings have been reported in successfully-treated nevus spilus studies. The 694-nm Q-switched ruby laser was used with a 40 ns pulse duration and fluences of 4.5 and 7.5 J/cm² for small and large lesions respectively. Initial improvement after two treatments in small lesions and one treatment in larger lesions at the higher fluence; however, there was a nearly complete return of background pigment observed at 1 year. [76] The 755-nm Q-switched alexandrite laser utilized with a spot size of 4 mm, pulse duration of 50 ns, and a fluence of 4–5 J/cm² was also less effective for nevus spilus because of repigmentation after transient bleaching. [83] Another report of the Q-switched ruby laser observed nearly complete clearance of the pigment from lesions in a small cohort of patients, notably with greater effectiveness than the Q-switched Nd:YAG laser in those patients. [84]

Nevus of Ito and Nevus of Ota are both characterized by dermal melanocytosis that appears as blue-gray discoloration of the skin. Nevus of Ota is most commonly seen in Asian and African-American populations, usually present as a unilateral, irregular blue-gray patch along area innervated by the first and second branches of the trigeminal nerve. [85] Greater than fifty percent of the lesion are present at birth, whereas 40% manifest during puberty. Nevus of Ito is patchy blue-gray discoloration of the skin occur elsewhere. [74] Given the depth of melanosis, pigmented lasers with longer wavelengths tend to clear lesions more quickly than those with shorter wavelengths. [86] Treatment with Q-switched ruby or Alexandrite lasers have shown to selectively destroy dermal melanocytes. [87,88] Using the 755-nm Q-switched alexandrite laser (pulse duration 100 ns and 4.75–7.0 J/cm² fluences) at 8–12 week intervals, Alster and Williams demonstrated 50% clinical clearance after two treatments and 100% after five treatments in most patients. [85] In another study of 15 patients between 6 and 52 years of age, using 694-nm Q-switched ruby laser with pulse duration of 40 ns and fluences 6–10 J/cm² showed complete clearing of the lesion in nearly 30% of patients and >50% lightening in the remaining patients. [86] In a larger study with 46 children, Q-switched ruby laser used in children produced complete clearance of the lesion faster than in adults, providing further support for early treatment of Nevus of Ota in the pediatric population. [89] Given the growing data on laser efficacy, Q-switched ruby laser is the best treatment option for lighter skin types while Q-switched Nd:Yag is for darker skin types. [86] The number of treatments required are dictated primarily by the depth and color of the lesion. [90,91]

Tattoos result from pigment deposition primarily in the dermis, either via professional application or trauma. Laser treatment for professional tattoos on adult patients will be discussed elsewhere in this book. Traumatic tattoos, such as those from the graphite from pencil tips, are the most frequently seen in the pediatric population. Traumatic tattoos is effectively treated with Q-switched ruby, Q-switched alexandrite or Q-switched Nd:YAG after single treatment.[26,74-76] In one report, Single treatment using the Q-switched ruby laser successfully cleared a traumatic tattoo from a pencil tip injury 1 year prior.[74] In another study reported successful outcome using the Q-switched alexandrite to treat traumatic tattoos from blacktop, surgical pen, gravel tattoos, and even fireworks.[75]

Congenital melanocytic nevi (CMN) are collections of melanocytes that may present as macular, papular, or plaque-like pigmented lesions in various shades of brown. Present at birth, CMN range in size from a few centimeters to 5–50% of the body surface area.[74] Laser treatment is very effective in improving the appearance of CMN by lightening or removing superficial cutaneous pigment without destroying melanocytes deeper in the skin.[92-94] Waldorf et al. demonstrated that Q-switched ruby laser effectively lightens and may clear pigmentation and eliminate superficial nevus cells from small and medium congenital nevi safely without scarring. In this study there was 57% clearance of pigmentation in all nevi by the fourth session and an average maximum clearance of 76% after approximately eight sessions. However, these results are not permanent and should not be considered definitive treatment.[94] Another report using the Q-switched ruby laser (694 nm, pulse duration 40–60 ns, fluence 7.5–8.0 J/cm^2, spot size 5 mm) or the normal-mode ruby laser (694 nm, pulse duration 3 ms, fluence 40 J/cm^2, spot size 7 mm) achieved a clinically visible decrease in pigment in over 50% of patients (age range 18–75 years), but they were unable to achieve complete removal of the lesions either clinically or histologically.[93] Combination therapy with laser surgery following epidermal ablation (CO$_2$ laser, pulse duration 1 ms, fluence 300 mJ/cm^2) was more effective than laser surgery with the QS alexandrite lasers alone.[95] Given the ongoing controversy in laser surgery treatment for CMN, there are no individual laser systems or settings among current lasers that is the standard of care for treatment.

Despite excellent results from laser treatment, whether to treat CMN is very controversial due to its malignant transformation potential. Most authors agree that the primary role of laser treatment is for cosmetically disfiguring and surgically unresectable lesions.[96]

Ablative Lasers in Children

Carbon dioxide (CO$_2$) laser
Erbium:Ytrium-Aluminum-Garnet (Er:YAG) laser

- Ablative lasers, including the CO2 and Er:YAG laser, have been utilized to treat a variety of lesions in the pediatric population, including a variety of nevi, acne scars, keloids, and epidermal nevi.

Ablative (or resurfacing) lasers were first designed for using in the adult population to remove or reduce wrinkles. They are now utilized to use in pediatric patients for many conditions, including acne scar, keloid, VV, epidermal nevus and inflammatory linear verrucous epidermal nevus (ILVEN), angiofibroma, and CMN.

Indications and Contraindications

- Indications
  - Epidermal Nevus
  - Scars (acne and keloid)
  - Congenital Melanocytic Nevus
  - Verrucae Vulgaris (Older Treatment Option)
  - Angiofibromas
- Contraindications
  - Patients with unrealistic expectations
  - Patients who tend to scar will be at a greater risk for this post-operative complication

Epidermal nevi (EN) are benign harmatomas of epidermis and papillary dermis, usually occur within the first year of life. Most lesions appear as well-circumscribed, hyperpigmented, papillomatous papules that are asymptomatic. Over time, the nevus may become more thickened and verrucous, developing into a significant cosmetic concern. Since topical therapies are of limited utility, most treatment methods attempt to ablate the lesion and decrease its thickness with resurfacing lasers, such as the CO$_2$ and Er:YAG lasers.[44] One such report of the pulsed 2,940-nm Er:YAG laser (0.4–0.45 J/cm^2, spot size 2 mm) demonstrated excellent clinical results for the treatment of superficial or small, discrete lesions which could be ablated accurately; however, they did not evaluate the efficacy of laser therapy for larger, thicker EN which may be more difficult to treat.[97] Additionally, CO$_2$ laser was effective in some of thicker EN not responsive to argon laser, but there was a high incidence of post-treatment hypertrophic scar.[98] Another group showed that the variable-pulsed Er:YAG laser (pulse duration 500 ms, fluence 7.0–7.5 J/cm^2) and the dual-mode Er:YAG laser (pulse duration 350 ms, fluence 6.3 J/cm^2) were effective, and safe for ILVEN with complete clearance 75% of patients in one treatment, although 25% did have a relapse within 1 year.[99] In summary, both CO_2 and Er:YAG lasers can be effective for the treatment of EN, and its efficacy depends on the size and thickness of the lesion.

Similarly, CMN can also be treated with ablative lasers. Ostertag et al. has shown that Er:YAG laser was effective to treat CMN in neonates. Overall, the treatment was well tolerated, with good clinical and histological results. Eighty percent of patients had minimal to no repigmentation clinically, and disappearance of heavily pigmented cells in the upper part of the dermis histologically as well.[100] CMN can also be effectively treated with CO_2 laser, but this application may be limited by the slightly higher incidence of observed hypertrophic scarring.[101] More recently, the use of Q-switched lasers has taken more prominent role in the treatment of CMN; and appears to be more effective when using in combination with ablative methods.

Ablative lasers have also been utilized as an alternative therapy for treatment resistant viral warts. Previous study in 2002 had shown that single treatment of recalcitrant lesions with CO_2 laser had response rates between 56% and 81%.[102] Another group evaluated the efficacy of CO_2 laser technique for recalcitrant warts in pediatric patients. In this study, the skin was cut in a circular fashion with 5 mm margins around the wart and then vaporized the base of the lesions. This technique provided a high success rate with no recurrence at 12 months and was well tolerated by the patients, however, hypopigmentation was noted in about 25% of the cases.[103]

Both CO_2 and Er:YAG lasers have been moderately useful in the treatment of keloids and hypertrophic scars. Specifically, the pulsed Er:YAG laser with a 2-mm handpiece at 500–1,200 mJ/pulse at 3.5–9 W was used with an improvement of more than 50% in hypertrophic, depressed and burn scars.[104]

There are a number of clinically conditions in the pediatric population that can be effectively treated with ablative laser therapy. As these lasers are improved, there may be even safer and more effective treatments in the future.

Special Considerations in Children

Preoperative Management

Laser treatment of children poses a unique challenge for a variety of reasons. The approach to a child prior to laser treatments is different than their adult counterparts. First, parents may be more apprehensive and have more questions about the procedure than if they themselves were the patient. Thus pre-treatment counseling sessions may be longer as both parent and child should have their questions answered. During the visit, the parent and the child should be told step by step what will happen on treatment day. Post-treatment effects and the risk of adverse events such as dyspigmentation and scarring should also be informed. Parental expectations should be explored and all questions are answered. Expected outcomes and usual number of treatments are discussed as well. Using before and after photographs of previously treated patients may help allay anxieties in parents.[44]

Secondly, laser treatment produces sufficient discomfort and may not be as easily tolerated by children. Laser treatments are painful and have been likened to the sensation of flicking a rubber band on the skin.[105] There is not one specifically known age at which you can plan that a child will sit still and cooperate with the procedure. The age at which a child will cooperate with such a procedure depends on a number of factors, including maturity level among other things. For example, a 3 year old child who has been in and out of surgeries for congenital heart disease may sit still for laser treatments while an immature 10 year old may be uncooperative. In general, rapid and limited treatments seem to be tolerated well in young infants and mature adolescents with no anesthesia at all, or with topical anesthesia alone.[44]

Some form of anesthesia should be considered for all children undergoing laser treatments. The kind of anesthetic and how it will be administered should be discussed in the pretreatment counseling session. At a minimum, a topical local anesthetic such as lidocaine 4% or 5% cream (LMX®) or eutectic mixture of local anesthetics (EMLA) should be applied to the area to be treated. EMLA, which is half lidocaine and half prilocaine, has been occasionally associated with local and systemic side effects in the pediatric population.[106-108] In addition, some groups discourage its use before laser treatment as it can vasoconstrict the target area. LMX® has a longer duration of anesthesia, does not require occlusion and does not have any reported side effects.[109] According to the package insert, to avoid systemic absorption, LMX should not be applied over an area greater than 100 cm^2 in a child less than 10 kg or to an area greater than 600 cm^2 in a child weighing 10–20 kg.[4] In our practice, we use LMX® 4% invariably for younger children and in older children with large lesions. The cream is applied with tegaderm or saran wrap occlusion to the target area by our medical staff when the patient first checks in to their appointment. They then wait 15–30 min in the waiting room prior to laser treatments. A dressing with gauze or a permeable bandage prevents optimal absorption of LMX® into the skin.[75] Our technique has been successful and we have had 6 year olds cooperate with procedure using LMX® only. Localized intradermal injections and local intradermal nerve block have also been used. In younger children who will not tolerate the discomfort associated with the procedure even with local anesthesia, then oral, intravenous and/or general anesthesia can be used.[73]

Although not routine, oral agents such as chloral hydrate, benzodiazepines and codeine have been used for light sedation during in office procedures. These agents carry the risk of respiratory depression and their duration of action are unpredictable and thus their use is unpopular. In addition, while these agents provide light sedation, they do not provide any anesthetic effect.

In children with large lesions who require prolonged treatment and in younger children when immobilization cannot be obtained, deep sedation with IV sedatives or general anesthesia should be considered. When preformed in a pediatric hospital with pediatric anesthesiologists present there is no increased risk of morbidity or mortality from deep or general sedation.[110,111] An increased complication risk with general anesthesia is seen in the first year of life with a greater risk in the first months of life.[112] Despite the low rate of complications, the added risk of general anesthesia needs to be considered versus the benefits of PDL treatments. Lesions that represent significant health risks, cause functional impairment or a deformity in which a superior cosmetic result would be obtained with early surgical intervention or which may impact significantly psychosocial development may necessitate early surgical intervention despite the added risk inherent in general anesthesia. In other cases, parents may choose to wait until the child is old enough to cooperate with the procedure as an outpatient.

Intra Operative Management

Even with local anesthesia and a seemingly cooperative, prepared child, secure positioning is of utmost importance when treating children with lasers. We believe a minimum of three personnel should be in the room when treating a child with a laser; one to perform the laser surgery, one at the head of the table, holding the head and eye protection in place, and one at the foot of the table (See Fig. 5). We often also include a parent on the opposite side of the laser to aid in holding the child and ease their anxiety.

Age-appropriate eye safety is also very important. The standard safety goggles may be too large and provide inadequate protection.[113] As an alternative, overlapping 2×2 in. pieces of white gauze can be used held in place by staff or medical personnel. These patches can absorb or reflect laser light. Smaller metal corneal shields can also be used. White gauze can also be used to cover an area within the spot size diameter that should not be treated or has already been adequately treated.[4]

Creativity comes into play when interacting with young children in the procedure room. Our group frequently uses distraction anesthesia where by children are distracted by a DVD or handheld game of their choice.[114] Another technique often used is the pinching of the skin prior to the injection of lidocaine to distract away from the initial sting. Other authors have suggested creating a "parent – child tent" such as with a

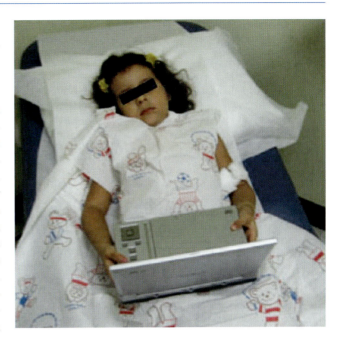

Fig. 5 Distraction anesthesia may be employed with the use of handheld DVD or gaming device of their choice

gown or a sheet,[115] this can be especially useful when the site to be treated is away from the face. Songs or counting can also be used. Dressing the surgical site with an age appropriate, child friendly dressing can help the patient feel more comfortable at the end of the procedure.[44]

Conclusions

Lasers can be safely and effectively used in children when the aforementioned special considerations are employed. Perhaps the most far-reaching example is the success in the treatment of PWS. Understanding the composition and natural history of pediatric skin lesions and the mechanics of skin and laser interactions is one step towards providing effective treatment for children. Laser surgery is an important part of the therapeutic armamentarium in children. We expect and are excited that with advancing technology in laser surgery, there will be an even greater role in the treatment of children.

References

1. Stier MF, Glick SA, Hirsch RJ. Laser treatment of pediatric vascular lesions: post wine stains and hemangiomas. *J Am Acad Dermatol*. 2008;58:261-285.
2. Railan D, Parlette EC, Uebelhoer NS, Rohrer TE. Laser treatment of vascular lesions. *Clin Dermatol*. 2005;24:8-15.

3. Hammes S, Roos S, Raulin C, et al. Does dye laser treatment with higher fluences in combination with cold air cooling improve the results of port-wine stains? *J Eur Acad Dermatol Venereol.* 2007;21:1229-1233.

4. Cantatore JL, Kriegel DA. Laser surgery: an approach to the pediatric patient. *J Am Acad Dermatol.* 2004;50:165-184.

5. van der Horst CM, Koster PH, de Borgie CA, et al. Effect of the timing of treatment of port-wine stains with the flash-lamp-pumped pulsed-dye laser. *N Engl J Med.* 1998;338(15):1028-1033.

6. Chapas AM, Eickhorsst K, Geronemus RG. Efficacy of early treatment of facial port wine stains in newborns: A review of 49 cases. *Lasers Surg Med.* 2007;39:563-568.

7. Reyes BA, Geronemus R. Treatment of port-wine stains during childhood with the flashlamp-pumped pulsed dye laser. *J Am Acad Dermatol.* 1990;23(6):1142-1148.

8. Goldman MP, Fitzpatrick RE, Ruiz-Esparza J. Treatment of port-wine stains (capillary malformation) with the flashlamp-pumped pulsed dye laser. *J Pediatr.* 1993;122(1):71-77.

9. Ashinoff R, Geronemus RG. Flashlamp-pumped pulsed dye laser for port-wine stains in infancy: earlier versus later treatment. *J Am Acad Dermatol.* 1991;24(3):467-472.

10. Morelli JG, Weston WL, Huff JC, Yohn JJ. Initial lesion size as a predictive factor in determining the response of port-wine stains in children treated with the pulsed dye laser. *Arch Pediatr Adolesc Med.* 1995;149(10):1142-1144.

11. Nguyen CM, Yohn JJ, Weston WL. Facial port wine stains in childhood: prediction of the rate of improvement as a function of the age of the patient, size and location of the port wine stain and the number of treatments with pulsed dye (585 nm) laser. *Br J Dermatol.* 1998;38:821-825.

12. Troilius A, Wragsjo B, Ljunggren B. Patients with port-wine stains and their psychosocial reactions after photo hermolytic treatment. *Dermatol Surg.* 2000;26:190-196.

13. Alster TS, Railan D. Laser treatment of vascular birthmarks. *J Craniofac Surg.* 2006;17:720-723.

14. Brownell CA, Zerwas S, Ramani GB. "So big": the development of body self-awareness in toddlers. *Child Dev.* 2007;78(5):1426-1440.

15. Kreuger DW. Body self. Development, psychopathologies, and psychoanalytic significance. *Psychoanal Study Child.* 2001;56:238-259.

16. Augustin M, Zschocke I, Wiek K, et al. Psychosocial stress of patients with port wine stains and expectations of dye laser treatment. *Dermatology.* 1998;197(4):353-360.

17. Hansen K, Kreiter CD, Rosenbaum M. Long-term psychological impact and perceived efficacy of pulsed-dye laser therapy for patients with port-wine stains. *Dermatol Surg.* 2003;29(1):49-55.

18. Anderson RR, Parrish JA. Selective photothermolysis: precise microsurgery by selective absorption of pulsed radiation. *Science.* 1983;220(4596):524-527.

19. Levine VJ, Geronemus RG. Adverse effects associated with the 577- and 585-nanometer pulsed dye laser in the treatment of cutaneous vascular lesions: a study of 500 patients. *J Am Acad Dermatol.* 1995;32(4):613-617.

20. Mahendran R, Sheehan-Dare RA. Survey of the practices of laser users in the UK in the treatment of port wine stains. *J Dermatolog Treat.* 2004;15(2):112-117.

21. Chang CJ, Nelson JS. Cryogen spray cooling and higher fluence pulsed dye laser treatment improve port-wine stain clearance while minimizing epidermal damage. *Dermatol Surg.* 1999;25(10): 767-772.

22. Renfro L, Geronemus RG. Anatomical differences of port-wine stains in response to treatment with the pulsed dye laser. *Arch Dermatol.* 1993;129(2):182-188.

23. Geronemus RG, Quintana AT, Lou WW, et al. High-fluence modified pulsed dye laser photocoagulation with dynamic cooling of port-wine stains in infancy. *Arch Dermatol.* 2000;136(7):942-943.

24. Kauvar AN, Geronemus RG. Repetitive pulsed dye laser treatments improve persistent port-wine stains. *Dermatol Surg.* 1995; 21(6):515-521.

25. Chowdhury MM, Harris S, Lanigan SW. Potassium titanyl phosphate laser treatment of resistant port-wine stains. *Br J Dermatol.* 2001;144(4):814-817.

26. Huikeshoven M, Koster PH, de Borgie CA, et al. Redarkening of port-wine stains 10 years after pulsed-dye-laser treatment. *N Engl J Med.* 2007;356(12):1235-1240.

27. Orten SS, Waner M, Flock S, et al. Port wine stains. An assessment of 5 years of treatment. *Arch Otolaryngol Head Neck Surg.* 1996;122(11):1174-1179.

28. Batta K, Goodyear HM, Moss C, et al. Randomised controlled study of early pulsed dye laser treatment of uncomplicated childhood hemangiomas: results of a 1-year analysis. *Lancet.* 2002; 360:521-527.

29. Kono T, Erocen AR, Nakazawa H, et al. Treatment of hypertrophic scars using a long-pulsed dye laser UIT cryogen-spray cooling. *Ann Plast Surg.* 2005;54(5):487-493.

30. Bruckner AL, Frieden IJ. Hemangiomas of infancy. *J Am Acad Dermatol.* 2003;48(4):477-493.

31. Drolet BA, Esterly NB, Frieden IJ. Hemangiomas in children. *N Engl J Med.* 1999;341(3):173-181.

32. Kono T, Sakurai H, Groff WF, et al. Comparison study of a traditional pulsed dye laser versus a long-pulsed dye laser in the treatment of early childhood hemangiomas. *Lasers Surg Med.* 2005;38:112-115.

33. Poetke M, Philipp C, Berlien HP. Flashlamp-pumped pulsed dye laser for hemangiomas in infancy: treatment of superficial vs mixed hemangiomas. *Arch Dermatol.* 2000;136:628-632.

34. Barlow RJ, Walker NP, Markey AC. Treatment of proliferative hemangiomas with 585 nm pulsed dye laser. *Br J Dermatol.* 1996;134:700-704.

35. Frieden IJ. Which hemangiomas to treat and how? *Arch Dermatol.* 1997;133:1593-1595.

36. David LR, Malek MM, Argenta LC. Efficacy of pulse dye laser therapy for the treatment of ulcerated hemangiomas: a review of 78 patients. *Br J Plast Surg.* 2003;56:317-327.

37. Witman PM, Wagner AM, Scherer K, et al. Complications following pulsed dye laser treatment of superficial hemangiomas. *Lasers Surg Med.* 2006;38(2):116-123.

38. Ulrich H, Baumler W, Hohenleutner U, et al. Neodymium-YAG for hemagiomas and vascular malformations – long term results. *J Dtsch Dermatol Ges.* 2005;3(6):436-440.

39. Karsai S, Roos S, Raulin C. Treatment of facial telangiectasia using a dual-wavelength laser system (595 and 1064 nm): a randomized controlled trial with blinded response evaluation. *Dermatol Surg.* 2008;34:702-708.

40. Achauer BM, Celikoz B, VanderKam VM. Intralesional bare fiber laser treatment of hemangioma of infancy. *Plast Reconstr Surg.* 1998;101:1212-1217.

41. Eichenfeld L, Wagner AM. Surgical techniques. In: Schachner LA, Hansen RC, eds. *Pediatric Dermatology.* 3rd ed. New York: Churchill Livingstone; 2003:175-187.

42. Roberts LJ. Use of lasers in pediatric skin disease. *Curr Probl Dermatol.* 2000;12:190-193.

43. Geronemus RG. Pulsed dye laser treatment of vascular lesions in children. *J Dermatol Surg Oncol.* 1993;19:303-310.

44. Chapas AM, Geronemus RG. Our approach to pediatric dermatologic laser surgery. *Lasers Surg Med.* 2005;37:255-263.

45. Tan E, Vinciullo C. Pulsed dye laser treatment of spider telangiectasia. *Australas J Dermatol.* 1997;38(1):22-25.

46. Cunningham BB. Laser therapy and dermatologic surgery. *Curr Opin Pediatr.* 1998;10:405-410.

47. Morelli JG. Use of lasers in pediatric dermatology. *Dermatol Clin.* 1998;16:489-495.

48. Kopera D. Verrucae vulgares: flashlamp-pumped pulsed dye laser treatment in 134 patients. *Int J Dermatol.* 2003;42:905-908.

49. Binder B, Weger W, Komericki P, et al. Treatment of molluscum contagiosum with a pulsed dye laser: pilot study with 19 children. *J Dtsch Dermatol Ges.* 2008;6(2):121-125 [Epub November 9].

50. Silverberg NB. Warts and molluscum in children. *Adv Dermatol.* 2004;20:23-73.

51. Ahmed I. Viral warts. In: Weston W, Lane A, Morelli J, eds. *Color Textbook of Pediatric Dermatology.* 3rd ed. St. Louis: Mosby Year-Book; 2002.

52. Kenton-Smith J, Tan ST. Pulsed dye laser therapy for viral warts. *Br J Plast Surg.* 1999;52(7):554-558.

53. Kauvar AN, McDaniel DH, Geronemus RG. Pulsed dye laser treatment of warts. *Arch Fam Med.* 1995;4(12):1035-1040.

54. Huilgol SC, Barlow RJ, Markey AC. Failure of pulsed dye laser therapy for resistant verrucae. *Clin Exp Dermatol.* 1996;21(2):93-95.

55. Park HS, Kim JW, Jang SJ, et al. Pulsed dye laser therapy for pediatric warts. *Pediatr Dermatol.* 2007;24(2):177-181.

56. Hughes PS. Treatment of molluscum contagiosum with the 595-nm pulsed dye laser. *Dermatol Surg.* 1998;24:229-230.

57. Hammes S, Greve B, Raulin C. Molluscum contagiosum: treatment with pulsed dye laser. *Hautarzt.* 2001;52(1):38-42.

58. Michel JL. Treatment of molluscum contagiosum with 585 nm collagen remodeling pulsed dye laser. *Eur J Dermatol.* 2004;14(2):103-106.

59. Kawecki M, Bernad-Wiśniewska T, Sakiel S, et al. Laser in the treatment of hypertrophic burn scars. *Int Wound J.* 2008;5(1):87-97.

60. Alster TS. Inflammatory linear verrucous epidermal nevus: treatment with the 585 nm flashlamp-pumped pulsed dye laser. *J Am Acad Dermatol.* 1994;31:513.

61. Eisen D, Alster TS. Use of a 585 nm pulsed dye laser for the treatment of morphea. *Dermatol Surg.* 2002;28:615-616.

62. Hoffman SJ, Waslh P, Morelli JG. Treatment of angiofibroma with pulsed tunable dye laser. *J Am Acad Dermatol.* 1993;29:790-791.

63. Sliger BN, Burk CJ, Alvarez-Connelly E. Treatment of granuloma annulare with the 595 nm pulsed dye laser in a pediatric patient. *Pediatr Dermatol.* 2008;25(2):196-197.

64. Weingold DH, White PF, Burton CS. Treatment of lymphangioma circumscriptum with tunable dye laser. *Cutis.* 1990;45:365-366.

65. Clark C, Cameron H, Moseley H, et al. Treatment of superficial cutaneous vascular lesions: experience with the KTP 532 nm laser. *Lasers Med Sci.* 2004;19(1):1-5.

66. Tanzi EL, Lupton JR, Alster TS. Lasers in dermatology: four decades of progress. *J Am Acad Dermatol.* 2003;49:1-31.

67. Uebelhoer NS, Bogle MA, Dover JS, et al. A split-face comparison study of pulsed 532-nm KTP laser and 595-nm pulsed dye laser in the treatment of facial telangiectasias and diffuse telangiectatic facial erythema. *Dermatol Surg.* 2007;33(4):441-448.

68. Tope WD, Kageyama N. "Hot" KTP-laser treatment of facial angiofibromata. *Lasers Surg Med.* 2001;29:78-81.

69. Hruza GJ, Geronemus RG, Dover JS, et al. Lasers in dermatology—1993. *Arch Dermatol.* 1993;129:1026-1035.

70. McBurney EI. Side effects and complications of laser therapy. *Dermatol Clin.* 2002;20(1):165-176.

71. Mariwalla K, Dover JS. The use of lasers in the pediatric population. *Skin Therapy Lett.* 2005;10(8):7-9.

72. Karsai S, Roos S, Hammes S, et al. Pulsed dye laser: what's new in non-vascular lesions? *J Eur Acad Dermatol Venereol.* 2007;21(7):877-890.

73. Anderson RR, Margolis RJ, Watenabe S, et al. Selective photothermolysis of cutaneous pigmentation by Q-switched Nd: YAG laser pulses at 1064, 532, and 355 nm. *J Invest Dermatol.* 1989;93(1):28-32.

74. Dohil MA, Baugh WP, Eichenfield LF. Vascular and pigmented birthmarks. *Pediatr Clin North Am.* 2000;47:783-812.

75. Ferguson RE Jr, Vasconez HC. Laser treatment of congenital nevi. *J Craniofac Surg.* 2005;16(5):908-914.

76. Taylor CR, Anderson RR. Treatment of benign pigmented epidermal lesions by Q-switched ruby laser. *Int J Dermatol.* 1993;32(12):908-912.

77. Kilmer SL, Wheeland RG, Goldberg DJ, et al. Treatment of epidermal pigmented lesions with the frequency-doubled Q-switched Nd:YAG laser. A controlled, single-impact, dose-response, multicenter trial. *Arch Dermatol.* 1994;130(12):1515-1519.

78. Kono T, Chan HH, Groff WF, et al. Long-pulse pulsed dye laser delivered with compression for treatment of facial lentigines. *Dermatol Surg.* 2007;33(8):945-950.

79. Grossman MC. What is new in cutaneous laser research. *Dermatol Clin.* 1997;15:1-8.

80. Tse Y, Levine VJ, McClain SA, Ashinoff R. The removal of cutaneous pigmented lesions with the Q-switched ruby laser and the Q-switched neodymium: yttrium aluminum garnet laser. A comparative study. *J Dermatol Surg Oncol.* 1994;20:795-800.

81. Graeme LM, Anderson RR. Lasers in dermatology. In: Freedberg EN, Eisen AZ, Wolff K, Austen KF, Goldsmith LA, Kats S, eds. *Fitzpatrick's Dermatology and General Medicine.* 6th ed. New York: McGraw-Hill Professional; 2003:2493-2509.

82. Johr RH, Schachner LS, Stolz W. Management of nevus spilus. *Pediatr Dermatol.* 1998;15:407-410.

83. Kagami S, Asahina A, Watanabe R, et al. Treatment of 153 Japanese patients with Q-switched alexandrite laser. *Lasers Med Sci.* 2007;22(3):159-163.

84. Grevelink JM, González S, Bonoan R, Vibhagool C, Gonzalez E. Treatment of nevus spilus with the Q-switched ruby laser. *Dermatol Surg.* 1997;23(5):365-369; discussion 369-370.

85. Alster TS, Williams CM. Treatment of nevus of Ota by the Q-switched alexandrite laser. *Dermatol Surg.* 1995;21:592-596.

86. Geronemus RG. Q-switched ruby laser therapy of nevus of Ota. *Arch Dermatol.* 1992;128:1618-1622.

87. Lu Z, Chen JP, Wang SX, et al. Effect of Q-switched alexandrite laser irradiation on dermal melanocytes of nevus of Ota. *Chin Med J.* 2000;113(l):49-52.

88. Lu Z, Chen JP, Wang XS, et al. Effect of Q-switched alexandrite laser irradiation on epidermal melanocytes in treatment of nevus of Ota. *Chin Med J.* 2003;116(4):597-601.

89. Kono T, Chan HH, Ercocen AR, et al. Use of Q-switched ruby laser in the treatment of nevus of ota in different age groups. *Lasers Surg Med.* 2003;32(5):391-395.

90. Ueda S, Isoda M, Imayama S. Response of naevus of Ota to Q-switched ruby laser treatment according to lesion colour. *Br J Dermatol.* 2000;142:77-83.

91. Kang W, Lee E, Choi GS. Treatment of Ota's nevus by Q-switched alexandrite laser: therapeutic outcome in relation to clinical and histopathological findings. *Eur J Dermatol.* 1999;9:639-643.

92. Imayama S, Ueda S. Long- and short-term histological observations of congenital nevi treated with the normal-mode ruby laser. *Arch Dermatol.* 1999;135:1211-1218.

93. Duke D, Byers HR, Sober AJ, Anderson RR, Grevelink JM. Treatment of benign and atypical nevi with the normal-mode ruby laser and the Q-switched ruby laser: clinical improvement but failure to completely eliminate nevomelanocytes. *Arch Dermatol.* 1999;135:290-296.

94. Waldorf HA, Kauvar AN, Geronemus RG. Treatment of small and medium congenital nevi with the Q-switched ruby laser. *Arch Dermatol.* 1996;132:301-304.

95. Alora MB, Anderson RR. Recent developments in cutaneous lasers. *Lasers Surg Med.* 2000;26:108-118.

96. Chong SJ, Jeong E, Park HJ, Lee JY, Cho BK. Treatment of congenital nevomelanocytic nevi with the CO_2 and Q-switched alexandrite lasers. *Dermatol Surg.* 2005;31(5):518-521.

97. Pearson IC, Harland CC. Epidermal naevi treated with pulsed erbium:YAG laser. *Clin Exp Dermatol.* 2004;29(5):494-496.

98. Hohenleutner U, Landthaler M. Laser therapy of verrucous epidermal naevi. *Clin Exp Dermatol.* 1993;18:124-127.

99. Park JH, Hwang ES, Kim SN, Kye YC. Er:YAG laser treatment of verrucous epidermal nevi. *Dermatol Surg.* 2004;30(3):378-381.

100. Ostertag JU, Quaedvlieg PJ, Kerckhoffs FE, et al. Congenital naevi treated with erbium:YAG laser (Derma K) resurfacing in neonates: clinical results and review of the literature. *Br J Dermatol.* 2006;154(5):889-895.

101. Horner BM, El-Muttardi NS, Mayou BJ. Treatment of congenital melanocytic nevi with CO_2 laser. *Ann Plast Surg.* 2005;55:276-280.

102. Hruza GJ. Laser treatment of epidermal and dermal lesions. *Dermatol Clin.* 2002;20:147-164.

103. Serour F, Somekh E. Successful treatment of recalcitrant warts in pediatric patients with carbon dioxide laser. *Eur J Pediatr Surg.* 2003;13(4):219-223.

104. Kwon SD, Kye YC. Treatment of scars with a pulsed Er:YAG laser. *J Cutan Laser Ther.* 2000;2:27-31.

105. Spicer MS, Goldberg DJ, Janniger CK. Lasers in pediatric dermatology. *Cutis.* 1995;55:270-272,278-280.

106. Calobrisi SD, Drolet BA, Esterly NB. Petechial eruption after the application of EMLA cream. *Pediatrics.* 1998;101(3 Pt 1): 471-473.

107. Chen BK, Eichenfield LF. Pediatric anesthesia in dermatologic surgery: when hand-holding is not enough. *Dermatol Surg.* 2001; 27:1010-1018.

108. Rincon E, Baker RL, Iglesias AJ, et al. CNS toxicity after topical application of EMLA cream on a toddler with molluscum contagiosum. *Pediatr Emerg Care.* 2000;16(4):252-254.

109. Friedman PM, Fogelman JP, Nouri K, et al. Comparative study of the efficacy of four topical anesthetics. *Dermatol Surg.* 1999;25(12): 950-954.

110. Keenan RL, Shapiro JH, Dawson K. Frequency of anesthetic cardiac arrests in infants: effect of pediatric anesthesiologists. *J Clin Anesth.* 1991;3:433-437.

111. Vespasiano M, Finkelstein M, Kurachek S. Propofol sedation: intensivists' experience with 7304 cases in a children's hospital. *Pediatrics.* 2007;120(6):e1411-e1417.

112. Cohen MM, Cameron CB, Duncan PG. Pediatric anesthesia morbidity and mortality in the perioperative period. *Anesth Analg.* 1990;70:160-167.

113. Eichenfield LF. Vascular lesion laser: practical techniques or some "light" suggestions. *Pediatr Dermatol.* 1999;16(4):332-334.

114. Burk CJ, Benjamin LT, Connelly EA. Distraction anesthesia for pediatric dermatology procedures. *Pediatr Dermatol.* 2007;4:419-420.

115. Yoo SS, Liggett J, Cohen BA. Use of parent-child tents in pediatric laser surgery. *Dermatol Surg.* 2003;29:399-401.

Dressings/Wound Care for Laser Treatment

Stephen C. Davis and Robert Perez

- Ablative and non-ablative lasers have different effects on the skin.
- Various postoperative treatments have been used, e.g., topical agents and/or dressings (open vs closed techniques).
- Additional research is needed to determine the optimal postoperative care after laser procedures.

Introduction

- The non-ablative lasers use longer wavelengths to infiltrate deeper into the dermis, however their efficacy compared to ablative techniques is not as significant.
- Thermal injury to the dermis after laser procedures results in the normal cellular and molecular cascade associated with injury.
- Varying degrees of erythema, swelling and crust formation are associated with thermal injury.

Laser procedures have increased drastically in the past decade. Advancing technology coupled with increasing environmental stressors, such as higher UV levels due to ozone depletion, have resulted in a large increase in laser procedures.[1] Lasers are an appealing form of therapy for acne scars, photodamage, wrinkles, and discoloration of the skin.[2] Ablative lasers (carbon dioxide – CO_2 and erbium:YAG) have been used effectively for years however with concerns of potential side effects and/or complications, the demand for ablative procedures has decreased with non-ablative techniques dramatically on the rise. The non-ablative lasers use longer wavelengths to infiltrate deeper into the dermis, however their efficacy compared to ablative techniques is not as significant.[3] With the rapid advances in laser technology there is a need to better examine the effects of these new devices on skin as well investigate optimal postoperative regimens. Since there are more complications with ablative techniques, we will focus the below discussion on ablative postoperative care.

In the skin, lasers function through basic photothermolitic principles.[4] With conventional ablative lasers, since water is the targeted chromophore, there is usually ablation of the entire epidermis with subsequent effects on the papillary dermis. Thermal injury to the dermis during this process results in the normal cellular and molecular cascade associated with injury. As part of this cascade, collagen is denatured, resulting in collagen shrinking and tightening of the tissue.[5] As a result, the treated skin regains some of its youthful elasticity and firmness.[6] Generally, lasers that can employ selective photothermolysis with minimal tissue damage are the most desirable.

Although multiple types of lasers are frequently employed using various pulsing techniques and cooling strategies, all skin rejuvenation procedures carry with them some risk of side effects, even in the hands of experts.[7] Most, if not all, laser procedures result in varying degrees of erythema, swelling and crust formation associated with thermal injury.[8] Dependant on the extent of ablation of the epidermis, pain can result due to exposed nerve endings. As with any surgical procedure, viral and bacterial infections are possible, particularly, early in the recovery process. Scarring, hypo-, and hyper-pigmentation also occur, although these effects are fairly uncommon.[9]

S.C. Davis (✉)
Department of Dermatology and Cutaneous Surgery,
University of Miami, Miller School of Medicine, Miami, FL, USA
e-mail: sdavis@med.miami.edu

Available Postoperative Treatments

> - Open techniques use topical agents only
> - Closed techniques use occlusive dressings (with or without topicals)
> - Moist wound healing is important for optimal healing
> - Ideal dressing or topical agent for post surgical care should: (1) stimulate healing, (2) reduce pain, (3) be easy to apply, (4) provide optimal cosmetic results

Various treatment options are available post laser therapy and these include occlusive, semi-occlusive dressings and/or the use of various topical agents. The use of topical agents only is commonly referred to the "open" technique, where the use of occlusive dressing is considered the "closed" technique. It has been well established that keeping wounds moist with an occlusive dressing allows faster epithelization, maintains growth factor viability, alleviates pain, and can reduce scar formation.[10–16] Different postoperative treatments can affect the quality of healing and an ideal dressing or topical agent for post surgical care should: (1) stimulate healing, (2) reduce pain, (3) be easy to apply and (4) provide optimal cosmetic results.[17] Because of the possibility of severe infection or disfiguration of the patient, postoperative therapy should be separated into phases based on the most immediate risks (Table 1). Care should be taken immediately after completion of the procedure to minimize the probability of scar formation and bacteria or viral infection. This is usually accomplished by using various cooling techniques to avoid the necrotic progression usually associated with thermal injury. Anti-inflammatory and antibiotics/antivirals can be used early in the recovery process to promote healing. Within the first 48 h, this can be accomplished by using cold water, corticosteroids, and water-soluble antibiotics. After 72 h, gentle moisturizers can be incorporated into the treatment regimen to enhance water retention in the healing tissue and to minimize the probability of scar formation. One week post-surgery, patients can begin using gentle cleansers to remove any crust or necrotic tissue which may remain in order to limit the nutrient available to pathogens. During the same time period, patients can begin using hypoallergenic make-up to cover any residual erythema. After the third week of recovery, patients can begin focusing on sun protection and conditioning masks to promote skin hydration. Treatment and make-up for residual erythema can be continued or intensified if needed. One month post-procedure, pigment correction can begin for either hypo- or hyper-pigmentation. Sun protection should be continued and scar treatment can begin, should it be necessary.[18]

Immediate Post-operative Treatment (0–48 h)

Immediately after completion of the procedure, ice packs can be applied to a patient to alleviate the burning sensation that is commonly experienced. Petrolatum can be applied to the treated area within 2 h of completion of the procedure.[19] Petrolatum provides some cooling and a moist environment conducive to proper healing. It is interesting to note that Eaglstein and Mertz found that vehicles, including different lots of petrolatum, can have a varied effect of the healing of acute partial thickness wounds.[20] It is also likely that different brands of petrolatum (or other moisturizers) may have varied effects after laser procedures. Petrolatum is sometimes replaced by the addition of an antibiotic cream. Gentamycin ointment is frequently recommended and sometimes combined with prednisone, or other corticoids, to reduce inflammation.[1] Antiseptic washes can be used to remove any remaining eschar and as a prophylactic. Dilute vinegar or chlorhexidine can be used to gently wash the area several times daily to prevent infection and to remove debris.[10] Interestingly, the rate of postoperative infections has also been shown not to be influenced by the use of prophylactic oral and/or intravenous antibiotics in the peri- or post-operative period.[21] Cautious use of antibiotics is suggested in high-risk patients, certain anatomic locations and the presence of infection.[22]

Table 1 Treatment schedule and indications for post-operative recovery

Time post operation	Treatment	Indication
0–48 h	Topicals/dressings Anti-inflammatory Antiseptic Cooling	Enhance healing Swelling Infection prevention
72 h–1 week	Moisturizers Antibiotics Antivirals	Minimize scarring Infection prevention
1–2 weeks	Cleansers Make-up Anti-erythema	Remove crusting Cover and treat erythema
3–4 weeks	Sunblock Anti-erythema	Sun protection Residual erythema
>4 weeks	Vitamins, colorants or bleaching agents	Pigmentation conditions

Anti-inflammatory Agents

- *Corticoids* – Corticosteroids play a major role in the stress response of the body. They serve to modulate the immune system and various inflammatory mechanisms. Corticoids can be used to suppress the inflammatory response due to laser injury but should be used with caution. Although, they have potent anti-inflammatory action, some corticoids can inhibit healing through their interactions with inflammatory cytokines, which are essential of adult mammalian healing.[23]
- *Alpha bisabolol* – Alpha bisabolol is a cyclic monosaturated sesquiterpinic alcohol isolated from the horse chestnut. The compound is more of an anti-irritant than an anti-inflammatory although it does have some anti-inflammatory activity.[24] The agent is highly vasoactive (constrictive) and reduces vessel permeability.[1] These activities are attributed to blockage of 5-lipoxygenase and cyclooxigenase in the arachadonic acid pathway.[25]
- *Enoxolone (glycyrrhetinic acid)* – Enoxolone has been used to reduce inflammation by ancient civilizations since the third century B.C. Evidence of its use has been found in China, Greece, Rome, and Egypt.[26] It is isolated from licorice root and was first described, in modern times, as a potent anti-inflammatory in 1958.[27] The compound functions as a non-steroidal anti-inflammatory but at high doses may induce swelling, redness, and edema by inhibiting 11-hydroxy-steroid-dehydrogenase.[15] At low concentrations, enoxolone has been shown to interfere with steroid metabolism in

renal tissues, resulting in global anti-inflammatory action.[28]

In addition to topical agents, various dressing materials have been used post operative for laser resurfacing. Occlusive dressings can provide a moist environment, protect the wound from bacterial invasion and depending on their composition influence the micro environment.[29–32] The fear of infection which is often associated with the use of occlusive dressings has made many practitioners avoid their use. However, studies have shown lower infection rates with wounds which are covered with certain types of occlusive dressings.[33] When used properly, dressings can enhance patient discomfort, simplify postoperative wound care and do not increase the risk of infection or contact dermatitis.[34]

Optimal postoperative treatment regimens have not been clearly defined. In studies conducted with partial thickness excisional wounds in swine, we found that in order to promote optimal epithelization using an occlusive polyurethane film, the dressings need to be applied within 2 h after wounding and should be kept in place for at least 48 h for optimal healing effects.[20] Whether this is true for laser procedures that have different effects on the tissue, remains to be seen. In another study, we have found that laser sites (porcine model) covered with different dressing materials all epithelized faster than untreated control sites. However, sites which had the least amount of inflammation, also had a "better" histologic appearance which may correlate to a better cosmetic result.[17] Below is a list of various dressing materials with a brief description and mention of potential benefits and disadvantages (Table 2).

Table 2 Dressings available after laser procedures

Dressing	Description/benefits/disadvantages	Example
Transparent films	Polymer sheets (most common – polyurethane) Easy to observe area through dressing Does not absorb exudate	Opsite, Tegaderm, Silon TSR
Foams	Foamed polymers (most common – polyurethane) Adheres to normal skin, absorbs exudate Cannot see through dressing material	Flexzan, Revitaderm
Hydrogel	Hydrophillic polymers (cross linked) Cooling effect for patient's pain Enhances healing of burn wounds Not adhesive to normal skin	Second skin, Vigilon
Polymer mesh	Partially transparent polyethylene or silicon polymers allow the passage of blood and fluids. Semi-occlusive Can be adhesive or non-adhesive to normal skin Does not provide optimal moist environment	N-Terface, Mepitel
Hydrocolloids	Estomeric, adhesive and gelling agents Absorbs exudate well and adheres to normal skin Cannot see through dressing material	DuoDerm
Alignates	Derived from seaweed – hydrophilic gelAbsorbs exudate, hemostatic Can be difficult to remove	Kaltostat

Early Post-operative Treatment (72 h to 1 Week)

During the first week of recovery, a darkening of the skin may be observed mostly due to remnant epidermal debris. While it is essential for optimal healing, the debris may provide a readily available nutrient source for bacteria. Therefore, antibiotic treatment should be continued to prevent infection. The treatment can be combined with moisturizers in order to soften the residual epidermal tissue and provide a moist environment for healing.

Moisturizers

- *Squalene oil (olive oil)* – Olive oil, high in squalene content has been used for centuries to treat burns and wounds in Mediterranean countries. Squalene is a triterpene and an intermediate in cholesterol biosynthesis.[35] Squalene-rich olive oil has been shown to have antioxidant properties and protect skin lipids from oxidation by UV radiation. High olive oil consumption is thought to play a role in the reduced rate of various types of cancers in Mediterranean societies.[36] In addition to its anti-cancer properties, squalene-rich olive oil has been implicated in accelerated wound healing.[1]
- *Hyaluronic acid* – Hyaluronic acid is a naturally occurring component of the skin. Higher amounts of hyaluronic acid in the skin, such as in the developing fetus,[37] have been associated with scarless healing or reduced scar formation.[38] The compound's structure provides it unique hygroscopic, rheological, elastic properties which contribute to the effects it has on the skin. As part of the extracellular matrix of skin, hyaluronic acid helps maintain moisture and elasticity.[39] Both characteristics may play essential roles in healing and in the relief of itching sometimes associated with laser procedures. Increases in the elasticity of the treated skin may result in enhanced results.
- *Bovine mucopolysaccharide-cartilage complex (MCC)* – Preparations of MCC have been used for over 25 years to treat chronic wounds originating from pressure, trauma, vascular insufficiency, or venous stasis. MCC has been shown to reduce inflammation and edema and enhance wound healing.[40,41] Cartilage is made primarily of collagen which, in a wound, provides a scaffold for chemotactic and cellular factors. The scaffolding allows migration and stabilization of granulocytes, macrophages, and fibroblasts, all of which play major roles in cutaneous healing.[42] A comparison of MCC to standard of care for Er:YAG treated skin showed a consistent reduction in the severity of erosion, edema, and inflammation in the MCC treated skin.[43]

- *Silicone ointment* – Silicone ointment can be used as a moisturizer for the first week of post-operative care. Silicone creates a barrier and prevents the skin's exudative process. The trap water is reabsorbed into the tissue and provides a moist environment for cellular migration.[1]

Intermediate Post-operative Treatment (1–2 Weeks)

The intermediate recovery period is a transitional period from active healing and modification in the skin to the remodeling period which will result in near final results. During this period, infection or healing issues should be addressed with more intensive therapies.[1] Usually, the previous treatment regimen can be maintained. However, should any erythema or edema remain, it is usually acceptable to incorporate hypoallergenic make-up as cover. These make-up preparations usually include some of the aforementioned anti-inflammatory agents.[44] Alpha bisabolol is particularly popular in the cosmetic industry for its anti-irritant effects.[14]

Late Post-operative Treatment (3–4 Weeks)

During and after the third week of recovery, the patient should be encouraged to incorporate photoprotective agents into any ongoing regimen. Protection from UV is highly recommended due to the depleted state of the skin following laser treatment. UV protection is a good precaution to avoid pigmentation problems as recovery continues. Because of the initial ablation of melanocytes, the skin may not be fully capable of photoprotection making it more susceptible to DNA damage. The increased vulnerability of the skin during this period may increase a patient's risk of skin cancer or pigmentation inconsistencies. Sun-blocks with micronized titanium dioxide, avobenzene, methoxycinnamate, or D-panthenol can all be used. However, sun blocks with moisturizers and equivalent UV-A and UV-B protection factors should be selected. Ideally, patients would incorporate hats and protective clothing for prolonged sun exposure since most, if not all, sun blocks have limited overall protection.[45]

Post-recovery Pigment Correction (>4 Weeks)

One of the least favorable outcomes in laser resurfacing is pigmentation irregularity. Hypo- and hyperpigmentation can cause serious psychosocial harm to a patient. While most pigmentation issues resolve themselves, some may need treatment or additional therapy to alleviate. In some instances, additional laser procedures or chemical treatments may be necessary to remedy the condition.[46]

- *Hydroquinone* – Hydroquinone is the fastest acting and most commonly used pigment correction agent.[29] In the skin, hydroquinone stops tyrosine action in the skin and interferes with melanosome development.[1]
- *Wildberry extract and kojic acid* – Both preparations contain active forms of hydroquinone, but may produce different results than synthetic hydroquinone due to slightly different modes of action. Wildberry extract contains hydroquinone glycosides which are a very powerful and stable form of the compound. Kojic acid contains a copper kelant which produces a powerful hydroquinone-like activity.[1]
- *Vitamin C* – Vitamin C is usually used in conjunction with depigmentating agents to enhance their activity. In addition, Vitamin C stimulates fibroblasts and protects skin from photodamage.[47]
- *Retinoic acid* – Retinoic acid is used as a bleaching agent for post-inflammatory hyperpigmentation. However, retinoic acid may be irritating and should be used in combination with anti-irritants.[48] Although the mode of action of retinoic acid has not been completely elucidated, some studies suggest that the compound functions by inhibiting the detoxification enzyme glutathione-S-transferase increasing melancytotoxicity.[49]

Scarring

Hypertrophic scarring is a serious, but rare side-effect of laser resurfacing. In addition to psychosocial implications, hypertrophic scars may cause significant pain and loss of function. Many factors can contribute to the development of scars. Poor surgical technique or inappropriate laser parameters can damage the deeper tissue resulting in extensive thermal necrosis and scarring. Some anatomical locations require more care or milder techniques for resurfacing. For example, the mandibular and anterior neck regions are more susceptible to scarring and should be treated with caution.[50] Post-operative infection, family history, previous dermabrasion, or isotretinoin treatment may contribute strongly to the likelihood of scar formation.[51]

- *Class I corticosteroids* – Corticosteroids modulate the bodies inflammatory and immune response. Topical and intralesional treatment may aid in halting scar progression. The treatment regimen should begin immediately upon detection of abnormal erythema with tissue induration.[31]

- *Silicone gel* – Silicone gels have been used successfully in the treatment of hypertrophic scars resulting from burn injury. Whether this is due to their occlusive properties or a unique characteristic of the silicone gel is unclear. Treatment moderately improved scar thickness and scar color.[52] Clinical trials have demonstrated the ability of silicon gels to stop the progression of and soften newly forming scars.[53] Trials on established scars have been equally as successful in reducing firmness and improving elasticity of 1–6 month old scars.[54]
- *Imiquimod 5% cream* – Imiquimod cream is a topical immune response modulator. Imiquimod stimulates proinflammatory cytokines, particularly interferon-α. This results in a cell mediated response which results in collagen break-down. Although treatments frequently results in some erythema, local pain, and pinpoint bleeding, imiquimod results in significant improvement in scar quality, elevation, and color.[55]

Conclusion

There are few well controlled studies that determine the optimal treatment regimen post laser therapy. Whether a specific combination of agents and/or dressings provide the best environment to allow beneficial cosmetic effects while reducing potential complications, remains to be seen. Since there is an increase in new lasers that are being developed for various procedures, there also needs to be additional research conducted to determine which postoperative care treatments have the most beneficial result. Although some of these studies can be performed in a controlled preclinical setting, well designed clinical trials are needed.

References

1. Chajchir A, Benzaquen I. Carbon dioxide laser resurfacing with fast recovery. *Aesthetic Plast Surg*. 2005;29:107-112.
2. Tanzi EL, Alster TS. Single-pass carbon dioxide laser versus multiple-pass Er:YAG laser skin resurfacing: a comparison of postoperative wound healing and side effects. *Dermatol Surg*. 2003; 29(1):80-84.
3. Sadick NS. Update on non-ablative light therapy for rejuvenation: a review. *Lasers Surg Med*. 2003;32:120-128.
4. Anderson RR, Parrish JA. Selective photothermolysis, precise microsurgery by selective absorption of pulsed radiation. *Science*. 1983;220:524-527.
5. Ross EV, McKinlay JR, Anderson RR. Why does carbon dioxide resurfacing work? a review. *Arch Dermatol*. 1999;135:444-454.
6. Kunzi-Rapp K, Dierickx CC, Cambier B, Drosner M. Minimally invasive skin rejuvination with erbium:YAG laser used in thermal mode. *Lasers Surg Med*. 2006;38:899-907.
7. Willey A, Anderson RR, Azpiazu JL, et al. Complications of laser dermatologic surgery. *Lasers Surg Med*. 2006;38:1-15.

8. Chan HHL, Lam L, Wong DSY, Wei WI. Role of skin cooling improving patient tolerability of Q-switched alexandrite (QS alex) laser in nevus of Ota treatment. *Lasers Surg Med.* 2003;32: 148-151.

9. Ho DD, London R, Zimmerman GB, Young DA. Laser-tattoo removal: a study of the mechanism and the optimal treatment strategy via computer simulations. *Lasers Surg Med.* 2002;30: 389-397.

10. Winter GD. Formation of the scab and the rate of epithelisation of superficial wounds in the skin of the young domestic pig. *Nature.* 1962;193:293-294.

11. Eaglstein WH, Mertz PM. New method for assessing epidermal wound healing: the effects of triamcinolone acetonide and polyethelene film occlusion. *J Invest Dermatol.* 1978;71:382-384.

12. Eaglstein WH. Effect of occlusive dressings on wound healing. *Clin Dermatol.* 1984;2(3):107-111.

13. Alvarez OM, Mertz PM, Eaglstein WH. The effect of occlusive dressings on collagen synthesis and re-epithelialization in superficial wounds. *J Surg Res.* 1983;35:142-148.

14. Ono I, Suda K, Iwatsuki K, Kaneko F. Evaluation of cytokines in donor site wound fluids. *Scand J Plast Reconstr Surg Hand Surg.* 1994;28(4):269-273.

15. Nemeth AJ, Eaglstein WH, Taylor JR, Peerson LJ, Falanga V. Faster healing and less pain in skin biopsy sites treated with an occlusive dressing. *Arch Dermatol.* 1991;127(11):1679-1683.

16. Eisenberg M. The effect of occlusive dressings on re-epithelializations of wounds in children with epidermolysis bullosa. *J Pediatr Surg.* 1986;21(10):892-894.

17. Davis SC, Badiavas E, Rendon-Pellerano MI, Pardo RJ. Histological comparison of postoperative wound care regimens for laser resurfacing in a porcine model. *Dermatol Surg.* 1999;25:387-393.

18. Berwald C, Levy JL, Magalon G. Complications of the resurfacing laser: a retrospective study of 749 patients. *Ann Chir Plast Esthét.* 2004;49:360-365.

19. Kilmer SL, Chotzen VA, Silva SK, McClaren ML. Safe and effective carbon dioxide laser skin resurfacing of the neck. *Lasers Surg Med.* 2006;38:653-657.

20. Eaglstein WH, Mertz PM. "Inert" vehicles do affect wound healing. *J Invest Dermatol.* 1980;74:90-91.

21. Walia S, Alster TS. Cutaneous CO_2 laser resurfacing infection rate with and without prophylactic antibioitics. *Dermatol Surg.* 1999;25: 857-861.

22. Messingham MJ, Arpey CJ. Update on the use of antibiotics in cutaneous surgery. *Dermatol Surg.* 2005;31:1068-1078.

23. Christian LM, Graham JE, Padgett DA, Glaser R, Kiecolt-Glaser JK. Stress and wound healing. *Neuroimmunomodulation.* 2006;13: 337-346.

24. Andersen F, Hedegaard K, Petersen TK, Bindslev-Jensen C, Fullerton A, Andersen KE. The hairless guinea-pig as a model for treatment of cumulative irritation in humans. *Skin Res Technol.* 2006;12:60-67.

25. Andersen F, Hedegaard K, Petersen TK, Bindslev-Jensen C, Fullerton A, Andersen KE. Anti-irritants I: dose-response in acute irritation. *Contact Dermatitis.* 2006;55:148-154.

26. Shibata S. A drug over the millennia: pharmacognosy, chemistry, and pharmacology of licorice. *Yakugaku Zasshi.* 2000;120: 849-862.

27. Finney RS, Somers GF. The antiinflammatory activity of glycyrrhetinic acid and derivatives. *J Pharm Pharmacol.* 1958;10: 613-620.

28. Schleimer RP. Potential regulation of inflammation in the lung by local metabolism of hydrocortisone. *Am J Respir Cell Mol Biol.* 1991;4:166-173.

29. Eaglstein WH, Davis SC, Mehle AL, Mertz PM. Optimal use of an occlusive dressing to enhance healing. *Arch Dermatol.* 1988;124(3): 392-395.

30. Mertz PM, Marshall DA, Eaglstein WH. Occlusive wound dressings to prevent bacterial invasion and wound infection. *J Am Acad Dermatol.* 1985;12:434-440.

31. Mertz PM, Davis SC, Cazzaniga A, Drosou A, Eaglstein W. Barrier and antibacterial properties of 2-octyl cyanoacrylate derived wound treatment films. *J Cutan Med Surg.* 2003;7(1):1-12.

32. Oliveria MF, Davis SC, Mertz PM. Can occlusive dressing composition influence proliferation of bacterial wound pathogens? *Wounds.* 1998;10(1):4-11.

33. Hutchinson JJ. Prevalence of wound infection under occlusive dressings: a collective survery of the literature. *Wounds.* 1989;1: 123-133.

34. Newman JP, Fitzberald P, Koch RJ. Review of closed dressings after laser resurfacing. *Dermatol Surg.* 2000;26:562-571.

35. Smith TJ. Squalene: potential chemopreventive agent. *Expert Opin Investig Drugs.* 2000;9:1841-1848.

36. Owen RW, Giacosa A, Hull WE, et al. Olive-oil consumption and health: the possible role of antioxidants. *Lancet Oncol.* 2000;1: 107-112.

37. Mast BA, Diegelmann RF, Krummel TM, Cohen IK. Scarless wound healing in the mammalian fetus. *Surg Gynecol Obstet.* 1992; 174:441-451.

38. Colwell AS, Longaker MT, Lorenz HP. Fetal wound healing. *Front Biosci.* 2003;1:s1240-s1248.

39. Chen WY, Abatangelo G. Functions of hyaluronan in wound repair. *Wound Repair Regen.* 1999;7:79-89.

40. Pudden JF, Allen J. The clinical acceleration of healing with a cartilage preparation. *J Am Med Assoc.* 1965;192:352-356.

41. King S. Catrix: an easy-to-use collagen treatment for wound healing. *Br J Community Nurs.* 2005;10:s31-s34.

42. Purna SK, Babu M. Collagen based dressings-a review. *Burns.* 2000;26:54-62.

43. Tanzi EL, Perez M. The effect of a mucopolysaccharide-cartilage complex healing ointment on Er:YAG laser resurfaced facial skin. *Dermatol Surg.* 2002;28:305-308.

44. Grassi A, Palermi G, Paradisi M. Study of tolerance and efficacy of cosmetic preparations with lenitive action in atopic dermatitis in children. *Clin Ter.* 2000;151:77-80.

45. Lautenschlage S, Wulf HC, Pittelkow MR. Photoprotection. *Lancet.* 2007;370:528-537.

46. Ke MS, Soriano T, Lask GP. Optimal treatments for hyperpigmentation. *J Cosmet Laser Ther.* 2006;8:7-13.

47. Gross RL. The effect of ascorbate on wound healing. *Int Ophthamol Clin.* 2000;40:51-57.

48. Alster T, Lupton JR. Treatment of complications of laser skin resurfacing. *Arch Facial Plast Surg.* 2000;2:279-284.

49. Kasraee B, Handjani F, Aslani FS. Enhancement of the depigmenting effect of hydroquinone and 4-hydroxyanisole by all-trans-retinoic acid (tretinoin): the impairment of glutathione-dependent cytoprotection? *Dermatology.* 2003;206:289-291.

50. Nanni CA, Alster TS. Complications of cutaneous laser surgery: a review. *Dermatol Surg.* 1998;24:209-219.

51. Katz BE, MacFarlane DF. Atypical facial scarring after isotretinoin therapy in a patient with previous dermabrasion. *J Am Acad Dermatol.* 1994;30:852-853. s.

52. Gold MH. Topical silicone gel sheeting in the treatment of hypertrophic scars and keloids. A dermatologic experience. *J Dermatol Surg Oncol.* 1993;19:912-916.

53. Fulton JJ. Silicone gel sheeting for the prevention and management of evolving hypertrophic and keloid scars. *Dermatol Surg.* 1995;21: 947-951.

54. Carney S, Cason CG, Gowar JP, Stevenson JH, McNee J, Groves AR. Cica-care gel sheeting in the management of hypertrophic scarring. *Burns.* 1994;20:163-167.

55. Zurada JM, Kriegel D, Davis IC. Topical treatments for hypertrophic scars. *J Am Acad Dermatol.* 2006;55:1024-1031.

Prevention and Treatment of Laser Complications

Rachael L. Moore, Juan-Carlos Martinez, and Ken K. Lee

- Lasers are useful for treating a variety of dermatologic conditions but have a number of potential complications associated with their use.
- A basic understanding of laser mechanics is paramount in preventing and troubleshooting complications.
- Wavelength, fluence, pulse duration and spot size can be varied to achieve the desired effect on tissue.
- The innovation of coupling surface cooling with laser treatment has allowed for the use of increased fluence to maximize treatment efficacy while minimizing damage to the overlying epidermis.
- Complications can be avoided by keeping the operating room safe. This includes the use of eye protection and smoke evacuators, when indicated. Operating suites should have well marked signs and restricted entry. Lasers should be kept in standby mode when not in use.
- Only adequately trained physicians should evaluate patients and determine their candidacy for laser treatment and select treatment parameters. This will help ensure that lasers are not being used inadequately to treat potentially hazardous indications such as skin cancers.
- Patients that give a history of pigmentary disorders, connective tissue diseases or abnormal scarring are at increased risk of having an adverse event following laser therapy. Those on certain medications or with dark or tanned skin are also at increased risk.

- Pain, erythema and edema, crusting and vesiculation, purpura, dyspigmentation and scarring are side effects caused by treatment with most dermatologic lasers to varying degrees. These side effects can be minimized or avoided entirely when proper precautions are taken.

Other side effects are unique to treatment of specific conditions. For example, tattoo removal can be associated with allergic contact dermatitis or paradoxical tattoo darkening, while resurfacing procedures pose an increased risk of infection.

Introduction

Dermatologic laser therapy was initially introduced in the 1960s; however, it was not until the theory of selective photothermolysis was introduced that their use became widespread. There are a variety of side effects and complications associated with laser therapy. Some of these are unavoidable but many are preventable. Understanding laser mechanics and how to vary wavelength, fluence, pulse duration and spot size to achieve the desired effect can help minimize or prevent adverse events. Cooling has allowed for the use of increased fluence to maximize treatment efficacy by protecting the epidermis from excess thermal damage.

R.L. Moore (✉)
Dermatologic and Laser Surgery, Oregon Health and
Sciences University, 3303 SW Bond Avenue CH16D,
Portland, OR 97239, USA
e-mail: moorerac@ohsu.edu

K. Nouri (ed.), *Lasers in Dermatology and Medicine*,
DOI: 10.1007/978-0-85729-281-0_29, © Springer-Verlag London Limited 2011

Since the introduction of lasers into the dermatologic field by Dr. Leon Goldman in 1963,[1] they have become both standard treatment for many dermatoses and a source of future innovations. While generally considered safe and well tolerated, their potential to cause adverse events should not be underestimated. A thorough understanding of lasers and their applications is paramount in managing predictable side effects and avoiding complications. This chapter will briefly outline laser mechanics, provide a detailed description of both common and uncommon complications, and discuss their prevention and treatment.

Laser Mechanics

The word *laser* is an acronym for *l*ight *a*mplification by the *s*timulated *e*mission of *r*adiation.[2] Laser light is unique in that it is composed of a single wavelength and all emitted photons are in the same phase. These properties are termed monochromatic and coherent, respectively. The wavelength of light is determined by the optical medium, which can be a solid (e.g., alexandrite), liquid (e.g., pulsed dye laser) or gas (e.g., carbon dioxide laser). When laser light hits the skin, it is absorbed, reflected, transmitted, or scattered. The desired treatment effect occurs when the light is absorbed and the energy is converted to heat (photothermal), acoustic waves (photomechanical) or used in chemical reactions (photochemical). The majority of dermatologic lasers employ photothermal reactions.

In 1983, the theory of selective photothermolysis was introduced, revolutionizing the application of lasers.[3] This theory posits that because each chromophore has a unique photoabsorption spectrum, it can be selectively targeted and destroyed using specific wavelengths. Endogenous chromophores include melanin, hemoglobin and water.[2] Tattoo ink is an exogenous chromophore frequently targeted with laser therapy.

A basic understanding of laser physics is required to troubleshoot complications and difficult-to-treat patients. By varying wavelength, fluence, pulse duration and spot size, the desired effect can be achieved (see Table 1 for definitions). The wavelength of light used determines which tissue chromophores will be targeted. The energy per area emitted by the laser is the fluence. High fluence can result in untoward damage to tissue, while insufficient fluence will lead to incomplete treatment. The concept of pulse duration is vital in minimizing damage to the surrounding tissue. The ideal pulse duration is generally the same[4] or shorter[2] than the thermal relaxation time (TRT) of the target. Immediately following photon absorption, the chromophore loses this newly absorbed energy in the form of heat. TRT is the time required for a chromophore to lose 50% of its heat to the surrounding tissue and is directly proportional to the square of its diameter. Thus, there is a positive relationship between pulse duration, TRT and diameter of the target. Destruction of targets with a small diameter, such as melanosomes, requires small pulse durations in order to limit damage to surrounding tissue. Those with a larger diameter, such as blood vessels, can be treated with longer pulse durations. For this reason, *Quality-* or Q-switched (QS) lasers (see Table 1 for definitions) are often used for pigmented lesions, while pulsed dye lasers (PDL), with pulse durations in the millisecond range, are used for vascular lesions.

Spot size and wavelength can each impact the depth of penetration of the laser. Depth of penetration is determined by both the amount of light absorption in the tissue and the scatter.[2] In general, larger spot sizes (10–15 mm) and longer wavelengths (1,000–1,200 nm) have less scatter than smaller spot sizes (3–5 mm) and shorter wavelengths (300–400 nm) and penetrate deeper into the tissue. However, when wavelengths exceed approximately 1,300 nm, such as the CO_2 resurfacing laser at 10,600 nm, depth is limited to the superficial epidermis due to absorption by water, the primary targeted chromophore in this range.

Cooling

The ideal laser settings will provide enough thermal energy and selectivity to damage the targeted chromophore while minimizing injury to the surrounding skin.[5] However, the energy required to damage the target often exceeds that which is needed to harm the overlying epidermis. In order to

Table 1 Common laser definitions

Term	Definition	Unit of measurement
Fluence	Energy delivered per unit area	J/cm^2
Pulse duration (pulse length or pulse width) • Q-switched • Long-pulsed	The time it takes a waveform to reach 50% of its full amplitude • Q-switch is an optical valve in a laser that allows for rapid energy build-up before it is open to allow light out	 • 10^{-9}–10^{-12} s • 10^{-3} s
Thermal relaxation time (TRT)	Time required for a target to lose 50% of its heat to the surrounding environment TRT $\propto$ (directly) target diameter^2	s
Spot size	The diameter of the opening through which the laser beam is emitted	cm

overcome this obstacle, cooling devices have been implemented. Many laser handpieces are now equipped with cryogen spray cooling or sapphire contact plates that cool the skin immediately prior to the laser pulse. The epidermis is then selectively cooled, raising the threshold for thermal damage, while temperatures for the intended (deeper) dermal targets are relatively unaffected. Pre-cooling with ice-packs, gel and aluminum rollers can also be used but these are generally not as effective as the incorporated cooling devices. In addition to increasing the treatment efficacy of lasers, cooling also plays a prominent role in providing anesthesia during therapy.

General Considerations

Safety in the operating suites, professional errors and certain patient factors should be initially considered to help limit adverse events. The operating suites should have well marked signs and restricted access, and lasers should be kept in standby mode when not in use. Use of eye protection and smoke evacuators should be employed when indicated. An appropriately trained physician should evaluate all patients to determine candidacy prior to laser treatment. This will limit improper laser treatment of various diseases, such as skin cancers. Laser parameters should also be set by the clinician. Patients with a history of pigmentary disorders, connective tissue disease or abnormal scarring may be at increased risk for laser treatment. Additionally, those with dark or tanned skin or taking certain medications may suffer from additional side effects.

Safety in the Operating Rooms

Lasers are useful medical devices but can be dangerous. The operating staff and patient are susceptible to a number of hazards, including burns, accidental fires, infection and ocular injury. General safety measures, such as a visible door sign when the laser is in use and controlled access into the laser areas, are important. All lasers should be kept in standby mode when not in use and have a rapid deactivation mode to prevent unintentional firing. To avoid accidental fires, the use of oxygen and alcohol-based cleansing methods should be minimized. Each laser should have its own outlet, limiting the use of extension cords. Since human papilloma virus (HPV)[6] and human immunodeficiency virus (HIV)[7] particles have been found in aerosolized material after laser therapy, a smoke evacuator should be employed when lasers with significant potential to splatter aerosolized particles (such as CO_2 resurfacing) are used.

Lasers can subject the unprotected eye to significant damage, including visual loss. The degree of ocular damage is determined by the wavelength of light as well as the amount and duration of energy exposure.[8] Within the eye, there is a broad absorption spectrum resulting from three primary chromophores: melanosomes, found in the retinal epithelium, iris, sclera and choroid; hemoglobin, found in retinal vasculature; and water, found primarily in the cornea and lens. The symptoms associated with damage to these ocular structures are summarized in Table 2. Especially important to remember is that absorption of light outside the visual spectrum is visually undetectable. Additionally, due to their lack of sensory innervation, absorption damage to the retina, iris, choroid and sclera can be painless. Thus, ocular exposure to wavelengths in the near infrared range (700–1,400 nm), which is primarily absorbed by these pigmented eye structures, can lead to pronounced injury without symptoms.[8,10]

To prevent untoward injury, wavelength-specific eye protection should be worn any time the laser is in operation. Metal contact lenses should be placed on the patient when treating periorbital skin, and metal goggles should be worn for the treatment of facial lesions. Plastic goggles should be avoided in these cases due to the risk of melting. Pediatric and smaller patients should have size-specific goggles; if these are not available, the use of a thick layer of white gauze (which non-specifically absorbs and reflects laser light) can be used.

Professional Errors

An appropriately trained physician should evaluate all patients prior to laser treatment to determine whether they will be

Table 2 Ocular structures at risk for laser injury[8-10]

Wavelength (nm)	Susceptible ocular structure	Chromophore	Mechanism	Associated symptoms
180–400	Cornea and lens	Tissue proteins	Photochemical	Pain
400–700	Retina, iris, choroid, sclera	Melanin	Photothermal	Color flash and afterimage
700–1,400	As above	As above	As above	No symptoms until significant visual loss
1,400–10,600	Cornea and lens	Water	As above	Immediate burning pain

Table 3 Medications potentially associated with increased risk of laser therapy complications

Medication	Possible associated complications	Recommendations
Blood thinning agents: • Aspirin • Coumadin • Vitamin E • Anti-platelet agents	Increased bruising, bleeding	Consider discontinuation if using laser with high bruising potential (e.g., PDL)
Indomethacin	Increased scarring potential shown in murine models[15]	Not good evidence for discontinuation, but may consider if high risk of scarring
Isotretinoin	Hypertrophic scarring reported after dermabrasion[16]; other studies have shown no increased risk[17,18]	Consider discontinuation 6 months prior, especially if using lasers with high scarring potential (e.g., ablative resurfacing)[19]; evidence for this, however, is weak
Drugs that induce pigmentation: • Minocycline • Amiodarone • Anti-malarials • Tricyclic anti-depressants (e.g., desipramine, imipramine)	Dyspigmentation	Consider discontinuation prior to procedure if there is increased risk of dyspigmentation (e.g., dark or tanned skin, ablative resurfacing procedures)
Gold (parenteral)	Localized chrysiasis after QS laser treatment[20]	Consider avoiding treatment in patients with history of parenteral gold therapy

appropriate candidates for therapy. Some patients are at increased risk of sustaining complications (see Patient Factors section below), and these factors should be considered prior to choosing laser parameters. In some cases these risk factors may prove to be contraindications to laser treatment, as the risk of complications may outweigh the benefits. Verbal and written informed consent, including an explanation of the potential risks and benefits, alternative treatment options, number of treatment sessions, and cost per session should be obtained prior to the planned procedure which can help avoid the patient feeling pressured into making a quick decision.[11]

The indication for laser therapy must be appropriate. While treatment of rhytides may seem straightforward, treatment of other lesions, such as those on photo-damaged skin, may present more challenges to the non-dermatologist. Often, only minor differences distinguish a solar lentigo from a melanoma, or an actinic keratosis from a nonmelanoma skin cancer. These subtleties may not be obvious to the untrained clinician. Any lesion in question should be biopsied prior to treatment.

Troubleshooting complications requires a firm understanding of laser mechanics. A skilled operator will not only choose appropriate laser settings, but will be attentive in monitoring the tissue reaction to the laser treatment. An immediate white/gray discoloration can indicate significant thermal damage requiring modification of laser settings. Ideally, test spots should be done at least 2 weeks prior to the planned procedure.

Patient Factors

Patient factors must be taken into account in the assessment of an individual's risk profiles. Patients with dark or tanned

skin are at increased risk of hypopigmentation if treated with lasers that target melanosomes. Any history of abnormal scarring, vasculopathy or vitiligo should be elicited, as these conditions may indicate a propensity toward hypertrophic scarring, bruising and dyspigmentation, respectively. Treatment should be avoided in areas with concurrent infection or inflammation as it can exacerbate these conditions. Connective tissue diseases, which can be a marker for photosensitivity, may be a contraindication to laser therapy.[12] One study reported new-onset discoid lupus erythematosus thought to be from thermal injury sustained after argon laser treatment for facial telangiectases.[13] Debate exists in the literature, however, as others have successfully treated discoid lupus with similar lasers.[14] Additionally, there are several medications (summarized in Table 3) that may confer an increased risk of complications. These should be considered and avoided if possible.[15,16,19,20]

General Laser Complications

Dermatologic lasers share a number of side effects that can be minimized or avoided when proper precautions are taken. Wavelength, fluence, pulse duration, spot size and cooling can all impact the degree of side effects experienced. Overlapping pulses and high fluences may help achieve a desired affect, but can increase the risk of complications. In general, ablative resurfacing procedures have an increased incidence of these complications compared with other laser modalities.

Prevention and Treatment of Laser Complications

Table 4 Commonly used lasers listed by indication

Vascular lesions	Pigmented lesions	Tattoo removal	Photoepilation	Resurfacing
PDL (585–600 nm)	QS Ruby (694 nm)	QS Ruby (694 nm)	LP Ruby (694 nm)	Carbon dioxide (10,600 nm)
LP Nd:YAG (1,064 nm)	QS Nd:YAG (532, 1,064 nm)	QS Nd:YAG (532, 1,064 nm)	LP Nd:YAG (1,064 nm)	Er:YAG (2,490 nm)
LP KTP (532 nm)	QS Alexandrite (755 nm)	QS Alexandrite (755 nm)	LP Alexandrite (755 nm)	Fractional (1540 nm)
IPL	IPL		LP Diode (800 nm)	
IPL			IPL	

Er:YAG erbium:yttrium aluminum garnet, *IPL* intense pulsed light, *KTP* potassium titanyl phosphate, *Nd:YAG* neodymium:yttrium aluminum garnet, *PDL* pulsed dye laser, *QS* Q-switched, *LP* long-pulsed

Lasers can be used to treat a wide variety of conditions and each laser has its own unique properties (Table 4). A complication, or adverse event, can be defined as any undesirable or unforeseen outcome after a particular treatment. This is to be distinguished from a side effect, which is expected after therapy. However, many side effects, if severe, can lead to complications.

The most common complications, which can occur with any laser, are pain, erythema and edema, crusting and vesiculation, purpura, dyspigmentation and scarring. Identifying the causative factor for each of these common complications can aid in their prevention and treatment. It is important to ask the following:

- *Am I treating the correct indication and patient with the correct laser?*
- *Was the fluence appropriate?*
- *Was the pulse duration appropriate?*
- *Was the correct spot size used?*
- *Was the cooling appropriate?*
- *Was there too much pulse overlap or stacking of passes?*

The purpose of this section will be to review each of these common side effects and discuss their prevention and management.

Pain

Risk Factors for Excess Pain

- Inadequate anesthesia
- High fluence
- Insufficient cooling

Although certain lasers are associated with more pain than others, some level of mild pain is an expected side effect of most laser therapy. Unexpected or excessive pain, however, can occur with inadequate anesthesia or inappropriate laser settings (excess fluence or insufficient cooling).

Prevention and Treatment

It is imperative to appropriately anesthetize patients, as needed, prior to their procedure. Some lasers (e.g., the PDL) often do not require pre-treatment anesthesia, while use of other lasers (e.g., resurfacing lasers) require significant pain control. Anesthetics can be injected subcutaneously to provide local relief, whereas regional nerve blocks can provide anesthesia over a larger area. For those patients unable to tolerate the pain from injection of local anesthetic, pre-cooling with aluminum rollers or ice-packs for several minutes or application of topical anesthetic compounds 1 h prior to needle insertion can minimize their discomfort. Pretreatment with Er:YAG pulses followed by topical lidocaine may minimize needle insertion pain even further.[21]

Anesthesia may also be achieved with only topical treatment. A randomized, placebo controlled trial with 30 patients found topical lidocaine/tetracaine (S-Caine) peels successful in adequately relieving pain associated with tattoo removal.[22] A set protocol with hot compresses, topical lidocaine and oral anxiolytics (vicodin, diazepam or ketorolac) provided adequate pain relief in 190 of 200 patients who underwent CO_2 resurfacing in a recent case series.[23] The disadvantage of using topical treatments, however, is the additional time required for the anesthetic to take effect.

Cooling devices have played a large role in minimizing pain and optimizing treatment of specific lesions. Decreased pain was associated with concomitant cooling in both the treatment of port-wine stains with the PDL[24] and pigmented lesions with the QS Alexandrite.[25] Pre-cooling (e.g., with aluminum rollers or ice packs) may also significantly reduce pain.[26]

Erythema and Edema

Risk Factors for Excess Erythema and Edema

- Pulse stacking, multiple passes
- High energy settings

- Location (periocular > other areas)
- Patient factors (fair skin > dark skin; history of acne rosacea)
- Use of topical tretinoin prior to procedure
- Inadequate post-treatment cooling

Erythema and edema are expected side effects of most laser therapies. Although these are usually transient, they can persist for months. A retrospective study of 500 patients who underwent CO_2 laser resurfacing found that all patients experienced post-operative erythema lasting an average of 4.5 months.[27] Prolonged erythema and edema occurs in preventable situations. Excess pulse stacking or passes,[28] treatment of periocular areas, and use of high energy settings can all lead to prolonged erythema and edema. Additionally, patients with fair skin or a history of acne rosacea may be predisposed to intense erythema. Use of irritating medications, such as topical tretinoin, may also worsen erythema.[29]

Prevention and Treatment

If possible, unnecessary risks should be avoided. However, treatment efficacy is often maximized with pulse stacking and use of high-energy settings. Ensuring the patient is aware of these risks and that their expectations are appropriate cannot be overemphasized. Management of erythema and edema is supportive: application of post-treatment cold-packs, head elevation and sun precautions are important. Topical or oral corticosteroids can be used in severe cases. Topical ascorbic acid may be effective in decreasing the post-operative severity and duration of erythema after ablative resurfacing procedures.[30]

Crusting and Vesiculation

Risk Factors for Excess Crusting and Vesiculation

- High fluence
- Insufficient cooling
- Small spot size
- Short wavelengths

Crusting and vesiculation are manifestations of epidermal damage that generally results from excess thermal injury. This is commonly due to high fluence and/or insufficient cooling. Additionally, treatment with small spot sizes and shorter wavelengths imparts a higher risk of epidermal damage due to shallower depth of penetration. It is important to keep in mind, however, that some superficial crusting is an expected side effect for many lasers.

Prevention and Treatment

Treatment is supportive. Keeping wounds moist with petrolatum may help speed the recovery process and minimize the risk of scarring. Use of over-the-counter antibiotic ointments should be avoided as neomycin and bacitracin are some of the most common causes of allergic contact dermatitis[31] and bacitracin has shown no wound healing benefit over white petrolatum.[32] Sun precautions are recommended. Patients should be instructed not to unroof blisters, if they form. Symptomatic bullae can be lanced in a sterile fashion.

Purpura

Risk Factors for Excess Purpura

- High fluence
- Long wavelengths
- Treatment with pulsed dye lasers (purpura mode)

Purpura results when there is damage to small vessels and subsequent extravasation of red blood cells. It is common following treatment with the PDL and is, in fact, a therapeutic endpoint when treating certain vascular lesions with short pulse durations and high fluences (so-called purpura-mode). Nevertheless, unexpected bruising can occur with use of other lasers if the fluence is set too high. Lasers with long wavelengths penetrate deeper and have a greater risk of damaging dermal blood vessels. Cooling, which primarily protects the epidermis, has little impact on the amount of damage to dermal blood vessels.

Prevention and Treatment

If possible, all patients should be off anti-coagulant and anti-platelet agents at least several days prior to the planned procedure. Discontinuing a medication, even if transiently, should always be discussed with the patient's prescribing physician first.

Lowering fluence and increasing pulse duration (in the PDL) can help minimize purpura.

Because many vascular lesions, such as port wine stains and hemangiomas, cannot be effectively treated with non-purpuric parameters, patients should be aware of the potential down-time post-treatment. This is particularly important for people with high cosmetic demands. In one study, 45% of patients with purpura after treatment of their port-wine stains reported significant restriction in activity, primarily due to the bruising.[33]

It has been suggested that the use of topical Vitamin K will help both prevent and minimize post-treatment bruising. A small randomized controlled study found decreased bruising severity with twice daily application of vitamin K cream for 2 weeks following laser treatment with the PDL.[34] However, the same study found that pre-treatment with vitamin K cream for 2 weeks did not seem to alter the bruising.

Arnica (*Arnica montana*) is an herbal remedy that has been purported both to help prevent the development and aid in the treatment of bruises. However, a randomized, double-blinded, placebo-controlled, split-face study with 19 patients found no difference in either 2-week pre-treatment or 2-week post-treatment application of arnica gel compared with placebo.[35]

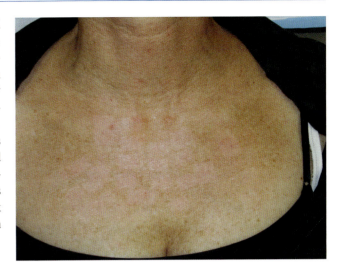

Fig. 1 Reticulated hypopigmentation after IPL treatment. This likely resulted from actinic bronzing that caused increased absorption of light. This is transient; with subsequent treatments the dyspigmentation will even out

Dyspigmentation

Risk Factors for Dyspigmentation

- High fluence
- Inadequate cooling
- Patients factors (dark, tanned > fair skin)
- Short wavelength
- Small spot size

Dyspigmentation can be transient or permanent and takes on two forms: hyper- or hypopigmentation. Hyperpigmentation is a common manifestation of post-inflammatory change in the tissue. Following resurfacing procedures, it is seen in one-third of all patients and nearly all of those with Fitzpatrick type IV-VI skin (reviewed in[29]). It generally appears 3–4 weeks post-operatively and spontaneously resolves over the next several months, though permanent hyperpigmentation can occur.

Hypopigmentation occurs when lasers inadvertently target melanin (Figs. 1 and 2). QS lasers and IPL often cause a transient hypopigmentation during treatment due to the absorption of light by melanin and subsequent injury to individual melanosomes (Fig. 1). Following resurfacing procedures, "relative hypopigmentation" can be seen where treated areas lie adjacent to untreated, photodamaged (darker) skin.[29] However, if the fluence is too high or cooling is inadequate, thermal injury can extend beyond the melanosome and damage melanocytes and other tissue structures, causing permanent hypopigmentation. Rarely, permanent hypopigmentation can appear 6–12 months after resurfacing procedures ("delayed hypopigmentation") due to thermal injury.

In general, patients with dark or tanned skin have a greater risk of dyspigmentation (Fig. 2). For such patients, treatment with lasers with shallower depths of penetration (i.e., shorter

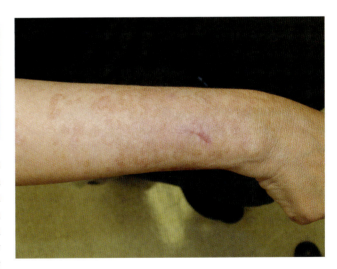

Fig. 2 Hypopigmentation and scar formation after IPL treatment. Treatment took place when the patient was tan, potentially leading to this complication

wavelengths and smaller spot sizes) confers greater injury to epidermal melanocytes and should be avoided.

Prevention and Treatment

Patients should be aware of dyspigmentation risks and have appropriate expectations. For those with darker skin types, lasers with longer wavelengths and larger spot sizes should be considered, as the depth of penetration will be greater and risk of injury to epidermal melanocytes smaller.[36] If these options are not available, treatment with lower fluences is prudent.

Caution should be used when treating patients who are tan. To prevent sun exposure to planned treatment areas, patients should be advised to keep tattoos or other sites covered, if possible, for 1 month prior to the procedure.[36] For areas such as the face, sun avoidance and regular use of sunscreen with an SPF >30 should be advocated prior to laser treatment. This is particularly important for resurfacing procedures where there is a high risk of dyspigmentation.[29]

Pre-treatment of dark skin with alpha-hydroxy acids or bleaching agents combined with a topical steroid may help reduce epidermal pigment and therefore prevent hypopigmentation due to laser therapy.[36] Additionally, many of these topical agents may cause minor inflammation that can hasten removal of dermal (tattoo) pigment.

For ablative resurfacing procedures, some authors advocate pre- and postoperative use of topical bleaching agents, tretinoin cream and steroid compounds to help minimize post-inflammatory hyperpigmentation.[37] However, a prospective study of 100 patients undergoing CO_2 laser resurfacing found no significant difference in the incidence of post-inflammatory hyperpigmentation between patients pretreated ≥ 2 weeks with glycolic acid cream or combination tretinoin/hydroquinone creams versus no pretreatment.[38]

Use of petrolatum and strict sun avoidance can hasten epidermal healing and help minimize post inflammatory dyspigmentation; however, correction of dyspigmentation, once it occurs, can be difficult. Bleaching creams, superficial chemical peels, kojic and retinoic acid may help blend lines of demarcation. These products should be avoided, however, in the first post-operative month after resurfacing procedures, as they can cause profound irritation and worsen hyperpigmentation. For hypopigmentation, use of topical PUVA (oxsoralen and UVA light therapy) has been used to induce melanogenesis.[29]

Scarring

Risk Factors for Excess Scarring

- High fluence
- Inadequate cooling
- Pulse stacking, multiple passes
- Wrong laser
- Patient factors (history of isotretinoin, keloid formation or radiation therapy)
- Location (mandible, anterior neck, infraorbital > other areas)
- Poor post-operative wound care regimen (for resurfacing procedures)
- Infection

Scarring is a rare but potentially severe side effect of laser therapy. The terminology in the literature can be confusing. For some, *textural change* describes a transient phenomenon where there is a change in the contour of the skin, truly differentiating it from a permanent scar.[39] However, others use *textural change* to describe a subtle, but potentially severe, reticular pattern of scarring. Because of this lack of consensus in terminology, many early articles underreported the incidence of scarring, listing the complication instead as textural change. It is the authors' opinion that the term *textural change* should be reserved for non-scarring processes only.

The most likely cause of scar formation following laser treatment is excessive thermal injury to the treated tissue. Pulse stacking or multiple passes,[40] high energy fluences or inadequate cooling can all precipitate thermal injury. Dermal depressions can be caused by vessel dissolution or thermal injury. Inadequate contact cooling (e.g., over the alar groove) or high fluences can lead to this finding. Selection of an appropriate laser and use of the correct treatment parameters, for a given indication, is paramount in avoiding excessive tissue damage and scarring. Patients with a history of recent isotretinoin therapy, keloid scar formation or radiation therapy may be at increased risk for hypertrophic scar formation following resurfacing procedures.[16] Additionally, post-operative resurfacing complications, such as infection and contact dermatitis, may also lead to scarring.

Treatment of certain anatomical locations, including the mandible, anterior neck and infraorbital areas are more likely to scar.[27] Reduced laser parameters are recommended in these areas.

Prevention and Treatment

A skilled clinician will monitor the skin for evidence of excessive thermal injury both during and after laser treatment. Marked erythema or graying of the epidermis during treatment may indicate significant damage and the need to discontinue treatment or adjust parameters. Multiple test spots with varying fluences and/or pulse durations can be performed prior to treatment, particularly in patients with an increased risk of scarring. These can often be performed at the time of initial consultation.

After resurfacing procedures, focal areas of erythema and induration often precede the formation of hypertrophic scars.[29] These areas should be cultured and the patient treated, if infection is suspected. If infection is ruled out, prompt application or intralesional injection of corticosteroids can halt the progression of hypertrophic scars. Silicone gel sheeting or topical imiquimod may also be useful in preventing and/or treating hypertrophic scar formation (reviewed in Zurada et al.[41]).

Intralesional steroids, 5-fluorouracil (5-FU) and laser therapy have proved beneficial in the treatment of hypertrophic scars.[42,43] PDL treatment has been reported to improve the symptoms, pliability and color and decrease the size of hypertrophic scars.[42,44] A recent single-blinded study with

69 patients compared treatment of hypertrophic scars with intralesional triamcinolone (TAC) alone or in combination with intralesional 5-FU or intralesional 5-FU and PDL therapy.[43] Combination therapy with TAC and 5-FU, both with and without PDL therapy, provided statistically significant improvement in the overall erythema, pruritus, pliability and size of the scars compared with TAC alone. Patients reported the most improvement with the triple TAC, 5-FU and PDL therapy, however.

Depressed scars may improve over a period of several months.[39] Ablative or non-ablative resurfacing procedures and dermal fillers can be used to correct the contour defects depending on their severity.

Idiosyncratic Complications

There are a number of complications unique to treating specific lesions. Perhaps the best known example of this is during removal of tattoos. Upon laser treatment, tattoo pigment is released extracellularly, exposing it to immunologic cells and oxidizing radicals, and can lead to allergic contact dermatitis or paradoxical darkening. Resurfacing procedures not only pose a risk of profound scarring (albeit rarely), but the loss of the epidermal barrier also makes one more susceptible to infection, acne and milia formation. Treatment of vascular and pigmented lesions and photoepilation are also associated with unique, though uncommon, side effects.

There are a handful of complications that are unique to treating specific dermatologic conditions with certain lasers. These complications and their management will be discussed in the following section.

Photoepilation

Hypertrichosis

Several studies have documented paradoxical hypertrichosis following laser hair removal.[45,46] This primarily occurs after several treatments have been performed on the face and neck of female patients with darker skin types. The mechanism that triggers the conversion of these vellus to terminal hairs is unknown, but may be related to inflammation induced by the laser therapy itself. Management of this uncommon complication is with further photoepilation.

Leukotrichia

Photoepilation is most commonly performed with the long-pulsed Ruby, Alexandrite and Diode lasers. Patients with darker skin tones may be treated with the long-pulsed Nd:YAG lasers. These lasers target melanin and penetrate deep enough to reach the hair follicle. By using millisecond instead of nanosecond pulse durations, thermal damage extends beyond the melanocytes to involve other structures within the follicle important for hair growth.[47] This leads to the desired destruction of the targeted follicle. With subtherapeutic fluence levels, follicular melanocytes may be destroyed in the absence of other follicular injury, resulting in leukotrichosis.

Reticulate Erythema

Persistent reticulate erythema has been described in at least 10 patients following hair removal with the Diode laser.[48] Pernio, and perhaps other connective tissue diseases, as well as high energy fluences seem to be potential risk factors. Most patients are female.

Urticarial-Like Plaques

Pruritic, urticarial-like plaques have been described following photoepilation.[12] Unlike urticaria, however, lesions may last several days to weeks. Topical and oral corticosteroids and anti-histamines can be used for symptomatic relief.

Pigmented Lesions

Leukotrichia

Melanin, located in the epidermis, dermis and follicular structures, is the primary chromophore targeted in the treatment of various pigmented lesions. Melanocytes within the hair follicle can be destroyed inadvertently when using high fluences and more deeply penetrating, longer, wavelengths. Permanent leukotrichia can result. Limiting the fluences and selecting lasers with shorter wavelengths, if possible, will minimize this complication.

Tissue Splatter and Pinpoint Bleeding

Tissue splatter and pinpoint bleeding are expected side effects of treatment with Q-switched lasers. When tissue targets are heated to destructive levels over nanosecond (QS) pulse

References

1. Goldman L, Blaney DJ, Kindel DJ Jr, et al. Pathology of the effect of the laser beam on the skin. *Nature*. 1963;197:912-914.
2. Tanzi EL, Lupton JR, Alster TS. Lasers in dermatology: four decades of progress. *J Am Acad Dermatol*. 2003;49:1-31; quiz 31-34.
3. Anderson RR, Parrish JA. Selective photothermolysis: precise microsurgery by selective absorption of pulsed radiation. *Science*. 1983;220:524-527.
4. Anderson RR. Lasers in dermatology – a critical update. *J Dermatol*. 2000;27:700-705.
5. Nelson JS, Majaron B, Kelly KM. Active skin cooling in conjunction with laser dermatologic surgery. *Semin Cutan Med Surg*. 2000; 19:253-266.
6. Sawchuk WS, Weber PJ, Lowy DR, et al. Infectious papillomavirus in the vapor of warts treated with carbon dioxide laser or electrocoagulation: detection and protection. *J Am Acad Dermatol*. 1989;21: 41-49.
7. Baggish MS, Poiesz BJ, Joret D, et al. Presence of human immunodeficiency virus DNA in laser smoke. *Lasers Surg Med*. 1991;11: 197-203.
8. Barkana Y, Belkin M. Laser eye injuries. *Surv Ophthalmol*. 2000;44: 459-478.
9. Isenhath S, Willey A, Bouzari N, et al. Complications in Dermatologic Surgery, Mosby Elsevier, Philadelphia, USA.
10. Sliney D, Aron-Rosa D, DeLori F, et al. Adjustment of guidelines for exposure of the eye to optical radiation from ocular instruments: statement from a task group of the International Commission on Non-Ionizing Radiation Protection (ICNIRP). *Appl Opt*. 2005;44: 2162-2176.
11. Greve B, Raulin C. Professional errors caused by lasers and intense pulsed light technology in dermatology and aesthetic medicine: preventive strategies and case studies. *Dermatol Surg*. 2002;28: 156-161.
12. Dawson E, Willey A, Lee K. Adverse events associated with nonablative cutaneous laser, radiofrequency, and light-based devices. *Semin Cutan Med Surg*. 2007;26:15-21.
13. Wolfe JT, Weinberg JM, Elenitsas R, et al. Cutaneous lupus erythematosus following laser-induced thermal injury. *Arch Dermatol*. 1997;133:392-393.
14. Kuhn A, Becker-Wegerich PM, Ruzicka T, et al. Successful treatment of discoid lupus erythematosus with argon laser. *Dermatology*. 2000;201:175-177.
15. Haedersdal M, Poulsen T, Wulf HC. Laser induced wounds and scarring modified by antiinflammatory drugs: a murine model. *Lasers Surg Med*. 1993;13:55-61.
16. Rubenstein R, Roenigk HH Jr, Stegman SJ, et al. Atypical keloids after dermabrasion of patients taking isotretinoin. *J Am Acad Dermatol*. 1986;15:280-285.
17. Khatri KA. Diode laser hair removal in patients undergoing isotretinoin therapy. *Dermatol Surg*. 2004;30:1205-1207; discussion 1207.
18. Khatri KA, Garcia V. Light-assisted hair removal in patients undergoing isotretinoin therapy. *Dermatol Surg*. 2006;32:875-877.
19. Alster T, Zaulyanov L. Laser scar revision: a review. *Dermatol Surg*. 2007;33:131-140.
20. Trotter MJ, Tron VA, Hollingdale J, et al. Localized chrysiasis induced by laser therapy. *Arch Dermatol*. 1995;131:1411-1414.
21. Baron ED, Harris L, Redpath WS, et al. Laser-assisted penetration of topical anesthetic in adults. *Arch Dermatol*. 2003;139: 1288-1290.
22. Chen JZ, Jacobson LG, Bakus AD, et al. Evaluation of the S-Caine peel for induction of local anesthesia for laser-assisted tattoo removal: randomized, double-blind, placebo-controlled, multicenter study. *Dermatol Surg*. 2005;31:281-286.

23. Kilmer SL, Chotzen V, Zelickson BD, et al. Full-face laser resurfacing using a supplemented topical anesthesia protocol. *Arch Dermatol*. 2003;139:1279-1283.
24. Waldorf HA, Alster TS, McMillan K, et al. Effect of dynamic cooling on 585-nm pulsed dye laser treatment of port-wine stain birthmarks. *Dermatol Surg*. 1997;23:657-662.
25. Chan HH, Lam LK, Wong DS, et al. Role of skin cooling in improving patient tolerability of Q-switched Alexandrite (QS Alex) laser in nevus of Ota treatment. *Lasers Surg Med*. 2003;32: 148-151.
26. Watanabe S, Kakigi R, Hoshiyama M, et al. Effects of noxious cooling of the skin on pain perception in man. *J Neurol Sci*. 1996;135: 68-73.
27. Nanni CA, Alster TS. Complications of carbon dioxide laser resurfacing. An evaluation of 500 patients. *Dermatol Surg*. 1998;24: 315-320.
28. Alam M, Omura NE, Dover JS, et al. Clinically significant facial edema after extensive treatment with purpura-free pulsed-dye laser. *Dermatol Surg*. 2003;29:920-924.
29. Alster TS, Lupton JR. Prevention and treatment of side effects and complications of cutaneous laser resurfacing. *Plast Reconstr Surg*. 2002;109:308-316; discussion 317-318.
30. Alster TS, West TB. Effect of topical vitamin C on postoperative carbon dioxide laser resurfacing erythema. *Dermatol Surg*. 1998;24:331-334.
31. Wetter DA, Davis MD, Yiannias JA, et al. Patch test results from the Mayo Clinic Contact Dermatitis Group, 1998–2000. *J Am Acad Dermatol*. 2005;53:416-421.
32. Smack DP, Harrington AC, Dunn C, et al. Infection and allergy incidence in ambulatory surgery patients using white petrolatum vs bacitracin ointment. A randomized controlled trial. *JAMA*. 1996;276:972-977.
33. Lanigan SW. Patient-reported morbidity following flashlamp-pumped pulsed tunable dye laser treatment of port wine stains. *Br J Dermatol*. 1995;133:423-425.
34. Shah NS, Lazarus MC, Bugdodel R, et al. The effects of topical vitamin K on bruising after laser treatment. *J Am Acad Dermatol*. 2002;47:241-244.
35. Alonso D, Lazarus MC, Baumann L. Effects of topical arnica gel on post-laser treatment bruises. *Dermatol Surg*. 2002;28:686-688.
36. Bernstein EF. Laser treatment of tattoos. *Clin Dermatol*. 2006;24: 43-55.
37. Ho C, Nguyen Q, Lowe NJ, et al. Laser resurfacing in pigmented skin. *Dermatol Surg*. 1995;21:1035-1037.
38. West TB, Alster TS. Effect of pretreatment on the incidence of hyperpigmentation following cutaneous CO_2 laser resurfacing. *Dermatol Surg*. 1999;25:15-17.
39. Willey A, Anderson RR, Azpiazu JL, et al. Complications of laser dermatologic surgery. *Lasers Surg Med*. 2006;38:1-15.
40. Ross EV, Barnette DJ, Glatter RD, et al. Effects of overlap and pass number in CO_2 laser skin resurfacing: a study of residual thermal damage, cell death, and wound healing. *Lasers Surg Med*. 1999; 24:103-112.
41. Zurada JM, Kriegel D, Davis IC. Topical treatments for hypertrophic scars. *J Am Acad Dermatol*. 2006;55:1024-1031.
42. Alster T. Laser scar revision: comparison study of 585-nm pulsed dye laser with and without intralesional corticosteroids. *Dermatol Surg*. 2003;29:25-29.
43. Asilian A, Darougheh A, Shariati F. New combination of triamcinolone, 5-Fluorouracil, and pulsed-dye laser for treatment of keloid and hypertrophic scars. *Dermatol Surg*. 2006;32:907-915.
44. Manuskiatti W, Wanitphakdeedecha R, Fitzpatrick RE. Effect of pulse width of a 595-nm flashlamp-pumped pulsed dye laser on the treatment response of keloidal and hypertrophic sternotomy scars. *Dermatol Surg*. 2007;33:152-161.
45. Alajlan A, Shapiro J, Rivers JK, et al. Paradoxical hypertrichosis after laser epilation. *J Am Acad Dermatol*. 2005;53:85-88.

46. Kontoes P, Vlachos S, Konstantinos M, et al. Hair induction after laser-assisted hair removal and its treatment. *J Am Acad Dermatol.* 2006;54:64-67.

47. Grossman MC, Dierickx C, Farinelli W, et al. Damage to hair follicles by normal-mode ruby laser pulses. *J Am Acad Dermatol.* 1996;35:889-894.

48. Lapidoth M, Shafirstein G, Ben Amitai D, et al. Reticulate erythema following diode laser-assisted hair removal: a new side effect of a common procedure. *J Am Acad Dermatol.* 2004;51:774-777.

49. Beeson WH, Rachel JD. Valacyclovir prophylaxis for herpes simplex virus infection or infection recurrence following laser skin resurfacing. *Dermatol Surg.* 2002;28:331-336.

50. Bellman B, Brandt FS, Holtmann M, et al. Infection with methicillin-resistant *Staphylococcus aureus* after carbon dioxide resurfacing of the face. Successful treatment with minocycline, rifampin, and mupiricin ointment. *Dermatol Surg.* 1998;24:279-282.

51. Alam M, Pantanowitz L, Harton AM, et al. A prospective trial of fungal colonization after laser resurfacing of the face: correlation between culture positivity and symptoms of pruritus. *Dermatol Surg.* 2003;29:255-260.

52. Sriprachya-Anunt S, Fitzpatrick RE, Goldman MP, et al. Infections complicating pulsed carbon dioxide laser resurfacing for photoaged facial skin. *Dermatol Surg.* 1997;23:527-535; discussion 535-536.

53. Walia S, Alster TS. Cutaneous CO_2 laser resurfacing infection rate with and without prophylactic antibiotics. *Dermatol Surg.* 1999;25:857-861.

54. Conn H, Nanda VS. Prophylactic fluconazole promotes reepithelialization in full-face carbon dioxide laser skin resurfacing. *Lasers Surg Med.* 2000;26:201-207.

55. Ashinoff R, Levine VJ, Soter NA. Allergic reactions to tattoo pigment after laser treatment. *Dermatol Surg.* 1995;21:291-294.

56. Bhardwaj SS, Brodell RT, Taylor JS. Red tattoo reactions. *Contact Dermatitis.* 2003;48:236-237.

57. Antony FC, Harland CC. Red ink tattoo reactions: successful treatment with the Q-switched 532 nm Nd:YAG laser. *Br J Dermatol.* 2003;149:94-98.

58. Dave R, Mahaffey PJ. Successful treatment of an allergic reaction in a red tattoo with the Nd-YAG laser. *Br J Plast Surg.* 2002;55:456.

59. Zemtsov A, Wilson L. CO_2 laser treatment causes local tattoo allergic reaction to become generalized. *Acta DermVenereol.* 1997;77:497.

60. Taylor CR. Laser ignition of traumatically embedded firework debris. *Lasers Surg Med.* 1998;22:157-158.

61. Anderson RR, Geronemus R, Kilmer SL, et al. Cosmetic tattoo ink darkening. A complication of Q-switched and pulsed-laser treatment. *Arch Dermatol.* 1993;129:1010-1014.

62. Ross EV, Yashar S, Michaud N, et al. Tattoo darkening and nonresponse after laser treatment: a possible role for titanium dioxide. *Arch Dermatol.* 2001;137:33-37.

63. Varma S, Swanson NA, Lee KK. Tattoo ink darkening of a yellow tattoo after Q-switched laser treatment. *Clin Exp Dermatol.* 2002;27:461-463.

64. Fitzpatrick RE, Lupton JR. Successful treatment of treatment-resistant laser-induced pigment darkening of a cosmetic tattoo. *Lasers Surg Med.* 2000;27:358-361.

65. Herbich GJ. Ultrapulse carbon dioxide laser treatment of an iron oxide flesh-colored tattoo. *Dermatol Surg.* 1997;23:60-61.

66. Dinehart SM, Flock S, Waner M. Beam profile of the flashlamp pumped pulsed dye laser: support for overlap of exposure spots. *Lasers Surg Med.* 1994;15:277-280.

Ethical Issues

Abel Torres, Tejas Desai, Alpesh Desai, and William Kirby

- Ethical behavior transcends legal implications, and represents the level of professionalism, humanity and morality a physician should possess in order to address his/her patient's care.
- If a physician upholds his/her ethical responsibility to a higher standard than a legal obligation, the patient's best interests may be addressed.
- The Hippocratic Oath may not address specific ethical problems unique to the utility of lasers, therefore many professional associations have devised tenets to follow.
- The simple acronym, "E-T-H-I-C-A-L" may help guide a physician to uphold the highest ethical standard when performing a laser procedure.
- Financial gain may entice a physician to not optimize care for a patient.
- It is ethical for a physician to remain honest about their experience and training.
- Full disclosure of pertinent information to the patient may be sensible so he/she may remain the autonomous decision-maker without physician biases.
- Unreported interests may not only be financially unethical but also may promote biased research and conclusions based on false pretenses.
- A patient should not be discriminated against except when laser treatment may negatively alter treatment for that patient.
- Advertising techniques are suitable as long as they are not fraudulent or misleading.
- A physician may report to peer-review authorities about unsafe laser practices of another practitioner if he/she presents a clear danger to the public.
- A practitioner's lack of action of not reporting inappropriate conduct taken by another physician may be considered unethical and unlawful.

A. Torres ✉
Department of Dermatology, Loma Linda University
School of Medicine, Loma Linda, CA, USA
e-mail: abelt@aol.com

In general, ethics can be considered the science of moral duty, of ideal human character, and of the ideal ends of human action.[1] Ethics is closely tied to morals, and it can be said that ethics is the science of morals, and morals are the practice of ethics.[1] The legal standard of care is usually the minimum required, while ethics usually pertains to a higher standard. If a physician upholds his/her ethical responsibility to a higher standard than a legal obligation, the patient's best interests may be addressed. It is a physician's ethical commitment to the patient, himself/herself and the profession of medicine that may guide a successful laser procedure.

Laser treatments in dermatology may create an ethical dilemma for physicians since some procedures are elective. Clinical endpoints for laser therapy can be difficult to objectively quantify, and patient satisfaction often becomes the cornerstone of treatment efficacy. Furthermore, cosmetic patients may have unrealistic expectations, and instilled in the public, is a media-driven mentality that lasers are generally safe devices without complications.

The continued, heightened controversy in recent years is the result of one looming question: is aging a physical illness?[2] Whether the aging face needs rejuvenation may spark dead-end debates even among colleagues in dermatology.[3] The Hippocratic Oath may not address specific problems unique to the utility of lasers, therefore many professional associations including the American Medical Association (AMA), American Society of Dermatologic Surgery (ASDS), American Academy of Dermatology (AAD), American Osteopathic College of Dermatology (AOCD), and American Society of Laser Medicine and Surgery (ASLMS) have established tenets in terms of patients' best interests, professionalism, and personal conduct. These guidelines serve to establish standards for non-medical care in an ever-changing, cosmetic world. In addition, physicians' ethical responsibilities sometimes differ from their legal ones.[4] They are not solely limited to clinical practice, but also include the moral treatment of human subjects in laser medicine and surgery research. Multiple issues may be encountered between a practitioner's moral duty and the patient's best interests. A simple acronym, "ETHICAL" (Economics, Training, Heart to Heart Discussion Between Physician and Patient, Interests, Contraindications, Advertising and Libel versus Letting

K. Nouri (ed.), *Lasers in Dermatology and Medicine*,
DOI: 10.1007/978-0-85729-281-0_30, © Springer-Verlag London Limited 2011

Authorities Know of Misconduct) can serve as a guide to help remind physicians of their ethical responsibilities to patients.

Economics

Financial gain may entice a physician to not optimize care for a patient. It is wise and ethical for the physician to uphold the dignity of the patient, and not exploit or abuse the relationship for financial matters. Gifts, kickbacks and other financial gain received in exchange for operating one laser brand over another may be considered unethical without the consent of the patient. The definition of equipment tampering is any safety bypassing allowing the unauthorized reuse of the product.[5] Approved equipment with replacing equipment that is not approved for use may result in negative outcomes for the patient. Furthermore, the resale of lasers to non-physicians is not advocated and may be subject to penalties under the labeling requirements of the Food Drug and Cosmetic Act.[5] This action may contribute to non-medical workers operating lasers on patients without the proper training. Moreover, economic bias may sometimes be difficult for physicians to preclude, when they may feel obligated to endorse a product because they receive monies for company lectures and/or research.

Training

It is ethical for a physician to remain honest about their experience and training. Formal procedural dermatology training can assist in demonstrating competency in selected laser procedures, including their proper use and management of complications. It is prudent to disclose to a patient when medical personnel and extenders will be part of the treatment, since some clinics have nurses or physician assistants operating lasers or light devices. A recent survey conducted by the ASDS showed that nearly 41% of responding dermasurgeons reported an increase in patients seeking treatment due to injury caused by untrained, non-physicians performing laser and light rejuvenation techniques.[5] Depending on the state, non-medical personnel may perform treatments provided that a physician is on site should a complication or issue arise. Non-physicians must have appropriate documented training in the physics, safety, and surgical techniques for each procedure performed.[5] The ASMLS recommends physician extenders complete a basic training program devoted to the principles of lasers, their instrumentation and safety issues.[6] A minimum 8–10 h is suggested by the American National Standards Institute (ANSI)

standards.[6] Furthermore 40% of the time should be allocated to practical sessions.[6] It is also recommended that such medical personnel spend time in a clinical setting or preceptorship.[6] It is encouraged for the novice to first perform procedures with the supervision by the expert if state law permits.[6] The issue of laser training is becoming a serious problem in some states because there are no legal requirements for training, no quality control measures, no official quality standards or guidelines.[7] One study showed that compared to non-medical, laser operators, dermatologists were more likely to support clinical regulations that placed licensed physicians in control.[8]

Heart to Heart Discussion Between Physician and Patient

Full disclosure of pertinent information to the patient may be sensible so he/she may remain the autonomous decision-maker without physician biases. This helps promote a lasting relationship, build patient trust and most of all, serves the patient to the fullest. Cosmetic dermatology using medical lasers provides patients with the anticipation of positive appearance, body image and good emotional health. This may elicit patient sensitivity and vulnerability and places physicians in an influential role. This physician-patient relationship is the central focus of all ethical concerns.[9] This relationship is unintentionally not equal because a physician has the knowledge of medicine and the patient does not.[1] If physicians only accommodate patients' wishes, then patients are left to dictate the physician's behavior, causing the patient to become an object of a business transaction.[7] Hence, an ethical strain may be placed on the physician–patient relationship. Moreover, the physician has the responsibility to put the emphasis back on the patient as the beneficiary of their liaison.

Interests

Conflicts of interest affect human behavior, sometimes unconsciously.[10] They may cause a physician to not utilize an optimal laser treatment for a patient. Unreported interests may not only be financially unethical but also may promote biased research and conclusions based on false pretenses. Relationships that permit or encourage product promotion using the names of academic medical centers and departments may be ethically unsound and should be avoided.[11] This may not only sacrifice the dignity of patients, but also the physician and his/her moral standard. Disclosure of conflicts of interest becomes more of an issue when clinical research is involved. The role of an institutional board review (IRB) is to evaluate both the risk-benefit ratio of the proposed study and the appropriateness of consent that is obtained from the voluntary research subjects.[12] An IRB should have little difficulty determining the appropriateness of dermatological surgical research consent.[12] However, judging the suitability of a cosmetic dermatologic study may be perplexing at times. Moreover, many currently available lasers receive nonspecific skin FDA clearance. One study by Perkins et al. demonstrated many physicians do not mention evidence of ethics review from an IRB. Out of 150 prospective studies submitted to the *Journal of American Academy of Dermatology* (JAAD), a whopping 36% had no mention, and when asked to resubmit IRB approval, 22% were withdrawn, 12% were never resubmitted, and 12% responded that ethical review was not obtained.[13] The JAAD clearly states in its instructions to authors, which adhere to the guidelines set forth by the International Committee of Medical Journal Editors, "studies involving live human subjects must have been approved by the author's IRB or its equivalent."[13] The driving force behind not reporting an ethics review was likely oversight in many cases, but in others approval may not have been obtained.[13] This study from Perkins implies that some physicians were not ethical about being ethical!

Contraindications

A patient should not be discriminated against except when laser treatment may negatively alter treatment for the patient. In these types of situations, a physician should fully discuss the reasons why the patient does not make a good candidate. The physician cannot abandon a patient that experiences a complication. Such behavior is not only unethical, but may have legal implications. Ethical personal conduct permits a physician to make sound therapeutic judgments regardless of what medical science has proven. If a patient is at risk for a known side effect, a physician should not allow his/her own economic bias to affect the decision. Clinical research furnishes data, but ultimately personal conduct dictates the level of patient care.

Advertising

Advertisements in cosmetic dermatology has become commonplace for laser procedures. They should not be intended to create unrealistic expectations, and physicians should have the ability to substantiate claims made in those ads.[5] Mechanisms such as photographs or patient testimonials are suitable as long as they are not fraudulent or misleading. It is unethical to promote non-FDA medical lasers or devices on advertisements. At the present time, no information has been submitted to the FDA that could constitute solid scientific evidence of the safety and effectiveness of medical laser devices for cosmetics and related conditions.[14] Therefore, all such laser devices are considered to be class III Investigational Devices limited to use in accordance with the Investigational Device Exemption (IDE) regulation.[14] The commercial promotion, distribution, sale, or use of these investigational devices with no IRB approval for non-significant risk devices, or without FDA approval of an IDE application for a significant risk device may be considered a violation.[14]

Libel Versus Letting Authorities Know of Unethical Conduct

A physician may report to peer-review authorities about unsafe laser practices of another practitioner if he/she presents a clear danger to the public. There are appropriate ways to report unacceptable behavior of a physician for practitioners that may feel reluctance about reporting a colleague. Or may be concerned about being accused of slander. In these circumstances, a practitioner's lack of action of not reporting inappropriate conduct by another physician may be considered unethical and unlawful. Such practice may also harm a patient. According to the AAD, when a member is convinced that another member is violating the Bylaws, Code of Ethics, other Administrative Regulations, or Board-approved policies, the member should send a confidential written form of communication to the Academy's Secretary-Treasurer or Executive Director.[9] Yet is also unacceptable for physicians to slander their competition if no wrongdoing has taken place. Instilling a negative image about another colleague or practice does not reflect ethical professionalism to colleagues or patients.

Medical ethics are not laws in the legal sense, but they are standards of conduct which physicians practice.[1] Ethics in laser medicine is intended to facilitate appropriate physician behavior, and not to be construed as legal advice. Ethical behavior transcends legal implications, and represents the level of professionalism, humanity and morality a physician should possess in order to address his/her patient's care. For more information on ethical issues regarding laser procedures, please visit www.aad.org, www.asds.net, and www.aslms.org.

References

1. Webster SB. Professionalism and medical ethics in dermatology-2000. *Arch Dermatol*. 2000;136(1):101-102.
2. Ringel E. The morality of cosmetic surgery for aging. *Arch Dermatol*. 1998;134:427-431.
3. Cantor J. Cosmetic dermatology and physicians' ethical obligations: more than just hope in a jar. *Semin Cutan Med Surg*. 2005; 24:155-160.
4. Finklestein D, Wu AW, Holtzman NA, et al. When a physician harms a patient by a medical error: ethical, legal and risk-management considerations. *J Clin Ethics*. 1997;8(4):300-335.
5. Guidelines for ethical patient safety practices in today's rapidly changing, complex environment. www.asds.net/GuidelinesFor EthicalPatientSafetyPractices.aspx.
6. Standards of perioperative clinical practice in laser medicine and surgery. www.aslms.org.
7. Raulin C, Greve B, Raulin S. Ethical considerations concerning laser medicine. *Lasers Surg Med*. 2001;28:100-101.
8. Wagner RF, Brown T, McCarthy EM, et al. Dermatologist and electrologist perspectives on laser procedures by nonphysicians. *Dermatol Surg*. 2000;26(8):723-727.
9. Administrative regulations: code of medical ethics for dermatologists. www.aad.org. 2006.
10. Williams HC, Naidi L, Paul C. Conflicts of interest in dermatology. *Acta Derm Venerol*. 2006;86(6):485-497.
11. Newburger A. Taking ethics seriously in cosmetic dermatology. *Arch Dermatol*. 2006;142:1641-1642.
12. Goldberg D. Dermatologic surgical research and the institutional review board. *Dermatol Surg*. 2005;31(10):1317-1322.
13. Perkins AC, Choi JM, Kimball AB. Reporting of ethical review of clinical research submitted to the Journal of the American Academy of Dermatology. *J Am Acad Dermatol*. 2007;56(2):279-284.
14. Sec. 393.200 Laser(s) as Medical Devices for Facelift, Wrinkle Removal, Acupuncture, Auricular Stimulation, etc. (CPG 7133.21). Revised March 1995. www.fda.gov/ora/compliance_ref/cpg/cpgdev/cpg393-200.html

Medicolegal Issues (Documentation/Informed Consent)

Abel Torres, Tejas Desai, Alpesh Desai, and William Kirby

- The number of elective laser and light procedures continues to grow eliciting a host of medicolegal issues.
- Informed consent involves a meeting of the minds as a result of a discussion between the provider and the patient.
- The risks, benefits and alternatives of a procedure should be disclosed to a patient and is paramount to an informed consent.
- Unique patient and physician concerns regarding the laser procedure should be documented.
- The informed consent process might benefit from supplementary modes of communication such as patient questionnaires to improve retention rates.
- Most laser procedures require for lasers individualized informed consents.
- Special considerations for lasers that may be included in an informed consent can be recalled by a simple acronym, "L-A-S-E-R-S."
- It is important that pediatric patients be a part of the consent discussion if they have the capacity to do so.
- Informed refusal by the physician may be warranted if the physician feels a treatment is more beneficial than another.
- A successful laser procedure starts with the informed consent process.

A. Torres ✉
Department of Dermatology, Loma Linda University School of Medicine, Loma Linda, CA, USA
e-mail: abelt@aol.com

According to the American Society of Dermatologic Society (ASDS), its members collectively have performed over 100 million laser and light source cosmetic procedures.[1] This number should continue to expand as life expectancy increases, causing a seemingly everlasting population desiring to achieve a more youthful appearance. Combining these numerous laser procedures with unrealized patient expectations may be a recipe for a legal disaster.

Since the vast majority of laser procedures in dermatology are elective, the importance of patient informed consent and documentation cannot be overemphasized. Educating the patient in layman terms, further explaining the risks, benefits and alternatives are wise actions even before test spot and/or treatment is attempted. Moreover, the nature, course and aim of treatment should be clearly stated to define the objectives for the patient and physician. This allows the patient to make a rational decision based on the pertinent information that has been presented to them. Informed consent in laser treatment not only protects the physician, but the patient as well.

Informed consent is not merely a piece of paper to be signed by the patient. A nonverbal protocol functioning as an informed consent does not fully protect a physician and does not serve the best interest of a patient. Informed consent involves a meeting of the minds as a result of a discussion between the provider and the patient. Written consent is merely a confirmation of what has been discussed. A patient's signature on a preprinted consent form, which has not been preceded by a discussion, does not grant free rein, and in the event of a legal dispute, such forms may be declared invalid.[2] Unique patient and physician concerns regarding the laser procedure should be documented as part of the informed consent. This can help identify and personalize the treatment plan for each specific patient. Identical informed consents without additional notes may sometimes appear like a reflex, rather than a communication between patient and physician.

The authors prefer to write a risk, benefit and alternatives (RBA) note together with a written informed consent. The note emphasizes the RBA that is especially pertinent to the patient. In this way, it is a reminder to the provider to discuss these issues with the patient, and supplies additional

K. Nouri (ed.), *Lasers in Dermatology and Medicine*,
DOI: 10.1007/978-0-85729-281-0_31, © Springer-Verlag London Limited 2011

documentation to the medical record. Such a note does not have to be lengthy or extensive. It can consist of a sentence. An example of this would be: "The RBA discussed with the patient emphasizing the potential risk of post-treatment, permanent dyschromia due to the patient's Fitzpatrick skin type."

Informed consent retention has been shown to be less than 50% in other fields of medicine.[3] In addition, in patients undergoing dermatologic surgery, one study showed an overall retention rate of 26.5% just 20 min after being informed of ten possible complications.[3] It is apparent from this study that informed consent might benefit from supplementary modes of communication to improve retention rates. When treatment is usually reserved for a future day, the overall retention rate for patients can be expected to drop even more. Patient pamphlets for education can complement written and verbal informed consent. Handouts can be noted in the medical record indicating an exchange took place on the day of the consultation. It is helpful when numerous modes of communication are involved in order for the patient to solidify his/her decision on a non-medical procedure. Some physicians like Dr. David Duffy, M.D. advocate using a questionnaire that the patient must answer to demonstrate comprehension of the consent.

It is wise to seek informed consent for each type of laser that is operated by the physician. Each laser system functions in a unique fashion. The same laser created by various competitors may differ in terms of treatment settings and potential side effects. For this reason, establishing a relationship with the laser company for support is advantageous for the physician. Furthermore, ensuring that the medical device is FDA approved for patient therapy could minimize liability.

Special considerations involving informed consent for laser therapy include type of anesthesia, permission for release of photographs, revocation of consent, observations, no guarantee clause, and waiver of liability.[4] These key elements may be forgotten, and provides useful information to the patient while adding pertinent documentation to the medical record. If preoperative anesthetic is part of the laser technique, its risks and benefits should be discussed. Photographs can be taken to measure improvement, but at times, may be a sensitive issue with certain patients. It is vital that pictures be confidential and without identification. This can be explained or added to the medical record as an informed consent note. A revocation of consent discussion can let a patient know that they can discontinue treatment at any time he/she wishes. It is useful under circumstances when discontinuation may alter the outcome. A "no guarantee" clause makes the patient aware that although the laser procedure is effective in most cases, no guarantees can be made that a specific patient will benefit from the laser treatment. Finally, informed consent may need to include a waiver of financial liability. A patient should understand that insurance companies (even Medicare)

Table 1 Key elements to be included on an informed consent

Liability waiver	A patient needs to be aware that their insurance company may not cover services rendered
Anesthesia type	Disclose the risks, benefits and type of anesthesia used
Surveillance	Observations, outcomes and side effects on the postoperative record documents treatment course in the best interest of the patient
Expectations	A no guarantee clause indicates that a patient needs to be aware a positive clinical outcome cannot be certain
Revocation of consent	Offer the option of letting the patient refuse treatment at any time especially if it alters outcome
Snapshot	Photographs kept confidential without identification

only pay for services they determine to be reasonable and necessary, otherwise, denial of payment may ensue.[4] The acronym "LASERS," representing *l*iability waiver, type of *a*nesthesia, *s*urveillance and observations, no *e*xpectation/guarantee clause, *r*evocation of consent, and *s*napshots/photographs can remind the physician of the particular elements to be included into the informed consent (Table 1). Additional documentation may be specifically geared towards the patient and/or the type of laser treatment they are receiving. For example, the informed consent could include the risks, benefits and alternatives of a postoperative antiviral if the patient is at risk for herpes labialis.

The pediatric cosmetic dermatologic patient poses different considerations to informed consent. The pediatric patient is usually not legally competent so a physician must obtain consent from the legal guardians/parents. Otherwise, it could be considered a battery irrespective of the result.[5] The patients' parents become the surrogate decision-makers, and their view of the child predominates as the primary clinical endpoint. Nevertheless, it is important that pediatric patients be a part of the consent discussion if they have the capacity to do so. If general anesthesia is required for children, consent should encompass the risks and benefits associated with it.

A competent patient may refuse a recommended laser treatment. Although most laser procedures are voluntary, the physician should document the refusal of a specific treatment if warranted. There is more validity to this statement when a recommended treatment is more beneficial than another laser procedure. Patients can be motivated to obtain a laser procedure for many reasons such as cost. Clinical outcomes may differ, and the physician is encouraged to clarify which treatment option offers the best results. If the patient chooses to undergo another laser treatment with inferior results, an informed refusal appended to the medical chart helps another practitioner understand the issues involved, and may provide a deterrent to litigation. Informed consent and informed refusal go hand in hand, except the latter explains to a patient about the potential negative implications of refusing a treatment.[6] This ultimately benefits the patient.

A successful laser procedure starts with the informed consent process, allowing the patient to have peace of mind before he/she receives treatment and to make an informed decision. In a cosmetic world, patients do not view laser treatments as medical care, but it is the physician's duty to assert his/her role during the course. Lasers and light therapies are complex procedures, and a medical problem may occur rather easily if one is not careful. Complications of laser and light procedures are not uncommon, especially with the number being performed. The appropriate level of documentation helps clarify the care rendered regardless of what occurs. Periodic audits for quality assurance may be beneficial in a laser-based practice. An in-house audit could address weaknesses in the informed consent process and minimize liability.

References

1. Goldberg D. Legal considerations in cosmetic laser surgery. *J Cosmet Dermatol.* 2006;5(2):103-106.
2. Greve B, Raulin C. Professional errors caused by lasers and intense pulsed light technology in dermatology and aesthetic medicine: preventive strategies and case studies. *Dermatol Surg.* 2002;28(2): 156-161.
3. Fleischman M, Garcia C. Informed consent in dermatologic surgery. *Dermatol Surg.* 2003;29(9):952-955.
4. Goldberg D. *Laser Dermatology.* 1st ed. The Netherlands: Springer; 2005.
5. Cohen SN, Lanigan SW. Audit cycle of documentation in laser hair removal. *Lasers Med Sci.* 2005;20(2):87-88.
6. Wagner RF, Torres A, Proper S. Informed consent and informed refusal. *Dermatol Surg.* 1995;21:555-559.
7. Lahti JG, Shahbshin U, Lewis AT, et al. Pediatric cosmetic dermatology. *Clin Dermatol.* 2003;21:315-320.

Psychological Aspects to Consider Within Laser Treatments

Dee Anna Glaser

- While body image dissatisfaction may motivate the pursuit of cosmetic medical treatments, psychiatric disorders may be relatively common among patients seen in dermatologic settings.
- Clinicians who acquire a basic understanding of common psychiatric conditions can properly screen their patients.
- Body dysmorphic disorder (BDD) patients seek out cosmetic medical treatments with great frequency. It is therefore important for dermatologists to be educated in BDD and be able to recognize it before unnecessary procedures are performed.
- The dermatologist should be wary of the patient that has come severely depressed or on an impulse for they may have mood disorders that mainly encompasses two categories: unipolar depression and bipolar disorder.
- Personality disorders may cause difficulties in maintaining a healthy doctor-patient relationship due to poor compliance, communication skills and trust issues.
- Anxiety disorders may cause concerns for a dermatologist, especially since they can commonly occur along with other mental illnesses.
- Evaluating a patient's psychological condition is essential since every patient is not an appropriate candidate for cosmetic procedures.

- The exam should also include a thorough review of the patient's family and medical histories, as well as past treatments, outcomes and complications.
- Patients should be able to express how they feel about their appearance and why they are considering the procedure.
- Laser therapy is very effective when treating children and teens, but the laser team must be prepared to deal with psychological issues of both the patient and parents.

- Body image dissatisfaction may motivate the pursuit of cosmetic medical treatments. Psychiatric disorders characterized by body image disturbances, such as BDD, mood, anxiety, and personality disorders, are relatively common among these patients.
- Understanding of psychiatric issues in laser surgery becomes important and may prevent potential problems.
- Embarrassment and shame often prevent sufferers from revealing their true degree of distress, not only to their family and peers, but to healthcare professionals as well.

D.A. Glaser
Department of Dermatology, Saint Louis University School
of Medicine, Saint Louis, MO, USA
e-mail: glasermd@slu.edu

K. Nouri (ed.), *Lasers in Dermatology and Medicine*,
DOI: 10.1007/978-0-85729-281-0_32, © Springer-Verlag London Limited 2011

Introduction

Cosmetic treatments have become increasingly popular over the past decade with the advent of new techniques and devices, such as lasers. According to recent statistics released by the American Society for Aesthetic Plastic Surgery (ASAPS), there were nearly 11.5 million surgical and nonsurgical cosmetic procedures performed in the United States in 2006. The majority were nonsurgical with over 2.2 million laser procedures performed for hair removal, skin resurfacing and treatment of leg veins. Approximately 93% of laser skin resurfacing procedures were performed with non ablative techniques.[1]

The increase in popularity may be attributed to several factors including the perception that a better appearance will lead to happiness and success, the greater availability of safer, minimally invasive procedures, and amplified mass media attention.[2]

The media has showered the American public with shows and information that glamorizes cosmetic enhancement. The constant exposure to images of what culture claims to be ideal may drive individuals to achieve unrealistic appearance standards. Physical attractiveness is often attributed with a sense of confidence and better self-esteem. A person whose appearance falls below the contemporary aesthetic standards runs the risk of being the target for prejudice and discrimination.

Health professionals have long been interested in understanding the motivations for seeking a change in physical appearance as well as the psychological outcomes of these treatments.[2] The earliest documented studies of the psychological characteristics of cosmetic surgery patients occurred during the 1950s and 1960s. They reported high rates of psychopathology, up to 70%, among cosmetic surgery patients.[3]

Additionally, available data suggests that psychological complications occur at higher rates than do physical complications in plastic surgical practices. Though surgical site pain and sleep disturbance were frequent physical complaints, depression and anxiety were the most prevalent post surgical complications. Patients with pre-existing psychological conditions were even at greater risk for such outcomes. This leads to delayed recuperative time, poor patient compliance, anxiety, dissatisfaction of the procedure, and hostility toward the clinician.[4]

Although laser surgery can be used for medical purposes such as port wine stains and hemangiomas, many laser procedures are performed for aesthetic enhancements. The focus of this chapter will be on the psychological issues associated with the latter. To date, there is minimal data published on the psychological aspects of laser surgery specifically, but there is a growing interest in psychiatric issues surrounding the practice of cosmetic procedures.

While body image dissatisfaction may motivate the pursuit of cosmetic medical treatments, psychiatric disorders characterized by body image disturbances, such as BDD, mood, anxiety, and personality disorders, may be relatively common among these patients. Therefore an understanding of psychiatric issues in laser surgery becomes important and may prevent potential problems.

Evaluation of the Patient

Evaluating a patient's psychological condition is essential. Some patients may have significant emotional and psychological instability and therefore are not suitable candidates for cosmetic laser treatment. Using a consistent screening method may help identify appropriate and inappropriate patients for such procedures (see Table 1).

Table 1 General psychiatric features to asses during initial evaluation

	Considerations	Possible causes
General appearance	Is the patient's dress provocative and alluring?	PD or mania
Mood/affect	Is there a flat affect? Are they overly emotional? Are they paranoid or suspicious of you? Do they avoid eye contact? Are they cooperative or oppositional? Are they overly anxious?	Depression, PD, or mania BDD, PD, or depression
Speech	Is the voice monotone or easily excitable? Is there pressured speech? Is there latency of response?	PD or mood disorder Mania depression
Thought process	Is there tangibility or flight of ideas?	Psychosis or mania
Cognition	Can they make rational decisions independently? What are their expectations of the outcome of procedure? Are they insightful?	

PD personality disorders, *BDD* body dysmorphic disorder

Consider the patient's general appearance, demeanor and behavior, is there intense sadness or despair, inappropriate seductiveness? Are symptoms of rapid speech and euphoria present? Are they extremely critical of their self-image, despite the fact there may be no noticeable disfigurement or defect? Deciding to pursue a cosmetic procedure on a whim may denote a manic impulse, or an excessive need for approval may indicate a BDD patient. Subtle signs like these may suggest the patient's true motives and conditions. There may be baseline patient anxiety on any initial cosmetic consultation but spending time and communicating with the patient should ease such apprehension.

The psychological assessment should also include a thorough review of the patient's family, medical, and surgical histories. Some psychological disabilities tend to run in families and evidence of multiple cosmetic enhancements may insinuate a patient suffering from BDD. Reviewing their medication list may allude to various medical conditions.

It is crucial that a thorough history also include all past consultations, treatments, outcomes and complications. A history of multiple physicians treating the same problem, or patients who claim they usually suffer from multiple complications or prolonged postoperative course should alert the practitioner that this patient may be challenging to satisfy. Indeed, many patients with psychiatric illness are still well suited for cosmetic measures and benefit from it, but it is important to recognize those patients that have unrealistic expectations of what cosmetic procedures can achieve.

Factors to Consider

A patient who speaks poorly of previous physicians will often be disappointed with all of their subsequent treatments and physicians. Anticipating potential troubles should help minimize or avoid prospective dilemmas and anxiety in one's practice.

It is advantageous for the physician to listen to the concerns of nursing staff who take care the patient. The patient may be very unreasonable or unruly with the staff but appear very well-mannered and respectful in front of the physician. In such instances, it is important to re-evaluate the patient before proceeding with cosmetic procedures because such finicky behavior can be very detrimental to the doctor-patient relationship and to the doctor-staff dynamics in the future.

Furthermore, it is vital that there is a clear understanding of exactly what the patient expects of the procedure and a detailed discussion on the fine points of a procedure, such as its risks and possible outcomes. Patients who continue to ask, "But *I* will get results, won't I?" or "But *I* won't have any complications, right?" will maintain their unrealistic expectations, and in such cases a consultation with another physician may be preferred.

Be aware of patients who are unable to verbalize their cosmetic issue or those that say "I just want to look younger," or "I just want to look better." They may be difficult patients to achieve good satisfaction since they frequently will be discontent with the results and even declare that the procedure made them look worse. Similarly, the patient who tries to isolate the smallest little scar or wrinkle that is so vague and challenging to find will usually be dissatisfied with the treatment. Occasionally, a patient may demand one particular treatment and be unwilling to consider other options suggested by the physician. This may give rise to unhappy outcomes or unforeseen complications that could have been avoided.

The physician should recognize one's own personality, strengths, and style. Some patients are excellent candidates for cosmetic treatments but may simply fare better with a different physician. Suggesting that a patient get a second consultation with a colleague for another opinion may be beneficial in such circumstances. Patients will usually respect your honesty and the fact that you truly value their welfare.

First impressions often prove useful for gauging the suitability of a cosmetic procedure, but cannot guarantee proper patient selection. Therefore, a thorough medical history, including a psychological assessment should help the physician recognize appropriate patients and avoid certain predicaments. In certain circumstances, a referral to a mental health professional may be warranted if a psychological comorbidity is noted that fosters an unhealthy communication and relationship between the patient and treating physician.

The following is a central description of select psychiatric disorders that may be encountered during an initial consultation for laser cosmetic surgery. Recognizing the presence of such conditions will allow for appropriate treatment.

Body Dysmorphic Disorder

BDD is a psychological condition that involves a preoccupation with a perceived physical defect.[5] Any body parts could be the focus of their obsession. Most sufferers are concerned about their face and skin problem such as hair thinning, acne, wrinkles, scars, and vascular markings. They may be troubled about a lack of symmetry or disproportionate body size.[6]

Individuals with BDD experience anxiety, shame, and depression about their appearance and much of their self-worth is related to how they feel about their body. The preoccupations with an imaginary flaw are difficult to control. The repetitive behaviors may take many hours per day and usually provide very temporary psychological relief.[6,7]

Such behaviors may include frequently checking their appearance in mirrors or reflective surfaces, elaborate grooming rituals, refusing to take pictures, wearing excessive makeup or clothing to conceal the perceived flaw, comparing their appearance with that of others, and asking for reassurance from others related to the imagined defect.[7]

Many sufferers with BDD may pick their skin or aggressively seek unnecessary and excessive medical procedures, in an attempt to correct what they consider to be an imperfection. Such attempts usually yield dissatisfaction and may even worsen the person's perception of the flaw, not to mention the increased risk of health complications.[7]

Avoiding social situations is common among individuals with BDD because they tend to feel anxious and self-conscious around others (social phobia) where their perceived flaw might be noticed. This can cause high levels of occupational and social impairment including unemployment, absenteeism, and relational or marital problems.[7] In the most severe cases, BDD may keep them housebound.

Patients with BDD are more prone to major depression. Phillips et al. noted[8] that in clinical settings, 60% of patients with BDD have major depression and the lifetime risk for major depression in these patients is 80%. Patients with these comorbidities are at risk for suicide. Nineteen percent of BDD sufferers reported suicidal ideation while 7% had attempted suicide according to one study.[9]

Patients with BDD may not respond to all treatments for depression and may instead respond preferentially to serotonin-reuptake inhibitors.[8] In addition, lengthier treatment trials than those required for depression may be needed to successfully treat BDD and comorbid depression.

The cause of BDD is still unclear, but several contributing factors appear to play a role in the development of BDD, which also might vary for each individual. There may be a genetic predisposition, as it tends to run in families. Additionally, the family environment and cultural influences during early development may be important in shaping body image.[7] Some evidence suggests a neurochemical deficiency of serotonin may provoke BDD, since selective serotonin reuptake inhibitors (SSRIs) improves the condition.[10]

The onset is usually during adolescence and may be gradual or sudden. Preliminary estimates suggest that BDD may be quite common, with a rate of 1–2% in the general population.[6] It occurs as frequently, if not more, in men than women.

Embarrassment and shame often prevent sufferers from revealing their true degree of distress, not only to their family and peers, but to healthcare professionals as well. This makes BDD extremely difficult to diagnose, and even misdiagnosed as obsessive compulsive disorder and/or social anxiety disorder. It is therefore important for dermatologists to be educated in BDD and be able to recognize it before unnecessary procedures are performed. Dr. Katherine Phillips, author

of *The Broken Mirror*[7] and expert in the field of BDD, has developed a Body Dysmorphic Disorder Questionnaire (BDDQ) that may make a rapid and useful in-office screening tool (see Table 2).

Dermatologists may often be the first physicians to see BDD patients since many of them focus on their skin, hair and body size.[6] The prevalence of patients with BDD in dermatology offices ranges from 8% to 12%, and they seek out cosmetic medical treatments with great frequency.[11,12] According to one study, 76% of 289 BDD patients had sought cosmetic enhancement and that 66% did receive treatment for their perceived defects.[13] However, the exact frequency of sufferers with BDD seeking laser treatments is unknown.

BDD sufferers can be difficult patients for dermatologists to treat. Being sympathetic to their urges of cosmetic enhancement will not alleviate their obsession and often BDD patients insist on repeated procedures.[14] Patients diagnosed with BDD should receive consultation with a psychiatrist or psychologist. Psychiatric/psychological treatment often improves BDD symptoms and the suffering it causes. The treatments that appear most effective are SSRIs, as mentioned previously, and a type of therapy known as cognitive-behavioral therapy (CBT).[10] SSRIs can

Table 2 The body dysmorphic disorder questionnaire (BBDQ), developed by Dr. Katherine Phillips[7]

BDD questionnaire
1. Are you very concerned about the appearance of some part(s) of your body that you consider unattractive? If you answered "YES": Do these concerns preoccupy you? That is, do you think about them a lot and wish you could think about them less? (*If you answered "NO" to the above questions, then you are finished with this questionnaire*)
2. Is your main concern with your appearance that you are not thin enough or that you might become too fat?
3. What effect has your preoccupation with your appearance had on your life? A. Has your defect(s) caused you a lot of distress, torment, or pain? B. Has it significantly interfered with your social life? C. Has the defect(s) significantly interfered with your school work, your job, or your overall ability to function? D. Are there things you avoid because of your defect(s)? E. Have the lives or normal routines of your family or friends been affected by your defect(s)
4. How much time do you spend thinking about your defect(s) per day on average? A. Less than 1 h a day B. 1–3 h a day C. More than 3 h a day *It is probable that you have body dysmorphic disorder if you answered "YES" to both parts of question 1, "YES" to any of the questions for question 3, and answered "B" or "C" for question 4*

significantly diminish bodily preoccupation, depression and emotional distress, often improving daily functioning.[8,15] They can also significantly increase control over one's thoughts and behaviors.

When used by trained therapists, CBT substantially improves BDD symptoms in a majority of people, diminishing preoccupations with their appearance and compulsive behaviors, depressive symptoms, and anxiety, and improving body image and self-esteem. Methods include systematic desensitization, exposure techniques, self-confrontational techniques, and cognitive imagery.[6,8,10]

For further resources of information on BDD, see Table 3.

Mood Disorders

Mood disorders mainly encompass two categories: unipolar depression (in this case focusing on major depression) and bipolar disorder.

Major Depression

Patients may develop exaggerated physical complaints when suffering from major depressive episodes. These can include changes sleep, interest, guilt, energy, concentration, appetite, psychomotor with suicidal ideation and overwhelming sadness. Major depression, as defined by the *Diagnostic and Statistical Manual of Mental Disorders, Fourth Edition* (*DSM-IV*), manifests with at least five of the nine symptoms, one being a depressed mood or loss of interests/pleasure, present daily for a minimum of 2 consecutive weeks.[5] (see Table 4).

There are several subtypes of major depression, such as major depression with psychotic features and seasonal affective disorder (SAD). In major depression with

Table 3 Body dysmorphic disorder resources

Resources on body dysmorphic disorder
Internet resources:
http://www.bodyimageprogram.com (last accessed 11/28/07) http://www.bddcentral.com (last accessed 11/28/07)
Books:
The Broken Mirror: Understanding and Treating Body Dysmorphic Disorder. Phillips KA. New York: Oxford University Press; 1996
The Adonis Complex: The Secret Crisis of Male Body Obsession. Pope HG, Phillips KA, Olivardia R. New York: The Free Press; 2000

Table 4 Major depression criteria[5]

Major depression criteria
A. Five or more of the following symptoms have been present nearly every day for at least 2 weeks and represents a change from previous functioning (*Note: Do not include symptoms that are clearly due to a general medical condition, or mood-incongruent delusions or hallucinations*)
At least one symptom is:
(a) Depressed mood (b) Loss of interest or pleasure in nearly all activities
Other symptoms may include:
(a) Significant weight loss while not dieting, weight gain, or decrease or increase in appetite (b) Insomnia or hypersomnia (c) Psychomotor agitation or retardation (d) Fatigue or loss of energy (e) Feelings of worthlessness or excessive or inappropriate guilt (f) Diminished ability to think or concentrate, or indecisiveness (g) Recurrent thoughts of death (not just fear of dying), recurrent suicidal ideation without a specific plan, or a suicide attempt or a specific plan for committing suicide
B. The symptoms do not meet criteria for a mixed episode C. The symptoms cause clinically significant distress or impairment in social, occupational, or other important areas of functioning D. The symptoms are not due to the direct physiological effects of substance or a general medical condition E. The symptoms are not better accounted for by bereavement, i.e., after the loss of a loved one, the symptoms persist for longer than 2 months or are characterized by marked functional impairment, morbid preoccupation with worthlessness, suicidal ideation, psychotic symptoms, or psychomotor retardation

psychosis, patients develop hallucinations, delusions and even paranoia.[5] While individuals with other mental illnesses, like schizophrenia, also experience these symptoms, those with psychotic depression are usually aware that these thoughts aren't true. They may be ashamed and try to hide them, sometimes making this variation difficult to diagnose. Risk of suicide is high among these patients. Patients with SAD have recurrent major depressive episodes in a seasonal pattern. The most common type of SAD usually begins in late fall or early winter and goes away by summer. SAD may be related to changes in the amount of daylight during different times of the year and therefore may respond to light therapy in addition to, or instead of, psychotherapy or medications.[16]

Patients with depression may have vague requests regarding the desired cosmetic results and request cosmetic treatment only to feel better rather than correct a physical imperfection. As mentioned previously, they also tend to have delayed recuperative time, poor patient compliance, and dissatisfaction of the procedure.[4]

The prevalence of major depression of those seeking cosmetic enhancement is unknown. Nonetheless, the prevalence of major depression in the general population is approximately 3–5% in males and 8–10% in females.[17-19]

Rates of depression are increased in patients with most major chronic medical and neurological disorders.[20-23] The prognosis of depression is worsened by the presence of significant medical comorbidity.

A dermatologist should keep in mind that a patient with BDD may simply present with depression therefore concealing the underlying condition.[7] Major depression may exist as a sole diagnosis, but is commonly concurrent with other psychiatric disorders such as BDD, personality and anxiety disorders making it more difficult to treat.[8,24,25]

It has been noted that only a limited number of physicians screen for major depression despite its importance. Psychiatric history is an essential component of the evaluation and it may be necessary to ask about suicidal ideation. Practices may feel that screening for depression is too time consuming. However, there exists a simple two-item screening tool that assesses depressed mood and anhedonia. Answering yes to either of the question is considered a positive screen[26-28] (see Table 5).

Treatment includes some types of CBT as well as medications such as SSRIs, tricyclics, and monoamine oxidase inhibitors (MAO inhibitors).[29] If other therapies have failed, electroconvulsive therapy is considered where a small amount of electricity is applied to the scalp in order to affect neurotransmitters in the brain.[30]

Bipolar Disorder

Bipolar disorder is another psychiatric condition that a dermatologist may be presented with. It is characterized by extreme mood swings, along with other specific symptoms and behaviors. The symptoms of a manic episode often include elevated mood, extreme irritable and anxious, pressured speech, excitability, decreased need for sleep, hypersexuality, and extravagance (i.e., financial, social, and recreational). Hallucinations and delusions are not uncommon during a manic episode nor is impulsivity.[31]

Bipolar disorder is divided into two categories. Bipolar I patients have episodes of sustained mania, and often experience depressive episodes. Patients with bipolar II disorder have one or more major depressive episodes, with at least one hypomanic episode.[5,31] Hypomania refers to a briefer duration of manic symptoms (at least 4 days), and is often has less severe symptoms. Psychosis does not occur with hypomania.

Bipolar I disorder affects men and women equally; bipolar II disorder is more common in women.[32] The age of onset is generally between 15 and 30 years of age.[33,34] Genetics play an important role in the pathogenesis of bipolar disorder as well.

The lifetime prevalence of bipolar disorder has been estimated at 2.6–6.5% though the true prevalence of bipolar disorder is uncertain since patients may present with depression while not disclosing evidence of prior manic episodes.[17,35] Patients with bipolar disorder are frequently misdiagnosed as having unipolar depression. Table 6 is a sample mood disorder questionnaire that can be used in the office as a screening tool. Answering "yes" to 7 out of 13 questions in part 1 and answering "yes" to parts 2 and 3 is a positive screen.[36]

The dermatologist should be wary of the patient that has come as an impulse. Patients with bipolar disorder do not usually recognize the psychological nature of their condition during a manic episode and may later regret having had procedures or spending their money once their mania has subsided. Since these patients also experience depressive episodes, they may request cosmetic laser treatment to simply improve their mood as mentioned earlier.

Typical treatment includes mood stabilizing agents such as lithium, valproate, and carbamazepine.[37-39] The choice of a mood stabilizer is often based upon previous history, side-effect profiles, and any coexisting medical illness. Antipsychotic medications have also been used in patients with acute mania.

Personality Disorders

Personality disorders are long-term patterns of thoughts and behaviors that are inflexible, maladaptive or antisocial. This can limit their ability to function in relationships and at work. As examples, they may endure physical injury from fights or accidents due to impulsive behavior and be at higher risk for suicide and substance abuse.[40-43]

Typically personality disorders are grouped into three clusters that share similar characteristics[5]:

- *Cluster A* includes personality disorders marked by odd, eccentric behavior, including paranoid, schizoid and schizotypal personality disorders.

Table 5 A rapid depression screening tool

Two-item depression scale
During the past month, have you felt down, depressed or hopeless?
During the past month, have you felt little interest or pleasure in doing things?

Adapted from American Psychiatric Association[5]

Table 6 Mood disorder questionnaire to be used as a screening tool. Answering "yes" to 7 out of 13 questions in part 1 and answering "yes" to parts 2 and 3 is a positive screen[58]

Mood disorders questionnaire
1. **Has there ever been a period of time when:** (*mark yes or no for each line please*)   You were not your usual self and (while not using drugs or alcohol)   You felt so good or so hyper that other people thought you were not your normal self, or you were so hyper that you got into trouble?   You were so irritable that you shouted at people or started fights or arguments?   You felt much more self-confident than usual?   You got much less sleep than usual and found you didn't really miss it?   You were much more talkative or spoke faster than usual?   Thoughts raced through your head or you couldn't slow you mind down?   You were so easily distracted by things around you that you had trouble concentrating or staying on track?   You had much more energy than usual?   You were much more active or did many more things than usual?   You were much more social or outgoing than usual; for example, you telephoned friends in the middle of the night?   You were much more interested in sex than usual?   You did things that were unusual for you or that other people might have thought were excessive, foolish, or risky?   Spending money got you or your family into trouble?
2. **If you checked YES to more than one of the above, have several of these ever happened during the *same period of time*?**
3. **How much of a *problem* did any of these cause you – like being unable to work; having family, money, or legal troubles; getting into arguments or fights?**   *No problem   Minor problem   Moderate problem   Serious problem*
4. **Have any of your blood relatives (i.e., children, siblings, parents, grandparents, aunts, uncles) had manic-depressive illness or bipolar disorder?**
5. **Has a health professional ever told you that you have manic-depressive illness or bipolar disorder?**

- *Cluster B* personality disorders are those defined by dramatic, emotional behavior, including histrionic, narcissistic, antisocial and borderline personality disorders.
- *Cluster C* personality disorders are characterized by anxious, fearful behavior and include obsessive-compulsive, avoidant and dependent personality disorders.

Dermatologists may come across these patients in laser cosmetic offices, therefore, it is useful to have an understanding of what to expect and a system of approaching patients with personality disorders. They tend to have difficulties in maintaining a healthy doctor–patient relationship due to poor compliance, communication skills and trust issues.[44] Angry outbursts and late night phone calls to their clinician are not uncommon occurrences with some of these personality types.

Psychiatric treatment of patients with personality disorders is difficult. Mood stabilizers, SSRIs, anxiolytics and antipsychotic drugs are prescribed by the psychiatrist to treat target symptoms.[45,46] From a dermatology perspective, it is important for these patients to feel comfortable discussing their concerns. This will improve compliance with treatment recommendations. If the patient's personality continues to interfere with developing a comfortable and effective professional rapport, it may be appropriate to advise against the procedure or refer them to a colleague for second opinion.

The following personality disorders are a select few that may be encountered more commonly in dermatology offices.

Borderline Personality Disorder

Patients with borderline personality disorder experience instability in their self image, mood states, interpersonal relationships, and impulse control.[5,47] They commonly have stormy relationships. For example, at one moment a friend or romantic partner may be viewed as a trusted confidant; a week later, this same individual may be viewed as cruel and betraying. This anger can be directed at the physician or staff as well.

They may experience repeated marked swings in mood throughout the course of a single day, sometimes resulting in an incorrect diagnosis of bipolar disorder, when these mood swings last weeks or months.[47] These patients are prone to view others as all good or all bad. This phenomenon is called "splitting."[5] They selectively attend to information in a way that confirms his or her current opinion.

Most of these patients will require psychiatric referral for consideration of psychotherapy and drug therapy. A workable doctor-patient relationship is usually possible as long as the physician understands not to be dismayed if the patient becomes impulsive or angry. A patient with borderline personality may interpret the fact that you don't return a phone call immediately as a sign that you wish he or she would find another doctor. If the patient is upset, it may be much more effective to wait until next appointment to discuss the treatment plan.

Some small studies suggest that the prevalence in the general population is approximately 1–3%.[5] The ratio of female to male cases is at least 2:1.[5]

Histrionic Personality Disorder

Individuals with histrionic personality disorder are often excessively emotional, (from laughing to crying easily), and seek constant attention. They have distorted self-images and their self-esteem depends on the approval of others.[5] Due to this overwhelming desire to be noticed, they often behave dramatically or inappropriately to get attention and to manipulate others. For instance, a person with histrionic personality disorder may be inappropriately seductive to try to solicit special services from the office. Patients with histrionic personality also tend to be noncompliant, disorderly, and nonpunctual.[5] During a consultation, patients may constantly seek reassurance, approval, or praise. They also have a style of speech that is excessively impressionistic and lacking in detail.[5]

Histrionic personality disorder is present in about 2–3% of the general population and it occurs more frequently in women than in men, although some feel it is simply more often diagnosed in women because attention-seeking and sexual forwardness is less socially acceptable for women.[5] There may be a genetic susceptibility to this personality disorder. However some child psychologists have suggested that a lack of criticism or punishment as a child and comments that bring positive reinforcement only upon completion of approved behaviors may predispose a patient to histrionic personality.[48]

A goal for treatment is to lessen the dramatic effects of the patient so that he or she may try to uncover true feelings and help improve their self-reliance. The use of antidepressant or anti-anxiety medication is of limited value.

Narcissistic Personality Disorder

Narcissistic personality disorder is characterized by extreme exaggerated sense of self-importance. Although people with narcissistic personality disorder have an exaggerated image of their own importance, they have vulnerable self-esteems.[49] Therefore, they seek attention that confirms their grandiosity. When feedback doesn't validate their exaggerated image, they tend to lash out or withdraw. And though they need constant admiration, they tend to lack empathy for other people.[49] This disorder may regularly interfere with a person's behavior and interactions with family, friends or co-workers.

Table 7 Criteria for narcissistic personality disorder. Patient must have at least five of the following criteria to diagnose narcissistic personality disorder

Narcissistic personality disorder
(a) Has a grandiose sense of self-importance
(b) Is preoccupied with fantasies of unlimited success, fame, brilliance, beauty, or ideal love
(c) Believes that he or she is "special" and unique and can only be understood by other special people
(d) Requires excessive admiration
(e) Strong sense of entitlement
(f) Takes advantage of others to achieve his or her own ends
(g) Lacks empathy
(h) Is often envious or believes others are envious of him or her
(i) Arrogant affect

According to the DSM-IV, at least five criteria must be met to diagnose narcissistic personality disorder as listed in Table 7.[5]

The prevalence of narcissistic personality is less than 1% of the general population and more frequently seen in men than women.[5] Evidence for heritability greater than that of other personality disorders has been reported.

The dermatologist should be suspicious of those who exaggerate their achievements and talents even to the point of lying and those that demand to be recognized as superior. Narcissists tend to use others to achieve their own ends and have expectations that they are entitled to unreasonable and priority treatments.[49] If their behaviors are not supported, they may become frustrated and angry fostering an unhealthy doctor-patient relationship.

Obsessive–Compulsive Personality Disorder

Obsessive–compulsive personality disorder OCPD is a condition characterized by a chronic preoccupation with perfectionism, orderliness, and control.[5] A person with OCPD becomes preoccupied with uncontrollable patterns of thought and action. Symptoms may cause extreme distress and interfere with a person's occupational and social functioning.[5]

Some common signs of OCPD include[5]: perfectionism, inflexibility, lack of generosity, reluctance to allow others to do things, excessive devotion to work, restricted expression of affection, and a preoccupation with details, rules, and lists.

They demand from themselves and from others perfection and an inordinate attention to minutia.[5] They are anxious about delegating tasks to others for fear that they won't be completed correctly. They place greater value on compiling and following rigid schedules and checklists than on the activity itself or its goals.[5] Yet, they are not very efficacious or productive.

Interpersonal relationships are difficult with OCPD patients because of the excessive demands placed on friends, romantic partners and children. Consequently, they are difficult to deal with and "stubborn."[50]

OCPD is often confused with obsessive-compulsive disorder (OCD) due to the similarities in the name. However the mindsets are typically very different and unrelated. Those who are suffering from OCPD do not generally feel the need to repeatedly perform ritualistic actions, a common symptom of OCD.[51,52] Instead, people with OCPD tend to stress perfectionism above all else, and feel anxious when they perceive that things are not right as they see it.

In a laser setting, they may be difficult patients to please since they may not be satisfied with the treatment result and possibly request repeated procedures in order to correct the perceived imperfection. They can be suitable candidates for surgery, as long as they are realistic enough to understand that treatment results may not precisely match their goals.

Anxiety Disorders

Anxiety disorders can be split into various categories including generalized anxiety disorder, social phobia, specific phobia, obsessive–compulsive disorder, and post-traumatic stress disorder with an estimated prevalence at around 18%.[5,18] These can commonly occur along with other mental illnesses as discussed earlier. Granted that most individuals may have some baseline anxiety toward any procedure, but patients with anxiety disorder have anxiety that is more intense than the situation warrants. Additionally, these patients frequently experience physical complaints that accompany their anxiety such as palpitations, tachycardia, dyspnea, sweating, dizziness, nausea, restlessness, and headaches.[5]

Anxiety disorders have also been noted to increase the risk of subsequent development of depression,[53] leading to greater symptom severity and higher rates of suicidal ideation.[24,25] A mental health professional becomes a vital resource in these instances.

Patients with anxiety disorders may have difficulty resolving feelings if there is an imperfect cosmetic result and in turn trigger a relapse of their disorder. Anti-depressants, such as SSRIs, and tricyclics, beta blockers, benzodiazepines and psychotherapy are the mainstay of treatment for these patients.[54] Seeing a good response to these medications is important before proceeding to any specific treatment so that the patient can make competent decisions, understanding the risks and benefits of the procedure.

Psychological Aspects of Laser Therapy for Children and Teens

Children and teens present a unique challenge for physicians and yet laser therapy is not uncommonly used in this population to treat conditions such as vascular malformations, hemangiomas,[55-57] acne, scarring (acne, varicella, traumatic), hair removal, and tattoo removal. Laser therapy can be very effective when treating children and teens, but clearly the laser team must be prepared to deal with the psychological issues of both the patient and parents.

In younger children, fear of pain can be paralyzing for all involved. A brief but honest discussion of expectations in simple language is appropriate. Of great importance is understanding the intensity and duration of the discomfort along with what will be done to help alleviate it. Many children are afraid of the dark and simply applying laser-safety eyewear can cause concern. Start with the laser team and then the parent, to let the child see everyone else wearing eye protection. Since this can sometimes stem from parents' fear, it can be helpful for some children, to have one or both parents out of the laser suite. For others, allowing a child to sit on the parent's lap can be comforting to both the child and parent. Allow a favorite toy, book, blanket, doll or music in the laser suite. We have found that performing a test spot on the parent can be very reassuring to some children. Another trick is to give a test spot on the child at very low fluences so that the child can get use to the light and sound associated with the laser treatment.

Since parents or guardians need to give consent for procedures performed on minors, there may be anguish with issues such as: "Is this the right procedure? Is it the right time to perform procedures? Will my child look worse or suffer?" It can be very helpful to have a time to meet with the parents alone to address these kinds of concerns.

Another problem that may be encountered by the laser surgeon is when the parent insists upon a procedure that the child does not wish to have. This is especially problematic with laser procedures since they usually have to be done over several treatment sessions. Ideally, the procedure should be postponed until the child is emotionally willing to cooperate. If the procedure should not be postponed, appropriate and thorough pain management strategies are usually required, possibly even general anesthesia.

Conclusion

In summary, a dermatologist should perform a psychological assessment during every initial consultation in order to decide suitable candidates for any cosmetic procedure. Ask how they feel about their appearance and why are they considering the procedure. See how they believe others see them, and how they'd prefer to look and feel. Ask what their expectations of the surgery are.

Pay attention to patients who consult with more than one physician since they may be very difficult to satisfy and they seek answers they want to hear. Observe patients who exaggerate a perceived defect and those with certain mood and personality disorders since they may hope for a cure that may not be physical but rather psychological. Clinicians who acquire a basic understanding of these psychiatric conditions can properly screen their patients and enhance the understanding of their patient's goals, hopefully avoiding inappropriate procedures.

However, when a patient presents with a psychological comorbidity or has a psychological complication postoperatively, a referral to a mental health professional is more than warranted. As physicians, striving to treat the whole person and asking help from colleagues in this pursuit will make aesthetic practices even more rewarding.

References

1. The American Society for Aesthetic Plastic Surgery. Cosmetic surgery national data bank page. Available at: http://www.surgery.org/download/2006stats.pdf. Accessed November 30, 2007.
2. Sarwer D, Crerand C. Body image and cosmetic medical treatments. *Body Image*. 2004;1:99-111.
3. Edgerton M, Jacobson W, Meyer E. Surgical-psychiatric study of patients seeking plastic (cosmetic) surgery: ninety-eight consecutive patients with minimal deformity. *Br J Plast Surg*. 1960;13:136-145.
4. Rankin M, Borah G. National plastic surgical nursing survey. *Plast Surg Nurs*. 2006;26(4):178-183.
5. American Psychiatric Association. *Diagnostic and Statistical Manual of Mental Disorders*. Washington, DC: American Psychiatric Association; 2000.
6. Phillips K, Dufresne RJ. Body dysmorphic disorder: a guide for primary care physicians. *Prim Care*. 2002;29:99-111.
7. Phillips K. *The Broken Mirror: Understanding and Treating Body Dysmorphic Disorder*. New York: Oxford University Press; 1996.
8. Phillips K. Body dysmorphic disorder and depression: theoretical considerations and treatment strategies. *Psychiatr Q*. 1999;70(4):313-331.
9. Rief W, Buhlmann U, Wilhelm S, Borkenhagen A, Brahler E. The prevalence of body dysmorphic disorder: a population based survey. *Psychol Med*. 2006;36(6):877-885.
10. Castle DJ, Phillips KA, eds. *Disorders of Body Image*. Hampshire: Wrightson Biomedical; 2002.
11. Vulink N, Sigurdsson V, Kon M, Bruijnzeel-Koomen C, Westenberg H, Denys D. Body dysmorphic disorder in 3-8% of patients in outpatient dermatology and plastic surgery clinics. *Ned Tijdschr Geneeskd*. 2006;150(2):97-100.
12. Phillips K, Dufresne RJ, Wilkel C, Vittorio C. Rate of body dysmorphic disorder in dermatology patients. *J Am Acad Dermatol*. 2000;42:436-441.
13. Phillips K, Grant J, Siniscalchi J, Albertini R. Surgical and nonpsychiatric medical treatment of patients with body dysmorphic disorder. *Psychosomatics*. 2001;42:504-510.

14. Veale D, Boocock A, Gournay K, et al. Body dysmorphic disorder: a survey of 50 cases. *Br J Psychiatry*. 1996;169(2):196-201.
15. Phillips K, Albertini R, Rasmussen S. A randomized placebo-controlled trial of fluoxetine in body dysmorphic disorder. *Arch Gen Psychiatry*. 2002;59:381-388.
16. Golden R, Gaynes B, Ekstrom R, et al. The efficacy of light therapy in the treatment of mood disorders: a review and meta-analysis of the evidence. *Am J Psychiatry*. 2005;162:656-662.
17. Kessler R, Berglund P, Demler O, Jin R, Merikangas K, Walters E. Lifetime prevalence and age-of-onset distributions of DSM-IV disorders in the National Comorbidity Survey Replication. *Arch Gen Psychiatry*. 2005;62:593-602.
18. Kessler R, Chiu W, Demler O, Merikangas K, Walters E. Prevalence, severity, and comorbidity of 12-month DSM-IV disorders in the National Comorbidity Survey Replication. *Arch Gen Psychiatry*. 2005;62:617-627.
19. Williams D, González H, Neighbors H, et al. Prevalence and distribution of major depressive disorder in African Americans, Caribbean blacks, and non-Hispanic whites: results from the National Survey of American Life. *Arch Gen Psychiatry*. 2007;64:305-315.
20. Robinson R. Poststroke depression: prevalence, diagnosis, treatment, and disease progression. *Biol Psychiatry*. 2003;54:376-387.
21. McDonald W, Richard I, DeLong M. Prevalence, etiology, and treatment of depression in Parkinson's disease. *Biol Psychiatry*. 2003;54:363-375.
22. Huffman J, Smith F, Blais M, Beiser M, Januzzi J, Fricchione G. Recognition and treatment of depression and anxiety in patients with acute myocardial infarction. *Am J Cardiol*. 2006;98:319-324.
23. Reiche E, Nunes S, Morimoto H. Stress, depression, the immune system, and cancer. *Lancet Oncol*. 2004;5:617-625.
24. Wittchen H, Kessler R, Pfister H, Lieb M. Why do people with anxiety disorders become depressed? A prospective-longitudinal community study. *Acta Psychiatr Scand Suppl*. 2000;406:14-23.
25. Merikangas K, Zhang H, Avenevoli S, Acharyya S, Neuenschwander M, Angst J. Longitudinal trajectories of depression and anxiety in a prospective community study: the Zurich Cohort Study. *Arch Gen Psychiatry*. 2003;60:993-1000.
26. Mahoney J, Drinka T, Abler R, et al. Screening for depression: single question versus GDS. *J Am Geriatr Soc*. 1994;42:1006-1008.
27. Arroll B, Khin N, Kerse N. Screening for depression in primary care with two verbally asked questions: cross sectional study. *BMJ*. 2003;327:1144-1146.
28. Whooley M, Avins A, Miranda J, Browner W. Case-finding instruments for depression. Two questions are as good as many. *J Gen Intern Med*. 1997;12:439-445.
29. Thase M. Evaluating antidepressant therapies: remission as the optimal outcome. *J Clin Psychiatry*. 2003;64(13):18-25.
30. Persad E. Electroconvulsive therapy in depression. *Can J Psychiatry*. 1990;35(2):175-182.
31. Keck PJ, McElroy S, Arnold L. Bipolar disorder. *Med Clin North Am*. 2001;85:645-661.
32. Benazzi F. Bipolar disorder–focus on bipolar II disorder and mixed depression. *Lancet*. 2007;369:935-945.
33. Suppes T, Dennehy E, Gibbons E. The longitudinal course of bipolar disorder. *J Clin Psychiatry*. 2000;61(9):23-30.
34. Hilty D, Brady K, Hales R. A review of bipolar disorder among adults. *Psychiatr Serv*. 1999;50:201-213.
35. Das A, Olfson M, Gameroff M, et al. Screening for bipolar disorder in a primary care practice. *JAMA*. 2005;293:956-963.
36. Hirschfeld R, Williams J, Spitzer R, et al. Development and validation of a screening instrument for bipolar spectrum disorder: the mood disorder questionnaire. *Am J Psychiatry*. 2000;157:1873-1875.
37. American Psychiatric Association. Practice guideline for the treatment of patients with bipolar disorder. Part A: Treatment

recommendations for patients with bipolar disorder. *Am J Psychiatry*. 2002;159:1-50.

38. Drugs for psychiatric disorders. *Treat Guide Med Lett*. 2006;4(46): 35-46.

39. Bowden C. Novel treatments for bipolar disorder. *Expert Opin Investig Drugs*. 2001;10:661-671.

40. Soloff P, Lis J, Kelly T, Cornelius J, Ulrich R. Risk factors for suicidal behavior in borderline personality disorder. *Am J Psychiatry*. 1994;151:1316-1323.

41. Skodol A, Oldham J, Gallaher P. Axis II comorbidity of substance use disorders among patients referred for treatment of personality disorders. *Am J Psychiatry*. 1999;156:733-738.

42. Cadoret R, Leve L, Devor E. Genetics of aggressive and violent behavior. *Psychiatr Clin North Am*. 1997;20:301-323.

43. Caspi A, Begg D, Dickson N, et al. Personality differences predict health-risk behaviors in young adulthood: evidence from a longitudinal study. *J Pers Soc Psychol*. 1997;73:1052-1063.

44. Gerstley L, McLellan A, Alterman A, Woody G, Luborsky L, Prout M. Ability to form an alliance with the therapist: a possible marker of prognosis for patients with antisocial personality disorder. *Am J Psychiatry*. 1989;146:508-512.

45. Markovitz P, Calabrese J, Schulz S, Meltzer H. Fluoxetine in the treatment of borderline and schizotypal personality disorders. *Am J Psychiatry*. 1991;148:1064-1067.

46. Soloff PH. Symptom-oriented psychopharmacology for personality disorders. *J Pract Psychiatry Behav Health*. 1998;4:3-11.

47. Lieb K, Zanarini M, Schmahl C, Linehan M, Bohus M. Borderline personality disorder. *Lancet*. 2004;364:453-461.

48. Histrionic personality disorder. Available at: http://www.cleveland-clinic.org/health/health-info/docs/3700/3795.asp?index=9743. Accessed November 30, 2007.

49. Britton R. Narcissistic disorders in clinical practice. *J Anal Psychol*. 2004;49(4):477-490.

50. Villemarette-Pittman N, Stanford M, Greve K, Houston R, Mathias C. Obsessive-compulsive personality disorder and behavioral disinhibition. *J Psychol*. 2004;138(1):5-22.

51. Fineberg N, Sharma P, Sivakumaran T, Sahakian B, Chamberlain S. Does obsessive-compulsive personality disorder belong within the obsessive-compulsive spectrum? *CNS Spectr*. 2007;12(6): 467-482.

52. Mancebo M, Eisen J, Grant J, Rasmussen S. Obsessive compulsive personality disorder and obsessive compulsive disorder: clinical characteristics, diagnostic difficulties, and treatment. *Ann Clin Psychiatry*. 2007;17(4):197-204.

53. Goodwin R. Anxiety disorders and the onset of depression among adults in the community. *Psychol Med*. 2002;32:1121-1124.

54. Brown T, O'Leary T, Barlow D. *Generalised Anxiety Disorder. Clinical Handbook of Psychological Disorders: A Step-by-Step Treatment Manual*. New York: Guilford; 2001.

55. Wirt S, Wallace V, Rogalla C. Laser therapy for patients with vascular malformations. *Plast Surg Nurs*. 1997;17(4):200-204.

56. Clymer M, Fortune D, Reinisch L, Toriumi D, Werkhaven J, Ries W. Interstitial Nd:YAG photocoagulation for vascular malformations and hemangiomas in childhood. *Arch Otolaryngol Head Neck Surg*. 1998;124(4):431-436.

57. Leaute-Labreze C, Boralevi F, Pedespan J, Meymat Y, Taieb A. Pulsed dye laser for Sturge-Weber syndrome. *Arch Dis Child*. 2002;87(5):434-435.

58. Hirschfeld R, Williams J, Spitzer R, et al. Development and validation of a screening instrument for bipolar spectrum disorder: the mood disorder questionnaire. *Am J Psychiatry*. 2000;157: 1873-1875.

Photography of Dermatological Laser Treatment

Ashish C. Bhatia, Shraddha Desai, and Doug Roach

- The art and science of photography has evolved tremendously in the past decade, providing the practitioner of cutaneous laser procedures with a versatile and useful set of tools to enhance this procedure, ultimately improving patient care.
- The use of photography in cutaneous laser therapy is extensive. It encompasses the documentation of before-and-after assessments and long-term reviews of various skin conditions treated via laser therapy, the monitoring of the treated lesions and/ or any complications that should arise after the procedure, and the communication between physicians regarding identification of lesions and the treatments performed.
- Additionally, photography is an invaluable tool in the education of trainees, peers, and the general public[7].

Introduction

The use of illustrations and imaging has always had an essential role in the practice of medicine. In the field of dermatology, where visual identification is imperative, the development of small film cameras not only simplified the description of lesions made by medical dermatologists, but also allowed for pre- and post-procedural depictions of interventions for surgical and cosmetic dermatologists[8]. Now, with the advent of digital cameras and its ongoing evolution, clinicians are able to apply this efficient technology to cataloging outcomes of cutaneous laser therapy.

The applications for digital photography in laser treatment are numerous. It can be used in the assessment of the before-and-after appearance of a lesion, thereby determining success rates and long-term reviews of various skin conditions treated via laser therapy. Photographs can also be used to monitor treated lesions for any complications that arise post-procedure. Moreover, they are routinely used to teach students, residents, patients, and staff about the outcomes; both favorable and unfavorable, of a laser procedure.[3]

In order to gain the benefits from digital photography, it is necessary to first know how to operate a digital camera. The science of photography, like medicine, is rapidly evolving as technological innovations continue. In spite of these advances, the fundamental principles of photography remain unchanged. Therefore, a proper understanding and implementation of photo-taking skills will continue to aid in the value of photographs used to document laser therapy.

Disclaimer: Please note that any mention of specific manufactured products in this chapter is included only for their value as examples at this time. There may very well be faster, less expensive, and easier to use equipment in the near future that will render moot any recommendations or brand-specific comments made here.

Photography Equipment

- Clinical photography relies on the recording of light, whether it is on film or via an electronic sensor.
- The required equipment for documenting laser procedures includes: a digital camera, a media card, a media card reader, and a computer.
- Cameras and other photographic equipment should be selected based upon the needs of the practice. Portability, image capacity, image quality, ergonomics, durability, and other subjective factors play into such a decision.[13] Generally, there are tradeoffs for every decision point.

A.C. Bhatia (✉)
Department of Dermatology, Northwestern University Feinberg School of Medicine, Chicago, IL, USA and
The Dermatology Institute of DuPage Medical Group, Naperville, IL, USA
e-mail: acbhatia@gmail.com

K. Nouri (ed.), *Lasers in Dermatology and Medicine*,
DOI: 10.1007/978-0-85729-281-0_33, © Springer-Verlag London Limited 2011

Regardless of the subject matter and photographic equipment used, there is one aspect of photography that remains universal – the capturing of light. Light has been reflected off of an object, passed through a lens, and then recorded on either light-sensitive film or by a digital sensor. In order for the image to be well-recorded, it is necessary to accurately resolve the image at the film plane or CCD (focus), measure and appropriately regulate the amount of light entering the lens, and to account for the color of the light. Good control of these three functions will result in a sharp, adequately exposed, and properly colored photograph.

Camera Types

- The main categories of digital cameras are single-lens-reflex (SLR) type, Compact/ Subcompact (point-and-shoot) type, and hybrid cameras. Because all offer various advantages and disadvantages, there is no one ideal camera type.
- The digital camera selected for clinical photography should reflect the needs of the clinician and the clinical setting.

In general, clinicians use what is called a 35 mm format camera for photographing patients in the exam room or surgical suite. This name is a misnomer, stemming from the days when the camera film measured 24×36 mm. It is still unknown how this initially translated to 35 mm; however the specifications for most digital cameras and lenses reference this standard. Current 35 mm format cameras come in two basic categories: single-lens-reflex (SLR) and compact (point-and-shoot). The SLR is the most versatile and some manufacturers refer to it as a digital single-lens-reflex (DSLR).[5] The advantage of this camera is that it has the capacity to vary lenses, which can be important when recording extreme close-up images or when using the camera in conjunction with other optical devices such as microscopes. The other 35 mm camera type is much smaller and can fit easily into a pocket (subcompact) or purse (compact).[5] Both SLRs and compacts have the ability to use the same recording media and produce sharp and well-exposed images when used correctly. Additionally, most are equipped with auto-focus technology which permits the cameras to make automatic exposures.

Single Lens Reflex

In the early and middle part of the twentieth century, most cameras consisted of two lenses that were vertically mounted to the front of the camera body. One lens enabled the operator to view the scene while the other recorded the image. Thus, these cameras were "twin lens" as opposed to "single-lens," made popular with the advent of 35 mm film. The single lens cameras were also given the name "reflex" in reference to a pentaprism and mirrors inside the camera that allow the photographer to reflexively view the image through the same lens that permits light passage to the film. At the instant of exposure, the main mirror in the camera body flips out of the way so that light can travel unimpeded onto the film plane. A disadvantage of SLR cameras is that due to the necessary movement of the mirrors, the camera body tends to be large and frequently heavy. Without an attached lens, these cameras typically weigh between 18 and 33 oz whereas subcompact cameras weigh between 4 and 7 oz and compact cameras weigh between 6 and 19 oz.[6] However, an advantage of this technology is that it allows for the use of a variety of lens and flash options. Several lenses, like the wide-angle zoom and macro (close-up) are easily attached to the SLR camera body and are useful for lesion characterization. Moreover, SLRs have also been favored in the past by those who require the ability to set the exposure manually in order to accommodate unique lighting situations. In regards to the new digital or DSLR cameras, many of the older lenses will still function with the new digital camera body as long as the manufacturer is the same. Still, there may be some minor formatting compromise due to the different field of view of the digital media. Some manufacturers, like Nikon™, Canon™, and Fuji™, have overcome this by introducing reliable and affordable digital SLR cameras that are compatible with their current non-digital gear. In general, the cost of good SLR and DSLR cameras ranges from $500 to $1,400 without lenses.

Compact/Subcompact

The other 35 mm format camera is the compact/subcompact or point-and-shoot. Several years ago, this camera was referred to as a "Rangefinder" since this was the focusing mechanism it employed. Currently, it is the overwhelming choice of digital camera purchasers in the world. The main advantages of this camera are its overall body size, LCD size, and economy. Because compacts do not rely on a mirror system, they are not limited to large body sizes and even when equipped with a zoom lens, a subcompact and some compacts will fit easily into a lab coat pocket – a feat that cannot be managed by an SLR. At times, the compact size can be problematic for clinicians with larger hands as buttons and dials on the camera are small. As a result, it is recommended that clinicians physically test cameras before purchase. They also have large LCD (liquid crystal displays) screens so that the photographer can preview and review a photograph. Often, LCD displays on the SLR cameras can only be used to review a picture taken, but they cannot be used for preview. Additionally, the average cost of subcompact and compact cameras tend to be much lower than that of SLRs. In general, they range in price from \$100 to \$450.[6,10] Likewise, with recent advances in the art of lens manufacture, many of the enhanced compact cameras now compare favorably with the single lens reflex models for most medical situations. This is especially true if the purpose of the image is to document relative sizes and locations of lesions or defects. The majority of these models come equipped with zoom lenses that can offer a range of different focal lengths thus emulating, if not equaling, the chief feature of SLRs.

One shortfall of compact cameras is their flash capability. Most have a very small "pop-up" flash built into the camera body. Therefore, when shooting very close to or more than 9 ft from the subject, the flash can result in overexposure of the image or be considerably underpowered in lowlight conditions. However, these situations can be avoided by using the optical zoom capabilities of the camera while standing at approximately 4–5 ft from the subject.

Several manufacturers also offer a hybrid DSLR/compact camera which is thought of as "SLR-like." This camera type is larger than most compacts due to the accommodation of a particularly un-compact-like lens. This lens, while larger and of a greater zoom capability than other compacts, is not interchangeable. Still, the larger lens may have a better close-up capability and the camera itself has an option for an auxiliary flash. Overall, the camera has the look of a DSLR without many of the inherent SLR disadvantages.

Lenses

- SLR cameras have the ability to exchange lenses for different purposes, while compact cameras generally have non-interchangeable lenses with versatile features.
- Due to the nature of dermatology and dermatologic surgery, macro or "close up" capability is a must when choosing a camera.
- With digital cameras, avoid using the "digital zoom" feature since it can degrade image quality.

No matter which type of digital camera is selected, it is helpful to have a simple familiarity with lenses. The choice of lens is generally determined by the purpose of the camera as well as budgetary and shooting space constraints. If the intent is to record full body images, it will be necessary to either have a good amount of room in which to physically back up, or to use a wide-angle zoom lens. Should the practice be confined to facial surgery for instance, a normal or short telephoto lens is adequate. Still, in nearly all practices the nature of the subject seems to require at least some macro or close-up capability.

Wide-Angle Zoom

Zoom lenses are often used in smaller examination rooms to take full-body photographs of patients. This type of lens is especially useful in displaying the distribution and pattern of a whole-body rash.[6] They are designed such that the internal elements can alter position and produce a variable field of view, thus capturing the entire area of focus. The majority of compact cameras come equipped with zoom lenses as standard equipment. Most SLRs, however, are sold with a normal lens and have the option of mounting other fixed focal length or specialty lenses like wide-angle zooms.

In general, most digital cameras contain both optical and digital zoom capabilities. An optical zoom is like that of an older film camera. The camera alters its focal length by changing the position of internal lens elements. The optical zoom is frequently favored over the digital zoom, because this camera utilizes high quality optic lens technology. What has commonly been referred to as "digital" zoom does not involve optics, but rather is an electronic cropping of the image in the camera's viewfinder followed by enlargement. This in turn results in a lower quality image than a photo taken with an optical zoom lens. Therefore, it is better not to rely on digital zoom, but instead, use the digital camera's optical zoom feature whenever possible.

Macro or "Close-Up" Lenses

Macro-lenses are used to focus the camera within millimeters of the lesion in question. This allows for certain characteristics such as texture and color to be visualized with great detail.[6] If the dermatologist's camera of choice does not have the mounting capability for different lenses (like SLRs), the built-in lens should be able to focus on up-close objects. Unfortunately, many lower-priced cameras are not manufactured with this capability.

For dermatologic surgery, it is most appropriate to have a macro-lens that can capture an image at a 1:1 (subject to film) ratio. At this setting, a photographed area would be reproduced at exactly the same size on the film or media card as in reality. For 35 mm film, the subject will cover an area that is 24×36 mm; adequate for recording a small lesion. However, not all close-focusing lenses have a 1:1 capability. Therefore, it is important to ask about this feature prior to purchasing a lens.

Note that a lens that has macro capability also functions as a regular lens that is dependent on its focal length. This length will determine how far away the photographer can be while taking both normally-focused and macro pictures. At our facilities, we've determined that the most appropriate macro-lens length for obtaining photographs of patients and surgeries is 105 mm. This length allows for close focus of images while the camera remains at a reasonable distance from the site of interest. This also makes the situation more comfortable for both the patient and surgeon.

Flash

- Using the camera flash (instead of relying on ambient lighting) allows for image consistency, adequate depth of field, good color, and proper exposure of photographs.
- A hot shoe is a port on a camera that allows for an external flash unit to be mounted. This flexibility is desirable if shooting in situations that require complex external flash setups.

Regardless of office quality or surgical suite lighting, it is best not to rely on these as primary light sources. Instead, use the camera flash. It facilitates image consistency, adequate field depth, improved color, and appropriate exposure. An electronic flash produces light that simulates daylight, so that color balance is not required. Many newer cameras come with a small flash unit that is adequate for this in most cases. However, for images requiring a more professional look, or for the flash to function farther than 9 ft for full-body shots, it will be necessary to supplement the camera with an additional flash unit. When shopping for a camera or flash, it is important to note that flashes are rated by their light output by a "guide number" (GN). A guide number of 80 or higher (at ISO 100) is adequate for most dermatology needs.

Flash Options

SLRs have the option to not only exchange lenses, but flashes as well. This is accomplished with the aid of a "hot-shoe." A hot-shoe is a flat, horizontally mounted, square-shaped socket on top of the camera that attaches to an external flash unit. Most of these units have a number of electrical contacts on the socket (metal dots) that mate with similar contacts on the flash that allow for communication between the flash and camera.

A ring flash is a unique flash unit that can be attached via the hot-shoe and has the ability to eliminate shadows by casting light in all directions. This can be quite effective if the intent is to evenly illuminate and record a flat field. It is also useful for photographing within deep surgical defects or cavities (like the oral cavity), since no shadow will be created by the depth. On the other hand, this even lighting can be a drawback if the intent is to illustrate a lesion or rash that has a subtle texture. The major disadvantage of the ring flash is

that the emitted lights are almost universally underpowered. As a result, illumination of a full human figure will often result in underexposure. Still, the ring flash remains adequate for taking close-focus photographs.

Another flash option is a point flash. Any flash that can be "pointed" at the field either by removing it from its mount or by using a movable flash head feature can be called a point flash. The advantage of this type of flash is that the angle of light in relation to the photographed object creates a slight shadow that reveals shape, contour, and topography. If it is important to display the depth, height, or texture of a dermatological feature, this type of flash is far superior to a ring flash.

Digital compact cameras do not have the ability to exchange flash units and instead contain a built-in flash that may not be able to produce adequately-exposed photographs. Additionally, many compact cameras require batteries, so in order to maintain these for a longer period of time; the flash often has to be reduced in size and output potential. In order to circumvent this, an auxiliary flash can be used.

An auxiliary flash can either be connected directly to the camera or can be triggered at the right instance by some other means. Since some lower-priced compacts and SLRs do not have a PC socket or hot-shoe for flash connection, one can use a photo cell as an auxiliary flash. A photo cell is comparable to a wireless remote, but instead of controlling a television set, it fires a flash of light when it senses another flash (the one built into the camera). Photography studios have done this for several years, and refer to it as a "slave" flash unit. Several manufacturers of slave units can provide the medical photographer with adequate lighting in virtually all scenarios. Note that many digital cameras use a series of rapid low-power "pre-flashes" in order to set the camera white balance for a shot and to reduce the "red-eye" effect. These pre-flashes can therefore trigger the slave flash at an inappropriate time. Be certain that the camera has a setting to disable the pre-flash, or that the slave flash has the ability to filter out the flashes from its triggering cycle.

White Balance

- Adjusting the white balance on the camera prior to taking photographs can compensate for the unnatural color in photographs from varying ambient light sources.

All light has color, but this often goes unnoticed as our brains color-correct light without any conscious effort on our part. Each light source produces a particular wavelength which is identified by degrees Kelvin and commonly referred to as the light's "color temperature." Digital cameras correct for color

Photography of Dermatological Laser Treatment

temperature with "white balance." Since daylight, or white light is the standard by which we measure color, yellow is usually seen as yellow, green as green, and so on and so forth. However, when an artificial light source is introduced, like fluorescent lighting in the office, the color of light takes on a green tinge, especially when viewing human skin. The camera unfortunately records this color very well. For this reason, we must make adjustments to the "white balance" setting of a camera if subjects are photographed under fluorescent lighting. The same holds true for tungsten lighting found in common filament light bulbs and for the tungsten/halogen hybrid bulbs found in many surgical rooms. Fortunately, an electronic flash is designed with a color temperature that approximates daylight so a flash photo is the most color-precise image when taken with a daylight white balance setting.

Most digital cameras come with menu preset options that change the color sensitivity of the camera for various lighting situations. These may be adequate for certain situations, but for the most effective and accurate recording of color, it is advisable to use the "custom white balance" option which *is explained in the camera manual*. If the custom white balance procedure is followed properly, there will be no need to repeat the process each time the same room and light source is used. Under no circumstances should one rely on a common setting called "Auto White Balance" or AWB. This option is not able to replicate daylight effectively and because color reproduction is critical to medical photography, AWB is not recommended.

Digital Media

- Images stored by a digital camera are recorded onto digital media.
- There is an assortment of digital media formats and technological advances ensure increasing memory capacity and newer designs.
- Digital cameras can typically only use specific types of digital media, so it is important to use the right variety.

When a photograph is taken with a digital camera, light passes through the lens onto the image capture device. This is commonly a charge coupled device (CCD). It is a film-sized wafer that is embedded with millions of light sensing units called pixels that filter red, blue, and green (primary colors) light. With exposure to light, the pixels transmit light data along with its position in the array to a micro-processor which then translates this information into a coded pattern. This pattern is called a file format and the information it contains is passed along to the memory module (media card) for storage. The media card is the "film" of digital cameras and its storage size ranges from 64 megabytes (MB) to 8 gigabytes (GB). The larger the storage size, the more photographs that can be stored. Presently, there are about eight memory card types that work in digital cameras. These include the compact flash (CF), secure digital (SD), memory stick, and xD cards. Most formats have a large range of capabilities and are more than adequate for recording photographic images. Remember that memory card types are not interchangeable. A single memory card can only be used in a camera that accepts that type of storage device. However, each card can be used repeatedly. And in order to do so, it will be necessary to empty the card or download the images into a computer once the memory card becomes full.

A useful downloading accessory for a digital camera is a memory card reader. These small devices connect to a computer USB port and can accommodate various memory cards. Once the card is inserted into the reader, the images can be downloaded into the computer. The advantage to downloading in this fashion as opposed to connecting the camera directly to the computer is that because the camera isn't required, its battery power is saved. Most memory card readers are also inexpensive and range in price from $10 to $50. The main disadvantage of using memory cards for downloading is the risk of damaging the card or reader contacts with repeatead insertion and removal of the card.

Mega-Pixels

- Mega-pixels reflect the amount of information or detail contained within an image.
- Larger mega-pixel images contain more detail, but also require longer transfer times for recording and greater space for storing the image.

Mega-pixel refers to how many "picture elements" (pixels) are on your CCD or complementary metal oxide semiconductor (CMOS) chip that are exposed to light reflected off of a subject. The prefix "mega" means "millions of," and each pixel is the smallest unit in the photograph that can be assigned a unique color. Increasing the number of pixels that makes up an image increases the detail but only up to a point. As the number of mega-pixels enlarges, so does the file size (the amount of space required to store the image) and the burden of handling it. Large file sizes can slow down the recording of the image onto a memory card, the transfer of the images into a computer, and the processing of images by editing software. Moreover, multi-mega-pixel digital cameras produce just as much detail as 35 mm format cameras of 10 years ago, and even high mega-pixel cameras (8 mega-pixels and higher) are not necessary to attain publisher quality images. For the purpose of dermatologic surgery and laser treatment, obtaining a 1.5–2.5 mega-pixel image will be more than adequate.

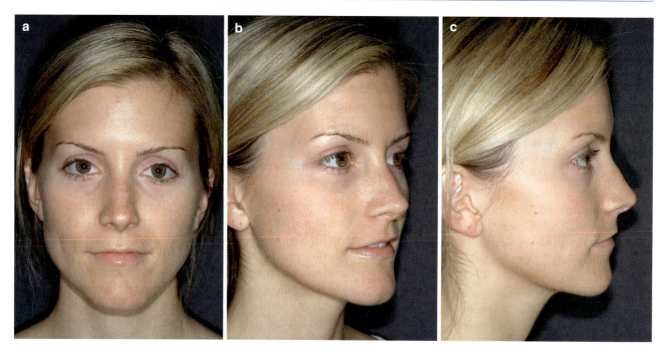

Fig. 1 Standard positioning for full facial photography. (**a**) Frontal view. (**b**) Oblique view (note nasal tip lined up with margin of posterior cheek). (**c**) Lateral view

self explanatory. However, the oblique view can be consistently captured using the technique where the tip of the nose should align with the most prominent edge of the distal cheek.

Surgical Photography

In surgery, there are concerns with keeping the field free of contaminating items such as cameras and lenses. Obviously, it would be most appropriate to have someone who is not scrubbed-in to handle the camera. This person should understand both how the camera works and what it is that needs to be photographed. Have appropriate stands & stools on hand for the camera operator to easily get above the field for the most effective angle. If the camera is equipped with an auxiliary flash and/or battery, the cords connecting these devices should be taped down prior to surgery so they do not fall into the field if the camera is positioned above it.

Make the first image of each procedure a shot that will identify the patient, such as the patient identification sticker or a card with this information printed on it.

Certain operating room lighting conditions are different than will be encountered in the office setting and may require some exposure compensation. For this reason, it is prudent to take some practice photographs prior to the procedure.

If gestures need be made in photos to point out a small artifact such as a stitch or tiny vessel, do not use fingers to do so. Keep the presence of hands to a minimum in photos and instead indicate the area with a straight clamp, pick-ups, or other such blunt but slim devices.

It is a sign of professionalism and pride if the field and any instruments or gloves that must be shown in a surgical photo are wiped clean of blood prior to taking a photograph. Also, if the periphery of the operating area is draped with blue towels, be sure that fresh clean ones are available to cover those that have been stained with fluids. Maintain suction in deep wounds right up until the image is made. Pools of blood are very distracting in photographs and can in fact obscure areas of interest. Similarly, if the wound is wet from irrigation or from wiping with wet sponges, quickly pat it dry just before the shot is taken in order to reduce the incidence of specular highlights.

When shooting excised or extracted gross specimens, use a clean blue towel as a background. Images of specimens should be photographed in their correct anatomical orientation and with at least one of the images including a size scale placed just far enough away from the tissue that it may be easily cropped out later if necessary.[10]

Final Thoughts

- Current digital camera technology has come to the threshold where it is now virtually indistinguishable from 35 mm image quality for most dermatologic purposes.
- If you purchase a good digital 6 or 7 mega pixel SLR camera system, you will soon recover your investment in film and processing costs as well as save on office expenses and personnel time.
- In dermatology perhaps more than any other medical discipline, well crafted imaging skills can enhance your career even as it helps you to be of greater value to your profession and your colleagues and of a greater service to your patients.

References

1. Lyon CC, Harrison PV, et al. A portable digital imaging system in dermatology: diagnostic and educational applications. *J Telemed Telecare*. 1997;3(Suppl 1):81-83.
2. Papier A, Peres MR, Bobrow M, Bhatia A, et al. The digital imaging system and dermatology. *Int J Dermatol*. 2000;39:561-575.
3. Berg D et al. A simple tool for teaching flap design with digital images. *Dermatol Surg*. 2001;27(12):1043-1045.
4. Kokoska MS, Currens JW, Hollenbeak CS, Thomas JR, Stack BC. Digital vs 35-mm photography. To convert or not to convert? Arch Facial Plast Surg. 1999;1(4):276-81.
5. Bhatia AC, Desai S, Brodell RT, Horvath MM. Digital Photography. eMedicine website. Available at: http://emedicine.medscape.com/article/1131303-overview. Accessed July 1, 2010.
6. Chilukuri S, Bhatia AC. Practical digital photography in the dermatology office. *Semin Cutan Med Surg*. 2008;27(1):83-85.
7. Sasson M, Schiff T, et al. Photography without film: low-cost digital cameras come of age in dermatology. *Int J Dermatol*. 1994;33(2):113-115.
8. Stone JL, Peterson RL, et al. Digital imaging techniques in dermatology. *J Am Acad Dermatol*. 1990;23(5 Pt 1):913-917.
9. Bhatia AC et al. The clinical image archiving clinical processes and an entire specialty. *Arch Dermatol*. 2006;142(1):96-98.
10. Lin BB, Taylor RS, et al. Digital photography for mapping Mohs micrographic surgery sections. *Dermatol Surg*. 2001;27(4):411-414.

Online Resources for Dermatologic Laser Therapies

Elizabeth E. Uhlenhake, Shraddha Desai, and Ashish C. Bhatia

- The internet is an abundant and easily accessible source of current health-related information for patients and physicians
- Physicians can harness the power of the internet to keep up-to-date on developments in their field and review the literature on a regular basis
- Physicians can also help direct patients to accurate and reliable information on the internet which is geared towards the general public
- Proper guidance of patients and their families can help make the internet a valuable tool for education

Introduction

The Internet has revolutionized the way in which both lay-people and health care professionals seek out and research information regarding health care topics and specific disease conditions.[1] A recent report states that approximately 80% of adult Internet users have conducted searches online for health or medical information.[2] With increasing accessibility to the internet and rising familiarity with search engines, this percentage continues to grow. Aside from accessibility and convenience, the Internet is superior to most paper-based medical

A.C. Bhatia (✉)
Department of Dermatology, Northwestern University
Feinberg School of Medicine, Chicago, IL, USA and
The Dermatology Institute of DuPage Medical Group,
Naperville, IL, USA
e-mail: acbhatia@gmail.com

resources due to the ease of updating information to reflect the most timely and current data.

The wealth of knowledge that can be obtained from the Internet however, has its drawbacks. Unfortunately, there is no control over what information can be accessed and anyone, from a physician to common layperson, can contribute information regardless of accuracy. This can lead to misinformation that ultimately results in mistakes and malpractice.[3] In order to prevent this from occurring, websites should be critically analyzed to determine their validity, reliability, and credibility. This holds true for anyone using such information from a website, but especially for physicians. It is imperative for physicians to provide their patients with a means of evaluating different websites and using only the most reliable and precise sources to prevent medical misunderstandings. In doing so, patients will get a sense of empowerment over their condition, knowing that only the most relevant information is being provided to them. Therefore, physicians should improve their patients' knowledge by supplying them with a list of highly reputable websites; an action commonly desired by patients according to recent studies.[4,5] The guidelines for evaluating websites that provide information on cutaneous laser therapies are reviewed here.

Internet Website Quality Evaluation

In evaluating the quality of a website, there are several indicators which can be used to measure the usefulness of the information presented. These include, but are not limited to: easy identification of the background and significance of the authors, the recent nature of information and its stability, the time since the last update of information, the completeness of the information and its ability to match the searcher's needs, the domain of the website, comparability with other resources, and the ease of use.[6,7] Table 1 highlights the important details which should be considered in each of these categories (Table 1).

K. Nouri (ed.), *Lasers in Dermatology and Medicine*,
DOI: 10.1007/978-0-85729-281-0_34, © Springer-Verlag London Limited 2011

Table 1 Consideration in the evaluation of laser related websites

Easy identification of the background and authority of the authors
- Check the authors' credentials
- Author's level of education
- Experience author has in the subject matter
- Previous list of publications

Current information/update
- When was the information published and/or uploaded onto the Internet
- When was the information last updated

Stability of the information
- Will the information remain on the site

Information contained matches the searcher's needs
- Focus on what you are looking for: laser therapy information, statistics, latest treatments, risks and benefits involved, procedural techniques, complications arising during laser procedures, costs involved

Domain of the website
- Check the URL to see if it is someone's personal page. If so, be sure to investigate the author thoroughly
- Is the website educational (.edu), nonprofit organizations (.org), commercial, or government (.gov, .mil, .us)

Comparability with other resources
- Look for a site with related links, explore other sites and publications by the author
- Check to see that the links to the other sources are on the same topic, well organized, and use the above criterion to evaluate them

Ease of use
- Easy navigation of site
- Check to see if the information is targeted toward the physician or the patient
- Check if the speed and connection of your Internet is compatible with that of patients visiting this website

Websites for Physicians

- Professional society websites offer valuable and reliable information for physicians in addition to links to other highly regarded sites
- Access to abstracts of peer-reviewed articles in medicine is readily available, providing a convenient way to keep abreast of the current literature

It is the physician's responsibility to his patients to be critical of any and all information that is retrieved from the internet. Consequently, suitable sites pertaining to laser therapies include those of well-known societies that deal specifically with these procedures. Such groups include the American Academy of Dermatology (AAD), Skin Care Physicians (from the AAD), the American Society of Dermatologic Surgeons (ASDS), and the American Society for Laser Medicine and Surgery (ASLMS).

The Journal of Investigative Dermatology Symposium Proceedings and Derm Net websites are also available options for information on laser interventions. Additionally, journal abstracts provided by PubMed, eMedicine, and the Cochrane Library are excellent sources of up-to-date information. The web addresses for these sites and others are provided in Table 2.

The AAD website is a practical site in which to begin researching laser treatments due to its extensive knowledge base and broad list of resources and links. Dermatologists also have the ability to learn about current issues like new

Table 2 Web addresses of useful websites for physicians and patients

Website	Information for the physician	Information for the patient
MedicineNet http://www.medicinenet.com		✓
Mayo Clinic http://www.mayoclinic.com/health		✓
The Hair Removal Journal http://www.hairremovaljournal.org/faqs.htm		✓
Derm Net http://www.dermnetnz.org/procedures/lasers.html	✓	✓
American Academy of Dermatology- http://www.aad.org	✓	✓
American Society for Laser Medicine & Surgery http://www.aslms.org/	✓	✓
American Society for Dermatologic Surgery http://www.asds.net	✓	✓
EMedicine http://www.emedicine.com	✓	✓
Skin Care Physicians (AAD) http://www.skincarephysicians.com	✓	✓
Skin Care Guide http://skincareguide.com	✓	✓
Journal of Investigative Dermatology Symposium Proceedings http://www.nature.com/jidsp/journal/v10/n3/full/5640219a.html	✓	
Cochrane Library http://www.cochrane.org/reviews/en/	✓	
PubMed http://www.pubmed.gov	✓	
Medscape Dermatology http://www.medscape.com	✓	
Skin Therapy Letter http://www.skintherapyletter.com	✓	

treatment options and management plans with Dermatology World Online. Additionally, the website contains links for the Journal of the American Academy of Dermatology (JAAD), the Dermatology Insights Journal (a patient-oriented journal), and the medical web guide. As a result, dermatologists can safely recommend the AAD website to their patients as a source of information on laser procedures, with close attention paid to the Dermatology Insights page and medical web guide that offer links for patient education material and support groups.

Another website created by the AAD is Skin Care Physicians which is geared specifically for patients and dermatologists to use as a resource for the latest information on the management of skin conditions including hair removal, photo rejuvenation, resurfacing, and vascular procedures. It is an excellent tool that provides patients with easy-to-understand explanations and basic information regarding laser procedures.

Another well-known group is the American Society for Dermatologic Surgery (ASDS) and their website is appealing to dermatologists for several reasons. First, it contains a physician discussion forum designed specifically to begin a dialog about laser procedures, including advances in the latest technology and research in the field. Dermatologists can also access recent information regarding dermatologic surgery procedures, guidelines, and upcoming educational events and meetings. The site also contains links to other websites providing additional information on dermatology and laser procedures, local research, and legislative advocacy groups. Members of the group are given access to the Journal of Dermatologic Surgery as well. Patients also gain benefit from this website. Here they can read reports about most dermatologic surgery procedures like laser or light therapy, laser hair removal, nonablative skin rejuvenation, resurfacing, and vascular treatment. The site also provides fact sheets for each procedure with before and after pictures and frequently asked questions. Finally, patients can use the site to search for a dermatologic surgeon by geographic region.

The American Society for Laser Medicine & Surgery (ASLMS) website is a physician and patient-friendly resource too. It offers physicians guidelines for office-based laser procedures, patient and procedure selection, patient safety, and quality assurance. It also addresses patient issues with a brief introduction to laser procedures, a physician locator feature, and safety tips for patients considering dermatologic laser and light-based device procedures, and includes a checklist of services each facility that performs such interventions should maintain.

The Journal of Investigative Dermatology Symposium Proceedings site has laser hair removal-specific information and provides the physician with an overview on the physiology of the hair follicle in order to discuss the latest strategies for photo-epilation. The website also contains a list of clinical guidelines that is useful to dermatologists.

The Derm Net website is another good source of valuable information on laser procedures and includes material for both physicians and patients. A patient information link leads the patient to data, including history, effectiveness, indications, complications, and adverse effects of various lasers. Under the doctors tab, the site features numerous quizzes and topics for laser discussions and offers an extensive list of resources available for more information.

Another valuable website for patients and dermatologists for continuing education is eMedicine. This particular website notes the history of laser procedures in addition to describing the various types of lasers that are currently and were historically used for laser hair removal, treatment of acquired and congenital vascular lesions, and non-ablative resurfacing. General principles and physics of laser therapy, indications, contraindications, clinical workup, follow-up protocols, outcomes, and alternative therapies are also discussed.

Finally, PubMed, a National Institute of Health (NIH) affiliate, offers an enormous amount of information that encompasses virtually all aspects of medicine. The information obtained on this site is in the form of medical articles obtained from peer-reviewed medical journals. Thus, the information is limited to physicians and not appropriate for patient use. Although searches can be made for any medical specialty and subject, dermatologists can specifically search for articles relating to laser therapy. Furthermore, many academic institutions offer specialized access to PubMed that allows users to view full text articles rather than abstracts for any subscribed journal.

Websites for Patients

- Many valuable online resources for physicians have sections geared towards patient education as well
- Guiding patients to appropriate resources can be an asset in laser procedure education. This also supplements any information given during routine office visits
- Patient-oriented websites are discussed below

Many of the aforementioned websites also provide useful knowledge for the patient population. The American Academy of Dermatology (AAD), Skin Care Physicians (AAD), eMedicine, the American Society of Dermatologic Surgeons (ASDS), and the American Society for Laser Medicine & Surgery (ASLMS) websites are of use to both physicians and patients. Patients, in particular, can access basic information about current laser treatments and follow helpful links to a number of other knowledgeable websites.

The Mayo Clinic also maintains a website for patient inquiries on health-related topics. Patients' questions regarding what the procedure entails, including pictures, prep work for the patient, risks and long term effects, eligibility for such treatments, and typical results from laser resurfacing and hair removal procedures, are all answered.

The Hair Removal Journal is also a great resource for patients considering hair removal with lasers. A frequently asked questions page contains information on almost every aspect of the process, including cost, where it can be performed, and the effect of color-treated hair and tanned skin on the process. This website is highly patient-oriented and provides a great deal of information in a simple and concise way. And like the other websites, it has links to related sites for more information.

Final Thoughts

The internet is an expansive source of information on numerous topics including laser treatment modalities. Because of its availability and low maintenance costs, it has become an attractive alternative to the more costly and time-consuming process of paper publishing. However, the ease of adding information in spite of its credibility also makes it a tool that must be used cautiously. Therefore, it is of utmost importance for physicians to critically assess the information obtained from websites not only for themselves but also for their patients. Using the above mentioned methods of analysis can make the internet an excellent resource for all that wish to learn more about laser therapies and other dermatologic procedures.

References

1. Fox S, Fallows D. *Internet Health Resources: Health Searches and Email Have Become More Commonplace, but There Is Room for Improvement in Searches and Overall Internet Access.* Washington, DC: Pew Internet and American Life Project; 2003:1-42.
2. Diaz JA, Griffith RA, et al. Patients' use of the Internet for medical information. *J Gen Intern Med.* 2002;17(3):180-185.
3. Murray E, Lo B, Pollack L, et al. The impact of health information of the Internet on health care and the physician-patient relationship: a national U.S. survey among 1,050 U.S. physicians. *J Med Internet Res.* 2003;5(3):e17.
4. Diaz JA, Sciamanna CN, Evangelou E, et al. Brief report: what types of Internet guidance do patients want from their physicians? *J Gen Intern Med.* 2005;20(8):683-685.
5. Murray E, Lo B, et al. The impact of health information on the Internet on health care and the physician-patient relationship: patient perceptions. *Arch Intern Med.* 2003;163(14):1727-1734.
6. Tillman HN. Evaluating quality on the net. http://www.hopetillman.com/findqual.html. Babson Park, 2006.
7. University of California Berkeley Library. Evaluating web pages: techniques to apply and questions to ask. http://www.lib.berkley.edu/teachinglib/guides/internet/evaluate.html. Berkley, 2006.

Starting a Laser Practice

Vic A. Narurkar

- Different types of lasers or light sources have specific functions for indicated treatments
- Treatment options are based on cost-effective methods
- Popularity of devices depends on histological data regarding pros and cons of treatment outcomes
- Laser or light options chosen by physician depend on practicality of device

Introduction

The field of energy based devices has witnessed an unparalleled growth in the last 10 years. The practicing physician is often overwhelmed and confused with the decision of how to integrate these devices into a practice. The marketing materials associated with these devices often override their actual clinical merits. Moreover, elaborate terms of financing these devices with unrealistic returns on investment (ROI) can further confuse the practicing physician. This chapter will review some fundamental aspects on how to integrate energy based devices in practical practice.

Integrating Energy Based Devices: A Systematic Approach

The question that one often asks when starting a practice is "what laser/light/energy" source should I choose that will benefit most clinical indications? Often, devices are touted

as "one size fits all," where one laser or light source may have a myriad of clinical indications. While this is an ambitious goal, it is far from realistic. The majority of devices do one or two things well, and other indications are suboptimal at best. Therefore, the first question one must ask is "What procedure do I foresee being the most in demand in my practice?" For example, in a dermatology practice, a significant number of patients seek care for vascular and pigmented lesions. In a plastic surgery practice, the emphasis is placed more on rhytids and laxity. Thus, the initial device that may be most optimal may reflect the specialty of the physician, as well as the clinical demographics of the practice. Vascular and pigmented lesion treatments are also often highly gratifying, as clinical improvement of these entities is quite remarkable with excellent photographic documentation showing efficacy. Examples of "workhorse" devices for vascular lesions include pulsed dye lasers, pulsed KTP lasers and pulsed light sources. Examples of "workhorse" devices for pigmented lesions include Q-switched lasers (532, 694, 755 nm) and pulsed light sources. Newer generation pulsed light sources and newer generation pulsed dye lasers are effective for the treatment of both vascular and pigmented lesions, and, therefore, may be a more cost-effective method for integrating a single device, as opposed to investing in multiple devices. Resurfacing devices include non ablative fractional lasers, ablative fractional lasers and traditional ablative lasers. For plastic surgery practices, resurfacing lasers are most likely the first device of choice. While traditional ablative resurfacing is highly effective, the downsides such as prolonged erythema, risks of hypopigmentation and limitation to facial areas, make these devices less popular in the twenty-first century. The advent of fractional laser resurfacing has reduced some of these risks. Thus, a fractional laser resurfacing device is often the ideal first device for a plastic surgery practice. After investing in the initial device, expansion to other devices in a systematic fashion is optimal. For dermatologists, a resurfacing device, should be the second device to integrate into a practice and for plastic surgeons, a vascular/pigmented lesion device fits this role. Afterwards, other devices can be integrated in a

V.A. Narurkar
Department of Dermatology, California Pacific Medical Center,
San Francisco, CA, USA
e-mail: vicnarurkar@yahoo.com, info@bayarealaserdr.com

K. Nouri (ed.), *Lasers in Dermatology and Medicine*,
DOI: 10.1007/978-0-85729-281-0_35, © Springer-Verlag London Limited 2011

step wise fashion based on economic returns on the first two. These include skin tightening devices, acne devices and body contouring devices. The question of hair reduction devices remains dubious. While this procedure is highly effective, it has now become much more commoditized and thus, should be considered as an adjunctive procedure in both dermatology and plastic surgery practices. Moreover, the advent of home held hair removal devices is further clouding the issue.

Costs of Devices: Direct and Indirect

When considering the purchase of an energy based device, one must account for all costs- direct and indirect. These include the cost of the capital equipment (usually defined as a direct cost) and the cost of consumables and service (usually defined as indirect costs). Often, the latter two are a significant portion of the overall cost of the device. Indirect costs are associated with all devices, regardless of the cost of "obvious" consumables. "Obvious" consumables include tips. Less obvious consumables include handpieces on light sources which expire, flashlamps, cryogen and parts of devices which expire. Finally, service costs are a component of any device. Therefore, inclusion of a service contract of reasonable terms is advisable in the initial purchase of a device. It is imperative to review the terms of the service contract to see what is included- similar to an automobile "bumper to bumper" warranty. The longevity of the device and the manufacturer should always be considered when making a purchase. Recently, several aesthetic companies have closed, leaving buyers with unserviceable devices or unattainable consumables.

Evidence Based Reviews and Peer Reviews

The purchase of a device should integrate evidence based review and a review by your peers. The first is often underwhelming for devices, as many devices may be a few years old. This should not preclude some evidence based review, as the markets are now mature and many devices have numerous peer reviewed publications to support their claims. "White papers" should not substitute for evidence based review, as these are usually sponsored marketing materials which should only be used to supplement evidence based publications. The next step after evidence based review, is to listen to your peers. Often, a manufacturer will provide names and testimonials from "experts" in the field. It is imperative to ask these references of their involvement with

the company (e.g., was the device gifted and what the terms were, was it a study, etc.). With mature device markets, it is now easier to get a true review by peers. This is more challenging when one is considering the purchase of a newer device with limited penetration in the field.

Rent Versus Lease Versus Purchase

Most manufacturers now provide in office demonstrations of their devices in the practice and many will leave the device in the office for a short period of time for physician evaluation. This is the optimal way of determining whether the device will be a "fit" into the practice. When this is not possible, renting devices is an excellent opportunity to see if these devices are indeed appropriate for the practice. Long term renting does not make sense, as scheduling becomes difficult and the long term costs of renting are much higher than leasing/purchasing the machine. Some devices are amenable to renting, such as tattoo removal devices or ablative devices, where it may be feasible to schedule patients on a restrictive basis. Whether to lease or purchase a piece of equipment is based on the financial health of the practice, the capital outlay and long term plans for the device. Used devices have very little value, and, like automobiles, once purchased the value declines significantly. A lease may be an easier way of integrating an expensive device without the initial capital outlay; but, as with all leases, one needs to review all of the terms very carefully to determine "the final costs" of the equipment. When purchasing/leasing the equipment, negotiation of a service contract within the initial cost of the equipment is highly advisable.

Marketing

The central dogma of marketing is internal marketing and is the most effective method for marketing your business. Therefore, for mature practices, when integrating a device into the practice, dissemination of the information of the device to the existing data base in the form of educational seminars, newsletters and web based information is a very cost effective method for marketing. New practices may benefit from investing in external marketing. Many device companies offer marketing incentives. Moreover, most device companies have sophisticated web based strategies such as "Find a doctor" which can assist physicians to grow their practices. It is imperative to link the physician website to the manufacturer website for streamlining patient referrals. Excessive external marketing is a waste of time and money. If external marketing is the main goal, target based external marketing is the best approach. Finally, if the staff of the physician can benefit from any of the device based procedures, they should be offered treatment so they can discuss the outcomes and benefits in a positive way to grow the practice. As the practice matures, marketing should be used primarily for branding, as new devices are integrated into the practice, the branding of the practice will enable existing and new patients to consider these procedures.

How to Avoid Common Mistakes

The single most common mistake is to obtain every single device on the market, buy every single handpiece on a platform model and to get the latest and the greatest. While it is tempting to be the first kid on the block to offer the latest laser procedure, this can be one of the greatest mistakes. Patients are looking for results and good outcomes. Disappointing outcomes and bad results can destroy the reputation of the physician and the practice. The second most common mistake is not accounting for all costs (direct and indirect) when considering devices. The true overhead costs of the device should include fixed and variable overhead. For example, if it takes 60 min to perform procedure X with device X and 30 min to perform procedure X with device Y, the fixed costs should be considered in the purchase price. A business plan with a "real" return on investment (ROI) should be included in all device based purchases. One should not rely on the manufacturer's ROI. Instead, the ROI should be based on the maturity of the practice, the demographics of the practice and the competition in the marketplace.

To Delegate or Not to Delegate

Energy based devices have rapidly become "delegated" procedures. In our practice, we do not delegate any energy based device treatments. This is not the norm in most practices. However, one needs to assess several parameters before deciding whether to delegate an energy based device procedure. First and foremost, is it safe for this device to be utilized by a non-physician? This is particularly true of ablative devices. They really should only be utilized by experienced physicians with a thorough understanding of the skin. Second, what are the state regulations of delegatable procedures? Third, what is the financial value of delegation? With the changing economy, many practices which relied highly on "delegating" procedures to non physicians are seeing a sharp decline, as patients get more conscious of spending

disposable income on procedures. Fourth, what is the possibility of the non physician going elsewhere and having those patients follow them to a competitor? While it may be impossible (as in our practice) to perform all of the procedures yourself, there are reasonable approaches. Before delegating any procedure to a non physician, the physician should master the energy based device and be aware of all of the complications and how to fix them. When delegating the procedure to a non-physician, direct supervision is optimal. Many states are now mandating direct supervision because of the plethora of complications from inexperienced users. Finally, when delegating procedures, one should never lose the relationship with the patient, as it is this critical bond that builds and sustains a practice.

Conclusions

The field of energy based devices (lasers, light sources, radiofrequency, and ultrasound) is undergoing a true revolution. The physician is bombarded with information touting the latest and the greatest device. It is imperative for the physician considering energy based devices to approach it in a stepwise fashion. This includes evidence based review, discussion with peers and assessment of the equipment in a real time fashion for choosing the optimal device for the practice. It should also include sound business decisions including direct and indirect costs of the equipment, marketing and sustainability of the device in the marketplace.

- The indirect/direct costs of the capital equipment and the cost of consumables and service should be considered at the time of purchase
- Journal and peer reviews are preferred over manufacturer's review since they resemble experience, not commercialism. Validity of new laser/light products can be evaluated by physician through sample trials. Renting, leasing or purchasing is dependent on physician's capital and demand for product
- Physician can attract patients to preferred treatment options by using targeted based marketing between manufacturer and physician website, providing cost-efficiency and effectiveness
- Results and good outcomes are preferred over new untested products. Poor reliability of device may ruin physician's reputation and practice
- Most efficiency of laser/light treatment is obtained by an experienced physician using a product that has been previously tested for efficacy

Research and Future Directions

Fernanda Hidemi Sakamoto and Richard Rox Anderson

The distinction between the past, present and future is only a stubbornly persistent illusion.

(Albert Einstein)

- What is next for fractionated laser treatments? New developments on microscopic patterns of injury and sparing using lasers and light sources.
- Photochemical tissue bonding (PTB), the next generation of tissue repair?
- Selective targeting using photodynamic therapy: development of new photosensitizers and clinical applications.
- Low-level light therapy: mechanisms and uses are emerging.
- Optical *in vivo* microscopy: approaching clinical use.

Introduction

In retrospect, it is interesting to realize the way technology and new developments are sometimes so obvious and simple. Looking back over the history of laser surgery, laser tissue ablation (removal) was developed over 40 years. It became popular in the 1980s and 1990s especially because of skin resurfacing, but faded at the end of 1990s due to side effects, and almost vanished from most clinical practices. In 2004, with the introduction of new fractionated methods of skin resurfacing, the same old lasers developed decades ago became popular again, by delivering their beams in microscopic patterns. The technology to make arrays of microscopic laser beams has been available for 40 years, but not used this

way in dermatology. The limiting factor is not the technology, but the way we look at it.

Future directions of laser surgery will depend mainly on medical needs and on the creativity of research to meet those needs. Lasers and light sources will probably be involved in developments of tissue engineering, gene therapy, "smart" devices that will be able to detect and treat at the same time, robots that may allow patients to perform safe self-treatment, light activated nanoparticles of selective targeting of cancer cells/infections, and/or combinations of all these and other technologies.

Which recently-developed technologies and strategies are closer to clinical practice? Here, we discuss the future of "fractionated" systems; photochemical tissue bonding, selective targeting using photodynamic therapy, the science behind low-level light therapy and *in vivo* optical microscopy. However, we do not know what the future holds.

Fractionated Treatments: What Is Next?

The use of microscopic patterns of injury and sparing described by Manstein et al.[1] created a new way of skin resurfacing and "photorejuvenation". Fractionated laser methods stimulate skin remodeling with rapid post-treatment healing, reducing down-time. Therefore, several varieties of "fractionated" systems suddenly became popular offering a number of different options: there are scanning to stamping mode devices, non-ablative and ablative systems. To date, all fractionated laser treatments utilize water as the primary chromophore, with consequent dermal remodeling. However, it is expected that in future, those devices will evolve to "smarter" versions that would be able to destroy specific targets, much as a "smart bomb" is guided to a target.

Biological pathways and responses involved in the fractionated treatments are not fully understood. Skin tightening has been well described,[2,3] but it is not known if fractionated treatments can reduce or expand the tissue. Fractional photothermolysis may, or may not, actually

R.R. Anderson (✉)
Department of Dermatology, Harvard Medical School,
Massachusetts General Hospital, 55 Fruit Street, BHX 630,
Boston, MA 02114, USA
e-mail: rranderson@partners.org

K. Nouri (ed.), *Lasers in Dermatology and Medicine*,
DOI: 10.1007/978-0-85729-281-0_36, © Springer-Verlag London Limited 2011

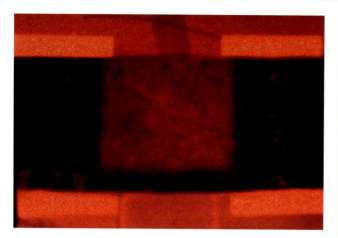

Fig. 1 Porphyrin fluorescence as a result of fractional ablative CO_2 laser-enhanced uptake of topical 20% aminolevulinic acid (ALA). An array of microscopic "laser-created" hole has dramatically increased uptake of ALA (Photo obtained by F.H. Sakamoto, MD, M. Wanner, MD, A.G. Doukas, PhD, W.A. Farinelli, B.S. and R.R. Anderson, MD, Wellman Center for Photomedicine, Massachusetts General Hospital, Harvard Medical School, Boston, MA)

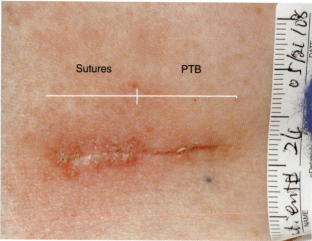

Fig. 2 Comparison of photochemical tissue bonding (PTB) (*right*) with conventional sutures (*left*) for superficial closure of skin excision wound. Photo was taken 2 weeks after surgery, immediately after suture removal. Surgery by S. Tsao, MD. PTB technology was developed in the laboratories of I.E. Kochevar and R.W. Redmond, Wellman Center for Photomedicine. Photo by M. Yao, M.D., Ph.D.

rejuvenate skin by forcing renewal and replacement of senescent tissue. Could fractionated treatments be used to treat or expand other solid organs? Could they be used to regenerate neurons, muscle, liver or any other vital cells? Remarkably, up to 50% of skin can be killed or ablated (vaporized) in a treatment session by fractionated treatment, with no apparent scarring or loss of functionality. It is not impossible that fractionated treatments could promote solid organ "rejuvenation".

Ablative fractional skin treatment may also provide drug delivery (Fig. 1). This has been described in a small pilot study using fractionated non-ablative laser to enhance photodynamic therapy benefits for skin rejuvenation.[4] Potentially, fractionated treatment could help treating any deep skin process including: tumors, recalcitrant hyperkeratotic psoriasis, granulomatous diseases, infections and deep mycosis or delivering vaccines.

Photochemical Tissue Bonding

Surgical sutures are the most common method for tissue reconstruction and repair. However, both common sutures and staples are not able to prevent fluid leakage, may cause foreign body reactions and scarring, and often require return visits for removal. Synthetic glues and electrical or laser-induced thermal welding may provide immediate tissue bonding but they can also induce scarring or foreign body reactions. Other types of sealants (fibrin and collagen-based) are expensive and not popular among clinicians.

Photochemical tissue bonding (PTB) has recently been created by Irene Kochevar and colleagues using rose-bengal as a photosensitizer and green light for photochemical activation (Fig. 2). The photosensitizer is totally reabsorbed into the body, causes little irritation and has no other known side effects. PTB causes collagen at tissue surfaces to cross-link during about 5 min of light irradiation, yielding a bond with less inflammation or scarring. Preclinical studies for blood vessel, nerve repair,[5] cornea,[6-8] and skin[9,10] have been presented. Interestingly, nerve repair with PTB in combination with human amniotic membrane was shown to be more efficacious than common suture for functional recovery. In comparison to standard sutures, the photochemically sealed amnion wrap also improved histological recovery.[5] This novel light-activated method of tissue repair may potentially produce better appearance and functional recovery.

Selective Targeting Using Photodynamic Therapy

Photodynamic therapy consist of delivering a light-activated drug or precursor, that after light irradiation reacts with oxygen producing free-radicals such as singlet oxygen and other reactive oxygen species (ROS). The ROS damage certain "targets" in tissue, by inducing apoptosis, necrosis, or activating local inflammatory/immune responses.

Many photosensitizers (PS) are currently available for medical use; in dermatology, psoralens, methylene-blue, aminolevulinic-acid (ALA) and its derivatives, porphyrins and porphyrin-derivatives are the most commonly used and studied for various conditions including actinic keratosis, cancer, vascular mal formations, inflammatory diseases, acne, infections, and more. The potential versatility of PDT is impressive.

The use of light with or without combination of a drug was used even by ancient civilizations in Egypt, India and China to treat skin diseases. Since then, photodynamic therapy (PDT) has become a popular modality of treatment in various systems and organs. However, even with increasing promise and many publications, the clinical impact of PDT has been modest. This is likely to change.

In order to increase efficacy and reduce side-effects, different approaches have been described to improve photosensitizer (PS) delivery and accumulation into targeted structures.[11] The development of PS that can penetrate easier into the plasma cell membrane is underway, e.g. by changing molecular physico–chemical properties, with consequent increased and faster local drug accumulation.[12] An example is the use of alkyl-esters of aminolevulinic acid (ALA) with higher lipophilicity such as the methyl, propyl and hexyl-esters of ALA[12]; or the use of liposome-encapsulated molecules, oil-dispersions or polymers.[13,14] Some of these new molecules are being studied in pre-clinical studies and in phase I and II clinical trials in the US and Europe.

Another strategy for selective PDT is by changing or modulating the target environment. For example, it is possible to inhibit the accumulation of PS in normal surrounding areas while increasing the amount of PS or its photodynamic effect within the targeted structures. When using ALA and ALA-derivatives to produce PDT, the drug has to be metabolized into porphyrins, especially protoporphyrin IX (PpIX). PpIX is the active PS. PpIX accumulation has been demonstrated to be dependant on heme synthesis enzymes, iron stores, and many other variables. By modulating those variables it is possible to control and produce selective targeting (Fig. 3). Table 1 summarizes different methods to modulate porphyrin-induced PDT that can be used to select tissue targeting.

One example is the use of temperature to control tissue targeting. Since most enzymes are temperature labile, Joe

Table 1 Mechanisms to produce targeted porphyrin-induced photodynamic therapy

1. Modification of ALA formulation:
   (a) Drug concentration
   (b) Delivery vehicle
   (c) Use of liposomes, nanoparticles, polymers, etc.
   (d) Chemically modified lipophilic ALA-derivatives

2. Modification of target tissue characteristics:
   (a) Use of chemicals to enhance drug penetration and metabolism: DMSO, EDTA,[15] propylene glycol,[16] glycolic acid, etc.
   (b) Use of physical methods to enhance drug penetration and metabolism: iontophoresis,[17] laser induced drug-delivery,[4] tape-stripping,[18] temperature modulation [19,20] microdermabrasion,[18,21] ultrasound, etc.
   (c) Use of chemicals to change heme synthesis: hydroxypyridinone (CP94) or desfferioxamine (iron chelators), or others
   (d) Change of molecular oxygen availability in the target tissue at the time of light exposure[22]
   (e) Induce target-cell differentiation[23-25]

3. Modification of ALA/ALA-derivatives and light delivery factors
   (a) Adequate incubation time of the drug in tissue prior to light exposure (time between drug application and light treatment) for each target[26]
   (b) Wavelength of light used in treatment
   (c) Adequate light fluence (also called "dose") in J/cm^2
   (d) Adequate light irradiance (rate at which the fluence is delivered, in W/cm^2; $1\ W/cm^2 = 1\ J/cm^2/s$)

et al. demonstrated local inhibition of PpIX accumulation when temperature is lower than about 20°C, and an increase in PS at temperatures above 37°C.[20] Thus, a simple temperature gradient in skin could possibly localize photosensitizer in target tissue and spare normal surrounding areas.

Finally, selective-PDT can be produced by a PS that will actively bind to specific cell-targets, for example, by combining a PS with monoclonal antibodies,[27] in a method called photoimmunotargeting (PIT).[11] PS can be synthetically conjugated to antibodies or aptamers that deliver the PS by binding to specific molecular markers. Those markers can be located on target cells (e.g. cancer), in cells involved in development of the disease, or in the cells effecting immune response. The use of these "new generation PS" could potentially enhance efficacy and reduce side-effects. However, new drugs often take a long time to reach clinical use.

In general, the simple understanding of the mechanisms of action of PDT and pharmacological aspects of PS can be used for selective targeting: by passive methods, by target modulation or by active targeting using conjugated PS into cell markers. The development of these techniques is promising and will create more efficient treatments.

Low-Level Light Therapy

The use of low-level light therapy (LLLT) has been described for pain treatment, anti-inflammatory effect, wound healing, infections and many other indications, amid certain skepticism

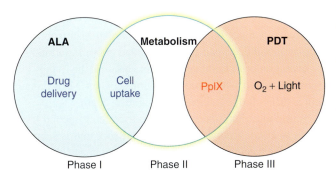

Fig. 3 Schematic figure representing three phases when porphyrin-induced PDT can be modulated. Phase I: by controlling drug-delivery methods; phase II: by controlling ALA metabolism into porphyrins (the active photosensitizer); phase III: by controlling light and porphyrins interaction during PDT

Table 2 Identified LLLT mitochondrial molecular targets and mechanisms of action

Cellular targets	Function	Wavelength	Mechanisms of action
Cytochrome c oxidase	Cell respiration	Red-NIR 630, 632.78, 650, 660, 725, 820 nm	Stimulatory effect[29] Increased RNA and protein synthesis[30] Increased proton electrochemical potential and ATP synthesis[31] Increase oxygen consumption[32,33]
Photoactive porphyrins	Heme synthesis	Visible ~410 nm ~500, 540, 585 nm 630 nm	Cell proliferation Tissue stimulation[34]
Flavoproteins[35]	Initiate free radical reactions	<500 nm	↓ Oxidative stress DNA repair Apoptosis

among scientists and clinicians. Recently, excellent studies have been published suggesting clinical efficacy and explaining some of the molecular biological mechanisms involved. So far, the exact response pathways are not completely known, but evidence points toward photochemical modification of mitochondrial functions. There are many variables involved such as light wavelength, irradiance, pulsing, and delivered light dose. The understanding of these factors is fundamental for choosing appropriate clinical indications and optimal parameters. It is also important to note that different cell types might respond differently to light.

There are many possible primary chromophores identified in the LLLT process, especially in mitochondria[28] (Table 2). Several mitochondrial signaling pathways can be changed such as: redox sensitive pathway, cyclic AMP-dependant signaling, nitric oxide control of respiration and other pathways.[28,36]

In dermatology, LLLT has been used but not yet well developed or optimized for given applications. Hopefully this will ensure based on great evidence.

In Vivo Optical Microscopy of Skin

Dermatology has mainly benefited, but in some ways suffered because skin is so available for inspection. In general, when a diagnosis based on examination is lacking, or cancer is a suspected diagnosis, a biopsy is performed. It is almost certain that taking a skin biopsy will be considered barbaric some day.

Since about 1990, biomedical research has been transformed by laser-based microscopic imaging methods including confocal microscopy and multi-photon fluorescence microscopy among others. These lend themselves easily for use in dermatology research, but have not had much clinical impact yet because of cost, lack of standardization, lack of verified diagnostic value, and lack of reimbursement for their use. The technology is rapidly progressing for small reliable lasers, fast beam scanning, optical components and high-speed computing – the things that underlie *in vivo* microscopy. As the cost and need for medical microscopy both increase, at some point laser-based skin imaging will become a mainstay. When it does, much of the practice of dermatology may change.

Confocal laser scanning microscopy (CM) of skin was first described by Rajadhyaksha et al. over a decade ago,[37,38] leading to commercialized devices cleared for human use, that are used mainly as research tools. CM can operate in either reflectance or fluorescence modes. Light returning from a tightly-focused laser beam is passed through a pinhole that eliminates out-of-focal-plane light, creating a virtual tissue section when the beam is scanned in a *conjugate focal* plane through live tissue. Melanin acts as a natural contrast agent for reflectance CM of human skin, which has been confirmed to offer valuable sensitivity and specificity for detection of melanoma and other pigmented lesions.[39-41] The depth of reflectance CM is about 0.3 mm, which includes epidermis, papillary dermis and upper reticular dermis. While no stains are used, the technique allows imaging of things than cannot be seen by conventional histopathology such as blood flow, cell movement, and most importantly – the evolution of a condition over time because the living skin is not destroyed with a biopsy. Fluorescence CM of human skin is difficult due to limited penetration depth.

Multiphoton microscopy (MPM) uses femtosecond laser pulses to excite fluorescence at a focal spot that is scanned through the tissue to create a virtual-section image. A femtosecond is 10^{-15} s – a very, very, very short time – during which more than one photon in a high power laser pulse can be absorbed without depositing enough energy to damage the tissue. The energy each photon delivers to a molecule is

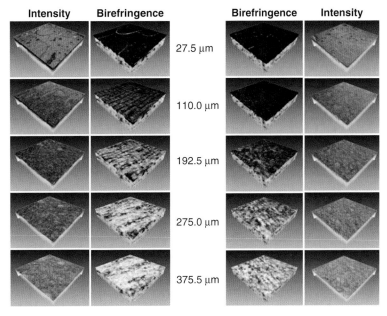

Fig. 4 An example of optical coherence tomography (OCT) of a 5 mm×5 mm×2 mm region of human forearm skin in vivo. Dermal collagen is highlighted in this version of OCT due to its birefringence (Courtesy of Prof. B. Hyle Park, Ph.D. [Department of Bioengineering, University of California Riverside, CA] and Prof. Johannes F. de Boer, Ph.D. [Vrije University, Amsterdam. Netherlands])

additive, which allows penetrating near-infrared light to excite the same natural tissue fluorescence we see with Wood's light or other ultraviolet sources. MPM has not been developed for clinical dermatology, but preliminary studies suggest great promise.[42-44] The fluorescence of mitochondria provide imaging of cell cytoplasm; elastin fibers can be specifically seen; collagen is easily imaged by the same instrument through process called second harmonic generation; and the same information of CM can be obtained. Depth of penetration with MPM is similar to CM, with the above advantages and resolution exceeding that of conventional histopathology.

Optical coherence tomography (OCT) was also invented and developed well over a decade ago, mainly for imaging of the retina. In live human skin, OCT creates vertical-section images of reflected light with lower resolution than CM or MPM, but much greater depth (Fig. 4). As the name implies, the wave coherence of light is used in OCT to detect light coming back from a specific depth in the tissue, conceptually similar to detecting the 'echo' of ultrasound waves for medical imaging. For many years, OCT images of skin were not very interesting because cells were not seen (low resolution), most structures were indistinct (low contrast), and images were grainy due to "speckle", a phenomenon of coherent wave imaging. These problems have been nearly eliminated, the speed of OCT has increased dramatically (tomography of the entire skin volume can be rapidly obtained over square centimeters of skin area), and versions that show microvasculature and/or extracellular matrix structure in exquisite detail have been demonstrated.[45-49] It is clear that tumors can be mapped in detail *in vivo*, but this has not yet been developed for dermatology. Other strategies for tumor margin detection such as polarized light imaging have also been demonstrated.[50-54]

Acknowledgements The authors would like to thank Prof. Irene Kochevar, PhD, Min Yao, MD, PhD (Wellman Center for Photomedicine, Massachusetts General Hospital, Harvard Medical School, Boston, MA) and Dr. Sandy Tsao, MD (Department of Dermatology, Massachusetts General Hospital, Harvard Medical School, Boston, MA), for providing the photograph and discussion about photochemical tissue bonding; Prof. Michael Hamblin, PhD and Aaron C-H Chen (Wellman Center for Photomedicine, Massachusetts General Hospital, Harvard Medical School, Boston, MA) for discussion about low-level light therapy; Prof. B. Hyle Park, PhD (Department of Bioengineering, University of California Riverside, CA) and Prof. Johannes F. de Boer, PhD (Vrije University, Amsterdam, Netherlands) for providing the photograph about optical coherence tomography.

References

1. Manstein D, Herron GS, et al. Fractional photothermolysis: a new concept for cutaneous remodeling using microscopic patterns of thermal injury. *Lasers Surg Med.* 2004;34(5):426-438.
2. Rahman Z, MacFalls H, et al. Fractional deep dermal ablation induces tissue tightening. *Lasers Surg Med.* 2009;41(2):78-86.
3. Sukal SA, Chapas AM, et al. Eyelid tightening and improved eyelid aperture through nonablative fractional resurfacing. *Dermatol Surg.* 2008;34(11):1454-1458.
4. Ruiz-Rodriguez R, Lopez L, et al. Enhanced efficacy of photodynamic therapy after fractional resurfacing: fractional photodynamic rejuvenation. *J Drugs Dermatol.* 2007;6(8):818-820.
5. Henry FP, Goyal NA, et al. Improving electrophysiologic and histologic outcomes by photochemically sealing amnion to the peripheral nerve repair site. *Surgery.* 2009;145(3):313-321.

6. Mulroy L, Kim J, et al. Photochemical keratodesmos for repair of lamellar corneal incisions. *Invest Ophthalmol Vis Sci.* 2000;41(11):3335-3340.

7. Proano CE, Azar DT, et al. Photochemical keratodesmos as an adjunct to sutures for bonding penetrating keratoplasty corneal incisions. *J Cataract Refract Surg.* 2004;30(11):2420-2424.

8. Proano CE, Mulroy L, et al. Photochemical keratodesmos for bonding corneal incisions. *Invest Ophthalmol Vis Sci.* 2004;45(7):2177-2181.

9. Chan BP, Kochevar IE, et al. Enhancement of porcine skin graft adherence using a light-activated process. *J Surg Res.* 2002;108(1):77-84.

10. Kamegaya Y, Farinelli WA, et al. Evaluation of photochemical tissue bonding for closure of skin incisions and excisions. *Lasers Surg Med.* 2005;37(4):264-270.

11. Solban N, Rizvi I, et al. Targeted photodynamic therapy. *Lasers Surg Med.* 2006;38(5):522-531.

12. Lange N. Pharmaceutical and biological considerations in 5-aminolevulinic acid in PDT. In: Hamblin MR, Mroz P, eds. *Advances in Photodynamic Therapy. Basic, Translational, and Clinical.* 1st ed. Norwood: Artech House; 2008:59-91.

13. Chen B, Pogue BW, et al. Liposomal delivery of photosensitizing agents. *Expert Opin Drug Deliv.* 2005;2(3):477-487.

14. Konan YN, Gurny R, et al. State of the art in the delivery of photosensitizers for photodynamic therapy. *J Photochem Photobiol B.* 2002;66(2):89-106.

15. Malik Z, Kostenich G, et al. Topical application of 5-aminolevulinic acid, DMSO and EDTA: protoporphyrin IX accumulation in skin and tumours of mice. *J Photochem Photobiol B.* 1995;28(3):213-218.

16. Steluti R, De Rosa FS, et al. Topical glycerol monooleate/propylene glycol formulations enhance 5-aminolevulinic acid in vitro skin delivery and in vivo protoporphyrin IX accumulation in hairless mouse skin. *Eur J Pharm Biopharm.* 2005;60(3):439-444.

17. Rhodes LE, Tsoukas MM, et al. Iontophoretic delivery of ALA provides a quantitative model for ALA pharmacokinetics and PpIX phototoxicity in human skin. *J Invest Dermatol.* 1997;108(1):87-91.

18. van den Akker JT, Iani V, et al. Topical application of 5-aminolevulinic acid hexyl ester and 5-aminolevulinic acid to normal nude mouse skin: differences in protoporphyrin IX fluorescence kinetics and the role of the stratum corneum. *Photochem Photobiol.* 2000;72(5):681-689.

19. Sakamoto FH, Doukas A, et al. Skin temperature can control ALA-Photodynamic therapy. American Society for Laser Medicine and Surgery, Twenty-Seventh Annual Meeting; 2007; Grapevine. Wiley-Liss, A Wiley Company.

20. Joe EK, Anderson RR, et al. Spatial confinement of 5-aminolevulinic acid-based photodynamic therapy by thermal and chemical inhibition. Fourth International Investigative Dermatology Meeting; 2003; Miami Beach.

21. Katz BE, Truong S, et al. Efficacy of microdermabrasion preceding ALA application in reducing the incubation time of ALA in laser PDT. *J Drugs Dermatol.* 2007;6(2):140-142.

22. Sitnik TM, Hampton JA, et al. Reduction of tumour oxygenation during and after photodynamic therapy in vivo: effects of fluence rate. *Br J Cancer.* 1998;77(9):1386-1394.

23. Li G, Szewczuk MR, et al. Effect of mammalian cell differentiation on response to exogenous 5-aminolevulinic acid. *Photochem Photobiol.* 1999;69(2):231-235.

24. Ortel B, Chen N, et al. Differentiation-specific increase in ALA-induced protoporphyrin IX accumulation in primary mouse keratinocytes. *Br J Cancer.* 1998;77(11):1744-1751.

25. Ortel B, Sharlin D, et al. Differentiation enhances aminolevulinic acid-dependent photodynamic treatment of LNCaP prostate cancer cells. *Br J Cancer.* 2002;87(11):1321-1327.

26. Sakamoto FH, Tannous Z, et al. Porphyrin distribution after topical aminolevulinic acid in a novel porcine model of sebaceous skin. *Lasers Surg Med.* 2009;41(2):154-160.

27. Oseroff AR, Ohuoha D, et al. Antibody-targeted photolysis: selective photodestruction of human T-cell leukemia cells using monoclonal antibody-chlorin e6 conjugates. *Proc Natl Acad Sci USA.* 1986;83(22):8744-8748.

28. Huang Y-Y, Chen A C-H, et al. Advances in low intensity laser and phototherapy. In: Tuchin VV, editor. *Advanced Biophotonics.* Taylor and Francis Books Inc, Boca Raton FL. 2010. ISBN 978-1-4398-0628-9.

29. Karu TI, Kolyakov SF. Exact action spectra for cellular responses relevant to phototherapy. *Photomed Laser Surg.* 2005;23(4):355-361.

30. Passarella S, Casamassima E, et al. Increase of proton electrochemical potential and ATP synthesis in rat liver mitochondria irradiated in vitro by helium-neon laser. *FEBS Lett.* 1984;175(1):95-99.

31. Passarella S, Ostuni A, et al. Increase in the ADP/ATP exchange in rat liver mitochondria irradiated in vitro by helium-neon laser. *Biochem Biophys Res Commun.* 1988;156(2):978-986.

32. Gordon MW. The correlation between in vivo mitochondrial changes and tryptophan pyrrolase activity. *Arch Biochem Biophys.* 1960;91:75-82.

33. Yu W, Naim JO, et al. Photomodulation of oxidative metabolism and electron chain enzymes in rat liver mitochondria. *Photochem Photobiol.* 1997;66(6):866-871.

34. Plaetzer K, Kiesslich T, et al. Characterization of the cell death modes and the associated changes in cellular energy supply in response to AlPcS4-PDT. *Photochem Photobiol Sci.* 2002;1(3):172-177.

35. Eichler M, Lavi R, et al. Flavins are source of visible-light-induced free radical formation in cells. *Lasers Surg Med.* 2005;37(4):314-319.

36. Borutaite V, Budriunaite A, et al. Reversal of nitric oxide-, peroxynitrite- and S-nitrosothiol-induced inhibition of mitochondrial respiration or complex I activity by light and thiols. *Biochim Biophys Acta.* 2000;1459(2–3):405-412.

37. Rajadhyaksha M, Gonzalez S, et al. In vivo confocal scanning laser microscopy of human skin II: advances in instrumentation and comparison with histology. *J Invest Dermatol.* 1999;113(3):293-303.

38. Rajadhyaksha M, Grossman M, et al. In vivo confocal scanning laser microscopy of human skin: melanin provides strong contrast. *J Invest Dermatol.* 1995;104(6):946-952.

39. Langley RG, Rajadhyaksha M, et al. Confocal scanning laser microscopy of benign and malignant melanocytic skin lesions in vivo. *J Am Acad Dermatol.* 2001;45(3):365-376.

40. Busam KJ, Charles C, et al. Morphologic features of melanocytes, pigmented keratinocytes, and melanophages by in vivo confocal scanning laser microscopy. *Mod Pathol.* 2001;14(9):862-868.

41. Busam KJ, Hester K, et al. Detection of clinically amelanotic malignant melanoma and assessment of its margins by in vivo confocal scanning laser microscopy. *Arch Dermatol.* 2001;137(7):923-929.

42. Koehler MJ, Konig K, et al. In vivo assessment of human skin aging by multiphoton laser scanning tomography. *Opt Lett.* 2006;31(19):2879-2881.

43. Konig K. Multiphoton microscopy in life sciences. *J Microsc.* 2000;200(2):83-104.

44. Konig K, Riemann I. High-resolution multiphoton tomography of human skin with subcellular spatial resolution and picosecond time resolution. *J Biomed Opt.* 2003;8(3):432-439.

45. de Boer JF, Milner TE, et al. Determination of the depth-resolved stokes parameters of light backscattered from turbid media by use of polarization-sensitive optical coherence tomography. *Opt Lett.* 1999;24(5):300-302.

46. Park BH, Saxer C, et al. In vivo burn depth determination by high-speed fiber-based polarization sensitive optical coherence tomography. *J Biomed Opt.* 2001;6(4):474-479.

47. Pierce MC, Sheridan RL, et al. Collagen denaturation can be quantified in burned human skin using polarization-sensitive optical coherence tomography. *Burns*. 2004;30(6):511-517.

48. Pierce MC, Strasswimmer J, et al. Birefringence measurements in human skin using polarization-sensitive optical coherence tomography. *J Biomed Opt*. 2004;9(2):287-291.

49. Pierce MC, Strasswimmer J, et al. Advances in optical coherence tomography imaging for dermatology. *J Invest Dermatol*. 2004; 123(3):458-463.

50. Tannous Z, Al-Arashi M, et al. Delineating melanoma using multimodal polarized light imaging. *Lasers Surg Med*. 2009;41(1):10-16.

51. Yaroslavsky AN, Barbosa J, et al. Combining multispectral polarized light imaging and confocal microscopy for localization of nonmelanoma skin cancer. *J Biomed Opt*. 2005;10(1):14011.

52. Yaroslavsky AN, Neel V, et al. Demarcation of nonmelanoma skin cancer margins in thick excisions using multispectral polarized light imaging. *J Invest Dermatol*. 2003;121(2):259-266.

53. Jacques SL, Ramella-Roman JC, et al. Imaging skin pathology with polarized light. *J Biomed Opt*. 2002;7(3):329-340.

54. Sterenborg NJ, Thomsen S, et al. In vivo fluorescence spectroscopy and imaging of human skin tumors. *Dermatol Surg*. 1995;21(9): 821-822.

Laser/Light Applications in Ophthalmology: Visual Refraction

Mahnaz Nouri, Amit Todani, and Roberto Pineda

- Refractive laser technology is used for correction of myopia, hyperopia and astigmatism.
- Laser vision correction can be performed on the surface the cornea after removing the epithelium or deeper into stroma under a hinged corneal flap.
- Proper candidate selection is essential to minimize the risk of complications.
- Corneal collagen cross-linking with ultraviolet light and riboflavin (a photo sensitizer) is a relatively new treatment modality for a variety of corneal keratectatic disorders.

History

Laser technology is only around half a century old. The first experimental laser, demonstrated by Maiman in 1960, was produced by a ruby crystal powered by a flashlamp.[1] However the first use of laser in the field of refractive surgery was demonstrated in 1983 by Trokel and Srinivasan who showed that argon-fluoride excimer laser of 193 nm could cleanly remove corneal stromal tissue with minimal damage to adjacent stroma.[2] This technology was developed for ophthalmic use after being applied to etch computer chips for IBM in the late 1970s. Initially, the laser was used to create radial keratotomy incisions[3,4]; later it was used to ablate the corneal tissue in the central visual axis. This later procedure was termed photorefractive keratectomy (PRK) by Trokel and Marshall. The first PRK in a seeing human eye was performed by Mc Donald and coworkers in 1988.[5] Since its inception, refractive laser technology has grown exponentially. In the US, The Food and Drug Administration (FDA) first approved the excimer laser for the treatment of mild to moderate myopia in October 1995. Later, it was approved for correction of hyperopia and astigmatism.

LASEK (laser-assisted subepithelial keratectomy) and epi-LASIK are modifications of the PRK procedure in which the corneal epithelium is preserved. The epithelium in such cases is displaced prior to the surface ablation, then replaced after laser application.

The term Laser (-assisted) in-situ keratomileusis (LASIK) was introduced by Ioannis Pallikaris and colleagues in 1988.[6] LASIK involves the creation of a hinged corneal flap followed by ablation and reshaping of the underlying stromal tissue with an excimer laser beam. In most settings, the hinged corneal flap is created by an automated keratome. The keratome-laser combination was reported in 1990 separately by two investigators, viz. Burrato, who performed photokeratomileusis (PKM), and by Pallikaris, who performed LASIK.[7] Burrato's technique involved fashioning of a free keratomileusis cap and performing PKM on the posterior (stromal) aspect of the cap and replacing it. Pallikaris' technique involved raising a hinged cap and treating the underlying stromal bed with an excimer laser.[7] While the results of PKM were not as promising as LASIK, the LASIK hinged corneal flaps were safer and resulted in more accurate flap realignment.

Surface Ablation – PRK (Photorefractive Keratectomy) /LASEK (Laser Subepithelial Keratomileusis)/Epi-LASIK

Surface ablation has traditionally referred to PRK and requires removal of the corneal epithelium. This can be performed mechanically (scraping), chemically with alcohol (15–20%), or with the excimer laser (transepithelial ablation). However, it is most commonly performed by using dilute alcohol (commonly 15–20% ethanol is used) to loosen up epithelial cells, removing the epithelium (sometimes as a sheet), followed by laser ablation of the subepithelial stroma. After the laser procedure is completed, the epithelial sheet is

M. Nouri (✉)
Boston Eye Group, Beacon Street, Brookline,
MA, USA
e-mail: mnouri2468@aol.com

K. Nouri (ed.), *Lasers in Dermatology and Medicine*,
DOI: 10.1007/978-0-85729-281-0_37, © Springer-Verlag London Limited 2011

either replaced (LASEK) or discarded (PRK). The theoretical advantages of LASEK over PRK include decreased postoperative discomfort, reduced risk of scarring and faster visual recovery. A study by Wissing et al. demonstrated reduced keratocyte loss with LASEK when compared to PRK in an animal study.[8] However, more clinical data is needed to conclusively demonstrate that LASEK has significant advantages over PRK. On the other hand PRK may be more advantageous than LASEK in situations like anterior basement membrane (Cogan's) dystrophy,[9] epithelial erosions or epithelial scaring, where it may be preferable to discard the diseased epithelium. In most cases, the choice of one procedure versus the other is largely dependant on surgeon preferences.

The principal advantage of surface ablation is the avoidance of flap-related LASIK complications, for e.g., flap dislocation, flap folds, button-hole formation, etc (discussed in details in section "Complications of Laser Refractive Surgery"). Moreover, surface ablation may be the preferred approach in certain situations. These include certain occupations in which the risk of flap trauma is persistently elevated, for e.g., in contact sports like basketball and rugby, military personnel, etc. Patients with a history of systemic herpetic infections (a relative contraindication) may be better suited for surface ablation, which theoretically severs less number of corneal nerves as compared to LASIK and may therefore have lesser propensity to reactivate the virus. For similar reasons, it is generally speculated that surface ablation has less of a tendency to induce dry eyes when compared to LASIK. Moreover, in patients with a prior history of flap abnormalities with attempted LASIK, it may be safer to perform surface ablation rather than run the risks of recutting the flap such as flap maceration and flap loss.[10] Several factors, such as lack of reproducibility of corneal flap thickness even when the same microkeratome is used[11] and variations in intensity and duration of microkeratome suction,[12] predispose to serious flap complications during recutting the flap.

The major advantages of LASIK over surface ablation are earlier post-operative visual recovery, less post-operative discomfort, less risk of haze esp. when associated with higher level of refractive error correction and shorter duration of post-operative steroid treatment.[9] Moreover, LASIK may be associated with less regression when compared to surface ablation for higher levels of correction.[9]

A variation of LASEK, termed epi-LASIK was applied by Pallikaris et al. who used an automated separator to remove the corneal epithelium mechanically, without the use of alcohol.[13] They suggested that this technique would provide increased post-operative comfort and decreased haze formation as compared to PRK. Histological studies seem to show better preservation of the epithelial sheet when compared to LASEK.[14]

LASIK

Laser in-situ keratomileusis (LASIK) is a two-step procedure that involves creation of a hinged corneal flap followed by ablation and reshaping of the underlying stromal tissue with an excimer laser ('excited dimer') beam. This is an argon fluoride (AFl) laser that operates at 193 nm in the ultraviolet spectrum and was first used for etching computer chips.[2] This laser wavelength allows ophthalmologists to surgically reshape the cornea through a series of mirrors and lenses in an attempt to circumvent the need for corrective lenses. There are three general types of delivery systems for the excimer lasers, depending on the size of the beam : broad beam, scanning slit, and small beam. The broad beam laser is the one more commonly used for corneal reshaping through an iris diaphragm. Due to the high energy per photon of the excimer laser beam, the ablation of the carbon-carbon bonds at the corneal surface allows for an accurate tissue removal of each layer with minimal penetration and therefore damage to adjacent tissues.

The first step in LASIK is creation of a hinged corneal disc (i.e., the 'flap'). This can be created by an automated microkeratome or more recently and with increased precision with the Intralase® femtosecond laser (Intralase Corp., Irvine, CA), an infrared YLF:glass (Nd:glass) laser which operates at 1053 nm[15] (Fig. 1).

Microkeratomes have greatly evolved in terms of ease of use, reliability and safety profile since the earlier original versions. Jose Ignacio Barraquer in 1958 unveiled his first manual microkeratome, which was designed for keratophakia and freeze keratomileusis.[16] Over time, this technique was evolved for obtaining a smoother technique to cut through the corneal stroma. Microkeratomes come in manual, semiautomated, and automated models. Some are even disposable. Typical components of a standard microkeratome include the motor for translational movement, head of the microkeratome bearing the blade, applanator lens to measure the diameter of the exposed cornea, vacuum fixation ring to secure the eye, flat stop ring to limit the movement of the microkeratome head through the fixation ring and a foot switch to operate the microkeratome movement. Although much improvement has been made since the earlier days in mirokeratome design, modern day microkeratomes are not devoid of complications. Most of the flap related complications during LASIK (discussed in section "Complications of Laser Refractive Surgery") are related to the use of microkeratomes. These complications depend on many factors, including surgeon experience and microkeratome safety features. Although there is a steep learning curve, complications decrease over time with increasing surgeon experience. Most modern microkeratomes have inbuilt safety features such as alarms, automatic shut down buttons and suction indicators.

Laser/Light Applications in Ophthalmology: Visual Refraction

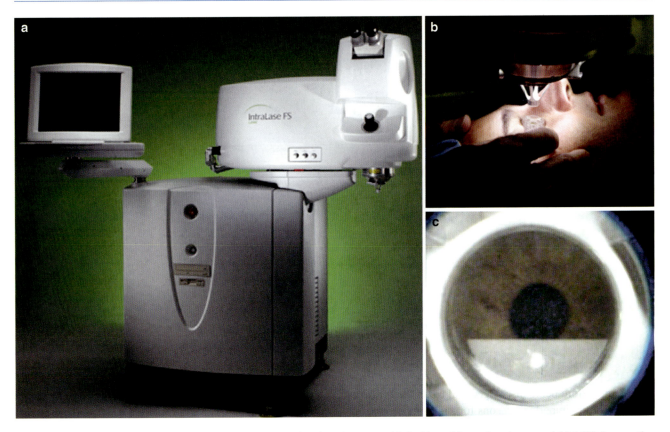

Fig. 1 (**a**) Intralase™ Femtosecond laser unit. (**b**) Intralase suction ring placement with docking of the applanation cone. (**c**) LASIK flap creation with Intralase™ using a raster scan pattern

With the advent of the femtosecond laser, creation of the LASIK flap has become much safer and simpler (Fig. 1). The flap can now be created optically with the near infrared laser, focused at a set depth within the corneal stroma. The laser fires at a rapid rate with pulse duration in the range of femtoseconds. This results in vaporization of corneal tissue by the process of photodisruption, leading to formation of plasma and shockwave. The expansion of plasma results in a resection plane which ultimately leads to creation of a lamellar flap. This flap still requires dissection of the lamellar plane prior to lifting the flap for treatment with the excimer laser. Thus, more uniform flaps with consistent thickness can be created. Also this laser system allows the refractive surgeon to fashion thinner flaps that have the advantage of preserving greater amounts of residual stromal bed. LASIK flap creation with femtosecond laser is growing in the U.S. and principally hindered by the cost of the laser.

Before the corneal lamellar flap is created, gentian violet surgical landmarks spanning the hinged flap and the peripheral cornea are placed and the flap is folded over to expose the stromal bed. The excimer laser (Fig. 2) is then used to reshape the corneal stroma to achieve the desired correction of refractive error. Both the size of the optical zone as well as the depth and profile of the laser ablation are important determinants of the correction achieved. Small or decentered ablation zones can result in problems of glare and haloes at night when the pupils may dilate beyond the functional optical zone. Deeper ablations can distort the corneal surface and can predispose to corneal flap striae or 'mudcracks.' In order to ensure adequate stromal hydration during LASIK, the laser treatment should be performed in a timely manner. Dehydration of the stroma can lead to overcorrection while over-hydration with BSS can dampen the effect of the laser. Most modern excimer lasers have a tracking mechanism (usually infrared cameras) based on the position of the pupil or the iris pattern in order to nullify the effect of torsion or slight movements of the eye during the time of laser treatment.

Once the ablation is complete, the undersurface of the flap along with the stromal bed is irrigated with balanced salt solution to remove any debris, and the flap repositioned onto the stromal bed. The interface is then allowed to dry for a few minutes. Proper adhesion of the flap is then confirmed. It is equally important to confirm adequate alignment of the flap with respect to the peripheral cornea using the pre-placed surgical landmarks as a guideline along with the configuration of the gutter between the flap and the peripheral cornea. At the end of the procedure, the patient should be re-examined under

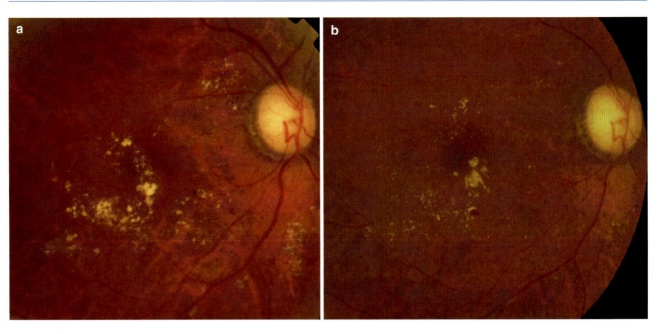

Fig. 4 60-year-old female with diabetic macular edema treated with focal argon laser. (**a**) Fundus photograph: clinically significant macular edema in the right eye. Yellow, hard exudates indicate areas of retinal thickening. (**b**) Fundus photograph: marked resolution of hard exudates 5 months after focal argon laser treatment

Macular Photocoagulation Study (MPS), a series of eight multicenter, randomized, prospective trials examining the use of argon and krypton laser for choroidal neovascular membranes was published.[9] This study evaluated the use of laser for extrafoveal and juxtafoveal lesions in three conditions: neovascular ARMD, presumed ocular histoplasmosis (POHS), and idiopathic choroidal neovascularization. One major drawback of these trials was the narrow eligibility criteria: no more than 15–20% of neovascular ARMD cases present with well-defined choroidal neovacularization as required by the trial.

In general, in all of the MPS trials, treatment did not decrease the patient's chance of maintaining stable visual acuity, but the proportion of eyes, treated or untreated, that maintained good or stable visual acuity was very small. The reason for this inadequate treatment effect is that despite treatment, many eyes continued to lose vision because of persistent or recurrent neovascularization that extended into the foveal center. Subfoveal recurrences were not treated with laser in these trials due to concerns about permanent central visual loss. Due to its deleterious effect on normal surrounding neural retina, the use of argon laser for choroidal neovascularization near the fovea sharply decreased with the advent of photodynamic therapy (see below) and anti-vascular endothelial growth factor therapies. However, argon laser does continue to have a rarely used but important role in that it is highly effective for extrafoveal isolated choroidal neovascular lesions. Patients should always be informed that this treatment induces a permanent scotoma.

Technique

Pan-Retinal Photocoagulation

Argon laser can be applied for PRP from a slit-lamp based or indirect ophthalmoscopic system (Fig. 5). The slit lamp-based system is used for a seated patient and consists of a

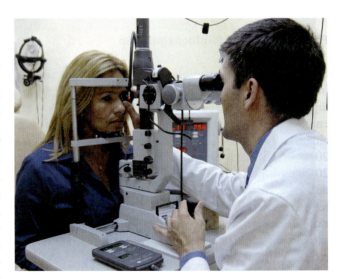

Fig. 5 Slit-lamp based delivery of argon laser photocoagulation. The patient is seen seated to the left with her face firmly placed in an ophthalmic microscope modified for laser delivery. The ophthalmologist views the retina and applies argon laser burns through a corneal contact lens seen in the physician's right hand

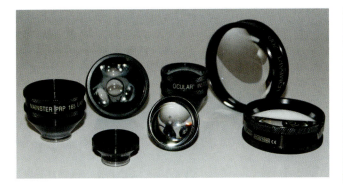

Fig. 6 Commonly employed ophthalmic lenses. A multitude of lenses can be used for argon laser treatment application depending on the desired magnification and field of view. Such lenses can be broadly categorized as either corneal contact lenses (five lenses located on the left: ocular Mainster 165, ocular three mirror, ocular Yannuzzi fundus, ocular Reichel-Mainster and ocular Mainster wide field) or indirect lenses (two lenses located on the right: 20-diopter and 28-diopter)

modified slit-lamp (specialized microscope for ophthalmoscopic exam) mounted on a table. The retina is visualized by using a wide-field contact lens (Fig. 6). The indirect system is composed of a headset worn by the ophthalmologist which emits the laser directly. For this system, the patient is typically reclined in an examining chair and the retina is visualized by using a 20-Diopter or 28-Diopter lens (Fig. 7).

The standard technique for PRP currently involves the placement of 800–1,600 laser burns with a 500 μm spot size, spaced 0.5 burn widths apart from each other with 0.1–0.2 s of duration.[10] Intensity is regulated so that mild white bleaching is obtained (Fig. 8). The treatment reaches from the temporal arcade to the equator, and up to 2 disc diameters temporal to the macular center. Typically one disc diameter or space is spared around the optic nerve to avoid central visual field defects.

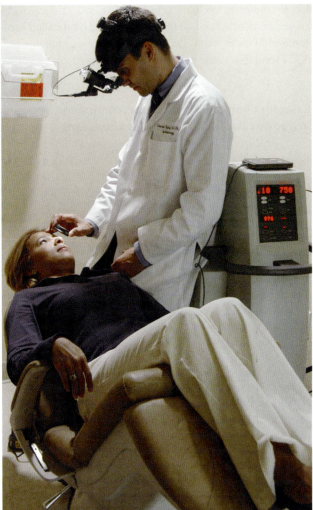

Fig. 7 Indirect-ophthalmoscopic based delivery of argon laser photocoagulation. The patient is seen reclined in an examining chair. The ophthalmologist applies argon laser spots using a headset-based laser and visualizes the retina using either a 20-diopter or a 28-diopter lens seen in the physician's right hand

Focal Argon Laser Photocoagulation

Focal laser is typically applied using a slit-lamp based system for a seated patient (Fig. 5). A magnifying contact lens is held by the ophthalmologist for detailed viewing of small retinal features (Fig. 6). Focal laser treatment typically consists of 50–100 μm laser burns of 0.05–0.1 s duration applied to microaneurysms between 500 and 3,000 μm from the center of the macula with the clinical endpoint defined as a color change to a mild whitening. For more diffuse macular edema, a grid pattern is typically applied in the following manner: 100–200 burns of a 50–200 μm spot size spaced 1 burn width apart within 2 disc areas of the fovea. In the ETDRS, an average of 3–4 treatment sessions 2–4 months apart were required.[7] The grid technique has been demonstrated in several more

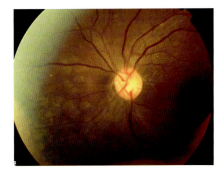

Fig. 8 42-year-old female with proliferative diabetic retinopathy underwent pan-retinal argon laser photocoagulation. Fundus photograph of retinal burns 3 h after application. Discrete, cream-colored round lesions are seen deep to the retinal vasculature. Over the ensuing weeks to months, these subtle lesions will evolve into more noticeable areas of retinal atrophy, often with associated pigment clumping, as seen in Figs. 1b and 2

recent studies to be more effective than milder focal techniques in reducing retinal thickening based on detailed measurements taken with the optical coherence tomography (OCT) and thus continues to be the standard of care.[11]

Laser for Choroidal Neovascular Membranes in Neovascular ARMD and Other Conditions

Laser for choroidal neovascular membranes is typically applied using a slit-lamp based system for a seated patient. A magnifying contact lens is held by the ophthalmologist for detailed viewing of small retinal features. In the MPS studies, argon laser was applied to cover the choroidal neovascular membrane (location judged on fluorescein angiogram) and 100 μm beyond the edge of the lesion, but was never applied closer than 200 μm from the center of the fovea. The laser was set initially at a 200 μm spot size, 0.2–0.5 s duration, and 100–200 mW power. The power was adjusted to achieve an intensity sufficient enough to produce a uniform whitening of the overlying retina.

Adverse Events

Pan-Retinal Photocoagulation

The complications of PRP in the DRS were generally mild and included a decrease in visual acuity of 1 or more lines in 11% and peripheral visual field loss in 5%.[12] The DRS and ETDRS also indicated that macular edema can be worsened by PRP leading to moderate visual loss.[4]

Focal Argon Laser Photocoagulation

The side effects and complications of focal laser in the ETDRS included: paracentral scotoma, transient increased edema/decreased vision, choroidal neovascularization, subretinal fibrosis, photocoagulation scar expansion over time, and inadvertent foveal burns.[4,7]

Laser for Choroidal Neovascular Membranes in Neovascular ARMD and Other Conditions

Complications from argon laser for choroidal neovascularization include: hemorrhage, perforation of Bruch's membrane, retinal pigment epithelial tear, and arteriolar narrowing.[9,13] Persistent or recurrent neovascularization is common: in the MPS, 34% of patients treated for new subfoveal neovascularization had persistent or new neovascularization over 3 years of follow-up[14]; 53% of eyes treated

for extrafoveal neovascularization in the MPS had recurrent neovascularization[15]; 32% of eyes treated for juxtafoveal neovascularization had persistent neovascularization, and an additional 42% had recurrent neovascularization at 5 years of follow-up.[9,13]

Future Directions

Pan-Retinal Photocoagulation and Focal Argon Laser Photocoagulation

The uses of PRP for proliferative diabetic retinopathy and focal laser for diabetic macular edema have been reliable mainstays of treatment for diabetic patients for decades. Pars plana vitrectomy (PPV) has also been used successfully for a decade for refractory diffuse macular edema which demonstrates a tractional component.[16] In the last several years, there has been an explosion of interest in the use of antivascular endothelial growth factors (anti-VEGF) formulated as intravitreal injections to serve as alternatives or supplements to laser treatments. Many early studies have found these agents to be beneficial for these conditions, especially in the short term.[17-19] Large scale randomized controlled prospective trials are currently underway in the United States and abroad to determine whether these agents are effective in the long term as single therapy or only as adjunctive therapy to traditional laser treatment.[20]

Laser for Choroidal Neovascular Membranes in Neovascular ARMD and Other Conditions

Argon laser photocoagulation is limited in its use for choroidal neovascularization due to narrow eligibility criteria, immediate visual loss due to scotoma, and high recurrence rates.[21] These shortcomings prompted research into other treatment modalities which have since proven to be safer and more effective in preserving and improving vision.

Photodynamic Therapy (PDT)

Indications

Ocular PDT was first introduced as a novel treatment for neovascular (wet) age-related macular degeneration (ARMD) and choroidal neovascularization in the mid to late 1990s. At the time, it was hoped that the narrow eligibility requirements and high recurrence rates of the MPS would be improved with PDT. Two large prospective multicenter randomized trials were completed with long-term follow-up examining its use for these conditions with extended follow-up, the Treatment of Age-Related Macular Degeneration with Photodynamic Therapy (TAP) study,[22] and the Verteporfin in Photodynamic Therapy Study Group (VIP) study.[23] The TAP study examined the use of PDT for certain subtypes of wet ARMD (those with some classic component on fluorescein angiography) and demonstrated benefit over placebo for patients with predominantly classic lesions. Vision in these patients remained stable with extended follow-up. In the VIP study, there were two arms: patients with choroidal neovascularization secondary to pathologic myopia and patients with wet ARMD with occult neovascularization. Patients in both arms had a visual benefit over placebo at 24 months, although subset analyses revealed a decrease in vision in treated patients over controls when the treated lesion size was large and baseline vision was better than 20/50.

Since the completion of the TAP and VIP trials, the off-label use of PDT has been reported in many small series for the treatment of many inflammatory, infections, trauma-related and idiopathic conditions associated with choroidal neovascularization including: idiopathic polypoidal choroidal vasculopathy (IPCV); inflammatory chorioretinitis including presumed ocular histoplasmosis syndrome (POHS), punctate inner choroidopathy (PIC), multifocal choroiditis; angioid streaks; chronic idiopathic central serous chorioretinopathy (ICSC); macular dystrophies; and choroidal rupture.[24] For many of these conditions, the advent of anti-VEGF pharmacotherapies has largely replaced the use of PDT over the past several years. PDT has also been reported in small case series for the treatment of intraocular tumors including: in tuberous sclerosis; choroidal hemangioma; capillary hemangioma; uveal melanoma; angiomas in Von Hippel Lindau disease; and squamous cell carcinoma of the conjunctiva.[25] Among these tumors, the largest body of evidence exists for the use of PDT for subretinal exudation and serous retinal detachment associated with choroidal hemangioma (Fig. 9). First reported by Barbazetto et al. in 2000,[26] there are now more than 10 small case series reporting its successful use including the largest series which had 19 patients.[27] Given its success with minimal complications, PDT has emerged as the new standard of care for this disease entity.

Technique

The protocol for the application of PDT was established in the TAP and VIP trials,[22,23] and generally a similar or identical protocol is used for off-label uses other than wet ARMD

or pathologic myopia. PDT is performed by using the photosensitizer verteporfin (Visudyne, Novartis Ophthalmics, Switzerland) which selectively targets vascular endothelial cells.[22] The procedure has two steps: first, the verteporfin is injected intravenously for 10 min (at a dose of 6 mg/m^2 body surface area). Five minutes later, selective activation of the dye in the target tissue is achieved by applying a diode laser emitting light at 689 nm to an area 1,000 µm larger than the greatest dimensions of the lesion of interest. The dose of light delivered is 50 J/cm^2 at an irradiance of 600 mW/cm^2 over 83 s. PDT's presumed mechanism of action is the selective vascular occlusion of the intraluminal portion of exposed vessels without damaging adjacent neural structures.[24]

Adverse Events

Minor adverse events reported in the TAP and TAP extension trials included: injection site inflammation, infusion-related back pain, allergic reactions, and photosensitivity reaction.[22] Rare ocular adverse events included vitreous hemorrhage and retinal capillary nonperfusion. Visual disturbance, defined as any visual complaint including visual field defect irrespective of its relationship to the treatment, occurred in 22% of treated patients versus 15% of controls at 24 months of follow-up.[28] Acute severe acuity visual decrease was extremely rare (<1%).

Future Directions

With the successful introduction of anti-VEGF, the use of PDT for wet ARMD has diminished dramatically. It will likely continue to be used as a secondary treatment option in patients who do not respond to anti-VEGF therapy and seek an alternative. It also continues to have a role in the treatment of other conditions such as choroidal hemangioma as outlined above, as well as other conditions which have not demonstrated a successful outcome after anti-VEGF therapy.

Diode Laser

Indications

The current primary application of diode laser in the posterior segment is the treatment of ocular tumors such as retinoblastoma, the most common primary intraocular malignant tumor in children, and uveal melanoma, the most common primary

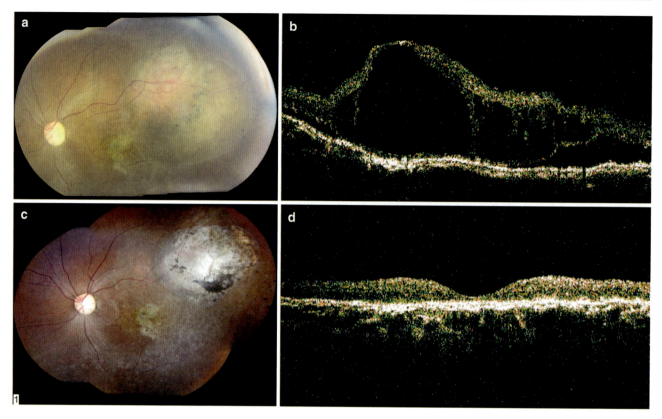

Fig. 9 45 year-old male with a large choroidal hemangioma, left eye. (**a**) Fundus photograph demonstrating the orange-red tumor at presentation. (**b**) Optical coherence tomography (*OCT*): vertically oriented scan with the retinal area located inferior to the fovea represented on the left and the retinal area located superior to the fovea represented on the right. There is a large amount of subretinal fluid (black cystic-appearing space under the retina) associated with the tumor. (**c**) Fundus photograph 9 months after photodynamic therapy (*PDT*). The tumor has regressed with associated chorioretinal scarring and atrophic changes in the retinal pigment epithelium. (**d**) OCT demonstrating resolution of the subretinal fluid

malignant intraocular tumor in adults. Guidelines and indications for the use of diode laser for these tumors are highly variable by center, and no clear standard has been established.

For retinoblastoma, laser treatment is most commonly used as an adjunctive therapy along with systemic chemotherapy. In the largest published study, 188 tumors in 80 eyes of 50 patients were treated with chemotherapy and laser, and 86% demonstrated regression.[29] In another study of 91 small tumors in 22 eyes of 24 patients treated with laser alone, 95% of tumors 1.5 disc diameters or smaller underwent long-term regression without any other treatment.[30]

For uveal melanoma, several groups of authors have reported the use of argon or diode laser in combination with plaque radiotherapy with the goal of ensuring better local tumor control, especially for tumors located near the optic nerve and fovea.[31-35] The largest of these studies examined the local tumor control rates in 270 patients treated with Iodine-125 plaque therapy followed by three sessions of transpupillary thermotherapy administered at plaque removal and at 4-month intervals.[33] Kaplan Meier estimates of tumor recurrence were 2% at 2 years and 3% at 5 years. These local control rates appear to be higher than those observed in the Collaborative Ocular Melanoma Study (10.3% failure at 5 years), but cannot be compared easily due to short follow-up time in the study. When compared with patients treated with radioactive plaque therapy alone, tumors treated with radioactive plaques and argon laser appear to regress faster but result in more short-term visual acuity loss.[35] Larger randomized prospective trials are needed comparing radioactive plaque therapy alone to plaque therapy with adjunctive laser and/or transpupillary thermotherapy.

Technique

For retinoblastoma, thermal energy is delivered from the 810 nm infrared lased by one of three techniques: (1) using an adaptor on the indirect ophthalmoscope and a 20-Diopter or 28-Diopter lens which delivers a large 1.6 mm spot size;

(2) using a pediatric laser gonioscopy lens and an adaptor on the operating room microscope which delivers a 3 mm spot size; or (3) using a transconjunctival diopexy probe which delivers a 1 mm spot size.[36] The laser is generally set on 350 mW to start the procedure and adjusted until a gray-white color change is noted in the tumor. Some centers utilize a method called transpupillary thermotherapy (TTT) which consists of modifications to the diode laser's hardware and software. Typically, the laser beam is aimed directly at the tumor, and the tumor surface is completely covered with overlapping laser spots to ensure that no areas are missed. The mechanism by which diode laser causes tumor cell death is thought to be different from the mechanism by which classic laser photocoagulation destroys tumors. The temperature of the diode laser is thought to be lower (45–60°C) and the thermal effect leads to direct apoptosis of the tumor cells. For this reason, the laser is directed at the tumor rather than at its feeder vessels.[36]

One controversy regarding the use of laser for retinoblastoma is whether to apply the laser directly to the macula. Some centers advocate the use of laser with avoidance of application directly to the fovea to decrease the risk of severe treatment-related central visual loss.[37] Other centers have reported results when using chemotherapy alone without and laser.[38] Our group recently published an analysis of our series of retinoblastoma patients treated with 4–9 cycles of three-drug chemotherapy and diode laser ablation.[39] All of the patients in this cohort had retinoblastoma presenting in the macula and each patient was treated aggressively with diode laser at every examination under anesthesia until the patient's tumor was noted to be inactive for at least 6 months (Fig. 10a–d). 100% of the patients with early stage disease and 83% of patients with advanced disease avoided external beam radiation and enucleation at 3 years. These tumor control rates far exceed those published at other centers. Furthermore, 57% of patients maintained 20/80 or better vision.

Adverse Events

Reported complications from diode laser include: focal iris atrophy, focal lens opacities, sector optic disc atrophy, retinal traction, optic disc edema, retinal vascular occlusion, serous retinal detachment, choroidal neovascular membrane, peripheral anterior synechiae, and corneal edema.[29,39] The most common side effect is focal iris atrophy which is associated with an increasing number of treatment sessions and an increasing tumor base diameter.[29]

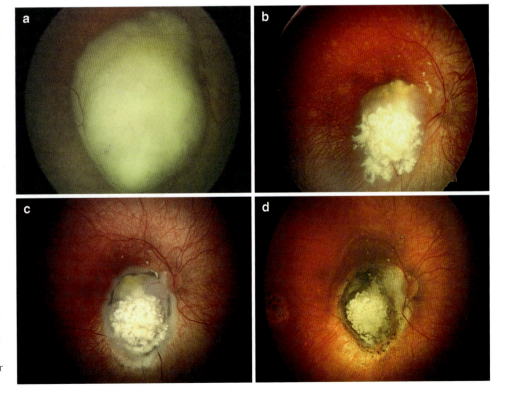

Fig. 10 Right eye of an 11 month-old male with advanced retinoblastoma, fundus photographs. (**a**) At presentation, the large tumor obscures the macula and optic nerve. (**b**) Dramatic shrinkage of the tumor is observed after 2 cycles of intravenous chemotherapy and 2 diode laser treatments. (**c**) Additional reduction in the size of the tumor is noted after 4 cycles of intravenous chemotherapy and 9 diode laser treatments. (**d**) Chorioretinal scarring and complete tumor regression with typical calcified appearance. The patient underwent a total of 6 cycles of intravenous chemotherapy and 9 diode laser application sessions. The patient developed an additional tumor focus temporal to the macula (left margin of photograph) that was treated with laser. The final visual acuity in this eye was 20/60 (Figures reproduced from Schefler et al.[39] With permission)

Future Directions

No standardized protocols have been established for the application of diode laser therapy for intraocular tumors. Optimal technique-related approaches, such as when and how often to treat, how much power to use, which areas of the tumor to treat, and whether to treat the fovea remain uncertain. Prospective standardized studies are essential in the future in order to establish the ideal treatment method and clinical standardization, especially for retinoblastoma given the current disparate tumor control rates at different institutions.

Endolaser for Vitreoretinal Surgery

Indications

First developed in 1979 by Charles, the introduction of endophotocoagulation was a significant advance in vitreoretinal surgery.[40] In his original system, he used a fiber optic probe attached to a portable xenon arc photocoagulator. The xenon arc was not ideal for surgery, however, and several years later, Peyman developed an argon laser probe that enabled more rapid firing, had a more comfortable and safe working distance, and didn't generate as much heat.[41] The argon green and diode lasers are currently used most frequently.

During vitrectomy procedures, the endolaser is used most commonly to create a laser barricade around retinal hole, surround retinectomy edges or giant retinal tear margins, and deliver scatter pan-retinal photocoagulation. For retinal holes, the goal is to achieve 360° of laser encircling the tear. In order to achieve an effective laser burn, subretinal fluid under the hole must be fully aspirated or the retinal pigment epithelium will not absorb the laser energy effectively. For retinectomies and giant retinal tears, laser spots are generally placed around large areas of detached retina or to wall off the area of prior detachment such as in cases or proliferative vitreoretinopathy or viral retinitis. Reattached retina is typically lasered overlying a scleral buckle which is typically a silicone band placed around the outside of the eye to maintain the reattached position of the retina. Endolaser can be placed through perfluorocarbon liquids which are often used to hold the retina in position. Afterword, perfluorocarbons are exchanged with air, reducing visibility and making lasering more difficult.

For panretinal laser photocoagulation, the goal is similar to pan-retinal photocoagulation performed using slit-lamp or indirect ophthalmoscopic systems. The endolaser typically enables easier access to more peripheral retina than the nonoperative systems, particularly if wide-angle intraoperative viewing systems are used.

Finally, endophotocoagulation can be applied to neovascular tissues prior to removing them or to retina prior to a retinectomy to minimize bleeding. The argon green laser is generally used for this purpose because it is best absorbed by blood. Diathermy can also be used.

Techniques

The standard endolaser probe is a 20-gauge instrument that is available in several forms including: straight or curved, blunt or tapered, simple or aspirating,[42] or illuminating (Fig. 11).[43] The straight probe with a blunt or tapered tip is used most commonly. The curved tip is useful for applying laser to the difficult-to-reach anterior superior retina or peripheral retina near the surgeon's dominant hand. The aspirating tip can be used to drain subretinal fluid or blood from the edge of retinal holes while lasering. The illuminating probe frees the opposite hand for use of another instrument.[44] More recently, thinner probes have been developed including 23-gauge and 25-gauge systems. These probes can be used in smaller sclerotomy incisions enabling a sutureless closure at the end of the surgery and enhanced post-operative comfort for the patient.

The initial settings of the argon laser are typically for 0.1–0.2 s with a power of 200 mW. For the diode laser, the settings are generally 0.2–0.3 s, and 200–300 mW. The power is typically adjusted gradually in 50 mW steps until a gray-white color change is noted. A continuous setting is helpful for treating active hemorrhage or around retinotomies.

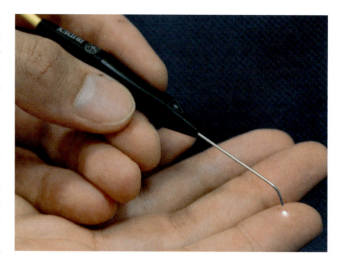

Fig. 11 Endocoagulation is performed using an argon laser probe. The fiber optic probe shown is a self-illuminating 20-gauge instrument with a curved tip. During vitrectomy, the probe is inserted through a sclerotomy. Common clinical indications for endolaser use include creating a laser barricade around a retinal hole, surrounding retinectomy edges or giant retinal tear margins, and delivering scatter pan-retinal photocoagulation

Adverse Events

Complications from endolaser are rare but can include: retinal tears, choroidal neovascularization, and retinal necrosis from overly intense treatment. Inadvertent overtreatment can occur by placing the probe too close to the retina or by not titrating the laser energy slowly upward based on a retinal color change.

Future Directions

The endolaser is a highly critical component of vitreoretinal surgery. When placed on proper settings and applied carefully, it can be performed safely with minimal risks. As smaller gauge systems have recently been developed, the number of available probes and configurations has increased, enabling greater choice and versatility for the surgeon. Endophotocoagulation will no doubt continue to be an integral aspect of vitreoretinal surgery for a long time.

Conclusions

Laser technology has been used for many years in ophthalmology with great success. Some previously common indications for the use of laser have become largely obsolete in recent years such as the use of argon laser for the treatment of juxtafoveal choroidal neovascular membranes. This shift in treatment approach has occurred due to the introduction of newer, more effective treatments. Nonetheless, the use of laser will no doubt continue to have an important role in ophthalmology. Given its accessibility and transparent media such as the cornea, aqueous, and vitreous, the eye remains an organ that is particularly amenable to this form of treatment. Direct inspection both during and after laser procedures enables easy assessment of the efficacy of laser use. Furthermore, the uveal tract, made up of the iris, ciliary body, and choroid, contains melanin pigment, allowing effective absorption of photothermal laser energy. As more clearly defined indications for the use of new pharmacotherapies such as anti-VEGF drugs are developed, laser procedures will likely develop an important combination therapy/adjunctive role for rare conditions such as intraocular tumors as well as for more common diseases such as proliferative diabetic retinopathy, diabetic macular edema, and choroidal neovascularization.

Disclaimer No conflict of interest or financial interest exists for any author.

References

1. Abramson DH. The focal treatment of retinoblastoma with emphasis on xenon arc photocoagulation. *Acta Ophthalmol Suppl.* 1989; 194:3-63.
2. Neubauer AS, Ulbig MW. Laser treatment in diabetic retinopathy. *Ophthalmologica.* 2007;221(2):95-102.
3. Diabetic Retinopathy Study Research Group. Photocoagulation treatment of proliferative diabetic retinopathy: the second report of diabetic retinopathy study findings. *Ophthalmology.* 1978;85(1): 82-106.
4. Early Treatment Diabetic Retinopathy Study Research Group. Early photocoagulation for diabetic retinopathy. ETDRS report number 9. *Ophthalmology.* 1991;98(5 Suppl):766-785.
5. The Diabetic Retinopathy Study Research Group. Preliminary report on effects of photocoagulation therapy. *Am J Ophthalmol.* 1976;81(4):383-396.
6. The Diabetic Retinopathy Study Research Group. Indications for photocoagulation treatment of diabetic retinopathy: Diabetic Retinopathy Study Report no. 14. *Int Ophthalmol Clin.* 1987; 27(4):239-253.
7. Early Treatment Diabetic Retinopathy Study Research Group. Focal photocoagulation treatment of diabetic macular edema. Relationship of treatment effect to fluorescein angiographic and other retinal characteristics at baseline: ETDRS report no. 19. *Arch Ophthalmol.* 1995;113(9):1144-1155.
8. Ferris FL 3rd, Davis MD, Aiello LM. Treatment of diabetic retinopathy. *N Engl J Med.* 1999;341(9):667-678.
9. Macular Photocoagulation Study Group. Laser photocoagulation for juxtafoveal choroidal neovascularization. Five-year results from randomized clinical trials. *Arch Ophthalmol.* 1994;112(4):500-509.
10. Preferred practice pattern: diabetic retinopathy. 2003. Accessed at http://www.aao.org/education/library/pppdr_new.cfm.
11. Fong DS, Strauber SF, Aiello LP, et al. Comparison of the modified Early Treatment Diabetic Retinopathy Study and mild macular grid laser photocoagulation strategies for diabetic macular edema. *Arch Ophthalmol.* 2007;125(4):469-480.
12. The Diabetic Retinopathy Study Research Group. Photocoagulation treatment of proliferative diabetic retinopathy. Clinical application of Diabetic Retinopathy Study (DRS) findings, DRS report number 8. *Ophthalmology.* 1981;88(7):583-600.
13. Macular Photocoagulation Study (MPS) Group. Evaluation of argon green vs krypton red laser for photocoagulation of subfoveal choroidal neovascularization in the macular photocoagulation study. *Arch Ophthalmol.* 1994;112(9):1176-1184.
14. Macular Photocoagulation Study Group. Persistent and recurrent neovascularization after laser photocoagulation for subfoveal choroidal neovascularization of age-related macular degeneration. *Arch Ophthalmol.* 1994;112(4):489-499.
15. Macular Photocoagulation Study Group. Argon laser photocoagulation for neovascular maculopathy. Five-year results from randomized clinical trials. *Arch Ophthalmol.* 1991;109(8):1109-1114.
16. Mason JO 3rd, Colagross CT, Vail R. Diabetic vitrectomy: risks, prognosis, future trends. *Curr Opin Ophthalmol.* 2006;17(3): 281-285.
17. Scott IU, Edwards AR, Beck RW, et al. A phase II randomized clinical trial of intravitreal bevacizumab for diabetic macular edema. *Ophthalmology.* 2007;114(10):1860-1867.
18. Ahmadieh H, Ramezani A, Shoeibi N. Intravitreal bevacizumab with or without triamcinolone for refractory diabetic macular edema; a placebo-controlled, randomized clinical trial. *Graefes Arch Clin Exp Ophthalmol.* 2008;246(4):483-489.
19. Avery RL, Pearlman J, Pieramici DJ, et al. Intravitreal bevacizumab (Avastin) in the treatment of proliferative diabetic retinopathy. *Ophthalmology.* 2006;113(10):1695. e1-e15.

20. Wu L, Martinez-Castellanos MA, Quiroz-Mercado H. Twelve-month safety of intravitreal injections of bevacizumab (Avastin(R)): results of the Pan-American Collaborative Retina Study Group (PACORES). *Graefes Arch Clin Exp Ophthalmol*. 2007;246(1):81-87.

21. Martidis A, Tennant MT. Age-related macular degeneration. In: Yanoff M, Duker JS, eds. *Ophthalmology*. 2nd ed. St. Louis: Mosby; 2004:925-933.

22. Treatment of age-related macular degeneration with photodynamic therapy (TAP) Study Group. Photodynamic therapy of subfoveal choroidal neovascularization in age-related macular degeneration with verteporfin: one-year results of 2 randomized clinical trials – TAP report. *Arch Ophthalmol*. 1999;117(10):1329-1345.

23. Verteporfin in Photodynamic Therapy Study Group. Photodynamic therapy of subfoveal choroidal neovascularization in pathologic myopia with verteporfin. 1-year results of a randomized clinical trial – VIP report no. 1. *Ophthalmology*. 2001;108(5):841-852.

24. Mennel S, Barbazetto I, Meyer CH, et al. Ocular photodynamic therapy – standard applications and new indications (part 1). Review of the literature and personal experience. *Ophthalmologica*. 2007; 221(4):216-226.

25. Mennel S, Barbazetto I, Meyer CH, et al. Ocular photodynamic therapy – standard applications and new indications. Part 2. Review of the literature and personal experience. *Ophthalmologica*. 2007; 221(5):282-291.

26. Barbazetto I, Schmidt-Erfurth U. Photodynamic therapy of choroidal hemangioma: two case reports. *Graefes Arch Clin Exp Ophthalmol*. 2000;238(3):214-221.

27. Jurklies B, Anastassiou G, Ortmans S, et al. Photodynamic therapy using verteporfin in circumscribed choroidal haemangioma. *Br J Ophthalmol*. 2003;87(1):84-89.

28. Bressler NM. Photodynamic therapy of subfoveal choroidal neovascularization in age-related macular degeneration with verteporfin: two-year results of 2 randomized clinical trials-tap report 2. *Arch Ophthalmol*. 2001;119(2):198-207.

29. Shields CL, Santos MC, Diniz W, et al. Thermotherapy for retinoblastoma. *Arch Ophthalmol*. 1999;117(7):885-893.

30. Abramson DH, Schefler AC. Transpupillary thermotherapy as initial treatment for small intraocular retinoblastoma: technique and predictors of success. *Ophthalmology*. 2004;111(5):984-991.

31. Kreusel KM, Bechrakis N, Riese J. Combined brachytherapy and transpupillary thermotherapy for large choroidal melanoma: tumor regression and early complications. *Graefes Arch Clin Exp Ophthalmol*. 2006;244(12):1575-1580.

32. Bartlema YM, Oosterhuis JA, Journee-De Korver JG, et al. Combined plaque radiotherapy and transpupillary thermotherapy in choroidal melanoma: 5 years' experience. *Br J Ophthalmol*. 2003;87(11): 1370-1373.

33. Shields CL, Cater J, Shields JA, et al. Combined plaque radiotherapy and transpupillary thermotherapy for choroidal melanoma: tumor control and treatment complications in 270 consecutive patients. *Arch Ophthalmol*. 2002;120(7):933-940.

34. Seregard S, Landau I. Transpupillary thermotherapy as an adjunct to ruthenium plaque radiotherapy for choroidal melanoma. *Acta Ophthalmol Scand*. 2001;79(1):19-22.

35. Augsburger JJ, Kleineidam M, Mullen D. Combined iodine-125 plaque irradiation and indirect ophthalmoscope laser therapy of choroidal malignant melanomas: comparison with iodine-125 and cobalt-60 plaque radiotherapy alone. *Graefes Arch Clin Exp Ophthalmol*. 1993;231(9):500-507.

36. Abramson DH, Schefler AC. Update on retinoblastoma. *Retina*. 2004;24(6):828-848.

37. Shields CL, Mashayekhi A, Cater J, et al. Macular retinoblastoma managed with chemoreduction. *Arch Ophthalmol*. 2005;123: 765-773.

38. Rodriguez-Galindo C, Wilson MW, Haik BG, et al. Treatment of intraocular retinoblstoma with vincristine and carboplatin. *J Clin Oncol*. 2003;21:2019-2025.

39. Schefler AC, Cicciarelli N, Feuer W, et al. Macular retinoblastoma: evaluation of tumor control, local complications, and visual outcomes for eyes treated with chemotherapy and repetitive foveal laser ablation. *Ophthalmology*. 2007;114(1):162-169.

40. Charles S. Endophotocoagulation. *Retina*. 1981;1(2):117-120.

41. Peyman GA, Grisolano JM, Palacio MN. Intraocular photocoagulation with the argon-krypton laser. *Arch Ophthalmol*. 1980;98(11): 2062-2064.

42. Peyman GA, D'Amico DJ, Alturki WA. An endolaser probe with aspiration capability. *Arch Ophthalmol*. 1992;110(5):718.

43. Peyman GA, Lee KJ. Multifunction endolaser probe. *Am J Ophthalmol*. 1992;114(1):103-104.

44. Awh CC, Schallen EH, De Juan E Jr. An illuminating laser probe for vitreoretinal surgery. *Arch Ophthalmol*. 1994;112(4): 553-554.

Laser/Light Application in Ophthalmology: Control of Intraocular Pressure

Ramez I. Haddadin and Douglas J. Rhee

- Glaucoma is a multifactorial optic neuropathy that results in progressive vision loss.
- The only treatable risk factor for glaucoma is elevated intraocular pressure (IOP).
- Diagnosis of glaucoma requires measurement of IOP, assessment of vision loss by visual field testing, and examination of the ocular fundus for signs of optic neuropathy such as cupping, and differentiation of open- and closed-angle glaucoma by gonioscopy.
- Treatment differs for closed-angle glaucoma (CAG) and open-angle glaucoma (OAG).
- Medications, laser procedures, and surgery are all critical to the management of glaucoma. How to treat a particular patient depends on the severity as well as the resistance to treatment of the glaucoma.
- Laser iridotomy is the creation of a microscopic hole through the iris that serves as an alternate route of aqueous drainage that bypasses the blockage at the pupil between the iris and the lens.
- Laser peripheral iridoplasty is a procedure that causes circumferential contraction of the iris away from the trabecular meshwork. Its main indication is CAG, and is often attempted when laser iridotomy fails or is not indicated because the pathophysiology does not involve pupillary block.

- Laser trabeculoplasty is the application of laser to the trabecular meshwork with the intention of increasing aqueous outflow. It is usually attempted after failed medical management but before a filtering surgical procedure is performed for OAG. Selective laser trabeculoplasty (SLT) is a new technique that seems to be equally effective to argon laser trabeculoplasty (ALT). Advantages of SLT include a potential benefit from treatment following ALT, and theoretically its use for multiple treatments.
- Both ALT and SLT are effective first-line agents for primary open-angle glaucoma.
- Cyclophotocoagulation is the use of laser to destroy ciliary body tissue in order to decrease aqueous humor production and reduce intraocular pressure. Because of its higher rate of side effects and complications, it is usually reserved for glaucoma refractory to all other treatment options. There are four approaches to cyclophotocoagulation: contact transscleral, noncontact transsceral, transpupillary, and endoscopic.
- There are a number of other applications for laser in glaucoma that are either adjuncts to or very similar to surgical procedures for glaucoma. These include laser sclerostomy, laser suture lysis, closure of cyclodialysis clefts, and goniophotocoagulation.

R.I. Haddadin (✉)
Department of Ophthalmology,
Massachusetts Eye & Ear Infirmary, Harvard Medical School,
Boston, MA, USA
e-mail: ramez_haddadin@meei.harvard.edu

K. Nouri (ed.), *Lasers in Dermatology and Medicine*,
DOI: 10.1007/978-0-85729-281-0_39, © Springer-Verlag London Limited 2011

Introduction

- Glaucoma is a multifactorial optic neuropathy that is initially asymptomatic but results in progressive visual field deficits.
- The prevalence of glaucoma increases with age, but can be seen at birth (i.e. congenital). Intraocular pressure (IOP) elevation is a major primary risk factor.
- The many types of glaucoma can be categorized into open-angle glaucoma (OAG) and closed-angle glaucoma (CAG).
- Diagnosis of glaucoma requires measurement of IOP, assessment of vision loss by visual field testing, and examination of the ocular fundus for signs of optic neuropathy such as cupping, and differentiation of OAG and CAG by gonioscopy.
- The only clinically proven treatment for glaucoma is lowering the IOP. This can be accomplished with medications, laser surgery, and/or incisional surgery.
- Laser surgery has become increasingly popular as a treatment modality for glaucoma because the risks are favorable in comparison to incisional surgery. A number of lasers are used, the most common being argon, neodymium:yttrium-aluminum-garnet (Nd:YAG), and diode lasers. The specific laser used depends on the desired effect on the tissue.

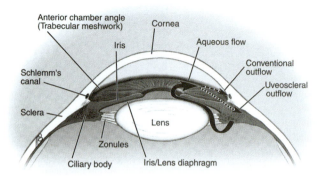

Fig. 1 Anterior segment anatomy and physiology

Definition, Classification, and Epidemiology

The term "glaucoma" refers to a group of disorders that share common phenotypes. There are over 20 different subtypes of glaucoma. The glaucomas are defined by a characteristic loss of retinal ganglion cell axons leading to a progressive optic neuropathy that is related to intraocular pressure (IOP). If untreated, glaucoma can cause visual disability and even blindness. Although elevated intraocular pressure (IOP) is no longer formally part of the definition, it is recognized as the major risk factor for progression of the disease.

The subtypes of glaucoma are categorized into open-angle glaucoma (OAG) or closed-angle glaucoma (CAG). The "angle" refers to the iridocorneal (iris-cornea) junction at the periphery of the anterior chamber (Fig. 1). The angle is the site of drainage for aqueous humor. OAGs and CAGs are further subclassified into 'primary,' when the cause of the dysfunctional IOP is unknown, or 'secondary,' when the cause of the elevated IOP is the result of a known disease process. Furthermore, glaucomas are classified by their onset – acute or chronic. The most common form of glaucoma in the United States is Primary Open-Angle Glaucoma (POAG).

With approximately three million Americans affected by glaucoma it is the second leading cause of blindness in the United States. Although it affects people of all ages, it is 6 times more common in those over 60 years of age than those 40 years of age. Annual medical costs for glaucoma services to glaucomatous patients and glaucoma suspects totals over 2.86 billion dollars.

Aqueous Physiology and Pathophysiology

Aqueous humor is a clear fluid that circulates in the anterior chamber of the eye to provide nutrients and remove metabolic waste from the avascular structures of the eye – namely the lens, cornea, and trabecular meshwork. The balance of aqueous secretion and drainage determines the IOP. Aqueous humor is produced by the ciliary processes, which are located behind the iris, through active secretion, ultrafiltration, and diffusion. Aqueous circulates within the posterior chamber, travels through the pupil, and exits the eye through the angle via one of two pathways (Fig. 1): (1) the conventional pathway through the trabecular meshwork, canal of Schlemm, intrascleral channels, and then episcleral and conjunctival veins; or (2) the uveoscleral pathway, through the ciliary body face, choroidal vasculature, and vortex or scleral veins. The conventional pathway is responsible for the majority of outflow, especially in older adults. CAG results from physical obstruction of these drainage tissues by approximation of the iris and cornea (Fig. 2). OAG occurs when aqueous drainage is impaired by increased resistance to aqueous drainage that is intrinsic to the outflow pathways (Fig. 3). Although it is possible that overproduction of aqueous humor could lead to an elevated IOP, all studies have shown that the pathophysiology is poor aqueous drainage. The average IOP is approximately 16 mmHg (2 mmHg standard deviation). An elevated IOP is defined as a value that is 2SD above the average (i.e., greater

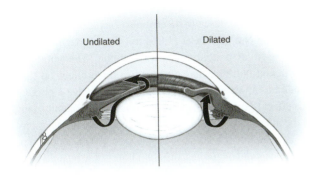

Fig. 2 Close-angle glaucoma due to pupillary block

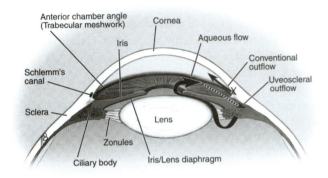

Fig. 3 Open-angle glaucoma

than 20 mmHg). There is a form of OAG, named "low-" or "normal-tension glaucoma," in which damage occurs within the average range (11–21 mmHg). Although IOP reduction is often effective treatment for this type of glaucoma, other etiologic factors such as vasospasm or ischemia are thought to have a larger role in the pathophysiology.

Symptoms

Vision loss from chronic glaucoma is usually painless and slowly progressive. Peripheral vision is usually affected first, and the deficits may be asymmetric. This results in delays in realization of vision loss.

Acute angle closure and a few secondary glaucomas present with symptoms, most commonly painful red eye, blurred central vision, and rapid progression of visual loss. The presence of non-visually related symptoms are due to the rapid change in IOP causing immediate ischemic compromise of several ocular tissues – principally, the cornea and optic nerve.

Diagnosis

Diagnosis of glaucoma requires a complete history and ocular examination including measurement of IOP, assessment of the anterior chamber angle by gonioscopy, quantification of vision loss by visual field testing, and examination of the ocular fundus for signs of optic neuropathy such as cupping (Fig. 4). Gonioscopy is examination of the iridocorneal angle with a slit-lamp and contact lens containing mirrors to visualize the angle. Measurement of an elevated IOP identifies a significant risk-factor but is neither necessary nor sufficient for the diagnosis of glaucoma. Visual field defects and optic nerve defects characteristic of glaucoma are strong support for the diagnosis but other causes of optic neuropathy such as optic neuritis need to be excluded.

Treatment

To date, lowering IOP is the only clinically proven treatment for the glaucomas. Glaucoma suspects may also be treated

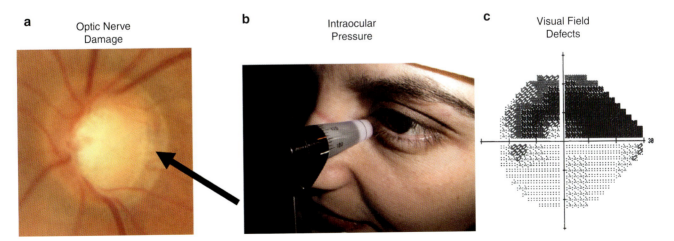

Fig. 4 Clinical triad of glaucoma, (**a**) optic nerve damage, (**b**) intraocular pressure, (**c**) visual field defects

depending on the presence of high risk characteristics and the individual risk aversion of the patient. The treatment approach differs between CAG and OAG. CAG treatment requires laser or surgery to bypass the mechanical blockage. OAG can be treated with topical medications, laser, and/or incisional surgery. Topical medication may decrease aqueous production or increase aqueous drainage. Laser trabeculoplasty attempts to enhance the drainage function of the trabecular meshwork. Laser peripheral iridotomy creates a secondary pathway to allow aqueous to bypass a potential blockage; in doing so, equalization of the pressure gradient between the spaces anterior and posterior to the iris often allows the angle to deepen. Laser iridoplasty directly alters the angle anatomy by moving the iris away from the drainage structures. Glaucoma that is refractory to the above treatments may require cyclodestructive procedures to destroy the ciliary body and decrease aqueous production. Incisional operations such as trabeculectomy and glaucoma drainage implant devices create a new pathway to drain aqueous from the anterior chamber to the subconjunctival space.

General Comments Regarding Lasers in Glaucoma

Many lasers are used in glaucoma management. Their use has increased because their less invasive nature and generally lower rates of complications appeal to surgeons. The most commonly used lasers are argon, diode, and neodymium:yttrium-aluminum-garnet (Nd:YAG). The argon laser (488–514 nm) has a thermal effect on tissues, which either results in coagulation or vaporization depending upon the power settings used. The diode laser (810 nm) also has a photocoagulative effect. The Nd:YAG laser (1,064 nm) has a coagulative effect when used in a continuous-wave mode. The short-pulsed q-switched Nd:YAG has a photodisruptive effect on tissues, which has an explosive effect. Other lasers have a photoablative effect that results in excision of tissue without any damage to the adjacent tissue. Photoablation has more applications for the cornea, but is also used in glaucoma. Besides the type of effect observed on tissues, different lasers may be used because they specifically target a certain type of tissue or because they have a desirable depth of penetration.

Laser Iridotomy

Iridotomy is the creation of a microscopic hole through the iris that provides an alternate route for aqueous to enter the anterior chamber (Fig. 5). Laser iridotomy is preferred over surgical iridotomy because it is safer, equally effective, and preferred by patients; however, surgical iridectomy serves as second-line treatment if laser iridotomy is unable to be performed (e.g. a patient who is unable to maintain position in the laser). The popularity of this established technological advancement is evidenced by utilization statistics. Although the total number of laser iridotomies and surgical iridectomies has increased in proportion to the aging population, the ratio of laser iridotomies to surgical iridectomies performed has increased from 15:1 in 1995 to 52:1 in 2004. The procedure is treatment for all forms of CAG that involve pupillary block. Patients with easily occludable angles may also require the procedure.

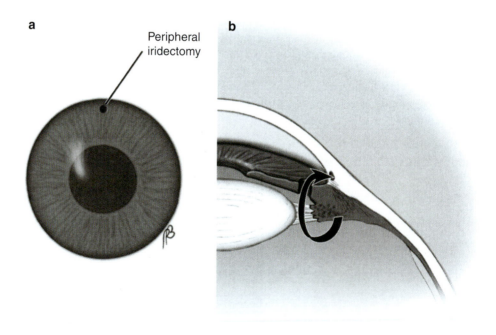

Fig. 5 Laser peripheral iridotomy, (**a**) shows clinical appearance of an iridotomy at the 12 o'clock position of the iris; (**b**) shows a secondary pathway to allow aqueous to bypass a potential blockage

Indications and Contraindications

Indications

- Closed-angle glaucoma with pupillary block
- Narrow angles with signs of glaucoma
- Narrow angles with positive provocative tests

Contraindications

- Opacified cornea
- Uncooperative patient who is unable to maintain position for the procedure

The primary indication for laser iridotomy is to relieve pupillary block that may progress to acute angle closure glaucoma or CAG. Mechanistically, pupillary block is caused by an increased resistance to aqueous flow through the pupil because of anatomic obstruction of the pupil by the lens or another anterior or posterior structure. Increased resistance leads to a pressure differential between the anterior and posterior chambers, which results in anterior bowing of the peripheral iris over the trabecular meshwork. Laser iridotomy is indicated if pupillary block has caused angle-closure or is in imminent threat of causing angle-closure. Angle-closure glaucoma may be acute, intermittent, or chronic; and all are indications for laser iridotomy. If narrow angles are identified, then the risks and benefits of treatment should be considered. For example, treatment would be indicated if there are signs of previous attacks or if the fellow eye has CAG. Additionally, patients with narrow angles can undergo tests to provoke angle-closure such as administration of a mydriatic agent, exposure to dark, or placement in the prone position. These tests may cause IOP elevation, and therefore may serve as an indication for treatment. Finally, in eyes where the clinician feels the angle is potentially occludable, laser iridotomy is indicated.

Specific causes of pupillary block include phacomorphic glaucoma (glaucoma caused by an excessively large lens), a dislocated lens, anterior protrusion of the vitreous face, occlusion by an artificial (pseudophakic) lens in the anterior chamber, posterior synechiae (adhesions of the central iris to the lens usually as a result of inflammation), or extreme miosis. This is in contrast to CAG without pupillary block such as vascular or inflammatory diseases that may cause peripheral anterior synechiae (adhesions of the peripheral iris to the cornea). However, patients with CAG without pupillary block may also be treated with laser iridotomy because some degree of pupillary block may be secondarily involved. Nanophthalmic (small eye) eyes frequently develop CAG because they have very small eyes relative to the size of their natural crystalline lens. Pupillary block related to an enlarged lens may be a contributing factor in these cases. The same reasoning may extend to patients with primarily an OAG. If a pupillary block component is suspected, the benefits of eliminating such a factor may outweigh the risks.

Contraindications to laser iridotomy are few and primarily include findings that increase the risk of complications from the procedure. Corneal burns may result from either (1) use of laser through an opacified cornea, or (2) use of laser in an eye with an extremely narrow angle. Acute CAG with pupillary block is ultimately treated with laser iridotomy; however, the procedure should ideally be done following the acute phase after the eye's inflammation has had a chance to subside and the cornea has cleared. However, this is not always possible and laser iridotomy is still indicated if the cornea is clear enough to perform the procedure. Topical and systemic anti-glaucoma medications can acutely lower the pressure.

Techniques

- Topical anesthesic and miotic medications are applied preoperatively.
- The argon, diode, or Nd:YAG laser is used to apply laser to the superior peripheral iris through a focusing iridotomy lens.
- The photocoagulative effect of argon laser is dependent upon pigmentation; therefore, techniques vary for irises of different colors.
- The Nd:YAG laser is photodisruptive and therefore does not dependent upon tissue pigmentation.
- IOP-lowering medications are used perioperatively. Corticosteroids may be temporarily used postoperatively to control inflammation.

Pre-operative Management

Topical proparacaine is sufficient to provide anesthesia. A miotic agent is applied topically to thin the iris and pull it away from the angle. This allows for easier penetration and minimizes corneal endothelial injury. An Abraham iridotomy lens will help stabilize the eye, keep the eyelids open, provide a magnified view, and minimize corneal burns by acting as a heat sink and increasing the power density of the laser at the iris. The iridotomy site should be made in a relatively thin region of the iris. Typically, the iridotomy site is between the 11 o'clock and 1 o'clock positions where the lid

Pre-operative Management

Topical proparacaine is sufficient to provide anesthesia. Pilocarpine is applied topically to constrict the pupil which will have the effect of thinning the iris tissue by virtue of spreading it over a larger area (i.e. place the iris under stretch). Apraclonidine or brimonidine is usually given before and after the procedure to reduce the risk of intraocular pressure elevations.

Description of the Technique

The argon laser is used for its coagulative effect to form contraction burns. The spot size is large (500 μm) with low power (200–400 mW) and long duration of delivery (0.5 s). The beam is aimed at the most peripheral iris to apply 20–24 spots are placed circumferentially, avoiding large radial vessels.

Post-operative Management

The peripheral anterior chamber should deepen immediately; therefore gonioscopy can be performed to confirm that the procedure was successful. Apraclonidine and topical steroid are given postoperatively to reduce the risk of intraocular pressure elevations and control inflammation. Topical anti-inflammatory treatment is continued for 3–5 days.

Adverse Events

- Side effects and complications are similar to those of laser iridotomy.
- Additionally, there is the risk of iris necrosis, which can be avoided with appropriate spacing of the laser spots.

Side Effects/Complications: Prevention and Treatment of Side Effects/Complications

Side effects include intraocular pressure elevations and inflammation. Their treatment is described above. Complications are similar to those of laser iridotomy. Additionally, *iris necrosis* may occur if the spots are placed too closely together. Spots should be spaced with 1–2 spot diameters apart.

Laser Trabeculoplasty

Laser trabeculoplasty is the application of laser to the trabecular meshwork with the intention of increasing aqueous outflow to reduce IOP in patients with OAG. It is usually attempted after failed medical management but before a filtering surgical procedure is performed. However, laser trabeculoplasty can be offered as the initial treatment for patients with open-angle glaucoma as an alternative to medications in patients with early stage disease or in patients who are unable to use topical medications.

The mechanism of increased aqueous outflow after laser trabeculoplasty is not well-understood. Three theories have been proposed to explain the efficacy of laser trabeculoplasty: mechanical, biologic, and cellular repopulation theories. The mechanical theory suggests that a thermal burn to the collagen results in local tissue contraction with mechanical stretch to the adjacent tissue. Presumably, the adjacent areas would have increased aqueous outflow. The biologic theory suggests that thermal energy stimulates trabecular endothelial cells to release matrix metalloproteinase enzymes, and recruits macrophages, which results in trabecular meshwork remodeling. The theory proposes that the resultant remodeling of extracellular matrix will increase aqueous outflow. The repopulation theory suggests that the laser energy stimulates trabecular endothelial cell division with downstream effects resulting in increased aqueous outflow.

The mechanisms above are potential explanations for the effect of laser trabeculoplasty performed with argon and diode lasers, techniques that were first proposed by Wise and Witter in 1979. Both of these types of lasers are equally effective in the long term (5 years); however, there are differing results in the short term (3 months), some suggesting a slight benefit to argon laser trabeculoplasty (ALT). ALT may also be technically easier since the end-point of laser application is more evident. A potential disadvantage of ALT is more post-laser pain and inflammation.

In 2001, a new technique called selective laser trabeculoplasty (SLT) was approved by the Food and Drug Administration. SLT uses a non-coagulative double frequency Nd:YAG laser to selectively target pigmented trabecular meshwork cells without causing a coagulative effect. The absence of thermal burns suggests that the mechanical theory does not play a role in SLT.

Laser trabeculoplasty has gained popularity in recent years. The number of laser trabeculoplasties performed decreased by 57% between 1995 and 2001 (perhaps as a result of the release of several new classes of topical anti-glaucoma medications during this time), and then doubled from 2001 to 2004.

Indications and Contraindications

> *Indications*
>
> - Insufficient IOP control with medication
> - Poor compliance with medical management
> - Adult open-angle glaucomas (with the exclusion of uveitic glaucomas)
>
> *Contraindications*
>
> - Poor visualization of the trabecular meshwork (e.g. Angle closure, peripheral anterior synechiae)
> - Hazy media
> - Corneal edema
> - Uveitic glaucoma
> - Juvenile glaucoma
> - Patients younger than 35 years unless their OAG is due to pigment dispersion syndrome
>
> *Relative Contraindications*
>
> - Patients with intraocular pressures >35 mmHg
> - ALT should be withheld in patients with very narrow angles due to the risk of peripheral anterior synechiae; SLT may be used in these situations

The general approach to managing primary and secondary open angle glaucomas is to use topical anti-glaucoma medications, such as topical prostaglandin analogs, beta-adrenergic antagonists, carbonic anhydrase inhibitors, and selective alpha2-adrenergic agonists, as first-line treatments, and laser trabeculoplasty in patients that remain inadequately controlled. Incisional filtering surgical procedures are generally used when all other measures have not successfully controlled the eye pressure. Studies suggest that ALT has similar efficacy as first-line treatment compared with the medications available at that time. The Glaucoma Laser Trial was a randomized control trial that followed patients treated with medication or ALT for 7 years. The final IOP in the ALT group was 1.2 mm Hg lower than the medically treated group, and their visual fields were slightly better concluding that ALT is at least as effective as medication as a first-line treatment. A Cochrane review concluded that laser trabeculoplasty controls IOP at 6 months and 2 years better than the medications used before the 1990s. Usually 180° of trabecular meshwork are treated initially, and if this fails to control IOP, the ophthalmologist may choose to treat the other 180°.

Smaller prospective randomized controlled studies have shown SLT is at least as effective as modern topical anti-glaucoma medications. SLT may have a larger role than ALT because mechanistically it does not cause as much tissue destruction. Hence, theoretically, SLT treatments can follow ALT treatments or SLT can be used exclusively for multiple treatments. The former has been investigated in a few studies, and results suggest that SLT is effective following both successful and failed ALT treatment. Whether multiple treatments with SLT is safe and effective has yet to be shown. Typically, 360° of trabecular meshwork are treated.

Laser trabeculoplasty should not be performed if laser cannot be applied to the trabecular meshwork safely. This includes corneal edema or any corneal opacities, hazy aqueous, or angle closure including peripheral anterior synechiae. Uveitic glaucoma is also a contraindication, as the laser trabeculoplasty is ineffective and may aggravate an existing inflammatory state.

Techniques

> - Topical anesthesic and miotic medications are applied preoperatively.
> - Argon or diode laser is typically applied to 180° of the trabecular meshwork circumference with power settings adjusted to produce minimal blanching.
> - Selective laser trabeculoplasty is typically applied to 360° of the trabecular meshwork circumference.
> - IOP-lowering medications are used perioperatively. IOP should be rechecked perioperatively, and again after 1–3 weeks to determine.

Pre-operative Management

Topical proparacaine is sufficient to provide anesthesia. Apraclonidine or brimonidine is usually given before and after the procedure to reduce the risk of intraocular pressure elevations.

Description of the Technique

A mirrored contact lens such as the Goldmann gonioscopy lens or Ritch lens is used to stabilize the eye and visualize the angle at the slit lamp (Fig. 7). The laser beam is focused at the junction of the posterior trabecular pigment band and the anterior meshwork (Fig. 8). The specifics of the laser application depend on the type of laser being used.

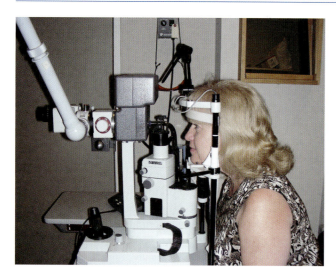

Fig. 7 Patient position at slit lamp-mounted laser

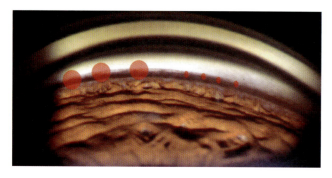

Fig. 8 Approximate sizes and locations of ALT (*left*) and SLT (*right*) laser spots

ALT and DLT generally require 40–50 spots over 180°. Power settings for ALT range from 400 to 1,200 mW with adjustment to produce blanching and occasional gas bubble formation. DLT power settings similarly range from 570 to 850 mW but blanching is usually less noticeable. As a result, the surgeon must be more attentive with regards to which portions of the meshwork have been treated. The spot size with ALT is typically 50 μm with 0.1 s exposures. DLT spot sizes range from 75 to 100 μm with exposures ranging from 0.1 to 0.5 s. With both ALT and DLT, one should try to space the application spots by 1–2 application spot widths apart.

SLT requires a similar technique to ALT and DLT but the 532 nm frequency-doubled q-switched Nd:YAG laser is used with very different parameters. Fifty-five to 65 spots are applied over 360°. Laser may be applied to 90°, 180°, or 360° of the meshwork, with guidelines still in evolution; in general, it is recommended to treat 180–360° with most practitioners treating 360°. Only a small fraction of the energy applied in ALT is needed for SLT treatment. The duration of exposure is 3 ns. The power setting is on the same order of magnitude; however, because of the short duration of exposure the energy applied is 1.2 mJ versus approximately 100 mJ for ALT. Moreover, the difference in energy density is even greater because the spot size used for SLT treatments is 400 μm (0.5 mJ/um^2 for ALT versus 10^{-5} mJ/um^2 for SLT). The application spots should be spaced approximately one to two application spot widths apart.

Post-operative Management

Glaucoma medications can be given post-operatively to reduce IOP elevations. IOP should be checked 30–120 min after the procedure and 1–2 weeks later. IOP reductions can be expected 4–6 weeks later, but can be seen as early as 2 weeks. If IOP reduction is inadequate, the remaining meshwork may be treated (for ALT and DLT or if only 180° of the meshwork were treated by SLT). There is no consensus on the treatment of post-operative inflammation following laser trabeculoplasty with some practitioners using topical corticosteroids, some using topical non-steroidal anti-inflammatories, and others using nothing (following SLT).

Adverse Events

- Transient and persistent IOP elevations may occur.
- Hyphema is rare and self-limited.
- Appropriate power settings and treatment locations will help avoid peripheral anterior synechiae.
- Mild iritis is common after ALT.

Side Effects/Complications: Prevention and Treatment of Side Effects/Complications

Transient as well as sustained *IOP elevations* may occur. *Hyphema* is rare and self-limited but can be treated by applying pressure to the globe with the goniolens or by photocoagulating with argon laser. *Peripheral anterior synechiae* are more common when areas posterior to the trabecular meshwork are treated. This should be avoided, and only the minimum power required to cause blanching should be used. Mild *iritis* is common after laser trabeculoplasty. Topical anti-inflammatories can control the inflammation. Laser trabeculoplasty is generally not helpful in patients with uveitic glaucoma and therefore should not be performed in most circumstances.

Cyclophotocoagulation

Cyclophotocoagulation is the use of laser energy to destroy ciliary body tissue usually in cases of refractory glaucoma. In contrast to all other procedures that have been described, the mechanism of IOP reduction for this procedure is a decrease in aqueous humor production. Cyclodestructive procedures are generally used as a last resort for refractory glaucomas because of their low success rates compared to filtration surgery and relatively high rates of complications and side effects. Cyclophotocoagulation has gained popularity over other cyclodestructive procedures such as cyclocryo-destruction because of its relatively lower rate of complications and side effects. The developmental trend with cyclophotocoagulation has been the use of lower power due to improved targeting; the lower power settings have improved the safety profile of these laser procedures. There are four approaches to cyclophotocoagulation: contact transscleral, noncontact transsceral, transpupillary, and endoscopic.

Indications and Contraindications

Indications

- Refractory glaucomas
- Open-angle glaucoma in which other treatments are contraindicated (e.g. neovascular glaucoma)
- Glaucomatous patients with low visual potential

Relative Contraindications

- Glaucomatous patients with high visual potential

Cyclophotocoagulation is usually for refractory glaucoma or glaucoma in which other treatments are contraindicated. Patients are already on maximal medication therapy with inadequate control. Filtering procedures have failed or may be high risk for the patient because of aphakic glaucoma, neovascular glaucoma, or perhaps glaucoma after penetrating keratoplasty. Such a less invasive procedure is also more appropriate for patients with low visual potential. Cyclophotocoagulation can also be a procedure of choice for eyes that have very distorted anatomy or eyes with an opaque cornea.

Techniques

- Retrobulbar anesthesia is administered preoperatively.
- Nd:YAG and diode lasers are the two most commonly used.
- The contact transscleral approach utilizes a fiber-optic probe to apply laser through the conjunctiva.
- The noncontact and transpupillary approaches utilize a slit lamp to apply the laser.
- Approximately 270° of the circumference of the ciliary processes are treated so as to reduce the risk of hypotony.
- Endoscopic delivery of laser for photoablation of the ciliary body is performed as an operative procedure due to the need to have an incision in the eye.

Pre-operative Management

Retrobulbar anesthesia is usually given for pain during and after the procedure. For the contact transscleral approach the eye is exposed with a speculum and the ocular surface is moistened with a saline solution before applying a fiber-optic probe to the conjunctiva. A slit lamp is used for noncontact transscleral and transpupillary approaches

Description of the Technique

There is no standardized protocol for cyclophotocoagulation procedures, and studies report varying success and complication rates. The two most commonly used lasers are Nd:YAG and diode lasers. A prospective study comparing the lasers found no significant difference in visual acuity or IOP reduction between the two lasers; therefore, the diode laser is often preferred because of its portability and lower energy requirements to achieve the same tissue result. A retrospective review of recent data from transscleral cyclophotocoagulation procedures concluded that the diagnostic category and age of the patients influence outcome more than the specific laser protocol or total energy used. Usually, approximately 270° of the circumference are treated. Treating more increases the risk of hypotony. Spot size is 100–400 µm with the 810 nm diode laser and 900 µm with the Nd:YAG laser. With the noncontact approach the laser is focused 3.6 mm beyond the surface of the globe; non-contact techniques are currently not favored. Pulse duration is 1–2 s at 1,750–2,000 mW with a total of 30–40 applications. The power setting is adjusted so that it is just below the power required to cause an audible 'pop.' The transpupillary approach may be used if the aqueous is clear and the pupil is sufficiently dilated so that ciliary epithelium can be directly visualized. The endoscopic approach will be described in the "Future Directions" section.

Post-operative Management

Antibiotic and steroid ointments are given and the eye is patched overnight for transscleral cyclophotocoagulation due to the use of a retrobulbar block anesthesia. Glaucoma medications are continued until IOP decreases, which may take several weeks. Retreatment may be necessary if IOP reduction is inadequate after weeks. It is not uncommon to require multiple treatments.

Adverse Events

> - Pain is usually managed with systemic acetamino-phen, ibuprofen, or cycloplegics depending on the source of the pain. Topical corticosteroid anti-inflammatory agents are also prescribed
> - Hypotony and phthisis are significant risks

Side Effects/Complications: Prevention and Treatment of Side Effects/Complications

Common side effects include *pain, inflammation, postoperative IOP increases, iritis, reduced vision.* Pain is usually managed with acetaminophen or ibuprofen. Pain secondary to iridocyclitis may be relieved with cycloplegics. *Hypotony* may develop after 6–36 months, and is one of the reasons that cyclodestructive procedures are a last resort. *Phthisis* is also a possible complication.

Miscellaneous Procedures

There are a number of other applications for laser in glaucoma that are either adjuncts to or very similar to surgical procedures for glaucoma.

Laser can be used to *cut subconjunctival sutures* placed in a number of different surgical procedures. The laser is preferred because the suture can cut the suture without having to incise the conjunctiva. Dark nylon or proline sutures that are too tight can be severed with argon laser. For example, trabeculectomy scleral flap sutures are usually placed tightly to avoid post-operative hypotony. To achieve the appropriate IOP reduction in the long-term, some of these sutures may be lysed with laser post-operatively.

Cyclodialysis clefts occur when ciliary muscle separates from the underlying sclera. This was once a treatment for glaucoma, but can also occur as a result of trauma or a complication of other surgeries. It results in hypotony and decreased vision. Use of the argon laser to deliver photocoagulative burns to the internal surface of the scleral in an attempt to scar these clefts closed has been described.

The iridocorneal angle may become vascularized eventually leading to neovascular glaucoma. This can result from a number of ischemic phenomena including diabetes mellitus and central retinal vein occlusion. Although panretinal photocoagulation is the primary treatment for these conditions because it is treating the source of the ischemic stimulus, *goniophotocoagulation* may be used as adjunctive treatment. Indications include anterior segment vascularization that is unresponsive to panretinal photocoagulation and cases in which angle vascularization is already present when panretinal photocoagulation is begun.

Laser sclerostomy is the use of laser to perforate the sclera at the iridocorneal angle has been investigated as an experimental treatment for glaucoma. Although not exactly the same, it can be thought of as the laser counterpart to a trabeculectomy, which is a guarded filtering surgery that is performed if glaucoma is not controlled with medication and laser trabeculoplasty. The laser can be applied externally with a goniolens or under a conjunctival flap, or internally. Numerous lasers have been studied and antifibrotic agents such as mitomycin C are sometimes used as adjunctive treatment; however, the role of laser sclerostomy in comparison to the well-known trabeculectomy surgery remains undetermined.

Future Directions

> - Laser-based procedures have become much more common in all areas of glaucoma treatments, in many cases replacing their surgical counterparts. Their less invasive nature and lower rates of complications are appealing and seem to be motivation for research to refine existing procedures and for continued innovation in the field.
> - Future studies should clarify differences between SLT and ALT. Moreover, the role of laser trabeculoplasty as a first- instead of second-line treatment for OAG as well as the effectiveness of repeated SLT requires further study.
> - Endoscopic cyclophotocoagulation is a newly developed cyclodestructive procedure which has several advantages over other forms of cyclophotocoagulation. Future studies will clarify whether the use ECP should also be limited to refractory glaucoma.
> - Goniopuncture is a new treatment for open-angle glaucoma that may have promise as a future treatment for glaucoma.

Laser-based procedures have been become much more common in all areas of glaucoma treatments. Their less invasive nature and lower rates of complications are appealing and seem to be motivation for research to refine existing procedures and for continued innovation in the field.

Selective laser trabeculoplasty is an exciting new methodology for laser trabeculoplasty. SLT seems to have similar efficacy and safety profiles to argon laser trabeculoplasty for the initial treatment. The theoretical potential for multiple retreatments is alluring but remains unstudied. Additionally, the roles of medical management and trabeculoplasty as first-line treatments may change.

Transscleral and transpupillary cyclophotocoagulation procedures have been described above. Cyclophotocoagulation has more recently been performed endoscopically through the anterior segment or pars plana. Endoscopic cyclophotocoagulation (ECP) has the advantage of direct visualization of the ciliary processes and application of laser. As a result, the surgeon is better able to titrate the total energy applied to the ciliary processes, and therefore reduce the rates of postoperative complications. There is a tendency to presume that ECP will have similar complications to the transscleral approach and cyclocryodestruction; however, further studies with larger sample sizes are needed. Some surgeons contend that ECP should be a candidate treatment for patients in earlier stages of glaucoma. Continued study of outcomes and refinement of the procedure parameters will help delimit its role in glaucoma management.

Goniopuncture is the creation of a hole in the trabecular meshwork that results in a direct connection between the anterior chamber and Schlemm's canal and therefore, theoretically, increased aqueous outflow facility. The technique was initially proposed in 1950 by Harold G. Scheie but has been more intensively studied in the last 10 years as a treatment for open angle glaucoma. An erbium:YAG laser is used endoscopically often in combination with phacoemulsification cataract surgery. The erbium:YAG laser is a 2.94 μm wavelength laser that has a photoablative effect on ocular tissues with minimal thermal damage. One study found IOP reductions after 1 year similar to those after trabeculectomy. Another study found comparable IOP reductions at 1–3 years. Such a new procedure will require studies with longer follow-up and standardization of the technique and laser settings before it is fully incorporated into glaucoma management.

Conclusion

Glaucoma is a multifactorial optic neuropathy resulting in potentially progressive vision loss. Although there are many modalities of treatment that can be successfully employed to slow or stop the progression of glaucoma, the major and only treatable risk factor for glaucoma is elevated intraocular pressure. Diagnosis of glaucoma requires measurement of intraocular pressure, evaluation of visual fields, funduscopy, and differentiation of closed-angle glaucoma (CAG) and open-angle glaucoma (OAG) by gonioscopy. The management differs for CAG and OAG. CAG with a pupillary block component is treated by laser iridotomy. CAG without pupillary block may benefit from peripheral laser iridoplasty. First-line treatment of OAG is usually medications. Laser trabeculoplasty has been traditionally reserved for those requiring additional, but modest, IOP reduction; however, studies suggest that it is equally effective in lowering IOP. If IOP remains inadequately controlled, filtration surgical procedures may be used. Cyclodestructive procedures such as cyclophotocoagulation are reserved for refractory glaucoma because of their relatively higher rates of side effects and complications.

Iridotomy is the creation of an artificial pupil in the iris that provides an alternate route for aqueous to enter the anterior chamber bypassing the space in-between the iris and lens on its way to the pupil. The procedure is treatment for all forms of closed-angle glaucoma that involve pupillary block (i.e. increased resistance through or total occlusion of the space between the iris and lens). Patients with easily occludable anterior chamber angles may also require an iridotomy. Contraindications include an opacified cornea, an extremely narrow angle, or an inflamed eye. A topical anesthesic and miotic medications are applied preoperatively. The argon, diode, or Nd:YAG laser is used to apply laser to the superior peripheral iris through a focusing iridotomy lens. Absorption of argon laser energy causes photocoagulation and is dependent upon pigmentation and therefore techniques vary for irises of different colors. On the other hand, the Nd:YAG laser is photodisruptive and therefore does not dependent upon tissue pigmentation. IOP-lowering medications are used perioperatively, and corticosteroids may be used postoperatively for inflammation. If the angle remains narrow after treatment, laser peripheral iridoplasty may be considered.

Argon laser peripheral iridoplasty causes circumferential contraction of the iris away from the trabecular meshwork. It is another treatment for closed-angle glaucoma, and is often attempted when laser iridotomy fails or is not indicated because the pathophysiology does not involve pupillary block. This includes plateau iris and anterior displacement of the iris by posterior structures such as an enlarging lens. The procedure may be performed prior to laser trabeculoplasty to deepen focal areas of angle narrowing, and prior to laser iridotomy if the eye is acutely inflamed. Severe corneal edema or peripheral anterior synechiae are contraindications. A topical anesthetic and miotic medications are applied preoperatively. Argon laser is applied circumferentially to the peripheral iris to cause contraction burns. The effect should be immediately evident. IOP-lowering medications are used perioperatively, and corticosteroids may be used postoperatively for inflammation. Adverse events are similar to those of laser iridotomy with the addition of iris necrosis, which can be avoided by appropriately spacing laser spots.

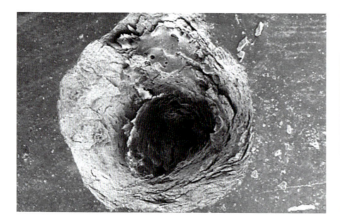

Fig. 22 Scanning electron micrograph of human enamel exposed to Er:YAG 2,940 nm laser energy. Note the fragmented margin and absence of thermal cracking. Magnification ×500

With the Erbium group of lasers the free-running micropulse emission mode results in rapid and expansive vaporisation of interstitial water and dissociation of the hydroxyl radical in the hydroxyapatite crystal causing an explosive dislocation of the gross structure[7–9] (Fig. 22).

Clinically, this is seen as ejection of micro-fragments of tooth tissue within the laser plume and the change in pressure in the immediately surrounding air results in an audible "popping" sound. In target tissue that has greater water content (caries > dentine > enamel), the popping sound is louder. With experience, this can aid the clinician in selectively ablating carious verses non-carious tissue. Compared to near infra-red wavelengths, the explosive outward effect of Erbium laser energy results in minimal thermal diffusion through the tooth structure. Co-axial with this laser is a water spray, to aid in dispersing ablation products and to provide cooling of the target site. The development of ultra-short pulse laser emissions of the Erbium group of wavelengths appears promising in reducing the conductive heat potential, whilst increasing the rates of tissue ablation.

Nonetheless, both laser wavelengths allow cavity preparation within acceptable clinical parameters.

Disadvantages of laser use on hard tissue when compared to rotary instruments may include the following:

- Laser use is contraindicated in the removal of existing amalgam and gold restorations
- Laser use on natural tooth tissue results in slower rates of cutting
- Laser delivery is axial and end-cutting and limits cutting procedures
- Lasers are contraindicated in the preparation of full-veneer crowns and bridges

Techniques

- Hard tissue management
- Tooth cavity preparation/removal of caries
- Hard tissue modification
- Surgical excision of bone

General Pre-operative Management

For all laser-assisted surgical dental procedures, the following should be followed:

- Secure operating room, define controlled area and place proper laser warning signs.
- Set up laser and test proper laser operation.
- Test fire laser, employing all safety measures, using minimum power settings and direct beam into an attenuating medium, e.g., water. The objective is to ensure correct laser operation, patency of delivery system and emission of cutting and aiming beams.
- Supplies dispensed, equipment and sterile instruments arranged.
- Patients information: review charting, x-rays, etc.
- Patients seated: review treatment plan and informed consent.
- Safety: eye protection placed, patient first followed by operating personnel.

Operating Techniques

Hard Tissue Management

Enamel is composed, by volume 85% mineral (predominately carbonated hydroxyapatite) 12% water and 3% organic proteins. The majority of free water exists within the peri-prismatic protein matrix. Of the major hard tissues, enamel exhibits greatest resistance to laser ablation and this is seen most in healthy, fluoridated, occlusal sites, where ablation rate is approximately 20% of that achieved with a turbine. Fluoridated enamel presents a greater resistance, due to the combined effects of a harder fluorapatite mineral and the replacement of the hydroxyl group by fluoride.

Dentine has a higher water content and less mineral density than enamel, being 47% by volume mineral (carbonated hydroxyapatite), 33% protein (mostly collagen) and 20% water. Consequently, ablation rates are faster than for enamel and power parameters can be correspondingly lower.

In Class III, IV and V cavity sites and certainly where prismatic density is less (as in deciduous teeth), the ablation rate in enamel is comparable to rotary instrumentation.[10,11] Anecdotally, the speed of laser cutting is maximised if the incident beam is directed parallel to the prismatic structure of the enamel to access the interstitial free water. In early research into the use of Er:YAG and enamel, it was shown that laser power parameters of approximately 350 mJ/2–4 pps (average power 0.7–1.4 W) would initiate enamel ablation in human teeth.[12] With the development of better co-axial coolant and shorter pulses, fast and efficient cavity preparation can be achieved with power levels of 400–700 mJ/10–20 pps (average power range 4–8 W) which, with adequate water cooling, does not cause pulpal damage. Clinical experience would suggest that with "harder" occlusal enamel, the use of higher energy-per-pulse and lower repetition rates provides for easier ablation. Where an etch-bonding technique is required, lower power levels (350–500 mJ/5–10 pps – Av. Power 1.75–3.5 W) should be employed. The concept of average power is more important in those lasers where the pulse rate is fixed.

With carious dentine there is a potential in gross caries for the laser beam to quickly pass through the surface layer, thus leading to dehydration in deeper layers. Where gross caries is present it is advisable to use an excavator to remove bulk volume, both to prevent heat damage and to expedite cavity preparation. Both Erbium lasers will leave a cut surface without a smear layer[13] and it is advisable to use a dentine protector on open tubules exposed by the ablation process.

Early study into the effect of the Er:YAG laser on bone showed that, as with enamel and dentine ablation, tissue cutting is a thermally induced explosive process.[14] As with other hard tissue interaction, it is essential to maintain a co-axial water spray to prevent heat damage which would delay healing. Studies into the rate of thermal denaturation of collagen, a major component of bone tissue, show that above a critical temperature (74°C) the rate of collagen denaturation rapidly increases causing coagulation of tissue.[15] At temperatures above 100–300°C there is an ascending dehydration, followed by carbonisation of proteins and lipids. The poor haemostatic effect of current Mid-Infra-Red lasers, with adjunctive water spray can be used to advantage in the ablation of bone, in ensuring blood perfusion of the surgical site.

However, the use of lasers in a bone ablation process results in a considerable splatter of blood and precautions (eye protection and mask) are recommended. An additional risk may be the creation of an air embolism in the tissue due to the air-induced water spray, although a review of the literature has not revealed any association. The use of erbium lasers in dento-alveolar surgery represents a less-traumatic experience for the patient, when compared to the intense vibration of the slow-speed surgical bur. Ablation threshold measurements of 10–30 J/cm^2 have been recorded for bone of varying density[15] and clinically, with maxillary alveolar bone, the speed of laser cutting is comparable with that of a bur and slightly slower in the mandible, reflecting the greater cortical bone composition. It is considered important that excessive power parameters are avoided, to reduce the "stall-out" effect of debris and minimise blood-spatter. Laser power values of 350–500 mJ/10–20 pps (average power range 3.5–7.0 W) with maximal water spray appear to effect good ablation rates.

The micro-analysis of the cut surface reveals little evidence of thermal damage and any char layer appears to be restricted to a minimal zone of 20–30 μm in depth.[15] Studies into the healing of lased bone would support the contention that the reduced physical trauma, reduced heating effects and reduced bacterial contamination, together with some claims to an osteogenic potential, lead to uncomplicated healing processes, when compared to conventional use of a surgical bur.[16,17]

Tooth Cavity Preparation/Removal of Caries

The classic approach to cavity design, as advocated by G.V. Black consisted of access, outline form, retention form and extension for prevention. This approach was in acknowledgement of the use of metal restorative materials and the prevalence of dental caries. With fluoridation and better hygiene and dietary measures, together with the emergence of non-metallic, ceramic-based resin materials, the need for large cavity design has been significantly reduced.

With laser-assisted cavity preparation, it is not possible to create sharp cavo-surface line angles and retention form has been addressed through the possibility of micro-retention of composite resin materials.

The cavity should be prepared using a near-contact approach with the delivery tip just above the tooth or cavity surface. Ablation of hard tissue and caries proceeds through a series of brush-strokes, allowing the laser energy to impact at 90° to the surface. Where hard intact enamel requires removal, it is better to align the laser tip parallel to the prismatic structure, as the inter-prismatic material has a higher water content. It is advisable to remove any un-supported enamel that over-hangs the carious lesion, either with the laser or a sharp had instrument. Gross caries can be excavated to prevent stall-out of the laser energy into dessicated soft debris. Removal of deeper caries will reveal a lightening of the surface colour as healthy tooth tissue is revealed and the louder sound of high-water content caries ablation may be lessened. Finally, the cavity should be lightly dried to ensure that the cavity margin has been correctly extended and an explorer used to detect any residual caries.[18,19]

Any potential for bacterial decontamination within the prepared cavity can be maximised through the use of a rubber dam to isolate the tooth.

Unlike rotary instrumentation, laser cavity preparation does not leave a dentine smear layer and it may be necessary to apply a dentine protector to minimise the possibility of post-treatment sensitivity.

There is some controversy over the marginal seal and stability of the composite restoration when the cavity has been prepared with a laser. Certainly, the gross appearance of the cavity margin when dried resembles an etch-like appearance, but this is due to the fragmentation of the tooth structure. A majority opinion exists to advocate the additional acid-etch of the cavity margins, although some studies have suggested that the strength of the seal is less than in conventionally-prepared restorations.[20,21] Consequently, there is some support for extending the acid-etch 1–2 mm beyond the cavity margin and into healthy enamel (Figs. 23–25).

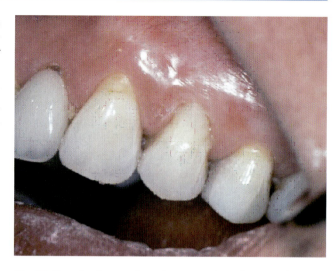

Fig. 25 Completed restoration using composite resin restorative

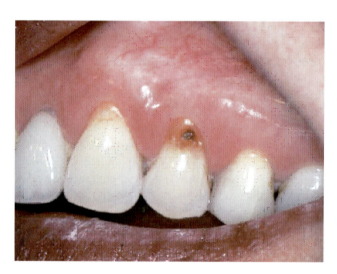

Fig. 23 Carious cavity buccal margin *upper left* bicuspid

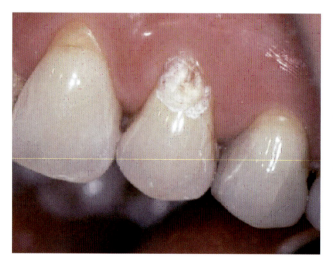

Fig. 24 Caries removed and cavity prepared using the Er:YAG 2,940 nm laser (800 μm sapphire tip/contact/350 mJ pp/10 Hz/Water spray/Av. Power 3.5 W)

Hard Tissue Modification

Clinical procedures that may be considered under this heading include fissure sealing, direct composite resin veneers and orthodontic bracket placement.

The prime requisite is to reduce the laser energy to a level that creates a surface dislocation of the enamel prismatic structure, but does not initiate deeper ablation. Using the Erbium YAG or Erbium Chromium YSGG laser, power parameters would be 350–450 mJ/pulse, 10 Hz with water spray and to draw the laser delivery tip away from the enamel surface to create a greater spot diameter and reduce the power density; by moving the tip back and forth from the surface, it is possible to define the amount of interaction of laser energy with the target tissue.

The use of a rotary bur in defining a labial surface preparation for a veneer will often produce a superficial smear layer in the enamel and this is very common with diamond burs. This layer can impede the development of acid-etch tags within the enamel. With laser energy the surface is left as a micro-retentive area and one that is devoid of proteinaceous contaminants that may impede bonding. Notwithstanding, there are two caveats; the prepared enamel still requires a conventional acid-etch stage[22,23] and it is advisable to limit the laser-ablated area to one within 1 mm of the veneer margin. In this way, the possibility of weakened enamel and possible marginal breakdown can be minimised.

The optimal conditions for fissure sealing are non-carious enamel, devoid of organic debris and a technique that allows the full depth of the fissure to be conditioned and sealed. Often, the use of an acid-etch technique alone fails to reach into the deeper areas of the fissure and the use of the Erbium laser allows exposure of all enamel surfaces, the removal of all organic material and sterilisation of the surface. Again, laser power parameters should be reduced to ensure that no breach of the amelo-dentinal junction occurs (Figs. 26–29).

Surgical Excision of Bone

The surgical removal of alveolar bone can form part of a range of treatments including surgical removal of teeth, tooth apical surgery, access to bony pathology and periodontal bone management. In all cases, there is a responsibility on the clinician to treat the area with care in order to prevent tissue over-heating and delayed or non-healing. The use of the Erbium lasers in bone ablation offers a less traumatic experience for the patient and the co-axial water spray

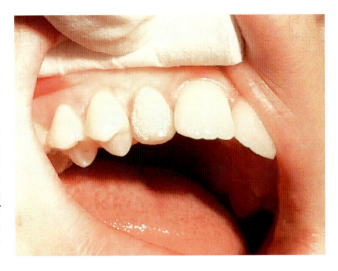

Fig. 28 Enamel "etched" using the Er:YAG 2,940 nm laser (800 μm sapphire tip/contact/300 mJ pp/10 Hz/Av. Power 3.0 W). Tooth surface dried

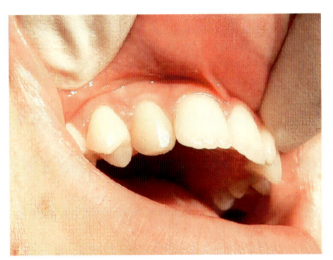

Fig. 26 *Upper right* cuspid prior to direct composite resin restoration

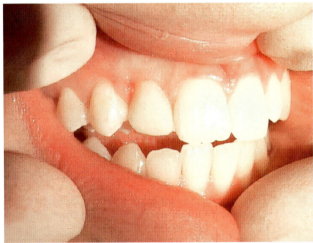

Fig. 29 Completed restoration

ensures temperature control and maintains the essential blood flow by preventing any coagulative effect.

The laser power parameters are similar to those used for tooth dentine ablation (350–500 mJ/ pulse, 10 Hz) and it should be remembered that the laser tip is end-cutting. As such a series of brush-strokes over the bone target should be employed, so that there is a successive surface ablation. The diameter of tips available (200–1,300 μm) allows a finer and more precise incision line and the prevention of heat and tactile damage to the tissue may account for anecdotal reports of less post-operative complications with laser ablation compared to rotary instrumentation.

An advantage of the fine diameter laser tips available allows a more precise removal or remodelling of crestal alveolar bone associated with periodontal pockets or crown lengthening procedures. With a closed flap approach to crown

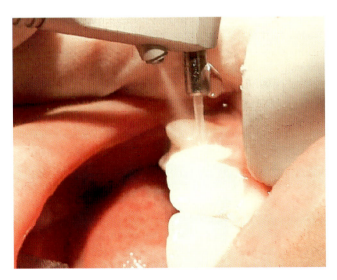

Fig. 27 Laser preparation using the Erbium 2,940 nm laser and water spray

lengthening, the end-cutting nature of the tip is an absolute advantage over rotary instrumentation and has led to a growth in this treatment modality; however, there is always the danger of not being able to visualise the target tissue and caution must be exercised in this respect (Figs. 30 and 31).

Post-operative Management

Following any form of laser use on dental had tissue, there is no specific management that would not apply to a similar procedure carried out with a rotary instrument. Post-operative bone surgery in whatever its' context, demands good wound debridement and, wherever possible or appropriate stable coverage of the bone through flap closure to prevent any bone necrosis.

Adverse Events

- Care must be observed when using a soft tissue laser in close approximation to a tooth, in order to avoid damage or conductive heat effects
- Excessive incident laser power may cause pulp sensitivity and post-operative pain
- Too little or no water spray will result in "stall out" and thermal damage to the tooth or bone
- Deep dentine ablation should be undertaken with reduced incident laser energy
- The ablation of bone is accompanied by a risk of blood-splatter and care should be exercised to protect the operator and assistant

Side Effects and Complications

The use of the Erbium laser wavelengths on dental hard tissue is considered by many clinicians as a treatment modality that poses least risk to either the integrity of the surrounding healthy tooth tissue or the vital pulp, provided the correct power parameters are employed. Where problems can arise may be summarised as the employment of too great an incident laser power setting, whereby pulp sensitivity may result, or where too little water spray is used. In such cases, there is a build up of ablation debris and thermal rise amounting to the phenomenon of "stall out". Here, the incident energy is absorbed by the tooth tissue or debris, which becomes dried and heat rise leads to possible carbonisation.

The possibility of post-operative tooth sensitivity is one that can always arise and is multi-factoral. The incidence of sensitivity that is wholly due to laser action is seen most often in deep cavities or large fresh cavities, where there is an increase in the number of large diameter dentinal tubules. In these cases, it may be prudent to reduce the laser parameters or apply the laser tip in a de-focussed mode together with the application of a calcium hydroxide liner or dentine protector, to protect the tubules.

Similar stall-out phenomena can occur during bone ablation and the use of the Erbium lasers in their free-running pulsed emission mode gives rise to considerable blood splatter. Consequently, the co-axial water spray must be maintained at adequate levels and high-speed suction closely

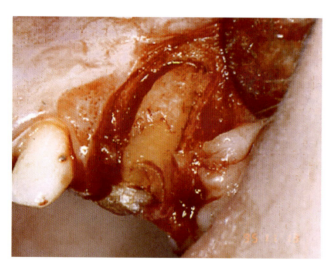

Fig. 30 Surgical removal of fractured *upper left* cuspid. Bone removal achieved using the Er:YAG 2,940 nm laser (1,000 μm sapphire tip/contact/450 mJ pp/10 Hz/Water spray/Av. Power 4.5 W). There is little haemostasis with the chosen laser parameters

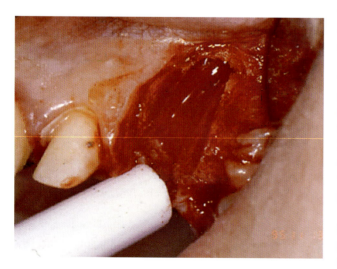

Fig. 31 Root removed, showing accuracy of laser cut

applied to the surgery site to minimise the splatter. Both operator and assistant should use suitable masks and face-shields for protection.

Future Directions

- Existing Erbium wavelengths interact well with tooth tissue and bone; faster ablation rates run the risk of increasing collateral thermal damage. Consequently, shorter pulse width delivery will allow this to be further developed.
- Ultra-violet lasers <350 nm have high absorption in water and offer little collateral damage. Research has shown good interaction with tooth tissue, but risks of ionising change and unit cost and reliability issues have prevented further advancement at this stage.
- Carbon dioxide exists as at least three distinct wavelengths that have been produced by laser hardware – 9,300, 9,600 and 10,600 nm. The latter is the most stable and has been produced as the conventional CO_2 laser during the past 30 years. Studies have shown very high absorption of the relatively stable 9,600 nm in hydroxyapatite and nano-second or shorter pulsing has addressed the problem of carbonisation that occurs in the CW 10,600 nm wavelength.
- The near future may see the emergence of a dedicated 9,600 nm ultra-pulsed CO_2 laser that will have application in restorative dentistry.

Use of Lasers in Anti-Bacterial Techniques Adjunctive to Dental Surgery: Laser Use in Periodontology, Endodontics, Implantology

Indications and Contraindications

- A major element of successful therapy in periodontology, endodontology and implantology is the elimination of pathogen bacterial strains.
- All bacterial strains have cellular structure that contains water and those longer IR laser wavelengths that are absorbed by water will prove advantageous in bacterial control.

- Shorter wavelengths will be absorbed by those bacterial strains that have pigmented cellular structure.
- The quartz optic fibre delivery of short IR laser wavelengths is ideal in being able to access root canals and periodontal pockets. Longer wavelengths can be employed through innovative fine-diameter wave-guides.
- Laser tips are end-emitting and do not allow the sides of periodontal pockets or root canals to be easily exposed to predictive energy levels.
- Laser techniques allow little if any tactile feedback and the accuracy of laser tissue interaction is distorted by the "blind" use of light energy within root canals and closed periodontal pockets.
- The use of laser energy of all wavelengths on implant surfaces must be exercised with caution to prevent heat build up, direct heat damage to the titanium structure and possible conductive heat effects to the surrounding bone.

There can be no compromise over the employment of thorough and evidence-based therapeutic measures in the dental specialties of periodontology endodontics and implantology. All aetiological and pre-disposing factors must be evaluated and applied against the presenting condition in order to define the scope, type and success of therapy. As such, the use of lasers should be seen as adjunctive and supplemental to established protocols.

The use of surgical lasers in periodontology can be seen in three areas of treatment: removal of diseased pocket lining epithelium, bactericidal effect of lasers on pocket organisms and the removal of calculus deposits and root surface detoxification. When integrated into a sound approach to pocket reduction, all current dental wavelengths have been advocated for the removal of diseased epithelium.[1-5] Added to the current wavelengths is the recent development of a frequency-doubled (wavelength halved) Nd:YAG laser at 532 nm, termed the KTP laser which has a range of action similar to that of the 810 nm diode. The haemostatic advantage of using laser energy confers a controlling factor that is beneficial to both clinician and patient. Conceptually, in a periodontal pocket that is essentially supra-bony, the removal of hyperplastic soft tissue together with a reduction in bacterial strains, renders the post-laser surgical site amenable to healing within normal limits. Where the pocket is infra-bony, a number of procedures have been advocated, including laser-ENAP (excisional new attachment procedure) where the Nd:YAG (1,064 nm) laser is used in a non-flap procedure to reduce pocket depths of several millimetres through a succession of treatment appointments.[6]

rotated and removed through a 20–40 s cycle. This cycle may be repeated three to four times, with a short interval.

Within the confines of the root canal, the use of laser wavelengths without water cooling can lead to a potential high rise in temperature. Risks associated include melting/cracking of dentine walls and trans-apical irradiation of the tooth socket. With short infrared and CO_2 lasers, if benefit is to be obtained, power levels of 0.75–1.5 W should be considered maximal. With water-assisted Erbium lasers, power values of 150–250 mJ/4–8 pps are considered suitable, but it is essential to allow water to reach the ablation site in order to prevent over-heating and cavitation of canal walls.

Following laser use, the canal can be obturated according to personal choice of materials and technique (Figs. 33 and 34).

Treatment of Peri-Implantitis

Careful assessment must be made as to causative factors and the scope for successful outcome. The many studies that have been carried out into the use of laser energy in the treatment of peri-implantitis would suggest that the prevailing caution is not to generate excessive heat within the metal or the surrounding bone; any temperature rise beyond 47°C will lead to changes in the bone structure and possible necrosis.

The implant is exposed through a muco-periosteal flap and granulation tissue must be carefully removed. It has been advocated that near IR wavelengths such as Diode (810–980 nm) can be used to ablate granulation tissue and it is advised that this should be done with a water spray. Alternatively, the Erbium YAG and Erbium Chromium YSGG lasers can be successfully employed with their co-axial water spray. The use of the carbon dioxide laser is not recommended.

With the implant threads exposed, it is possible to use the laser to decontaminate the surface. The levels of laser energy must be controlled to limit any damage or excess heating and parameters may be 0.7–1.0 W, CW (Diode) or 150–250 mJ/4–8 pps, plus water (Erbium group). The accessible implant surface should be treated in a series of brush-strokes during a period of 1–2 min. Following this, the bone defect may be repaired using a suitable matrix and membrane and primary closure of the flap obtained (Figs. 35–37).

Post-operative Management

Within the general use of laser energy in the adjunctive bacterial decontamination of periodontal, endodontic and implant

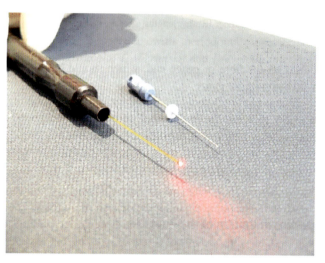

Fig. 33 The 320 μm diameter quartz optic fibre compared to a ISO #15 hand file

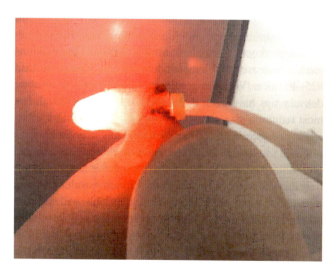

Fig. 34 320 μm diameter quartz optic fibre inserted into a root canal. The *red aiming beam* shows the extent of light distribution that might be expected with IR laser energy

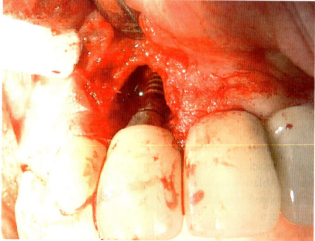

Fig. 35 Peri-implantitis associated with *upper* anterior implant fixture. *Lesion* shows the amount of bone destruction. Soft granulation tissue removed

Adverse Events

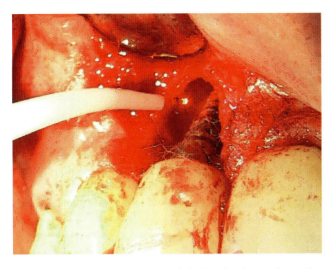

Fig. 36 Bacterial decontamination of titanium implant surface using the Diode 810 nm laser (320 μm fibre/non-contact/1.0 W CW)

- The use of laser energy must be adjunctive to and supplemental to established conventional treatment protocols
- In many treatment sites, the use of the laser is compromised by a "blind" approach and care must be exercised to prevent unwanted effects
- Wherever possible, low energy levels must be used and care taken to minimise the risk of thermal damage or exposure of delicate healthy tissue to laser energy

sites, there are no specific measures that need apply in the immediate post-operative period. Where the periodontal pocket has been treated, the patient should refrain from toothbrushing during 24–36 h after treatment and flossing during a 5 day period. Instead, the patient should be instructed to use a proprietary chlorhexidine mouthwash. The treated pockets should not be probed for 3 months to allow good healing.

In the treatment of peri-implantitis, the stability of the sutured soft tissue flap should be maintained during 10 days, at which time any remaining sutures should be removed.

Side Effects and Complications

Provided appropriate laser wavelength is chosen and correct power parameters employed, both within the framework of accepted general treatment protocols, there should be no side effects or complications. There is some concern as to the long-term efficacy of laser use in bacterial decontamination where a possibility may exist of re-infection, although such concerns surround more conventional therapies.

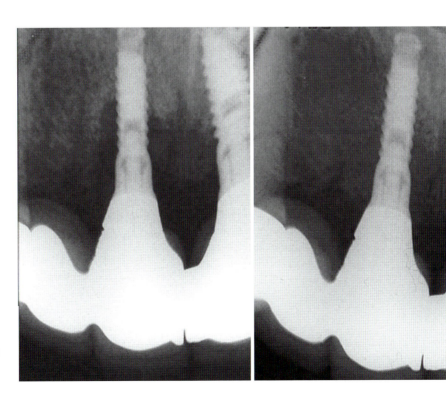

Fig. 37 Peri-apical radiographs of the affected implant. *Left*: the extent of the bone destruction, *Right*: following surgery and use of bone graft matrix, healing at 3 months

Future Directions

- Soft tissue surgery will continue to develop as part of the general dentist's remit in delivering care.
- Minor surgery of benign pathology will become more common amongst those dentists who have lasers.
- With the growth in demand for cosmetic dentistry, the use of lasers in delivery of smile augmentation, including soft tissue re-contouring will grow.
- The development of smaller laser units and the ability to deliver longer wavelengths through diode array will allow a greater market penetration of soft tissue lasers.

Low-Level Laser Use in Dental Surgery

Indications and Contraindications

- Low level laser therapy (LLLT) involves the use of laser energy at sub-ablative levels.
- LLLT when applied to soft tissue may stimulate cellular and biochemical groups through a process known as photo-biomodulation; a number of clinical conditions affecting the teeth and jaws may be amenable to low-level laser therapy.
- LLLT when applied to mineral hard tissue (enamel and dentine) will cause a natural fluorescence that can be employed in caries detection.
- LLLT when applied to a chosen chemical mediator can result in the production of singlet oxygen that is cyto-toxic to bacterial strains. This may be employed in periodontal, endodontic and restorative procedures to destroy pathogens.
- Other uses of low level lasers in dentistry include composite curing and scanning of tooth preparations in restorative dentistry.
- Photo-biomodulation may be difficult to quantify in terms of dosage and patient treatment. Few double-blind studies have been carried out and anecdotal reports of success abound.

A number of applications of low-level laser light have emerged, which utilise either the specific wavelength/ chromophore relationship or the inherent accuracy of a collimated beam.

Low-Level Laser Therapy (Photobiostimulation)

This involves the use of visible red and near-infrared light with tissue in order to stimulate and improve healing, as well as reduce pain. The incident wavelength determines the effect – visible light is transmitted through the superficial cellular layers. Light waves in the near-infrared range potentially penetrate several millimetres and these wavelengths are used to stimulate deep cellular function. Light energy is absorbed within living tissue by cellular photoreceptors, e.g., cytochromophores. The incident electromagnetic energy is converted by cellular mitochondria into ATP (adenosine triphosphate).[1] Consequently, the stimulated increase in ATP production would suggest an increased cellular activity in e.g., fibroblasts involved in tissue healing.[2] In addition, the conversion of some of the incident energy into heat would suggest an increase in local micro-circulation through vasodilation.

The stimulatory effects of LLLT include the following[3–6]:

- Proliferation of macrophages
- Proliferation of lymphocytes
- Proliferation of fibroblasts
- Proliferation of endothelial cells
- Proliferation of keratinocytes
- Increased cell respiration/ATP synthesis
- Release of growth factors and other cytokines
- Transformation of fibroblasts into myofibroblasts
- Collagen synthesis

In addition, there is evidence to support the analgesic effects of LLLT, through an enhanced synthesis of endorphins and bradykinins, decreased c-fibre activity and an altered pain threshold. Therapeutic analgesic effects may also occur, through the release of serotonin and acetylcholine centrally and histamine and prostaglandins peripherally.[7,8]

Reported effects of LLLT photo-biomodulation in clinical dentistry include the following[9–14]:

- Dentine hypersensitivity
- Post-extraction socket/post-trauma sites
- Viral infections: herpes labialis, herpes simplex
- Neuropathy: trigeminal neuralgia, paraesthesia
- Aphthous ulceration
- TMJDS
- Post-oncology: mucositis, dermatitis, post-surgery healing

Composite Resin Curing

One of the major emission wavelengths of argon lasers is the 488 nm 'blue'. This wavelength coincides with the absorption peak of camphoroquinone, a photo-initiator used in composite resin restorative materials. The early work carried out on the effectiveness of a high density prime wavelength light source suggested that the depth of curing and hardness of the set composite offered advantages over contemporary light curing systems.[15-17] The intensity of the incident laser beam, using low power levels (150–300 mW) offered a light source that would enhance desired restorative properties without excessive pulpal temperature rise. Unfortunately, the duality of emission wavelengths of the argon active medium required selective filtering of the longer, 514 nm 'green' (soft tissue ablative) wavelength, together with the limitation of the hardware required to restrict emission light energy. Consequently, argon laser curing units were expensive and rendered suitable only for composite curing and some laser whitening uses. In addition, the simultaneous development of more powerful curing systems (e.g., plasma-arc curing lights) offered similar results without the cost and peripheral safety requirements of the laser unit.

Caries Detection

The use of fluorescence in caries detection was first suggested more than a century ago, but received greater significance with introduction of laser technology into dentistry. In the 1980s, a clinically applicable visual detection method, focussing on the natural green fluorescence of tooth tissue was developed.[18,19] The technique used a 488 nm excitation wavelength from an argon-ion laser to discriminate bright green fluorescing of healthy tooth tissue from poorly fluorescing carious lesions. The technique was developed further in the early 1990s into what is now known as quantitative light-induced fluorescence (QLF), where the digitisation of fluorescence images is used to quantify the measure of mineral loss.[20]

Around that time, a red fluorescence method emerged. The red fluorescence, excited either using long UV (350–410 nm) or red (550–670 nm) wavelengths, was observed in advanced caries as well as plaque and calculus on teeth. As opposed to the green fluorescence loss observed in caries, a substantial red fluorescence occurs between 650 and 800 nm in caries lesions and this is much brighter than that found with sound enamel or dentine.[21,22] The first commercially available unit using a red laser was manufactured by Kavo (Kavo GmbH) in 1998, with an emission wavelength of 655 nm.

The unit, which offers a reproducible analogue scoring of site examination, allows a degree of objective assay of those suspect areas of caries that are subject to on-going review as to treatment. Primarily, the use of this modality has been to detect occlusal or flat surface defects, although some interstitial caries can be recorded. The effectiveness of this system is deemed to be best incorporated as an adjunct to other diagnostic methods (tactile, visual, radiographic), to limit the possibility of 'false positive' results.

Other quantitative light-induced fluorescence units have been developed as a highly sensitive method for determining short-term changes in lesions in the mouth.[23] In one, the control unit consists of an illumination device and imaging electronics.

The argon ion laser was replaced in 1995 by a xenon based arc-lamp and the light from this lamp is filtered by a blue-transmitting filter. A light-guide transports the blue light to the teeth in the mouth and a dental mirror provides uniform illumination of the area to be recorded. The excitation wavelength around 405 nm produced by the system allows visualisation and quantification of both the dental tissues' intrinsic green fluorescence as well as the red fluorescence from bacterial origin as observed in calculus, plaque and (advanced) caries. The green fluorescence loss observed from demineralised enamel as well as natural carious lesions is strongly correlated with mineral loss. The red fluorescence offers insight into oral hygiene levels, allows visualisation of leaking margins of sealants and restorations and is furthermore suggested for use during caries excavation.[24-28]

Current research in the USA centres on the use of polarisation-sensitive optical coherence tomography (PS-OCT). Preliminary studies have proved successful at imaging hard and soft tissue in the oral cavity and a numerical analysis of the optical properties of the surface and subsurface enamel can be obtained. At research levels, using a near infrared beam (λ 1,310 nm), caries detection is possible at both surface level and under composite restorations and sealants.[29,30]

Photo-Activated Disinfection (PAD)

The concept of light-activated drug-therapy is well-established in medicine in the form of photo-dynamic therapy. Photo-activated disinfection is a development over and above the conventional use of chemicals to achieve bacterial decontamination in restorative dentistry. As opposed to chemicals that are spontaneously interactive with cellular structures, PAD employs a photo-activated liquid, a solution of tolonium chloride. Exposure of this chemical to low-level visible red light (635 nm) releases singlet oxygen that ruptures bacterial cell walls.[31] Investigations in the early 1990s, notably by Wilson and Pearson at the Eastman Dental Institute, London, determined the susceptibility to PAD of *Streptococcus mutans* when the organism was present in a collagen matrix – an environment similar to that which would exist within a carious tooth.[32] If bacterial contamination of the prepared cavity could be rendered sterile, the hypothesis suggested that the potential for recurrent caries might be significantly reduced. The concept has also been expanded to consider a more-interceptive treatment of demineralised, but otherwise intact enamel surfaces, where bacterial elimination and fluoride therapy might prevent development of a more significant carious cavity.[33] Recent *in vitro* and *in vivo* studies into the use of PAD in endodontics[34,35] have demonstrated the effectiveness of this therapy against a number of anaerobic bacterial strains associated with endodontic infections (*Fusobacterium nucleatum*, *Peptostreptococcus micros*, *Prevotella intermedia* and *Streptococcus intermedius*). In addition, PAD has been shown to be effective against *Enterococcus faecalis*.[36] This research has ultimately led to the production of a commercial unit for use in dental surgery.

Laser-Assisted Tooth Whitening

Differing treatment modalities have been developed to address the phenomenal growth in demand for tooth whitening. Originally, the Argon 488 nm laser wavelength was marketed to provide intense photonic energy to assist the action of hydrogen peroxide on stained enamel and dentine, but the cost of the unit together with the safety requirements led to its decline in use.[37] Other techniques emerged, ranging from the use of LED and plasma-arc lights to home-use kits, using a pre-formed custom tray system.

The present resurgence in laser-assisted tooth whitening has been the development of a diode-based KTP (Potassium Titanyl Phosphate) 532 nm laser. This laser interacts with bleaching gel containing carbamide peroxide in a photo-activated way, as opposed to the longer (Diode 810 nm, CO_2 10,600 nm) wavelengths, which act in a photothermal way to provide heat to the gel and consequently accelerate the chemical reaction.[38]

Home-based methods use gels with either carbamide peroxide or hydrogen peroxide as the active ingredients. These gels are typically acidic preparations with hygroscopic properties. Thus, tooth sensitivity and rebound of color change often occur due to remineralisation and rehydration when using this technique.[39]

With the KTP laser technique a red gel, containing Rhodamine B and hydrogen peroxide is applied to the tooth and exposed to the laser energy. The Rhodamine B molecule has its maximal absorption at 539 nm. When this dye is exposed to 532 nm light, it absorbs photons of energy with subsequent electron transition to the singlet excited state.

The molecule may then undergo reactions with molecular oxygen, resulting in the production of hydroxyl radicals, superoxide ions, peroxides, labile singlet oxygen, or reactive oxygen species. In this way, the interaction between the KTP laser energy and the dye is a photochemical process.[39]

A portion of the KTP laser energy aborbed into the Rhodamine B dye is also transferred from the excited molecule into the bleaching gel in the form of thermal energy. This transfer results in controlled heating of the gel and not the tooth, minimising the possibility of thermal damage to the pulp. This superficial heating of the gel accelerates the breakdown of hydrogen peroxide, which furter boosts the overall yield of perhydroxyl radicals over a given time.[39]

Apart from extrinsic staining due to lifestyle factors, a common source of intrinsic staining is due to the administration of tetracycline antibiotics during tooth formation. Such staining has been shown to be resistant to chemical bleaching agents that produce oxidising radicals, whereas the tetracycline molecule can be photo-oxidised with the 532 nm laser.[40]

Other Low-Level Laser Uses in Dentistry

The development of laser-based measuring devices (e.g., the confocal micrometer), utilising beam-splitting of a low-energy laser and an optical detector, has enabled accurate replication of the morphology of dental and oral structures and materials used in restorative dentistry. The earliest use of laser scanning was in the field of orthodontics and facial development to provide 3D imaging and recording of pre- and post-treatment of deformities.[41–43] Scanned data was linked to computer software using CAD (computer-assisted design). This concept has been expanded during the last decade, to enable the scanning of restorative cavities prior to the production of cast or milled indirect restorations and the recording of oral and facial swellings.[44,45]

The development of laser Doppler flowmetry into applications in dentistry has allowed detailed analysis of pulpal and gingival blood flow, to assist in treatment planning.[46–48]

An additional associated use of laser light in oral medicine is through Raman spectroscopy. A Raman spectrum represents the scattering of incident laser light by molecular or crystal vibrations. Such vibration is quite sensitive to the molecular composition of samples being investigated, and areas of research include the *in vitro* and *in vivo* study of disease processes such as cancer, atherosclerosis and bone disease. With regard to the latter, Raman spectroscopic analysis *in vivo* of mineral and matrix changes has been shown to be useful in mapping early changes in bone tissue.[49]

Laser/Light Application in Dental Procedures

Techniques

- Low-level laser therapy (photobiostimulation)
- Composite resin curing
- Caries detection
- Photo-activated disinfection (PAD)
- Laser-assisted tooth whitening

General Pre-operative Management

Low level lasers are classified as lower than surgical lasers, spanning groups II through IIIB depending on their output and MPE values. Correspondingly, general pre-operative measures to safeguard the patient and staff may not be as rigorous as with Class IV lasers. For all Class IIIM and IIIB lasers, which include photo-biomodulation units, composite curing, tooth whitening and photo-activated disinfection laser units, the following should be followed:

- Secure operating room, define controlled area and place proper laser warning signs.
- Set up laser and test proper laser operation.
- Supplies dispensed, equipment and sterile instruments arranged.
- Patients information: review charting, x-rays, etc.,
- Patients seated: review treatment plan and informed consent.
- Safety: eye protection placed, patient first followed by operating personnel.

Operating Techniques

With photo-biomodulation treatment, the dosimetry of low-level laser light is crucial to the infra-surgical effects of the wavelengths used. In clinical practice, low-level laser therapy delivers fluence of 2–10 J/cm^2, depending on the target tissue[50] as follows: oral epithelium and gingival tissue – 2–3 J/cm^2, trans-osseous irradiation 2–4 J/cm^2 and extra-oral muscle groups/TMJ 6–10 J/cm^2. Most LLLT units are hand-held devices or use a pod that can be charged prior to use. The affected area is selected and the laser energy applied either directly or occasionally at a remote location, according to the clinical guide manual. It is common practice to carry out treatment during a number of sessions, depending on reported improvements in the presenting symptoms (Fig. 38).

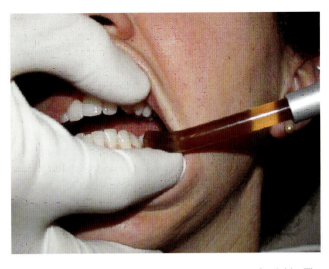

Fig. 38 Low-level laser probe in use in the treatment of pulpitis. The laser device is hand-held

Caries detection should be complementary to conventional visual, tactile and radiographic examination of individual tooth sites. The advantage of these units is the analogue score which can be used as an objective benchmark in monitoring suspect areas of decalcification or caries.[51] It is important that a strict protocol is followed whereby the unit is calibrated where possible, prior to each use, the tooth site is cleaned of debris, otherwise possible false-positive readings may not be excluded.[52] At this time, only those lesions not associated with existing restorations should be scanned and it is essential that the incident laser beam is perpendicular to the lesion (Fig. 39).

PAD techniques have been determined by the manufacturer and involve the placement of a freshly mixed solution of tolonium chloride into the treatment site (tooth cavity,

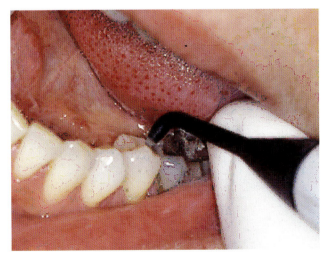

Fig. 39 Use of the DiagnDent (Kavo, Germany). The tip is applied to the tooth surface and findings recorded using the analogue score

periodontal pocket or root canal). The object of the procedure is to destroy pathogens and it is necessary to carry out all preparatory treatment and to isolate the area from oral fluids. The solution is exposed to the laser probe and the visible red light allows easy visualisation. Exposure time is approximately 1 min, after which the solution is washed with distilled water, the area dried where possible and the restoration placed in a conventional manner. With restorative and endodontic treatment, the desired procedure is completed, which will seal the area, but with periodontal PAD techniques, it may be necessary to repeat the treatment at 2–3 month intervals, according to the needs of the periodontal disease.

With laser-assisted tooth whitening it is essential to protect the gingival tissues in order that the peroxide gel does not cause a chemical burn. The teeth are polished, an initial shade taken and isolated from saliva. A protective light-activated silicone paste is applied to the gingival margins, after which the peroxide gel is freshly mixed and applied to the teeth to be whitened.

Power levels for the KTP laser are usefully determined through pre-sets on the laser control panel and are approximately 1 W with the tooth site exposed for a period of 30 s. This process can be repeated three to four times. After this any remaining gel is washed off and the silicone barrier is removed (Figs. 40 and 41).

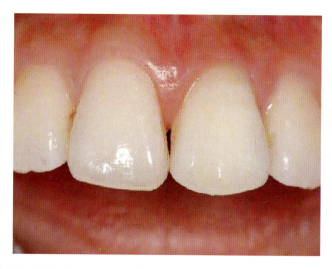

Fig. 41 Tooth appearance after laser tooth whitening

- PAD should be used in accordance with the manufacturers recommendation and current treatment protocols. The possibility of bacterial re-colonisation of treatment sites must be borne in mind
- Care must be exercised in laser-assisted tooth whitening to protect soft tissues, apply the correct bleaching gel and only use laser parameters recommended for the procedure

Adverse Events

- Laser use in Low level photo-biostimulation, composite curing and caries detection have no side effects, provided its use is evidence-based and correct laser parameters are employed

Future Directions

- The use of low level lasers in diagnostics has spanned the past 10 years and developments will continue to make this an integral instrument in everyday dental examinations.
- One major laser manufacturer already has incorporated the 655 nm DiagnoDent technology as a co-axial beam to the Erbium YAG laser. This allows even greater precision in the selective ablation of dental caries.
- More structured research into the use of LLLT in dentistry and oral surgery will continue. At least this will be in response to the growing use of these instruments worldwide.
- The observed "LLLT effect" that is thought to occur along the thermal gradient during surgical ablation of soft tissue will be the subject of further research.
- The development of a diode-based KTP laser capable of both tooth whitening and supra-ablative soft tissue surgery may allow this unit to become more attractive to the general dentist.

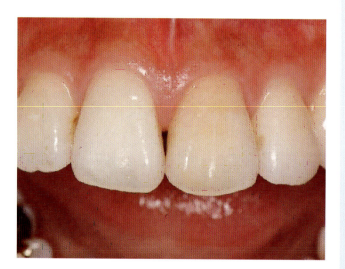

Fig. 40 Non-vital *upper left* central incisor prior to bleaching

Conclusion

The use of lasers in dentistry has witnessed phenomenal growth during the past 15 years, having previously been viewed with some scepticism by a majority of dental professionals . Certainly, the introduction of lasers into this clinical speciality lagged behind similar introduction in many other areas of medicine, but this was due in part to the predominance of long-standing clinical dogma of clinical techniques, the size and power of early lasers and the reluctance of individual clinicians to pay the large expense involved.

The first "dental" laser was an off-shoot of an existing ophthalmic laser and the promotion of this laser in 1989 implied an application in treating dental caries that was shown through experience to be over-optimistic and misleading. The original Nd:YAG has been showed to be an excellent soft tissue laser, but it's worth to the general dentist in the early 1990s was small. The 810 nm Diode, introduced in 1992 demonstrated excellent soft tissue capabilities in an affordable unit – a concept that has recently resulted in a flood of similar machines into the dental market.

The real expansion in laser use began with an acknowledgement of the need for a hard tissue laser and a marketing strategy that recognised the ability of the dentist to afford these machines. The Erbium YAG laser was introduced in 1995 and with the similar Erbium Chromium YSGG, went a long way to meeting the demand for an alternative to the rotary drill.

Dental care maintains a "high street" image in the eyes of the patient; ideally, painless and non-intrusive on-going maintenance of natural teeth and gums is provided in an aesthetically-pleasing way to the ambulatory and conscious patient, affording them little if any disturbance to their daily lives. Any instrumentation that helps maintain this role will have a positive appeal to the patient. In addition, the current shift in treatment provision to a patient-centred approach, demands of the clinician a greater emphasis on matching the patient's expectation. Correspondingly, laser use has increased among those dentists who seek to market their practice.

There is an often cynical reflection in the dental profession that, due to the close association between the delivery of restorative care and the perception of the patient, the "commercialisation" of dentistry has led to a "quick-fix" mentality, intrinsically linked to a pain-free experience in order to seek greater patient approval. Laser technology, although several decades old continues to conjure irrational perceptions of being able to surpass unpleasant aspects of dentistry and this extends to patients and dentists alike. The understanding of basic elements of laser-tissue interaction can help to dispel such assumptions, but also account for the ways in which such instruments can be beneficial in the delivery of dental care.

Research into laser – tissue interaction in the mouth has defined an evidence-base that allows predictable clinical outcomes and has led to objective investigation of the use of laser energy in all areas of clinical dentistry. As most of this research has been carried out in universities and centres of influence, the concept of lasers complementing conventional clinical techniques is beginning to enter undergraduate teaching.

Laser manufacturers have reacted to the growth in potential of lasers in dentistry by developing a wide range of wavelengths that have useful applications in everyday practice. Laser delivery hand-pieces now provide comfort for the clinician and allow access to difficult areas of the mouth. Above all, recognition of the particular needs of the dental professional will now lead to bespoke dental lasers that will enhance and maintain the progress that has occurred during the past two decades.

References

Background

1. Maiman TH. Stimulated optical radiation in ruby. *Nature*. 1960; 187:493-494.
2. Myers TD, Myers WD, Stone RM. First soft tissue study utilising a pulsed Nd:YAG dental laser. *Northwest Dent*. 1989;68:14-17.
3. Hibst R, Keller U. Experimental studies of the application of the Er:YAG laser on dental hard substances: 1. Measurement of ablation rate. *Lasers Surg Med*. 1989;9:338-344.
4. Moshonov J, Stabholz A, Leopold Y, Rosenberg I, Stabholz A. Lasers in dentistry. Part B – interaction with biological tissues and the effect on the soft tissues of the oral cavity, the hard tissues of the tooth and the dental pulp. *Refuat Hapeh Vehashinayim*. 2001;18: 21-28, 107-108.

Use of Lasers with Oral Soft Tissue

1. Bayat A, Arscott G, Ollier WE, McGrouther DA, Ferguson MW. Keloid disease: clinical relevance of single versus multiple site scars. *Br J Plast Surg*. 2005;58:28-37.
2. Funato N, Moriyama K, Baba Y, Kuroda T. Evidence for apoptosis induction in myofibroblasts during palatal mucoperiosteal repair. *J Dent Res*. 1999;78:1511-1517.
3. Kaminer R, Liebow C, Margarone JE 3rd, Zambon JJ. Bacteremia following laser and conventional surgery in hamsters. *J Oral Maxillofac Surg*. 1990;48:45-48.
4. Nanami T, Shiba H, Ikeuchi S, Nagai T, Asanami S, Shibata T. Clinical applications and basic studies of laser in dentistry and oral surgery. *Keio J Med*. 1993;42:199-201.
5. Fisher SE, Frame JW, Browne RM, Tranter RM. A comparative histological study of wound healing following CO_2 laser and conventional surgical excision of canine buccal mucosa. *Arch Oral Biol*. 1983;28:287-291.
6. Spencer P, Cobb CM, Wieliczka DM, Glaros AG, Morris PJ. Change in temperature of subjacent bone during soft tissue laser ablation. *J Periodontol*. 1998;69:1278-1282.
7. Pogrel MA, McCracken KJ, Daniels TE. Histologic evaluation of the width of soft tissue necrosis adjacent to carbon dioxide laser incisions. *Oral Surg Oral Med Oral Pathol*. 1990;70:564-568.

8. Spencer P, Cobb CM, Wieliczka DM, Glaros AG, Morris PJ. Change in temperature of subjacent bone during soft tissue laser ablation. *J Periodontol.* 1998;69:1278-1282.

9. Hall RR. The healing of tissues incised by a carbon dioxide laser. *Br J Surg.* 1971;58:222-225.

10. Wyman A, Duffy S, Sweetland HM, Sharp F, Rogers K. Preliminary evaluation of a new high power diode laser. *Lasers Surg Med.* 1992;12:506-509.

11. Hall RR, Hill DW, Beach AD. A carbon dioxide surgical laser. *Ann R Coll Surg Engl.* 1971;48:181-188.

12. Esen E, Haytac MC, Oz IA, Erdogan O, Karsli ED. Gingival melanin pigmentation and its treatment with the CO_2 laser. *Oral Surg Oral Med Oral Pathol Oral Radiol Endod.* 2004;98:522-527.

13. Tal H, Oegiesser D, Tal M. Gingival depigmentation by erbium:YAG laser: clinical observations and patient responses. *J Periodontol.* 2003;74:1660-1667.

14. Yousuf A, Hossain M, Nakamura Y, Yamada Y, Kinoshita J, Matsumoto K. Removal of gingival melanin pigmentation with the semiconductor diode laser: a case report. *J Clin Laser Med Surg.* 2000;18:263-266.

15. Lanning SK, Waldrop TC, Gunsolley JC, Maynard JG. Surgical crown lengthening: evaluation of the biological width. *J Periodontol.* 2003;74:468-474.

16. Gracis S, Fradeani M, Celletti R, Bracchetti G. Biological integration of aesthetic restorations: factors influencing appearance and long-term success. *Periodontol 2000.* 2001;27:29-44.

17. Adams TC, Pang PK. Lasers in aesthetic dentistry. *Dent Clin North Am.* 2004;48:833-860. vi.

Use of Lasers with Oral Hard Tissue

1. Bassi G, Chawla S, Patel M. The Nd:YAG laser in caries removal. *Br Dent J.* 1994;177:248-250.

2. Harris DM, White JM, Goodis H, et al. Selective ablation of surface enamel caries with a pulsed Nd:YAG dental laser. *Lasers Surg Med.* 2002;30:342-350.

3. Cox CJ, Pearson GJ, Palmer G. Preliminary in vitro investigation of the effects of pulsed Nd:YAG laser radiation on enamel and dentine. *Biomaterials.* 1994;15:1145-1151.

4. Yamada MK, Watari F. Imaging and non-contact profile analysis of Nd:YAG laser- irradiated teeth by scanning electron microscopy and confocal laser scanning microscopy. *Dent Mater J.* 2003;22:556-568.

5. Srimaneepong V, Palamara JE, Wilson PR. Pulpal space pressure and temperature changes from Nd:YAG laser irradiation of dentin. *J Dent.* 2002;30:291-296.

6. Lan WH, Chen KW, Jeng JH, Lin CP, Lin SK. A comparison of the morphological changes after Nd-YAG and CO_2 laser irradiation of dentin surfaces. *J Endod.* 2000;26:450-453.

7. Takamori K, Furukawa H, Morikawa Y, Katayama T, Watanabe S. Basic study on vibrations during tooth preparations caused by high-speed drilling and Er:YAG laser irradiation. *Lasers Surg Med.* 2003;32:25-31.

8. Glockner K, Rumpler J, Ebeleseder K, Stadtler P. Intrapulpal temperature during preparation with the Er:YAG laser compared to the conventional burr: an in vitro study. *J Clin Laser Med Surg.* 1998;16:153-157.

9. Pelagalli J, Gimbel CB, Hansen RT, Swett A, Winn DW 2nd. Investigational study of the use of Er:YAG laser versus dental drill for caries removal and cavity preparation – phase I. *J Clin Laser Med Surg.* 1997;15:109-115.

10. Belikov AV, Erofeev AV, Shumilin VV, Tkachuk AM. Comparative study of the 3um laser action on different hard tissue samples using free running pulsed Er-doped YAG, YSGG, YAP and YLF lasers. *Proc SPIE.* 1993;2080:60-67.

11. Mercer C, Anderson P, Davis G. Sequential 3D X-ray microtomographic measurement of enamel and dentine ablation by an Er:YAG laser. *Br Dent J.* 2003;194:99-104.

12. Hibst R, Keller U. Mechanism of Er:YAG laser-induced ablation of dental hard substances. *Proc SPIE.* 1993;1880:156-162.

13. Corona SA, de Souza AE, Chinelatti MA, Borsatto MC, Pécora JD, Palma-Dibb RG. Effect of energy and pulse repetition rate of Er:YAG laser on dentin ablation ability and morphological analysis of the laser-irradiated substrate. *Photomed Laser Surg.* 2007;25(1):26-33.

14. Hibst R. Mechanical effects of erbium:YAG laser bone ablation. *Lasers Surg Med.* 1992;12:125-130.

15. Thomsen S. Pathologic analysis of photothermal and photomechanical effects of laser-tissue interactions. *Photochem Photobiol.* 1991;53:825-835.

16. Fried NM, Fried D. Comparison of Er:YAG and 9.6-microm TEA CO_2 lasers for ablation of skull tissue. *Lasers Surg Med.* 2001;28:335-343.

17. Sasaki KM, Aoki A, Ichinose S, Ishikawa I. Ultrastructural analysis of bone tissue irradiated by Er:YAG laser. *Lasers Surg Med.* 2002;31:322-332.

18. Wang X, Zhang C, Matsumoto K. In vivo study of the healing processes that occur in the jaws of rabbits following perforation by an Er,Cr:YSGG laser. *Lasers Med Sci.* 2005;20:21-27.

19. Walsh JT Jr, Deutsch TF. Er:YAG laser ablation of tissue: measurement of ablation rates. *Lasers Surg Med.* 1989;9:327-337.

20. Chinelatti MA, Ramos RP, Chimello DT, Borsatto MC, Pecora JD, Palma-Dibb RG. Influence of the use of Er:YAG laser for cavity preparation and surface treatment in microleakage of resin-modified glass ionomer restorations. *Oper Dent.* 2004;29:430-436.

21. Corona SA, Borsatto MC, Pecora JD, De SA Rocha RA, Ramos TS, Palma-Dibb RG. Assessing microleakage of different class V restorations after Er:YAG laser and bur preparation. *J Oral Rehabil.* 2003;30:1008-1014.

22. Niu W, Eto JN, Kimura Y, Takeda FH, Matsumoto K. A study on microleakage after resin filling of class V cavities prepared by Er:YAG laser. *J Clin Laser Med Surg.* 1998;16:227-231.

23. Gutknecht N, Apel C, Schafer C, Lampert F. Microleakage of composite fillings in Er,Cr:YSGG laser-prepared class II cavities. *Lasers Surg Med.* 2001;28:371-374.

Use of Lasers in Anti-Bacterial Techniques Adjunctive to Dental Surgery: Laser Use in Periodontology, Endodontics, Implantology

1. Rossmann JA, Cobb CM. Lasers in periodontal therapy. *Periodontol 2000.* 1995;9:150-164.

2. Israel M, Rossmann JA, Froum SJ. Use of the carbon dioxide laser in retarding epithelial migration: a pilot histological human study utilizing case reports. *J Periodontol.* 1995;66:197-204.

3. Williams TM, Cobb CM, Rapley JW, Killoy WJ. Histologic evaluation of alveolar bone following CO_2 laser removal of connective tissue from periodontal defects. *Int J Periodontics Restor Dent.* 1995;15:497-506.

4. Wilder-Smith P, Arrastia AA, Schell MJ, Liaw LH, Grill G, Berns MW. Effect of Nd:YAG laser irradiation and root planing on the root surface: structural and thermal effects. *J Periodontol.* 1995;66:1032-1039.

5. Rizoiu IM, Eversole LR, Kimmel AI. Effects of an erbium, chromium:yttrium, scandium, gallium garnet laser on mucocutane-

ous soft tissues. *Oral Surg Oral Med Oral Pathol*. 1996;82:386-395.

6. Yukna RA, Evans G, Vastardis S, Carr RL. Human periodontal regeneration following laser assisted new attachment procedure. Paper presented at: IADR/AADR/CADR 82nd General Session; March 10–13, 2004; Honolulu.

7. Harris DM, Yessik M. Nd:YAG better than diode. *Lasers Surg Med*. 2004;35:206-213.

8. Grassi RF, Pappalardo S, Frateiacci A, et al. Antibacterial effect of Nd:YAG laser in periodontal pockets decontamination: an in vivo study [article in Italian]. *Minerva Stomatol*. 2004;53:355-359.

9. Moritz A, Schoop U, Goharkhay K, et al. Treatment of periodontal pockets with a diode laser. *Lasers Surg Med*. 1998;22:302-311.

10. Coffelt DW, Cobb CM, MacNeill S, Rapley JW, Killoy WJ. Determination of energy density threshold for laser ablation of bacteria. An in vitro study. *J Clin Periodontol*. 1997;24:1-7.

11. Folwaczny M, Mehl A, Haffner C, Benz C, Hickel R. Root substance removal with Er:YAG laser radiation at different parameters using a new delivery system. *J Periodontol*. 2000;71:147-155.

12. Frentzen M, Braun A, Aniol D. Er:YAG laser scaling of diseased root surfaces. *J Periodontol*. 2002;73:524-530.

13. Eberhard J, Ehlers H, Falk W, Acil Y, Albers HK, Jepsen S. Efficacy of subgingival calculus removal with Er:YAG laser compared to mechanical debridement: an in situ study. *J Clin Periodontol*. 2003;30:511-518.

14. Aoki A, Ando Y, Watanabe H, Ishikawa I. In vitro studies on laser scaling of subgingival calculus with an erbium:YAG laser. *J Periodontol*. 1994;65:1097-1106.

15. Siqueira Junior JF. Strategies to treat infected root canals. *J Calif Dent Assoc*. 2001;29:825-837.

16. Piccolomini R, D'Arcangelo C, D'Ercole S, Catamo G, Schiaffino G, De Fazio P. Bacteriologic evaluation of the effect of Nd:YAG laser irradiation in experimental infected root canals. *J Endod*. 2002;28:276-278.

17. Rooney J, Midda M, Leeming J. A laboratory investigation of the bactericidal effect of a Nd:YAG laser. *Br Dent J*. 1994;176:61-64.

18. Fegan S, Steiman H. Comparative evaluation of the antibacterial effects of intracanal Nd:YAG laser irradiation: an in vitro study. *J Endod*. 1995;21:415-417.

19. Moritz A, Gutknecht N, Gohrakhay K, Schoop U, Wernisch J, Sperr W. In vitro irradiation of infected root canals with a diode laser: results of microbiologic, infrared spectrometric, and stain penetration examinations. *Quintessence Int*. 1997;28:205-209.

20. Le Goff A, Dautel-Morazin A, Guigand M, Vulcain JM, Bonnaure-Mallet M. An evaluation of the CO_2 laser for endodontic disinfection. *J Endod*. 1999;25:105-108.

21. McKinley I, Ludlow M. Hazards of laser smoke during endodontic therapy. *J Endod*. 1994;20:558-559.

22. Hardee M, Miserendino L, Kos W, Walia H. Evaluation of the antibacterial effects of intracanal Nd:YAG laser irradiation. *J Endod*. 1994;20:377-380.

23. Schoop U, Kluger W, Moritz A, Nedjelik N, Georgopoulos A, Sperr W. Bactericidal effect of different laser systems in the deep layers of dentin. *Lasers Surg Med*. 2004;35:111-116.

24. Jha D, Guerrero A, Ngo T, Helfer A, Hasselgren G. Inability of laser and rotary instrumentation to eliminate root canal infection. *J Am Dent Assoc*. 2006;137:67-70.

25. Mombelli A. Etiology, diagnosis, and treatment considerations in peri-implantitis. *Curr Opin Periodontol*. 1997;4:127-136.

26. Leonhardt A, Renvert S, Dahlen G. Microbial findings at failing implants. *Clin Oral Implants Res*. 1999;10:339-345.

27. Martins MC, Abi-Rached RS, Shibli JA, Araujo MW, Marcantonio E Jr. Experimental peri-implant tissue breakdown around different dental implant surfaces: clinical and radiographic evaluation in dogs. *Int J Oral Maxillofac Implants*. 2004;19:839-848.

28. Shibli JA, Martins MC, Lotufo RF, Marcantonio E Jr. Microbiologic and radiographic analysis of ligature induced peri-implantitis with different dental implant surfaces. *Int J Oral Maxillofac Implants*. 2003;18:383-390.

29. Kourtis SG, Sotiriadou S, Voliotis S, Challas A. Private practice results of dental implants. Part I: survival and evaluation of risk factors – Part II: surgical and prosthetic complications. *Implant Dent*. 2004;13:373-385.

30. Oh TJ, Yoon J, Misch CE, Wang HL. The causes of early implant bone loss: myth or science? *J Periodontol*. 2002;73:322-333.

31. Augthun M, Tinschert J, Huber A. In vitro studies on the effect of cleaning methods on different implant surfaces. *J Periodontol*. 1998;69:857-864.

32. Buchter A, Meyer U, Kruse-Losler B, Joos U, Kleinheinz J. Sustained release of doxycycline for the treatment of peri-implantitis: randomised controlled trial. *Br J Oral Maxillofac Surg*. 2004;42:439-444.

33. Klinge B, Gustafsson A, Berglundh T. A systematic review of the effect of anti-infective therapy in the treatment of peri-implantitis. *J Clin Periodontol*. 2002;29(Suppl 3):213-225.

34. Tang Z, Cao C, Sha Y, Lin Y, Wang X. Effects of non-surgical treatment modalities on peri-implantitis. *Zhonghua Kou Qiang Yi Xue Za Zhi*. 2002;37:173-175.

35. Bunetel L, Guerin J, Agnani G, et al. In vitro study of the effect of titanium on *Porphyromonas gingivalis* in the presence of metronidazole and spiramycin. *Biomaterials*. 2001;22:3067-3072.

36. Haas R, Dörtbudak O, Mensdorff-Pouilly N, Mailath G. Elimination of bacteria on different implant surfaces through photosensitization and soft laser. *Clin Oral Implants Res*. 1997;8:249-254.

37. Kato T, Kusakari H, Hoshino E. Bactericidal efficacy of carbon dioxide laser against bacteria-contaminated implants and subsequent cellular adhesion to irradiated area. *Lasers Surg Med*. 1998;23:299-309.

38. Kreisler M, Kohnen W, Marinello C, et al. Bactericidal effect of the Er:YAG laser on dental implant surfaces: an in vitro study. *J Periodontol*. 2002;73:1292-1298.

39. Miller RJ. Treatment of the contaminated implant surface using the Er,Cr:YSGG laser. *Implant Dent*. 2004;13:165-170.

40. Ichikawa T, Hirota K, Kanitani H, Miyake Y, Matsumoto N. In vitro adherence of *Streptococcus constellatus* to dense hydroxyapatite and titanium. *J Oral Rehabil*. 1998;25:125-127.

Low-Level Laser Use in Dental Surgery

1. Passarella S. Increase of proton electrochemical potential and ATP synthesis in rat liver mitochondria irradiated in vitro by helium-neon laser. *FEBS Lett*. 1984;175:95-99.

2. Karu T. Photobiological fundamentals of low powered laser therapy. *IEEE J Quantum Electron*. 1987;23:1703-1717.

3. Dube A, Bansal H, Gupta PK. Modulation of macrophage structure and function by low level He-Ne laser irradiation. *Photochem Photobiol Sci*. 2003;2:851-855.

4. Stadler I, Evans R, Kolb B, et al. In vitro effects of low-level laser irradiation at 660 nm on peripheral blood lymphocytes. *Lasers Surg Med*. 2000;27:255-261.

5. Kovacs IB, Mester E, Gorog P. Stimulation of wound healing with laser beam in the rat. *Experientia*. 1974;30:1275-1276.

6. Enwemeka CS, Parker JC, Dowdy DS, Harkness EE, Sanford LE, Woodruff LD. The efficacy of low-power lasers in tissue repair and pain control: a meta-analysis study. *Photomed Laser Surg*. 2004;22:323-329.

7. Laakso EL, Cramond T, Richardson C, Galligan JP. Plasma ACTH and β-endorphin levels in response to low level laser therapy for myofascial trigger points. *Laser Ther*. 1994;3:133-142.

8. Montesinos M. Experimental effects of low power laser in encephalon and endorphin synthesis. *J Eur Med Laser Assoc.* 1988;1:2-7.

9. Kimura Y, Wilder-Smith P, Yonaga K, Matsumoto K. Treatment of dentine hypersensitivity by laser: a review. *J Clin Periodontol.* 2000;27:715-721.

10. Taube S, Piironen J, Ylipaavalniemi P. Helium-neon laser therapy in the prevention of post-operative swelling and pain after wisdom tooth extraction. *Proc Finn Dent Soc.* 1990;86:23-27.

11. Schindl A, Neuman R. Low intensity laser therapy is an effective treatment for recurrent herpes simplex infection: results from a randomised double-blind placebo controlled study. *J Invest Dermatol.* 1999;113:221-223.

12. Pinheiro AL, Cavalcanti ET, Pinheiro TI, Alves MJ, Manzi CT. Low-level laser therapy in the management of disorders of the maxillofacial region. *J Clin Laser Med Surg.* 1997;15:181-183.

13. Howell RM, Cohen DM, Powell GL, Green JG. The use of low energy laser therapy to treat aphthous ulcers. *Ann Dent.* 1988;47: 16-18.

14. Wong SF, Wilder-Smith P. Pilot study of laser effects on oral mucositis in patients receiving chemotherapy. *Cancer J.* 2002;8: 247-254.

15. Kelsey WP, Blankenau RJ, Powell GL, Barkmeier WW, Stormberg EF. Power and time requirements for use of the argon laser to polymerize composite resins. *J Clin Laser Med Surg.* 1992;10: 273-278.

16. Powell GL, Blankenau RJ. Effects of argon laser curing on dentin shear bond strengths. *J Clin Laser Med Surg.* 1996;14:111-113.

17. Blankenau RJ, Kelsey WP, Powell GL, Shearer GO, Barkmeier WW, Cavel WT. Degree of composite resin polymerization with visible light and argon laser. *Am J Dent.* 1991;4:40-42.

18. Bjelkhagen H, Sundström F. A clinically applicable laser luminescence method for the early detection of dental caries. *IEEE J Quantum Electron.* 1981;17:266-270.

19. Bjelkhagen H, Sundström F, Angmar-Månsson B, Ryden H. Early detection of enamel caries by the luminescence excited by visible laser light. *Swed Dent J.* 1982;6:1-7.

20. de Josselin de Jong E, Sundström F, Westerling H, Tranaeus S, ten Bosch JJ, Angmar-Månsson B. A new method for in vivo quantification of changes in initial enamel caries with laser fluorescence. *Caries Res.* 1995;29:2-7. doi:de Josselin de Jong E.

21. Hibst R, Gall R. Development of a diode laser-based fluorescence detector. *Caries Res.* 1998;32:294.

22. Lussi A, Megert B, Longbottom C, Reich E, Francescut P. Clinical performance of a laser fluorescence device for detection of occlusal caries lesions. *Eur J Oral Sci.* 2001;109:14-19.

23. Stookey GK. Optical methods – quantitative light fluorescence. *J Dent Res.* 2004;83(Suppl):C84-C88.

24. Heinrich-Weltzien R, Kühnisch J, van der Veen M, de Josselin de Jong E, Stosser L. Quantitative light-induced fluorescence (QLF) – a potential method for the dental practitioner. *Quintessence Int.* 2003;34:181-188.

25. Hafström-Björkman U, Sundström F, de Josselin de Jong E, Oliveby A, Angmar-Månsson B. Comparison of laser fluorescence and longitudinal microradiography for quantitative assessment of in vitro enamel caries. *Caries Res.* 1992;26:241-247.

26. Emami Z, Al-Khateeb S, de Josselin de Jong E, Sundström F, Trollsås K, Angmar-Månsson B. Mineral loss in incipient caries lesions quantified with laser fluorescence and longitudinal microradiography. A methodologic study. *Acta Odontol Scand.* 1996; 54:8-13.

27. Ando M, van Der Veen MH, Schemehorn BR, Stookey GK. Comparative study to quantify demineralized enamel in deciduous and permanent teeth using laser - and light induced fluorescence techniques. *Caries Res.* 2001;35:464-470.

28. Lennon AM, Buchalla W, Switalski L, Stookey GK. Residual caries detection using visible fluorescence. *Caries Res.* 2002;36:315-319.

29. Fried D, Xie J, Shafi S, Featherstone JD, Breunig TM, Le C. Imaging caries lesions and lesion progression with polarization sensitive optical coherence tomography. *J Biomed Opt.* 2002;7: 618-627.

30. Jones RS, Staninec M, Fried D. Imaging artificial caries under composite sealants and restorations. *J Biomed Opt.* 2004;9: 1297-1304.

31. Soukos NS, Wilson M, Burns T, Speight PM. The photodynamic effects of toluidine blue on human oral keratinocytes and fibroblasts and Streptococcus sanguis evaluated in vitro. *Lasers Surg Med.* 1996;18:253-259.

32. Williams JA, Pearson GJ, Colles MJ, Wilson M. The photo-activated antibacterial action of toluidine blue O in a collagen matrix and in carious dentine. *Caries Res.* 2004;38:530-536.

33. Vlacic J, Meyers IA, Walsh LJ. Combined CPP-ACP and photoactivated disinfection (PAD) therapy in arresting root surface caries: a case report. *Br Dent J.* 2007;203(8):457-459.

34. Williams JA, Pearson GJ, John Colles M. Antibacterial action of photoactivated disinfection {PAD} used on endodontic bacteria in planktonic suspension and in artificial and human root canals. *J Dent.* 2006;34:363-371.

35. Bonsor SJ, Nichol R, Reid TM, Pearson GJ. Microbiological evaluation of photo-activated disinfection in endodontics (an in vivo study). *Br Dent J.* 2006;200:337-341.

36. Lee MT, Bird PS, Walsh LJ. Photo-activated disinfection of root canals: a new role for lasers in endodontics. *Aust Endod J.* 2004;30:93-98.

37. Goldstein RE. In-office bleaching: where we came from, where we are today. *J Am Dent Assoc.* 1997;128(Suppl):11S-15S.

38. Zhang C, Wang X, Kinoshita J, et al. Effects of KTP laser irradiation, diode laser, and LED on tooth bleaching: a comparative study. *Photomed Laser Surg.* 2007;25(2):91-95.

39. Walsh LJ, Liu JY, Verheyen P. Tooth discolorations and its treatment using KTP laser-assisted tooth whitening. *J Oral Laser Appl.* 2004;4:7-21.

40. Walsh LJ, Liu JY, Verheyen P. Tooth discolorations and its treatment using KTP laser-assisted tooth whitening. *J Oral Laser Appl.* 2004;4:7-21.

41. McCance AM, Moss JP, Wright WR, Linney AD, James DR. A three-dimensional soft tissue analysis of 16 skeletal class III patients following bimaxillary surgery. *Br J Oral Maxillofac Surg.* 1992;30:221-232.

42. McCance AM, Moss JP, Fright WR, James DR, Linney AD. A three dimensional analysis of soft and hard tissue changes following bimaxillary orthognathic surgery in skeletal III patients. *Br J Oral Maxillofac Surg.* 1992;30:305-312.

43. Commer P, Bourauel C, Maier K, Jager A. Construction and testing of a computer-based intraoral laser scanner for determining tooth positions. *Med Eng Phys.* 2000;22:625-635.

44. Denissen HW, van der Zel JM, van Waas MA. Measurement of the margins of partial-coverage tooth preparations for CAD/CAM. *Int J Prosthodont.* 1999;12:395-400.

45. Harrison JA, Nixon MA, Fright WR, Snape L. Use of hand-held laser scanning in the assessment of facial swelling: a preliminary study. *Br J Oral Maxillofac Surg.* 2004;42:8-17.

46. Kocabalkan E, Turgut M. Variation in blood flow of supporting tissue during use of mandibular complete dentures with hard acrylic resin base and soft relining: a preliminary study. *Int J Prosthodont.* 2005;18(3):210-213.

47. Gleissner C, Kempski O, Peylo S, Glatzel JH, Willershausen B. Local gingival blood flow at healthy and inflamed sites measured by laser Doppler flowmetry. *J Periodontol.* 2006;77(10):1762-1771.

48. Strobl H, Moschen I, Emshoff I, Emshoff R. Effect of luxation type on pulpal blood flow measurements: a long-term follow-up of luxated permanent maxillary incisors. *J Oral Rehabil.* 2005; 32(4):260-265.

49. Tarnowski CP, Ignelzi MA Jr, Wang W, Taboas JM, Goldstein SA, Morris MD. Earliest mineral and matrix changes in force-induced musculoskeletal disease as revealed by Raman microspectroscopic imaging. *J Bone Miner Res*. 2004;19:64-71.

50. Bjordal JM, Couppe C, Ljunggren A. Low level laser therapy for tendinopathies: evidence of a dose-related pattern. *Phys Ther Rev*. 2001;6:91-100.

51. Toraman Alkurt M, Peker I, Deniz Arisu H, Bala O, Altunkaynak B. In vivo comparison of laser fluorescence measurements with conventional methods for occlusal caries detection. *J Dent*. 2007;35(8): 679-682.

52. Silva BB, Severo NB, Maltz M. Validity of diode laser to monitor carious lesions in pits and fissures. *Lasers Med Sci*. 2007;35(8): 679-682.

Laser/Light Applications in Otolaryngology

Vanessa S. Rothholtz and Brian J. F. Wong

Introduction

- History of laser use in Otolaryngology – Head and Neck Surgery
- Laser safety
- Laryngology
- Otology
- Oropharyngeal surgery
- Rhinology
- Pediatric otolaryngology
- Conclusions

History of Laser Use in Otolaryngology

Historically, in otolaryngology, the laser was used like a scalpel or cautery to incise, cauterize, and coagulate tissue in a precise fashion. Contemporary laser use in the head, neck, and upper airway now focus upon treating for a wide range of clinical applications. By selecting the correct laser wavelength and selecting appropriate dosimetry parameters, surgeons can control both the temporal and spatial evolution of heat within the target site, creating different tissue effects depending upon the desired clinical outcome. Light is variably absorbed and scattered as it propagates through tissue, and the distribution of light in tissue determines the nature of the specific interaction.[1] As in dermatology, the selection of the appropriate laser in head and neck applications is critically important. The selection of a specific device and

B.J.F. Wong (✉)
Division of Facial Plastic and Reconstructive Surgery,
Department of Otolaryngology Head and Neck Surgery,
Department of Biomedical Engineering, Department of Surgery
and The Beckman Laser Institute, University of California,
Irvine, CA, USA
e-mail: bjwong@uci.edu

mode of delivery are just as important as wavelength and dosimetry.

The Otolaryngologist – Head and Neck surgeon frequently works in areas that are either difficult to access using classic methods or require extreme precision, and in these circumstances laser technology can be of immense value. For example, during microsurgery of the larynx or ear, a micromanipulator or microscope-mounted scanner, is needed to precise focus and translate a laser beam as small as 100 µm across minute target sites. In surgery of the subglottis and trachea, flexible optical fibers (fiberoptics) or waveguides are used to deliver laser light to these remote locations. In minimally invasive laryngeal cancer operations, high power CO_2 lasers are needed to cut tissue while maintaining hemostasis.

Frequently Used Lasers in Otolaryngology

The workhorse in Otolaryngology – Head and Neck Surgery is the carbon dioxide laser. It is used extensively in surgery of the larynx and ear because it can cut tissue precisely, seal small blood vessels and also ablate bone. In cancer surgery, CO_2 lasers may seal lymphatics, potentially reducing the spread of disease. Since infrared light is invisible, the CO_2 laser is always used with a visible aiming beam. The potassium-titanyl phosphate (Neodymium-doped:Yttrium-Aluminum-Garnet), KTP(Nd:YAG), laser is also used in laryngotracheal surgery as well as surgery of the oropharynx and nose. The KTP(Nd:YAG) laser is most frequently used for vascular lesions because of its absorption by oxyhemoglobin. In the nose, the KTP(Nd:YAG) laser is most frequently used for treatment of hereditary hemorrhage telangiectasias (Osler-Weber-Rendu disease). This is a visible wavelength laser and hence easily transmitted using low-cost optical fibers. It can be made to produce a pulsed output beam, also known as giant pulse laser or Q-switching, that allows for the delivery of nanosecond pulses, which lead to less tissue injury.[2] Nd:YAG lasers are used in otolaryngology as well, however the deep penetration depth of this wavelength has

K. Nouri (ed.), *Lasers in Dermatology and Medicine*,
DOI: 10.1007/978-0-85729-281-0_41, © Springer-Verlag London Limited 2011

resulted in limited use; though in contact mode, this laser has applications as a precise cutting device.[3-6]

The Argon laser is also used for nasal and middle ear surgery. It is absorbed by hemoglobin and melanin and is generally used in continuous-wave mode. The Holmium:YAG (Ho:YAG) laser is a mid-infrared laser wavelength that is moderately absorbed by water, its principal chromophore. It is valuable because it has a relatively shallow optical penetration depth like the carbon dioxide laser, but can be transmitted using low-cost silica fibers. Its use in otolaryngology has been very limited thus far due to the lack of availability of these devices in most medical centers. The Erbium:YAG laser is used for both nasal surgery, in rhinophyma, and cosmetically for skin resurfacing. It has high absorption in bone and minimal thermally-induced peripheral damage. It also has a tolerable photoacoustic wave effect in the surrounding tissue.[7] Pfalz, Fisch and others have developed Erbium:YAG lasers for middle ear surgery, but the high cost of these systems severely limited adoption. There currently is no commercial manufacturer of Erbium:YAG laser systems designed for middle ear surgery (Table 1).

Laser Safety in Otolaryngologic Applications

As in dermatology, laser safety needs to be considered for the patient, surgeon and surgical staff. The use of a laser near the eyes and in the airway warrants the diligent practice of laser safety at all times. Blindness, burns to the skin, airway injury and death may result if precautions are not taken to prevent these devastating events. The safety precautions and measures to prevent eye injury in head and neck surgery are identical to those used in dermatology, with the exception that the laser dosimetry is often significantly more powerful than that used to treat the skin. Eye protection measures are reviewed elsewhere.

The use of lasers in surgery in the airway presents a major challenge that is unique to otolaryngology – head and neck surgery. Flammable anesthetic gases such as nitric oxide and halothane increase the risk of fire and explosion during airway surgery, particularly when using a high laser power in the presence of flammable endotracheal tubes that may serve as an initiator for combustion in an oxygen rich environment.[10] Specialized laser-safe endotracheal tubes (Fig. 1)

Table 1 Laser applications in otolaryngology[8-10]

Laser type	Wave length	Penetration depth	Delivery methods	Indications/applications
Argon	514 nm	0.8 mm	Fiber Micromanipulator Focusing handpiece	Ear – stapes surgery Nose – telangiectasias

CO_2	10,600 nm	30 μm	Articulated arm
			Micro-manipulator hollow
			wave-guide scanner
			Focusing handpiece
				Glottis/subglottis/larynx/
				oropharynx
				  Benign/malignant
				  Therapeutic/diagnostic
				Tonsils
				  Lingual
				Oral cavity/tongue
				  Benign/malignant
				  Therapeutic/diagnostic
				Nose
				  Turbinate hypertrophy

Erbium: YAG	2,940 nm	3 μm	Articulated arm
			sapphire fiber
				Nose
				  Rhinophyma
				Cosmetic
				  Laser resurfacing

Holmium:YAG	2,120 nm	0.4 mm	Fiber/bare fiber contact
			Handpiece
				Nose
				  Sinus surgery
				  Turbinate hypertrophy

KTP (Nd:YAG)	532 nm	0.9 mm	Fiber/bare fiber contact
			Side-fire
			Focusing handpiece
			Diffuser tip
			Micromanipulator
				Nose
				  Polyps
				  Epistaxis
				Oropharynx/palatine tonsils
				  Obstructive sleep apnea
				Vascular malformations
				Nose
				  Telangiectasias
				Trachea
				  Stenosis
				  Subglottic hemangioma

Nd:YAG	1,064 nm	4 mm	Fiber/bare fiber Contact tips	Vascular malformations Tumor removal (contact mode) Turbinate surgery

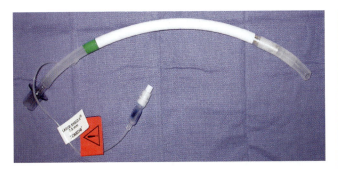

Fig. 1 Laser-specific endotracheal tube wrapped with reflective metallic tape. Laser-Shield II® Endotracheal Tube – Medtronic

exhibit prolonged mean times to ignition in comparison to standard endotracheal tubes. Reflective metallic tape wrapped around the endotracheal tube is shown to reduce the risk of ignition of all tubes.[11,12]

Foth has extensively studied the safety of endotracheal tube use in laser surgery. He evaluated the increase in temperature of both the external and internal aspects of a variety of endotracheal tubes that are commonly used in anesthesia. He found that, in comparison to a metallic tube, the temperatures measured in the compound tube were much lower and that a significant difference was observed between the temperatures inside and outside of the compound tube.[13-16]

Laser Safety Protocol (Adapted from[12])

I. Eye protection
  A. Patient
    1. Tape patient's eyes shut
    2. Double layer of saline-saturated eye pads placed over the patient's eyes
  B. Operating room personnel
    1. Wear appropriate protective glasses with side protectors
    2. Surgeon does not require protective glasses when working with the operating microscope or when endonasal using a Hopkins rod endoscope
  C. Warning signs
    1. Placed outside of all entrances in the operative room where the laser is used
    2. Caution persons entering the room that the laser is in use and that protective glasses are required
  D. Limited access
    1. Limit traffic into the operating room when the laser is in use
    2. Keep doors to the operating room closed when laser is in use

II. Skin protection
  A. Use a double layer of saline-saturated surgical towels, surgical sponges or lap pads to cover all exposed skin and mucous membranes of the patient outside of the surgical field
    1. Keep this protective layer wet during the case
    2. Do not forget to protect the teeth, when exposed
  B. When microlaryngeal surgery is performed, the patient's face and peri-oral area is completely draped with saline-saturated towels
III. Smoke evacuation
  A. Aspirate laser-induced smoke from the operative field
  B. Have two separate suction set-ups available in the operating room
    1. One suction for laser-induced smoke and steam
    2. One suction for blood and mucous
  C. Use filters in the suction lines for laser-induced smoke and steam
IV. Anesthetic considerations
  A. Use of nonflammable general anesthetic
  B. Limit oxygen concentration to maximum of 30% when the laser is in use
    1. Mix oxygen with helium, nitrogen or air – do not use nitrous oxide
    2. Mix oxygen with helium
  C. Use a laser-specific endotracheal tube wrapped with reflective metallic tape (e.g., Rusch red rubber tube - Hudson RCI, Temecula, California; Laser-Shield II® Endotracheal Tube - Medtronic Jacksonville, FL)
  D. Protection of the endotracheal tube cuff
    1. Use saline-saturated cottonoids to protect the endotracheal tube cuff
      (a) Keep the cottonoids moist
      (b) Count the cottonoids
    2. Inflate the cuff with methylene blue colored saline
  E. Instrument selection
    1. Use a wide-bore microlaryngoscope
    2. Choose instruments with a non-reflective surface

Laryngology

Jako and Strong pioneered the use lasers in laryngeal surgery in the 1970s. They were among the first to describe the laser excision of an early laryngeal cancer.[17-19] Lasers gained popularity in the 1980s for removal of benign laryngeal lesions such as recurrent respiratory papillomatosis.[20] During this time, Steiner began his seminal work expanding the scope of laryngeal laser surgery to treat more extensive malignant tumors of the larynx and upper-aerodigestive tract. His pioneering work is perhaps the greatest contribution to organ sparing laryngeal surgery over the past 20 years and demonstrated the advantages of utilizing microsurgical laser techniques in the treatment of laryngeal cancer and its equivalency to open techniques for specific stage disease.[21]

The CO_2 laser was the first wavelength used in laryngeal surgery and remains the laser of choice for the majority of laryngeal operations requiring this technology. Recent advances in laser technology, anesthesia, and surgical instrumentation have made minimally invasive laryngeal procedures more common. These new approaches have led to better organ preservation rates, improved post-operative functionality and reduced recovery time. It is important to remember that endoscopic examination under general anesthesia is typically performed prior to definitive treatment in order to ensure that comprehensive therapeutic decisions can be made.

Lasers provide surgeons with a precision cutting tool. Using a micromanipulator coupled surgical laser (Fig. 2) at 25× to 40× magnification can negate intention and physiologic tremor of the surgeon and also allow for simultaneous use of both hands and the laser (Fig. 3). The laser can also reach areas that are otherwise difficult to access without performing an open procedure (neck incision, pharyngotomy, laryngectomy, etc.). Presently, commercially available hollow waveguides and fiberoptics continue to expand the role of lasers in airway surgery.

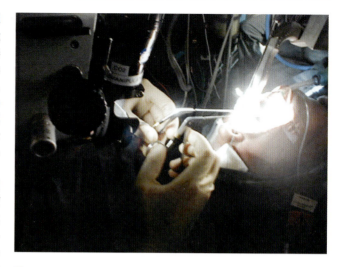

Fig. 3 Micromanipulator coupled surgical laser. Note the bimanual instrumentation allowed by placing the patient in suspension (Photograph provided courtesy of Dr. Brian Wong)

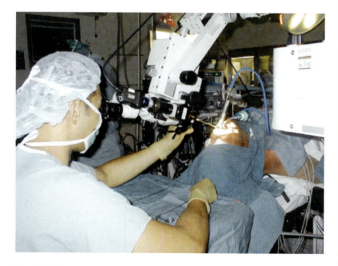

Fig. 2 Micromanipulator coupled surgical laser with patient placed in suspension (Photograph provided courtesy of Dr. Brian Wong)

Indications and Contraindications

- Indications
  - Malignant Lesions
    - Glottic carcinoma – Early stages
    - Supraglottic carcinoma
    - Hypopharyngeal carcinoma
    - Palliative therapy (tumor debulking)
  - Benign Lesions
    - Polyps
    - Papillomatosis
    - Hemangiomas and Vascular Malformations
  - Laryngomalacia
  - Vocal Cord Paralysis
  - Reinke's Edema
- Contraindications
  - Abnormal anatomy that precludes suspension laryngoscopy
  - Malignant Lesions
    - Glottic – Late stages III / IV
      - Extension into surrounding tissues
      - Recurrent disease after radiation therapy
    - Hypopharyngeal carcinoma
  - Benign Lesions
    - Lesions located at the anterior commissure
    - Lesions located at the free edge of the vocal cord
    - Cricoid cartilage stenosis

Malignancy

Transoral endoscopic laser laryngeal microsurgery depends upon the ability of the surgeon to determine the extent of tumor invasion prior to excision via detailed physical examination performed under general anesthesia and imaging studies. The primary objective is to achieve complete resection of the cancer with clear margins, while maintaining as much organ function as possible (e.g., swallowing, speech, etc.). While transoral laser laryngeal microsurgery (TLM) has many advantages such as decreased post-operative morbidity, reduced recovery time and the potential for organ preservation, recurrence or incomplete resection are significant risks. Hence, the procedure requires skill and sound clinical judgment. It is generally contraindicated in patients with known extensive invasion into other structures and recurrent cancer in previously irradiated areas.[22]

Glottic Carcinoma

The glottis is the area of the larynx that includes the vocal cords. Use of the laser to excise glottic cancer is well established for lesions staged at T1 and early T2. For all T2a carcinomas of the glottis, laser excision is recommended regardless of the pattern of the spread of the tumor.[19,23,24] Provided the tumor is superficial, it is of limited significance whether the disease involves the supraglottis, subglottis or the anterior commissure. The superficial location of the tumor in T1 and early T2 disease allows it to be excised by partial mucosectomy. Laser-assisted endoscopic excision of T3 and T4 laryngeal carcinomas is controversial. Most experts in the field reject the idea of laser microsurgical excision of these advanced tumors unless a classic laryngectomy is not an option due to underlying co-morbid disease. Patients with T3 or T4 laryngeal lesions require the widest possible endoscopic excision followed by post-operative radiotherapy to the primary site and surrounding groups of lymph nodes; however they more often undergo a classic open total or partial laryngectomy.[25,26] Steiner groups patients with T3 ($n = 17$) and T4 ($n = 6$) lesions in the same category as patients with T2b glottic and supraglottic lesions and routinely treats these tumors with laser-assisted endoscopic surgery.[25]

Supraglottic Carcinoma

Supraglottic tumors typically occur either in the suprahyoid epiglottis and false cord area or in the infrahyoid/epiglottic area. It is relatively rare that small, well-circumscribed tumors are diagnosed in the supraglottic area because the tumors only produce symptoms, and therefore are brought to the attention of a physician, when they are much larger. Only a few reports have been published on the laser resection of early stage supraglottic carcinomas.[27-31] Tumors in the suprahyoid epiglottis and false cord area are easily removed. Laser excision is indicated because wide margins can be taken without the concern of adversely affecting function.

Infrahyoid epiglottic cancers are difficult to assess preoperatively even with imaging studies and are at risk for infiltrating the pre-epiglottic space. There are conflicting opinions regarding endoscopic laser resection of carcinoma that involves the pre-epiglottic space. Iro urges caution and restraint in treatment of T3 staged supraglottic cancers with transoral laser surgery.[32] Whereas Rudert believes that these supraglottic cancers that invade the pre-epiglottic space are candidates for endoscopic laser resection.[33] If endoscopic excision is performed and margins remain positive, salvage radiotherapy will not be sufficient, and classic laryngectomy may be required.

Hypopharyngeal Carcinoma

Pre-resection analysis of the airway during surgical endoscopy under general anesthesia may not be able to identify the true extent of hypopharyngeal tumors. Imaging studies can aid in this endeavor. Tumors involving the piriform sinuses usually involve the thyroid cartilage, arytenoids, paraglottic and pre-epiglottic space as well as other soft tissues of the neck with little or no evidence seen on endoscopy. Because of these factors, the majority of laryngologists agree that partial pharyngo-laryngeal resection utilizing only a laser is insufficient for complete eradication of disease and cannot be justified. Classic open surgery (i.e., laryngectomy, laryngopharyngectomy) remains the standard of care.

Palliative Therapy

The laser is a useful tool in debulking tumors that obstruct the upper airway and may be an alternative to tracheostomy.[34,35] Avoiding a tracheostomy greatly improves a patient's quality of life. Palliative airway surgery requires judgment. If too little tumor is resected, the obstruction will persist and ultimately lead to a tracheostomy. However, aggressive resection of tumor may lead to aspiration and the need for a tracheostomy to protect the airway and provide pulmonary toilet. Laccourreye published a 10-year experience describing the use of the CO_2 laser to debulk obstructing endolaryngeal carcinomas in 42 patients for the avoidance of a tracheostomy. Ninety-three percent or 39 of 42 patients avoided tracheostomy.[36]

Recanalizing the upper digestive tract by ablating hypopharyngeal and esophageal outlet tumors poses a serious risk of hemorrhage and will only provide temporary improvement in swallowing. Placement of a percutaneous gastrostomy tube (PEG) tube is a safer and better option for these head and neck cancer patients with dysphagia. If palliative laser surgery is considered, one should aim for sustainable symptomatic relief.

Benign Disease

The CO_2 laser has a firmly established role in the treatment of benign laryngeal disorders such as papillomas, polyps, vascular malformations and strictures. Since Jako and Strong first introduced the CO_2 laser in 1970, several groups, including those led by Shapshay, Zeitels, Ossoff, Steiner, Motta and Rudert, have published extensively on their experiences with laser surgery in benign laryngeal disease.[37] The use of other lasers such as the KTP(Nd:YAG) laser, the pulsed dye laser and the diode laser has also been reported, but their use has not been as widespread due to lack of availability in most medical centers. Therefore, the carbon dioxide laser remains largely the laser of choice.

Polyps

The vocal cords have a delicate subepithelial tissue layer that can be damaged as a result of repetitive collisions and shearing forces. Vocal cord polyps are generally unilateral, sessile and appear to be spherical and well circumscribed. They typically originate at the free edge and on the anterior two thirds of the vocal cord. (Fig. 4) Voice abuse and chronic inflammation from tobacco smoke irritation are common causes of injury to the vocal cord epithelium and lead to damage within the epithelial basement membrane. A large percentage of patients with polyps are heavy smokers or are exposed to a large amount of secondary tobacco smoke. When conservative methods (i.e., voice rest, speech therapy, etc.) fail, treatment is surgical removal. It is important to always send the excised polyps for histology to exclude an early malignancy or to diagnose a benign tumor. For this reason, these polyps should never be vaporized with the laser.

Papillomas

Laryngeal Papillomas are typically caused by HPV types 6 and 11 and can affect any age group (Fig. 5). The virus causes formation of benign epithelial papillomas of the larynx. Diagnosis is made with flexible fiberoptic laryngoscopy or microlaryngoscopy. Although papillomas most commonly occur on the vocal cords, the larynx, esophagus and trachea must be comprehensively examined during endoscopy because the papillomas can occur anywhere along the aerodigestive system. While the CO_2 laser is still used to ablate these lesions, the concern over aerosolization of viral particles has made mechanical laryngeal microdebriders an increasingly more common treatment approach. The recent availability of waveguides for CO_2 has lead to renewed interest in the laser for use in office-based laryngeal surgery for papillomas without the need for general anesthesia.[38]

Hemangiomas and Vascular Malformations

Subglottic hemangiomas present with persistent cough, hoarseness or stridor, and manifest as reddish, well-circumscribed masses during surgical endoscopy. Surgery involves primarily vaporization and ablation rather than excision.[39] The CO_2, KTP or Nd:YAG laser is used with low power settings (1–3 W), as high power settings can lead to tracheal perforation, pneumothorax or intractable bleeding.

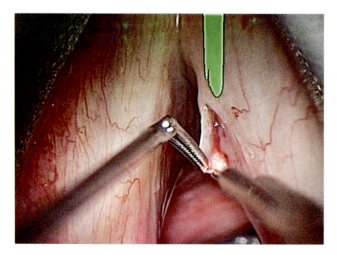

Fig 4 Pulsed 532 nm KTP laser assisted subepithelial resection of fibrovascular mass (hemorrhagic polyp) on the middle 2/3 of the left true vocal cord. The green area is refraction from the laser light (Photograph provided courtesy of Dr. Steven Zeitels)

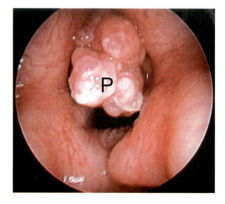

Fig. 5 Laryngeal papilloma (P) at the level of the glottis (Photograph provided courtesy of Dr. Gupreet S. Ahuja)

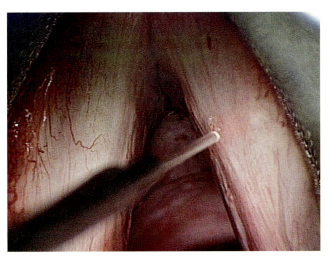

Fig. 6 Pulsed 532 nm KTP laser assisted photoangiolysis of ectatic blood vessels in a singer (Photograph provided courtesy of Dr. Steven Zeitels)

Vascular malformations typically are located in the supraglottic area and are generally asymptomatic. Symptoms of a laryngopharyngeal vascular malformation may include foreign body sensation or mild stridor of unknown origin. Carbon dioxide laser excision or Nd:YAG coagulation is the treatment of choice, though other wavelengths can be used as well with appropriate dosimetry. Use of the Nd:YAG laser has a higher rate of postoperative scarring and stenosis due to the deeper penetration depth of this wavelength, but is extremely valuable in treating large vascular malformations where volumetric heating of large regions of tumor are required. These extensive tumors are more commonly found in the oropharynx and oral cavity.[40] Ectatic blood vessels along the vocal cord surface (Fig. 6) may alter the pitch and timbre of the voice and can be problematic for singers and other professionals. They are commonly treated using pulse dye laser and other laser devices.

Laryngomalacia

Stridor in children is most commonly caused by laryngomalacia, and 60–75% of childhood cases of stridor are associated with laryngomalacia.[19] Approximately 20% of these cases do not resolve spontaneously and will require surgical intervention. Dysphagia, apnea and respiratory distress are all indicators for surgical intervention. Laryngomalacia will be discussed in a later section along with subglottic hemangiomas.

Vocal Cord Paralysis

Patients that have bilateral vocal cord paralysis may develop severe respiratory distress and airway obstruction from the diminished patency of the glottic airway. Vocal cord paralysis commonly presents following surgery where the recurrent laryngeal nerve is inadvertently injured (i.e., during thyroid tumor surgery). In the immediate post-operative period the patient develops stridor and respiratory insufficiency. Acutely, treatment may involve intubation and tracheostomy. For long-term treatment, CO_2 lasers can be used to enlarge the glottic chink and increase airway patency.[41] This is challenging surgery because it is important to strike a balance between airway patency and voice quality when enlarging the glottis.

Reinke's Edema

Reinke's edema is a reactive sub-epithelial fluid accumulation of unknown etiology; although it is frequently associated with smoking and other activities that produce chronic vocal cord inflammation. Submucosal edema seen on endoscopy is a characteristic feature of the disease. Symptoms of Reinke's edema include hoarseness and other voice changes. The pulsed dye laser at 585nm wavelength can be used to successfully treat this condition. Certain other disorders can mimic the appearance of Reinke's edema. For example, Reinke's edema may mimic the chronic inflammatory changes that are associated with early laryngeal carcinoma. Therefore, the surgeon should have a low threshold to biopsy suspicious lesions.

Contraindications for Surgery of Benign Airway Lesions

There are few contraindications to Transoral Laser Microsurgery (TLM) for benign lesions. One important rule is that surgeons should avoid unnecessary disruption or excision of the anterior commissure and the free edge of the vocal cords. Disruption of the anterior commissure may result in extensive scar formation and an anterior glottic web. TLM is also contraindicated in cricoid cartilage stenosis.[42] Most contraindications are related to the relative risks of anesthesia or sedation.

Techniques

- Pre-Operative Management
  - Imaging and Vocal cord mobility assessment
  - Laser parameters
- Description of Technique
  - Suspension microlaryngoscopy
  - Laser Delivery / Devices
  - Malignant Lesions
  - Benign Lesions
- Post-Operative Management

Pre-operative Management

In the pre-operative evaluation, patients always undergo an indirect mirror or a flexible fiberoptic laryngoscopy examination to determine the extent of the lesion and vocal cord mobility. Video stroboscopy of the vocal cords may be included in the pre-operative evaluation to determine the dynamics of vocal cord movement. Some patients may undergo diagnostic imaging (CT or MRI of the neck) to determine the extent of disease. Vocal cord polyps warrant a trial of speech therapy for vocal coaching and training in proper voice use prior surgery. Patients with carcinoma of the larynx, recurrent papillomatosis and Reinke's edema must be strongly encouraged to quit smoking.

The most common parameters for the CO_2 laser beam using a micromanipulator is a 250 μm spot size with a working distance of 350 mm. Laser power is usually below 8 W. In the superpulse mode, where exposure time is 0.1 s or less, a low power setting of 2–3 W is used. The superpulse mode is useful in achieving maximum ablation through minimal penetration and maximum energy absorption at the surface of interest. There is almost no charring due to the minimal thermal diffusion in the surrounding areas around the target. In preparation for incision of epithelium in cases such as Reinke's edema, microvascular coagulation is required. The laser is typically set for a 0.05 s pulse of 1 W of power using an unfocused beam.[20] Recently, flash scanner technological originally developed for use in dermatologic applications has been re-purposed and adapted for use in laryngeal microsurgery. These devices allow creation of user-defined ablation patterns and cuts under precise computer control. The high cost of these systems has limited the broad adoption of this technology (Acublade-SurgiTouch system, Lumenis, Santa Clara, CA).

Description of Technique

Suspension microlaryngoscopy provides a method in which the surgeon is able to directly visualize the larynx and its surrounding structures. Gustav Killian was among the first to describe suspension laryngoscopy in 1912 and later developed the Killian-Lynch suspension laryngoscope along with Robert Clyde Lynch. Zeitels showed effective use of suspension laryngoscopy in 120 cases in a prospective assessment.[43] Suspension allows for bimanual direct laryngoscopic surgery.[44] Furthermore, suspension laryngoscopy permits the use of a laryngoscope with a larger bore thereby enhancing exposure. Figure 7 demonstrates the positioning of a patient in suspension, and Fig. 8 shows the normal anatomy of the larynx as visualized under suspension microlaryngoscopy.

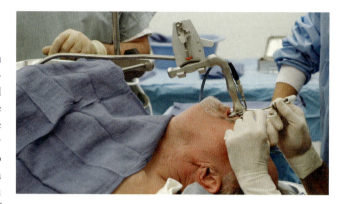

Fig. 7 Suspension laryngoscopy (Photograph provided courtesy of Dr. Roger Crumley)

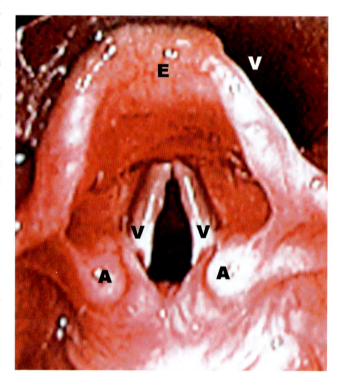

Fig. 8 View of the glottis through the laryngoscope. *A* arytenoids, *E* epiglottis, *V* (*black*) vocal cords, *V* (*white*) vallecula (Photograph provided courtesy of Dr. Gupreet S. Ahuja)

With the patient anesthetized and lying supine, the head is fully extended. A rigid laryngeal endoscope is introduced through the oral cavity and past the epiglottis into the larynx until the desired endolaryngeal structures are visualized. The vocal cords should be clearly visualized from the anterior commissure to the vocal process on both sides. The rigid laryngoscope is then stabilized and secured using a suspension arm. Surgery is performed using a microscope with a 400 mm focal length lens or using a Hopkins rod endoscope inserted thru the laryngoscope bore. There are several instances that make suspension microlaryngoscopy very difficult or even impossible. Abnormal anatomy such as a short, stiff neck, long or protruding maxillary teeth, displaced larynx and lesions or a mass at the base of tongue may limit and prevent suspension laryngoscopy in these patients.[42]

Suspension laryngoscopy provides a direct airway in which anesthesia may be administered either through an endotracheal tube that is inserted parallel to the laryngoscope or via jet ventilation. This direct airway also provides an unimpeded path for the surgeon to access the vocal cords and other structures in the larynx. The rigid laryngoscope also prevents collapse of the pharynx and hypopharynx that would then obstruct the surgeon's view. The greatest advantage that suspension laryngoscopy provides is that it allows for a minimally invasive approach to laryngeal surgery where traditional approaches have involved large external incisions and significant morbidity.

Lasers and Laser Devices

Since Jako coupled the carbon dioxide laser to the operating microscope in 1972 for laryngeal surgery, the CO_2 laser has been the wavelength of choice. The CO_2 laser is used in the majority of operations because of its widespread availability in most medical centers and its efficiency in simultaneously cutting tissue and maintaining hemostasis. Other commonly used lasers in otolaryngology include the KTP(Nd:YAG) laser and the argon laser. In laryngeal surgery, the CO_2 laser is generally coupled to a micromanipulator attached to the microscope. This allows the surgeon to use microsurgical instruments and the laser at the same time. It also provides maximum surgical field visualization with high magnification and an unobstructed view of the lesion. The CO_2 laser has several advantages over conventional surgical instruments that cut or cauterize in that traditional devices may obstruct the field of view or amplify the surgeon's intention tremor via a lever arm of up to 20 cm. Furthermore, post-operative edema is less with CO_2 laser endoscopic surgery compared to non-laser methods, and thus reduces the risk of post-operative airway obstruction and subsequent tracheostomy. Diminishing the amount of edema also improves the patient's post-operative swallowing function. The thermal damage zone when using micromanipulators introduces limited artifact into the histological assessment, and it coagulates small blood vessels and seals lymphatic channels thus minimizing the incidence of metastases.[20] The diameter of the laser beam, pulse duration and irradiance can be adjusted to produce different tissue effects. Spot sizes between 1 to 4 mm are used for tissue ablation and 0.2–1 mm used for cutting with powers varying anywhere from 2 to 10 W. Some micromanipulators further focus the beam down to an even smaller spot size, and combined with short pulse durations or

flash scanner technology, can ablate tissue with minimal to no charring just as in skin resurfacing.[45] Morbidity of using the CO_2 laser when appropriate is far less than cold surgery, and the cost effectiveness is much greater.[46]

In certain cases where lesions extend out of the surgeon's visual field, the CO_2 laser can be delivered by a flexible hollow waveguide. However there are limitations with the use of the hollow waveguide due to its limited angulation, the diameter of the laser spot and the significant and variable loss of power during transmission.[20] Regardless, recent techniques using hollow fiber technology are evolving.[47-51]

Malignant Lesions

Glottic Carcinoma

T1 and T2a carcinomas of the glottis are typically resected en bloc and clear margins of 1–3 mm are obtained. However with laser surgery, it is possible to maintain more narrow margins that allow for preservation of vocal function and reduction in post-operative edema.

Transoral Laser Microsurgery (TLM) has yielded good functional results and low rates of recurrence from multiple groups since the 1990 s. Studies have shown that it is possible to preserve the larynx in over 92% of cases with a 5 year local control rate that ranges from 80% to 94%.[27,52] Treatment of early glottic cancer with TLM has a distinct advantage over other procedures in that it maintains the availability of all treatment options for patients with local or secondary tumor recurrence including laser re-excision, radiation therapy or open partial laryngectomy.[53,54]

T2b and T3 carcinoma of the glottis typically involves the vocal cords with supraglottic or subglottic extension. The operative technique using lasers for these tumors involves subdividing the tumor into several pieces for removal. Resection of these tumors may involve the cricoid and thyroid cartilage, the arytenoids, the cricothyroid ligament and any involved laryngeal soft tissue.

The application of laser assisted endoscopic surgery via suspension laryngoscopy draws comparisons to Mohs surgery because resections are driven by frozen section histology. One of the greatest differences between endoscopic laryngeal surgery and cutaneous Mohs surgery lies in the fact that Mohs surgery aims to achieve the best cosmetic result as possible while attempting to remove as little tissue as possible without compromising the tumor resection. In laryngeal surgery, functionality remains essential post-operatively in laryngeal cancer patients. Laser assisted endoscopic laryngeal surgery has potential to allow surgeons to excise cancer piecemeal with frozen section guidance. Frozen section guidance of surgical resections in the larynx is difficult due intubation or forceful endoscopic suspension can easily chip, loosen, or fracture teeth if the surgeon is not careful with the orientation of the laryngoscope in the oral cavity. In a study of 339 microlaryngoscopy patients, 75% were found to have small mucosal lesions of the oral cavity, oropharynx and lip.[57] Though the injuries were minor, they were a source of major complaints for the patients but resolved over a period of several days. Other complications associated with laser microsurgery include lingual and hypoglossal nerve palsy. Prolonged displacement of the tongue can cause severe contusion and swelling that often leads to dysphagia and sometimes-permanent dysesthesia (sensory disturbance) in the tongue.

There are many general safety considerations involving the use of surgical lasers in surgery that were discussed earlier in this chapter. In particular to laryngeal surgery where high-powered lasers are used in small confined areas with flammable gas, the use of caution cannot be emphasized enough. Stray laser light is not a rare event and is capable of causing burns in unwanted areas. It is recommended practice to cover areas beyond the target site to protect from unwanted burns. Control of oxygen content, inhalation agents, and use of special laser endotracheal tubes in these procedures is important.

Though TLM rarely requires tracheotomy post operatively, it is nevertheless a real possibility in the intermediate and advanced cases. Surgeons must always be aware of certain indicators for tracheotomy. Prolonged compression of the tongue during TLM can cause lingual edema that can lead to airway compromise. Sudden secondary hemorrhage is a major risk in TLM and often necessitates a tracheotomy. Large arteries and vessels should not only be cauterized but clipped as well to avoid sudden secondary hemorrhage.

TLM typically causes the formation of large granulomas if cartilage is exposed by the surgical procedure. These granulomas are perpetuated by small osseocartilaginous sequestrae unless they are removed.[22] TLM involving the anterior commissure often results in a round anterior glottic effect, and this often leads to breathiness and hoarseness.[58]

Laser surgery for benign lesions in the larynx is relatively safe compared to most other treatment modalities. It is a minimally invasive technique with almost no complications attributed to the laser itself.

Future Directions

- Omni Guide Beampath
- Tissue welding
- Office based procedures with lasers
- Femto-second lasers

Future directions of laser use in laryngology involves new devices for delivery, office based laser applications, the use of the laser for welding tissue and the creation of lasers that are even more precise than those which are currently available. A recent technological advance (Omni Guide, Boston, MA) has provided surgeons the use of CO_2 lasers through a flexible fiber. The Omni Guide Beam Path uses a hollow "photonic band gap fiber." The fiber is placed in a handpiece coupled with a suction that eliminates the need for a micromanipulator and allows the surgeon to have the freedom of a laser cutting tool in his or her hand. The Omni Guide Beam Path has proven useful in the surgery of both benign and malignant lesions.[59]

Awake office based laser surgery is gaining popularity in the treatment of benign laryngeal lesions because of the relative safety of lasers and the quick recovery period post procedure. Though the CO_2 laser has traditionally been the laser of choice for laryngeal surgery, different lasers have been reported to be useful in office-based surgery. In the office, new technologies such as distal chip endoscopy and rare-earth doped fiber lasers have allowed for creative and innovative surgical techniques. Typical diseases treated with these new techniques are dysplasias and papillomas. A 585 nm pulsed dye laser was originally the laser of choice for vascular lesions; however the 532 nm pulsed KTP laser has proven to be superior. The use of the 2,013 nm Thulium laser which mimics the CO_2 laser closely may become useful as an office based laser as well.[60-64] Even though otolaryngologists are performing more office procedures that incorporate lasers, the breadth of procedures remains limited for important reasons such as airway compromise, which is poorly handled in the office setting.

Otology

Indications and Contraindications

- Indications
  - External auditory canal lesions
  - Eustachian tube dysfunction
  - Perforated tympanic membrane
  - Exostoses
  - Debulking of Tumors
  - Acoustic Neuroma
  - Cholesteatoma Resection
  - Otosclerosis
  - Vertigo
  - Facial Nerve Paresis / Paralysis
- Contraindications
  - Anatomic, clinical and physiologic limiting factors
  - Large skull base tumors

Laser applications in otology include the treatment of vascular lesions in the external auditory canal (EAC), exostoses (bony outgrowths) in the EAC, the debulking of inoperable tumors, Eustachian tube dysfunction, myringotomy/tympanostomy in otitis media, graft fixation in tympanoplasty, stapedectomy/stapedotomy in otosclerosis, tympanosclerosis, removal of cholesteatoma, cochleostomy, labyrinthectomy in benign paroxysmal positional vertigo, endolymphatic hydrops and facial nerve decompression.[65]

The use of the laser in middle ear surgery is one of the most elegant examples of laser technology use and applications. Perkins pioneered the use of the argon laser in middle ear surgery in the late-1970s performing the first laser stapedotomy for otosclerosis. One of the first uses of the laser in the field was in patients with otosclerosis. The disease is now one of the most common indications for laser use in otologic surgery. Otosclerosis is a localized disorder of bone resorption and deposition (remodeling) in the middle and inner ear that causes progressive unilateral or bilateral conductive hearing loss that typically begins in the third to fifth decade of life. This defect in bone remodeling in the vicinity the stapes footplate and oval window leads to reduced mobility of the stapes and hearing loss. Mechanical causes of hearing loss, also known as conductive hearing loss, can be entirely corrected through surgery.[66,67] Patients with otosclerosis benefit from the argon laser through its precise vaporization of the stapedial tendon, mobilizing the posterior crus of the stapes and in stapes footplate fenestration.[68,69] This procedure is called a stapedectomy or stapedotomy, and is performed in order to recreate ossicular chain mobility and decrease conductive hearing loss. Knowledge of middle ear anatomy is critical in obtaining good post-operative results with minimal complications. Avoidance of injury to the facial nerve and the chorda tympani nerve is the standard of care.[65,68,70-83]

DiBartolomeo described other uses of the argon laser in the field of otology. He utilized this laser in the tympanoplasty (repair of the tympanic membrane), stapedectomy, lysis of adhesions and myringotomy (placement of a hole in the tympanic membrane). He describes the "spot welding" technique of the laser that allows for the adherence of a fascial graft placed in substitution of the tympanic membrane onto the soft tissue annulus.[84] The use of the argon laser in otologic surgery is precise, safe and effective. Delivery of a laser to the ear and temporal bone can be either via a fiber (KTP and argon) or via a micro-manipulator such as those used with CO_2 lasers.[65]

Eustachian tube dysfunction is a common ear disorder in which patients may experience chronic recurrent ear infections or difficulty in clearing a blocked sensation of their middle ear. A laser myringotomy may be performed to equalize the pressures between the middle and outer ear, and to assist the ear in draining fluid.[85-89] Laser Eustachian tuboplasty (LETP) is the practice of utilizing a diode or an argon laser to vaporize select areas of hypertrophic mucosa and submucosa tissue along the length of the Eustachian tube. In a 2-year follow-up study of 13 adults, Poe et al. found that medical management combined with LETP on a select group of patients can be successful in eliminating chronic middle ear effusions.[90]

A cholesteatoma is a collection of keratinized epithelium that is located in an abnormal location at the external auditory canal, middle ear, petrous bone or mastoid. It is either congenital in etiology or is acquired due to repeated infection. It is not invasive, but it is destroys the bones of the middle ear leading to a conductive hearing loss. It can also erode the mastoid bone and tegmen can possible lead to a cerebral spinal fluid leak. Therefore, the cholesteatoma needs to be removed in its entirety.[91] Excision is associated with a high rate of recurrence. The use of a laser in this surgery may assist the surgeon in removing the mass in more difficult to reach areas of the middle ear and mastoid.[92,93]

Contraindications to laser use for otologic applications include performing a stapedectomy in the presence of active otitis media, an only-hearing ear that responds well to amplification, vertigo and endolymphatic hydrops, certain inner ear malformations or an overhanging facial nerve that completely obstructs access to the oval window niche. Laser stapedectomy in patients with a perforated tympanic membrane must be postponed until the perforation is fixed. In the case of an overlying facial nerve, preservation of the facial nerve is most important, and conventional instruments are used to perform the operation rather than the laser.

Techniques

- Pre-Operative Management
  - Laser Selection
  - Laser Doppler Vibrometry
- Description of Technique
  - Stapedectomy / Stapedotomy
  - Cholesteatoma Excision
  - Myringotomy / Tympanostomy
  - Tympanoplasty
  - Labrinthectomy
- Post-Operative Management

Pre-operative Management and Laser Selection

Pre-operative management of patients undergoing laser assisted otologic surgery includes a full history and physical, an audiogram and likely non-contrast computer tomography (CT) imaging of the temporal bone and internal auditory canal. When choosing a laser to use near a neurosensory organ like the ear, it is important to consider the potential collateral damage. The thermal and photoacoustic effects in laser use are a function of dosimetry and tissue optical and thermal properties. Bone has substantially smaller water content than skin or other soft tissues and visible wavelengths are not well absorbed. In the absence of any distinct chromophore, using an argon or a KTP(Nd:YAG) laser to ablate bone requires the use of an initiator. An initiator absorbs laser light and undergoes pyrolysis. In middle ear surgery, a small droplet of blood or charred tissue placed on the laser target serves this purpose. Accordingly, there is a risk of thermal injury, as considerable temperature elevations occur within this region, and ablation occurs with at best modest thermal confinement.[82] In contrast, infrared wavelengths are well absorbed by both the hydroxyapatite crystals in bone and the interwoven collagen fibers. Ablation proceeds by the classical mechanisms just as in skin, though photoacoustic transients may be generated leading to audible pops. These mechanical transients may propagate through the inner ear and may result in injury to the delicate neuroepithelium.

In general, shorter laser pulse durations lead to less thermal injury provided the conditions for thermal confinement are met.[94,95] However, repeated pulses in rapid succession may lead to the build up of heat in the target site; hence successive pulses should be separated by a sufficient amount of time to allow for complete thermal relaxation. Short pulse laser systems (e.g., Erbium:YAG) generate an acoustic pressure wave that leads to a vibration of the ossicular chain which may result in "noise trauma". The heat generated by the laser may also cause "convection currents" that also lead to vibratory stimulations. Both of these stimulations can cause acoustic injury and should be controlled by appropriate dosimetry selection. Regardless, the mechanical transients produced during laser ablation are comparable or even less harmful than the vibratory effects produced using conventional methods to perform surgery.[7,65,82,96,97]

Description of Technique

In addition to the argon laser, the CO_2 laser, the KTP laser and more recently, the erbium-YAG laser are used to perform a stapedectomy or stapedotomy in patients with otosclerosis. In the stapedectomy and stapedotomy, the stapedial tendon is vaporized with the laser, then the incudostapedial joint is disarticulated using mechanical instrumentation, and the posterior crus is severed with the laser (Fig. 11a, b). The anterior crus of the stapes is then fractured manually without the laser and the stapes superstructure is removed.

The laser is then used to place a single large hole or a set of smaller holes generating a "rosette" type pattern in the stapes footplate to accommodate the prosthesis (Fig. 11c). A mobile prosthesis is put into place.[65,68,70-83] No study to date has demonstrated which laser among the three most commonly used in stapes surgery (argon, KTP and CO_2) is best. Recently, erbium:YAG lasers have been developed for use in performing this operation, however the high cost of these lasers has limited broad adoption.[71,98] The success of laser stapes surgery is based on audiometric analysis (hearing tests) and complication rates. Audiometric results after laser stapedotomy in relation to mean differences in the bone conduction auditory thresholds show improvements of 0.53–5.6 dB in those thresholds regardless of the laser system utilized.[70,99]

Smaller cholesteatomas and residual tissue in previously attempted excisions of cholesteatoma have been vaporized with the CO_2, Argon and KTP lasers with some reports of lower recurrence rates.[65] Laser use is particularly beneficial when removing cholesteatoma from the delicate bones of the middle ear such as the stapes or in removing disease that traverses the obturator foramen of the stapes. When using the laser in this application, its energy is absorbed more by the cholesteatoma than by the bony surroundings.[92,93]

Use of the laser in myringotomy and tympanoplasty is a boutique interest in otolaryngology, primarily due to costs. Myringotomy is performed by using either an Argon laser or a KTP laser directed by a fiber delivery system to create an incision in a patient's ear drum for tympanostomy tube placement, for fluid removal or to gain access to the middle ear. It most often performed in patients with chronic otitis media with effusion. Use of the laser instead of a myringotomy knife has shown to be beneficial by preventing the necessity of tympanostomy tube placement; however laser myringotomy without tube placement only creates a temporary hole in the tympanic membrane that lasts less than 6 weeks, and therefore patients with recurrent or persistent episodes of otitis media with effusion may need tube placement at a later date. Office-based laser assisted tympanic membrane fenestration with a hand-held otoscope combined with the CO_2 flashscanner laser, OtoLAM (ESC/Sharplan, Yokneam, Israel) and placement of a pressure equalization tube under local anesthesia has been described as well. Outcomes have shown improvement in hearing and reduced incidence of tube plugging, however this was performed in a non-randomized population.[85-89,100]

Tympanoplasty is the repair of a defect in the eardrum by placing fascia or perichondrium over the defect. In this application, the KTP laser can be used to weld the collagen fibers together along their edges.[92,93,101-103] While promising, neither laser application of myringotomy nor

Laser/Light Applications in Otolaryngology

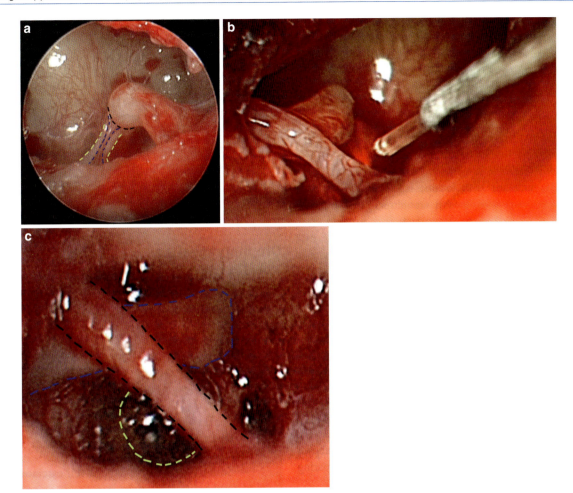

Fig. 11 (**a**) In stapedectomy, the stapes tendon (*blue dashed line*) is vaporized with the laser and the incudostapedial joint (*black dashed line*) is disarticulated. The posterior crus (*yellow dashed line*) is then severed with the laser. (Photograph provided courtesy of Dr. Hamid Djalilian). (**b**) Intraoperative image of an argon laser directed at the posterior crus of the stapes after having displaced the chorda tympani nerve from the line of fire. (Photograph provided courtesy of Dr. Hamid Djalilian) (**c**) Intraoperative image of the oval window after laser stapedectomy. Notice the charred appearance of where the stapes was located (*yellow dashed line*). Also note the preservation of the chorda tympani nerve (*black dashed line*). The long process of the incus (*blue dashed line*) is still intact above and will be used to anchor the stapes prosthesis (Photograph provided courtesy of Dr. Hamid Djalilian)

tympanoplasty been widely adopted due to the extensive cost of the system.

CO_2 laser use in acoustic neuroma surgery has shown to be advantageous due to its precision in cutting and coagulating around the facial nerve. The use of KTP and Argon lasers for acoustic neuroma excisions have also been noted, but are not widely used. Laser use is limited by the size of the tumor, approach to the lesion and the surgeon's experience. For smaller tumors (2–3 cm), stereotactic radiation is beneficial in preventing further growth of the mass and preserving facial nerve function and hearing.[65,104,105] Laser use in endolymphatic hydrops[106] and labyrinthectomy for benign paroxysmal positional vertigo (BPPV) been described, but not been adopted due to their potentially high rate of hearing loss compared to traditional surgery.[107-109] Laser use in the decompression of the facial nerve has also been successfully performed.[110]

Post-operative Management

The majority of patients are sent home on the same day of surgery. They are told to keep their ear canal and surgical site water free. Packing is frequently left in the external auditory canal for up to 2 weeks for removal by the surgeon at a post-operative visit. A repeat audiogram is performed at approximately 6 weeks post-operatively. Patients who undergo cholesteatoma surgery are followed approximately every 4–6 months or more frequently to monitor for recurrence and to adequately maintain the cleanliness of the mastoid bowl.

of the cricopharyngeus muscle. More recently, the endoscopic use of the CO_2 laser to take down the wall is emerging as a comparable treatment.[37,143,144] Almost 90% of patients report normal swallowing function after undergoing the procedure.

Post-operative Management

Patients with either extensive resections of SCCA in the oral cavity or those who have SCCA involving the base of tongue are kept in an intensive care unit setting overnight for airway monitoring. Occasionally, if swelling is severe, the patient remains intubated and is administered steroids until the edema subsides. Rarely, a tracheotomy is necessary if the patient cannot be intubated or if the airway obstruction is anticipated to be long-term.

Any patient with surgery performed in the oral cavity is placed on a liquid diet post-operatively and slowly advanced to a soft diet on which he or she remains for at least 2 weeks. The oral mucosa heals quickly, and patients are encouraged to drink as much fluids as they can handle to decrease xerostomia, infection and post-operative pain. Patients who have undergone a Zenker's diverticulectomy are placed on a full liquid diet for at least 2 weeks and watched closely for a symptoms that may indicate a dehiscence of the operative site including chest pain, shortness of breath or the return of dysphagia.

Adverse Events

- Uncontrolled Pain
- Recurrence of condition
- Mediastinitis
- Airway obstruction

Side Effects/Complications

Complication rates are significantly higher (90%) in patients with oral SCCA who have been previously irradiated than those who have not had radiation treatments (10%).[145] Complications reported in patients who have received radiation therapy include uncontrolled pain, bleeding, infection, delayed healing and edema.[146] As discussed above, patients may have post-operative edema of the tongue and oral cavity soft tissue leading to airway obstruction. When obstruction is severe enough, intubation or a temporary tracheostomy may be warranted.

Post-operative bleeding in any oral cavity laser procedure is rare, but may be insidious in onset. If suspected, the patient must be carefully examined, and if found, the patient must be brought back to the operating room to control the bleeding.

Complications of both open and endoscopic Zenker's diverticulectomy include post-operative fever with or without mediastinitis, esophageal injury and need for re-operation. However generally, the use of the laser is less morbid than an open procedure.[143,147,148]

Prevention and Treatment of Side Effects/Complications

Complications can be minimized by obtaining good visualization of the surgical field and by obtaining adequate hemostasis intraoperatively. Encouraging fluid intake by mouth is important in preventing post-operative pain and dehydration. Airway obstruction may be minimized with post-operative steroids, however the primary concern is in preventing an emergent situation. This is averted by thorough preparation and close monitoring of the patient in the immediate post-operative period.

Future Directions

- Interstitial laser therapy
- Photodynamic therapy

Currently, the use of the laser in head and neck SCCA is limited by the size, location and stage of the disease. Future therapeutics that may lead to the improved treatment of advanced head and neck cancer include interstitial laser therapy (ILT) with the Nd:YAG laser. Laser use in the involved tissues leads to an increase in thermal energy at the site. Chemotherapeutic agents, such as cisplatin are activated by this thermal energy and create a more precise and minimally invasive technique to ablate higher-staged or unresectable neoplasms.[149-151]

Photodynamic therapy (PDT) has been proposed as a potential adjuvant treatment of head and neck cancers and pre-cancerous lesions. PDT takes advantage of energy that has been created by the absorption of laser light in that it can induce specifically directed photochemical changes in tissue. Photosensitizers are administered to a patient, accumulate in targeted tissues and undergo light-induced chemical reactions that may lead to selective tissue necrosis and cell death. To date, in the field of otolaryngology, photodynamic therapy has been attempted in patients with soft palate squamous cell carcinoma, recurrent nasopharyngeal carcinoma and laryngeal papillomatosis. Dosing and distribution of the photosensitizer has been difficult to track and quantify. Additionally, patients may experience symptoms of overstimulation such as anaphylaxis if exposed to daylight or neon light during treatment. However, the pilot studies show potentially promising results.[152-159]

Rhinology

Indications and Contraindications

- Indications
  - Hereditary hemorrhagic telangiectasia
  - Recurrent epistaxis
  - Functional endoscopic sinus surgery
  - Rhinophyma
  - Choanal atresia
  - Chronic nasal obstruction
- Contraindications
  - Refractory epistaxis
  - Large sinonasal tumors

The area in which lasers are most commonly and successfully used in nasal surgery are in patients who have persistent recurrent epistaxis due to intranasal hereditary hemorrhagic telangiectasias (HHT). HHT is an autosomal dominant condition of the vascular tissue that presents in a person at the ages of 20–40. Friable angiodysplastic lesions that easily bleed and are millimeters in size can present anywhere, but often are located on the mucosa of the nasal cavity, tongue, lips and cheeks. Patients frequently present with epistaxis as the first sign of the disease.[160]

Other areas of rhinology that are utilizing lasers, albeit in a limited fashion, include functional endoscopic sinus surgery (FESS), rhinophyma reduction, inferior nasal turbinate reduction, choanal atresia and laser cartilage reshaping.

Choanal atresia can be either bilateral or unilateral. Bilateral conditions are typically addressed within the first few days of life because the neonate is unable to breath via his or her nares due to the closed nasal passages. This obstruction can be remedied with laser ablation.[161-163] Hyperplastic inferior nasal turbinates can cause uncomfortable nasal congestion, a closed nasal airway and obligate oral breathing that may lead to obstructive sleep apnea and snoring. Along with LAUP described above, some patients may also undergo laser reduction of the inferior turbinates with a KTP, Nd:YAG or Ho:YAG laser.[164-169]

Contraindications of laser use in nasal surgery include refractory nasal epistaxis and large sinonasal tumors. A relative contraindication is the presence of severe recurrent bilateral nasal epistaxis and its simultaneous treatment. Laser cauterization of bilateral septal lesions may lead to necrosis of the septum and the creation of a septal perforation.

Techniques

- Pre-Operative Management
- Description of Technique
  - Hereditary hemorrhagic telangiectasia
  - Functional endoscopic sinus surgery (FESS)
  - Rhinophyma
  - Choanal atresia
- Post-Operative Management

Pre-operative Management

Patients with chronic recurrent epistaxis undergo a thorough work-up for coagulopathic disease prior to surgery. A full history and physical are performed which includes looking for cutaneous and intra-oral telangiectasias that may need to be addressed. Prior to undergoing FESS, patients obtain a computerized tomography (CT) scan of the paranasal sinuses to determine the extent of the disease and for anatomic surgical planning.

Technique

In HHT, the argon, KTP(Nd:YAG), and more recently, diode lasers can be used to photocoagulate these telangiectasias. Low power settings are used for each laser wavelength so that irradiation creates blanching and coagulation of the lesion. While patients often report improvement after one treatment, recurrent treatments are often necessary and more often the rule rather than the exception. Lasers can also be used in recurrent epistaxis due to other causes, and the most frequent site of bleeding in patients without HHT is Kiesselbach's plexus, located on the anterior septum. Figure 12 illustrates the use of a KTP(Nd:YAG) laser and side-firing fiber aimed at a telangectasia on the anterior nasal septum.[170-175]

Functional endoscopic sinus surgery is a procedure that is performed most commonly in patients with chronic sinusitis or nasal polyposis. Caution must be observed when working within the paranasal sinuses because of the close proximity to the globe, optic nerve, carotid arteries and skull

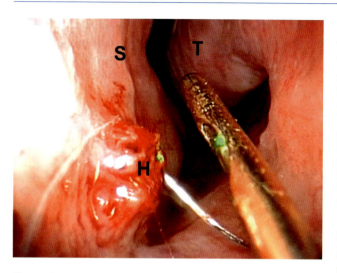

Fig. 12 Laser vaporization and hemostasis of a Hereditary Hemorrhagic Telangiectasia (H) along the septum (S). The inferior turbinate (T) can be seen along the lateral wall of the nasal cavity (Photograph provided courtesy of Dr. Brian Wong)

base. When compared to cold or hot steel techniques in rhinophyma reduction, laser use leads to less intraoperative and postoperative bleeding, easier procedures and less discomfort.[176,177]

Unilateral choanal atresia is often treated anywhere from several weeks after birth up to age 12. After the atretic area is opened, a nasal stent is placed and left in for weeks to months. The KTP(Nd:YAG) and the Holmium:YAG lasers have been used to treat this condition. While the CO_2 laser was the first to be described, it has fallen out of favor for this application due to the challenge of inserting a relatively large handpiece into the posterior nasal cavity. Reports have found lasers to be beneficial in the treatment of choanal atresia due to the decreased rates of re-obstruction and diminished risk of complications associated with the procedure.[161-163]

Adverse Events

- Nasal septal perforation
- Need for re-operation
- Synechiae

Side Effects/Complications/Prevention

A possible complication of laser treatment of hereditary hemorrhagic telangiectasias is the creation of a nasal septal perforation. To avoid this, laser irradiation is not targeted on adjacent septal surfaces in the left and right nasal cavity simultaneously, and treatment may be broken up into multiple separate operations. In any intranasal procedure in which a laser is used, stenosis due to scarring or synechiae may occur, this can be prevented by conservative use of the laser when treating adjacent septal and lateral nasal wall lesions.

Future Directions

- Laser cartilage reshaping

Laser use in surgery involving the septum has thus far been limited due to the potential risk of septal perforation. Ablative procedures have been performed and work well for septal spurs and other obstructive deformities.[178] Recently, laser cartilage reshaping (LCR) has been developed as a non-ablative way to reshape nasal septal deformities. The benefits of laser use in reshaping the cartilage of the ear in otoplasty has also been explored.[179] LCR involves the use of photo-thermal heating both the septal mucosal and cartilage without the need for incisions. In laser cartilage reshaping, specimens are held in mechanical deformation and then heated using laser radiation. Heat generation accelerates the process of mechanical stress relaxation, which allows tissue to remain in stable new shapes and geometries. Although the mechanisms underlying laser cartilage reshaping have not been completely identified, numerous animal studies have investigated the various biophysical mechanisms underlying shape change, and this method is showing great promise in the field of otolaryngology.[180,181]

Pediatric Otolaryngology

Indications and Contraindications

- Indications
  - Laryngomalacia
  - Subglottic hemangioma
  - Juvenile onset recurrent respiratory papillomatosis
  - Choanal atresia
  - Vallecular Cyst
- Contraindications
  - Congenital subglottic stenosis

As discussed previously, choanal atresia is a condition present in neonates that can be treated by using a laser directed toward the imperforate area. The treatment of juvenile onset recurrent respiratory papillomatosis with a CO_2 laser has also been described in a previous section.[182] Other conditions that are present in the neonate and pediatric populations that may be treated with a laser include laryngomalacia, vallecular cysts, subglottic stenosis and subglottic hemangioma.

Laryngomalacia most often presents in the neonate as "noisy breathing". The classification falls under three types. Type I is the most common and least serious. It is characterized by the intermittent prolapse of redundant supraglottic mucosa. Type II laryngomalacia is defined by shortened aryepiglottic folds, and type III is identified by a posteriorly displaced epiglottis. Types I and II can be treated with a CO_2 laser.

Congenital subglottic stenosis is the membranous or cartilaginous narrowing of the larynx at the cricoid area without previous intubation or trauma and may present with biphasic stridor, dyspnea, recurrent croup or other airway difficulties during the first few months of life. The use of the carbon dioxide laser to treat congenital subglottic stenosis is mostly historical due the development of restenosis at the initial site or at a more distal site. In Fig. 13a, the airway obstruction produced by the stenotic airway segment (subglottis) is readily apparent. The CO_2 laser was used to excise portions of this obstructive lesion to improve airway patency (Fig. 13b).[183-186] Vallecular cysts may also present with noisy breathing and airway obstruction. Their etiology is unknown. Laser excision of vallecular cysts (Fig. 14a) is routinely practiced with a high success rate. Typically, a CO_2 laser is used to cut the margins of the cyst, facilitating either removal or marsupialization (Fig.14 b).

Subglottic hemangioma presents in a similar fashion to subglottic stenosis with stridor, hoarseness, cough, failure to thrive secondary to dysphagia and cyanosis. Cutaneous hemangiomas are present in 50% of patients with subglottic disease, and therefore suspicion should be high in any patient with these symptoms and a history of a cutaneous lesion. A subglottic hemangioma enlarges rapidly as it undergoes proliferation. It appears as a smooth spherical and often blue-hued mass on the subglottic wall (Fig.15a). They present twice as often in girls compared to boys and are typically diagnosed in the first few months of life. While they do spontaneously involute, subglottic hemangiomas have a potential for airway obstruction. To prevent airway compromise, aggressive treatment is warranted, and the laser plays an integral role in this.

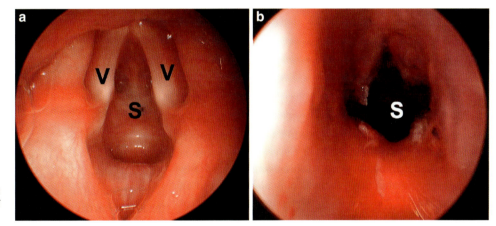

Fig. 13 Subglottic stenosis (S) in a pediatric patient before (**a**) and after laser excision from a subglottic view (**b**). *V* vocal cords (Photograph provided courtesy of Dr. Gupreet S. Ahuja)

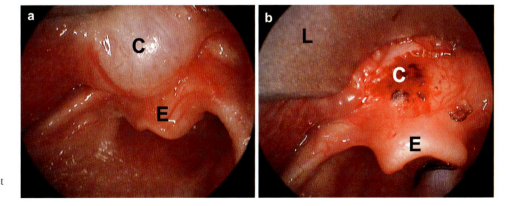

Fig. 14 Vallecular cyst (C) in a pediatric patient before (**a**) and after (**b**) laser excision. *E* epiglottis, *L* Blade of laryngoscope (Photograph provided courtesy of Dr. Gupreet S. Ahuja)

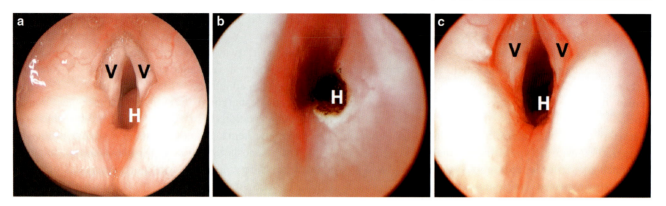

Fig. 15 Subglottic Hemangioma (H) in a pediatric patient before (**a**), after laser excision from a subglottic view (**b**) and after laser excision from a supraglottic view (**c**). Note how the airway has increased patency and that the lesion was not circumferential. *V* vocal cords (Photograph provided courtesy of Dr. Gupreet S. Ahuja)

Techniques

- Pre-Operative Management
- Description of Technique
  - Laryngomalacia
  - Subglottic hemangioma
- Post-Operative Management

Pre-operative Management

Laryngomalacia in a neonate is most often diagnosed using flexible fiberoptic laryngoscopy. Some neonatess might require nasogastric tube feedings due to the risk of aspiration that is associated with this condition. Severe laryngomalacia may necessitate intubation while awaiting surgery due to frequent oxygen desaturations. Patients may also be placed on peri-operative H2 blockers or proton pump inhibitors for treatment of gastroesophageal reflux disease, a frequent co-morbid condition.

Techniques

In type I laryngomalacia, the CO_2 laser is used to perform a supraglottoplasty and excise or reduce the aryepiglottic folds. Type II laryngomalacia may be treated by using the CO_2 laser to divide the aryepiglottic folds.[185,187,188]

The CO_2, Nd:YAG and KTP(Nd:YAG) lasers have been suggested as possible methods to remove hemangiomas in the subglottis (Fig. 15a) due to their ability to excise and coagulate these vascular lesions. The KTP(Nd:YAG) laser is favored in this application because it is more easily delivered to the area via flexible fiberoptics and is readily absorbed by hemoglobin. Figure 15b is an image of the subglottic region after laser treatment of a hemangioma. Figure 15c is a panoramic image of the larynx showing both the supra- and subglottic airway after the hemangioma was removed. Most treatment methods produce some degree of subglottic stenosis. However, the stenosis grade is typically mild such that patients are asymptomatic and do not require tracheotomy.[184-186,189-191]

Post-operative Management

All pediatric patients who undergo laser surgery of the airway are sent to the pediatric or neonatal intensive care unit post-operatively for airway observation. Whereas patients who undergo subglottic hemangioma excision via an open approach often receive a tracheostomy, those in whom a laser is used for ablation often do not. Steroids are given to reduce the formation of edema in the airway mucosa. Frequent serial examination with flexible fiberoptic laryngoscopy is performed to monitor for supraglottic edema, stenosis and hemangioma recurrence.

Adverse Events

- Tracheal stenosis
- Tracheal granulomas
- Airway compromise
- Aspiration
- Pneumonia
- Subcutaneous emphysema
- Mediastinitis
- Malnutrition

Side Effects/Complications

Possible adverse events that may occur when treating both laryngomalacia and subglottic hemangiomas include tracheal stenosis, granuloma formation and airway compromise. All of these events may lead to intubation of the patient post-operatively and in extreme circumstances, tracheostomy is necessary. Other complications include aspiration, pneumonia, subcutaneous emphysema, bleeding that may require re-exploration and mediastinitis. Additionally, subglottic hemangiomas or stenosis may recur post-operatively. In the immediate post-operative period, patients may experience dysphagia leading to malnutrition and require a feeding tube for supplementary alimentation.

Prevention of Side Effects/Complications

Tracheal stenosis may be prevented by performing excision of subglottic lesions in a quadrant approach thereby minimizing the chance of circumferential scar formation. An airway emergency is prevented by preparation and monitoring in an ICU setting post-operatively. To prevent aspiration and malnutrition, a prophylactic nasogastric feeding tube is placed intra-operatively and remains in place until the patient demonstrates safe and adequate consumption of food and drink.

Future Directions

- Laser myringotomy
- Cholesteatoma Excision

Both laser myringotomy and cholesteatoma excision hare been described in previous sections. Laser myringotomy with or without placement of pressure equalization tubes under local anesthesia will reduce the risk of general anesthesia that is typically employed in this procedure. Laser use in creating a myringotomy may also decrease the incidence of tube plugging, persistent bleeding and other complications associated with this procedure. However, these observations have yet to be demonstrated in a large randomized prospective study. Cholesteatoma excision may be assisted routinely by the use of lasers in the areas that are anatomically difficult to access.

Conclusion

- Laser safety
- Laryngology
- Otology

- Oropharyngeal surgery
- Rhinology
- Pediatric otolaryngology

Laser applications in otolaryngology – head and neck surgery are extensive and diverse. While most commonly used in laryngology and otology, laser applications are being developed for use in all areas of the head and neck including oropharynx, nose, paranasal sinuses, cranial base, and in the pediatric population. As new devices and delivery systems are developed, new applications will evolve. One element that is critical in all areas of application is laser safety, and this should take the utmost importance when planning and undertaking any procedure. Lasers are used to treat both malignant and benign laryngeal diseases ranging from cancer to vocal cord paralysis. Middle ear applications have focused on primarily treating otosclerotic disease (stapes surgery), though in recent times new applications include the treatment of Eustachian tube dysfunction and cholesteatoma. Lasers are used to excise tumors in the oropharynx and oral cavity because they precisely cut and coagulate tissue. In rhinology, treatment of hereditary hemorrhagic telangiectasias is commonplace and an elegant example of laser therapy for noncutaneous vascular lesions. In children, the laser may be used to ablate subglottic hemangiomas, correct laryngomalacia and excise atretic choanae. Laser applications in otolaryngology continually develop and evolve, and a plethora of new devices, procedures and applications are emerging each year.

References

1. Jacques SL. Role of tissue optics and pulse duration on tissue effects during high-power laser irradiation. *Appl Opt.* 1993;32:2447-2454.
2. Ries WR. Cutaneous applications of lasers. *Otolaryngol Clin North Am.* 1996;29(6):915-930.
3. Janda P, Sroka R, Mundweil B, Betz CS, Baumgartner R, Leunig A. Comparison of thermal tissue effects induced by contact application of fiber guided laser systems. *Lasers Surg Med.* 2003;33(2):93-101.
4. Vagnetti A, Gobbi E, Algieri GM, D'Ambrosio L. Wedge turbinectomy: a new combined photocoagulative Nd:YAG laser technique. *Laryngoscope.* 2000;110(6):1034-1036.
5. Brown DH. The versatile contact Nd:YAG laser in head and neck surgery: an in vivo and clinical analysis. *Laryngoscope.* 2000;110(5 Pt 1):854-867.
6. Midgley HC 3rd. Nd:YAG contact laser surgery. The scalpel of the future? *Otolaryngol Clin North Am.* 1990;23(1):99-105.
7. Li ZZ, Reinisch L, Van de Merwe WP. Bone ablation with Er:YAG and CO_2 laser: study of thermal and acoustic effects. *Lasers Surg Med.* 1992;12(1):79-85.
8. Garrett CG, Ossoff RH, Reinisch L. Laser Surgery: basic principles and safety considerations. In: Cummings CW, Flint PW, Haughey BH, Robbins KT, Thomas JR, Harker LA, Richardson MA, Schuller DE,

editors. *Cummings Otolaryngology: Head and Neck Surgery.* 4th ed. Philadelphia: Elsevier Mosby; 2005.

9. Reinisch L. Laser physics and tissue interactions. *Otolaryngol Clin North Am.* 1996;29(6):893-914.

10. Philipp CM, Berlien HP. Basic principles of medical laser technology. In: Huttenbrink K, ed. *Lasers in Otorhinolaryngology.* New York: Thieme; 2005:1-20.

11. Ossoff RH, Karlan MS. Safe instrumentation in laser surgery. *Otolaryngol Head Neck Surg.* 1984;92(6):644-648.

12. Ossoff R. Laser safety in otolaryngology – head and neck surgery: anesthetic and educational considerations for laryngeal surgery. *Laryngoscope.* 1989;99(8):1-26.

13. Foth H-J. Endotracheal tubes for laser surgery: temperature rise and clinical experiences. *SPIE Proc Med Appl Lasers III.* 1996;2623:522-529.

14. Ungemach J. New laser tracheal tube. *SPIE Proc Lasers Med Dent Diagn Treat.* 1996;2887:129-132.

15. Foth HJ. Laser resistance of endotracheal tubes I: experimental results of a compound tube in comparison to a metallic tube. *Lasers Med Sci.* 1998;13(4):242-252.

16. Foth HJ. Laser resistance of endotracheal tubes II: observed temperature rise and theoretical explanation. *Lasers Med Sci.* 1999;14(1):24-31.

17. Strong MS, Jako GJ. Laser surgery in the larynx. Early clinical experience with continuous CO_2 laser. *Ann Otol Rhinol Laryngol.* 1972;81(6):791-798.

18. Strong MS, Jako GJ, Polanyi T, Wallace RA. Laser surgery in the aerodigestive tract. *Am J Surg.* 1973;126(4):529-533.

19. Steiner W, Ambrosch P. *Endoscopic Laser Surgery of the Upper Aerodigestive Tract.* Stuttgart: Thieme; 2000.

20. Oswal VH. *Laser Surgery for Benign Laryngeal Pathology.* The Hague: Kugler Publications; 2002.

21. Steiner W. Experience in endoscopic laser surgery of malignant tumours of the upper aero-digestive tract. *Adv Otorhinolaryngol.* 1988;39:135-144.

22. Pearson BW, Salassa JR, Hinni ML. Transoral laser micro resection of advanced laryngeal tumors. In: Cummings CW, Flint PW, Haughey BH, Robbins KT, Thomas JR, Harker LA, Richardson MA, Schuller DE, editors. *Cummings Otolaryngology: Head and Neck Surgery.* 4th ed. Philadelphia: Elsevier Mosby; 2005.

23. Rudert H. Larynx and hypopharynx cancers – endoscopic surgery with laser: possibilities and limits. *Arch Otorhinolaryngol Suppl.* 1991;1:3-18.

24. Eckel HE, Thumfart WF. Laser surgery for the treatment of larynx carcinomas: indications, techniques, and preliminary results. *Ann Otol Rhinol Laryngol.* 1992;101(2 Pt 1):113-118.

25. Steiner W, Pfalz R. Laser surgery. *HNO.* 1993;41(8):A19-A20.

26. Motta G, Esposito E, Cassiano B, Motta S. T1-T2-T3 glottic tumors: fifteen years experience with CO_2 laser. *Acta Otolaryngol Suppl.* 1997;527:155-159.

27. Ambrosch P, Kron M, Steiner W. Carbon dioxide laser microsurgery for early supraglottic carcinoma. *Ann Otol Rhinol Laryngol.* 1998;107(8):680-688.

28. Zeitels SM, Davis RK. Endoscopic laser management of supraglottic cancer. *Am J Otolaryngol.* 1995;16(1):2-11.

29. Zeitels SM. Surgical management of early supraglottic cancer. *Otolaryngol Clin North Am.* 1997;30(1):59-78.

30. Davis RK, Kelly SM, Hayes J. Endoscopic CO_2 laser excisional biopsy of early supraglottic cancer. *Laryngoscope.* 1991;101(6 Pt 1):680-683.

31. Eckel HE. Endoscopic laser resection of supraglottic carcinoma. *Otolaryngol Head Neck Surg.* 1997;117(6):681-687.

32. Iro H, Waldfahrer F, Altendorf-Hofmann A, Weidenbecher M, Sauer R, Steiner W. Transoral laser surgery of supraglottic cancer: follow-up of 141 patients. *Arch Otolaryngol Head Neck Surg.* 1998;124(11):1245-1250.

33. Rudert HH, Werner JA, Hoft S. Transoral carbon dioxide laser resection of supraglottic carcinoma. *Ann Otol Rhinol Laryngol.* 1999;108(9):819-827.

34. Vaughan CW. Transoral laryngeal surgery using the CO_2 laser: laboratory experiments and clinical experience. *Laryngoscope.* 1978;88(9 Pt 1):1399-1420.

35. Vaughan CW, Strong MS, Jako GJ. Laryngeal carcinoma: transoral treatment utilizing the CO_2 laser. *Am J Surg.* 1978;136(4):490-493.

36. Laccourreye O, Lawson G, Muscatello L, Biacabe B, Laccourreye L, Brasnu D. Carbon dioxide laser debulking for obstructing endolaryngeal carcinoma: a 10-year experience. *Ann Otol Rhinol Laryngol.* 1999;108(5):490-494.

37. Eckel HE. Lasers for benign diseases of the larynx, hypopharynx and trachea. In: Huttenbrink K, ed. *Lasers in Otorhinolaryngology.* New York: Thieme; 2005:96-105.

38. Koufman JA, Rees CJ, Frazier WD, et al. Office-based laryngeal laser surgery: a review of 443 cases using three wavelengths. *Otolaryngol Head Neck Surg.* 2007;137(1):146-151.

39. Pransky SM, Canto C. Management of subglottic hemangioma. *Curr Opin Otolaryngol Head Neck Surg.* 2004;12(6):509-512.

40. Waner MaSJID. *Hemangiomas and Vascular Malformations of the Head and Neck.* New York: Wiley; 1999.

41. Crumley RL. Endoscopic laser medial arytenoidectomy for airway management in bilateral laryngeal paralysis. *Ann Otol Rhinol Laryngol.* 1993;102(2):81-84.

42. Werner JA. *Transoral Laryngeal Surgery.* Tuttlingen: Endo-Press; 2004.

43. Zeitels SM, Franco RA Jr, Dailey SH, Burns JA, Hillman RE, Anderson RR. Office-based treatment of glottal dysplasia and papillomatosis with the 585-nm pulsed dye laser and local anesthesia. *Ann Otol Rhinol Laryngol.* 2004;113(4):265-276.

44. Killian G. Die schwebelaryngoskopie. *Arch Laryngol Rhinol.* 1912;26:277-317.

45. Braun M. Intense pulsed light versus advanced fluorescent technology pulsed light for photodamaged skin: a split-face pilot comparison. *J Drugs Dermatol.* 2007;6(10):1024-1028.

46. Courey MS, Ossoff RH. Laser applications in adult laryngeal surgery. *Otolaryngol Clin North Am.* 1996;29(6):973-986.

47. Cheon MS, Juhn JW, Hwang YS. Design of stark-tuned far-infrared laser with circular hollow waveguide. *Appl Opt.* 2006;45(27):7131-7136.

48. Narita S, Matsuura Y, Miyagi M. Tapered hollow waveguide for focusing infrared laser beams. *Opt Lett.* 2007;32(8):930-932.

49. Sato S, Shi YW, Matsuura Y, Miyagi M, Ashida H. Hollow-waveguide-based nanosecond, near-infrared pulsed laser ablation of tissue. *Lasers Surg Med.* 2005;37(2):149-154.

50. Soljacic M, Ibanescu M, Johnson SG, Joannopoulos JD, Fink Y. Optical bistability in axially modulated OmniGuide fibers. *Opt Lett.* 2003;28(7):516-518.

51. Stalmashonak A, Zhavoronkov N, Hertel IV, Vetrov S, Schmid K. Spatial control of femtosecond laser system output with submicroradian accuracy. *Appl Opt.* 2006;45(6):1271-1274.

52. Steiner W, Ambrosch P, Hess CF, Kron M. Organ preservation by transoral laser microsurgery in piriform sinus carcinoma. *Otolaryngol Head Neck Surg.* 2001;124(1):58-67.

53. Steiner W, Fierek O, Ambrosch P, Hommerich CP, Kron M. Transoral laser microsurgery for squamous cell carcinoma of the base of the tongue. *Arch Otolaryngol Head Neck Surg.* 2003;129(1):36-43.

54. Brandenburg JH. Laser cordotomy versus radiotherapy: an objective cost analysis. *Ann Otol Rhinol Laryngol.* 2001;110(4):312-318.

55. Davis RK, Shapshay SM, Strong MS, Hyams VJ. Transoral partial supraglottic resection using the CO_2 laser. *Laryngoscope.* 1983;93(4):429-432.

56. Zeitels SM, Vaughan CW, Domanowski GF. Endoscopic management of early supraglottic cancer. *Ann Otol Rhinol Laryngol.* 1990;99(12):951-956.

57. Klussmann JP, Knoedgen R, Wittekindt C, Damm M, Eckel HE. Complications of suspension laryngoscopy. *Ann Otol Rhinol Laryngol.* 2002;111(11):972-976.

58. Pearson BW, Salassa JR. Transoral laser microresection for cancer of the larynx involving the anterior commissure. *Laryngoscope.* 2003;113(7):1104-1112.

59. Jacobson AS, Woo P, Shapshay SM. Emerging technology: flexible CO_2 laser WaveGuide. *Otolaryngol Head Neck Surg.* 2006;135(3): 469-470.

60. Franco RA Jr, Zeitels SM, Farinelli WA, Faquin W, Anderson RR. 585-nm pulsed dye laser treatment of glottal dysplasia. *Ann Otol Rhinol Laryngol.* 2003;112(9 Pt 1):751-758.

61. Burns JA, Zeitels SM, Akst LM, Broadhurst MS, Hillman RE, Anderson R. 532 nm pulsed potassium-titanyl-phosphate laser treatment of laryngeal papillomatosis under general anesthesia. *Laryngoscope.* 2007;117(8):1500-1504.

62. Zeitels SM, Akst LM, Burns JA, Hillman RE, Broadhurst MS, Anderson RR. Office-based 532-nm pulsed KTP laser treatment of glottal papillomatosis and dysplasia. *Ann Otol Rhinol Laryngol.* 2006;115(9):679-685.

63. Zeitels SM, Anderson RR, Hillman RE, Burns JA. Experience with office-based pulsed-dye laser (PDL) treatment. *Ann Otol Rhinol Laryngol.* 2007;116(4):317-318.

64. Zeitels SM, Burns JA. Office-based laryngeal laser surgery with local anesthesia. *Curr Opin Otolaryngol Head Neck Surg.* 2007; 15(3):141-147.

65. Jovanovic S. Lasers in otology. In: Huttenbrink K, ed. *Lasers in Otorhinolaryngology.* New York: Thieme; 2005:21-52.

66. Chole R. Pathophysiology of otosclerosis. *Otol Neurotol.* 2001;22(2):249-257.

67. Schuknecht H. Cochlear otosclerosis: fact or fantasy. *Laryngoscope.* 1974;84(5):766-782.

68. Perkins R, Curto FS Jr. Laser stapedotomy: a comparative study of prostheses and seals. *Laryngoscope.* 1992;102(12 Pt 1):1321-1327.

69. Perkins RC. Laser stapedotomy for otosclerosis. *Laryngoscope.* 1980;90(2):228-240.

70. Jovanovic S. CO_2 laser stapedotomy with the "one shot" technique – clinical results. *Otolaryngol Head Neck Surg.* 2004;131:750-757.

71. Arnoldner C, Schwab B, Lenarz T. Clinical results after stapedotomy: a comparison between the erbium: yttrium-aluminum-garnet laser and the conventional technique. *Otol Neurotol.* 2006;27(4):458-465.

72. Buchman CA, Fucci MJ, Roberson JB Jr, De La Cruz A. Comparison of argon and CO_2 laser stapedotomy in primary otosclerosis surgery. *Am J Otolaryngol.* 2000;21(4):227-230.

73. Keck T, Burner H, Rettinger G. Prospective clinical study on cochlear function after erbium:yttrium-aluminum-garnet laser stapedotomy. *Laryngoscope.* 2005;115(9):1627-1631.

74. McGee TM. The argon laser in surgery for chronic ear disease and otosclerosis. *Laryngoscope.* 1983;93(9):1177-1182.

75. McGee TM. Laser applications in ossicular surgery. *Otolaryngol Clin North Am.* 1990;23(1):7-18.

76. McGee TM, Diaz-Ordaz EA, Kartush JM. The role of KTP laser in revision stapedectomy. *Otolaryngol Head Neck Surg.* 1993;109(5): 839-843.

77. Poe DS. Laser-assisted endoscopic stapedectomy: a prospective study. *Laryngoscope.* 2000;110(5 Pt 2 Suppl 95):1-37.

78. Sedwick JD, Louden CL, Shelton C. Stapedectomy vs stapedotomy. Do you really need a laser? *Arch Otolaryngol Head Neck Surg.* 1997;123(2):177-180.

79. Silverstein H, Rosenberg S, Jones R. Small fenestra stapedotomies with and without KTP laser: a comparison. *Laryngoscope.* 1989;99(5):485-488.

80. Vernick DM. A comparison of the results of KTP and CO_2 laser stapedotomy. *Am J Otol.* 1996;17(2):221-224.

81. Wiet RJ, Kubek DC, Lemberg P, Byskosh AT. A meta-analysis review of revision stapes surgery with argon laser: effectiveness and safety. *Am J Otol.* 1997;18(2):166-171.

82. Wong BJ, Lee J, Hashisaki GT, Berns MW, Neev J. Thermal imaging of the temporal bone in CO_2 laser surgery: an experimental model. *Otolaryngol Head Neck Surg.* 1997;117(6):610-615.

83. Lesinski SG, Newrock R. Carbon dioxide lasers for otosclerosis. *Otolaryngol Clin North Am.* 1993;26(3):417-441.

84. DiBartolomeo J. The argon laser in otology. *Laryngoscope.* 1980;90:1786-1796.

85. Brodsky L, Cook S, Deutsch E, et al. Optimizing effectiveness of laser tympanic membrane fenestration in chronic otitis media with effusion. Clinical and technical considerations. *Int J Pediatr Otorhinolaryngol.* 2001;58(1):59-64.

86. Deutsch ES, Cook SP, Shaha S, Brodsky L, Reilly JS. Duration of patency of laser-assisted tympanic membrane fenestration. *Arch Otolaryngol Head Neck Surg.* 2003;129(8):825-828.

87. Jassir D, Odabasi O, Gomez-Marin O, Buchman CA. Dose-response relationship of topically applied mitomycin C for the prevention of laser myringotomy closure. *Otolaryngol Head Neck Surg.* 2003;129(5):471-474.

88. Silverstein H, Kuhn J, Choo D, Krespi YP, Rosenberg SI, Rowan PT. Laser-assisted tympanostomy. *Laryngoscope.* 1996;106(9 Pt 1): 1067-1074.

89. Valtonen HJ, Poe DS, Shapshay SM. Experimental CO_2 laser myringotomy. *Otolaryngol Head Neck Surg.* 2001;125(3):161-165.

90. Poe DS, Grimmer JF, Metson R. Laser eustachian tuboplasty: two-year results. *Laryngoscope.* 2007;117(2):231-237.

91. Semaan M. The pathophysiology of cholesteatoma. *Otolaryngol Clin North Am.* 2006;39:1143-1159.

92. Nishizaki K, Yuen K, Ogawa T, Nomiya S, Okano M, Fukushima K. Laser-assisted tympanoplasty for preservation of the ossicular chain in cholesteatoma. *Am J Otolaryngol.* 2001;22(6):424-427.

93. Saeed SR, Jackler RK. Lasers in surgery for chronic ear disease. *Otolaryngol Clin North Am.* 1996;29(2):245-256.

94. Jacques S. Time-resolved propagation of ultra-short laser pulses within turbid tissues. *Appl Opt.* 1989;28:2223-2229.

95. Anderson R, Beck H, Bruggemann U, Farinelli W, Jacques SL, Parrish JA. Pulsed photothermal radiometry in turbid media: internal reflection of back-scattered radiation strongly influences optical dosimetry. *Appl Opt.* 1989;28:2256-2262.

96. Gherini S, Horn KL, Causse JB, McArthur GR. Fiberoptic argon laser stapedotomy: is it safe? *Am J Otol.* 1993;14(3):283-289.

97. Gherini S, Horn KL. Laser stapedotomies. *Laryngoscope.* 1990; 100(2 Pt 1):209-211.

98. Pfalz R, Hibst R, Bald N. Suitability of different lasers for operations ranging from the tympanic membrane to the base of the stapes. *Adv Otorhinolaryngol.* 1995;49:87-94.

99. Lesinski SG. Lasers for otosclerosis – which one if any and why. *Lasers Surg Med.* 1990;10(5):448-457.

100. Brodsky L, Brookhauser P, Chait D, et al. Office-based insertion of pressure equalization tubes: the role of laser-assisted tympanic membrane fenestration. *Laryngoscope.* 1999;109(12):2009-2014.

101. Gerlinger I, Rath G, Szanyi I, Pytel J. Myringoplasty for anterior and subtotal perforations using KTP-532 laser. *Eur Arch Otorhinolaryngol.* 2006;263(9):816-819.

102. Kakehata S, Futai K, Sasaki A, Shinkawa H. Endoscopic transtympanic tympanoplasty in the treatment of conductive hearing loss: early results. *Otol Neurotol.* 2006;27(1):14-19.

103. Pyykko I, Poe D, Ishizaki H. Laser-assisted myringoplasty – technical aspects. *Acta Otolaryngol Suppl.* 2000;543:135-138.

104. Nissen AJ, Sikand A, Welsh JE, Curto FS. Use of the KTP-532 laser in acoustic neuroma surgery. *Laryngoscope.* 1997;107(1):118-121.

105. Glasscock ME 3rd, Jackson CG, Whitaker SR. The argon laser in acoustic tumor surgery. *Laryngoscope.* 1981;91(9 Pt 1):1405-1416.

106. Adamczyk M, Antonelli PJ. Selective vestibular ablation by KTP laser in endolymphatic hydrops. *Laryngoscope.* 2001;111(6): 1057-1062.

107. Anthony PF. Laser applications in inner ear surgery. *Otolaryngol Clin North Am.* 1996;29(6):1031-1048.

108. Antonelli PJ, Lundy LB, Kartush JM, Burgio DL, Graham MD. Mechanical versus CO_2 laser occlusion of the posterior semicircular canal in humans. *Am J Otol.* 1996;17(3):416-420.

109. Nomura Y. Argon laser irradiation of the semicircular canal in two patients with benign paroxysmal positional vertigo. *J Laryngol Otol.* 2002;116(9):723-725.

110. Kelly J. Laser decompression of the facial nerve. *Otolaryngol Clin North Am.* 1996;29(6):1049-1061.

111. Vernick MD. Laser applications in ossicular surgery. *Otolaryngol Clin North Am.* 1996;29(6):931-941.

112. Wilson L, Lin E, Lalwani A. Cost-effectiveness of intraoperative facial nerve monitoring in middle ear or mastoid surgery. *Laryngoscope.* 2003;113(10):1736-1745.

113. Wiegand DA, Mertz PS, Latz B. Detection of intraoperative laser injury to the facial nerve by electromyographic monitoring of facial muscles. *Laryngoscope.* 1991;101(7 Pt 1):771-774.

114. Kujawski OB, Poe DS. Laser eustachian tuboplasty. *Otol Neurotol.* 2004;25(1):1-8.

115. Ambrosch P. Lasers for malignant lesions in the upper aerodigestive tract. In: Huttenbrink K, ed. *Lasers in Otorhinolaryngology.* New York: Thieme; 2005:131-134.

116. Burkey BB, Garrett G. Use of the laser in the oral cavity. *Otolaryngol Clin North Am.* 1996;29(6):949-972.

117. Davis RK. Laser surgery for oral cavity and oropharyngeal cancer. In: Davis RK, ed. *Lasers in Otolaryngology: Head and Neck Surgery.* Philadelphia: Saunders Company; 1990:132-144.

118. Eckel HE, Volling P, Pototschnig C, Zorowka P, Thumfart W. Transoral laser resection with staged discontinuous neck dissection for oral cavity and oropharynx squamous cell carcinoma. *Laryngoscope.* 1995;105(1):53-60.

119. Schuller DE. Use of the laser in the oral cavity. *Otolaryngol Clin North Am.* 1990;23(1):31-42.

120. Carruth JA. Resection of the tongue with the carbon dioxide laser: 100 cases. *J Laryngol Otol.* 1985;99(9):887-889.

121. Duncavage JA, Ossoff RH. Use of the CO_2 laser for malignant disease of the oral cavity. *Lasers Surg Med.* 1986;6(5):442-444.

122. Strong MS, Vaughan CW, Jako GJ, Polanyi T. Transoral resection of cancer of the oral cavity: the role of the CO_2 laser. *Otolaryngol Clin North Am.* 1979;12(1):207-218.

123. Stevens RH, Davis RK. Laser surgery for benign conditions in the oral cavity. In: RK Davis, ed. *Lasers in Otolaryngology: Head and Neck Surgery.* Philadelphia: Saunders Company; 1990:121-131.

124. Ducic Y, Marsan J, Olberg B, Marsan S, Maclachlan L, Lamothe A. Comparison of laser-assisted uvulopalatopharyngoplasty to electrocautery-assisted uvulopalatopharyngoplasty: a clinical and pathologic correlation in an animal model. *J Otolaryngol.* 1996;25(4):234-238.

125. Han S, Kern RC. Laser-assisted uvulopalatoplasty in the management of snoring and obstructive sleep apnea syndrome. *Minerva Med.* 2004;95(4):337-345.

126. Hanada T, Furuta S, Tateyama T, Uchizono A, Seki D, Ohyama M. Laser-assisted uvulopalatoplasty with Nd:YAG laser for sleep disorders. *Laryngoscope.* 1996;106(12 Pt 1):1531-1533.

127. Krespi YP, Kacker A. Laser-assisted uvulopalatoplasty revisited. *Otolaryngol Clin North Am.* 2003;36(3):495-500.

128. Laranne J, Lagerstedt A, Pukander J, Rantala I, Hanamure Y, Ohyama M. Immediate histological changes in soft palate after uvulopalatopharyngoplasty with CO_2, contact Nd:YAG or combined CO_2 and Nd:YAG laser beams. *Acta Otolaryngol Suppl.* 1997;529:206-209.

129. Terris DJ. Comparing uvulopalatopharyngoplasty and laser-assisted uvulopalatoplasty. *Arch Otolaryngol Head Neck Surg.* 1997;123(3):278-279.

130. Terris DJ, Wang MZ. Laser-assisted uvulopalatoplasty in mild obstructive sleep apnea. *Arch Otolaryngol Head Neck Surg.* 1998;124(6):718-720.

131. Vaidya AM, Petruzzelli GJ, Walker RP, McGee D, Gopalsami C. Identifying obstructive sleep apnea in patients presenting for laser-assisted uvulopalatoplasty. *Laryngoscope.* 1996;106(4):431-437.

132. Fujita S, Woodson BT, Clark JL, Wittig R. Laser midline glossectomy as a treatment for obstructive sleep apnea. *Laryngoscope.* 1991;101(8):805-809.

133. Bier-Laning, Adams GL. Patterns of recurrence after carbon dioxide laser excision of intraoral squamous cell carcinoma. *Arch Otolaryngol Head Neck Surg.* 1995;121:1239-1244.

134. Panje WR, Scher NN, Karnell M. Transoral carbon dioxide laser ablation for cancer, tumors and other diseases. *Arch Otolaryngol Head Neck Surg.* 1989;115:681-688.

135. Williams SR, Carruth JA. The role of the carbon dioxide laser in treatment of carcinoma of the tongue. *J Laryngol Otol.* 1988;102(12):1122-1123.

136. Wang CP, Chang SY, Wu JD, Tai SK. Carbon dioxide laser microsurgery for tongue cancer: surgical techniques and long-term results. *J Otolaryngol.* 2001;30(1):19-23.

137. Strong MS, Vaughan CW, Healy GB, Shapshay SM, Jako GJ. Transoral management of localized carcinoma of the oral cavity using the CO_2 laser. *Laryngoscope.* 1979;89(6 Pt 1):897-905.

138. Ben-Bassat M, Kaplan I, Shindel Y, Edlan A. The CO_2 laser in surgery of the tongue. *Br J Plast Surg.* 1978;31(2):155-156.

139. Ishii J, Fujita K, Komori T. Clinical assessment of laser monotherapy for squamous cell carcinoma of the mobile tongue. *J Clin Laser Med Surg.* 2002;20(2):57-61.

140. Riley RW, Powell NB, Li KK, Weaver EM, Guilleminault C. An adjunctive method of radiofrequency volumetric tissue reduction of the tongue for OSAS. *Otolaryngol Head Neck Surg.* 2003;129(1):37-42.

141. Powell NB, Zonato AI, Weaver EM, et al. Radiofrequency treatment of turbinate hypertrophy in subjects using continuous positive airway pressure: a randomized, double-blind, placebo-controlled clinical pilot trial. *Laryngoscope.* 2001;111(10):1783-1790.

142. Li KK, Powell NB, Riley RW, Troell RJ, Guilleminault C. Radiofrequency volumetric reduction of the palate: an extended follow-up study. *Otolaryngol Head Neck Surg.* 2000;122(3):410-414.

143. Chang CW, Burkey BB, Netterville JL, Courey MS, Garrett CG, Bayles SW. Carbon dioxide laser endoscopic diverticulotomy versus open diverticulectomy for Zenker's diverticulum. *Laryngoscope.* 2004;114(3):519-527.

144. Lippert BM, Folz BJ, Rudert HH, Werner JA. Management of Zenker's diverticulum and postlaryngectomy pseudodiverticulum with the CO_2 laser. *Otolaryngol Head Neck Surg.* 1999; 121(6):809-814.

145. Frame JW, Morgan D, Rhys-Evans PH. Tongue resection with the CO_2 laser: the effects of past radiotherapy on postoperative complications. *Br J Oral Maxillofac Surg.* 1988;26:464-471.

146. Christiansen H, Hermann RM, Martin A, et al. Long-term follow-up after transoral laser microsurgery and adjuvant radiotherapy for advanced recurrent squamous cell carcinoma of the head and neck. *Int J Radiat Oncol Biol Phys.* 2006;65(4):1067-1074.

147. Miller FR, Bartley J, Otto RA. The endoscopic management of Zenker diverticulum: CO_2 laser versus endoscopic stapling. *Laryngoscope.* 2006;116(9):1608-1611.

148. Zbaren P, Schar P, Tschopp L, Becker M, Hausler R. Surgical treatment of Zenker's diverticulum: transcutaneous diverticulectomy versus microendoscopic myotomy of the cricopharyngeal muscle with CO_2 laser. *Otolaryngol Head Neck Surg.* 1999; 121(4):482-487.

149. Luukkaa M, Aitasalo K, Pulkkinen J, Lindholm P, Valavaara R, Grenman R. Neodymium YAG contact laser in the treatment of cancer of the mobile tongue. *Acta Otolaryngol.* 2002;122(3):318-322.

150. Paiva MB, Blackwell KE, Saxton RE, et al. Nd:YAG laser therapy for palliation of recurrent squamous cell carcinomas in the oral cavity. *Lasers Surg Med.* 2002;31(1):64-69.

151. Graeber IP, Eshraghi AA, Paiva MB, et al. Combined intratumor cisplatinum injection and Nd:YAG laser therapy. *Laryngoscope.* 1999;109(3):447-454.

152. Biel MA. Photodynamic therapy and the treatment of head and neck cancers. *J Clin Laser Med Surg.* 1996;14(5):239-244.

153. Biel MA. Photodynamic therapy in head and neck cancer. *Curr Oncol Rep.* 2002;4(1):87-96.

154. D'Cruz AK, Robinson MH, Biel MA. mTHPC-mediated photodynamic therapy in patients with advanced, incurable head and neck cancer: a multicenter study of 128 patients. *Head Neck.* 2004;26(3):232-240.

155. Biel M. Advances in photodynamic therapy for the treatment of head and neck cancers. *Lasers Surg Med.* 2006;38(5):349-355.

156. Mioc S, Mycek MA. Selected laser-based therapies in otolaryngology. *Otolaryngol Clin North Am.* 2005;38(2):241-254.

157. Essex RW, Qureshi SH, Cain MS, Harper CA, Guymer RH. Photodynamic therapy in practice: a review of the results of the first 12 months experience with verteporfin at the Royal Victorian Eye and Ear Hospital. *Clin Exp Ophthalmol.* 2003;31(6):476-481.

158. Ofner JG, Schlogl H, Kostron H. Unusual adverse reaction in a patient sensitized with Photosan 3. *J Photochem Photobiol B.* 1996;36(2):183-184.

159. Davis RK. Photodynamic therapy in otolaryngology-head and neck surgery. *Otolaryngol Clin North Am.* 1990;23(1):107-119.

160. Lippert BM. Lasers in rhinology. In: Huttenbrink K, ed. *Lasers in Otorhinolaryngology.* New York: Thieme; 2005:54-73.

161. Pototschnig C, Volklein C, Appenroth E, Thumfart WF. Transnasal treatment of congenital choanal atresia with the KTP laser. *Ann Otol Rhinol Laryngol.* 2001;110(4):335-339.

162. Tzifa KT, Skinner DW. Endoscopic repair of unilateral choanal atresia with the KTP laser: a one stage procedure. *J Laryngol Otol.* 2001;115(4):286-288.

163. Healy GB, McGill T, Jako GJ, Strong MS, Vaughan CW. Management of choanal atresia with the carbon dioxide laser. *Ann Otol Rhinol Laryngol.* 1978;87(5 Pt 1):658-662.

164. Levine HL. The potassium–titanyl phosphate laser for treatment of turbinate dysfunction. *Otolaryngol Head Neck Surg.* 1991;104(2):247-251.

165. Oswal VH, Bingham BJ. A pilot study of the holmium YAG laser in nasal turbinate and tonsil surgery. *J Clin Laser Med Surg.* 1992;10(3):211-216.

166. Janda P, Sroka R, Baumgartner R, Grevers G, Leunig A. Laser treatment of hyperplastic inferior nasal turbinates: a review. *Lasers Surg Med.* 2001;28(5):404-413.

167. Lippert BM, Werner JA. Reduction of hyperplastic turbinates with the CO_2 laser. *Adv Otorhinolaryngol.* 1995;49:118-121.

168. Lippert BM, Werner JA. Comparison of carbon dioxide and neodymium: yttrium-aluminum-garnet lasers in surgery of the inferior turbinate. *Ann Otol Rhinol Laryngol.* 1997;106(12):1036-1042.

169. Lippert BM, Werner JA. Long-term results after laser turbinectomy. *Lasers Surg Med.* 1998;22(2):126-134.

170. Velegrakis GA, Prokopakis EP, Papadakis CE, Helidonis ES. Nd:YAG laser treatment of recurrent epistaxis in heredity hemorrhagic telangiectasia. *J Otolaryngol.* 1997;26(6):384-386.

171. Lennox PA, Harries M, Lund VJ, Howard DJ. A retrospective study of the role of the argon laser in the management of epistaxis secondary to hereditary haemorrhagic telangiectasia. *J Laryngol Otol.* 1997;111(1):34-37.

172. Bergler W, Riedel F, Baker-Schreyer A, Juncker C, Hormann K. Argon plasma coagulation for the treatment of hereditary hemorrhagic telangiectasia. *Laryngoscope.* 1999;109(1):15-20.

173. Ben-Bassat M, Kaplan I, Levy R. Treatment of hereditary haemorrhagic telangiectasia of the nasal mucosa with the carbon dioxide laser. *Br J Plast Surg.* 1978;31(2):157-158.

174. Ducic Y, Brownrigg P, Laughlin S. Treatment of haemorrhagic telangiectasia with the flashlamp-pulsed dye laser. *J Otolaryngol.* 1995;24(5):299-302.

175. Harries PG, Brockbank MJ, Shakespeare PG, Carruth JA. Treatment of hereditary haemorrhagic telangiectasia by the pulsed dye laser. *J Laryngol Otol.* 1997;111(11):1038-1041.

176. Har-El G, Shapshay SM, Bohigian RK, Krespi YP, Lucente FE. The treatment of rhinophyma. 'Cold' vs laser techniques. *Arch Otolaryngol Head Neck Surg.* 1993;119(6):628-631.

177. Goon PK, Dalal M, Peart FC. The gold standard for decortication of rhinophyma: combined erbium-YAG/CO_2 laser. *Aesthet Plast Surg.* 2004;28(6):456-460.

178. Kamami YV, Pandraud L, Bougara A. Laser-assisted outpatient septoplasty: results in 703 patients. *Otolaryngol Head Neck Surg.* 2000;122(3):445-449.

179. Trelles MA, Mordon SR. Correction of ear malformations by laser-assisted cartilage reshaping (LACR). *Lasers Surg Med.* 2006;38(7):659-662. Discussion 658.

180. Ovchinnikov Y, Sobol E, Svistushkin V, Shekhter A, Bagratashvili V, Sviridov A. Laser septochondrocorrection. *Arch Facial Plast Surg.* 2002;4(3):180-185.

181. Wong BJ, Milner TE, Harrington A, et al. Feedback-controlled laser-mediated cartilage reshaping. *Arch Facial Plast Surg.* 1999;1(4):282-287.

182. Hartnick CJ, Boseley ME, Franco RA Jr, Cunningham MJ, Pransky S. Efficacy of treating children with anterior commissure and true vocal fold respiratory papilloma with the 585-nm pulsed-dye laser. *Arch Otolaryngol Head Neck Surg.* 2007;133(2):127-130.

183. Bagwell CE. CO_2 laser excision of pediatric airway lesions. *J Pediatr Surg.* 1990;25(11):1152-1156.

184. Bent JP. Airway hemangiomas: contemporary management. *Lymphat Res Biol.* 2003;1(4):331-335.

185. Ahmad SM, Soliman AM. Congenital anomalies of the larynx. *Otolaryngol Clin North Am.* 2007;40(1):177-191. viii.

186. Karamzadeh AM, Wong BJ, Crumley RL, Ahuja G. Lasers in pediatric airway surgery: current and future clinical applications. *Lasers Surg Med.* 2004;35(2):128-134.

187. Crockett DM, Strasnick B. Lasers in pediatric otolaryngology. *Otolaryngol Clin North Am.* 1989;22(3):607-619.

188. Whymark AD, Clement WA, Kubba H, Geddes NK. Laser epiglottopexy for laryngomalacia: 10 years' experience in the west of Scotland. *Arch Otolaryngol Head Neck Surg.* 2006;132(9):978-982.

189. Nicolai T, Fischer-Truestedt C, Reiter K, Grantzow R. Subglottic hemangioma: a comparison of CO_2 laser, Neodym-Yag laser, and tracheostomy. *Pediatr Pulmonol.* 2005;39(3):233-237.

190. Madgy D, Ahsan SF, Kest D, Stein I. The application of the potassium-titanyl-phosphate (KTP) laser in the management of subglottic hemangioma. *Arch Otolaryngol Head Neck Surg.* 2001;127(1):47-50.

191. Ishman SL, Kerschner JE, Rudolph CD. The KTP laser: an emerging tool in pediatric otolaryngology. *Int J Pediatr Otorhinolaryngol.* 2006;70(4):677-682.

Laser/Light Applications in Gynecology

Cornelia de Riese and Roger Yandell

- Several non-invasive neoplastic and infectious conditions of the external female genitalia are amenable to treatment with a variety of ablative lasers.
- Ablative laser treatment of the vulva, vagina and cervix provides a relatively fast treatment modality and results in healing with little scar formation and excellent cosmetic and functional results, as well as fairly uncomplicated postoperative recovery.
- Intra-abdominal uses of different lasers are valuable alternatives to other thermal or mechanical cutting instruments.
- Severe side effects and complications of laser use can be minimized by careful patient selection, using the most appropriate instruments, proper surgical technique, and meticulous postoperative care.
- Good candidates for laser ablative procedures are generally considered to be individuals who have been refractory to medical and/or chemical treatment, and those presenting with extensive disease, as well as patients in whom a single surgical procedure is indicated for medical, psychological, or social reasons.
- With ongoing advancements in laser technology and techniques, improved clinical outcomes with minimal postoperative recovery will be realized.

C. de Riese (✉)
Obstetrics and Gynecology, Texas Tech University
Health Sciences Center, Lubbock, TX, USA
e-mail: cornelia.deriese@ttuhsc.edu

Introduction

- Gynecologists first used laser in 1979 and have used CO_2, KTP-532, Argon, and Nd:YAG to treat lower genital tract, intrauterine, and intra-abdominal disease.

The use of CO_2 laser in the treatment of uterine cervical intraepithelial lesions is well established and indications, as well as techniques, have changed very little for over 30 years. The Cochrane Systematic Review from 2000 suggests no obviously superior technique. CO_2 laser ablation of the vagina is also established as a safe treatment modality for VAIN (Vaginal Intraepithelial Neoplasia), and has been used extensively in the treatment of VIN (Vulvar Intraepithelial Neoplasia) and lower genital tract condylomata acuminata. CO_2 laser permits treatment of lesions with excellent cosmetic and functional results. The treatment of heavy menstrual bleeding by destruction of the endometrial lining using various techniques, including Nd:YAG laser ablation, has been the subject of a 2002 Cochran Database Review. Among the compared treatment modalities are modified laser techniques. The conclusion by reviewers is that outcomes and complication profiles of newer techniques compare favorably with the gold standard of endometrial resection. Myoma coagulation or myolysis with Nd:YAG laser through the laparoscope or hysteroscope is a conservative treatment option for women who wish to preserve their child bearing potential. The ELITT diode laser system is one of the new successful additions to the European armamentarium. CO_2 laser is the dominant laser type used with laparoscopy for ablation of endometriotic implants. The KTP-532 nm laser also has been used for essentially all of the previously mentioned applications of carbon dioxide. It is less widely available, but does offer certain distinct advantages which will be discussed further.[1]

K. Nouri (ed.), *Lasers in Dermatology and Medicine*,
DOI: 10.1007/978-0-85729-281-0_42, © Springer-Verlag London Limited 2011

History of Procedures

> - In 1973 laser was first used in gynecology by Kaplan for vaporization of infected cervical tissue.
> - The use of the laser through a laparoscope was first described by Bruhat in 1979.
> - Goldrath first described intrauterine procedures using the Nd:YAG in 1981.
> - The media used in gynecologic surgeries are CO_2 and argon gases, as well as KTP, Nd:YAG crystals, and diode lasers.

Albert Einstein postulated his idea of stimulated emission of radiation in 1917,[2] but it took 40 more years for this idea to be converted into a practical device. In 1958 Arthur L. Schawlow and Charles H. Townes published their initial article covering the basic principles of the laser in the *American Physical Society's Physical Review*.[3,4] This was followed by their first proposal of gas lasers excited by electrical discharge. In 1960 Ali Javan, William Bennett, and Donald Herriott constructed a helium neon laser, the first laser to generate a continuous beam of light.[2] In 1961 the first continuous operation of an optically pumped solid-state laser $Nd:CaWO_4$ by L.F. Johnson, G.D. Boyd, K. Nassau, and R.R. Soder was reported.[2] C.K.N. Patel developed the first CO_2 laser in 1964.[5] The same year the Nd:YAG laser was introduced by J.F. Geusic and R.G. Smith.[2] The first experimental medical application was reported in 1965.[6]

In 1973 laser was first used in gynecology by Kaplan for vaporization of infected cervical tissue.[7] The following year Bellina reported the first definitive procedures done on the vulva, vagina and cervix using the CO_2.[8] Over the next decade, hundreds of articles were published discussing the techniques of the use of carbon dioxide laser and the treatment of intraepithelial neoplasia and condyloma of the lower genital tract. In 1989 Yandell presented information regarding excisional cone biopsy of the cervix using the argon, KTP-532, and the Nd:YAG lasers, touting marked improvement in hemostasis and application of the energy using the shorter wavelength fiber optic instrumentation.[1]

Intra-abdominal and intrauterine applications were also explored. Bruhat first described use of carbon dioxide layer through the laparoscope in 1979.[9] Three years later, Keye reported on the use of argon laser for the treatment of endometriosis.[10] This was followed very shortly by introduction of the KTP-532 and the Nd:YAG lasers laparoscopically. In 1981 Goldrath first described the use of Nd:YAG laser in the endometrial cavity for the destruction of the endometrium and later, for resection of the uterine septa, submucous myomata, and excision of polyps.[11] In 1984, Rettenmaier first published data on the treatment of gynecologic tumors of the vagina and vulva using photoradiation with hematoporphyrin dyes.[12]

Epidemiology of Human Papillomaviruses

Human papilloma virus (HPV) infections, and genital HPV in particular, are serious public health concerns, not just due to their immediate impact on quality of life, but also due to the tremendous economic burden to the affected patient and the public.[13] In the USA, close to $3.5 billion are spent annually for the treatment of HPV-related conditions.

Classification of Virus Types

Human papilloma viruses only have affinity to the human body. Almost 200 different types have been identified to date. They are subcategorized according to tissue tropism: cutaneous versus mucosal, and oncogenic potential. Depending on the host's immuno competence, these infections may be transient or persistent.[14]

Emphasis in this chapter will be placed on anogenital tract infections. There are about 10–15 low-risk types, with types 6 and 11 being most prominent, which are responsible for genital wart growth. There are 15–20 high risk or oncogenic types, which are responsible for precancerous and cancerous transformation of genital epithelial tissues. The most prevalent high risk types are 16, 18, 31, 33, 35, 39, 45, 51, and 52.[15-18]

Risk Factors

Genital HPV infections are predominately sexually transmitted. Vertical transmission from delivering mother to newborn is confirmed for respiratory papillomatosis.[17] The risk for virus acquisition is directly correlated with the number of sexual partners.[14,19-22] Smoking is an additional risk factor, as may be the use of contraceptive pills in women.[23] Condom use appears to provide incomplete protection due to the involvement of uncovered genital contact sites.

Incidence and Prevalence

Estimates of the infection rate within populations are challenging because of the unpredictability of the natural history, the lack of requirements to report the disease, and the large variations between different populations and age groups.

The overall risk of infection is ultimately related to sexual behavior and risk factors. HPV is considered the leading sexually transmitted infection in the USA. According to data from the Centers for Disease Control (CDC) and the National Health and Nutrition Examination Survey (NHANES), at least 50% of sexually active men and women will acquire HPV infections at some point in their lives.[24] Not surprisingly, adolescents and young adults show the highest incidence numbers.[21,25] HPV infections in men are less extensively studied, but infection rates appear similar to those found in women and are estimated to be as high as 73%.[23,26] Male circumcision appears to decrease the risk of infection for the male and probably the risk of transmission of the virus.[27]

Studies on the distribution of different virus types within 11 countries from Africa, Europe, and South America demonstrated geographic variation, with the HPV 16 type being more prominent in Europe.[28]

Tissue Tropism and Clinical Infections

Several HPV types have a propensity to infect keratinizing epithelium and cause cutaneous warts, such as common warts and plantar warts (types 1,2,4), butcher's warts (types 2 and 7), and flat warts (type 3 and 10).[29,30] Bowen's disease is a form of squamous cell carcinoma in situ from which numerous virus types have been isolated: 16, 18, 31, 32, 34 and others.[18,29,31,32]

Several of the above mentioned virus types also infect non-keratinizing epithelial surfaces, especially within the anogenital region, but also within the mouth and pharynx. Condylomata acuminata are the best known genital warts and affect at least 1% of the sexually active population, with the peak prevalence in the young adult age group.[19,20,22,32] Subclinical infections are very common and constitute a major challenge for the treating physician. Colposcopy and acetic acid are required tools for detection of these latent stages.

There is now ample evidence that links persistence of high risk HPV types to the development of cervical cancer and other surface cancers of anal, vulvar, penile, and oropharyngeal origin.[18,33-36] In the past, cervical cancer was the most frequent malignancy among women in developing countries, but it now ranks second after breast cancer.[18]

Outlook

The introduction of the quadrivalent papilloma virus vaccine for adolescent and young adult females in 2006 will positively impact the epidemiology of immunized women in the decades ahead, but generations of already infected women will need attention for many years to come.

Laser Use on Vulva, Vagina, and Cervix

Indications and Contraindications

- Indications
  - Intraepithelial Neoplastic Disease
  - Condyloma acuminata refractory to medical and chemical treatment.
  - Cervical Stenosis
  - Extensive Disease including extension into anus and urethra/bladder of condyloma acuminatum.
- Contraindications
  - Patients in whom invasive cancer has not been ruled out.

Since the instruments first became available to gynecologists, laser has been used in the treatment of pre-malignant (dyplastic) lesions of the lower genital tract. These include cervical intraepithelial neoplasia (CIN), vaginal intraepithelial neoplasia (VAIN), and vulvar intraepithelial neoplasia (VIN).

The vast majority of these intraepithelial neoplasias are of the uterine cervix, with the incidence rising dramatically over the last four decades. This increase parallels the rise in infection rates of human papilloma virus in the young female population. At birth, the squamo-columnar junction between the vagina and the endocervical columnar epithelium lies at the outer aspects of the ectocervix. At menarche, the vaginal pH drops substantially from 7.2 to 4.5. This, coupled with a marked effect on the vaginal flora, causes the onset of metaplastic change over the columnar epithelium that is exposed to the vaginal environment. During the course of metaplastic change, this exposed endocervical tissue is covered by a pseudo-stratified squamous epithelium with small infoldings in the surfaces down to the level of the original columnar tissue. These infoldings are frequently, and incorrectly, described as glands or crypts, for lack of a better term. The entire process takes approximately 8–10 years, and during this time the tissues of this transformation zone are extremely susceptible to the virus. Once the HPV is incorporated into the cells, they may undergo neoplastic transformation or simply remain infected, depending on the specific viral subtype. The body may recognize the virus as foreign and mount an immune response, but in many cases, it does not, allowing persistent infection or neoplastic change, which can then advance in severity. The lesion spreads over the cervical surface and as it does so, it also moves down into these "glands" of the newly formed transformation zone.

When the patient presents, usually following an abnormal pap smear, the work up includes colposcopy with biopsy of the most suspicious areas, to determine the severity of the disease. Because the lesion is intraepithelial, destruction of the epidermis is adequate for treatment of the neoplastic lesion; however, it is known that large areas of the normal appearing transformation zone are infected by the virus despite no visible lesions being present on colposcopic exam. The other concern regarding treatment is that because of the infolding of the epithelium, the dysplastic lesion may extend several millimeters below the surface, and into the endocervical canal. With this in mind, the generally accepted treatment is destruction of the entire transformation zone to the depth of 5–7 mm.

Treatment methods used in the past were diathermy, and later cryotherapy. Neither of these modalities allows the physician to discern the depth of destruction at the time of the procedure. The use of laser, however, allows very accurate vaporization or ablation of the transformation zone down to the desired depth, with extension of that vaporization further up into the endocervical canal to visibly and measurably treat the entire extent of the tissue involved.

Evaluation and treatment of vaginal and vulvar intraepithelial neoplasia is similar, and in some ways simpler, because the epithelium involved is completely exposed, unlike that of the uterine cervix. Care must be taken, especially in the vagina, to not destroy more than the effected epithelium, which generally is less than 1 mm in thickness. Problems also arise in treating the portion of vulva in which there is hair because of the spread of the disease down into the follicles. Another concern with VIN is that it tends to be multifocal, requiring very careful colposcopic exams and frequently several biopsies in order to identify the extent of lesions.

Of paramount importance is insuring that there is no invasive disease prior to using local destructive treatments. Any suspicion of invasion requires further excisional tissue diagnosis. For many years, excisional cone biopsy was performed using the "cold" knife, or "hot" electrocautery. This is a markedly inaccurate procedure which removes the entire ectocervix and the distal and middle portion of the endocervical canal for tissue evaluation. The "Cold knife" cone is fraught with potential complications including excessive blood loss; inadequate incision depth, which may make it difficult to discern whether the lesion is invasive or microinvasive if it is incompletely excised; and excessive tissue removal, resulting in incompetent cervix and subsequent second trimester pregnancy loss. Because of their precision and hemostatic characteristics, lasers have been used for excisional cone biopsies by many surgeons for the last 20 years.

The other major indication for the use of laser of the lower genital tract is the treatment of condyloma accuminata. These lesions are generally first treated conservatively using cytotoxic agents such as podophylin, immune modulators such as imiquimod, or acids such as TCA for the destruction of specific early disease. Cryocautery may also be used for destruction. However, in most cases, each of these requires multiple treatments which can be fairly painful and irritating. The use of cryocautery may also be complicated by excessive destruction into the dermis, which causes scarring and may result in ulceration and infection. Because large areas of skin are infected with the virus and appear normal at the time of initial treatments, it is very common for secondary lesions to become apparent around lesions which have been previously treated. In some cases the local treatment itself may not be adequate to cause destruction of the primary lesions. Frequently patients present with extensive disease involving large areas of the lower genital tract and local treatment using medical or chemical means is simply impractical. These patients are generally treated primarily with laser in the operating room for the best results. In a significant number of these cases, the condylomata extend into the anal canal and may also extend into the urethra and bladder neck. The KTP-532 laser may be used inside the bladder and urethra for precise destruction of lesions in a fluid environment.

One known complication of conventional cone biopsy of the cervix is stenosis of the cervical os. In this situation, hypertrophic scarring of the surgical defect essentially closes the endocervical canal to the point that menstrual flow may be obstructed, or secondary infertility becomes an issue. The best treatment for this condition is CO_2 vaporization of the scar tissue which has occluded the canal. Following this procedure, the endocervical columnar epithelium typically grows outward as the squamous tissue grows in from the exocervix, creating a more normal patent opening.

Techniques

- Adequate preoperative patient evaluation and education.
- Timing of the procedure to closely follow the menstrual cycle.
- Mechanical bowel prep is indicated in the majority of cases.
- Antibiotics are rarely indicated if the appropriate depth of destruction is maintained.
- The Carbon Dioxide and KTP-532 lasers are both used for the treatment of lower tract disease.
- Although the CO_2 laser is the most commonly used, the KTP-532 offers the important benefit of substantially less post-operative pain, which is the single most significant morbidity encountered.
- Care must be taken not to ablate too deeply, especially in the vagina and over opposing vulvar surfaces.
- Early postoperative evaluation is the key to avoiding major complications.

Preoperative Management

There is no consensus among laser experts regarding the most appropriate preoperative regimen for laser use in gynecology. Adequate preoperative patient evaluation and education are paramount because of the relatively long and sometimes painful postoperative course, and the relatively high persistence and recurrence rates of both intraepithelial neoplasia and HPV. It is always best to time the procedure just after the menstrual period to allow the longest time possible for healing before the next menses. In some instances it is appropriate to postpone menstruation by using hormonal therapy such as injectable depomedroxyprogesterone or oral contraceptive suppression.

It is always advantageous to administer a mechanical bowel prep prior to any extensive procedure. This will decrease exposure of the surgical field to bowel flora. The prep should be administered the day before surgery, as enemas given on the same day tend to increase contamination during the procedure.

Due to the moist, de-epithelialized state of ablative laser-treated skin and the possibility of bacterial contamination and overgrowth over the vulva and vagina, some gynecologic laser surgeons advocate oral or topical antibiotic prophylaxis. This practice remains controversial, due to the lack of results of controlled studies, and has not been used by this author. Antibiotics have not been used for laser procedures on the cervix. The one exception to this is the patient who is found to have Bacterial Vaginosis at the preoperative evaluation. Because of the high bacterial count of anaerobic organisms in the vagina, this condition should always be treated with metronidazole or clindamycin before surgery.

Description of the Technique

Laser in the Treatment of Cervical Disease

When laser was first introduced as a tool for the gynecologist, it was the CO_2 laser which was used for treatment of cervical disease.[7] In the early reports of laser surgery, Baggish and Dorsey helped to define and establish the techniques used in CO_2 laser therapy. They described using a 0.5–1 mm spot size and power of 25–50 W, resulting in a power density of 2,500–20,000 W/cm^2 to cut, versus a 2–3 mm spot size and 20–25 W for vaporization which has a corresponding power density of approximately 500–800 W/cm^2. This was done under colposcopic guidance with the laser coupled via a micromanipulator. In 1982, they reported a series of over 400 cases with CIN treated by laser with an overall cure rate of almost 96% at about 1-year follow-up.[37] The only significant changes since then have been the use of slightly higher

power densities. However moving above the 1,500 W/cm^2 range frequently results in the beam cutting into vessels without first coagulating them and may cause significant bleeding. The higher power density does result in less thermal damage to the specimen, and offers a superior specimen for pathologic evaluation. There are very few current publications on this subject. *Cochrane Systematic Reviews* published on surgery for CIN and compared seven surgical techniques. They concluded that the Loop Electrosurgical Excision Procedure (LEEP) appeared to provide the more reliable specimen for pathology but the overall morbidity was lower with the laser conization. The limited evidence suggests that there is no obviously superior surgical technique for CIN.[38]

The KTP-532 laser has also been used for excisional and ablative procedures of the cervix, although there is little published data. The fiber is passed through a 9 in. hand piece with a 30° curve at the tip. This allows a free hand excision of the surgical specimen using 10–15 W (power density of 3,600–5,000 W/cm^2). The most significant benefit is the marked decrease in bleeding encountered, which is generally the most difficult complication to deal with when using other modalities, including the carbon dioxide laser. This is explained by the high photochemical absorption of the 532 nm wavelength in the hemoglobin molecule. The beam passes through the relatively clear vessel wall, coagulating the blood before cutting it. Because of the forward penetration of this wavelength, the fiber is angled toward the patient and away from the specimen to decrease coagulation artifact and increase hemostasis during the incision of tissue. This author has used the KTP-532 preferentially for the past 15 years and found it allows for almost bloodless excisional cone biopsies[1] see Fig. 1.

The Nd:YAG laser has also been used for excisional procedures, but because it must be coupled with a sapphire tip to do incisional work, it is somewhat more costly and difficult to manipulate inside the confined space of the vagina. It is, however, extremely hemostatic because of this wavelength's intrinsic coagulation of protein.

Some authors suggest that combining LEEP with additional laser treatment of the cut margins and wound bed may improve long term success.[39,40] Microscopically guided laser vaporization or laser excisional cone may be a less aggressive, and certainly more controllable, treatment modality than a traditional "cold knife cone (CKC)" and therefore, may be the choice for young women interested in preservation of fertility.[41-43]

In addition to the previously mentioned complications of CKC, it may result in the removal of too much or all of the endocervical glands resulting in cervical factor infertility and/or cervical stenosis, which precludes the passage of menstrual tissue. In the case of cervical stenosis, the CO_2 laser is the instrument of choice to vaporize the scar tissue which is occluding the canal. A higher power density is used

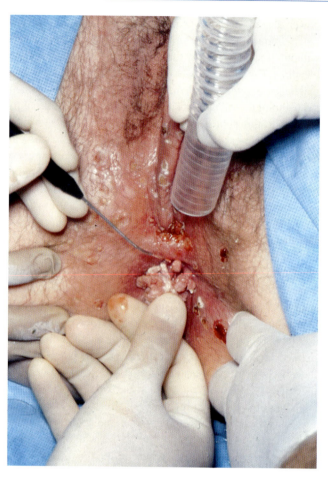

Fig. 1 The flexible quartz fiber of the KTP-532 laser is seen passing through a hand piece which allows a 30° angle at the tip. This allows the surgeon to apply the beam parallel to the skin surface for vulvar and vaginal procedures and is advantageous when performing excisional cone biopsies of the cervix

in the range of 5,000 W/cm² to decrease thermal damage of the surrounding area, and allow the normal tissues to grow back into place.

The use of lasers has significantly decreased the complications, which have been historically encountered with the traditional cold knife cone.

Laser in the Treatment of Vaginal Disease

The treatment of vaginal dysplasia and condyloma remain challenging, regardless of treatment modalities. Since the vaginal epithelium is less than a millimeter thick, ablation has to be very superficial. Traditionally, the procedure was done in similar fashion to cervical laser vaporization, under colposcopic supervision with the micromanipulator. A 2 mm spot size is chosen at a 20–30 W power setting.[6,44] Duane Townsend was among those establishing the technique. Because of the sharp tangential angulation of the impact beam delivered to the vaginal wall from a colposcopic delivery system, many surgeons today prefer to use a hand held device. This is incrementally better, but because of the bulky nature of the CO_2 hand piece, it is still difficult to deliver a beam at 90° to the surface. The use of a fiber-optic laser such as the KTP-532 delivered through a hand piece with an angled tip as previously described, can allow the surgeon to deliver the beam with a more even distribution of energy to the surgical site. This is done using 10 W and short exposure times to compensate for the increased penetration of this wave length into the underlying tissue. With either technique it is very important not to overlap exposure applications in order to protect the underlying dermis.

The bulk of the available literature is from the 1980s to the mid-1990s. Uniformly, recurrence or persistence rates in the 30–50% range are reported after the first laser treatment. Even after the second and third treatment courses, 20% relapse or persist. This disease is considered multifocal in the majority of cases. In the case of VAIN III involving the vaginal cuff angles after hysterectomy, upper vaginectomy is proposed over plain laser ablation. Additional superficial lasing of the surrounding vagina is generally recommended.[45-52] The main advantage of the laser procedure in comparison to conventional surgery or the use of cytotoxic agents, is the preservation of the anatomic integrity of the vagina, even after repeated laser courses.[49] The recommended curative and safe depth to be achieved with the laser treatment is only 1.5 mm, which allows for reepithelialization without scarring.[53]

In the case of larger exophytic condyloma, the lesions are vaporized down to a level consistent with the surrounding vaginal wall before the adjacent normal appearing epithelium is treated. Because of the high recurrence rates, it is assumed that substantial areas of this normal appearing epithelium are in fact infected by HPV. In many cases of extensive disease, the correct plane of the original vaginal wall may be extremely difficult to determine. In this case, it is better to err in the direction of removing less tissue and, in some cases, to only treat part of the affected area. In many instances in which only partial vaporization is completed, the post-operative inspection reveals complete clearance of the condyloma. It is believed that these patients' immune systems are stimulated to recognize the HPV as a result of the surgery and develop an immune response to the virus resulting in clearing of the untreated lesions.

Laser in the Treatment of Vulvar Disease

CO_2 laser treatment for vulvar lesions was introduced about the same time as that of the cervix. The first reports were again by Baggish and Dorsey.[54,55] They established the technique still in use, which employs a spot size of 2–3 mm and power settings of 15–30 W.

The goal is to confine the damage to the epidermis and upper papillary dermis; however, stacking of laser pulses by treating an area with multiple passes in rapid succession or by using a high overlap setting on a scanning device can lead to excessive thermal injury with subsequent increased risk of scarring. This untoward effect can be avoided by moving the beam in a serpentine fashion or in ever increasing concentric circles while avoiding overlap. The depth of ablation correlates directly with the cumulative amount of time × wattage, or work measured in joules, applied to a specific location. Using a power density of $800–1,000$ W/cm^2 is generally considered ideal, and should result in instantaneous boiling of the water in the epithelium, causing a vapor pocket above the dermis with elevation of the superficial layer. A power density, which is too high, results in deep vaporization into the dermis, which should be avoided. However this affect is time sensitive and as the skill and speed of the surgeon increase, a somewhat higher power density may be employed. If the power density is too low, an ablative plateau is reached with less effective tissue ablation and accumulation of thermal injury. This effect is most likely caused by reduced tissue water content after initial desiccation, resulting in less selective absorption of energy. The avoidance of pulse stacking and incomplete removal of partially desiccated tissue is paramount to prevention of excessive thermal accumulation with any laser system. The objective of ablative laser treatment is to destroy tissue down to the papillary dermis. Limiting the depth of penetration decreases the risk for scarring and permanent pigmentary alteration. When choosing treatment parameters, the surgeon must consider factors such as the anatomic location and proximity to vital organs. To reduce the risk of excessive thermal injury, partially desiccated tissue should be removed manually with wet gauze after each laser pass to expose the underlying dermis.

This technique is very reliable when treating the non-hairy vulvar surfaces. In areas containing hair, the method must be altered in an attempt to treat intraepithelial neoplastic disease, which progresses toward the base of the follicle. In most cases this is best done by making a second pass over this tissue after the superficial epithelium has been removed. This characteristic of VIN is felt to be one of the primary causes of persistent disease in cases which have otherwise been adequately treated by laser, and is perhaps the main reason some gynecologists still advocate excision in these areas. When cosmesis is a priority, the laser is still preferable, and the patient must be informed that she must commit to close follow-up and the possibility that further treatment may be needed. Unfortunately, because of the high recurrence rates in all VIN cases, this is more or less true for all patients.

When treating condyloma, the same techniques are generally applicable, but must be modified for larger exophytic lesions. The smaller condylomata may be simply vaporized or excised, but only to the level of the skin with care being taken not to coagulate the deeper dermis. The surrounding normal appearing epithelium is then treated in the same fashion as described above to a distance of $1–2$ cm from the original wart. If this is not done, recurrence rates are very high.

For the larger pedunculated lesions, several techniques may be employed to decrease bleeding, which may occur if the CO_2 laser is being used. Although the carbon dioxide laser is generally regarded as a very hemostatic instrument, it does so by thermal coagulation of vessels as the tissue is vaporized at the impact site, unlike the KTP-532 and Nd:YAG wavelengths which actually pass through water and coagulate by direct absorption in hemoglobin and protein respectively. When larger vessels are encountered, the CO_2 may cut into the wall before the more rapidly moving blood is coagulated, creating bleeding. Further attempts to seal the vessel are then hampered by the complete absorption of the energy at the surface of the emerging blood, which does not allow heat to penetrate to the vessel below. The blood must be cleaned away while pressure is applied to the vessel in order to tamponade the bleeding to allow further progress. Alternatively, pedicles may be coagulated circumferentially before attempting excision. This is more productive if the blood flow can be stopped by pressure at the base. In some cases, it is better to use a much lower power density in the range of $200–400$ W/cm^2 to essentially cook the tissue initially. The wattage may be decreased or the spot size increased to accomplish the change. This can however, result in thermal spread into the dermis. In some instances, ectrocautery or sutures may be needed.

The KTP-532 laser, although much less widely available, may also be used in the treatment of these diseases, and offers significant advantages once the technique is mastered. Because this wavelength is not absorbed in water, there is deeper penetration ($1–2$ mm) than seen with the CO_2. In order to decrease damage to the dermis, a higher power density ($2,000–5,000$ W/cm^2) is used with a shorter application time, resulting in a more immediate coagulation of the epidermis, and less thermal spread. The outcome is somewhat different, because the effect will be desiccation and coagulation, with little or no vaporization. The treated epidermis is then wiped away using a gauze pad. The incidence of bleeding is much lower because of the extremely high absorption of the 532-nm wavelength in hemoglobin, and the ability to move through vessel walls, which are mainly water, before cutting into them. Should bleeding be encountered, the hand piece is backed away a few centimeters which will rapidly increase the spot size secondary to the $15°$ divergence of the beam from the fiber tip, resulting in a much lower power density for coagulation purposes. See Fig. 2a and b.

The most significant advantage to this wavelength is a marked decrease in postoperative pain compared to the CO_2 laser. Significant and prolonged pain is the most common morbidity of vulvar laser treatment. Because the CO_2 has

Fig. 2 (**a**) Patient with extensive condylomata acuminata of the vagina, vulva, and peri-anal skin. (**b**) Same patient following treatment using the KTP-532 laser. There is marked edema forming in the clitoral hood and labia minora before the entire procedure is completed. Note the absence of pitting into the dermis and the extended treatment area around all previously visible lesions

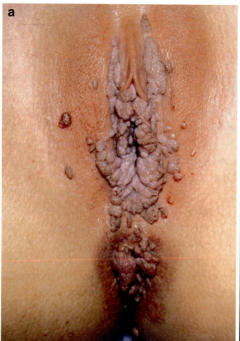
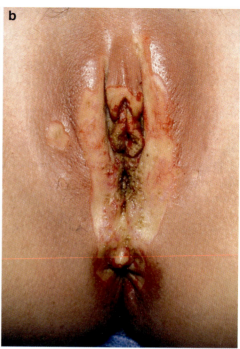

very little forward scatter, the equivalent of a second degree burn is being created, with the intact sensory nerves exposed. Although the exact mechanism is uncertain, it is postulated that the 532 nm wavelength is absorbed in these nerve endings, essentially decreasing their response to stimuli for a short time during the healing process. There does not appear to be any long term effect. The increased depth of penetration may also be beneficial in treating VIN in skin containing hair follicles, although this has not yet been substantiated.

Laser therapy of vulvar intraepithelial neoplasia and condyloma results in excellent cosmetic and functional healing, but carries the risk of recurrent and persistent disease. Repeated treatments may be necessary. In light of the multifocal nature of these disease processes in the majority of patients, laser, with its ease of technique and low morbidity, is the treatment of choice, especially for younger women.[5,44,56,57] For extensive VIN III, excisional laser surgery of the more suspicious areas combined with vaporization of the surrounding "normal" epithelium provides a histologic specimen and appears to be more effective than pure vaporization.[57]

Post-operative Management

The post-operative management of the lower genital tract largely centers around the treatment and prevention of pain and bleeding. Following excisional or vaporization cone biopsy of the cervix, the most common complication is delayed bleeding. This occurs as the escar falls away at 10–14 days. Because of this, the base of the excision site may be coagulated at a very low power density to further seal vessels. This is followed by placing Monsel's solution (Ferrous Sub-Sulfate) on the treated surface to decrease the risk of bleeding.

Following vaginal and vulvar procedures, the management and follow up is more complicated due to the variety of symptoms and complications encountered. The most common problem is pain following vulvar procedures. The most significant complication is that of opposing denuded surfaces of the vagina and labia scarring together. Some gynecologists have routinely coated the treated surfaces with silver sulfadiazine 1% (Silvadene) as is commonly used in severe burn patients to deter infection and stimulate tissue regeneration. The incidence of infection is extremely low after these procedures without using any type of antimicrobial compound. Because of the expense of Silvadene and assuming the depth of destruction is appropriate, the author prefers to use triamcinolone cream applied immediately after the surgery is completed. The steroid cream blocks a substantial amount of the edema and pain associated with the immediate post-operative period and physically separates the denuded tissues, preventing adhesion formation. Application of either of these medications may continue for 1–3 days if they are deemed helpful.

Because of the high incidence of significant pain following vulvar procedures, these patients should routinely be discharged with substantial amounts of oral pain medication, even when compared to major gynecologic surgeries. The expectation is that the most significant discomfort will occur at 7–14 days post-operatively. It is not recommended that

Laser/Light Applications in Gynecology

lidocaine ointment be used secondary to the relatively short time of pain relief it offers and because there may be significant systemic absorption and toxicity. Sitz baths are encouraged two to three times daily, using a physiologic electrolyte solution, which can be easily made by adding a salt water aquarium preparation mixture, which is available at most pet stores, to bath water. The patient is told to keep the area as dry as possible by using a hair dryer with low heat, and by avoiding underwear to keep the area exposed to air. It is also of note that Preparation H, which is marketed for the symptomatic relief of hemorrhoids, has been found anecdotally to offer significant pain relief in these cases.

These patients should have frequent post operative exams to insure that significant scarring or adhesions are not forming and to evaluate pain control. In patients being treated for condyloma accuminata, evaluation for new lesions should also be done at each visit. These may be found very early following surgery and should be treated locally as soon as they become apparent.

Adverse Events

- Severe scarring and contracture of the vagina is a known complication.
- Attempts to treat the entire lower genital tract in an attempt to rid the area of HPV is futile and frequently results in major complications.
- The most important preventative factor is the avoidance of excessive depth of destruction.

Side Effects/Complications

Pain, bleeding, and persistence of HPV are the most common problems encountered following laser therapy of the lower genital tract, as was previously discussed. These issues are present to a greater or lesser degree in the majority of cases. The more serious complication of vaginal and vulvar scarring and contracture are much less common today than in the past, but require constant diligence and attention to detail during surgery to be avoided. During the 1980s there was a period in which it was believed that laser treatment of the skin and mucosa of the entire lower genital tract could eradicate human papilloma virus entirely. As a result of such attempts, and almost certainly coupled with an excessive depth of destruction, there were a number of cases in which the patient's vagina scarred/contracted down to a fraction of the original size. In the cases referred to this author for treatment of these problems, the patients generally had very

severe post-operative pain and had not been examined until several weeks after their surgery. This complication can take on several different presentations. If the upper vagina scars to the contralateral side it can completely occlude the cervix from the vagina thus obstructing menstrual flow. If similar scarring occurs at the introitus, the vaginal opening may be closed to the point of precluding intercourse. In the worst case senario, the entire length of the vagina may react similar to the skin following third-degree burns with extensive fibrosis and contracture. In all of these situations, the treatment as discussed below is lengthy, usually requiring one or more plastic surgeries, and frequently does not result in a good outcome.

Prevention and Treatment of Side Effects/ Complications

The most important aspect of prevention of side effects revolves around having an experienced surgeon who is tedious about maintaining the depth of tissue damage at the level of the basement membrane. As previously alluded to, the use of inherently hemostatic wavelengths, which also tend to seal off exposed nerves such as the KTP-532, is advantageous but not widely available. The treatment of the minor side effects was previously discussed under post-operative management and must be individualized.

The prevention of the vast majority of severe complications noted above can be accomplished through education and mentoring of physicians regarding surgical technique. The concept that multiple procedures and longer term treatments are preferable to these types of complications is paramount. Despite the best efforts, these severe complications will continue to be encountered occasionally secondary to hypertrophic scarring, infection, and idiopathic responses. Treatment may be dramatically affected if the problems associated with excessive depth of tissue destruction and abnormal scarring are identified early in the post-operative course. Estrogen cream and steroids may be employed to increase epithelialization and decrease scarring. There is frequently an indication for manual dilation and the placement of vaginal obturators to counteract contracture formation. Obviously infectious processes, although rare, may be dealt with much better if identified early.

Once the scarring has matured, the effect of vaginal dilators is slow and usually very uncomfortable. Obturators are usually progressively enlarged over prolonged intervals, if possible. They are generally kept in place constantly except for cleansing. If the scarring occludes menstrual flow, or if no progress can be made using dilators, relaxing incisions and at times grafting must be considered. The overall treatment course can be protracted and in some cases the patient protoporphyrine absorbs the light resulting in the formation of triplet protoporphyrine IX and free oxygen radicals, which lead to cell destruction within the illuminated tissue areas.[87-89] Photodynamic therapy is well established for the treatment of Barrett's esophagus[84,90] and certain skin conditions such as psoriasis.[84,91] PDT using topically applied ALA (trademark Levulan, Berlex/DUSA Pharmaceuticals, Inc., MA) was registered by the FDA for the treatment of actinic keratoses of the skin in 2000. There are also several case studies and series that report complete or partial response in patients treated for external anal dysplasia low and high grade.[92-94] Similar results have been reported for the treatment of dysplastic and cancerous vulvar,[95-98] vaginal[99,100] and uterine cervical[101] disease. In the treatment of vulvar intraepithelial neoplasia (VIN) the lesions are typically irradiated with 75–150 J/cm2 of laser light at a wavelength of 635 nm (argon or KTP/YAG ion pumped dye laser) about 2–3 h after sensitizing drug application.[10,95,102] The treatment time varies between 10 and 40 min.[99,102] In Europe, PDT is usually performed on the awake patient, after pretreatment with a systemic non-steroidal or narcotic pain medication or sedative. Despite this being a "cold" laser application, most patients complain about severe burning sensations at the site during the first several minutes of the treatment cycle. Following the procedure only mild burning is reported, and depending on skin complexion, a pronounced erythema is noted.[102] Photodynamic treatment has also been used for non-dysplastic vulvar conditions such as lichen sclerosis.[102] The decreased recurrence rate for VIN and condylomata following PDT is attributed to a specific immune mechanism which is stimulated by this unique procedure. It may, in part, also be secondary to the improved visibility and subsequent destruction of subclinical lesions.[100] Skinfolds, hyperkeratosis and marked pigmentation can block the illumination and lead to failure.[100] It should be noted that research is ongoing to perfect this methodology for the treatment of the intraperitoneal spread of ovarian and other malignancies by delivery of the light laparoscopically.

In summary, photodynamic therapy is a minimally invasive procedure that provides unique properties especially suited for the local treatment of superficial epithelial lesions in different organ systems, including the genital tract. There is evidence that it is well tolerated and at least as effective as other conventional modes of treatment.

Conclusion

The literature of the past decade was reviewed for outcome data and put into perspective by integrating the personal clinical experience of the authors. The result is this conclusion on the current state of the art use of lasers in gynecologic surgery. Unchanged from the laser's introduction as a tool in gynecologic surgery, differences in penetration, absorption, and suitable delivery media for the different laser wavelengths dictate their clinical application. The use of CO_2 laser in the treatment of cervical intraepithelial lesions is well established, and indications and techniques have not changed considerably over the past 20 years. The KTP laser may also be used for this procedure and may offer some advantages in hemostasis and application, but is not widely available. Randomized controlled trials comparing the CO_2 laser to other treatment modalities are scarce. The Cochrane Systematic Review from 2000 suggests that there is no obvious superior technique. The recent literature and personal observation suggest that laser treatment appears to be less complicated by infection and bleeding and is the preferred method for young females who desire future fertility. Persistence and recurrence rates are in the 10% range and independent of clear surgical margins.

CO_2 laser ablation for vaginal intraepithelial neoplasia is also an established, as well as safe, treatment modality. Repeated treatment may be necessary, since persistent disease is not infrequent, particularly when treating multifocal disease. In case of VAIN III at the vaginal cuff after hysterectomy, upper vaginectomy appears to be the treatment of choice and is often combined with CO_2 laser ablation of surrounding vaginal tissue. CO_2 laser surgery permits treatment of vulvar condyloma and vulvar intraepithelial neoplasia with excellent cosmetic and functional results. Again, persistent and recurrent disease in the 20% range is a known problem and close follow-up and retreatment are frequently indicated. VIN III may be better treated with laser excision than pure laser vaporization. Other benign lesions of the vulva can also be treated with laser, but published data are scarce. The KTP laser offers the significant advantage of decreased pain, especially when applied to vulvar procedures.

The treatment of abnormally heavy menstrual bleeding by destruction of the endometrial lining using various techniques has been the subject of a 2002 Cochrane Systematic Database Review. Among the compared treatment modalities are also newer and modified laser techniques. The conclusion of the reviewers is that outcomes and complication profiles of newer techniques compare favorably with the gold standard of endometrial resection via the hysteroscope. The majority of new destruction techniques are performed in a blind fashion. The ELITT diode laser system is one of the new successful additions in Europe. It is not yet FDA approved in the United States.

CO_2 laser is also the dominant laser type used with laparoscopy for ablation of endometriotic implants, although the KTP laser offers several advantages because of its preferential absorption in hemoglobin and hemosiderin, and ease of application. Recurrence rates are known to be as high as 50%. With endometriomas, excision of the capsule appears to be more beneficial than simple coagulation or vaporization. Myoma coagulation or myolysis with Nd:YAG laser through the laparoscope or hysteroscope is the most recent addition to the armamentarium of the gynecologic surgeon. Even MRI guided percutaneous approaches have been described. No long term data are available yet.

Laser is a well accepted treatment modality among patients and physicians. Disadvantages are the high cost involved and the sophistication of equipment and maintenance. Decreasing expenses, increasing safety and ease of application will further support the use of laser in gynecology.

References

1. Yandell RB et al. Evaluation of the KTP-532 nm laser for excisional cone biopsy of the cervix. Abstract presented at the Proceedings of the Combined Clinical Meeting of the American Society for Colposcopy and Cervical Pathology, and Gynecology Laser Society; April 1998.
2. http://www.bell-labs.com/history/laser/contrib.html
3. Schawlow AL. *Sci Am*. 1963;209:36.
4. Schawlow AL, Townes CH. *Physiol Rev*. 1985;112:1940.
5. Patel CKN. High-power carbon dioxide lasers. *Sci Am*. 1968; 219:23.
6. Dorsey J. Application of laser in gynecology. In: *TeLinde's Operative Gynecology*. 7th ed. Philadelphia: Lippincott; 1992:499.
7. Kaplan I et al. The treatment of erosions of the uterine cervix by means of the CO_2 laser. *Obstet Gynecol*. 1973;41(5):795-796.
8. Bellina JH. Gynecology and the laser. *Contrib Gynecol Obstet*. 1974;5.
9. Bruhat MA. et al. Use of the CO_2 laser via laparoscopy. In: Kaplan I, ed. Proceedings of the 3rd International Society for Laser Surgery. Tel Aviv: International Society for Laser Surgery; 1979:275.
10. Keye WR, Dixon J. Photocoagulation of endometriosis by the argon laser through the laparoscope. *Obstet Gynecol*. 1983;62:383.
11. Goldrath M et al. Laser photo-vaporization of endometriosis for the treatment of menorrhagia. *Am J Obstet Gynecol*. 1981;140:14.
12. Rettenmaier MA et al. Photoradiation therapy of gynecologic malignancies. *Gynecol Oncol*. 1984;17:206.
13. Insinga RP et al. The healthcare costs of cervical human papillomavirus-related disease. *Am J Obstet Gynecol*. 2004;191(1):114-120.
14. Ho GY. Natural history of cervicovaginal papillomavirus infection in young women. *N Engl J Med*. 1998;338:423.
15. Munoz N et al. Epidemiologic classification of human papillomavirus types associated with cervical cancer. *N Engl J Med*. 2003; 348:518.
16. Bosch FX et al. Prevalence of human papillomavirus in cervical cancer: a worldwide perspective. International biological study on cervical cancer (IBSCC) study group. *J Natl Cancer Inst*. 1995;87:796.
17. Bonnez W, Reichman R. Papillomaviruses. In: Mandell, Douglas, Bennett, eds. *Principles and Practice of Infectious Diseases*. 6th ed. Philadelphia, PA: Churchill Livingstone; 2005:1841-1856.
18. Franco EL et al. Cervical cancer: epidemiology, prevention and the role of human papillomavirus infection. *CMAJ*. 2001;164:1017.
19. Burk RD et al. Declining prevalence of cervicovaginal human papillomavirus infection with age is independent of other risk factors. *Sex Transm Dis*. 1996;23(4):333-341.
20. Winer RL et al. Genital human papillomavirus infection: incidence and risk factors in a cohort of female university students. *Am J Epidemiol*. 2003;157:218.

21. Tarkowski TA et al. Epidemiology of human papillomavirus infection and abnormal cytological test results in an urban adolescent population. *J Infect Dis*. 2004;189:46.
22. Koutsky L. Epidemiology of genital human papillomavirus infection. *Am J Med*. 1997;102:3.
23. Baseman JG, Koutsky LA. The epidemiology of human papillomavirus infections. *J Clin Virol*. 2005;32(suppl 1):S16-S24.
24. Centers for Disease Control and Prevention Fact Sheet. Genital HPV Infection. www.edc.govlhvpl.
25. Dunne EF et al. Prevalence of HPV infection among females in the United States. *JAMA*. 2007;297:813.
26. Dunne EF et al. Prevalence of HPV infection among men: a systematic review of the literature. *J Infect Dis*. 2006;194:1044.
27. Castellsague X et al. Male circumcision, penile human papillomavirus infection, and cervical cancer in female partners. *N Engl J Med*. 2002;346(15):1105-1112.
28. Clifford GM et al. Worldwide distribution of human papillomavirus types in cytologically normal women in the International Agency for Research on Cancer HPV prevalence surveys: a pooled analysis. *Lancet*. 2005;366:991.
29. Carr J, Gyorfi T. Human papillomavirus. Epidemiology, transmission, and pathogenesis. *Clin Lab Med*. 2000;20:235.
30. Bonnez W, Reichman RC. Papillomaviruses. In: Mandell GL, Bennett JE, Dolin R, eds. *Principles and Practice of Infectious Diseases*. 5th ed. Philadelphia: Churchill Livingston; 2000:1630.
31. Mackenzie-Wood A et al. Imiquimod 5% cream in the treatment of Bowen's disease. *J Am Acad Dermatol*. 2001;44:462.
32. Fazel N et al. Clinical, histopathologic, and molecular aspects of cutaneous human papillomavirus infections. *Dermatol Clin*. 1999;17:521.
33. Llewellyn CD et al. Risk factors for squamous cell carcinoma of the oral cavity in young people – a comprehensive literature review. *Oral Oncol*. 2001;37:401.
34. Uobe K et al. Detection of HPV in Japanese and Chinese oral carcinomas by in situ PCR. *Oral Oncol*. 2001;37:146.
35. Sonnex C. Human papillomavirus infection with particular reference to genital disease. *J Clin Pathol*. 1998;51:643.
36. Sedlacek TV. Advances in the diagnosis and treatment of human papillomavirus infections. *Clin Obstet Gynecol*. 1999;42:206.
37. Baggish MS. Management of cervical intraepithelial neoplasia by carbon dioxide laser. *Obstet Gynecol*. 1982;60:378-384.
38. Martin-Hirsch PL et al. Surgery for cervical intraepithelial neoplasia. *Cochrane Database Syst Rev*. 2000;2:CD 001318.
39. Bar-Am A et al. Combined colposcopy, loop conization, and laser vaporization reduces recurrent abnormal cytology and residual disease in cervical dysplasia. *Gynecol Oncol*. 2000;78(1):47-51.
40. Hullberg L et al. Menstrual blood loss: a population study. *Acta Obstet Gynecol Scand*. 1966;45:320-351.
41. Martel P et al. Utilization of CO_2 lasers in continuous or pulsed mode for conizations: apropos of 230 cases. *Gynécol Obstét Fertil*. 2000;28(7–8):537-546.
42. Moriyama M et al. CO_2 laser conization for cervical intraepithelial neoplasia: a comparison with cold knife conization during pregnancy. *Clin Laser Med Surg*. 1991;9(2):115-120.
43. Van Rooijen M et al. Pregnancy outcome after laser vaporization of the cervix. *Acta Obstet Gynecol Scand*. 1999;78(4):346-348.
44. Townsend DE et al. Treatment of vaginal carcinoma in situ with the carbon dioxide laser. *Am J Obstet Gynecol*. 1982;143:565-568.
45. Campagnutta E et al. Treatment of vaginal intraepithelial neoplasia (VAIN) with the carbon dioxide laser. *Clin Exp Obstet Gynecol*. 1999;26(2):127-130.
46. Curtin JP et al. Treatment of vaginal intraepithelial neoplasia with the CO_2 laser. *J Reprod Med*. 1985;30:942-944.
47. Diakomanolis E et al. Vaginal intraepithelial neoplasia: report of 102 cases. *Eur J Gynaecol Oncol*. 2002;23(5):457-459.

48. Diakomanolis E et al. Treatment of vaginal intraepithelial neoplasia with laser ablation and upper vaginectomy. *Gynecol Obstet Invest.* 2002;54(1):17-20.
49. Diakomanolis E et al. Conservative management of vaginal intra-epithelial neoplasia (VAIN) by laser CO_2. *Eur J Gynaecol Oncol.* 1996;17(5):389-392.
50. Hoffman MS et al. Laser vaporization of grade 3 vaginal intraepithelial neoplasia. *Am J Obstet Gynecol.* 1991;165:1342-1344.
51. Woodman CB et al. The management of vaginal intraepithelial neoplasia after hysterectomy. *BJOG.* 1984;91:707-711.
52. Yalcin OT et al. Vaginal intraepithelial neoplasia: treatment by carbon dioxide laser and risk factors for failure. *Eur J Obstet Gynecol Reprod Biol.* 2003;106(1):64-68.
53. Benedet JL. Epidermal thickness measurements in vaginal intraepithelial neoplasia. *J Reprod Med.* 1992;37:809-812.
54. Baggish MS, Dorsey JH. CO_2 laser for the treatment of vulvar carcinoma in situ. *Obstet Gynecol.* 1981;57:371-375.
55. Baggish MS. Treating viral venereal infections with the CO_2 laser. *Reprod Med.* 1982;27(12):737-774.
56. Hoffman MS et al. Laser vaporization for vulvar intraepithelial neoplasia III. *J Reprod Med.* 1992;37:135-137.
57. Sideri M et al. Evaluation of CO(2) laser excision or vaporization for the treatment of vulva intraepithelial neoplasia. *Gynecol Oncol.* 1999;75:277-281.
58. Vessey MP et al. The epidemiology of hysterectomy: findings in a large cohort study. *Br J Obstet Gynaecol.* 1992;99:402-407.
59. Lethaby A, Hickey M. Endometrial destruction techniques for heavy menstrual bleeding. *Cochrane Database Syst Rev.* 2002;2:CD 001501.
60. Jones K et al. Endometrial laser intrauterine thermotherapy for the treatment of dysfunctional uterine bleeding: the first British experience. *Br J Obstet Gynaecol.* 2001;108:749-753.
61. Donnez J et al. Endometrial laser intrauterine thermotherapy: the first series of 100 patients observed for 1 year. *Fertil Steril.* 2000;74(4):791-796.
62. Bhattacharya S et al. A pragmatic randomized comparison of transcervical resection of the endometrium with endometrial laser ablation for the treatment of menorrhagia. *Br J Obstet Gynaecol.* 1997;104:601-607.
63. Phillips G et al. Risk of hysterectomy after 1000 consecutive endometrial laser ablations. *Br J Obstet Gynaecol.* 1998;105(8):897-903.
64. Goldfarb HA. Myoma coagulation (myolysis). *Obstet Gynecol Clin North Am.* 2000;27(2):421-430.
65. Nisolle M et al. Laparoscopic myolysis with the Nd:YAG laser. *J Gynecol Surg.* 1993;9:95.
66. Chapman R. Low power interstitial photocoagulation of uterine leiomyomas by KTP/YAG laser. *Lasers Med Sci.* 1994;9:37-46.
67. Chapman R. Low power interstitial photocoagulation of uterine leiomyomas by KTP/YAG laser: a review of 50 consecutive cases. *SPIE Proc Med Appl Lasers II.* 1994;2327:304-312.
68. Chapman R. Treatment of uterine leiomyomas by interstitial hyperthermia. *Gynaecol Endosc.* 1993;2:227-234.
69. Penna C et al. CO_2 laser surgery for vulvar intraepithelial neoplasia. *J Reprod Med.* 2002;47:913-918.
70. Phillips DR et al. Experience with laparoscopic leiomyoma coagulation and concomitant operative hysteroscopy. *J Am Assoc Gynecol Laparosc.* 1997;4(4):425-433.
71. Goldfarb HA. Laparoscopic coagulation of myoma (myolysis). *Obstet Gynecol Clin North Am.* 1995;22(4):807-819.
72. Chapman R. Treatment of large uterine fibroids. *Br J Obstet Gynaecol.* 1997;104:867-871.
73. Hindley JT et al. Clinical outcomes following percutaneous magnetic resonance image guided laser ablation of symptomatic uterine fibroids. *Hum Reprod.* 2002;17(10):2737-2741.
74. Law P et al. Magnetic resonance-guided percutaneous laser ablation of uterine fibroids. *J Magn Reson Imaging.* 2000;12(4):565-570.

75. Visvanathan D et al. Interstitial laser photocoagulation for uterine myomas. *Am J Obstet Gynecol.* 2002;187(2):382-384.
76. Keckstein J. Laser techniques in gynaecology. *Endosc Surg Allied Technol.* 1994;2(3–4):176-180.
77. Donnez J. CO_2 laser laparoscopy in infertile women with adhesions or endometriosis. *Fertil Steril.* 1987;48:390-394.
78. Nezhat C et al. Surgical treatment of endometriosis via laser laparoscopy. *Fertil Steril.* 1986;45:778-783.
79. Donnez J, Nisolle M. *An Atlas of Operative Laparoscopy and Hysteroscopy.* 2nd ed. New York/London: Parthenon Publishing; 2001.
80. Vercellini P et al. Coagulation or excision of ovarian endometriomas? *Am J Obstet Gynecol.* 2003;188(3):606-610.
81. Jacobson TZ et al. Laparoscopic surgery for pelvic pain associated with endometriosis. *Cochrane Database Syst Rev.* 2001;4:CD 001300.
82. Divaris D et al. Phototoxic damage to sebaceous glands and hair follicles of mice after systemic administration of 5-aminolevulinic acid correlates with localized protoporphyrin-IX fluorescence. *Am J Pathol.* 1990;136:891-897.
83. Kennedy JC et al. Photodynamic therapy with endogenous protoporphyrin IX: basic principles and present clinical experience. *J Photochem Photobiol B.* 1990;1–2:143-148.
84. Kennedy JC, Pottier RH. Endogenous protoporphyrin IX, a clinically useful photosensitizer for photodynamic therapy. *J Photochem Photobiol B.* 1992;4:275-292.
85. Peng Q et al. 5-Aminolevulinic acid-based photodynamic therapy: principles and experimental research. *Photochem Photobiol.* 1997;65:235-251.
86. Hillemanns P et al. Photodynamic therapy in women with cervical intra-epithelial neoplasia using topically applied 5-aminolevulinic acid. *Int J Cancer.* 1999;81:34-38.
87. Tromberg BJ et al. In vivo tumor oxygen tension measurements for the evaluation of the efficiency of photodynamic therapy. *Photochem Photobiol.* 1990;2:375-385.
88. Foote CS. Definition of type I and type II photosensitized oxidation. *Photochem Photobiol.* 1991;5:659.
89. Ochsner M. Photophysical and photobiological processes in the photodynamic therapy of tumours. *Photochem Photobiol.* 1997;39:1-18.
90. Fan KFM et al. Photodynamic therapy using 5-aminolevulinic acid for premalignant and malignant lesions of the oral cavity. *Cancer.* 1996;78:1374-1383.
91. Wolf P et al. Topical photodynamic therapy with endogenous porphyrins after application of 5-aminolevulinic acid. An alternative treatment modality for solar keratoses, superficial squamous cell carcinomas, and basal cell carcinomas? *J Am Acad Dermatol.* 1993;1:17-21.
92. Scholefield JH. Treatment of grade III anal intraepithelial neoplasia with photodynamic therapy: report of a case. Dis Colon Rectum, 2003; 46(11):1555-1559. *Tech Coloproctol.* 2004;8:200.
93. Webber J, Fromm D. Photodynamic therapy for carcinoma in situ of the anus. *Arch Surg.* 2004;139:259-261.
94. Hamdan KA et al. Treatment of grade III anal intraepithelial neoplasia with photodynamic therapy: report of a case. *Dis Colon Rectum.* 2003;46:1555-1559.
95. Hillemanns P et al. Photodynamic therapy of vulvar intraepithelial neoplasia using 5-aminolevulinic acid. *Int J Cancer.* 2000;85:649-653.
96. Fehr MK et al. Photodynamic therapy of vulvar intraepithelial neoplasia III using topically applied 5-aminolevulinic acid. *Gynecol Oncol.* 2001;80:62-66.
97. Morton CA et al. Comparison of photodynamic therapy with cryotherapy in the treatment of Bowen's disease. *Br J Dermatol.* 1996;5:766-771.
98. Martin-Hirsch PL. Photodynamic treatment for lower genital tract intraepithelial neoplasia [letter]. *Lancet.* 1998;351:1403.

99. Lobraico RV, Grossweiner LI. Clinical experiences with photodynamic therapy for recurrent malignancies of the lower female genital tract. *J Gynecol Surg*. 1993;9:29-34.

100. Fehr MK et al. Photodynamic Therapy of vulvar and vaginal condyloma and intraepithelial neoplasia using topically applied 5-aminolevulinic acid. *Lasers Surg Med*. 2002;30:273-279.

101. Wierrani F et al. 5-Aminolevulinic acid-mediated photodynamic therapy of intraepithelial neoplasia and human papillomavirus of the uterine cervix–a new experimental approach. *Cancer Detect Prev*. 1999;23:351-355.

102. Hillemanns P et al. Photodynamic therapy of vulvar lichen sclerosus with 5- aminolevulinic acid. *Obstet Gynecol*. 1999;93:71-74.

Laser/Light Applications in General Surgery

Raymond J. Lanzafame

- Lasers and light source technologies have been applied to a wide variety of open and laparoscopic procedures in general surgery and other disciplines.
- The ability to produce highly precise and controllable effects on tissues, and the potential to facilitate complex dissection make these devices a welcome addition to the armamentarium of the surgeon.
- Each laser wavelength has a characteristic effect on tissue and it is the combination of the laser tissue interaction and the selection of the appropriate delivery systems and laser parameters that determine the ultimate effects of laser use during surgery.
- This chapter will review the array of laser technologies available for both open and laparoscopic surgical use and will discuss the relative merits and disadvantages of each.

Introduction

- A wide variety of lasers and light-based sources are available for use in both open and minimally invasive surgical procedures.
- Proper selection of wavelength, delivery devices, and the use of appropriate surgical technique provides several advantages in the care of the surgical patient.

- Proper use can reduce blood loss, decrease postoperative discomfort, reduce the chance of wound infection, decrease the spread of some cancers, minimize the extent of surgery in selected circumstances, and result in better wound healing, if they are used appropriately by a skilled and properly trained surgeon.
- The general surgeon encounters a wide and varied array of clinical conditions and operative scenarios in daily practice.
- Many different surgical skills and modalities are required to achieve acceptable outcomes for the patient.
- There are oftentimes several treatment options and surgical procedures that are equally efficacious for a particular disease process.
- Any surgical procedure can be performed using lasers.
- General surgeons use a wide variety of laser wavelengths and laser delivery systems to cut, coagulate, vaporize or remove tissue.
- The majority of "laser surgeries" actually use the laser device in place of other instruments to accomplish a standard procedure.
- Lasers are used in both contact and non-contact modes depending on the wavelength and the particular clinical application. These devices are interchangeable to some degree, assuming that the proper delivery device and laser parameters are selected.

Lasers have occupied the fancy of the lay public, scientists and clinicians alike. These technologies have been applied to a wide variety of open and laparoscopic procedures in a variety of disciplines including general surgery.[1-85] The ability to produce highly precise and controllable effects on tissues, improved hemostasis, easy adaptability to fiberoptic and minimally invasive delivery systems, and the potential to

R.J. Lanzafame
e-mail: raymond.lanzafame@gmail.com

K. Nouri (ed.), *Lasers in Dermatology and Medicine*,
DOI: 10.1007/978-0-85729-281-0_43, © Springer-Verlag London Limited 2011

facilitate complex dissection make these devices a welcome addition to the armamentarium of the surgeon.

The general surgeon encounters a wide and varied array of clinical conditions and operative scenarios in daily practice. Many different surgical skills and modalities are required to achieve acceptable outcomes for the patient. There are oftentimes several treatment options and surgical procedures that are equally efficacious for a particular disease process. One need only consider the options available to treat breast cancer as an example of this phenomenon. Surgeons often differ as to what particular instruments are the most useful during the conduct of specific technical aspects of surgical procedures. While the motto of the Stanley Tool Corporation (Bridgeport, CT.) "The right tool for the right job" is apropos; surgeons will differ in their definition of the right tool. Such decisions are often based on preference rather than on necessity. Any surgical procedure can be performed using lasers. However, there are no general surgical procedures for which the laser is *sine qua non*.

General surgeons use a wide variety of laser wavelengths and laser delivery systems to cut, coagulate, vaporize or remove tissue. The majority of "laser surgeries" actually use the laser device in place of other tools such as scalpels, electrosurgical units, cryosurgery probes or microwave devices to accomplish a standard procedure like mastectomy or cholecystectomy.[2-57] Lasers allow the surgeon to accomplish more complex tasks. Proper use can reduce blood loss, decrease postoperative discomfort, reduce the chance of wound infection, decrease the spread of some cancers, minimize the extent of surgery in selected circumstances, and result in better wound healing, if they are used appropriately by a skilled and properly trained surgeon. They are useful in both open and laparoscopic procedures. Lasers are used in both contact and non-contact modes depending on the wavelength and the particular clinical application. These devices are interchangeable to some degree, assuming that the proper delivery device and laser parameters are selected. However, the visible light and Nd: YAG lasers should not be used for skin incisions, since they are less efficient than the carbon dioxide laser and result in excessive thermocoagulation of the wound edges.

Laparoscopic cholecystectomy can be credited with fueling a revolution in surgical thinking and application. Surgeons initially had an intense interest in lasers and laser technology for use during laparoscopic cholecystectomy.[3,4,9,16-19,21-28] Nearly 80% of all cholecystectomies performed in the United States during 1992 were performed laparoscopically, with only 4% being performed with laser technology.

The majority of general surgeons rapidly discarded "the laser" for electrosurgical devices and "conventional" instruments as they grappled with mastering new techniques and procedures with unfamiliar laparoscopes, video cameras and skills which they had never seen or used previously. The initial enthusiasm and interest in the use of lasers in minimally invasive surgery from the general surgeon's perspective can be traced to the work of Reddick, Schultz, Saye and McKernan.[20,22-26] It must be understood however that the advent of video endoscopy, specific laparoscopic instrumentation for cholecystectomy and other procedures along with the development of multiple-load endostaplers have done much to simplify minimally invasive surgery for the skilled laparoscopist.

This chapter will review the array of laser technologies available for both open and laparoscopic surgical use and will discuss the relative merits and disadvantages of each.

Lasers Versus Other Technologies

- Advantages of other technologies
  - Electrosurgical devices are much more familiar, ubiquitous in the operating room.
  - Capital equipment expenditures are less for many of these devices and some disposables used with them.
  - These devices are "faster" since the surgeon is much more conversant with electrosurgical technology and its appropriate application.
  - The main advantages of electrosurgical devices are the ubiquity of them in the operating room and the fact that no additional training or safety considerations need be implemented.
  - These factors, when coupled with the average surgeon's comfortability with using them, make them the technology of choice for many surgeons. devices.
- Disadvantages of electrosurgical devices
  - The main disadvantages of electrosurgical devices rest on the relative imprecision of the delivery of energy to the desired target.
  - The build-up of char and debris on the electrode surface can result in the delivery of energy to areas adjacent to the desired target rather than to the target itself.
  - Electrosurgical devices work poorly in the presence of blood, edema and irrigating solutions.
  - The majority of insulated laparoscopic hand instruments have relatively large exposed electrode surfaces. A large electrode may result in damage to adjacent structures.
  - Capacitance coupling can occur with monopolar devices.
  - The tips of bipolar or harmonic scalpel devices can become hot during use and can damage tissues contacted after use.

- Advantages of laser technology
  - Proponents of laser technology list the high degree of precision possible with these devices and the ability to control the tissue effect at the desired target as being the main advantages of these devices.
- Disadvantages of laser technology
  - Opponents often cite the acquisition expense of laser machinery and accessories in addition to an increased operative time as the main disadvantages of lasers.
  - Additional training and attention to safety are necessary.

One must consider whether any laser adds anything to the surgeon's armamentarium. Electrosurgical devices are much more familiar, ubiquitous in the operating room, "less expensive" from perspective of capital equipment expenditures and for some disposables, and "faster" particularly since the surgeon is much more conversant with electrosurgical technology and its appropriate application. Other alternatives including bipolar cautery and the harmonic scalpel are becoming increasingly popular alternatives to both monopolar cautery and lasers. The skills required to use these newer technologies are also more easily acquired since they are closely akin to the repertoire of the surgeon.

The main advantages of electrosurgical devices are the ubiquity of them in the operating room and the fact that no additional training or safety considerations need be implemented. These factors, when coupled with the average surgeon's comfortability with using them, make this the technology of choice for many surgeons.[2-13,16-21,28] Both monopolar and bipolar instrumentation is available for both open and laparoscopic use and the majority of "routine" laparoscopic instrumentation is insulated to permit their use with electrosurgical devices. The main disadvantages of electrosurgical devices rest on the relative imprecision of the delivery of energy to the desired target. The build-up of char and debris on the electrode surface can result in the delivery of energy to areas adjacent to the desired target rather than to the target itself. Electrosurgical devices work poorly in the presence of blood, edema and irrigating solutions. The majority of insulated laparoscopic hand instruments have relatively large exposed electrode surfaces. A large electrode may result in damage to adjacent structures, particularly in close spaces. Capacitance coupling is also a potential problem. Bipolar devices and harmonic scalpels avoid the issues of stray current injuries. However, the instrument tips can become hot during use and can damage tissues contacted after use.

An array of laser technology is available for use during laparoscopy for incisional purposes. Currently, this includes the argon, CO_2, holmium, KTP and Nd: YAG lasers. More recently, high power diode laser technology has become available for use in soft tissue applications. New entrants in this arena are likely. Laser technology is also available for lithotripsy. We will discuss each of these wavelengths and technologies in some detail below. Several points bear mention prior to the consideration of specific technologies.

Proponents of laser technology list the high degree of precision possible with these devices and the ability to control the tissue effect at the desired target as being the main advantages of these devices.[3-6,9,10,16-34] Opponents often cite the acquisition expense of laser machinery and accessories in addition to an increased operative time as the main disadvantages of lasers in general. Although these issues are often raised, few recognize that the "cost" of a technology is not necessarily correlated with the actual price of the technology and that the price has little to do with the charge or the reimbursement. It must be understood that the net or global effect of a technology may be to lower the total cost of an illness when one considers factors such as the length of hospitalization, the degree and length of disability and the ability of the patient to return to normal productivity.

Surgical "speed" evolves and improves and the "length of the procedure" declines after the "learning curve" and once the surgeon becomes experienced and facile with the technique and the technology used to accomplish a procedure. It should be recognized that a laser may be used for only a small portion of a procedure and several other factors also impact the operative time.

The surgeon should have a complete working understanding of lasers, their delivery systems and their tissue effects prior to attempting to apply them to laparoscopic or other procedures. The surgeon should attend specific hands-on laser training programs if laser education and the opportunity to use these devices during the course of an approved residency training program were not available or if the surgeon is not familiar with a particular device or delivery system. Clearly, the house officer is in the ideal position to acquire the intellectual and manual skills necessary to use lasers and other technologies properly if this opportunity is provided as a part of the residency training program. Postgraduate continuing medical education programs are useful for those who did not have formal training elsewhere. It is imperative that the surgeon continue to develop these newly acquired skills in an ongoing, graded fashion. This requires the gradual incorporation of the use of laser technology into clinical practice by tackling the simpler procedures and tasks first, followed by more difficult problems later, after the surgeon has developed a sense of comfortability with the technology. One should have a working understanding of the limits and advantages of lasers in one's own hands. The surgeon must be aware that all lasers and delivery systems are not alike and that attention to the selection of the proper wavelength, the proper delivery system and the proper laser parameters are central to achieving the desired clinical endpoint given the appropriate technical expertise.

The above point cannot be neglected by the surgeon. The selection of a laser device, delivery system or any other instrument during the course of a procedure is critical to the conduct and outcome of that procedure. The selection of instrumentation for procedures involves a number of variables as we have already discussed. However, the preference of the surgeon is a major determinant in this process. Preference depends on availability, skill, judgment, experience and the sense that a particular tool "feels right" or "works well" for a particular task in the hands of a particular surgeon. One needs only to examine the back table during an operative procedure to realize that several alternatives exist for the surgeon's execution of a particular task.

Laser Characteristics/ General Considerations

- Adequate preoperative patient evaluation and education.
- Antibiotic prophylaxis as indicated.

Several different laser wavelengths and laser delivery systems are available for use during surgery.[2-57] Each laser wavelength has a characteristic effect on tissue and it is the combination of the laser tissue interaction and the selection of the appropriate delivery systems and laser parameters that determine the ultimate effects of laser use during surgery. This presumes that the surgeon has the appropriate skill and technique. Thus, it is possible to precisely select and control the degree of tissue injury during surgery.

The ability to achieve the desired effect on the target tissue is also dependent on the surgeon's understanding about the relationship between Power Density (PD) and the laser tissue interaction. Power density represents a concentration function and is defined as:

$$PD = Power/\pi * r^2 = W/cm^2$$

The power is the selected output power of the laser given in watts and r represents the radius of the beam's spot. It can be seen that given this relationship, the spot size or beam diameter has a significant influence on the power density relative to a given power output of a laser. The length of exposure of a target tissue to the laser energy is the fluence that is measured in Joules per centimeter squared and which is defined as follows:

$$FLUENCE = (Power/\pi * r^2) * (time\ in\ seconds)$$
$$= W\ sec/cm^2 = J/cm^2$$

The surgeon generally endeavors to use the highest power density that can be safely controlled, thereby minimizing the duration of the exposure and unwanted tissue injury by conductive heating of the tissue during contact with the laser beam.

The primary result of the laser tissue interaction produces the classical histology of injury. The center of the wound is the zone of ablation, where tissue is vaporized or removed given a sufficiently high power density. This is followed by a zone of irreversible injury or necrosis, which is followed by a zone of reversible injury. Minimizing the duration of laser exposure will optimize the tissue effects for most applications by reducing conductive thermal injury to the tissues adjacent to the area of exposure to the laser beam.

Laser Use in Minimally Invasive Surgery

- Laser utilization offers several advantages during operative laparoscopy.
- These devices can provide substantial convenience and time savings for the surgeon by enhancing precision, control, and hemostasis, while decreasing the need for instrument swapping.
- Virtually all laser wavelengths have found some utility in laparoscopic procedures.
- The KTP: YAG, holmium and Nd: YAG lasers are the most versatile and are the least intrusive on endoscopic visualization.
- These versatile devices have many justifiable uses during surgery.
- The surgeon should have a thorough understanding of the procedure to be performed as well as the laser device, its delivery systems and safety considerations.
- Practice and continued use of these devices will lead to improved outcomes.

We will first discuss laser utilization in laparoscopic and endoscopic surgery. The types of laser technology available for laparoendoscopic use are listed in Table 1. We will describe these laser wavelengths in more detail and consider the applications and shortfalls for each. Specific laser parameters for open surgery are presented in Tables 2, 3, and 4. The reader may find it useful to refer to this

Laser/Light Applications in General Surgery

Table 1 Lasers available for laparoscopic use and their properties

Laser	λ	Power max	Absorption chromophore	Tissue necrosis
CO_2	10.6 μ	150 W	Water	200 μ–0.5 mm
Holmium	2.1 μ	150 W	Water	300 μ–2 mm
Argon	488, 514 nm	30 W	Pigment, hemoglobin	300 μ–4 mm
KTP	532 nm	80 W	Pigment, hemoglobin	400 μ–4 mm
Nd:YAG	1.064 μ	120 W	Pigment, proteins	200 μ–2 cm
Dye	508–690 nm	20 W	Pigment	300 μ–1 mm
Diode	905 nm	30 W	Pigment, proteins	500 μ–1 mm

Table 2 Parameters for the CO_2 laser

Tissue type/tasks	Power	Spot diameter
Skin incision	15–25–40 W continuous (CW)	0.2 mm
Subcutaneous tissue/fat incision	60 W CW[c]	0.2–0.4 mm
Dissection of breast tissue/creation of flaps	60 W CW[c]	0.2–0.4 mm
Muscle incision/ transection	60–80 W CW	0.4 mm
Dissection clavipectoral fascia	40 W–60 W[f] CW	0.4 mm
Axillary dissection[b]	40 W–60 W[f] CW	0.4 mm
Laser sterilization[d]	40 W CW	10–20 mm
Tissue vaporization/ ablation[e]	15–100 W CW or pulsed	0.2–20 mm

Wavelength: 10,600 nm; Mode: TEMoo; Handpiece: 125 mm lens[a] (0.2 mm spot diameter)

[a]The 125 mm lens is the most convenient for use for most applications. The 50 mm lens with a spot diameter of 0.09 mm achieves the same power density with 25% of the wattage. For example, the 10 W with a 50 mm lens in-focus produces the same power density as 40 W with a 125 mm lens in-focus. However, the 50 mm lens is more cumbersome and difficult to use for non-cutaneous applications

[b]This procedure requires the use of an optical backstop such as the Köcher bronchocele sound, which permits precise dissection without damaging adjacent or underlying structures

[c]Using settings higher than 60 W CW increase the likelihood of causing a flash fire due to ignition of aerosolized fat in the plume

[d]Laser sterilization is accomplished by defocusing the laser and gently heating the wound surface. The tissue should be heated just to the point of dessication and slight shrinkage of the wound. Blanching and charring of the wound is indicative of excessive irreversible damage to the wound

[e]Vaporization or ablation of tissues is most efficient when a high power density is used with a large spot diameter. This permits the surgeon to cover a large area expeditiously

[f]Use powers no greater that 40 W until you become proficient and are comfortable with the higher powers. However, 60 W is more efficient and hemostatic

Table 3 Parameters for the KTP laser

Wavelength[a]	532 mm
Output	1–40 W[c]
Delivery system	Fiberoptic, 0.2 mm, 0.3 mm, 0.4 mm, 0.6 mm diameter fibers. Microstat® probes are formed to an appropriate configuration for the desired task.
Incision[b]	10–20 W continuous wave or pulsed
Coagulation	1–20 W continuous wave or pulsed
Vaporization/ablation[d]	10–20 W continuous wave or pulsed

[a]The KTP/YAG system delivers both the 532 nm (KTP) wavelength and the 1,060 nm Nd:YAG wavelength but, at this time, not the two simultaneously. The Nd:YAG can be operated at power settings from 1 to 6 W. It is a more efficient photocoagulator than is the 532 nm wavelength at higher powers

[b]The KTP laser is used with the cleaved fiber in direct contact with the tissue for most uses. Near-contact use is analogous to defocusing the laser beam. Skin incisions are usually not made with the KTP laser because of the extent of lateral tissue damage (burn). However, some users do prefer to make incisions in the anoderm with the laser. Blackened instruments and optical backstops are helpful

[c]Higher energies can be used in aqueous environments, but open and laparoscopic procedures generally do not require settings above 20 W CW. Higher powers will result in frequent damage to the fiber's tip

[d]Vaporization is best accomplished by using the fiber in a defocused position. Pulsing the laser or using continuous wave mode for brief intervals reduces the likelihood of flaming and burning of the fiber tip. If fiber burnout does occur, the fiber is easily recleaved and the cladding is stripped, making it again ready for use

information as a rough guide for laparoendoscopic applications as well.

Laser utilization offers several advantages during operative laparoscopy. These devices can provide substantial convenience and time savings for the surgeon by enhancing precision, control, and hemostasis, while decreasing the need for instrument swapping. Dissection and hemostasis in areas of inflammation and scar can be facilitated and the potential for stray energy damage, which is a known hazard of electrosurgery, can be minimized. Although virtually all laser wavelengths have found some utility in laparoscopic procedures, the KTP: YAG, holmium and YAG laser are the most versatile and are the least intrusive on endoscopic visualization.[3-7,9-12,14,16-28,30-33]

All of the fiber capable lasers can be used under water or saline irrigation and are effective in cases with edema. These properties provide substantial advantages over monopolar electrosurgical devices. However, the surgeon must understand the laser tissue interaction for the particular wavelength and delivery system chosen in order to minimize the potential for iatrogenic injury.

Table 4 Parameters for use of the Nd:YAG laser

Delivery system	Incision	Coagulation	Vaporization/ablation
Lens[a]	NR	20–120 W	20–120 W
Polished fiber[b]	NR	20–120 W	20–120 W
Sapphire tip[c]	5–25 W	5–25 W	5–25 W
Sculpted/power fiber[d]	5–35 W	5–35 W	NR
Cleaved bare fiber[e]	10–55 W	20–120 W	20–120 W

Wavelength: 1,060 nm; Output: 1–120 W; Delivery Systems: Fiberoptic, usually with 0.4 mm or 0.6 mm fibers; varies with type of application and terminal delivery system apparatus. Common delivery systems are: lens or polished fiber, sapphire tip, sculpted or "power fiber," cleaved bare fiber
NR not recommended
[a]The lens system was one of the first applications of the Nd:YAG laser. The laser energy cuts poorly due to extensive forward and back scattering in tissue. The main applications of the lens system was for coagulation or for tissue vaporization
[b]Polished fiber applications are mainly for endoscopic coagulation or vaporization techniques. It is poor for making incisions
[c]Sapphire tips function as a "laser-assisted" device with a large portion (up to 80%) of the laser input being converted to heat and only a small percentage (approximately 20%) being transmitted by the distal third of the tip. This explains the lack of increased response with increasing laser power and also explains why the sapphire tip permits the laser to incise tissues with zones of injury which resemble other lasers and electrocautery (i.e., 300–1,000 μ). Skin incision is not recommended
[d]These recent developments are touted to transmit 81% of laser energy when held in contact with tissue. The fibers which have recently been placed on the market are said to transmit 81% of laser energy when held in contact with tissue. There are no published data which verifies this statement. When we tested one fiber, it did not produce coagulation of pigmented meat when held in water in near contact with the meat. They produce effects that are similar to sapphire tips on tissue but the surgeon can increase incisional speed and effect with increasing power input. Some manufacturers recommend these fibers for skin incision, but many surgeons do not prefer this
[e]Cleaved fibers (bare fibers) can be used for cutting, coagulation or vaporization. This mode of delivering of YAG energy is extremely dangerous if optical backstops are not used due to the 10° angle of divergence of energy from an optical fiber and due to the extreme forward and backscatter of YAG energy in biological tissues

CO_2 Laser

- CO_2 lasers have been used extensively for gynecologic laparoscopic applications but have been rarely utilized for other minimally invasive surgical procedures.
- This wavelength is intensely absorbed by cellular water.
- The CO_2 laser wavelength is carried via hollow tubes, waveguides and mirrors. Flexible fiberoptics are being developed for clinical use.
- The focusing cube and waveguide systems require a direct line of sight or the use of angled mirrors.

CO_2 lasers have been used extensively for an array of gynecologic laparoscopic applications but have been rarely utilized for laparoscopic cholecystectomy and other minimally invasive surgical procedures.[6,7,9,10,19] The energy of the CO_2 laser (wavelength = 10,600 nm) is in the far-infrared portion of the electromagnetic spectrum. This wavelength is intensely absorbed by cellular water. This property results in "superficial" injury to tissues and enables the sealing of blood vessels and lymphatics that are up to 0.5–1.0 mm diameter. The potential for inadvertent injury to deeper structures is minimal. The zone of necrosis is approximately 100–300 μ, when the CO_2 laser is used at appropriate fluences in a cutting mode. This most closely resembles the histology of an incision created by the scalpel. This wavelength is absorbed independently of the color of the tissue. Thus, the clinical effect seen in soft tissues is relative to the water content of the target tissue. The local infiltration of tissue with saline or anesthetic solutions will protect or insulate them from injury by the laser beam until the fluid has been vaporized. This laser is the most efficient modality available for ablation or vaporization of large volumes of tissue such as tumor nodules or endometriomas.

The CO_2 laser wavelength is carried via hollow tubes, waveguides and mirrors. Flexible fiberoptics are being developed for clinical use. The Omniguide® fiber is a flexible chalcogenide glass fiber optic that has been utilized for neuro-surgical and otolaryngological surgeries. The potential exists for broader clinical use, including various general surgical procedures. The laparoscopic use of this wavelength is possible with the use of a focusing cube and an operative laparoscope or with a variety of waveguides designed for multi-puncture laparoscopic applications. The focusing cube permits the use of the CO_2 laser in a free beam mode for cutting, vaporization and coagulation of tissue. The focusing cube also is capable of transmitting an aiming beam. This feature makes it easier for the surgeon to direct the laser energy to the desired target. A variety of procedures such as myomectomy, partial oophorectomy, resection and ablation of endometriomas, adhesiolysis, and even cholecystectomy have been accomplished successfully with this delivery system. Cholecystectomy requires a McKernan-type approach. The successful use of this approach requires knowledge and facility with the operative laparoscope and the surgeon's ability to visualize the desired target and maneuver a micromanipulator or joy stick. The surgeon can alter the tissue effect by focusing or defocusing the laser beam as well as varying the laser wattage selected.

Laser waveguides are hollow tubes with mirror-like surfaces which reflect the CO_2 wavelength. Waveguides are available in both rigid and flexible versions, and can be used to achieve a spot size (i.e., burn or incision) which is in the range of 0.8–2.2 mm. However, laser waveguides, particularly those capable of carrying high powers are increasingly difficult to obtain today. As a general principle, the waveguide is used in a non contact fashion, particularly since tissue contact can obstruct the waveguide and liquid can be drawn into the waveguide by capillary action. The resultant of these events is the irreversible destruction of the waveguide.

The successful use of this laser for dissection and hemostasis requires that the surgeon be facile and expert with the laser as this will affect the ability to dissect tissues and achieve an adequate degree of hemostasis. Both the focusing cube and waveguide systems require a direct line of sight or the use of angled mirrors. This further complicates the maneuverability of these devices more so than fiber capable lasers and conventional instruments. Both configurations require flowing gas to cool the system and to prevent vaporized tissue plume from being thrown into the device. The most frequently used purge gases are argon and carbon dioxide. High CO_2 gas flow rates can actually absorb the laser energy and reduce its efficiency (i.e., the transmission of energy from the laser to the tissue). Therefore, lower flow rates (i.e., 1 L/min.) are suggested. Some laser systems are equipped with a nitrogen purge gas system. The surgeon should NOT use nitrogen during laparoscopy as its absorption from the peritoneum can cause "the bends."

The optimal use of the CO_2 laser for laparoscopic or open use is achieved when the beam is oriented perpendicular to the desired target. Hemostasis is enhanced by tissue compression, the use of epinephrine containing local anesthetic solutions and the ability of the operator to recognize the presence of a vessel prior to its division. Under these conditions, the surgeon defocuses the laser (i.e., moves the handpiece, waveguide or operating laparoscope farther away from the target) and then applies short bursts of energy to the vessel in the area to be divided. This maneuver heats and coagulates the vessel, thereby enabling its division by the focused beam. The surgeon should use the highest power setting with which he/she is comfortable as this will enable more efficient cutting, better hemostasis and less thermal injury to the wound edges by minimizing conductive and radiative heat loss into the wound. Intermittent evacuation of the vaporized tissue plume or the use of a re-circulating filtration system assure a clear field of view and prevents absorption of toxic products of combustion by the patient. This problem is identical in magnitude and toxicity to vaporized tissue plume created by any electrosurgical, thermal or laser source. Similarly the "smoke" should not be vented into the operating room as it should be considered hazardous for physician OR personnel. OSHA/NIOSH has written regulations which require that physician OR staff be protected from vaporized tissue plume regardless of its source.[1,52,56,57]

Argon Laser

- The argon laser has been used extensively for gynecologic laparoscopic procedures.
- Visible light wavelengths can be passed through water, enabling the argon laser to be used in aqueous environments such as the bladder and in the presence of irrigating fluids as is routinely encountered during abdominal and pelvic procedures.
- Both free-beam and conventional fiberoptic applications are utilized during operative laparoscopy.
- White or lightly colored tissue will not cut efficiently and will not be vaporized (ablated) unless they are first painted with India ink, indigo carmine dye or another exogenous chromophore.
- One of the main drawbacks of the argon laser is the camera/eye safety filter which must block the six wavelengths produced by the laser. These filters are usually a deep orange color and absorb 30–60% of the visible spectrum, resulting in color distortion of the image.

The argon laser has been used extensively for gynecologic laparoscopic procedures.[10,11,16-21,26] This laser produces light in the visible portion of the spectrum. This laser actually produces six lines (wavelengths). However, the majority of the laser output is in the blue-green spectrum (wavelengths = 488, 514 nm). This energy is intensely absorbed by hemoglobin and melanin although other exogenous chromophores will absorb these wavelengths efficiently. Visible light wavelengths can be passed through water, enabling the argon laser to be used in aqueous environments such as the bladder, during hysteroscopy, arthroscopy and in the presence of irrigating fluids as is routinely encountered during abdominal and pelvic procedures. This property enables the surgeon to photocoagulate a bleeding area while irrigating to locate the source of the bleeding.

Both free-beam and conventional fiberoptic applications are utilized during operative laparoscopy. A Microslad unit may be coupled with the operative laparoscope. A gimbaled mirror and joy stick allow the surgeon to maneuver the beam in the surgical field. The fiber can be used in both a contact and non-contact mode.

Argon laser light penetrates and scatters in tissues. The resultant damage can be as much as 6 mm depending upon the tissue exposed. When used in an incisional mode, the speed of incision and the degree of hemostasis are adequate. Blood vessels on the order of 2 mm diameter can be divided and coagulated with this wavelength. Although some authors have reported successful hemostasis with vessels as large as 3–4 mm diameter, delayed re-bleeding may occur. Therefore the surgeon would do well to use ligature and Hemo-clip methods for hemostasis in these instances. The etiology of the delayed bleeding is necrosis of photocoagulated tissue and resultant tissue slough. This condition also occurs after use of the Nd: YAG laser in a free beam mode on similar tissues.

The contact or fiber optic method is much more easily mastered than is the free beam approach since the surgeon has direct tactile feedback from the tissue. The speed of incision and the degree of hemostasis are adequate and the more selective absorption of the wavelength in hemoglobin enables the surgeon to photocoagulate vessels prior to their division by bringing the fiber away from the tissue surface. This maneuver is similar to defocusing the free beam. The defocused mode is used to vaporize endometriomas. Some manufacturers produce a variety of sculpted fibers and metal-jacketed fiber delivery systems. These fibers are constructed to be more durable and work "more like a scalpel" due to absorption of some of the laser energy in the fiber resulting in heating of the fiber. This produces an optically driven cautery effect. So-called bare or urologic fibers are easily used and are cleaved and stripped as the fiber end degrades with use. Optimal cutting occurs by using the tip of the fiber either end-on or oblique to the plane of the dissection.

Since these wavelengths are color dependent, the surgeon should note that white or lightly colored tissue such as meniscus and tumor implants will not cut efficiently and will not be vaporized (ablated) unless they are first painted with India ink, indigo carmine dye or another exogenous chromophore. A droplet of blood placed on the surface is sometimes effective for this purpose. Blackened or ebonized instruments and the use of optical backstops are required to prevent beam reflection and iatrogenic injury.

One of the main drawbacks of the laparoscopic use of the argon laser is the camera/eye safety filter. The eye and camera filters must block the six wavelengths produced by the laser. These filters are usually a deep orange color and absorb 30–60% of the visible spectrum. As a result, the color balance of the image is distorted and the need for a high powered light source is critical to the surgeons' ability to visualize the operative field. Many laser systems have intermittent shutter mechanisms which place the filter in the visual field only while the laser is actually being fired. The surgeon must be an expert at the local anatomy and the details of the procedure prior to attempting to work with this laser. These factors make the use of the argon laser a rarity today.

Nd: YAG Laser

- This wavelength is carried via conventional fiberoptics and, like visible light lasers; the energy will be transmitted through water.

- The energy can be applied to tissues with a wide array of delivery systems including: cleaved bare fibers, GI fibers, sapphire tips, sculpted fibers, as well as free beam via a micromanipulator or Microslad® unit.
- The energy of the Nd: YAG laser is intensely absorbed by tissue protein and chromophores and is highly scattered in tissue. These properties result in deep penetration of the energy and much greater damage below the tissue than can be appreciated at the surface.
- Use of the bare fiber for dissection has been practiced safely by surgeons having a detailed understanding of anatomy and by orienting the fiber in a plane which is tangential to the line of incision to limit the forward scattering of the energy into the tissues.
- The YAG wavelength is a poor ablating wavelength, particularly when compared to the CO_2, KTP or holmium wavelengths whose rates of ablation are significantly faster.

The neodymium YAG laser produces near infrared light at a wavelength of 1,060 nm. This wavelength is carried via conventional fiberoptics and, like visible light lasers; the energy will be transmitted through water. The energy can be applied to tissues with a wide array of delivery systems including: cleaved bare fibers (i.e., urologic fibers), polished GI fibers, sapphire tips (i.e., the delivery device which is marketed as the Contact Laser®), sculpted fiber (e.g., Microcontact® tip and various other proprietary versions of this technology), as well as free beam via a micromanipulator or Microslad® unit.[3,5,6,10-12,16-21,26-28] The energy of the Nd: YAG laser is intensely absorbed by tissue protein and chromophores, and is highly scattered in tissue. These properties result in deep penetration of the energy and much greater damage below the tissue than can be appreciated at the surface. This makes non contact (i.e., GI fiber, free beam) and bare fiber applications of the Nd: YAG laser extremely dangerous unless the surgeon has a thorough understanding of the laser-tissue interaction and orients the beam in a direction which would reduce the likelihood of damaging nearby structures. The Nd: YAG laser is a poor cutting instrument when it is used in a non contact mode. The development of sapphire tips and sculpted fiber technologies facilitated use of this laser in contact with tissue. Free-beam type applications can result in damage to as much as 1–2 cm of liver tissue and the photocoagulation of vessels up to 4 mm in diameter.

Sapphire tip technology creates a combined thermal and optical interaction with tissue. Much of the Nd: YAG energy is absorbed by the sapphire or fiber tip and converted to heat.

The result is to produce optically driven cautery.[16-20] The temperature of the tip can be tightly regulated for some applications. These instruments improve the cutting ability of the laser, but the tissue damage and the extent of coagulation are reduced dramatically. The histology of these devices is quite similar to the results produced by electrosurgical devices. Since their main tissue interaction is thermal cautery, the rate of incision and the degree of hemostasis can be reduced when these devices are used in the presence of irrigating fluids or in the aqueous environment of the bladder or joint space. The surgeon adjusts the laser parameters accordingly in order to achieve the desired effect. Sapphire tips are fragile and are expensive in comparison to other delivery systems. They remain hot for a short while after the laser has been turned off, which can cause damage or adherence to adjacent structures upon accidental contact. The sapphire tip may become disconnected from the fiber while operating and may be lost. When these devices are used in vascular and aqueous conditions such as the bladder, prostate or uterus, the fibers must NEVER be cooled with air or gas as embolism of gas has proven fatal. Fiber cooling with saline or other irrigating fluids is quite safe however. Sapphire tip technology is seldom used today due to these issues with their use and since other, less expensive alternatives are available.

Sculpted fibers have been developed with many of the same properties as the sapphire tip, but without the liability of the tip remaining hot for an appreciable period of time after lasing has ceased and with less fragility of the tip. Some types of sculpted fibers transmit a sufficient quantity of laser energy to permit the coagulation of bleeders by using the fiber in a non contact mode. Sculpted fibers are good compromise for many laparoscopic applications. However, many of the currently available fiber designs are much stiffer than conventional fibers, which make them somewhat less pliable and somewhat more fragile than conventional silica-silica and quartz fibers.

Surgery with sapphire tips and sculpted fibers is facilitated by using them at an oblique angle relative to the plane of dissection. This technique enhances hemostasis by taking advantage of the heated mass of sapphire (or fiber tip), which coagulates the tissues prior to their division by the much hotter tip portion.

Use of the bare fiber for dissection has been practiced safely by several experienced surgeons. However, the surgeon must have an intimate understanding of anatomy and should orient the fiber in a plane which is tangential to the line of incision to limit the forward scattering of the energy into the tissues. The use of ebonized instruments and optical backstops are mandatory.

Hemostasis with the YAG laser is best accomplished by using the laser (fiber, beam) in a defocused mode and delivering short bursts of energy to the area and its immediate periphery. It is generally better to deliver a few pulses and then wait for a few minutes to observe the area rather than attempting to lase continuously as the latter practice will increase tissue damage unnecessarily and may actually result in the vaporization of the clot and re-bleeding.

The Nd: YAG laser has been used for the vaporization (ablation) of tumors.[16,47,53,56,57] Typically, the surgeon will orient the beam parallel to the long axis of hollow viscera to avoid iatrogenic injury or perforation. Most of these procedures are performed in stages. In other words, the tumor is treated, allowed to slough, and then is treated as needed in subsequent sessions after debridement or natural sloughing of the photocoagulated tissue. The YAG wavelength is actually a poor ablating wavelength, particularly when compared to the CO_2, KTP or holmium wavelengths whose rates of ablation are significantly faster. Lightly colored tissues require substantially more energy to initiate tissue ablation. Ablation does not proceed until an area becomes desiccated and/or carbonized. The carbon then absorbs the laser energy and "catalyzes" the ablation of the subjacent tissue. Painting the tissue with India ink, Methylene blue, blood or other chromophores makes the process much more efficient and safer by dramatically reducing the total amount of energy required to photoablate a given volume of tissue.

KTP Laser

- The KTP laser is a frequency-doubled YAG laser which produces pure lime green light at a wavelength of 532 nm.
- The KTP wavelength is intensely absorbed by hemoglobin and melanin. Its absorption by hemoglobin is quite efficient as it is very near the hemoglobin absorption peak at 540 nm.
- This wavelength is easily transmitted through water and is carried via conventional fiberoptics.
- The KTP laser is capable of incision, coagulation and vaporization of tissue. This wavelength is much more efficient than the argon laser for these functions and surpasses the Nd: YAG laser as regards cutting and vaporization functions.
- This laser is quite versatile for laparoscopic procedures.

The KTP laser is a frequency-doubled YAG laser which produces pure lime green light at a wavelength of 532 nm. The 532 nm wavelength is also available using crystals other than potassium-titanyl-phosphate. The version manufactured by Laserscope (San Jose, CA) is capable of delivering both the 532 nm KTP wavelength and the 1,060 nm, Nd: YAG wavelength. The surgeon can switch between these wavelengths depending upon the needs of the procedure. Laserscope currently offers refurbished units for sale. The KTP wavelength is intensely absorbed by hemoglobin and melanin. Its absorption by hemoglobin is quite efficient as it is very near the hemoglobin absorption peak at 540 nm. This wavelength is easily transmitted through water and is carried via conventional fiberoptics. Typically, a cleaved and stripped bare fiber is used with a suction-irrigation instrument. Free-beam applications are possible with a micromanipulator or Microslad®.

The KTP laser is capable of incision, coagulation and vaporization of tissue.[10,12,15-17,19-25] This wavelength is much more efficient than the argon laser for these functions and surpasses the Nd: YAG laser as regards cutting and vaporization functions. These properties make this laser quite versatile for laparoscopic procedures. Vessels of up to 2 mm diameter are easily coagulated. The hemoglobin selectivity of this wavelength enables the surgeon to defocus the beam (i.e., move the fiber away from the tissue surface) and preferentially coagulate a vessel prior to its division. Bleeders such as those encountered in the gallbladder bed during cholecystectomy are dealt with by irrigating the area with saline, using the laser in a defocused mode and delivering short bursts of energy. Persistent bleeding can be dealt with by switching to the Nd: YAG laser output, if a dual wavelength laser is available.

As with the argon and Nd: YAG lasers, the KTP laser requires eye safety filters, camera filters, and optical backstops along with ebonized instruments to prevent damage from stray light or beam reflection hazards. Since the KTP laser produces a single line of visible light, interference filters are available. Interference filters protect the camera and the eyes from injury by blocking the transmission of the 532 and 1,060 nm wavelengths. This causes little if any color distortion. The CCD camera and monitor are easily adjusted to compensate for the filtered color. The tip of the fiber is the portion emitting laser energy and is therefore the part which incises and/or coagulates the tissue. Therefore the surgeon must position the fiber either perpendicularly or obliquely relative to the plane of dissection.

A high power KTP laser system capable of delivering 80 W to tissue has been developed for laser ablation of the prostate.[14,15,22] This laser produces an effect similar to a traditional TURP, with significantly reduced perioperative bleeding and with shorter operative times relative to its counterpart. It is likely that further developments of this technology will be spun off to other endoscopic and laparoscopic applications in the future.

Holmium Laser

- The holmium laser produces infrared light at a wavelength of 2,100 nm and is intensely absorbed by water.
- The highly efficient absorption of this wavelength by water permits cutting and ablation of bone and cartilage.

- This laser can be used in an aqueous environment due to the development of a cavitation bubble between the fiber and the tissue.
- The laser output is pulsed and high fluences may produce significant splattering and sputtering of tissue from the target area. This can coat the laparoscope and obscure the view.
- This laser is the most efficient wavelength for meniscectomy and percutaneous laser disc decompression (PLDD), and lithotripsy of urinary calculi. It is infrequently used by general surgeons.

The holmium laser produces infrared light at a wavelength of 2,100 nm. This wavelength is intensely absorbed by water. The holmium laser wavelength can be carried via conventional fiberoptics unlike the CO_2 wavelength. The fiber is usually encased in a metallic sheath for single puncture use or for use in combination with a suction-irrigation probe. This delivery system is quite durable and tends to be "self-cleaning." Bare fiber delivery systems are also widely available for use.[16,17,19,20]

The highly efficient absorption of this wavelength by water permits cutting and ablation of bone and cartilage. Despite its water absorption, this laser can be used in an aqueous environment due to the development of a cavitation bubble between the fiber and the tissue. This "Moses effect" transmits the laser energy to the tissue. Current systems can achieve outputs of 80 W. The laser output is pulsed and high fluences may produce significant splattering and sputtering of tissue from the target area. This can coat the laparoscope and obscure the view. This problem can be minimized by selecting an appropriate power output and repetition rate as well as viewing the surgical site at a slightly greater distance than one would normally use with other modalities.

The incisional and ablative speed of this laser is somewhat slower than many of the other wavelengths available for laparoscopic use, particularly at lower fluences. However, this is offset by the ease of use and durability of the fiberoptics. The zone of coagulation is similar to that seen with electrosurgical devices and sculpted fibers. This laser is the most efficient wavelength for meniscectomy and percutaneous laser disc decompression (PLDD), and lithotripsy of urinary calculi. It is infrequently used by general surgeons for the most part.

Diode Laser Technology

- The promise of these systems is their compact size, easy portability and the potential for lower capital and maintenance costs.

> • The typical wavelengths are carried by conventional fiber optics and are most frequently applied with sculpted or bare fiber technology.

High powered diode laser systems are becoming available for clinical use.[19,20] The promise of these systems is their compact size, easy portability and the potential for lower capital and maintenance costs. The Diomed® laser (Diomed Inc., The Woodland TX) was the first such unit approved for surgical use. This laser produces near-infrared light at 805 nm. The wavelength is carried by conventional fiber optics and is most frequently applied with sculpted fiber technology. Wound histology and the incisional speed of this device are quite similar to that observed with the Nd: YAG laser. It is likely that other diode laser devices will become available in the future. Eye safety and intraoperative measures to prevent iatrogenic injury are similar to those described for the Nd: YAG laser. However, this wavelength scatters less in tissue and therefore the depth of penetration of the free beam is shallower than the free beam YAG laser.

Lithotripsy Devices

> • Laser and non laser based technologies have both been applied for laparoscopic common duct exploration and lithotripsy as well as for use in the urinary tract.
> • A variety of wavelengths including: pulsed dye lasers, alexandrite, and holmium laser devices are available for clinical use at the present time.
> • These lasers generate photoacoustic shock waves at the surface of the calculus at the point of the laser's impact that jackhammers and disintegrates the stone into small particles which can be flushed from the duct.

The surgeon had a limited number of options as regards management of the patient with choledocholithiasis during the early years of laparoscopic cholecystectomy. As surgeons became more facile with minimally invasive surgical techniques and as smaller diameter fiberscopes and glide-wires became available, it became possible to perform common duct exploration and stone extraction laparoscopically.

Stone extraction with baskets and forceps proceeds in a manner that is similar to that of open common duct exploration. However, these procedures can be difficult in the presence of large stones or stones which have become impacted

at the ampulla. These patients can be successfully managed with a variety of lithotripsy techniques. Laser and non laser based technologies have both been applied for laparoscopic common duct exploration and lithotripsy.[4,19,20] Electrohydraulic or spark gap lithotripsy devices were developed several years ago along with the development of flexible choledochoscopy. These devices relied on a piezoelectric or spark-gap device implanted at the distal end of the catheter to generate shock waves which would then fragment the calculus. These catheters were relatively inexpensive as compared to other devices. However, they were relatively large in diameter which made them impractical for use with small diameter flexible fiber choledochosopes.

Laser based lithotripsy devices are available for laparoscopic and ureteroscopic use. A variety of wavelengths have been tested including: pulsed dye lasers, alexandrite, holmium and excimer lasers. Of these, pulsed dye laser, alexandrite and holmium laser devices are available for clinical use at the present time. These lasers generate photoacoustic shock waves at the surface of the calculus at the point of the laser's impact. This jackhammers and disintegrates the stone into small particles which can be flushed from the duct. A cleaved fiber is placed in contact with the stone and a cavitation bubble develops as the laser is fired. Absorption of laser energy at the proper fluence and duty cycle causes the bubble to vibrate and fragment the stone. These devices are quite simple to use. They can be applied under direct vision with a fiberscope, or they can be placed percutaneously or threaded into the common bile duct or ureter "blindly." A characteristic cracking or snapping sound is audible as the stone is contacted and as fragmentation occurs. Matching of the wavelengths and the relatively low fluences required for this photoacoustic effort enables destruction of the calculus without damage to the tissues of the common duct or ureter. Holmium laser units are more frequently used since they are typically found in the urology department.

Practical Tips for Laser Use in Minimally Invasive Surgery

> • The surgeon should have an intimate understanding of the details of the procedure as well as the laser technology and delivery systems selected for use.
> • Learn the procedure and become comfortable with it after having successfully accomplished it using so-called "conventional" devices prior to attempting it with laser technologies.
> • The surgeon should practice with the laser devices as much as possible prior to using them clinically.

- A thorough understanding of tissue effects and the ability to assemble and troubleshoot the instrumentation is critical.
- It is helpful to work with the instrumentation in a pelvic trainer and then gradually introduce laser technology into clinical procedures.
- The operative port should be positioned such that the laser fiber can easily reach the intended surgical site end on. This is particularly important for direct fiber systems such as bare fibers for KTP, holmium or argon lasers, or waveguides for CO_2 lasers.
- Sculpted fibers and contact tips (sapphire tips) cut and coagulate optimally when they can be dragged obliquely across the tissues rather than using them end-on.
- The rate of movement of the fiber should be deliberately slow enough to allow the tissue to be cut through completely prior to advancing the fiber. The fiber should not be visibly bowed.

We have considered the various laser technologies and delivery systems available for laparoscopic use. This section will discuss various practical tips to optimize the clinical results from these devices.

It must again be emphasized that the surgeon should have an intimate understanding of the details of the procedure as well as the laser technology and delivery systems selected for use. It is preferable to learn the procedure and become comfortable with it after having successfully accomplishing it using so-called "conventional" devices prior to attempting it with laser technologies. The surgeon should practice with the laser devices as much as possible prior to using them clinically. A thorough understanding of tissue effects and the ability to assemble and troubleshoot the instrumentation is critical.[12,13,17,19-21,28,32] It is helpful to work with the instrumentation in a pelvic trainer and then gradually introduce laser technology into clinical procedures.

Trocar placement should be well-thought and should be based on the needs of the procedure as well as the habitus of the patient. As a general principle, the operative port should be positioned such that the laser fiber (and other instruments) can easily reach the intended surgical site end on. This is particularly important for direct fiber systems such as bare fibers for KTP, holmium or argon lasers or waveguides for CO_2 lasers. Sculpted fibers and contact tips (sapphire tips) cut and coagulate optimally when they can be dragged obliquely across the tissues rather than using them end-on. Therefore the trocar placement may need to be modified for the specific laser and delivery system which is to be utilized.

The assistant surgeon should provide steady countertraction in order to distract the line of incision, facilitate exposure, optimize the efficiency and efficacy of laser use.

The tissues should be incised in fluid, complete strokes as this too will increase the efficiency of the dissection and enable the dissection to proceed with better hemostasis. Staccato and repetitive passage of the laser fiber over the same area tends to produce a more irregular incision and frequently causes bleeding as vessels become injured at multiple points in the irregular wound.

Typically the fiber capable lasers are applied by placing the fiber into a suction-irrigation cannula. The fiber should be positioned such that it is easily visualized and such that the proposed line of incision is not obstructed by the suction irrigator. An optimal distance is often 1–2 cm for fiber extension. This permits visualization and maneuverability of the fiber and the surgical site without having the a floppy fiber as a result of having too much fiber length protruding from the suction irrigator. It is also critical that the fiber be retracted completely within the instrument when the instrument is being removed or inserted into the abdomen (or other site). This maneuver prevents fiber breakage or iatrogenic injury. The foot pedal for the laser and the electrosurgical device should be within easy reach while the monitor is viewed and the instrumentation is manipulated. Ideally, the surgeon should only have access to one pedal at one time in order to prevent inadvertent triggering of the wrong device.

Several devices are available which bend or angulate the bare fiber and thereby permit the surgeon to optimize the position of the fiber relative to the topography of the dissection. Again, the fiber should be permitted to enhance visualization and minimize fiber breakage.

The surgeon should learn to use a light touch when using laser fibers. The rate of movement of the fiber should be deliberately slow enough to allow the tissue to be cut through completely prior to advancing the fiber. The fiber should not be visibly bowed as this indicates undue pressure or too deep a placement of the fiber into the wound. These conditions reduce efficiency and increase the likelihood of fiber breakage.

Sapphire tips and sculpted fibers should be used in a similar fashion to the method suggested for bare fibers. However, the tip or probe should be oriented more obliquely or tangential to the line of incision. This optimizes the coagulative effect of the laser and facilitates the dissection.

Laser Injury and Its Prevention During Laparoscopic Surgery

- The surgeon should understand and implement safety procedures as recommended by the ANSI Standard (ANSI Z136.3, 2005) and other appropriate regulatory bodies to prevent injury to patients and personnel.

- The use of ebonized surfaces is helpful in the case of visible light and near infrared lasers.
- Instruments will become hot as they are absorbing the laser's energy. Therefore, inadvertent contact with adjacent structures must be carefully avoided to prevent secondary burns.
- Accidental injuries from inadvertent activation of the laser foot pedal can be avoided by placing only a single foot pedal in the surgeon's proximity and by placing the laser in stand-by mode when it is not in use.
- Any site of stray burn or contact with a heated instrument should be inspected carefully and should be handled as if it were a frank perforation. This is particularly important when using the Nd: YAG laser.
- The patient that has symptoms beyond those expected for the procedure, or the patient with ileus or "doing poorly" postoperatively should be suspected of having an iatrogenic injury and should be managed accordingly.

We have discussed the various wavelengths available for use during minimally invasive procedures and have considered some of the techniques to prevent injury. The surgeon would do well to understand and implement safety procedures as recommended by the ANSI Standard (ANSI Z136.3, 2005) and other appropriate regulatory bodies.[1,52] Implementation of these guidelines will prevent injury to patients and personnel.

The primary risk of injury during laparoscopy is to the patient's intraabdominal and pelvic structures due to the closed nature of the surgery and the proximity of adjacent structures.[2,3,8,12-14,19-21,28,29,33] Several methods have been developed to minimize the risk of potential injuries due to reflection of energy from the surface of surgical instruments. These methods are designed to scatter the beam or absorb the incident laser energy. It should be remembered that the CO_2 laser wavelength is color independent. Therefore, ebonized surfaces are not helpful in this case. Instruments should have brushed beaded or sand-blasted surfaces. Titanium is preferable as a back stop material. The use of ebonized surfaces is helpful in the case of visible light and near infrared lasers. However, the surgeon must remember that these instruments will become hot as they are absorbing the laser's energy. Therefore, inadvertent contact with adjacent structures must be carefully avoided to prevent secondary burns.

The surgeon should orient the laser fiber and beam such that the possibility of past-pointing is avoided. This too can result in damage to nearby structures, particularly if back-stops are not in use during the dissection. Accidental injuries from inadvertent activation of the laser foot pedal can also occur. These potential problems are best avoided by placing only a single foot pedal in the surgeon's proximity and by placing the laser in stand-by mode when it is not in use.

The bowel and bladder should always be checked for perforation injuries or potential burns, particularly after extensive dissections or vaporizational procedures. Such a practice is prudent irrespective of the technology that has been used during the conduct of the case. Several strategies have been used including filling the area with irrigation fluid, insufflating the bowel with air, and/or the instillation of betadine, methylene blue, indigo carmine or other dyes and observing the tissue for any leaks or staining. Leaks or suspected areas of injury should be oversewn or closed using good surgical technique.

Any site of stray burn or contact with a heated instrument should be inspected carefully and should be handled as if it were a frank perforation. This is particularly important when using the Nd: YAG laser since the degree of damage is grossly underestimated by visualization of the surface.

As should be the case with any minimally invasive procedure, the patient that has symptoms beyond those expected for the procedure, or the patient with ileus or "doing poorly" postoperatively should be suspected of having an iatrogenic injury and should be managed accordingly.

Summary

We have discussed the tissue effects and delivery systems available for laser utilization during minimally invasive surgical procedures. These versatile devices have many justifiable uses during surgery. The surgeon should have a thorough understanding of the procedure to be performed as well as the laser device, its delivery systems and safety considerations. Practice and continued use of these devices will lead to improved outcomes.

Laser Use in Open Surgical Procedures

- Lasers are also applicable to open surgical procedures.
- Common surgical uses include wound debridement and ulcer excision, breast surgery, cholecystectomy, hernia repair, bowel resection, hemorrhoidectomy, solid organ surgery, and treatment of pilonidal cysts.
- The carbon dioxide laser remains a surgical mainstay for these applications.
- It is preferable to consider how best to utilize lasers rather than whether to use a laser for a particular procedure.

> - The experienced laser surgeon will soon recognize that many different laser wavelengths and delivery systems are useful and interchangeable for most operations. Certain applications will require a specific wavelength or delivery system.

Lasers are also applicable to open surgical procedures. Common surgical uses include wound debridement and ulcer excision, breast surgery, cholecystectomy, hernia repair, bowel resection, hemorrhoidectomy, solid organ surgery, and treatment of pilonidal cysts.[16,34-58] Lasers are used on a routine basis by a relative minority of general surgeons today. The majority of them use lasers for wound debridements and special cases. The carbon dioxide laser remains a surgical mainstay for these applications.

Like all surgical instruments, there are some uses for which lasers are indispensable and other uses where their merit is relative. Electrocautery and lasers enable the surgeon to incise tissues, obtain hemostasis and dissect with a single instrument. Unlike electrocautery, these devices enable the vaporization or ablation of large volumes of tissues (e.g., tumors) and permit the sterilization of contaminated wounds (e.g., decubitus ulcer) without the transmission of thermal or electrical energy to distant sites via neurovascular routes.

It is preferable to consider how best to utilize lasers rather than whether to use a laser for a particular procedure. As with any new technique or deviation from the routine, the use of the laser may result in an increase in operative time initially, but repeated use usually results in streamlining the procedure and reduction in operative time as the user become more comfortable and experienced.

It is helpful to have an assistant who is familiar with the laser(s). The lack of proper assistance might prove disastrous. When possible, the surgeon and surgical assistants should work together frequently and should practice with their hospital's equipment prior to attempting a major procedure for the first time. These practice sessions can be accomplished in the laboratory or after hours. Meat, fruit and vegetables provide sufficient material for the surgical team to familiarize themselves with the technology. Practice, when coupled with an adequate understanding of what a particular laser wavelength and delivery system is capable of accomplishing, enables the surgeon to select the appropriate laser (if any) for a given procedure.

The experienced laser surgeon will soon recognize that many different laser wavelengths and delivery systems are useful and interchangeable for most operations. However, certain applications will require a specific wavelength or delivery system.

Laser Parameters for Open Surgery

> - Surgery will proceed more efficiently and with less thermal damage to adjacent tissues when the surgeon uses the maximum power density (fluence) that he/she is able to control comfortably.
> - Guidelines are presented for parameters typically useful when using lasers for open surgical procedures.

Let us begin our discussion of "how" to use lasers optimally with some suggested guidelines for use of the CO_2, KTP and Nd: YAG lasers. The reader should recognize that the tables, which follow, represent a series of parameters, which we have found to be the most useful. They are not intended to be absolute, but are intended to be suggestions, which should be tailored for the individual procedure to be performed. Modification of the suggested parameters should be based on the skill and experience of the surgeon. It should be noted that surgery will proceed more efficiently and with less thermal damage to adjacent tissues when the surgeon uses the maximum power density (fluence) that he/she is able to control comfortably.

Table 2 presents guidelines for the CO_2 laser. Parameters for the KTP laser are presented in Table 3. Table 4 lists suggested guidelines for the use of the Nd: YAG laser.

Preparation of the Operative Site and Surgical Retractors

> - Some special considerations are in order when lasers are used during surgery.
> - Wound scrubs and paints should be aqueous or non-flammable.
> - Draping and gown materials should be flame retardant or non-flammable.
> - The wound itself should be surrounded with moistened towels or sponges, or should have gel lubricants layered around the wound, particularly when one first begins using lasers.
> - Retractors may be wrapped with wet gauze or stockingette material if a significant risk of beam reflection exists.
> - One must maintain constant vigilance when using lasers.

- The procedure must be conducted with a continuous awareness of the three-dimensional topography and anatomy of the operative site.
- Adjacent structures should be protected at all times to prevent inadvertent injury.
- Appropriate optical backstops for the particular laser in use should be employed whenever possible.

Some special considerations are in order when use of the laser is contemplated.[1,41,52] Wound scrubs and paints should be aqueous or non-flammable. Considerable debate arises with respect to the prudence of using Hibiclens® (chlorhexidine gluconate) as a surgical prep due to the fact that the solution contains alcohol. In fact, the preparation contains 4% alcohol and is not flammable. This solution may therefore be used safely. It is still an excellent practice to ensure that no surgical prep solution is allowed to puddle or collect on or around the patient. Draping and gown materials should be flame retardant or non-flammable. Cooling blankets must not contain alcohol or other flammable coolants.

The wound itself should be surrounded with moistened towels or sponges, particularly when one first begins using the laser. This reduces the possibility of fire. Alternatives include the use of gel lubricants, which can be placed in layers around the wound. Recently, sheets of gel wound protectant have become available for use. This material can be trimmed to conform to the surgical site. It adheres much like electrocautery grounding pads and provides wound protection without the inconvenience of a wet field.

Many so-called laser retractors, which feature blackened or ebonized surfaces, are available. Such specialized instruments may be helpful when working in confined spaces, particularly when one is using visible light lasers (e.g., KTP and Argon) and near infrared lasers (e.g., Nd: YAG). These instruments do not absorb the longer infrared wavelength of the CO_2 laser. Instruments with a beaded or matte surface or those with special coatings are required to prevent significant reflection of the CO_2 laser beam. For the most part, these specialized instruments are unnecessary. Retractors may be wrapped with wet gauze or stockingette material if a significant risk of beam reflection exists. Plastic and acrylic retractors are also useful and inexpensive.[37,41] However, extreme caution must be exercised to avoid striking them with the laser beam, as they will melt or burn and can cause injury to the patient.

Acrylic blocks are serviceable as inexpensive, but effective retractors. Quarter-inch (6 mm) acrylic sheet material can be cut into $8 \times 15 \times 0.6$ cm sections, packaged and presterilized for use. They can be resterilized or may be discarded after a single use. They cost about 20 cents each.[37,41] These retractors facilitate the application of steady traction on the wound, making incision and dissection more efficient. Wide malleable retractors may be wrapped with a moistened Miculicz pad or stockingette material as an alternative to the acrylic blocks. These retractors have the advantage of being capable of being formed, which facilitates their use in deeper wounds.

One must maintain constant vigilance when using lasers. The procedure must be conducted with a continuous awareness of the three-dimensional topography and anatomy of the operative site. Adjacent structures should be protected at all times to prevent inadvertent injury. Moistened Miculicz pads or towels are used to pack the wound and adjacent areas. Appropriate optical backstops for the particular laser in use should be employed whenever possible. Examples of these include the Köcher bronchocele sound, glass rods, titanium rods, and saline.

Practical Tips for Laser Use

- All lasers function most efficiently when appropriate power densities (fluences) are used in conjunction with proper technique.
- Tissue should be held under constant tension to distract the tissues, thereby exposing the plane of dissection and maintaining good exposure.
- Cutting should be done in a single pass of the laser, with care being taken to avoid rapid, back and forth type motions, which create multiple planes of dissection and undue bleeding.
- Liquefied fat should be aspirated or blotted.
- "Water is your friend" is important when using the CO_2 laser. Delicate dissection around nerves, tendons, vessels and other structures can be accomplished safely by infiltrating local anesthetic or saline into the tissue plane below the intended target.
- A similar technique is useful when using the KTP and Nd: YAG lasers. These wavelengths are easily transmitted through water. An opaque optical backstop should be used.

All lasers will function most efficiently when appropriate power densities (fluences) are used in conjunction with proper technique. Tissue should be held under constant tension to distract the tissues, thereby exposing the plane of dissection and maintaining good exposure. This requires about twice the amount of "pull" or force, as that is required for conventional surgical techniques.

Cutting should be done in a single pass of the laser, with care being taken to avoid rapid, back and forth type motions, which create multiple planes of dissection and undue bleeding. The full thickness of tissue to be cut should be incised by advancing the beam (i.e., your hand) slowly along the proposed line of incision.

Liquefied fat should be aspirated or blotted. This prevents flash flaming of the liquefied fat (in the case of the CO_2 laser), reduces the transmission of thermal energy to the tissues and permits more efficient incision by enabling more direct interaction between the laser and the tissues to be incised.

The concept that "water is your friend" is important when using the CO_2 laser. Delicate dissection around nerves, tendons, vessels and other structures can be accomplished safely by infiltrating local anesthetic or saline into the tissue plane below the intended target. This forms a natural barrier to penetration by the laser beam until or unless the surgeon vaporizes this layer. This principle may be coupled with the use of solutions containing epinephrine to enhance the hemostatic effect of the laser by promoting local vasoconstriction. This technique is useful when performing hemorrhoidectomy. The varix is ligated proximally (i.e., crown ligature) and the tissue is infiltrated with 0.25% Bupivacaine with epinephrine. This maneuver separates the varix from the sphincter muscles, produces vasoconstriction, and prevents the inadvertent sectioning of the sphincter. A similar technique is useful when performing hemorrhoidectomy with the KTP and Nd: YAG lasers. However, these wavelengths are easily transmitted through water or saline. Therefore, an opaque optical backstop should be used. The surgeon should also recognize that absorption of laser energy by the backstop can heat these instruments and result in thermal damage if they are used carelessly or for prolonged periods without stopping to permit them to cool.

Practical Considerations

- The CO_2 laser is useful for the incision, excision and vaporization of tissues.
  - The surgeon should generally select the minimum spot size and the highest fluence that can be managed safely.
  - A 125 mm hand-piece is the most commonly used delivery device for free-hand application.
  - The main advantages of electrosurgical devices are the ubiquity of them in the operating room and the fact that no additional training or safety considerations need be implemented.

- It is important to divide tissues completely in a V-shaped plane in order to achieve the maximum speed and efficiency.
  - Generally, these devices should be used at 25–40 W for skin incisions and 60 W for incision of fat, muscles and other tissues.
  - Liquefied fat should be aspirated to increase efficiency and present flash fires due to the diesel effect.
- The Nd: YAG laser is capable of photocoagulating as much as 2 cm tissue when applied in a free-beam mode, with much of the photothermal coagulation occurring 4 mm beneath the target surface.
  - A contact tip or sculpted fiber results in much of the laser energy being absorbed at the tip of the instrument. This produces zones of coagulation similar to these seen with electrosurgical devices or with use of the KTP/532 laser.
  - Contact YAG laser procedures are generally performed at 10–25 W.
  - Bare fiber applications for solid organ surgeries are more efficient at energies of 50–60 W.
  - Tumor ablation is generally performed at energies of 40–100 W. The surface needs to be desiccated or carbonized in order to provide a nidus for the ablation to begin, particularly if the lesion is not deeply pigmented.
- The KTP laser is a versatile tool for both open and laparoscopic procedures.
  - It cuts, vaporizes and coagulates tissues efficiently, with a zone of injury that is intermediate between a CO_2 laser and electrosurgical unit used in coagulation mode.
  - KTP laser incision is efficient over power outputs between 8 and 25 W.
  - The fiber capable lasers are easier to learn to use since the surgeon is able to maintain tactile feedback as the fibers contact the tissues.
  - These lasers should generally not be used for skin incision and are best used on tissues deep to the dermis.
- Pulsed dye lasers are used for the management of common duct stones and for the fragmentation of renal and ureteral calculi.

A CO_2 laser is useful for the incision, excision and vaporization (ablation) of tissues.[34-44,53,55,57] The surgeon should generally select the minimum spot size and the highest fluence that can be managed safely. This increases the efficiency and speed of the procedure and enhances hemostasis. A 125 mm hand-piece is the most commonly used delivery device for free-hand application. Using the beam in focus will produce optimal results for skin incisions and fine dissection of tissues. Defocusing the beam permits greater transfer of heat to the underlying tissues and improves hemostasis during the division of muscular and parenchymatous organ tissues. Tissues should be maintained under constant traction to facilitate the dissection and the surgeon should maintain a relatively slow, steady hand speed. It is also important to divide tissues completely in a V-shaped plane in order to achieve the maximum speed and efficiency. Generally, these devices should be used at 25–40 W for skin incisions and 60 W for incision of fat, muscles and other tissues. It is generally helpful to use not more than 60 W for soft tissue incision since the laser is more difficult to control and since the potential for a flash fire in the wound due to aerosolization of liquefied fat exists. Liquefied fat should be aspirated to increase efficiency and present flash fires due to the diesel effect. CO_2 lasers capable of generating outputs greater that 60 W can be used for effective and efficient ablation of bulky lesions and expeditious debridements of large areas.

CO_2 laser waveguides are available for both open uses. Flexible waveguides are more practical and are typically used at outputs of 30 W or less. They are available with some laser systems, including models marketed for dental office use. These delivery systems are not practical for skin incisions but have been used for numerous other applications.

The CO_2 laser sterilizes as it cuts and vaporizes in a nontouch fashion. It is useful for wound debridements and in situations where decreasing or eliminating wound contamination is desirable. Use of this laser in either a freehand mode or with scanners facilitates hemostasis during surface debridements such as in cases of burn wound care or management of decubitus ulcers. Recent developments with erbium laser delivery systems may make the Er: YAG laser an attractive alternative for these procedures in the future, although these devices are more common in dermatology, dental, and plastic surgical applications.

The Nd: YAG laser is capable of photocoagulating as much as 2 cm tissue when applied in a free-beam mode, with much of the photothermal coagulation occurring 4 mm beneath the target surface.[34,47,53-57] This occurs due to forward and back scattering of light in the tissue. Using a contact tip or sculpted fiber results in much of the laser energy being absorbed at the tip of the instrument (delivery device). This produces zones of coagulation similar to these seen with electrosurgical devices or with use of the KTP/532 laser. Contact YAG laser procedures are generally performed at 10–25 W. However, bare fiber applications for solid organ surgeries are more efficient at energies of 50–60 W. Tumor ablation is generally performed at energies of 40–100 W. The surface needs to be desiccated or carbonized in order to provide a nidus for the ablation to begin, particularly if the lesion is not deeply pigmented. The surface can be "doped" by applying a droplet of blood, India ink, methylene blue or another chromophore to start the ablation process by enabling surface absorption of the YAG laser energy.

The KTP laser is a versatile tool for both open and laparoscopic procedures.[16,54,56,57] This wavelength is intensely absorbed by hemoglobin, myoglobin and melanin and the laser is capable of both contact and noncontact use. It cuts, vaporizes and coagulates tissues efficiently, with a zone of injury that is intermediate between a CO_2 laser and electrosurgical unit used in coagulation mode. KTP laser incision is efficient over power outputs between 8 and 25 W.

Generally speaking, the fiber capable lasers are easier to learn to use initially, since the surgeon is able to maintain tactile feedback as the fibers contact the tissues. These lasers should generally not be used for skin incision and are best used on tissues deep to the dermis. The power densities, and hence speed of action of argon, KTP and holmium lasers may be increased by using smaller fibers if desired. Contact Nd: YAG tips and sculpted fibers behave most like optically-driven cautery with cutting speed and efficiency reaching a plateau once the tip is heated. The surgeon should remember that these tips can remain quite hot for several seconds after the beam is deactivated. Iatrogenic injury or adherence to the wound can occur at this time if careless tissue contact occurs.

Pulsed dye lasers are also used in general surgical procedures, particularly for the management of common duct stones at the time of cholecystectomy or during perioperative ERCP. These laser systems are also quite helpful in the fragmentation of renal and ureteral calculi.[4,16,56,57]

Lasers have been useful in the palliation of obstructing esophageal, bronchial and colonic lesions both with and without photosensitizing agents such as Photofrin®. Most of these procedures are performed using flexible or rigid endoscopes. Both laser and other light sources are used for these applications.[34,47,50,57]

Some surgeons reserve lasers for special procedures such as tumor resections including, nonanatomic resection of liver metastasis, procedures on patients with bleeding disorders, and in the treatment of infected or contaminated wounds. These versatile instruments can provide many advantages and are a useful addition to the armamentarium of the surgeon, who is conversant with their tissue effects and delivery systems. However, it is unlikely that lasers will completely replace scalpels, electrosurgical devices and other "standard" instruments. Some procedures such as laparoscopic herniorrhaphy and many parts of "laser surgeries" are better performed without one. Nonetheless, surgeons would do well to become comfortable with laser technology and use it is clinical practice. Beginners will achieve better results and improved outcomes by graded use of these devices on simple procedures initially and tackling more complex procedures as operative experience increases.

The CO_2 laser represents an excellent modality for surgery of the breast.[34-36,41,47,48,55,57] The laser permits the precise creation of flaps with significant reduction in operative blood loss, postoperative drainage, and postoperative seroma formation. Both the volume and duration of postoperative drainage is significantly reduced in patients treated with the laser. These factors can be used to advantage particularly in the case of immediate reconstruction wherein postoperative seroma formation could predispose the patient to wound infection. Experimental studies have demonstrated that the laser results in a tenfold reduction in local recurrence as compared to scalpel or cautery treatment particularly when laser excision is combined with sterilization of the wound. This suggests that the CO_2 laser should be the modality of choice for the surgical treatment of carcinoma of the breast.

Axillary dissection may be accomplished successfully with the YAG, KTP, or CO_2 lasers. However, the use of the Nd: YAG laser with sapphire contact probe or a sculpted fiber delivery systems does not require the use of optical backstops as is the case for the KTP and CO_2 lasers. Laser use permits the precise definition of anatomic structures as a result of enhanced hemostasis and clear definition of the planes of dissection. Experimental evidence suggests that lasers are useful in reducing the likelihood of tumor implantation at the time of surgery and may reduce local recurrence in human breast carcinoma.[35,36,39,41-43,48,55,57] It is noteworthy that lasers seal blood vessels and lymphatics and therefore reduce the volume and duration of postoperative drainage.

The YAG laser permits precise bloodless dissection in surgery of the head and neck, using a sculpted fiber or sapphire contact tip in these dissections. Contact Nd: YAG delivery systems provide a great margin of safety due to the small percentage of laser energy which actually reaches the tissue beyond the tip.[47,48,55,57] Other laser wavelengths such as the CO_2 laser and KTP laser also have been used quite successfully. However, these systems require the use of optical backstops and an expert understanding of the laser's capability and the surgical anatomy.

Hemorrhoidectomy may be accomplished with a variety of laser wavelengths and techniques. The use of lasers has been documented to reduce the perioperative morbidity of surgical hemorrhoidectomy. Significant reductions in the incidence of urinary retention and delayed bleeding are noted. In addition, the patients generally resume their normal activity in approximately one half the time required by their conventionally treated counterparts. The incidence of post-hemorrhoidectomy strictures is greatly reduced.[41,48,53,57]

Lasers are quite useful for herniorrhaphy and are particularly useful for recurrent hernia repair. Hemostasis is excellent and scar tissue from previous repairs can be divided easily. The majority of hernioplasties are performed with local anesthesia and conscious sedation. Laser use permits excellent hemostasis without the use of electrocautery. This is particularly advantageous because the patient may find electrocoagulation to be painful due to conduction of electrical current along neurovascular bundles and away from the wound site, despite an adequate local block. Additional advantages are significant reduction in postoperative edema, ecchymosis, and discomfort. Patients resume normal activities much sooner than their conventionally treated counterparts.

Lasers are quite helpful in the performance of herniorrhaphy and procedures such as breast biopsy, particularly under local anesthesia. Patient comfort is enhanced during the performance of the procedure as well as postoperatively. A clear, dry operative field is obtained and the procedure is accomplished more rapidly since less time is spent in obtaining hemostasis. A variety of wavelengths can be used interchangeably in the performance of herniorrhaphy. Postoperative discomfort is reduced due to the reduction in edema and induration of laser wounds.

The CO_2 laser is extremely effective in the ablation of large volumes of tissue. This is particularly useful in the case of local recurrence of carcinoma. Some large tumors may be quite vascular. Hemostasis may be enhanced by the use of epinephrine containing local anesthetics injected at the periphery of the lesion. Another approach is the combined use of free beam YAG laser energy as a means of coagulating the tumor mass followed by its immediate ablation with the CO_2 laser.

Photobiomodulation

- Low Level Laser Therapy (LLLT) is currently being used to treat various conditions based on the principles of photobiomodulation.
- These therapies are based on the observation that photostimulatory effects are generally observed at fluences between 1 and 10 J/cm2, while photoinhibitory effects are typically observed at higher fluences.
- Light sources including lasers, light emitting diodes, superluminous diodes, and other noncoherent sources are employed both clinically and experimentally. The most effective wavelengths appear to be clustered in the red and near infrared portions of the electromagnetic spectrum.

Low Level Laser Therapy (LLLT) is currently being used to treat various conditions based on the principles of photobiomodulation.[58-72] Several in vitro and in vivo studies have demonstrated that LLLT has a significant influence on a variety of cellular functions and clinical conditions.[56-81] However, other studies have concluded that LLLT had little or no effect on treatment outcomes.[63]

The traditional application of photobiomodulation in clinical and experimental models is based on the observation that photostimulatory effects are generally observed at fluences between 1 and 10 J/cm^2, while photoinhibitory effects are typically observed at higher fluences. Treatments are generally administered on a daily or every other day basis, and usually three to four times per week.[58] Several different light sources including lasers, light emitting diodes, superluminous diodes, and other noncoherent sources are employed both clinically and experimentally. The most effective wavelengths appear to be clustered in the red and near infrared portions of the electromagnetic spectrum.

Work from several investigators has demonstrated that photobiomodulation influences a variety of biological processes, including the acceleration of wound healing,[69,71,77,79,80] increased mitochondrial respiration and adenosine triphosphate (ATP) synthesis,[66,68,70,75,76] cell proliferation,[67-69,74,81] enhancement and promotion of skeletal muscle regeneration following injury[70] and a variety of other effects. Photobiomodulation enhances collagen synthesis in the wound area, thereby increasing wound tensile strength.[71] Stimulation of cell proliferation results from an increase in mitochondrial respiration and ATP synthesis.[66,72-74]

Recent work from our laboratory has demonstrated that in vitro cell proliferation and metabolism can be influenced by varying the dose frequency or treatment interval.[80,85] Our results suggested that a unique dose frequency regime may exist for tissues and cell lines and that the determination of that treatment paradigm is necessary in order to achieve maximal stimulation of cellular metabolism and proliferation. The data also demonstrated that the use of other treatment regimes results in bioinhibition, despite the delivery of the same total energy.[80] We found that two treatments per day were more effective than once daily therapy in some cases. Therefore, the empiric use of a single treatment per day dosing frequency as a treatment strategy for all cell lines and tissues might explain why conflicting results demonstrating both positive and negative effects have been published and why the efficacy of LLLT remains controversial. Long exposures using 670 nm light at low intensities were ineffective in accelerating wound healing in an experimental pressure ulcer model.[85] This finding, in conjunction with data from other studies indicates that a certain threshold must be reached, although it is unknown whether delivering the light in a pulsed fashion with higher peak powers but the same time course would yield the same results. Our experimental findings demonstrate that identification of the proper treatment parameters for the particular cell line or tissue is crucial to achieve photobiostimulation.

This form of therapy holds great promise for the treatment of both acute and chronic wounds. It is likely that improved delivery devices and treatment paradigms will be available in the near future.

Conclusion

This chapter has presented a synopsis of the use of lasers and light sources in general surgery.

These devices are used in both open and laparoscopic procedures. A wide variety of wavelengths and delivery systems can be applied in both routine and complex surgical procedures. Lasers and light sources can yield improved outcomes and allow the surgeon to work more efficiently, given proper selection of wavelength, delivery systems, laser parameters and the use of appropriate technique. The appropriately trained and skilled surgeon, who is conversant with the anatomy and technical details of the procedure at hand, will find these devices a welcome addition to the surgical armamentarium.

References

1. American National Standards Institute. *American National Standard for Safe use of Lasers in Medical Facilities (ANSI Z136.3-2005)*. Orlando: The Laser Institute of America; 2005:62 pp.
2. Bakri YN, Sundin T, Mansi M. Ureteral injury secondary to laparoscopic CO_2 laser. *Acta Obstet Gynecol Scand*. 1994;73:665-667.
3. Norderlon BM, Hobday KA, Hunter JG. Laser vs electrosurgery in laparoscopic cholecystectomy. A prospective randomized trial. *Arch Surg*. 1993;128(2):33-36.
4. Carroll B, Chandra M, Papaioannou T, et al. Biliary lithotripsy as an adjunct to laparoscopic common bile duct stone extraction. *Surg Endosc*. 1993;7(4):356-359.
5. Corbitt JDJR. Laparoscopic cholecystectomy: laser versus electrocautery. *Surg Laparosc Endosc*. 1991;1(4):268-269.
6. Crowgey SR, Adamson GD. Endoscopic energy: laser. In: Adamson GD, Martin DC, eds. *Endoscopic Management of Gynecologic Disease*. Philadelphia: Lippincott-Raven Publishers; 1996:27-41.
7. Diamond MP, Daniell JF, Feste J, et al. Initial report of the carbon dioxide laser laparoscopy study group: complications. *J Gynecol Surg*. 1989;5:269-272.
8. Grainger DA, Soderstrom RM, Schiff SF, Glickman MD, DeCherney AH, Diamond MP. Ureteral injuries at laparoscopy: insights into diagnosis management, and prevention. *Obstet Gynecol*. 1990; 75:839-843.
9. Hersman MJ, Rosin RD. Laparoscopic laser cholecystectomy: our first 200 patients. *Ann R Coll Surg Engl*. 1992;74(4):242-247.
10. Hinshaw JR, Daykhovsky L, Glantz G, et al. Current controversies in laparoscopic cholecystectomy: a roundtable discussion. *J Laparoendosc Surg*. 1990;1(1):17-29.
11. Hulka JF, Reich H. *Textbook of Laparoscopy*. 3rd ed. Philadelphia: WB Saunders Co; 1998:548 pp.
12. Hunter JG. Exposure, dissection, and laser versus electrosurgery in laparoscopic cholecystectomy. *Am J Surg*. 1993;165(4):492-496.
13. Kim AK, Adamson GH. Laparoscopic laser injury. In: Kavic MS, Levinson CJ, Wetter PA, eds. *Prevention and Management of Laparoscopic Surgical Complications*. Miami: Society of Laparoendoscopic Surgeons; 1999:21-28.

14. Kollmorgan TA, Malek RA, Barrett DM. Laser prostatectomy: two and a half years' experience with aggressive multifocal therapy. *Urology.* 1996;48:217-222.

15. Kuntzman TA, Malek RA, Barrett DM. High-power potassium titanyl phosphate laser vaporization prostatectomy. *Mayo Clin Proc.* 1998;73:798-801.

16. Lanzafame RJ. Applications of lasers in laparoscopic cholecystectomy. *J Laparoendosc Surg.* 1990;1(1):33-36.

17. Lanzafame RJ. Applications of laser in laparoscopic cholecystectomy: technical considerations and future directions. *SPIE.* 1991; 1421:189-196.

18. Lanzafame RJ, Brien T, Rogers DW, et al. Comparison of sapphire contact scalpels for surgery. *Lasers Surg Med.* 1990;2(Suppl):9.

19. Lanzafame RJ. Laser utilization in minimally invasive surgery: applications and pitfalls. In: Lanzafame RJ, ed. *Prevention and Management of Complications in Minimally Invasive Surgery.* New York: Igaku-Shoin; 1996:30-42.

20. Lanzafame RJ. Laser energy for minimally invasive surgery. In: Wetter PA, Kavic MS, Levinson CJ, eds. *Prevention and Management of Laparoendoscopic Surgical Complications.* 2nd ed. Miami: Society of Laparoendoscopic Surgeons; 2005:61-72.

21. Laycock WS, Hunter JG. Electrosurgery and laser application. In: MacFayden BV, Ponsky JL, eds. *Operative Laparoscopy and Thoracoscopy.* Philadelphia: Lippincott-Raven; 1996:79-91.

22. Malek PA, Kuntzman RS, Barrett DM. High power potassium-titanyl phosphate laser vaporization prostatectomy. *J Urol.* 2000; 163:1730-1733.

23. Reddick EJ, Olsen DO. Laparoscopic laser cholecystectomy. A comparison with mini-lap cholecystectomy. *Surg Endosc.* 1989; 3(3):131-133.

24. Reddick EJ, Baird D, Daniel J, et al. Laparoscopic laser cholecystectomy. *Ann Chir Gynaecol.* 1990;79(4):189-191.

25. Reddick EJ, Olsen D, Alexander W, et al. Laparoscopic laser cholecystectomy and choledocholithiasis. *Surg Endosc.* 1990;4(3):133-134.

26. Schultz LS, Hickok DF, Garber JN, et al. The use of lasers in general surgery. A preliminary assessment. *Minn Med.* 1987;70(8):439-442.

27. Schwartz RO. Complications of laparoscopic hysterectomy. *Obstet Gynecol.* 1993;81:1022-1024.

28. Smith EB. Complications of laparoscopic cholecystectomy. *J Natl Med Assoc.* 1992;84(10):880-882.

29. Soderstrom RM. Bowel injury litigation after laparoscopy. *J Am Assoc Gynecol Laparosc.* 1993;1:74-77.

30. Spaw AT, Reddick EJ, Olsen DO. Laparoscopic laser cholecystectomy: analysis of 500 procedures. *Surg Laparosc Endosc.* 1991;1(1):2-7.

31. Steger AC, Moore KM, Hira N. Contact laser or conventional cholecystectomy: a controlled trial. *Br J Surg.* 1988;75(3):223-225.

32. Unger SW, Edelman DS, Scott JS, et al. Laparoscopic treatment of acute cholecystitis. *Surg Laparosc Endosc.* 1991;1(1):14-16.

33. Williams IM, Lewis DK, Shandall AA, et al. Laparoscopic cholecystectomy: laser or electrosurgery. *J R Coll Surg Edinb.* 1994;39(6):348-349.

34. Apfelberg DB, ed. *Evaluation and Installation of Surgical Laser Systems.* New York: Springer; 1986:324.

35. Lanzafame RJ, Rogers DW, Naim JO, DeFranco C, Ochej H, Hinshaw JR. Reduction of local tumor recurrence by excision with the CO_2 laser. *Lasers Surg Med.* 1986;6(5):439-441.

36. Lanzafame RJ, Rogers DW, Naim JO, Herrera HR, DeFranco C, Hinshaw JR. The effect of CO_2 laser excision on local tumor recurrence. *Lasers Surg Med.* 1986;6(2):103-105.

37. Lanzafame RJ, Hinshaw JR, Pennino RP. Cost-effective retractors for laser surgery. *AORN J.* 1986;43(6):1218-1219.

38. Lanzafame RJ, McCormack CJ, Rogers DW, Naim JO, Hinshaw JR. Effects of laser sterilization on local recurrence in experimental mammary tumors. *Surg Forum.* 1986;7:480-481.

39. Hinshaw JR, Herrera HR, Lanzafame RJ, Pennino RP. The Use of the carbon dioxide laser permits primary closure of contaminated and purulent lesions and wounds. *Lasers Surg Med.* 1987; 6(6):581-583.

40. Lanzafame RJ, Herrera HR, Jobes HM, et al. The influence of "hands-on" laser training on usage of the CO_2 laser. *Lasers Surg Med.* 1987;7:61-65.

41. Lanzafame RJ, Hinshaw JR, eds. *Color Atlas of CO_2 Laser Techniques.* St. Louis: Ishiyaku EuroAmerica, Inc; 1988:294 pp.

42. Lanzafame RJ, McCormack CJ, Rogers DW, Naim JO, Herrera HR, Hinshaw JR. Mechanisms of the reduction of tumor recurrence with the carbon dioxide laser in experimental mammary tumors. *Surg Gynecol Obstet.* 1988;167:493-496.

43. Lanzafame RJ, Qui K, Rogers DW, et al. A comparison of local tumor recurrence following excision with the CO_2 laser, Nd:YAG laser, and Argon Beam Coagulator. *Lasers Surg Med.* 1988;8(5):515-520.

44. Lanzafame RJ, Naim JO, Rogers DW, Hinshaw JR. A comparison of continuous wave, chop wave, and super pulse laser wounds. *Lasers Surg Med.* 1988;8(2):119-124.

45. Lanzafame RJ. Cholecystectomy with lasers. *Laser Med Surg News Adv.* 1988;6(6):31-36.

46. Pennino RP, O'Connor T, Lanzafame RJ, Hinshaw JR. Tissue sculpturing: potential new applications and techniques of CO_2 laser surgery. *Laser Med Surg News Adv.* 1988;6(5):20-23.

47. Joffe SN, ed. *Lasers in General Surgery.* Baltimore: Williams & Wilkins; 1989:319 pp.

48. Lanzafame RJ, Pennino RP, Herrera HR, Hinshaw JR. Breast surgery with the CO_2 laser. In: Joffe SN, ed. *Lasers in General Surgery.* Baltimore: Williams & Wilkins, Inc.; 1989:25-33.

49. Lanzafame RJ. New instruments for laser surgery. *Lasers Surg Med.* 1990;10:595-596.

50. Lanzafame RJ, Wang MJ, Naim JO, Rogers DW. The effect of preoperative laser hyperthermia and laser excision on local recurrence in mammary tumors. *Surg Forum.* 1990;41:481-483.

51. Apfelberg DB, ed. *Atlas of Cutaneous Laser Surgery.* New York: Raven Press; 1992:483 pp.

52. Sliney DH, Trokel SI. *Medical Lasers and Their Safe Use.* New York: Springer; 1992:230 pp.

53. Daly CJ, Grundfest WS, Johnson DE, Lanzafame RJ, Steiner RW, Tadir Y, Graham MW, eds. *Lasers in Urology, Gynecology, and General Surgery. Progress in Biomedical Optics.* Vol 1879. S.P.I.E; 1993:248 pp.

54. Lanzafame RJ. Techniques for the simultaneous management of incarcerated ventral herniae and cholelithiasis via laparoscopy. *J Laparoendosc Surg.* 1993;3(2):193-201.

55. Lanzafame RJ. Applications of laser technology in breast cancer therapy. *Semin Surg Oncol.* 1995;11:328-332.

56. Lanzafame RJ. *Prevention And Management Of Complications In Laparoscopic Surgery.* New York: Igaku-Shoin Medical Publishers, Inc.; 1996:368 pp.

57. Lanzafame RJ. General surgery. In *Manual for Laser Biophysics and Safety,* Professional Medical Education Association. MedicalEducation@Compuserve.com.

58. Tunér J, Hode L. *Laser Therapy. Clinical Practice and Scientific Background.* Sweden: Grangesberg; Prima Books; 2002:571 pp.

59. Hopkins JT, McLodat TA, Seegmiller JG, Baxter GD. Low-level laser therapy facilitates superficial wound healing in humans: a triple-blind, sham-controlled study. *J Athl Train.* 2004;39(3):223-229.

60. Schindl A, Schindl M, Schindl L. Successful treatment of a persistent radiation ulcer by low power laser therapy. *J Am Acad Dermatol.* 1997;37(4):646-648.

61. Schindl M, Kerschan K, Schindl A, Schön H, Heinzl H, Schindl L. Induction of complete wound healing in recalcitrant ulcers by low-intensity laser irradiation depends on ulcer cause and size. *Photodermatol Photoimmunol Photomed.* 1999;15(1):18-21.

62. Kujawa J, Zavodnik L, Zavodnik I, Buko V, Lapshyna A, Bryszewska M. Effect of low-intensity (3.75-25 J/cm^2) near-infrared (810 nm) laser radiation on red blood cell ATPase activities and membrane structure. *J Clin Laser Med Surg*. 2004;22(2):111-117.

63. Basford JR. The clinical and experimental status of low-energy laser therapy. *Crit Rev Phys Rehabil Med*. 1989;1:1-9.

64. Mester E, Mester AF, Mester A. The biomedical effects of laser application. *Lasers Surg Med*. 1985;5(1):31-39.

65. Yu W, Naim JO, McGowan M, Ippolito K, Lanzafame RJ. Photomodulation of oxidative metabolism and electron chain enzymes in rat liver mitochondria. *Photochem Photobiol*. 1997;66(6):866-871.

66. Lam TS, Abergel RP, Castel JC, Dwyer RM, Lesavoy MA, Uitto J. Laser stimulation of collagen synthesis in human skin fibroblast cultures. *Lasers Life Sci*. 1986;1:61-77.

67. Passarella S, Casamassima E, Molinari S, et al. Increase of proton electrochemical potential and ATP synthesis in rat liver mitochondria irradiated in vitro by helium-neon laser. *FEBS Lett*. 1984;175(1):95-99.

68. Conlan MJ, Rapley JW, Cobb CM. Biostimulation of wound healing by low-energy laser irradiation. A review. *J Clin Periodontol*. 1996;23(5):492-496.

69. Morimoto Y, Arai T, Kikuchi M, Nakajima S, Nakamura H. Effect of low-intensity argon laser irradiation on mitochondrial respiration. *Lasers Surg Med*. 1992;15(2):191-199.

70. Stadler I, Lanzafame RJ, Evans R, et al. 830-nm irradiation increases the wound tensile strength in a diabetic murine model. *Lasers Surg Med*. 2001;28(3):220-226.

71. Karu TI. *The Science of Low Power Laser Therapy*. London: Gordon and Breach Science Publishers; 1998:14-33, 53-94, 95-121.

72. Karu TI. Primary and secondary mechanisms of action of visible to near–IR radiation on cells. *J Photochem Photobiol B*. 1998;49(1):1-17.

73. Vladimiorv IA, Klebanov GI, Borisenko GG, Osipov AN. Molecular and cellular mechanisms of the low intensity laser radiation effect. *Biofizika*. 2004;49(2):339-350.

74. Eells JT, Wong-Riley MT, VerHoeve J, et al. Mitochondrial signal transduction in accelerated wound and retinal healing by near-infrared light therapy. *Mitochondrion*. 2004;4(5–6):559-567.

75. Silveira PC, Streck EL, Pinho RA. Evaluation of mitochondrial respiratory chain activity in wound healing by low-level laser therapy. *J Photochem Photobiol B*. 2007;86(3):279-282.

76. Prado RP, Liebano RE, Hochman B, Pinfildi CE, Ferreira LM. Experimental model for low level laser therapy on ischemic random skin flap in rats. *Acta Cir Bras*. 2006;21(4):258-262.

77. Hawkins D, Houreld N, Abrahamse H. Low level laser therapy (LLLT) as an effective therapeutic modality for delayed wound healing. *Ann NY Acad Sci*. 2005;1056:486-493.

78. Stadler I, Lanzafame RJ, Oskoui P, Zhang RY, Coleman J, Whittaker M. Alteration of skin temperature during low level laser irradiation at 830 nm in a mouse model. *Photomed Laser Surg*. 2004;22(3):227-231.

79. Lanzafame RJ, Stadler I, Coleman J, et al. Temperature-controlled 830 nm LLLT of experimental pressure ulcers. *Photomed Laser Surg*. 2004;22(6):483-488.

80. Brondon P, Stadler I, Lanzafame RJ. A study of the effects of phototherapy dose interval on photobiomodulation of cell cultures. *Lasers Surg Med*. 2005;36(5):409-413.

81. Karu TI. Low power laser therapy. In: Vo-Dinh T, ed. *Biomedical Photonics Handbook*, 48. London: CRC Press; 2003:1-25.

82. Schindl A, Rosado-Schlosser B, Trautinger F. The reciprocity rule in photobiology - a review. *Hautarzt*. 2001;52(9):779-785. also at www.photobiology.com.

83. Liu TCY, Jiao JL, Xu XY, Liu XG, Deng SX, Liu SH. Photobiomodulation: phenomenology and its mechanism. *SPIE Proc*. 2004;5632:185-191.

84. Stadler I, Zhang RY, Oskoui P, Whittaker MS, Lanzafame RJ. Development of a simple clinical relevant murine model of pressure ulcer. *J Invest Surg*. 2004;17:221-227.

85. Lanzafame RJ, Stadler I, Kurtz AF, et al. Reciprocity of exposure time and irradiance on energy density during photoradiation on wound healing in a murine pressure ulcer model. *Lasers Surg Med*. 2007;39(6):534-542.

Laser/Light Applications in Urology

Nathaniel M. Fried and Brian R. Matlaga

- Summary of laser-tissue interactions in urology.
- Holmium:YAG and FREDDY laser lithotripsy.
- Laser treatment of benign prostatic hyperplasia using high-power Holmium:YAG and KTP (Greenlight) lasers.
- Laser incision of urethral and ureteral strictures.
- Other laser applications in urology for treatment of penile carcinoma, partial nephrectomy, tissue welding,…etc.

Introduction

- Lasers have had a major impact in urology especially for the treatment of urinary stone disease and benign prostatic hyperplasia.

Medical laser systems have had a reputation for being large, difficult to use, and expensive. However, recent technological advances have resulted in the commercial availability of clinical lasers that are more compact, powerful, affordable, and user-friendly. Clinical expertise in laser surgery has also improved, and as a result, the impact of lasers on the practice of urology has been significant.

Solid-state lasers, such as the potassium-titanyl-phosphate (KTP) or frequency-doubled neodymium yttrium-aluminum-garnet (Nd:YAG) laser, and holmium:YAG (Ho:YAG) lasers, have replaced older gas and dye lasers for soft tissue procedures and laser lithotripsy. Continued development of flexible endoscopes combined with the availability of small, flexible, biocompatible, inexpensive, and disposable optical fibers, have also created new opportunities for minimally invasive laser procedures in the urological tract.

Laser procedures in urology are based on a wide range of mechanisms for laser-tissue interactions, including photothermal, photomechanical, and photochemical (Table 1). Examples of photothermal applications include laser ablation of soft tissues for treatment of benign prostate hyperplasia (BPH), strictures, bladder cancer, laser tissue welding, and long-pulse laser lithotripsy. Photomechanical applications include short-pulse laser lithotripsy, and photochemical applications include photodynamic therapy (PDT) for treatment of bladder and prostate cancer.

This article reviews in detail the two most common clinical applications of lasers in urology - laser lithotripsy for fragmentation of urinary stones and laser ablation of the prostate for treatment of benign prostatic hyperplasia (BPH), and also covers other laser applications such as incision of strictures and tissue welding. The development of new experimental laser technologies for potential use in urology is also discussed.

Laser Lithotripsy

Introduction

- Holmium:YAG laser is the most common lithotripter for fragmenting urinary stones located in the ureter, kidney, and bladder, and is a multiple-use laser in urology.
- FREDDY laser represents a compact, solid-state alternative to the older dye laser for short-pulse, photomechanical-based lithotripsy.

The first laser to be used for the fragmentation of urinary calculi was the continuous wave ruby laser, the subject of in vitro experiments in the 1960s.[1] The ruby laser destroyed

N.M. Fried (✉)
Department of Physics and Optical Science,
University of North Carolina, Charlotte, NC, USA
e-mail: nmfried@uncc.edu

K. Nouri (ed.), *Lasers in Dermatology and Medicine*,
DOI: 10.1007/978-0-85729-281-0_44, © Springer-Verlag London Limited 2011

Table 1 Mechanisms of laser-tissue interaction

Interaction	Mechanism	Lasers	Applications
Photothermal	Light → heat	Holmium:YAG, KTP, Neodymium:YAG	Benign prostatic hyperplasia, bladder tumors, strictures, long-pulse lithotripsy, soft tissue coagulation, tissue welding
Photomechanical	Light → shock wave	Dye, FREDDY	Short-pulse lithotripsy
Photochemical	Light → chemical reaction	Dye, diode	Photodynamic therapy for bladder and prostate cancer

kidney stones by a photothermal effect, as stones were simply heated until their melting point was reached. As a consequence, extreme heat was generated at the stone surface, making the ruby laser impractical for clinical use. Subsequent development of the pulsed dye laser marked the beginning of the clinical use of lasers to fragment urinary calculi.[2] The application of pulsed energy to the stone surface yields a finite zone of energy density, with little heat dissipation into the surrounding fluid and tissue.

The first widely available pulsed dye laser was the coumarin laser, which relied on the excitation of green coumarin dye by light energy. The coumarin laser was a significant advancement in the field of laser lithotripsy, as it could fragment stones of all composition except for cystine, and the energy could be transmitted through small, 200 μm, quartz fibers. Although success rates of 80–95% were reported, the coumarin laser had a number of drawbacks, including the high initial cost of the device, disposal of the toxic coumarin dye, and cumbersome eye protection.

The Holmium:Yttrium-Aluminum-Garnet (Ho:YAG) laser was developed to replace the pulsed dye laser, and is now generally considered to be the standard laser for stone fragmentation (Table 2). The holmium laser is a solid-state device, and is smaller, less costly to operate, and requires less maintenance than the previous pulsed-dye lasers. The holmium laser has a long pulse duration of approximately 500 μs which promotes stone fragmentation by two mechanisms: photomechanical, via shock wave generation, as well as photothermal, via heat generation. The primary mechanism of stone fracture is the photothermal effect.[3] The holmium laser wavelength is strongly absorbed by water, and its depth of penetration is relatively shallow; consequently, the laser can be discharged at a distance of even 0.5–1 mm from soft tissue with no resultant collateral damage.[4]

The frequency doubled double-pulse Neodymium:YAG (FREDDY) laser is the result of efforts to reduce the size, cost, and maintenance of clinical laser systems (Table 2). The FREDDY laser incorporates a KTP crystal into the resonator of a Nd:YAG laser, so that when the device is activated two laser pulses are produced simultaneously. The stone fragmentation mechanism is photomechanical, as one laser pulse generates a plasma bubble and the second laser pulse excites to violently collapse and release a shockwave at the surface of the stone. Although initial work with the FREDDY laser was encouraging, more recent evidence suggests that certain types of calculi do not respond well to this technology.[5] For this reason, the FREDDY laser has not achieved the widespread utilization of the holmium laser.

Indications and Contraindications

> Indications
>
> • Urinary stones less than 1.0–1.5 cm in diameter
>
> Contraindications
>
> • Presence of untreated infection.

In general, any stone within the urinary tract may be treated with the holmium laser. However, holmium laser lithotripsy as a treatment modality for renal calculi is sensitive to stone size, and for large stone burdens the procedure's efficacy can be markedly reduced. For upper urinary tract calculi less than 1.0–1.5 cm, ureteroscopic holmium laser lithotripsy is a reasonable treatment option.[6] However, when the stone burden increases beyond this size limit, the likelihood of achieving a stone-free outcome is reduced, and such patients may be best approached in a percutaneous fashion using a rigid lithotrite. For patients with bladder calculi, the holmium laser can be used to fragment stones of any size. In general the treatment of bladder stones is more efficient, as larger laser fibers can be used, which allow the transmission of greater amounts of energy.

Table 2 Technical specifications for lasers currently used for lithotripsy

Laser parameters	Holmium:YAG	KTP/Nd:YAG
Wavelength (nm)	2,120	532/1,064
Operation mode	Long-pulse	Short-pulse
Pulse energy (J)	0.4–3	0.160
Pulse length (μs)	350–700	1.2
Repetition rate (Hz)	5–20	1–20
Average power (W)	30	3.2
Electrical specifications	110 V, 15 A	110 V, 6 A
Weight (kg)	84	45

The only true contraindication to holmium laser lithotripsy of urinary calculi is the presence of untreated infection, as life-threatening sepsis may result. Otherwise, there are no other specific contraindications to holmium laser lithotripsy. Indeed, even patients receiving anti-coagulation therapy have been reported to have successfully undergone holmium laser treatment of urinary calculi.[7]

Technique

Fiber Selection

- 550 or 1,000 μm fiber for use with rigid cystoscope in bladder.
- 365 μm fiber for use with rigid ureteroscope in ureter.
- 200 μm fiber for use with flexible ureteroscope in kidney.

Energy Settings

- Pulse energies of 0.6–1.2 J.
- Pulse rates of 5–15 Hz.

Prior to fragmenting a stone with the holmium laser, the treating physician must first select the appropriate fiber for delivery of the laser energy as well as the proper energy settings of the laser itself.[8,9] Holmium laser fibers are typically available in 200, 365, 550, and 1,000 μm diameters, either in end- or side-firing configuration. Laser lithotripsy is most effective with an end-firing fiber rather than a side-firing fiber. The diameter of the fiber to be used typically depends on the location of the targeted stone and the endoscope used to access the stone. For patients with stones in the urinary bladder, a rigid cystoscopic instrument is used to visualize the stone, and either a 550 or 1,000 μm laser fiber is used to deliver the laser energy to the stone. The larger fiber size enables greater energy transmission to the stone, and irrigation flow through the cystoscopic instruments is not affected by these larger fibers. Ureteroscopes are much more miniaturized, and irrigation flow through these endoscopes is more sensitive to the size of the laser fiber. In general, a 365 μm fiber can be easily passed through a rigid ureteroscope with minimal effect on the flow of irrigant. However, a 365 μm fiber will attenuate the flow of irrigation through a flexible ureteroscope, as well as impair the deflection of the flexible endoscope. For these reasons, a 200 μm fiber should be used when a flexible ureteroscope is required to access the stone, and a 365 fiber should be used when a rigid ureteroscope is required to access the stone.

Lithotripsy with the holmium laser depends on both the pulse energy as well as the pulse rate. For the fragmentation of stones, pulse energies of 0.6–1.2 J and pulse rates of 5–15 Hz are necessary. To maximize the laser's margin of safety, treatment usually begins with a pulse energy of 0.6 J and only increases as needed to fragment the stone. The laser fiber should be applied to the targeted stone in a paintbrush fashion, which vaporizes the stone rather than drilling into it. The endpoint of laser lithotripsy is generally either when stone fragments are small enough that they might be expected to pass spontaneously or until they can be safely extracted with a basket or grasping device.

Adverse Events

- Injury to urothelial tissue and tissue perforation.

In general, the Holmium laser is one of the safest intracorporeal lithotrites available for stone fragmentation. The most significant adverse event is injury of the urothelial tissue adjacent to the treated stone. The depth of tissue penetration of the Holmium laser is 0.5–1.0 mm, so in most cases such injuries may be managed conservatively, although a ureteral stricture may be a long term consequence of such an event. The Holmium laser does produce a weak shockwave, so in some cases stone fragments can be retropulsed and migrate away from the endoscope, which may increase the complexity of the procedure. Eye protection is required for operators of the Holmium laser, although at the energy levels used for the fragmentation of calculi the operator's cornea would be damaged only if it was positioned at less than 10 cm from the laser fiber. A theoretical side effect of holmium laser lithotripsy is the production of cyanide when uric acid stones are treated, although this has never been encountered in clinical experience.

Future Directions

- Development of smaller (150 μm) fibers that are more flexible and do not impede endoscope bending.
- More rapid and efficient fragmentation of larger urinary stones using novel solid-state and fiber lasers (e.g., Erbium:YAG and Thulium fiber lasers).

The field of laser lithotripsy is advancing in two different directions: improvements to the existing Holmium laser platform, and development of novel laser platforms. The most significant improvement in Holmium laser lithotripsy will likely come from improved delivery fibers. At present, the smallest fiber in widespread use, the 200 μm fiber, impedes deflection of a flexible ureteroscope by up to 20°. As smaller laser fibers, such as 150 μm fibers, are produced, it is likely that this effect on endoscope deflection will be further reduced. The fracture of a laser fiber inside of an endoscope can result in a catastrophic failure of the scope, and when this occurs the fiber-optic bundles that transmit images and light are generally destroyed. Future efforts towards maximizing fiber durability may reduce these events.

The Erbium:YAG laser has recently been tested for fragmentation of urinary calculi.[10] The erbium laser wavelength of 2,940 nm is more strongly absorbed by water than that of the holmium laser wavelength at 2,120 nm, which has translated to a 2–3 fold increase in efficiency for fragmenting urinary stones in an in vitro setting. However, there are several limitations of the erbium laser that prevent its immediate use in the clinic. The erbium laser wavelength cannot be transmitted through standard low-OH silica fibers, and mid-infrared fibers are needed which are typically less flexible, more expensive, and less biocompatible than silica fibers. The high-power thulium fiber laser has also been tested for lithotripsy, and, unlike the erbium laser, it may be used with standard silica fibers.[11] The thulium fiber laser has several potential advantages over the solid-state holmium laser, including more efficient operation, more flexible operating parameters, and a smaller beam diameter for easier coupling into small optical fibers for use in flexible endoscopes.

Benign Prostatic Hyperplasia

Introduction

- Holmium:YAG and Frequency-doubled Neodymium:YAG (KTP or "Greenlight") are most commonly used lasers for treatment of BPH.
- Higher power Holmium:YAG (100 W) and KTP (120 W) lasers have recently become available for more rapid treatment of BPH.

As the population ages, the prevalence of BPH, and its accompanying voiding symptoms, is increasing.[12] The natural history of BPH is often one of progression, with mild symptoms becoming more bothersome over time. Indeed, among 50-year-old men, the lifetime incidence of surgical or medical intervention for BPH is estimated to be 35%. Transurethral resection of the prostate has historically been the most common surgical intervention for men with the

Table 3 Technical specifications for lasers used in treatment of BPH

Laser parameters	Holmium	KTP
Wavelength (nm)	2,120	532
Operation mode	Pulsed	CW
Pulse length (μs)	<600	–
Repetition rate (Hz)	5–50	–
Average power (W)	100	120
Electrical specifications	220 V, 30 A	220 V, 30 A
Weight (kg)	155	152

symptoms of BPH. Over the past decade, several laser based technologies have been developed for the treatment of men suffering from BPH.

In general, the popularly utilized laser platforms for the treatment of BPH are the KTP laser and the Holmium:YAG laser (Table 3), both of which rely on an ablative mechanism of action in which prostate tissue is removed either through incision or vaporization by elevating the tissue temperature well above 100°C. The 532 nm wavelength of the KTP laser is more strongly absorbed by blood, resulting in a shallow optical penetration depth in the tissue (approximately 0.8 mm) (Fig. 1), and efficient tissue ablation with a thermal coagulation zone of approximately 1–2 mm. The KTP laser procedure, pioneered by Malek and associates,[13] is termed Photoselective Vaporization of the Prostate (PVP) because the laser wavelength is not absorbed by water, but rather selectively absorbed by hemoglobin in the tissue, resulting in direct vaporization of the prostate. During PVP, a cavity is created after laser tissue vaporization, which is similar to TURP. With the recent commercial availability of higher power, 80 W KTP lasers, such as the "Greenlight" laser, higher tissue vaporization rates have been achieved in a virtually bloodless procedure. Operative times have decreased significantly compared to earlier studies with the lower power 40 W and 60 W KTP lasers. As a result, this procedure has recently become one of the preferred methods for laser

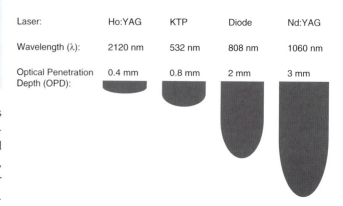

Fig. 1 Optical penetration depths in soft tissue as a function of wavelength for several common lasers used in urology

treatment of BPH, and early studies have demonstrated results equivalent to TURP.[14,15] The long-term effectiveness of the procedure has yet to be determined. The most recent version of the KTP laser provides even more power, 120 W, although long-term evaluations of its clinical performance have not yet been reported.

The application of the Holmium:YAG laser to BPH has evolved in stages. Initially, holmium laser vaporization of the prostate (HoLAP) was developed using low-power holmium lasers, but it was found to be a time-consuming procedure limited to use in smaller prostates. Holmium laser resection of the prostate (HoLRP) was then developed, but the technique was difficult to learn. During HoLRP, the holmium laser with a wavelength of 2,120 nm is used to provide precise tissue cutting with an optical penetration depth of only 0.4 mm, thus producing a thin coagulation zone. The prostatic lobes are resected and removed with a syringe or grasping loop. This procedure is also slow, requires long laser irradiation times, and is not practical for large prostates.

However, with the recent introduction of higher power holmium lasers with output powers up to 100 W, HoLAP has been re-explored, as procedure times could be reduced so that they are comparable to KTP laser ablation. As of yet, however, there are no published studies directly comparing the 80 W KTP and the 100 W Ho:YAG lasers for vaporization of prostate tissue, so it is unclear which technology provides an advantage for this type of procedure. Further complicating matters, both lasers operate based on different mechanisms of laser-tissue interaction. The KTP laser radiation can be transmitted easily through water in a noncontact mode, because the laser radiation is selectively absorbed by the hemoglobin in the tissue. On the contrary, the holmium laser radiation is highly absorbed by the water in the tissue, and although it can be used in noncontact mode due to the "Moses effect" (a cavitation bubble forms at the end of the fiber tip due to the short laser pulse and effectively "parts the waters"), the efficiency of tissue vaporization may be reduced.

The most recent evolution of the holmium laser procedure is termed Holmium laser enucleation of the prostate (HoLEP) and was pioneered by Gilling and colleagues.[16] This procedure was developed because it was found that HoLRP was too slow during earlier studies using lower power holmium lasers. HoLEP involves laser resection of large prostate lobes into chunks that are pushed up into the bladder, mechanically morcellated into smaller pieces, and then flushed out of the urinary system. Unlike HoLRP, this technique can be used on extremely large prostate glands of >70–100 g. Randomized studies comparing HoLEP and TURP have shown that HoLEP provides better relief of bladder outflow obstruction in small prostates, and it is at least equivalent to TURP in improving symptoms and flow rates in larger prostates.[16-19] Recent studies have also demonstrated that the holmium laser is also effective for treating patients receiving anticoagulant

Table 4 Comparison of laser procedures for treatment of BPH

Laser/procedure	Advantages	Disadvantages
Holmium (HoLEP)	Multiple-use laser Tissue for histology Symptom scores Peak flow rates Low morbidity Low blood loss Short catheterization Low re-treatment rate	Steep learning curve Cost of laser + morcellator Operation time
KTP (PVP)	No blood loss Simple procedure Symptom scores Peak flow rates	Cost of fibers

therapy or with bleeding disorders.[20] However, the HoLAP technique requires significant capital investment in a 100 W holmium laser and a mechanical morcellator. The procedure is also considered more difficult to learn than PVP and has longer procedural times and a longer learning curve. However, unlike the KTP laser, the holmium laser can be used for other soft and hard tissue procedures, including incision of strictures, ablation of tumors, and laser lithotripsy, thus offsetting some of the capital equipment costs and making the holmium laser the most versatile laser for use in urology. A summary of the advantages and disadvantages of each laser technique for treatment of BPH is provided in Table 4.

Indications and Contraindications

Indications

- Moderate to severe lower urinary tract symptoms due to BPH.
- Complications, such as urinary retention, due to BPH.
- KTP laser vaporization for men with small to medium size prostates.
- Holmium laser enucleation for men with larger prostates.

Contraindications

- None.

The American Urological Association's Guidelines on Benign Prostatic Hyperplasia recommend surgery for any man with moderate to severe lower urinary tract symptoms due to benign enlargement of the prostate, or for any man who has developed complications, such as urinary retention, as a result of BPH. The choice of surgical approach is a technical consideration, and electrosurgical resection, as well as laser therapies, are all reasonable treatment options. Nonetheless, the KTP and the holmium lasers each have unique attributes which make them more appropriate for certain patients.

The KTP laser achieves its ultimate result by the high power, rapid photothermal ablation of vascular tissue, which leads to vaporization of prostate tissue. Although obstructing prostate tissue can be removed in this way, the speed of tissue removal is limited, and for exceptionally large prostates the operative times can be quite long. Follow-up studies have found that the reduction in both prostate size and PSA levels are not more than 30–44% following KTP laser ablation of the prostate.[12] Therefore, KTP laser ablation may be most appropriately performed on men with small to medium sized prostates.

Holmium laser ablation of the prostate is an almost identical procedure to the KTP laser ablation, as both modalities rely on the vaporization of prostate tissue. The Holmium laser achieves its end result as intracellular water within the prostate tissue rapidly absorbs laser energy and the constituent cells are ablated. Again, just as with KTP laser ablation, holmium laser ablation is limited by the size of the prostate, and is most effective for men with small to medium sized prostates. For men with large prostates, holmium laser enucleation may be the most appropriate laser intervention, as it permits the treatment of larger prostates with either holmium laser resection of the prostate or holmium laser enucleation of the prostate.

Technique

- Equipment includes laser, continuous irrigation cystoscope, and side-firing fiber.
- Ho: YAG laser is strongly absorbed by water component in the tissue and used to enucleate the prostate.
- KTP laser is strongly absorbed by hemoglobin in tissue and used to vaporize the prostate.
- Ho:YAG laser enucleation of prostate (HoLEP) is considered more difficult to learn and a longer procedure, however, there is longer follow-up data, and it is a multiple-use laser that can be used for lithotripsy and other soft tissue procedures as well.
- KTP laser beam more rapidly vaporizes prostate tissue and can be transmitted through a fluid environment, since the wavelength is not strongly absorbed by water.
- Both Ho:YAG and KTP lasers provide sufficient thermal damage for hemostasis.

Laser ablation, whether it is performed with a KTP laser or a holmium laser, utilizes the same basic technique. Equipment needs are modest, and in general the only equipment needed in addition to the laser is a continuous irrigation cystoscope and a side-firing laser fiber. The laser is used in a near contact mode, as the fiber is placed approximately one half millimeter from the surface of the prostate. Ablation begins at the bladder neck, and is carried down to the verumontanum, the distal boundary of ablation. The laser fiber is swept laterally to the right and left, creating a channel within the prostatic urethra. Once the median lobe has been ablated, attention is turned to the lateral lobes, and in a similar sweeping fashion this tissue is ablated. Ablation is carried down to a depth of the prostatic capsule, which is evident when transcese fibers are encountered underneath the ablated tissue. Bleeding points can be controlled by defocusing the laser fiber, or moving it away from the surface of the prostatic tissue.

Holmium laser resection and holmium laser enucleation of the prostate are more complex operations. For patients with an enlarged median lobe, this structure is generally enucleated or resected first. A groove is created with the laser at either side of the median lobe, from the bladder neck to the vermontanum, and carried to the depth of the prostate capsule. The median lobe is then undermined just proximal to the verumontanum and enucleated in a retrograde fashion. Dissection of the lateral lobes occurs at a plane between the surgical capsule and the prostate adenoma, as the laser is used to free the attachments of these two structures, and the beak of the resectoscope is used to provide upward traction creating a further space of separation. Once the dissection has proceeded to the anterior aspect of the prostate, a groove is created at the extreme anterior aspect and joined to the plane of dissection. The lobe is then separated from the capsule and pushed into the bladder, morcellated, and evacuated. The contralateral lobe is treated in the same fashion.

Adverse Events

- Small probability of bleeding, bladder neck contracture.

Laser treatment of the prostate, whether in the form of ablation or enucleation, is generally considered to be a virtually bloodless procedure. However, there are certain cases in which bleeding may be more likely, such as those patients with particularly large prostates. Although even in such cases the risk of blood transfusion remains low. Other adverse events associated with laser ablation of the prostate include bladder neck contracture, or scarring at the bladder neck.

This delayed complication is rare, particularly with HoLEP, and if it does occur generally can be treated with a holmium laser incision of the bladder neck.

Future Directions

- Development of higher power Holmium:YAG and KTP lasers.
- Novel laser sources (e.g., Thulium:YAG and Thulium fiber lasers).
- Photodynamic therapy (PDT) as a non-thermal method of treatment.

New experimental and clinical lasers have recently been introduced for treatment of BPH. Most recently, a solid-state Thulium:YAG laser has been introduced for clinical use as a potential alternative to the holmium laser for soft tissue applications (Table 5). The thulium laser operates in continuous-wave (CW) mode at a wavelength of 2,010 nm and may provide improved tissue cutting and hemostasis without the mechanical damage caused by the pulsed holmium laser. Like the holmium and KTP lasers, the power output of the thulium laser has been steadily increased from 50 to 70 W to provide more rapid tissue ablation. The thulium laser is currently being studied in urology for resection of the prostate.[21,22] However, the clinical use of this technology in urology is very new, and few studies have been published to date, so evaluation of the efficacy of this laser is not yet possible.

The Thulium fiber laser has also been tested in the laboratory for vaporization of the prostate (Table 5). Preliminary laboratory experiments using a 110-W Thulium fiber laser have demonstrated that it is capable of rapidly vaporizing prostate tissue, ex vivo, while also producing sufficient thermal coagulation zones to achieve hemostasis during the procedure.[23] However, further pre-clinical studies have yet to be performed to properly assess the efficacy of this new experimental technology for potential clinical use in treatment of BPH.

The use of photodynamic therapy (PDT) for treatment of BPH has been previously proposed, but few studies have been performed.[24] During PDT, which is currently also being tested for treatment of bladder and prostate cancer, a photosensitizing drug is delivered intravenously to the patient. The compound is selectively absorbed by cells, and then typically a few days after administration of the drug, the tissue is exposed locally to low levels of laser energy using a light source, resulting in tissue necrosis in the exposed area. Active research in PDT is ongoing on several fronts. Improved photosensitizing agents are being developed, some of which absorb at longer laser wavelengths, providing deeper optical penetration of the laser radiation in the tissue, and thus more uniform treatment of larger tissue volumes, such as the prostate. Some of the newer PDT drugs can also be applied locally, or clear more rapidly from the body, and have fewer side effects (e.g., reduced skin photosensitization) as well. Optimization and real-time monitoring of treatment dosimetry is also being conducted to minimize complications from PDT. Most recently, early clinical trials are in progress using transurethral photodynamic therapy (PDT) and an experimental light-activated drug (Lemuteporfin, QLT, inc., www. qltinc.com) for treatment of BPH.[24]

Strictures

Introduction

- Urethral and ureteral strictures can occur as a result of trauma.
- Cold knife incision and balloon dilation have widely variable success rates.
- Surgical reconstruction is gold standard but carries with it high cost and morbidity.
- Holmium:YAG laser has been used for treating strictures with some success.

Strictures can occur at two locations in the urinary tract: ureteral strictures, and urethral strictures. Both types of stricture generally occur as a response to trauma, be it as a result of surgical instrumentation or injury, radiotherapy, infection, or stone passage. Although surgical reconstruction remains the most definitive repair, such an approach can be morbid. Consequently, minimally invasive treatment of stricture disease, including balloon dilation, cold knife incision, electrocautery, and holmium laser incision have all been explored.[25]

Table 5 New clinical and experimental lasers for use in treatment of BPH

Laser parameters	Thulium	Thulium fiber
Wavelength (nm)	2,010	1,908 or 1,940
Average power (W)	5–70	<150
Operation mode	CW or long-pulse	CW or long-pulse
Pulse length (ms)	50 - CW	arbitrary
Electrical requirements	220 V, 10 A	115 V, 15 A for <60 W
		220 V, 10 A for >60 W
Weight (kg)	150	40–120

Indications/Contraindications

> Indications
>
> - Short strictures less than 2 cm length.
>
> Contraindications
>
> - Long strictures greater than 2 cm length.

The most important predictor of success or failure of a minimally invasive laser-based therapy is the length of the stricture. Therefore, the most appropriate patients for endoscopic laser urethrotomy or ureterotomy are those with a small stricture. For both urethral and ureteral strictures, a length greater than 2 cm portends a poor outcome, and patients with such strictures should not undergo a laser-based treatment approach.[25,26]

Technique

> Ureteral Strictures
>
> - Full thickness incisions with Holmium laser settings of 1.2 J and 15 Hz.
> - Ureteral stent left indwelling for 4–6 weeks.
>
> Urethral strictures
>
> - Incisions at 6 and 12 o'clock.
> - Placement of Foley catheter for several days

Laser incision of ureteral strictures is generally approached ureteroscopically. In all cases a safety guidewire is placed across the incision. In patients with proximal ureteral strictures, the posterolateral wall should be incised with the laser, whereas for patients with distal ureteral strictures the anteromedial aspect should be incised. The incision should be full thickness, and carried into normal appearing ureter on both the proximal and distal margins. Standard laser settings are an energy of 1.2 J and a rate of 15 Hz. In most cases a balloon catheter is deployed at the conclusion of the laser incision, to confirm complete incision of the stricture. A ureteral stent is generally left indwelling for 4–6 weeks.

Urethral strictures are generally approached in a cystoscopic fashion. Again, a safety wire is placed across the stricture, and internal urethrotomies are created in the 12 o'clock position, between the corpora cavernosa. If a single urethrotomy is inadequate, a second incision may be required, typically at the 6 o'clock location. The duration of Foley catheter drainage is variable, although most clinicians leave the catheter for several days.

Adverse Events

> Hemorrhage from incision of vascular tissue.

Laser urethrotomy or ureterotomy is a safe procedure. Intraoperatively, the most significant complication is hemorrhage. When incising the urethra, significant hemorrhage may be encountered should the incision be carried into vascular structures, such as those found within the corpora cavernosa. In most cases such events may be managed with urethral catheter drainage, which will tamponade the bleeding vessel. Similarly, hemorrhage may occur during laser incision of the ureter, should a peri-ureteral vessel be encountered; in most cases hemorrhage should be amenable to conservative management.

Future Directions

> - Erbium:YAG laser for more precise incision of strictures.

Experimental and investigational clinical studies have recently been reported utilizing the Erbium:YAG laser for precise incision of urethral tissues with minimal peripheral thermal damage as a potential alternative to the holmium laser.[27,28] The high-temperature water absorption coefficient at the erbium laser wavelength of 2,940 nm is about 30 times higher than that of the holmium laser wavelength at 2,120 nm. This difference has translated into a reduction of peripheral thermal damage during incision of urethral and ureteral tissues from 300 μm at 2,120 nm to 10–30 μm at 2,940 nm. However, there are several limitations of the erbium laser that prevent its immediate use for clinical applications in urology. The erbium laser does not induce sufficient thermal damage to produce thermal coagulation and hemostasis of highly vascular tissues. Therefore, use of the erbium laser should be limited to use in incision of scar tissue, such as strictures. The erbium laser wavelength also cannot be transmitted through standard silica fibers, and mid-infrared fibers are needed which are typically less flexible, more expensive, and less biocompatible than silica fibers.

Other Applications of Lasers in Urology

Other applications of lasers in urology include Ho:YAG laser ablation of superficial transitional cell bladder tumors,[29] Nd:YAG and CO_2 laser ablation of penile carcinoma,[30] Nd:YAG and Ho:YAG laser incision of ureteroceles,[31] Nd:YAG and diode laser ablation of urethral hair,[32] Ho:YAG laser extraction of encrusted ureteral stents,[33] and laser partial nephrectomy.[34] Laser tissue welding has also been investigated for vasovasostomy, ureteral repair, pyeloplasty, urethral reconstruction, and hypospadias repair. Potential advantages of laser welding include fluid-tight closure, reduced probability of infection, and reduced operative repair time. Clinical applications of tissue welding have been limited, however, due to weak and inconsistent weld strengths.[35] Several experimental approaches to laser tissue welding are currently being explored, including both photothermal and photochemical methods of tissue closure (Table 6). Two approaches to photothermal welding include "laser soldering" and "laser welding". Laser soldering involves the topical application of a solder in the form of a biological adhesive and a light absorbing dye. The solder is heated by the laser and welded to the surface of the tissue incision, creating a "thermal band-aid" that will stay closed and prevent leakage of fluids, until the wound healing has progressed to a stage where the tissue is strong enough to remain closed on its own. During laser tissue welding, the laser energy is directly absorbed by the cut tissue edges at the weld site, resulting in tissue temperatures above 50°C, thermal denaturation of collagenous tissue, and the creation of non-covalent tissue bonds. The objective is to achieve a strong, full-thickness weld. During photochemical welding, low power laser irradiation and activation of a chemical cross-linking agent creates covalent tissue bonds at the weld site. The advantage of this technique over photothermal welding is that strong, covalent bonding of tissue may be achieved in the absence of thermal damage. However, close approximation of the cut tissue edges through applied pressure is necessary to produce these strong bonds.

Conclusions

In summary, urologists use lasers for both soft and hard tissue applications, including most commonly laser incision or vaporization of the prostate for treatment of benign prostatic hyperplasia and fragmentation of urinary stones during laser lithotripsy. Other applications include incision of urethral and ureteral strictures, treatment of bladder cancer, bloodless partial nephrectomy, treatment of penile carcinoma, tissue welding, and photodynamic therapy of bladder and prostate cancer.

Overall, the future of lasers in urology looks bright. New laser systems continue to enter the urology clinic that are more powerful, more compact, more versatile, and less expensive than the previous lasers, providing the urologist with the means to develop new minimally invasive laser applications in urology and improve on existing applications. For example, the recent introduction of higher power solid state lasers, such as the 100 W Ho:YAG and 120 W KTP lasers, has resulted in more rapid and efficient incision or vaporization of prostate tissue during treatment of benign prostatic hyperplasia. On the horizon, even more compact and efficient laser technologies, such as fiber lasers, may replace current solid state lasers for use in BPH treatment, and photodynamic therapy may also represent a promising alternative to the photothermal laser ablation techniques currently used in the clinic for treatment of BPH. Applications of the high-power KTP laser will expand beyond BPH, to other procedures requiring excellent hemostatic properties during laser incision, such as laparoscopic partial nephrectomy.

While several new lasers are being tested for lithotripsy, issues with cost (e.g., thulium fiber laser), the fiber delivery system (e.g., erbium laser), or lack of multiple-use applications (e.g., FREDDY laser) will need to be overcome before the holmium laser can be replaced. Development of more

Table 6 Comparison of laser tissue welding techniques

	Photothermal		Photochemical
	Laser soldering	Laser welding	
Objective	Thermal band-aid	Full-thickness weld	Heat-free weld
Interface	Solder-tissue	Tissue-tissue	Tissue-dye-tissue
Wavelength	808 nm	450–1,300	470 nm
Mode	CW	CW or pulsed	CW
Irradiance	High power	High power	Low power
Irradiation time	Short (15 s–10 min)	Short (15 s–10 min)	Long (>10 min)
Dye	Indocyanine green	With or without dye	Naphthalimides/riboflavin
Adhesive	Albumin or fibrinogen	None	None
Advantages	Fluid-tight closure	Strong welds	No thermal damage
Disadvantages	Variable solder-tissue adhesion	Thermal damage, inconsistent welds	Variable tissue apposition, longer irradiation times

flexible hollow waveguides for the delivery of pulsed carbon dioxide and erbium laser energy through flexible endoscopes may allow these laser wavelengths to be used in the upper urinary tract for more efficient laser lithotripsy.

The results for laser treatment of strictures have been disappointing, although more precise lasers for tissue incision with minimal thermal insult to healthy tissue (e.g., erbium laser) may provide better results. There remains a fundamental need to better understand the wound healing method before strictures can be eliminated.

Laser tissue welding is ideal for urology, which has many applications needing rapid, microsurgical, fluid-tight tissue closure. However, the field has progressed slowly and faces competition from more validated, lower-cost, and easy-to-use tissue closure techniques (e.g., sutures, staples, biological adhesives). Although numerous scientific laser tissue welding studies have been conducted, few of these studies have advanced to the stage of clinical testing.

In the field of photodynamic therapy, photosensitizing drugs will continue to be developed with longer activation wavelengths for destruction of larger tissue volumes such as the prostate gland. These drugs will have shorter clearance times, they will be taken immediately prior to light activation, and they will not have the side effects usually associated with the early photosensitizing drugs, such as skin photosensitization.

Technological advances in diagnostic imaging and robotics will allow these minimally invasive laser procedures in urology to be performed with even more precision and control, and with real-time monitoring, thus improving the efficacy and safety of the procedure.

References

1. Mulvaney WP, Beck CW. The laser beam in urology. *J Urol.* 1968;99:112-115.
2. Watson GM, Wickham JE. Initial experience with a pulsed dye laser for ureteric calculi. *Lancet.* 1986;1:1357-1358.
3. Chan KF, Vassar GJ, Pfefer TJ, et al. Holmium:YAG laser lithotripsy: a dominant photothermal ablative mechanism with chemical decomposition of urinary calculi. *Lasers Surg Med.* 1999;25:22-37.
4. Santa-Cruz RW, Leveillee RJ, Krongrad A. Ex vivo comparison of four lithotripters commonly used in the ureter: what does it take to perforate? *J Endourol.* 1998;12:417-422.
5. Yates J, Zabbo A, Pareek G. A comparison of the FREDDY and holmium lasers during ureteroscopic lithotripsy. *Lasers Surg Med.* 2007;39:637-640.
6. Galvin DJ, Pearle MS. The contemporary management of renal and ureteric calculi. *BJU Int.* 2006;98:1283-1288.
7. Watterson JD, Girvan AR, Cook AJ, et al. Safety and efficacy of holmium: YAG laser lithotripsy in patients with bleeding diatheses. *J Urol.* 2002;168:442-445.
8. Nazif OA, Teichman JM, Glickman RD, Welch AJ. Review of laser fibers: a practical guide for urologists. *J Endourol.* 2004;18(9): 818-829.

9. Knudsen BE, Glickman RD, Stallman KJ, et al. Performance and safety of holmium: YAG laser optical fibers. *J Endourol.* 2005;19(9):1092-1097.
10. Lee H, Kang HW, Teichman JMH, Oh J, Welch AJ. Urinary calculus fragmentation during Ho:YAG and Er:YAG lithotripsy. *Lasers Surg Med.* 2006;38:39-51.
11. Fried NM. Thulium fiber laser lithotripsy: an in vitro analysis of stone fragmentation using a modulated 110-watt thulium fiber laser at 1.94 μm. *Lasers Surg Med.* 2005;37(1):53-58.
12. Kuntz RM. Laser treatment of benign prostatic hyperplasia. *World J Urol.* 2007;25:241-247.
13. Malek RS, Kuntzman RS, Barrett DM. High power potassium-titanyl-phosphate laser vaporization prostatectomy. *J Urol.* 2000; 163:1730-1733.
14. Malek RS, Kuntzman RS, Barrett DM. Photoselective potassium-titanyl-phosphate laser vaporization of the benign obstructive prostate: observations on long-term outcomes. *J Urol.* 2005;174 (4 Pt 1):1344-1348.
15. Bachmann A, Ruszat R, Wyler S, et al. Photoselective vaporization of the prostate: the basel experience after 108 procedures. *Eur Urol.* 2005;47(6):798-804.
16. Tan AH, Gilling PJ, Kennett KM, Frampton C, Westenberg AM, Fraundorfer MR. A randomized trial comparing holmium laser enucleation of prostate with transurethral resection of prostate for treatment of bladder outlet obstruction secondary to benign prostatic hyperplasia in large glands (40–200 grams). *J Urol.* 2003;170: 1270-1274.
17. Kuntz RM, Ahyai S, Lehrich K, Fayad A. Transurethral holmium laser enucleation of the prostate versus transurethral electrocautery resection of the prostate: a randomized prospective trial in 200 patients. *J Urol.* 2004;172(3):1012-1016.
18. Kuntz RM, Lehrich K, Ahyai S. Transurethral holmium laser enucleation of the prostate compared with transvesical open prostatectomy: 18-month follow-up of a randomized trial. *J Endourol.* 2004;18(2):189-191.
19. Wilson LC, Gilling PJ, Williams A, et al. A randomised trial comparing holmium laser enucleation versus transurethral resection in the treatment of prostates larger than 40 grams: results at 2 years. *Eur Urol.* 2006;50(3):569-573.
20. Elzayat E, Habib E, Elhilali M. Holmium laser enucleation of the prostate in patients on anticoagulant therapy or with bleeding disorders. *J Urol.* 2006;175(4):1428-1432.
21. Xia SJ, Zhuo J, Sun XW, Han BM, Shao Y, Zhang YN. Thulium laser versus standard transurethral resection of the prostate: a randomized prospective trial. *Eur Urol.* 2008;53(2):382-389.
22. Bach T, Herrmann TR, Ganzer R, Burchardt M, Gross AJ. RevoLix vaporesection of the prostate: initial results of 54 patients with a 1-year followup. *World J Urol.* 2007;25(3):257-262.
23. Fried NM. High-power laser vaporization of the canine prostate using a 110 W thulium fiber laser at 1.91 μm. *Lasers Surg Med.* 2005;36:52-56.
24. Perez-Marrero R, Goldenberg SL, Shore N, et al. A phase I/II dose-escalation study to assess the safety, tolerability, and preliminary efficacy of transurethral photodynamic therapy with lemuteporfin in men with lower urinary tract symptoms due to benign prostatic hyperplasia. *J Urol.* 2005;173(4):421-422 (A1556).
25. Jordan GH, Schlossberg SM, Devine CJ. Surgery of the penis and urethra. In: Walsh PC, Retik AB, Vaughan ED, Wein AJ, eds. *Campbell's Urology*, vol. 3. 7th ed. Philadelphia: WB Saunders; 1998:3341-3347.
26. Razdan S, Silberstein IK, Bagley DH. Ureteroscopic endoureterotomy. *BJU Int.* 2005;95(Suppl 2):94-101.
27. Varkarakis IM, Inagaki T, Allaf ME, et al. Comparison of erbium:yttrium-aluminum-garnet and holmium:yttrium-aluminum-garnet lasers for incision of urethra and bladder neck in an in vivo porcine model. *Urology.* 2005;65(1):191-195.

28. Munoz JA, Riemer JD, Hayes GB, Negus D, Fried NM. Er:YAG laser incision of urethral strictures: early clinical results. *Proc SPIE*. 2007;6424:64241F-64244F.

29. Syed HA, Biyani CS, Bryan N, Brough SJ, Powell CS. Holmium:YAG laser treatment of recurrent superficial bladder carcinoma: initial clinical experience. *J Endourol*. 2001;15(6): 625-627.

30. Windahl T, Andersson SO. Combined laser treatment for penile carcinoma: results after long-term followup. *J Urol*. 2003;169(6): 2118-2121.

31. Marr L, Skoog SJ. Laser incision of ureterocele in the pediatric patient. *J Urol*. 2002;167:280-282.

32. Crain DS, Miller OF, Smith LJ, Roberts JL, Ross EV. Transcutaneous laser hair ablation for management of intraurethral hair after hypospadias repair: initial experience. *J Urol*. 2003;170:1948-1949.

33. Bukkapatnam R, Seigne J, Helal M. 1-step removal of encrusted retained ureteral stents. *J Urol*. 2003;170:1111-1114.

34. Anderson JK, Baker MR, Lindberg H, Cadeddu JA. Large-volume laparoscopic partial nephrectomy using the potassium-titanyl-phosphate (KTP) laser in a survival porcine model. *Eur Urol*. 2007;51(3):749-754.

35. Kirsch AJ, Cooper CS, Gatti J, et al. Laser tissue soldering for hypospadias repair: results of a controlled prospective clinical trial. *J Urol*. 2001;165(2):574-577.

Lasers in Cardiology and Cardiothoracic Surgery

Pritam R. Polkampally, Allyne Topaz, and On Topaz

Introduction

- History and rationale for laser in the treatment of cardiovascular diseases
- Early applications, growing expectations and the development of realistic perspectives
- Current indications and applications: coronary, peripheral, TMR, EP
- Technique of lasing and catheter technology
- Adverse outcomes
- Future potential

History

Lasers were first introduced to cardiovascular medicine in the 1980s. In light of the laser's avid absorption in atherosclerotic material, the aim was to treat a variety of coronary and peripheral occlusions that were considered "non ideal" for standard balloon angioplasty.[1] Initial studies predicted that laser would render coronary bypass surgery an unnecessary operation as preliminary experience reported successful plaque removal.[2-4]

Early Experience

Publication of several large scale successful clinical trials during early experience with laser led to a conviction that laser had established a prominent role in interventional

O. Topaz (✉)
Duke University School of Medicine, Division of Cardiology,
Charles George Veterans Affairs Medical Center,
Asheville, NC, USA
e-mail: on.topaz@va.gov

cardiology.[5,6] However, the application of the device in cardiac catheterization laboratories was fraught with technical difficulties. The devices were very large, cumbersome to handle and necessitated lengthy warm up and calibration time. The laser catheters were also very rigid and lasing technique with rapid advancement of the catheters across the target lesions was frequently utilized. This technique did not allow adequate absorption of the laser energy within the irradiated plaque. Consequently, laser induced spasm, thrombosis, dissections and perforations became a significant concern.[7,8] Eventually, refinements in catheter design involving smaller laser generators[9] and introduction of safe lasing techniques emphasizing slow debulking and concomitant injections of saline[10,11] led to significant improvement in clinical outcomes.[12] With better understanding of laser as a treatment modality, numerous indications were established for utilization within the field of cardiovascular medicine. At present, laser is used percutaneously in the cardiac catheterization suite for treatment of coronary and peripheral atherosclerotic vascular disease, and surgically for Trans-myocardial revascularization and for pacemaker/AICD lead removal in electrophysiology laboratories.

Current Indications and Applications

Table 1 presents the current indications for use of laser in cardiovascular medicine. Careful case selection is integral to ensuring successful laser procedures. In acute ischemic coronary syndrome caused by obstructive plaque and associated thrombus, restoration of normal antegrade coronary flow is crucial for preservation of the myocardium. As the laser devices interact uniquely with plaque and thrombus, they can be successfully applied in select patients who sustain unstable angina pectoris (Fig. 1) or acute myocardial infarction.[13] The target vessel in these clinical scenarios is either a native coronary artery or an old saphenous vein graft. An important advantage of the laser is its safe

K. Nouri (ed.), *Lasers in Dermatology and Medicine*,
DOI: 10.1007/978-0-85729-281-0_45, © Springer-Verlag London Limited 2011

Table 1 Current indications for use of laser in cardiovascular medicine

1. Acute coronary and peripheral ischemic syndromes
2. Symptomatic patients with evidence of coronary and peripheral atherosclerotic disease
3. Treatment of complex coronary and peripheral atherosclerotic lesions – thrombotic, concentric, eccentric, sub-total and total occlusions
4. Revascularization of native coronary and peripheral arteries and old saphenous vein grafts
5. Extraction of pacemaker and defibrillator leads
6. TMLR for treatment of refractory, debilitating angina

activation in patients with depressed left ventricular ejection fraction presenting with acute ischemic coronary syndromes. Both holmium:YAG[14] and excimer laser have been demonstrated to be successful revascularization modalities for compromised ventricular function. When the outcome of excimer laser assisted angioplasty and stenting was compared in patients with depressed ejection fraction (mean LVEF = 28 ± 6%) versus those with preserved ejection fraction (LVEF = 53 ± 8%), a successful debulking and thrombus removal occurred regardless of baseline ventricular function.[15]

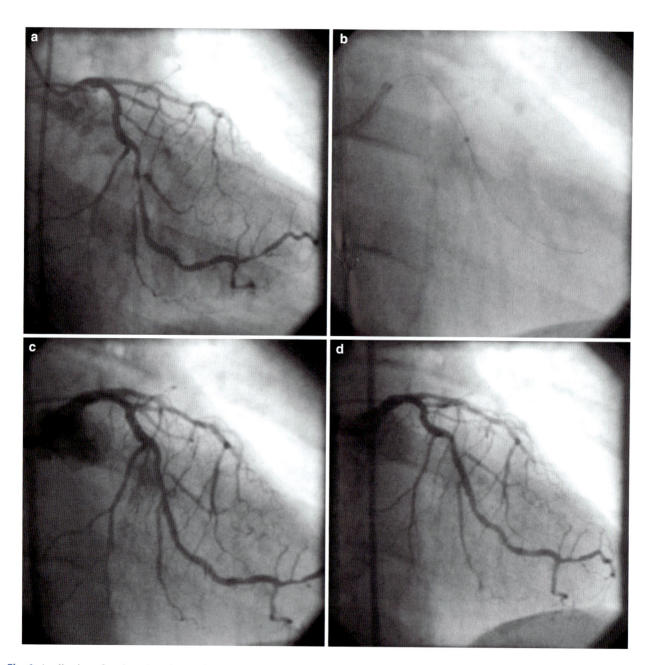

Fig. 1 Application of excimer laser in a patient with unstable angina pectoris. (**a**) Angiogram demonstrating a 95% eccentric, thrombotic stenosis at the middle portion of a large obtuse marginal branch of the Circumflex artery. (**b**) A 1.4 mm COS excimer laser (Spectranetics, Colorado Springs, CO) at the target lesion. (**c**) Results post successful antegrade and retrograde laser debulking along the stenosis. (**d**) Final angiogram following adjunct stenting with a drug eluting stent. There is complete patency of the target vessel. The patient recovered clinically

Contraindications

Lack of informed consent, unavailability of surgical coverage and unprotected left main disease (a relative contraindication) are considered coronary contraindications. As for peripheral laser applications, the presence of poor flow in a sole remaining vessel to the lower limb constitutes a contraindication.

The Specific Effects of Laser on Thrombus

Thrombus is commonly found in patients with unstable angina or acute myocardial infarction. The presence of intracoronary thrombus is associated with an increased complication rate both during and after percutaneous interventions. Laser energy interacts with two essential components of thrombus: fibrin and platelets. Pulsed wave lasers such as the mid infrared holmium:YAG and the ultraviolet excimer create acoustic shock waves that propagate along the irradiated vessel. These waves carry a dynamic pressure front toward the fibrin mesh within the thrombus. This process disrupts and breaks the fibrin fibers resulting in fibrinolysis and thereby reduces thrombus size.[16] Clinically, the excimer laser has been found to be a useful interventional tool for targeted thrombus removal strategy.[17] This laser also alters the aggregation kinetics of platelets leading to reduced platelet force development and inhibition of platelet activity. This phenomenon of platelets stunning is dose dependent and most pronounced at high fluence levels such as 60 mJ/mm^2.[18]

Laser in Acute Myocardial Infarction

Patients who sustain acute myocardial infarction and continue to experience persistent chest pain frequently exhibit an unstable hemodynamic condition. These patients commonly present after a failed response to thrombolytic pharmacotherapy or have contraindications to these medications. In such circumstances, a rescue intervention is indicated for preservation of myocardial tissue. The interest in excimer laser as a potentially beneficial revascularization modality in these patients stems from recognition of its potential for thrombus removal and concomitant plaque debulking. The CARMEL (Cohort of Acute Revascularization of Myocardial infarction with Excimer Laser) multicenter study enrolled 151 patients with acute myocardial infarction and large thrombus burden was present in the infarct related vessel in 75% of the patients. The excimer laser restored an abnormally low baseline coronary TIMI flow in the infarct related vessel (native coronary artery or a saphenous vein graft) to a normal level (Grade 3 TIMI flow) of antegrade perfusion. It also successfully debulked and decreased the target stenosis which was followed by adjunct stenting. An overall 91% procedural success rate, 95% device success rate and 97% angiographic success rate were reported.[19] A low rate (8.6%) of major adverse coronary events was recorded. Specifically, 3% dissection and only 0.6% distal embolization rates were encountered. There were no laser induced perforations. Death occurred only among 30% of the patients presenting with cardiogenic shock. Importantly, maximal laser effect was observed in lesions laden with a heavy thrombus burden. Separate analysis of the study's data base demonstrated maximal laser gain among those patients who presented with an already established Q wave myocardial infarction, an ongoing ST segment elevation and large-extensive thrombus burden in the infarct related vessel.[20] Altogether, the excimer laser is capable of removing as much as 80% of the thrombus burden from the treated targets.[21]

Application of Laser in Specific Target Lesions

Left main disease: Until recently left main coronary artery disease was considered a contraindication for percutaneous intervention. However with a recent paradigm shift from surgical approach to percutaneous revascularization, a defined role for laser in such a strategy has emerged. In a series of 20 symptomatic patients with severe left main disease, the excimer laser was used for pre-stent debulking (Fig. 2). Traditionally, performing a safe percutaneous intervention in the left main coronary artery requires at least partial myocardial protection by patent bypass grafts. However, in this experience patent grafts were present in only 20% of these patients while the majority had no protection or poor protection by a diseased graft. Nevertheless, successful intervention was achieved in 95% of the patients. The investigators concluded that small size laser catheters, when used with proper lasing technique and adjunct stenting can lead to successful debulking strategy in select patients with left main stenosis.[22]

Undilatable or uncrossable lesions: Excimer laser can be very useful in the treatment of atherosclerotic lesions which cannot be crossed with conventional balloon systems. It can also be effectively applied in lesions that fail to yield to the displacement forces induced by balloon angioplasty. The success rate in uncrossable or undilatable stenoses is high, approaching 90%. However, when these targets are calcified, the response is less favorable to laser debulking than that of non calcified lesions (79% vs. 96%, p < 0.05).[23]

Calcified lesions: Balloon angioplasty frequently produces suboptimal results in these lesions. In the past, lasers utilizing a wide range of wavelengths encountered difficulties in recanalization of these stenoses. However, following Rentrop's invention of a high energy level excimer laser catheter (capable of producing up to 80 mJ/mm^2 at 80 Hz

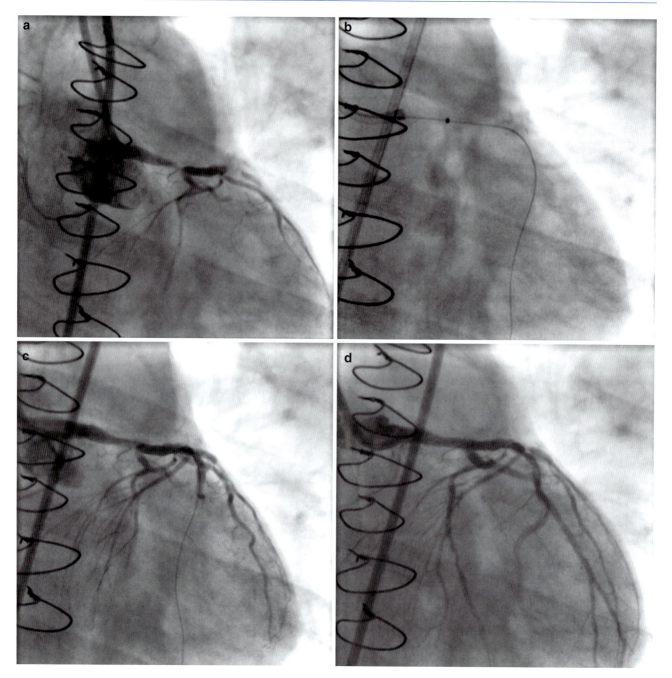

Fig. 2 Application of excimer laser in left main coronary artery disease in a patient with unstable angina. The patient underwent coronary bypass surgery just 4 weeks earlier but two saphenous vein grafts occluded with only the left internal mammary artery remaining patent. (**a**) The critical stenosis at the distal segment of the left main coronary artery. (**b**) Activation of a 0.9 mm X-80 excimer laser (Spectranetics, Colorado Springs, CO) catheter (the tip of the catheter is radiologically opaque) along the plaque. (**c**) Adequate recanalization post laser debulking. (**d**) Final angiographic results post adjunct stenting: patent left main artery is present with adequate flow into the Circumflex artery. The patient's symptoms were completely relieved

energy fluence) for calcified lesions, the device was introduced to the field as the 0.9 mm X-80 catheter. Improved results have been reported with this technology.[24] The unique capability of the excimer laser to debulk underlying calcium is also demonstrated in the critical scenario of a non-dilatable coronary stent. In such challenging cases calcium impinges on the stent struts and obstructs their full expansion during deployment. Laser ablation either softens or removes the calcium, thus enabling subsequent complete deployment and proper expansion of a stent.[25]

Total occlusions: These challenging atherosclerotic stenoses are frequently difficult to traverse with a guide wire, respond unfavorably to balloon angioplasty and resist stent deployment. A laser catheter or a laser wire can penetrate these lesions and facilitate adjunct balloon and stenting.[26] A success rate of 86–90% for the excimer laser has been reported in these occlusions.[27] Total occlusions are mostly long standing lesions that contain layers of old, well organized thrombus within calcified and fibrotic plaques. In the setting of acute myocardial infarction, however, they can present a specific revascularization challenge because of a large, fresh thrombus burden as imposed on an underlying plaque material. In such instances the laser can be used successfully for recanalization of the total occlusion.[28]

Aorto-ostial lesions: These resistant atherosclerotic obstructions are usually focal and often calcified. Precise laser debulking enables subsequent stenting. The success rate with laser and adjunct balloon angioplasty in two series of patients were reported as high as 94%,[29,30] thus, far exceeding the relatively low 74–80% success rate for standard balloon angioplasty.

Saphenous vein grafts lesions: Occlusions in old saphenous vein grafts frequently consist of diffuse or multifocal plaques and thrombus. These lesions are degenerative and prone to distal embolization. Despite the presence of a large thrombus burden within these vessels, a success rate of 94% was reported with both the ultraviolet excimer laser and mid-infrared holmium:YAG laser.[31,32] The considerable capability of laser to provide safe debulking of these grafts even in the setting of acute myocardial infarction and in the presence of a heavy thrombus burden has been documented.[33] Furthermore, the remarkably low rate of distal embolization during excimer laser debulking of old bypass grafts (1–5%) precludes the need for adjunct protection systems in most cases where the excimer laser is used.

Stent restenosis: Stent restenosis is attributed to localized or diffuse tissue growth. Laser debulking of stent restenosis is a preferred treatment over tissue displacement by standard balloon angioplasty.[34] Mehran et al. compared excimer laser and adjunct balloon dilations to balloon treatment alone and concluded that no complications were associated with the use of laser. The laser application resulted in greater luminal gain, ablation of intimal hyperplasia, and a tendency toward less frequent subsequent target vessel revascularization.[35] In cases of focal or severe diffuse stent restenosis within old vein grafts, laser debulking and removal of the obstructive regrowth tissue and its associated thrombus facilitates adjunct balloon angioplasty (Fig. 3).

Trans Myocardial Laser Revascularization (TMLR)

This unique revascularization concept is based on the diversion of arterial blood flow onto regions of the myocardium which do not receive adequate perfusion secondary to atherosclerotic coronary arterial disease. The attempts to reperfuse ischemic myocardium by direct myocardial recanalization predate coronary bypass grafting and coronary balloon angioplasty.[36] The TMLR procedure aims to create multiple 1 mm intramyocardial laser channels (TMLR) within the ischemic viable myocardium. The creation of these channels is expected to promote angiogenesis with growth of microvessels that provide fresh blood supply to the myocardium.[37] The increase in microvessels significantly correlates with the expression of matrix metalloproteinases-2 and platelet-derived endothelial cell growth factor.[38] A specific indication of the TMLR is for patients with refractory angina pectoris who are unable to undergo coronary bypass surgery for pain relief. TMLR has also been incorporated as an adjunct surgical treatment for those who undergo coronary bypass surgery but need further intraoperative revascularization of myocardial regions that cannot be reached with bypass grafts. The TMLR application involves application of specially designed laser catheters under direct vision or under fluoroscopy guidance. These catheters are placed in direct contact against the epicardium and activated with emission of laser fluence inward toward the myocardium. Various laser sources such as CO_2, excimer and holmium:YAG have been used for TMLR either surgically or percutaneously for treatment of patients with refractory angina.[39] TMLR has been shown in randomized studies to improve subjective symptoms of[40,41] promote increased exercise time[42] and improve quality of life as compared with maximal medical therapy.[43] Recently it has been proposed that combining TMLR with cell therapy delivered through direct myocardial injections is a safe strategy which may act synergistically to reduce myocardial ischemia and improve functional capacity.[44] However, despite a certain level of success TMLR remains quite an enigma as the exact functional mechanism of angina relief is unclear and the relief of angina may be short lived in many.[45] The prevailing theory of laser induced thermal damage to cardiac nerves resulting in cardiac denervation has been refuted.[46] Furthermore, whether TMLR results in improved cardiac function remains a controversial issue.

Laser for Revascularization of Heart Transplant Allograft Vasculopathy

Coronary allograft vasculopathy is a leading cause of late death in heart transplant recipients. As these patients are frequently not considered to be good candidates for repeat heart transplant, the endovascular treatment is a practical management option. However, this strategy has encountered certain difficulties: balloon angioplasty, directional atherectomy, and direct stenting have all been applied although the results have been disappointing.[47] The low profile laser catheters

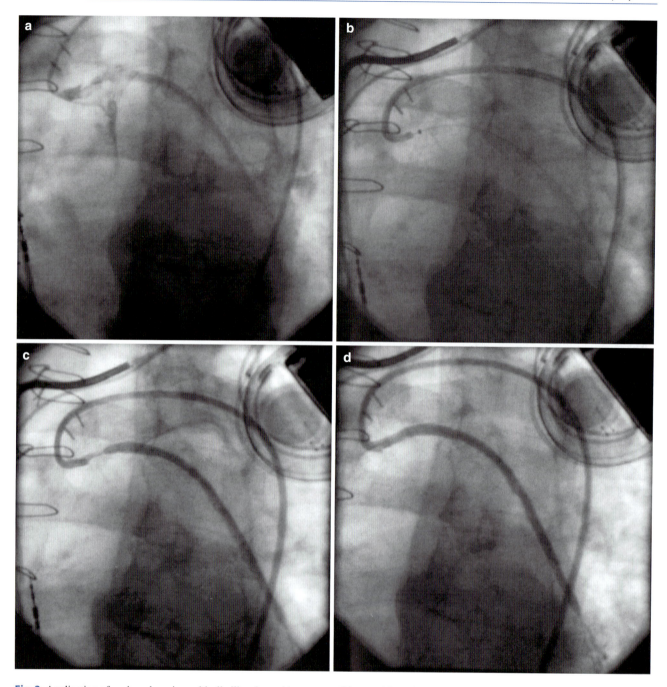

Fig. 3 Application of excimer laser in a critically ill patient with severe angina, marked anterior –lateral ischemia, unstable hemodynamic condition, impaired renal function and depressed left ventricular function. Initial angiography demonstrated critical disease in two old saphenous vein grafts to the obtuse marginal branch of the Circumflex artery and to the left anterior descending artery, respectively. A third bypass graft to the right coronary artery was totally occluded for several years. Of note, this patient underwent coronary bypass surgery twice in the past. A third open heart surgery was not considered a treatment option. Revascularization of the graft to the obtuse marginal artery: (**a**) A 99% stenosis of the proximal graft. (**b**) 0.9 mm X-80 excimer laser catheter at the stenosis. (**c**) Creation of a "pilot channel" along the target lesion. (**d**) Adequate results following adjunct stenting with a drug eluting stent

appear to provide a unique advantage for revascularization in these challenging target lesions.[48,49] As long term reduction of restenosis is not expected from the laser alone, adjunct stenting with drug eluting stents is indicated (Fig. 4).

Laser for congenital heart disease: In certain congenital cardiac defects, the laser can provide means of critical revascularization. For example, the prognosis of infants with pulmonary atresia and intact ventricular septum is poor and presents a major management challenge. Mechanical penetration of the atretic pulmonary valve is an applicable option for decompression of the right ventricle to reduce critically high pressure and improve overall left ventricular function.

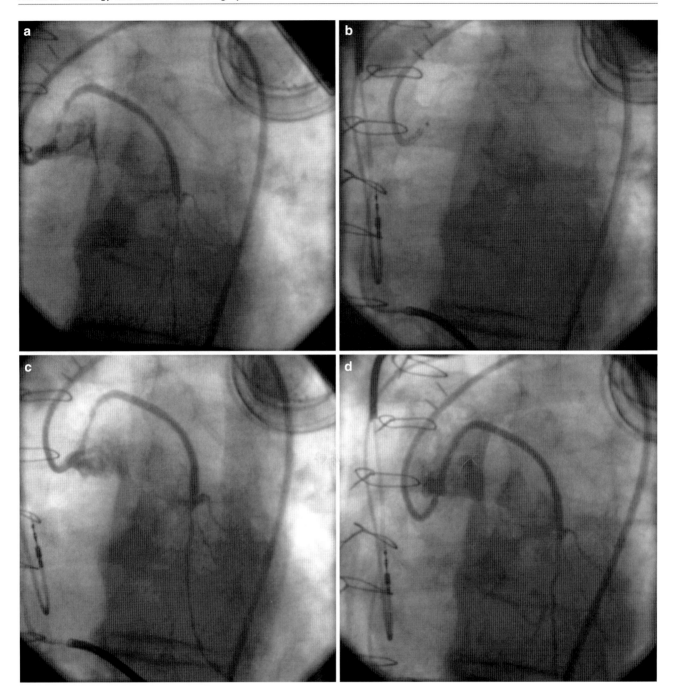

Fig. 4 Revascularization of the graft to the left anterior descending artery: (**a**) Angiogram of the saphenous vein graft demonstrating two tight proximal lesions within a previously placed stent. This represents severe stent restenosis accompanied by compromised flow along the graft. (**b**) A 0.9 mm X-80 laser catheter at the target. (**c**) Post laser debulking created an adequate recanalization which enabled deployment of balloon angioplasty. (**d**) Final results demonstrating marked patency of the treated stent. Normal antegrade flow was restored along the graft and the patients exhibited clinical improvement

Percutaneous excimer laser induced ablation of the atretic pulmonary valve can be accomplished safely by a "step by step" technique whereby the tip of the laser catheter is advanced before a guide wire. This recanalization then enables insertion and deployment of a peripheral balloon leading to life saving reopening of the main pulmonary artery. The laser fluence does not damage the surrounding cardiac tissue along this application.[50]

Laser in peripheral revascularization: Peripheral atherosclerotic arterial disease is a major cause of lower extremity ischemia and limb loss. While several lasers have been investigated for peripheral revascularization (Holmium:YAG,

Nd:YAG and excimer), initial experience by Isner and Rosenfield revealed more favorable clinical results with the ultraviolet excimer laser.[51] Over the last decade, the excimer laser has gained a recognized role in the treatment of superficial femoral occlusions, popliteal artery stenoses and infra popliteal lesions. These targets cause chronic or critical limb ischemia, claudication and non-healing ulcers. The laser provides safe and efficacious debulking, thrombus removal and facilitates stenting in such targets.[52-54] As for the technique of peripheral lasing Biamino and colleagues have utilized a gradual "step by step" approach for arterial recanalization with excimer laser. The long occlusions are reached by a guide wire and an over the wire laser catheter. The lesion is traversed by the laser catheter while the guide wire inside the catheter provides stable support. Then as the laser catheter debulks a portion of the obstructive plaque, the guide wire is advanced a few millimeters distally into the occlusion and the laser is reactivated to follow it with debulking. Then the process is repeated until the entire length of the lesion is recanalized.[55]

Laser in electrophysiology: Until recently the only option for removal of intracardiac pacemaker or defibrillator leads were either by surgical procedure or traction; however both approaches carried significant risk and complications. Currently, the excimer laser sheath technology (Spectranetics, Colorado Springs, CO) delivers ultraviolet light whereby the energy interacts with the encasing fibrotic tissue. The laser energy ablates the tissue surrounding the pacemaker or defibrillator leads making extraction of the entire lead possible without disruption of the myocardium and vascular structures. This results in a very high success rate and markedly low complication rate.[56] A certain limitation for the laser extraction method is the presence of heavily calcified adhesions.

Technique of lasing and catheter technology: For coronary applications with excimer laser, rapid exchange eccentric and concentric catheters are available in diameters of 0.9–2 mm. Most catheters contain the optimally spaced optic fibers.[57] Initial catheter selection depends on baseline stenosis severity whereby the greater the stenosis the smaller the initial catheter size.[58] Eccentric laser catheters are frequently used for revascularization of diffuse stent restenosis as they can be turned in increments of 90° thus providing three to four quadrants tissue ablation. Laser safety is important; the cardiac catheterization laboratory or operation room personnel and the patient must wear special protective goggles whenever the laser is activated. Since the depth of the excimer laser penetration is shallow (35–50 μm) the laser catheter is advanced slowly (0.5 mm/s) along the target lesion to provide adequate absorption and ablation of the atherosclerotic plaque and thrombus. Upon completion of several trains of emission along antegrade laser propagation the laser catheter should perform retrograde lasing. Saline flashes accompany all stages of the procedure to reduce adverse augmentation of acoustic shock waves from interaction between the contrast media and the laser light.[59]

Laser Induced Complications and Adverse Outcome

Several procedural and clinical complications can occur with either percutaneous or surgical laser application. These complications, though rare, relate almost without exception to faulty lasing techniques and mistakes in judgment by the operators.[8] Perforation, dissection, acute closure thrombosis, distal embolization and spasm have been reported.

Future Potential

Renal artery interventions: Since the excimer laser effectively removes coronary and peripheral plaques, conceptually it could also be applied for renal artery stenosis. In an early experience, this technology was found safe and effective in debulking of severe-critical renal artery stenosis. The application of laser energy facilitated adjunct stenting and preserved renal integrity. Improved hypertension control and management of congestive heart failure were observed. This was accompanied by preservation of renal function.[60]

Stroke: Thrombus plays a crucial role in the pathophysiology of intracranial stroke. As lasers enhance the effect of thrombolytic agents and favorably interact with thrombus and platelets they may become a unique treatment option for enhanced thrombolysis in selected acute stroke patients.[61]

Venous system: based on the abovementioned description of the favorable interaction between laser light and thrombus and fibrotic tissues, conceivably, selected patients with acute or chronic venous obstructions or thrombosis will benefit from laser treatment.

Summary

Cardiovascular lasers with various wavelengths produce intense electromagnetic energy. This dedicated revascularization strategy is aimed at ablation and removal of coronary and peripheral atherosclerotic plaques. The ultraviolet pulsed wave excimer laser (308 nm wavelength) is currently the only laser approved by the FDA for peripheral and coronary interventions in the context of acute and chronic ischemic syndromes. This laser can effectively debulk atherosclerotic and fibrotic plaques and remove associated thrombus burden. The holmium:YAG laser is currently approved for surgical TMLR. Careful case selection, proper utilization of the laser equipment and incorporation of a safe, efficacious lasing technique plays a crucial role in successful laser interventions.

References

1. Cook SI, Iegler NL, Shefer A, et al. Percutaneous excimer laser coronary angioplasty of lesions not ideal for balloon angioplasty. *Circulation*. 1991;84:632-643.
2. Grundfest WS, Litvack F, Goldenberg T, et al. Pulsed ultraviolet lasers and the potential for safe laser angioplasty. *Am J Surg*. 1985;150:220-226.
3. Abela GS, Normann SJ, Cohen DM, et al. Laser recanalization of occluded atherosclerotic arteries: an in vivo and in vitro study. *Circulation*. 1985;71:403-411.
4. Forrester JS, Litvack F, Grundfest WS. Laser angioplasty and cardiovascular disease. *Am J Cardiol*. 1986;57:990-992.
5. Bittl JA, Sanborn TA, Tcheng JE. Clinical success, complications and restenosis rates with excimer laser coronary angioplasty. *Am J Cardiol*. 1992;70:1553-1559.
6. Geschwind HJ, Dubois-Rande JL, Zelinsky R, et al. Percutaneous coronary mid-infrared laser angioplasty. *Am Heart J*. 1991;122: 552-558.
7. Bittl JA, Ryan TJ, Keaney JF. Coronary artery perforation during excimer laser coronary angioplasty. *J Am Coll Cardiol*. 1993;21: 1158-1165.
8. Topaz O. Editorial. Whose fault is it? Notes on "true" versus "pseudo" laser failure. *Cathet Cardiovasc Diagn*. 1995;36:1-4.
9. Taylor K, Reiser C. Large eccentric laser angioplasty catheter. In Proceedings of lasers in surgery: advanced characterization, therapeutics and systems. *SPIE*. 1997;2970:34-41.
10. Tcheng JE. Saline infusion in excimer laser coronary angioplasty. *Semin Interv Cardiol*. 1996;1:135-141.
11. Topaz O. A new safer lasing technique for laser facilitated coronary angioplasty. *J Interv Cardiol*. 1993;6:297-306.
12. Topaz O. Coronary laser angioplasty. In: Topol EJ, ed. *Textbook of Interventional Cardiology*. Philadelphia: WB Saunders; 1995: 235-255.
13. Topaz O, Bernardo NL, Shah R, et al. Effectiveness of excimer laser coronary angioplasty in acute myocardial infarction or in unstable angina pectoris. *Am J Cardiol*. 2001;87:849-855.
14. Topaz O, Rozenberg EA, Luxenberg MG, Schumacher A. Laser assisted coronary angioplasty in patients with severely depressed left ventricular function: quantitative coronary angiography and clinical results. *J Interv Cardiol*. 2005;8:661-669.
15. Topaz O, Minisi AJ, Bernardo NL, Alimar R, Ereso A, Shah R. Comparison of effectiveness of excimer laser angioplasty in patients with acute coronary syndromes in those with and without normal left ventricular function. *Am J Cardiol*. 2003;91(7):797-802.
16. Topaz O, Minisi AJ, Morris C, Mohanty PK, Carr ME Jr. Photoacoustic fibrinolysis: pulsed-wave, mid infrared laser-clot interaction. *J Thromb Thrombolysis*. 1996;3:209-214.
17. Dahm JB, Topaz O, Woenckhaus C, et al. laser facilitated thrombectomy: a new therapeutic option for treatment of thrombus–laden coronary lesions. *Catheter Cardiovasc Interv*. 2002;56: 365-372.
18. Topaz O, Minisi AJ, Bernardo NL, et al. Alterations of platelet aggregation kinetics with ultraviolet laser emission: the "stunned platelet" phenomenon. *Thromb Haemost*. 2001;86:1087-1093.
19. Topaz O, Ebersole D, Das T, et al. Excimer laser angioplasty in acute myocardial infarction (the CARMEL multicenter study). *Am J Cardiol*. 2004;93:694-701.
20. Topaz O, Ebersole D, Dahm JB, et al. Excimer laser in myocardial infarction: a comparison between STEMI patients with established Q-Wave versus patients with non-STEMI. *Lasers Med Sci*. 2008;23:1-10.
21. Topaz O, Shah R, Mohanty PK, McQueen RA, Janin Y, Bernardo NL. Application of excimer laser angioplasty in acute myocardial infarction. *Lasers Surg Med*. 2001;29:185-192.
22. Topaz O, Polkampally PR, Mohanty PK, Rizk M, Bangs J, Bernardo NL. Excimer laser debulking for percutaneous coronary intervention in left main coronary artery disease. *Lasers Med Sci*. 2009;24(6):955-960.
23. Bittl JA. Clinical results with excimer laser coronary angioplasty. *Semin Interv Cardiol*. 1996;1:129-134.
24. Bilodeau L, Fretz EB, Taeymans Y, Koolen J, Taylor K, Hilton DJ. Novel use of a high energy excimer laser catheter for calcified and complex coronary artery lesions. *Catheter Cardiovasc Interv*. 2004;62:155-161.
25. Sunew J, Chandwaney RH, Stein DW, et al. Excimer laser facilitated percutaneous coronary intervention of a nondilatable coronary stent. *Catheter Cardiovasc Interv*. 2001;53:513-517.
26. Topaz O. Laser for total occlusion recanalization. In: Waksman R, Saito S, eds. *Chronic Total Occlusions: A Guide to Recanalization*. Oxford: Blackwell Publishing; 2009.
27. Holmes DR Jr, Forrester JS, Litvack F, et al. Chronic total obstructions and short term outcome: the excimer laser angioplasty registry experience. *Mayo Clin Proc*. 1993;68:5-10.
28. Dahm JB, Ebersole D, Das T, et al. Prevention of distal embolization and no-reflow in patients with acute myocardial infarction and total occlusion in the infarct-related vessels. *Catheter Cardiovasc Interv*. 2005;64:67-74.
29. Tcheng JE, Bittl JA, Sanborn TA, et al. Treatment of aorto-ostial disease with percutaneous excimer laser coronary angioplasty. *Circulation*. 1992;86(Suppl 1):1-512A.
30. Eigler NL, Weinstock B, Douglas JS, et al. Excimer laser coronary angioplasty of aorto-ostial stenosis: results of the excimer laser coronary angioplasty (ELCA) registry in the first 200 patients. *Circulation*. 1993;88:2049-2057.
31. Bittl JA, Sanborn TA, Yardley DE, et al. Predictors of outcome of percutaneous excimer laser coronary angioplasty of saphenous vein bypass lesions. *Am J Cardiol*. 1994;74:144-148.
32. Topaz O. Holmium laser angioplasty. *Semin Interv Cardiol*. 1996;1:149-161.
33. Ebersole DG. Excimer laser for revascularization of saphenous vein grafts. *Lasers Med Sci*. 2001;16:78-83.
34. Dahm JB. Excimer laser coronary angioplasty for diffuse in stent restenosis: beneficial long-term results after sufficient debulking with a lesion-specific approach using various laser catheters. *Lasers Med Sci*. 2001;16:84-89.
35. Mehran R, Mintz GS, Satler LF, et al. Treatment of in-stent restenosis with excimer laser coronary angioplasty: mechanisms and results compared to PTCA alone. *Circulation*. 1997;96:2183-2189.
36. Topaz O. Myocardial revascularization the role of the Vineberg operation and related procedures. In: Abela George S, ed. *Myocardial Revascularization – Novel Percutaneous Approaches*. New York: Wiley-Liss; 2002:3-12.
37. Spanier T, Smith CR, Burkhoff D. Angiogenesis: a possible mechanism underlying the clinical benefits of transmyocardial laser revascularization. *J Clin Laser Med Surg*. 1997;15:269-273.
38. Li W, Chiba Y, Kimura T, et al. Transmyocardial laser revascularization induced angiogenesis correlated with the expression of matrix metalloproteinases and platelet –derived endothelial cell growth factor. *Eur J Cardiothorac Surg*. 2001;19:156-163.
39. Canestri F. Thermal lesions produced by CO2 laser beams: new findings to improve the quality of minimally invasive and transmyocardial laser revascularization protocols. *J Clin Laser Med Surg*. 2000;18:49-55.
40. Horvath KA, Cohn LH, Cooley DA, et al. Transmyocardial laser revascularization: results of a multicenter trial with transmyocardial laser revascularization used as sole therapy for end–stage coronary artery disease. *J Thorac Cardiovasc Surg*. 1997;113:645-653.
41. Allen KB, Dowling RD, Fudge TL, et al. Comparison of transmyocardial revascularization with medical therapy in patients with refractory angina. *N Engl J Med*. 1999;341:1029-1036.

42. Aaberge L, Nordstrand K, Dragsund M, et al. Transmyocardial revascularization with CO2 laser in patients with refractory angina pectoris. *J Am Coll Cardiol*. 2000;35:1170-1177.

43. Van Der Sloot JAP, Huikeshhoven M, Tukkie R, et al. Transmyocardial revascularization using an XeCL excimer laser: results of a randomized trial. *Ann Thorac Surg*. 2004;78:875-881.

44. Godwak LH, Schettert IT, Rochitte CE. Transmyocardial laser revascularization plus cell therapy for refractory angina. *Int J Cardiol*. 2008;127:295-297.

45. Hayat N, Shafie M, Gumaa MK, Khan N. Transmyocardial revascularization: is the enthusiasm justified? *Clin Cardiol*. 2001;24: 321-324.

46. Minisi AJ, Topaz O, Quinn SM, Mohanty LB. Cardiac nociceptive reflexes after transmyocardial laser revascularization: implications for the neural hypothesis of angina relief. *J Thorac Cardiovasc Surg*. 2001;122:712-719.

47. Topaz O, Cowley MJ, Mohanty PK, Vetrovec GW. Percutaneous revascularization modalities for heart transplant recipients. *Catheter Cardiovasc Interv*. 1999;46:227-237.

48. Topaz O, Bailey NT, Mohanty PK, et al. Application of solid state pulsed wave mid infrared laser for percutaneous revascularization in heart transplant recipients. *J Heart Lung Transplant*. 1998;17:505-510.

49. Topaz O, Janin Y, Bernardo N. Coronary revascularization in heart transplant recipients by excimer laser angioplasty. *Lasers Surg Med*. 2000;26:425-431.

50. Moskowitz WB, Titus JL, Topaz O. Excimer laser ablation for valvular angioplasty in pulmonary atresia and intact ventricular septum. *Lasers Surg Med*. 2004;35:327-335.

51. Isner JM, Rosenfield K. Redefining the treatment of peripheral artery disease: role of percutaneous revascularization. *Circulation*. 1993;84:1534-1557.

52. Das TS. Percutaneous peripheral revascularization with excimer laser: equipment, technique and results. *Lasers Med Sci*. 2001; 16:101-107.

53. Boccalandro F, Muench A, Sdringola S, et al. Wireless laser-assisted angioplasty of the superficial femoral artery in patients with critical limb ischemia who have failed conventional percutaneous revascularization. *Catheter Cardiovasc Interv*. 2004;63:7-12.

54. Topaz O. Editorial. Rescue excimer laser angioplasty for treatment of critical limb ischemia. *Catheter Cardiovasc Interv*. 2004;63: 13-14.

55. Biamino GC, Ragg JC, Struk B, et al. Long occlusions of the superficial femoral artery: success rate and 1 year follow-up after excimer laser assisted angioplasty. *Eur Heart J*. 1994;15(Suppl 1):147.

56. Gilligan DM, Dan D. Excimer laser for pacemaker and defibrillator lead extraction: techniques and clinical results. *Lasers Med Sci*. 2001;16:113-121.

57. Topaz O, Lippincott R, Bellendir J, et al. Optimally spaced excimer laser coronary catheters: performance analysis. *J Clin Laser Med Surg*. 2001;19:9-14.

58. Topaz O, Safian RD. Excimer laser coronary angioplasty. In: Safian RD, Freed MS, eds. *Manual of Interventional Cardiology*. 3rd ed. Royal Oaks: Physicians Press; 2001:681-691.

59. Topaz O. Laser. In: Topol EJ, ed. *Textbook of Interventional Cardiology*. 3rd ed. Philadelphia: WB Saunders; 1998:615-633.

60. On Topaz MD, Pritam R. Polkampally MD, Allyne Topaz BS, Jessica Jara MD, Majid Rizk MD, Chudamani R. Polkampally MD, Kara McDowell RN, George Feldman MD. Utilization of excimer laser debulking for critical lesions unsuitable for standard renal angioplasty. *Lasers Surg Med*. 2009;41:622-627.

61. Topaz O. Editorial. The quest for laser thrombolysis. *Lasers Med Sci*. 2001;16:232-235.

Laser/Light Applications in Neurology and Neurosurgery

Marlon S. Mathews, David Abookasis, and Mark E. Linskey

- Applications of light in neurology and neurosurgery can be diagnostic or therapeutic.
- Neurophotonics is the science of photon interaction with neural tissue.
- Photodynamic therapy (PDT) has been attempted to destroy infiltrative tumor cells in tissue.
- Spatially modulated imaging (MI) is a newly described non-contact optical technique in the spatial domain. With this technique, both quantitative mapping of tissue optical properties within a single measurement and cross sectional optical tomography can be achieved rapidly.
- The ability to control the activity of a defined class of neurons has the potential to advance clinical neuromodulation.

Introduction

Applications of light in neurology and neurosurgery can be diagnostic or therapeutic. While the therapeutic effects of light are dependent mainly on the ablative power of photon energy in lasers, the diagnostic use of light has mainly been in the near infrared (NIR) domain. This is because NIR light has better tissue penetration than visible light, as well as its ability to obtain physiologic information based on differential absorption and scattering of NIR light during different physiological states. In this chapter we review the diagnostic and therapeutic applications of light in neurology and neurosurgery. In the last section we give a brief overview of novel and promising optical technologies of neurologic interest in development.

M.S. Mathews (✉)
Department of Neurosurgery, University of California,
Irvine, CA, USA
e-mail: mmathews@uci.edu

Neurophotonics

Neurophotonics is the science of photon interaction with neural tissue. Four major types of photon-neural interactions characterize neurophotonics[1]: (a) absorption (energy of the photon is transferred to the tissue, may be re-emitted or transformed in the form of heat), (b) phosphorescence (energy of the photon is released by the tissue with a delay in the form of a photon with similar or lower energy), (c) fluorescence (energy of the photon is released in part in the form of a lower energy photon, the rest being dissipated as heat or as another lower energy photon), and (d) scattering (the photon remains of the same energy and is merely deviated in its trajectory). Some photons proceed less disturbed in their trajectory and transmission of light through tissue is observed.

All these types of interactions occur to some degree in the brain and in other living tissues; however, for NIR light, the dominant events are scattering and absorption (Fig. 1). For both scattering- and absorption-type interactions, the frequency of occurrence may change as a function of neuronal activity.

Changes in light scattering in relationship to action potentials were described by Cohen in 1972 and later by Stepnoski et al. in 1991.[2,3] They are typically attributed to changes in the neuronal membrane reflectance due to the reorientations of molecules in the membrane and/or to volumetric changes that are determined by the movement of ions and water across and around the membrane. Changes in scattering and absorption properties are also likely to occur in the dendrites and soma during postsynaptic potentials. At the macroscopic level, the postsynaptic potentials, reflecting the activity of a much more extended portion of the neurons and integrating the activity over longer periods of time, are likely to dominate the measures. Several studies indicate that neural tissue becomes more transparent (i.e., less scattering) when it is activated and probably less transparent (i.e., more scattering) when it is inhibited, in a manner that appears very similar in time course to the local field potential recorded from the same area.[4-6]

Unlike scattering, changes in light absorption are, for the most part, directly related to the changes in the blood oxygenation levels and flow that occur with regional neural activation.

K. Nouri (ed.), *Lasers in Dermatology and Medicine,*
DOI: 10.1007/978-0-85729-281-0_46, © Springer-Verlag London Limited 2011

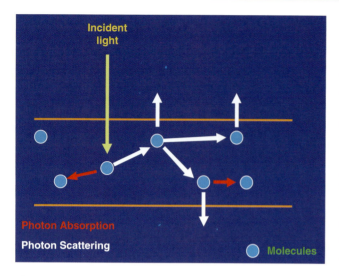

Fig. 1 Schematic showing the basic interaction of photons with tissue. Photon flux incident on tissue, when interacting with molecules can get partially absorbed leading to decreased flux (shown as *thinning of arrows*). The photons can also get multiply scattered before leaving the tissue giving rise to diffused light, which is a function of photon absorption and scattering and therefore depends on distance from the incident light. Transmitted light contains ballistic (*not scattered*) as well as snake photons (*weakly scattered*)

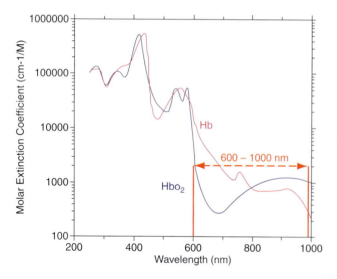

Fig. 2 Graph showing the molar extinction coefficients of oxy (HbO_2) and deoxy (Hb) hemoglobin. Between wavelengths of 600–1,000 nm the extinction coefficients of the two states of hemoglobin show low absorption with distinct spectral features. This provides a spectral window of good tissue penetrance of photons as well as allows better resolution of their individual chromophore concentrations from the Beer-Lambert Law

Both oxy- and deoxy-hemoglobin have very characteristic and distinct absorption spectra that correspond to the different colors of arterial and venous blood (Fig. 2). This makes it possible to use a spectroscopic approach to measure changes in the concentration of oxy- and deoxy-hemoglobin as a function of neural activity.[7,8]

An example is a small increase in deoxy-hemoglobin concentration occurring within 1–1.5 s from the onset of neural activity (reflecting the increased oxygen consumption of active neural tissue), which is soon followed by a decrement in deoxy-hemoglobin concentration and a much larger increase in the oxy-hemoglobin concentration. This leads to the Blood Oxygen Level Dependent (or BOLD) functional MRI (fMRI) signal dependent on vasodilation.[8]

The relative changes in absorption and scattering during neural activity result from different physiologic phenomena.[9] The hemodynamic-related absorption changes are much easier to observe than the neuronal phenomena. However, the scattering changes are a direct indication of neural activity, and therefore possess better temporal and spatial resolution, and more direct functional significance, than the hemodynamic phenomena. Different types of measurement methods may bias the recording system more toward one or the other of the two signals, which have been exploited in the development of novel optical modalities and imaging techniques described below.

Neurodiagnostic Applications of LASER and Light

NIRS and Photon Migration

Since Jobsis described the *in vivo* application of near-infrared spectroscopy (NIRS) to detect changes in cerebral hemoglobin oxygenation, several types of NIRS instruments have been developed.[10] NIRS is widely used for the noninvasive monitoring of changes in chromophores such as oxy- and deoxy hemoglobin, lipid, and water from changes in the reflected light intensity. In the NIR region, the absorption spectra of these primary chromophores are different (Fig. 2). With determination of tissue absorption coefficients at multiple wavelengths (600–1,000 nm) and using appropriate modeling, information about absolute chromophore concentrations can be obtained (diffuse optical spectroscopy or DOS).

In this wavelength band, NIR light can penetrate the adult skull and propagate within the brain.[1] Photons that propagate in the brain are strongly scattered elastically as they traverse several millimeters of tissue. Elastic scattering is characterized by the fact that the photon energy does not change. Since photons undergo multiple scattering events before they reach the detector, their trajectories are not straight lines; rather they resemble random walks. Multiple scattering of light which occurs as a consequence of spatial variation in refractive index influenced by cellular and extracellular optical densities, complicates quantitative measurements of light absorption in the NIR range. This complexity is a consequence of the uncertainty in optical path traveled by any given photon. Hence, a simple Beer's law technique for deducing chromophore concentration cannot be simply applied. However, by using time-resolved or frequency-domain instruments, which effectively can be used, with appropriate selection of a model of light propagation, to deduce the average path length of detected photons, the effects of scattering can be separated from absorption. Thus absolute concentrations of tissue chromophores can subsequently be estimated in a given region of interest by application of the Beer-Lambert Law[11] to the absorption coefficient. These techniques can provide quantitative measurements of optical and functional contrast between healthy and diseased tissue.[20] NIRS offers an inexpensive and safe bedside monitoring tool.

Photon migration allows gathering information from relatively deep structures in highly scattering media. The light emitted from a source(s) diffuses in a random fashion through the scattering medium. However, because of statistical properties, the photons picked up by the detectors are more likely to have followed certain paths than others through the medium. If enough photons are used, the entire process of migration of photons from the sources to the detectors can be described accurately using mathematical formulations related to the diffusion process. This makes it possible to go beyond images of the first interaction of photons with the medium and produce images of structures that are up to a few centimeters deep into the medium.[12]

Frequency Domain Photon Migration

The frequency domain NIR system uses diode lasers as a light source with intensities modulated in the kHz to MHz range. In a typical embodiment, the brain is illuminated by one or more optical fibers. The reflected (diffusive) light is received by a detecting optical fiber, located at a small (several mm), well defined distance from the incident light source point and coupled to a silicon photodiode (Fig. 3). By solving the inverse problem for the diffusion equation for the light that travels through the tissue from source to detector, the optical properties and hence chromophore concentrations of the intervening tissue can be deduced.[11] Alternative methods for recovering similar information have been developed and applied that rely on steady-state, non-modulated sources and multiple source-detector pairs, each pair separated by a well defined distance.[13]

Time Domain Photon Migration

In the time domain, sometimes know as time-resolved spectroscopy (TRS), source and detector are used and chromophore changes determined by calculating the emerging photon time

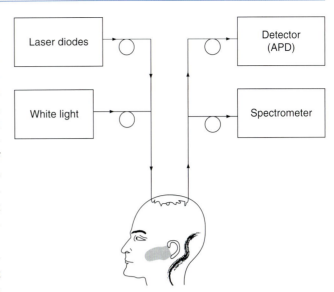

Fig. 3 Example of a broadband diffuse optical spectroscopy (b-DOS) system used to determine the optical properties (i.e. absorption and scattering) of brain tissue. This system combines Frequency domain (FD) photon migration (laser diodes and *APD*) and steady-state (*white light and spectrometer*) techniques. The system employs six laser diodes in the NIR range and avalanche photo diode (*APD*) detector. The APD detects the intensity-modulated diffuse reflectance signal at modulation frequencies after propagation through the brain. The optical properties are measured directly at each of the six laser diode wavelengths by using the frequency-dependent phase and amplitude data

of flight distribution.[14] In this domain, ultrashort (picosecond) pulsed laser light is incident on the tissue. The detection process requires high speed, high sensitivity detector, which may be a time-correlated single-photon counting (TCSPC) system or a streak camera. Absorption results in a reduction of transmitted amplitude and pulse-width whereas scattering predominantly results in pulse broadening. These effects can be accounted for using an appropriate model of light propagation such as the diffusion equation, which allows the tissue optical properties to be separated and quantified.

Recently, spatial domain photon migration (spatially modulated imaging) has been introduced that enables quantitative wide-field spectral imaging of tissue structure and function.[15] This technology is new and promising and may be particularly useful as an adjunct intraoperative imaging tool for cerebrovascular and neuro-oncologic surgery. A schematic diagram of spatial frequency domain imaging (SFDI) is shown in Fig. 4. The SFDI system is a relatively new concept that requires further validation. In principle, this method provides similar information to that provided by traditional DOS techniques, however it is able to do this in an imaging sense, using relatively inexpensive consumer grade electronics. Further description of the spatial frequency domain imaging is presented in section"Spatial Domain Imaging".

Several studies have been published on clinical applications of NIRS. Among other findings, these studies have described

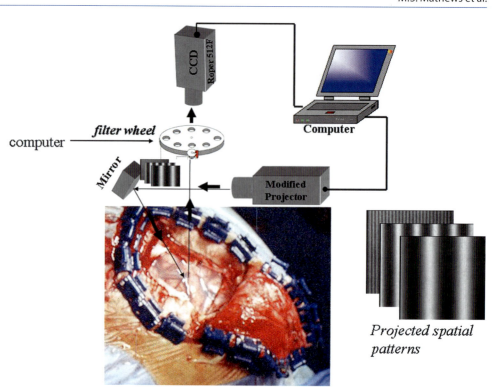

Fig. 4 Schematic diagram showing the intraoperative use of spatially modulated imaging. Periodic illumination patterns of various spatial frequencies with a 120° phase shifting between three adjacent patterns are projected onto the brain from a conventional projector controlled by a computer. The diffusely reflected pattern (the deformed fringe pattern) passes through near infrared (NIR) bandpass filters and is captured by *CCD camera* interfaced to a *PC computer*. The diffusion solution is then used as a model function in an inversion algorithm for determining separately the optical properties namely, absorption and reduced scattering coefficients over a wide spectrum range. Quantitative chromophore maps are then generated providing real time feedback to the surgeon

decrease in activation of the prefrontal cortex in traumatic brain injury patients,[16] detection of cerebral ischemia during cerebrovascular and endovascular surgery,[17-19] and measurement of cerebral hemodynamic response in infants.[126]

Intrinsic Signal Optical Imaging

Intrinsic Signal Optical Imaging (ISOI) is widely used for studying the hemodynamic response of the brain to stimulation. It is a functional neuroimaging technique that can map a large region of the cortex with high spatiotemporal resolution. The method uses a simple configuration containing a light source such as a light-emitting diode (LED) and a CCD camera to image the optical reflectance at this wavelength. The LED light in ISOI systems uses wavelengths (for instance 630 nm) that are maximally absorbed by the deoxygenated state of hemoglobin (Fig. 5). Hence, a decrease in reflected light indicates an increased absorption by deoxyhemoglobin. Therefore, ISOI provides relative changes in the local concentration of deoxyhemoglobin as a surrogate marker for neuronal activity.

Recently, a triphasic component has been described with a second increase in local deoxyhemoglobin concentration following the BOLD signal.[21] The triphasic component constitutes an initial dip, overshoot and undershoot in light reflectance. The initial dip is from increased local deoxyhemoglobin secondary to neural oxygen metabolism from activation. In contrast, the overshoot is dominated by increase in oxyhemoglobin from neurovascular coupling. This signal is analogous to the BOLD signal observed and measured with fMRI. The undershoot signal represents the effort of the brain to come back to its normal state. IOSI studies in epilepsy have shown the presence of an epileptic dip analogous to the initial dip seen with functional activation.[22] While ISOI's main role has been in functional brain imaging in animals, it has potential in intraoperative functional mapping during neurosurgical procedures.[23]

Optical Coherence Tomography

Optical Coherence Tomography (OCT) is a novel imaging system analogous to ultrasound except that imaging is performed with light instead of acoustic waves. OCT measures light reflected from turbid structures. OCT is based on principles of low-coherence interferometry which allows detection of back scattered near-infrared photons from selected depths and rejection of photons being scattered from other layers. It is structurally based on the Michelson's interferometer[1] (Fig. 6). As for the reflection method, it is based on the first interaction (back-scattering) of photons in tissue. Unlike

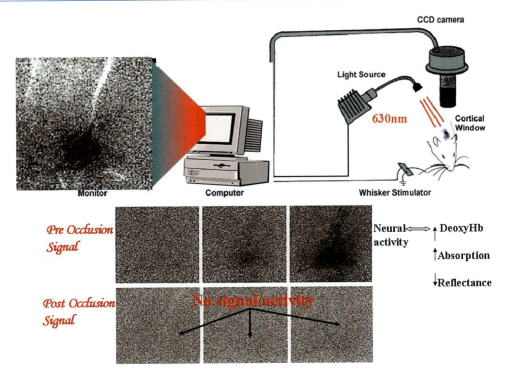

Fig. 5 Schematic diagram of an intrinsic optical imaging system (IOSI). Light is projected from a LED at wavelengths sensitive to the absorption of deoxyhemoglobin (e.g., 630 nm). Reflected light is captured on a *CCD camera*. Since, the amount of reflected light is inversely related to the regional deoxy hemoglobin concentration, functional activity can be mapped in the cortex. The tripanel *grayscale* figures show the results of IOSI in the rat barrel cortex during the first 1.5 s following contralateral whisker stimulation. Functional cortical activation (preocclusion) seen as the initial dip (*darkening* of the *upper* panel on the third image from *left* to *right*) is lost following MCA occlusion

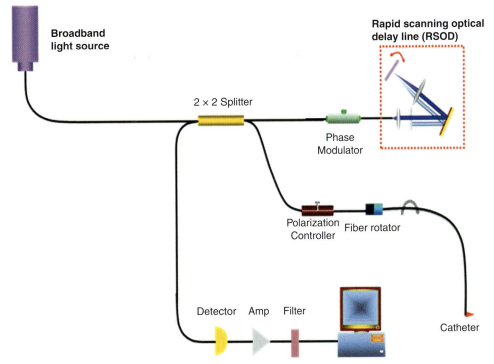

Fig. 6 Schematic diagram of a high speed, high resolution spectral domain OCT system which reconstructs vessel structure image. The system is constructed along the lines of a Michelson interferometer. Eighty percent of the incident power is coupled into sample arm while 20% is fed into a reference arm by a 1×2 fiber coupler. The reference power is attenuated by an adjustable neutral density attenuator for maximum sensitivity. Two circulators are used in both reference and sample arms to redirect the back-reflected light to the second 2×2 fiber coupler (50/50 split ratio) for balanced detection. The signal collected by a photodetector is digitized with an analog-digital acquisition card and transferred to a computer for processing

the reflection measures, however, it directly visualizes the depth at which this first interaction occurs.

In combination with scanning methods, OCT provides three-dimensional information about the scattering properties of living tissue. The spatial resolution that can be reached is near-histologic (micron scale), which makes OCT suitable for *in vivo* optical biopsy, allowing for the visualization of tissue cross-sectional microstructure even without a contrast agent or dye. Because signals from different depths are separated by the measurement approach, OCT can detect deeper events more easily than a reflection approach. The dependence on the first interaction of photons with the medium imposes maximum penetration limits on the technology that are incompatible with using this approach to study the human brain in a noninvasive manner.

OCT has the potential to provide new imaging, visualization, and quantification capabilities for a wide range of investigations in neuroscience and neuroimaging. Research has demonstrated its potential in the areas of developmental neurobiology, retinal imaging, cellular imaging, brain tumor imaging, and image-guided surgery for the repair of peripheral nerves.[20] By incorporating OCT technology into an endoscope Bohringer et al. were able to visualize tissue lining the walls of the third ventricle such as peri-aqueductal tissue, floor of the third ventricle, as well as the rostral wall of the basilar artery in a cadaveric study.[24] The same group also analyzed human brain tumor biopsies as well as an orthotopic mouse glioma model using time domain and spectral domain OCT and found good correlation of OCT findings of normal brain, tumor infiltrative brain and tumor with histology.[25] OCT has been used to visualize retinal hamartomas in patients with tuberous sclerosis,[26] to measure the retinal nerve fiber layer thickness in patients with mild cognitive impairment and Alzheimer's disease and multiple sclerosis.[27,28] Cadaveric studies have shown the potential of OCT for providing navigational guidance of deep brain stimulation probes.[29] Recently, the authors of this chapter have used a catheter based OCT system for *in vivo* cerebrovascular imaging in patients [unpublished].

Neurotherapeutic Applications of LASER and Light

Light Amplification by Stimulated Emission of Radiation (LASER) is monochromatic, coherent and collimated light that when shone into tissue, acts therapeutically, typically by generating heat. Its therapeutic effects rely on the ablative power of photon energy. Laser interaction with tissue has high spatial and temporal selectivity.

Spinal Applications

Laser Discectomy

Minimally invasive techniques have markedly improved the surgical treatment of herniated intervertebral discs and reduced morbidity and hospital stay. Distinct procedures have been developed to perform percutaneous discectomy with the use of lasers.[30-33] Choy et al. reported on percutaneous laser discectomies in 12 patients using a Nd:YAG laser introduced through an 18-gauge-needle. Five of these

underwent open surgery subsequently. Mayer et al. used a Nd:YAG laser delivered using optical fibers from a flexible endoscope to perform discectomies in six patients.[30] Due to lack of an obvious benefit of laser assisted over microsurgical procedures, the clinical use of percutaneous laser discectomy is extremely limited.

Lipomas

Lipomas often wrap around the conus medullaris and nerve roots, and have poorly defined borders with them. The use of lasers in patients with spinal lipomas and lipomeningoceles is to untether the spinal cord and nerve roots from these lesions. The CO_2 laser has been quite effective in achieving this through the vaporization of fat. McLone and Maidich reported on 50 cases of pediatric lipomas treated with CO_2 laser and found that the use of laser reduced the length of operation, intraoperative blood loss and degree of manipulation of spinal cord and nerve roots.[34] They also reported on improved postoperative neurologic function in these patients including recovery from urinary incontinence and improved motor function. Similarly, Maira et al. reported on the efficacy of the CO_2 laser to remove large spinal lipomas in two adults patients.[35]

Intramedullary Tumors

CO_2 and argon lasers have been utilized in the excision of intramedullary spinal cord tumors.[36-38] Lasers can be used for the myelotomy as well as the subsequent vaporization of tumor tissue. While theoretically attractive, its benefits over conventional surgical techniques are unclear.

Cerebrovascular Applications

Laser Assisted Vascular Anastomosis

Laser assisted vascular anastomosis was first performed by Yahr and colleagues in the mid 1960s.[39] Initially reported on microvessels (0.7–2 mm diameter) this procedure has subsequently been performed on larger vessels (3–8 mm diameter). Jain and Gorisch in 1979 reported on repair of small blood vessels (0.3–1 mm diameter) in the rat using Nd:YAG laser.[40] Frazier et al. in 1985, compared end-to-end anastomoses of femoral arteries (1.6 mm diameter) done with CO_2 laser versus conventional microvascular suture anastomosis in miniature swine.[41] He found that laser anastomosis took less time (20 versus 30 min) and had higher patency rates. In 1986 Quigley et al.

reported that intimal hyperplasia was reduced in laser assisted compared with surgical anastomosis.[42] He also reported on aneurysm formation in laser anastomosed vessels.[43] In 1989, Shapiro et al. reported that following successful end-to-side anastomosis of rat carotid arteries using Nd:YAG laser, 86% remained patent but 23% developed aneurysms in the anastomotic site.[44]

This high rate of laser induced aneurysm formation and the effectiveness of conventional microsurgical anastomosis have dampened the enthusiasm for clinical use of laser assisted anastomosis in neurosurgery. However since than Tulleken and colleagues have described a novel high flow bypass procedure using an excimer laser to revascularize the ischemic brain that has shown excellent patency without aneurysm formation.[45-47] The exact mechanism of laser welding of blood vessels is unclear but has been attributed to denaturation of collagen in the blood vessel walls.[41,48] Other potential cerebrovascular applications include use of lasers in reversing cerebral vasospasm.[49-51]

Neuro-Oncologic Applications

Meningiomas

In 1980, Takizawa et al. reported on the treatment of meningiomas with the CO_2 laser.[52] Beck described 51 cases of meningiomas treated with Nd:YAG laser, although he did not report the outcome.[53] Roux et al. reported on the combination of the CO_2 and Nd. YAG laser in treating 17 meningiomas.[54] They reported that the combined laser had greater tissue penetration power, with Nd. YAG contributing towards hemostasis. Lombard et al. studied 220 meningiomas reoperated on with laser vs. conventional techniques.[55] While patients in both groups improved after surgery, outcome was better in patients with meningiomas in eloquent areas that were treated with laser. Desgeorges et al. studied 164 meningiomas treated with various lasers over a 6 year period and found that complete tumor removal was documented in 83% of cases with 3% mortality.[56] They particularly commented on the ability of lasers to remove deep meningiomas that might be difficult to remove with conventional microsurgery.

Additionally, laser treatment had the advantages of reduced brain retraction, small exposures, reduced mechanical manipulation, and decreased intraoperative blood loss. Waidhauser et al. reported on 43 patients with frontobasal meningiomas, treated using Nd:YAG lasers.[57] They were able to obtain contact-free shrinkage of tumor, lysis of dural and bony attachments, and coagulation. They opined that Nd:YAG laser assisted surgery facilitated microsurgical dissection and reduced blood loss.

Vestibular Schwannomas

Laser assisted excision of vestibular schwannomas has been previously reported.[38,58] Preservation of cranial nerve function is important. Irrigation with suction of the laser plume has been used to minimize thermal injury to structure around the tumor. In 1993, Eiras et al. compared 12 giant vestibular schwannomas excised with CO_2 laser to 12 similar tumors operated microsurgically.[58] They found that, in their hands, preservation of facial nerve function was better in laser treated patients, although the duration of surgery was longer. Because of poor handling of the tumor-nerve interface and the potential for thermal injury to the nerves the use of lasers is no longer popular in vestibular schwannoma surgery and is more of historic interest.

Pituitary Tumors

In 1982, Takeuchi et al. were the first to report the use of Nd:YAG laser to penetrate the sellar floor during transsphenoidal pituitary surgery.[59] Oekler et al. subsequently reported on 15 cases of pituitary adenomas operated similarly, with laser use minimizing capsular bleeding.[60] Powers et al. reported using an Argon laser to open the sellar floor, cut through the duramater and vaporize a fibrous prolactinoma.[38] Laser use in pituitary surgery is particularly risky due to the possibility of thermal injury to adjacent structures such as the optic nerves, optic chiasm, and the internal carotid artery.

Intra-Axial Brain Tumors

Despite early enthusiasm for the use of lasers for intra-axial brain tumor resection, there remains no clear advantage of this technique over conventional microsurgery. Optical techniques may be more useful for surgical guidance during surgery for intra-axial brain tumors and for photodynamic therapy to the resection cavity for microinvasive disease. Intraoperative measurements have shown that white matter in the brain in distinctly higher in optical scattering of NIR light compared to glioma tissue.[61]

Laser-induced fluorescence (LIF) spectroscopy and imaging have been used to distinguish neoplastic tissue from normal brain, since normal brain has a characteristic pattern of fluorescence when exposed to light.[62,63] This is due to autofluorescence from endogenous fluorophores. Lin et al. combined tissue fluorescence with diffuse reflectance spectroscopy to distinguish normal brain from infiltrating tumor margin and reported a sensitivity and specificity of 100% and 76% respectively.[62] Amharref et al. described the use of fourier transform infrared microspectroscopy to distinguish normal brain tissue from tumor and tumor infiltrative brain based on tissue lipid concentrations.[64] Leppert et al. described multiphoton excitation to distinguish glioma from normal tissue using autofluorescence decay.[65]

Fluorescence Guided Resection and Photodynamic Therapy

The extent of surgical resection of gliomas correlates with increased survival.[66] However, complete resection of these tumors is often not possible because tumor margins are not readily distinguished from normal brain tissue. In order to further demarcate this, exogenous fluorophores have been administered that preferentially localize in brain tumors. These include Phthalocyanine tetrasulfonate, hematoporphyrin derivative (HPD), and 5-Amino Levulenic Acid (ALA).[67-69] Fluorescence guided resection (FGR) of tumors using ALA has been reported to have a sensitivity and specificity of 85% and 100% respectively.[70] In an interim analysis of a randomized control trial for FGR of gliomas, Stummer et al. reported complete resection of contrast enhancing tumor in 65% of patients assigned 5-aminolevulinic acid compared with 36% assigned white light.[71] Patients allocated 5-aminolevulinic acid had higher 6-month progression free survival than did those allocated white light (41.0% vs. 21.1%), with no difference in short term adverse effects.

Despite the ability of FGR to visualize tumor margins, resection cannot be carried out safely when the tumor has infiltrated brain tissue vital for survival or tissue responsible for important functions (eloquent brain). Photodynamic therapy (PDT) has been attempted to destroy infiltrative tumor cells in tissue.[72] In PDT, a photosensitizer is administered systemically that preferentially localizes within tumor cells in microscopically infiltrating tumor tissue. Laser light is then administered into the tissue of interest with spatial localization that excites the photosensitizer, releasing singlet oxygen within tumor cells. Single oxygen being toxic selectively kills tumor cells where it localizes.

The most common photosensitizers used for PDT are HPD and ALA. Clinical studies in patients with recurrent gliomas have demonstrated that PDT can increase survival in these patients and survival appears to correlate with light energy delivered.[73,74] The most common cause of PDT treatment failure is local recurrence, which is likely related to limited tissue penetration of light at 630 nm wavelength.[75] In general, longer wavelengths of light penetrate the brain better. However since light absorption by HPD and ALA is limited above 630 nm, newer photosensitizers in the future may allow longer activating wavelengths to be delivered possibly improving local control rates.

Benzoporphyrin derivative (BPD) is a newer photosensitizer that can be excited by 680 nm light and thus may have better potential of preventing local recurrence.[76] Animal studies with BPD indicated that increased tissue penetration does not result in increased toxicity.[76] Encouraging results have been obtained with FGR and PDT in brain tumors. The development of cheaper diode lasers and photosensitizers that absorb light at longer wavelengths for FGR and PDT could potentially improve survival rates from previous studies. Since PDT has been administered in patients only in the acute intraoperative setting, optimal dosing regimen has not been clinically studied. In vitro models have shown that administering PDT in repetitive[77,78] and chronic low fluence (metronomic)[78,79] doses as well as combinations with ionizing radiation,[80] hyperthermia[81] and radiosensitizers[82] may have superior therapeutic effects compared to single acute PDT treatment alone. Administering repetitive and chronic PDT in patients will require special devices such as indwelling balloon applicators previously described by Hirschberg and colleagues.[83]

Interstitial Laser Thermotherapy

Hyperthermia has been used as an adjunctive therapy for malignant brain tumors.[84,85] The severity of lesions created using laser ablation is proportional to the energy delivered on application time. Interstitial laser thermotherapy using Nd:YAG laser as a thermal source has been studied in animal models and humans.[86] Conical sapphire tipped optical fibers delivering a point source of Nd:YAG laser energy can be flexibly directed at any point within a tumor cavity.[87-90] Despite initial encouraging results in the treatment of malignant gliomas,[85] the role of hyperthermia in clinical neurosurgery is currently limited.

Stereotactic and Functional Neurosurgical Applications

Lasers have been utilized in neurosurgical operations for frameless stereotactic registration. Marmulla et al. described the use of frameless stereotactic laser registration of the auricles for lateral skull base surgery.[91] Schicho et al. compared laser surface scanning to fiducial marker-based registration in frameless stereotaxy with comparable results in four cadaveric heads.[92] Sinha et al. used laser ranges scanning for intraoperative cortical surface characterization in eight patients with brain tumors and mesial temporal epilepsy.[93]

In 1986 Kelly et al. described the results of CO_2 laser integration into a computer assisted volumetric stereotactic system for brain tumor resection.[94] It involved reconstruction of tumor volume from CT and MRI imaging data followed by a computer-monitored stereotactically directed laser to vaporize intracranial tumor. The position of the laser with respect to reformatted planar slices through the tumor was monitored on a computer terminal. In a separate report the same year they reported on 83 computer assisted stereotactic laser procedures in 78 tumor patients.[95] Although the authors mention that the stereotactic laser technique was particularly useful in aggressive resection of deep seated tumors within eloquent brain regions, no direct comparison was performed to standard microsurgical techniques. In 1989 Kelly et al. reported on excision of 12 colloid cysts of the third ventricle using stereotactic laser application with excellent results.[96]

Neuroablative lasers have been utilized in functional neurosurgery particularly in dorsal root entry zone (DREZ) lesions and commissural myelotomies.[97-99] DREZ lesions are primarily used for intractable pain following spinal cord injury, brachial plexus avulsions, post herpetic neuralgia, and phantom limb pain.[100]

Lasers have been used adjunctively in the management of epileptic syndromes. Kelly et al. reported in 18 patients with medically intractable epilepsy that underwent stereotactic amygdalohippocampectomy using a CO_2 laser.[101] Later they reported on stereotactic laser treatment of epileptogenic lesions associated with tuberous sclerosis.[102] While effective, it is unclear whether laser assisted techniques have advantages over conventional microsurgery in the treatment of epileptic lesions.

Neuroendoscopic and Pediatric Applications

Endoscopic applications of lasers in neurosurgery have been mainly in the management of hydrocephalus. Bucholz and Pittman used a Nd:YAG laser to endoscopically coagulate the choroid plexus in an infant with hydrocephalus.[103] Vandertop et al. performed reported endoscopic third ventriculostomy with a Nd. YAG laser and a new-generation laser diode in 33 patients and reported no morbidity.[104] Powers used an Argon laser to perform endoscopic fenestration in two infants with compartmentalization of the lateral ventricles secondary to ventriculitis.[105] Zammorano et al. integrated image-guided stereotaxis with rigid-flexible endoscopy and the Nd-YAG laser (endoscopic laser stereotaxis) and found this system useful in cystic and intraventricular lesions.[106] Otsuki et al. used a stereotactic guiding tubes and endoscopes to deliver laser irradiation to deep seated brain tumors.[107]

Peripheral Nerve Applications

Due to the limitations of microsurgical nerve repair such as scar formation, fascicle mismatching, neuroma formation, inflammatory response to suture material, researchers have been interested in the use of lasers for nerve repair.[108] This application is termed "laser neurorrhaphy."

Laser neurorrhaphy was first reported in 1984 by Almquist et al. with the use of argon laser to repair peripheral nerves in rats and monkeys.[109] Fischer et al. reported using CO_2 lasers for sciatic nerve repair in rats.[110] Seifert and Stoke demonstrated feasibility of microsurgical CO_2 laser assisted repair of the oculomotor nerve in cats.[111] Bailes et al. compared CO_2 laser with 9-0 nylon microsurgical neurorrhaphy in a primate model of sural to peroneal nerve graft and found comparable nerve conduction velocities (NCV) and histologic findings at 5, 8 ,10 and 12 months.[112] Huang et al. compared microsuture technique to CO_2 laser repair of sciatic nerves in rats and found the EMG and NCV studies to be comparable[113] although Maragh et al. compared laser neurorrhaphy to standard microsurgical nerve repair in rat sciatic nerves and found that nerve conduction velocities were better in the latter group.[114] Campion et al. reported improved neuromuscular function of argon laser neurorrhaphy compared to microsurgical epineural surgical repair in rabbits.[115] Korff et al. found similar amounts of regeneration in severed rat sciatic nerves repaired with suture or laser, at 2 months.[116] Menovsky and Beek compared CO_2 laser assisted nerve repair with fibrin glue or absorbable sutures in transected rat sciatic nerves and found no significant differences in motor function at 16 weeks and no histological differences.[117]

Preclinical studies of have demonstrated the advantages and disadvantages of laser neurorrhaphy. Advantages include shorter repair time as well as reduced neuroma and scar formation. Disadvantages include inferior tensile strength and higher costs. These studies have demonstrated the feasibility of laser assisted nerve repair. However until outcome studies demonstrate a clear advantage over conventional microsurgical techniques the clinical use of laser assisted repairs is likely to be limited.

Emerging Optical Technologies in Neurology and Neurosurgery

Spatial Domain Imaging

Spatially modulated imaging (MI) is a newly described non-contact optical technique in the spatial domain.[15] With this technique, both quantitative mapping of tissue optical properties within a single measurement and cross sectional optical tomography can be achieved rapidly. While compatible with time or frequency domain optical platform assessments, MI predominantly works in the spatial domain with optical information obtained using spatially-modulated illumination for imaging of tissue constituents.

With the MI scheme, periodic illumination patterns of various spatial frequencies with a 120° phase shifting between three adjacent patterns are projected onto the brain from a conventional projector controlled by a computer (Fig. 4). The diffusely reflected pattern (the deformed fringe pattern) passes through near infrared (NIR) bandpass filters and is captured by CCD camera interfaced to a PC computer. The diffusion solution is then used as a model function in an inversion algorithm for determining the optical properties namely, absorption and reduced scattering coefficients over a wide spectrum range.

The ability to separate optical absorption from scattering distinguishes MI from conventional planar reflectance imaging methods. Absorption and scattering maps can, in turn, be used to characterize tissue biochemical composition and structure. Measurement of the changes in absorption in the NIR spectral region (600–1,000 nm), and the knowledge of the molar extinction coefficients of individual chromophores, allows one to detect and measure changes in the oxyhemoglobin, deoxyhemoglobin, and oxygen saturation in the brain and map these changes spatially across a surface. The transformation of the mean optical absorption coefficients into tissue chromophore concentrations is achieved by using the modified Beer-Lambert law. Tomographic information can be obtained by varying the spatial frequency; low spatial frequency present deeper information while high spatial frequency provides surface information. Hence, by tuning the spatial frequency one can control the penetration depth in the tissue.

Projection of spatially modulated light can thus provide quantitative spatiotemporal maps of tissue optical properties and tomography, while being safe (the radiation is non-ionizing), portable, and relatively inexpensive. Spatially modulated imaging has been used to quantitatively map absorption, scattering, and hemodynamic changes following Middle Cerebral Artery occlusion,[118] cerebral edema, and seizures (unpublished data) in rodents. Spatially modulated imaging can be incorporated into a standard operating microscope with relative ease for intraoperative feedback to the surgeon.

Controlling Neural Activity with Light

While traditionally light applications in the neurosciences have been in neurodiagnostics and therapeutics, recent advances have made it possible to modulate or control neural activity with light. Mentioned below are two methods to control neural activity with light.

Photothermal Laser Nerve Stimulation

In vivo laser nerve stimulation of peripheral nerves at nontoxic energy levels was first described by Jonathan Wells and colleagues in 2005 in the sciatic nerves of leopard frogs and rats.[119] With this technique infrared (2.1–6.1 μm) pulses of energy from a tunable free electron laser were used to directly illuminate exposed sciatic nerves producing compound nerve and muscle action potentials (CNAP, CMAP). Later they reproduced the same findings with a Holmium:YAG laser. The activation of nerves using lasers was later described to be related to a photothermal effect resulting in activation of transmembrane ion channels.[120] Histologic examination of nerves activated optically at activation thresholds showed no evidence of tissue damage.[119,121]

Optical nerve stimulation overcomes several of the limitations of conventional electrical stimulation. Optical stimulation methods are noncontact, damage free and generated by energies well below tissue ablation thresholds. They are also spatially precise with little spread of stimulation energy and free of stimulation artifacts. Photothermal laser nerve stimulation is currently in research phase and is being tested for neural applications such as cochlear implants where spatially precise nerve stimulation is not only important, but necessary.

Light Gated Ion Channels

In the past, light has been used to control neuronal cells/tissues primarily by uncaging chemically-modified signaling molecules[122] (e.g., glutamate). However, as glutamate receptors are expressed almost ubiquitously in the central nervous system, glutamate uncaging in a 3D tissue volume cannot have selectivity to one cell type. It is also possible to attach a photoswitch (consisting of a photoisomerizable azobenzene group, covalently attached to a potassium channel antagonist) to generate light-activated forms of the Shaker potassium channel.[123] The azobenzene arm can be switched between *cis* and *trans* isomers by changing the light wavelength from long (580 nm) to short (380 nm), and thus toggling the ligand in and out of the protein's target site. In this method, the azobenzene compound must be supplemented during intact-tissue studies thus posing challenges similar to uncaging methods. In contrast, genetic manipulations can introduce natural light-sensitive proteins such as rhodopsins (no need for exogenous chemicals) which allow selective targeting of genetically defined classes of neurons in a tissue volume.

Recently, newly developed neuroengineering tools based on microbial opsins such as channelrhodopsin-2 (ChR2) and halorhodopsin (NpHR) have been described that enable the investigation of neural circuit function with cell-type-specific, temporally accurate and reversible neuromodulation.[71,124] ChR2 first cloned by Nagel and colleagues,[124] is a cation channel that allows cations to enter the cell following exposure to blue light (~470 nm) causing depolarizations. NpHR is a chloride pump that activates upon illumination with yellow light (~580 nm) resulting in cellular hyperpolarization.

As the activation maxima of these two proteins are over 100 nm apart, they can be controlled independently to either drive action potential firing or suppress neural activity in intact tissue and together may modulate neuronal synchrony.[125] Both proteins have fast temporal kinetics, on the scale of milliseconds, making it possible to drive reliable trains of high frequency action potentials *in vivo* using ChR2 and suppress single action potentials within high frequency spike trains using NpHR.[125]

Nerve stimulation using light gated ion channels holds great promise in clinical neurology.[124] ChR2 or NpHR expression can be restricted to cells that are synaptically connected to a previously-identified relevant population, in order to determine which connections are most important to disease symptoms. For example, it is possible to use viral delivery to retrogradely label neurons with ChR2 or NpHR based on their projection patterns. With this approach, it may be possible to stimulate only the cells in a particular brain region that connect to cells in another brain region of interest, and to determine how these connections are altered in a disease state. This approach may be especially useful in diseases such as schizophrenia and depression, where the implicated cell types receive input from and make functional connections with neurons in heterogeneous regions of the brain (such as the hippocampus and neocortex).

The ability to control the activity of a defined class of neurons has the potential to advance clinical neuromodulation.[124] Existing electrode-based Deep Brain Stimulation methods indiscriminately stimulate all neurons within a given volume, including cells that are not implicated in the disease state, thus leading to unwanted side-effects and even reduced efficacy as opposing excitatory and inhibitory cell types are affected by the electrodes. Genetic control makes it possible to develop more precise therapies by restricting the excited or inhibited neurons to the disease-relevant population. Moreover, the ability to simultaneously record electrical activity during optical stimulation without electrical artifacts makes it possible to engage in responsive neuromodulation by dynamically adjusting the stimulation or inhibition intensity based on feedback from the activity state in the brain. This feature may be especially useful for diseases characterized by sporadic fluctuations in electrical activity such as epilepsy. The combination of recording and optical control could also be used to bridge severed connections, for example to relay information from the brain to distal limbs in the case of severed spinal cord.

Summary

Laser and light based (optical) technologies have many potential applications in neurology and neurosurgery. These tools can accurately, safely, and minimally invasively provide diagnostic information. They can form the basis for therapeutic and intraoperative tools complementary to existing technologies. While few of these tools have to date percolated into the realm of everyday clinical neurologic practice, they have already found wide application in neuroscience research. Further research and development of optical techniques for clinical use require the education and interest of clinicians who are the major driving force behind clinically useful technologies. Neurophotonics is one of the major new frontiers in translational research in the "bench-to-bedside" move towards useful clinical application.

Acknowledgement The authors of this chapter are grateful to Samarendra K. Mohanty, Ph.D. and Professor Anthony J. Durkin, Ph.D., for their insightful discussions and comments.

References

1. Gratton G, Fabiani M, Elbert T, Rockstroh B. Seeing right through you: applications of optical imaging to the study of the human brain. *Psychophysiology.* 2003;40(4):487-491.
2. Cohen LB. Changes in neuron structure during action potential propagation and synaptic transmission. *Physiol Rev.* 1972;53: 373-417.
3. Stepnoski RA, LaPorta A, Raccuia-Behling F, Blonder GE, Slusher RE, Kleinfeld D. Noninvasive detection of changes in membrane potential in cultured neurons by light scattering. *Proc Natl Acad Sci U S A.* 1991;88:9382-9386.
4. Frostig RD, Lieke EE, Ts'o DY, Grinvald A. Cortical functional architecture and local coupling between neuronal activity and the microcirculation revealed by in vivo high-resolution optical imaging of intrinsic signals. *Proc Natl Acad Sci U S A.* 1990;87:6082-6086.
5. Rector DM, Harper RM, George JS. In vivo observations of rapid scattered-light changes associated with electrical events. In: Frostig RD, ed. *In Vivo Optical Imaging of Brain Function.* Boca Raton: CRC Press; 2002:93-112.
6. Rector DM, Poe GR, Kristensen MP, Harper RM. Light scattering changes follow evoked potentials from hippocampal Schaeffer collateral stimulation. *J Neurophysiol.* 1997;78:1707-1713.
7. Grinvald A, Lieke E, Frostig RD, Gilbert CD, Wiesel TN. Functional architecture of cortex revealed by optical imaging of intrinsic signals. *Nature.* 1986;324:361-364.
8. Malonek D, Grinvald A. Interactions between electrical activity and cortical microcirculation revealed by imaging spectroscopy: implications for functional brain mapping. *Science.* 1996;272:551-554.
9. Franceschini MA, Fantini S, Thompson JH, Culver JP, Boas DA. Hemodynamic evoked response of the sensorimotor cortex measured noninvasively with near-infrared optical imaging. *Psychophysiology.* 2003;40:548-560.
10. Jöbsis FF. Noninvasive, infrared monitoring of cerebral and myocardial oxygen sufficiency and circulatory parameters. *Science.* 1977;198:1264-1267.
11. Wyatt JS, Cope M, Delpy DT, et al. Quantitation of cerebral blood volume in human infants by near-infrared spectroscopy. *J Appl Physiol.* 1990;68(3):1086-1091.
12. Gratton G, Sarno AJ, Maclin E, Corballis PM, Fabiani M. Toward non-invasive 3-D imaging of the time course of cortical activity: investigation of the depth of the event-related optical signal (EROS). *Neuroimage.* 2000;11:491-504.

13. Fantini S, Hueber D, Franceschini MA, et al. Non-invasive optical monitoring of the newborn piglet brain using continuous-wave and frequency-domain spectroscopy. *Phys Med Biol.* 1999;44(6):1543-1563.

14. Brady KM, Lee JK, Kibler KK, et al. Continuous time-domain analysis of cerebrovascular autoregulation using near-infrared spectroscopy. *Stroke.* 2007;38(10):2818-2825 [Epub ahead of print].

15. Cuccia DJ, Bevilacqua F, Durkin AJ, Tromberg BJ. Modulated imaging: quantitative analysis and tomography of turbid media in the spatial-frequency domain. *Opt Lett.* 2005;30(11):1354-1356.

16. Hashimoto K, Uruma G, Abo M. Activation of the prefrontal cortex during the Wisconsin card sorting test (Keio version) as measured by two-channel near-infrared spectroscopy in patients with traumatic brain injury. *Eur Neurol.* 2007;59(1-2):24-30.

17. Moritz S, Kasprzak P, Arlt M, Taeger K, Metz C. Accuracy of cerebral monitoring in detecting cerebral ischemia during carotid endarterectomy: a comparison of transcranial Doppler sonography, near-infrared spectroscopy, stump pressure, and somatosensory evoked potentials. *Anesthesiology.* 2007;107(4):563-569.

18. Calderon-Arnulphi M, Alaraj A, Amin-Hanjani S, et al. Detection of cerebral ischemia in neurovascular surgery using quantitative frequency-domain near-infrared spectroscopy. *J Neurosurg.* 2007;106(2):283-290.

19. Bhatia R, Hampton T, Malde S, et al. The application of near-infrared oximetry to cerebral monitoring during aneurysm embolization: a comparison with intraprocedural angiography. *J Neurosurg Anesthesiol.* 2007;19(2):97-104.

20. Boppart SA. Optical coherence tomography: technology and applications for neuroimaging. *Psychophysiology.* 2003;40(4):529-541.

21. Chen-Bee CH, Agoncillo T, Xiong Y, Frostig RD. The triphasic intrinsic signal: implications for functional imaging. *J Neurosci.* 2007;27(17):4572-4586.

22. Bahar S, Suh M, Zhao M, Schwartz TH. Intrinsic optical signal imaging of neocortical seizures: the 'epileptic dip'. *NeuroReport.* 2006;17(5):499-503.

23. Pouratian N, Cannestra AF, Martin NA, Toga AW. Intraoperative optical intrinsic signal imaging: a clinical tool for functional brain mapping. *Neurosurg Focus.* 2002;13(4):e1.

24. Bohringer HJ, Lankenau E, Rohde V, Huttmann G, Giese A. Optical coherence tomography for experimental neuroendoscopy. *Minim Invasive Neurosurg.* 2006;49(5):269-275.

25. Bohringer HJ, Boller D, Leppert J, et al. Time-domain and spectral-domain optical coherence tomography in the analysis of brain tumor tissue. *Lasers Surg Med.* 2006;38(6):588-597.

26. Soliman W, Larsen M, Sander B, Wegener M, Milea D. Optical coherence tomography of astrocytic hamartomas in tuberous sclerosis. *Acta Ophthalmol Scand.* 2007;85(4):454-455.

27. Paquet C, Boissonnot M, Roger F, Dighiero P, Gil R, Hugon J. Abnormal retinal thickness in patients with mild cognitive impairment and Alzheimer's disease. *Neurosci Lett.* 2007;420(2):97-99.

28. Sepulcre J, Murie-Fernandez M, Salinas-Alaman A, Garcia-Layana A, Bejarano B, Villoslada P. Diagnostic accuracy of retinal abnormalities in predicting disease activity in MS. *Neurology.* 2007;68(18):1488-1494.

29. Jafri MS, Farhang S, Tang RS, et al. Optical coherence tomography in the diagnosis and treatment of neurological disorders. *J Biomed Opt.* 2005;10(5):051603.

30. Mayer HM, Brock M, Berlien HP, Weber B. Percutaneous endoscopic laser discectomy (PELD). A new surgical technique for non-sequestrated lumbar discs. *Acta Neurochir Suppl (Wien).* 1992;54:53-58.

31. Boult M, Fraser RD, Jones N, et al. Percutaneous endoscopic laser discectomy. *Aust N Z J Surg.* 2000;70(7):475-479.

32. Choy DS, Hellinger J, Tassi GP, Hellinger S. Percutaneous laser disc decompression. *Photomed Laser Surg.* 2007;25(1):60.

33. Choy DS. Percutaneous laser disc decompression: a 17-year experience. *Photomed Laser Surg.* 2004;22(5):407-410; Review.

34. McLone DG, Naidich TP. Laser resection of fifty spinal lipomas. *Neurosurgery.* 1986;18(5):611-615.

35. Maira G, Fernandez E, Pallini R, Puca A. Total excision of spinal lipomas using CO2 laser at low power. Experimental and clinical observations. *Neurol Res.* 1986;8(4):225-230.

36. Heppner F, Ascher PW, Holzer P, Mokry M. CO2 laser surgery of intramedullary spinal cord tumors. *Lasers Surg Med.* 1987;7(2):180-183.

37. Ascher PW, Heppner F. CO2-Laser in neurosurgery. *Neurosurg Rev.* 1984;7(2-3):123-133.

38. Powers SK, Edwards MS, Boggan JE, et al. Use of the argon surgical laser in neurosurgery. *J Neurosurg.* 1984;60(3):523-530.

39. Yahr WZ, Strully KJ, Hurwitt ES. Non-occluise small arterial anastomosis with a neodymium laser. *Surg Forum.* 1964;15:224-226.

40. Jain KK, Gorisch W. Repair of small blood vessels with the neodymium-YAH laser: a preliminary report. *Surgery.* 1979;85:684.

41. Frazier OH, Painvin GA, Morris JR, Thomsen S, Neblett CR. Laser-assisted microvascular anastomoses: angiographic and anatomopathologic studies on growing microvascular anastomoses: preliminary report. *Surgery.* 1985;97(5):585-590.

42. Quigley MR, Bailes JE, Kwaan HC, Cerullo LJ, Block S. Comparison of myointimal hyperplasia in laser-assisted and suture anastomosed arteries. A preliminary report. *J Vasc Surg.* 1986;4(3):217-219.

43. Quigley MR, Bailes JE, Kwaan HC, Cerullo LJ, Brown JT. Aneurysm formation after low power carbon dioxide laser-assisted vascular anastomosis. *Neurosurgery.* 1986;18(3):292-299.

44. Shapiro S, Sartorius C, Sanders S, Clark S. Microvascular end-to-side arterial anastomosis using the Nd: YAG laser. *Neurosurgery.* 1989;25(4):584-588; discussion 588-589.

45. Tulleken CA, van Dieren A, Verdaasdonk RM, Berendsen W. End-to-side anastomosis of small vessels using an Nd:YAG laser with a hemispherical contact probe. Technical note. *J Neurosurg.* 1992;76(3):546-549.

46. Tulleken CA, Verdaasdonk RM, Berendsen W, Mali WP. Use of the excimer laser in high-flow bypass surgery of the brain. *J Neurosurg.* 1993;78(3):477-480.

47. Tulleken CA, van der Zwan A, van Rooij WJ, Ramos LM. High-flow bypass using nonocclusive excimer laser-assisted end-to-side anastomosis of the external carotid artery to the P1 segment of the posterior cerebral artery via the sylvian route. Technical note. *J Neurosurg.* 1998;88(5):925-927.

48. White RA, Kopchok GE, Donayre CE, et al. Mechanism of tissue fusion in argon laser-welded vein-artery anastomoses. *Lasers Surg Med.* 1988;8(1):83-89.

49. Teramura A, Macfarlane R, Owen CJ, et al. Application of the 1-microsecond pulsed-dye laser to the treatment of experimental cerebral vasospasm. *J Neurosurg.* 1991;75(2):271-276.

50. Macfarlane R, Teramura A, Owen CJ, et al. Treatment of vasospasm with a 480-nm pulsed-dye laser. *J Neurosurg.* 1991;75(4):613-622.

51. Kaoutzanis MC, Peterson JW, Anderson RR, McAuliffe DJ, Sibilia RF, Zervas NT. Basic mechanism of in vitro pulsed-dye laser-induced vasodilation. *J Neurosurg.* 1995;82(2):256-261.

52. Takizawa T, Yamazaki T, Miura N, et al. Laser surgery of basal, orbital and ventricular meningiomas which are difficult to extirpate by conventional methods. *Neurol Med Chir (Tokyo).* 1980;20(7):729-737.

53. Beck OJ. The use of the Nd-YAG and the CO2 laser in neurosurgery. *Neurosurg Rev.* 1980;3(4):261-266.

54. Roux FX, Leriche B, Cioloca C, Devaux B, Turak B, Nohra G. Combined CO2 and Nd-YAG laser in neurosurgical practice. A 1st experience apropos of 40 intracranial procedures. *Neurochirurgie.* 1992;38(4):235-237.

55. Lombard GF, Luparello V, Peretta P. Statistical comparison of surgical results with or without laser in neurosurgery. *Neurochirurgie.* 1992;38(4):226-228.

56. Desgeorges M, Sterkers O, Ducolombier A, et al. Laser microsurgery of meningioma. An analysis of a consecutive series of 164 cases treated surgically by using different lasers. *Neurochirurgie.* 1992;38(4):217-225.

57. Waidhauser E, Beck OJ, Oeckler RC. Nd:YAG-laser in the microsurgery of frontobasal meningiomas. *Lasers Surg Med.* 1990; 10(6):544-550.

58. Eiras J, Alberdi J, Gomez J. Laser CO2 in the surgery of acoustic neuroma. *Neurochirurgie.* 1993;39(1):16-21.

59. Takeuchi J, Handa H, Taki W, Yamagami T. The Nd:YAG laser in neurological surgery. *Surg Neurol.* 1982;18(2):140-142.

60. Oekler RTC, Beck HC, Frank F. Surgery of the sellar region with the Nd:YAG laser. *Fortschr Med.* 1984;9:218-220.

61. Bevilacqua F, Piguet D, Marque P, Gross JD, Tromberg BJ, Depeursinge C. In vivo local determination of tissue optical properties: applications to human brain. *Appl Opt.* 1999;38:4939-4950.

62. Lin WC, Toms SA, Johnson M, Jansen ED, Mahadevan-Jansen A. In vivo brain tumor demarcation using optical spectroscopy. *Photochem Photobiol.* 2001;73(4):396-402.

63. Toms SA, Lin WC, Weil RJ, Johnson MD, Jansen ED, Mahadevan-Jansen A. Intraoperative optical spectroscopy identifies infiltrating glioma margins with high sensitivity. *Neurosurgery.* 2005;57 (4 suppl):382-391.

64. Amharref N, Beljebbar A, Dukic S, et al. Brain tissue characterisation by infrared imaging in a rat glioma model. *Biochim Biophys Acta.* 2006;1758(7):892-899.

65. Leppert J, Krajewski J, Kantelhardt SR, et al. Multiphoton excitation of autofluorescence for microscopy of glioma tissue. *Neurosurgery.* 2006;58(4):759-767.

66. Simpson JR, Horton J, Scott C, et al. Influence of location and extent of surgical resection on survival of patients with glioblastoma multiforme: results of three consecutive Radiation Therapy Oncology Group (RTOG) clinical trials. *Int J Radiat Oncol Biol Phys.* 1993;26(2):239-244.

67. Poon WS, Schomacker KT, Deutsch TF, Martuza RL. Laser-induced fluorescence: experimental intraoperative delineation of tumor resection margins. *J Neurosurg.* 1992;76(4):679-686.

68. Hebeda KM, Wolbers JG, Sterenborg HJ, Kamphorst W, van Gemert MJ, van Alphen HA. Fluorescence localization in tumour and normal brain after intratumoral injection of haematoporphyrin derivative into rat brain tumour. *J Photochem Photobiol B.* 1995; 27(1):85-92.

69. Stummer W, Pichlmeier U, Meinel T, et al. Fluorescence-guided surgery with 5-aminolevulinic acid for resection of malignant glioma: a randomised controlled multicentre phase III trial. *Lancet Oncol.* 2006;7(5):392-401.

70. Stummer W, Stocker S, Wagner S, et al. Intraoperative detection of malignant gliomas by 5-aminolevulinic acid-induced porphyrin fluorescence. *Neurosurgery.* 1998;42(3):518-525; discussion 525-526.

71. Soliman GSH, Truper HG. Halobacterium pharaonis: a new, extremely haloalkaliphilic archaebacterium with low magnesium requirement. *Zentralbl Bakteriol A.* 1982;3:318-329.

72. Madsen SJ, Angell-Petersen E, Spetalen S, Carper SW, Ziegler SA, Hirschberg H. Photodynamic therapy of newly implanted glioma cells in the rat brain. *Lasers Surg Med.* 2006;38(5):540-548.

73. Muller PJ, Wilson BC. Photodynamic therapy for recurrent supratentorial gliomas. *Semin Surg Oncol.* 1995;11(5):346-354.

74. Popovic EA, Kaye AH, Hill JS. Photodynamic therapy of brain tumors. *Semin Surg Oncol.* 1995;11(5):335-345.

75. Muller PJ, Wilson BC. An update on the penetration depth of 630 nm light in normal and malignant human brain tissue in vivo. *Phys Med Biol.* 1986;31(11):1295-1297.

76. Schmidt MH, Reichert KW 2nd, Ozker K, et al. Preclinical evaluation of benzoporphyrin derivative combined with a light-emitting diode array for photodynamic therapy of brain tumors. *Pediatr Neurosurg.* 1999;30(5):225-231.

77. Hirschberg H, Sorensen DR, Angell-Petersen E, et al. Repetitive photodynamic therapy of malignant brain tumors. *J Environ Pathol Toxicol Oncol.* 2006;25(1-2):261-279.

78. Mathews MS, Sun C, Madsen SJ, Hirschberg H. Comparing the effects of repetitive and chronic PDT in human glioma spheroids. *Proc SPIE.* 2007;6424(D):D1-D9.

79. Bisland SK, Lilge L, Lin A, Rusnov R, Wilson BC. Metronomic photodynamic therapy as a new paradigm for photodynamic therapy: rationale and preclinical evaluation of technical feasibility for treating malignant brain tumors. *Photochem Photobiol.* 2004;80: 22-30.

80. Madsen SJ, Sun CH, Tromberg BJ, Yeh AT, Sanchez R, Hirschberg H. Effects of combined photodynamic therapy and ionizing radiation on human glioma spheroids. *Photochem Photobiol.* 2002;76(4):411-416.

81. Hirschberg H, Sun CH, Tromberg BJ, Yeh AT, Madsen SJ. Enhanced cytotoxic effects of 5-aminolevulinic acid-mediated photodynamic therapy by concurrent hyperthermia in glioma spheroids. *J Neurooncol.* 2004;70(3):289-299.

82. Mathews MS, Sanchez RC, Sun C, Madsen SJ, Hirschberg H. The Effect of motexafin gadolinium on ALA photodynamic therapy in glioma spheroids. *Proc SPIE.* 2008;6842:68422N1-68422N7.

83. Hirschberg H, Madsen S, Lote K, Pham T, Tromberg B. An indwelling brachytherapy balloon catheter: potential use as an intracranial light applicator for photodynamic therapy. *J Neurooncol.* 1999; 44(1):15-21.

84. Salcman M, Samaras GM. Hyperthermia for brain tumors: biophysical rationale. *Neurosurgery.* 1981;9(3):327-335.

85. Sneed PK, Stauffer PR, McDermott MW, et al. Survival benefit of hyperthermia in a prospective randomized trial of brachytherapy boost +/− hyperthermia for glioblastoma multiforme. *Int J Radiat Oncol Biol Phys.* 1998;40(2):287-295.

86. Sugiyama K, Sakai T, Fujishima I, Ryu H, Uemura K, Yokoyama T. Stereotactic interstitial laser-hyperthermia using Nd-YAG laser. *Stereotact Funct Neurosurg.* 1990;54–55:501-505.

87. Sakai T, Fujishima I, Sugiyama K, Ryu H, Uemura K. Interstitial laser-thermia in neurosurgery. *J Clin Laser Med Surg.* 1992;10(1):37-40.

88. Nowak G, Rentzsch O, Terzis AJ, Arnold H. Induced hyperthermia in brain tissue: comparison between contact Nd:YAG laser system and automatically controlled high frequency current. *Acta Neurochir (Wien).* 1990;102(1–2):76-81.

89. Terzis AJ, Nowak G, Mueller E, Rentzsch O, Arnold H. Induced hyperthermia in brain tissue in vivo. *Acta Neurochir Suppl (Wien).* 1994;60:406-409.

90. Menovsky T, Beek JF, van Gemert MJ, Roux FX, Bown SG. Interstitial laser thermotherapy in neurosurgery: a review. *Acta Neurochir (Wien).* 1996;138(9):1019-1026.

91. Marmulla R, Eggers G, Muhling J. Laser surface registration for lateral skull base surgery. *Minim Invasive Neurosurg.* 2005;48(3):181-185.

92. Schicho K, Figl M, Seemann R, et al. Comparison of laser surface scanning and fiducial marker-based registration in frameless stereotaxy. Technical note. *J Neurosurg.* 2007;106(4):704-709.

93. Sinha TK, Miga MI, Cash DM, Weil RJ. Intraoperative cortical surface characterization using laser range scanning: preliminary results. *Neurosurgery.* 2006;59(4 suppl 2):ONS368-ONS376; discussion ONS376-ONS377.

94. Kelly PJ, Kall BA, Goerss S, Cascino TL. Results of computer-assisted stereotactic laser resection of deep-seated intracranial lesions. *Mayo Clin Proc.* 1986;61(1):20-27.

95. Kelly PJ, Kall BA, Goerss S, Earnest F 4th. Computer-assisted stereotaxic laser resection of intra-axial brain neoplasms. *J Neurosurg.* 1986;64(3):427-439.

96. Abernathey CD, Davis DH, Kelly PJ. Future perspectives in stereotactic neurosurgery: stereotactic microsurgical removal of deep brain tumors. *J Neurosurg Sci.* 1989;33(1):149-154.

97. Powers SK, Barbaro NM, Levy RM. Pain control with laser-produced dorsal root entry zone lesions. *Appl Neurophysiol.* 1988; 51(2-5):243-254.

98. Fink RA. Neurosurgical treatment of nonmalignant intractable rectal pain: microsurgical commissural myelotomy with the carbon dioxide laser. *Neurosurgery.* 1984;14(1):64-65.

99. Powers SK, Adams JE, Edwards MS, Boggan JE, Hosobuchi Y. Pain relief from dorsal root entry zone lesions made with argon and carbon dioxide microsurgical lasers. *J Neurosurg.* 1984;61(5): 841-847.

100. Nashold BS Jr. Current status of the DREZ operation: 1984. *Neurosurgery.* 1984;15(6):942-944.

101. Kelly PJ, Sharbrough FW, Kall BA, Goerss SJ. Magnetic resonance imaging-based computer-assisted stereotactic resection of the hippocampus and amygdala in patients with temporal lobe epilepsy. *Mayo Clin Proc.* 1987;62(2):103-108.

102. Bebin EM, Kelly PJ, Gomez MR. Surgical treatment for epilepsy in cerebral tuberous sclerosis. *Epilepsia.* 1993;34(4):651-657.

103. Bucholz RD, Pittman T. Endoscopic coagulation of the choroid plexus using the Nd:YAG laser: initial experience and proposal for management. *Neurosurgery.* 1991;28(3):421-426; discussion 426–427.

104. Vandertop WP, Verdaasdonk RM, van Swol CF. Laser-assisted neuroendoscopy using a neodymium-yttrium aluminum garnet or diode contact laser with pretreated fiber tips. *J Neurosurg.* 1998; 88(1):82-92.

105. Powers SK. Fenestration of intraventricular cysts using a flexible, steerable endoscope and the argon laser. *Neurosurgery.* 1986;18(5): 637-641.

106. Zamorano L, Chavantes C, Dujovny M, Malik G, Ausman J. Stereotactic endoscopic interventions in cystic and intraventricular brain lesions. *Acta Neurochir Suppl (Wien).* 1992;54:69-76.

107. Otsuki T, Jokura H, Yoshimoto T. Stereotactic guiding tube for open-system endoscopy: a new approach for the stereotactic endoscopic resection of intra-axial brain tumors. *Neurosurgery.* 1990; 27(2):326-330.

108. Menovsky T, Beek JF, Thomsen SL. Laser(-assisted) nerve repair. A review. *Neurosurg Rev.* 1995;18(4):225-235.

109. Almquist EE, Nachemson A, Auth D, Almquist B, Hall S. Evaluation of the use of the argon laser in repairing rat and primate nerves. *J Hand Surg Am.* 1984;9(6):792-799.

110. Fischer DW, Beggs JL, Kenshalo DL Jr, Shetter AG. Comparative study of microepineurial anastomoses with the use of CO2 laser and suture techniques in rat sciatic nerves: Part 1. Surgical technique, nerve action potentials, and morphological studies. *Neurosurgery.* 1985;17(2):300-308.

111. Seifert V, Stolke D. Laser-assisted reconstruction of the oculomotor nerve: experimental study on the feasibility of cranial nerve repair. *Neurosurgery.* 1989;25(4):579-582; discussion 582-583.

112. Bailes JE, Cozzens JW, Hudson AR, et al. Laser-assisted nerve repair in primates. *J Neurosurg.* 1989;71(2):266-272.

113. Huang TC, Blanks RH, Berns MW, Crumley RL. Laser vs. suture nerve anastomosis. *Otolaryngol Head Neck Surg.* 1992;107(1): 14-20.

114. Maragh H, Hawn RS, Gould JD, Terzis JK. Is laser nerve repair comparable to microsuture coaptation? *J Reconstr Microsurg.* 1988;4(3):189-195.

115. Campion ER, Bynum DK, Powers SK. Repair of peripheral nerves with the argon laser. A functional and histological evaluation. *J Bone Joint Surg Am.* 1990;72(5):715-723.

116. Korff M, Bent SW, Havig MT, Schwaber MK, Ossoff RH, Zealear DL. An investigation of the potential for laser nerve welding. *Otolaryngol Head Neck Surg.* 1992;106(4):345-350.

117. Menovsky T, Beek JF. Laser, fibrin glue, or suture repair of peripheral nerves: a comparative functional, histological, and morphometric study in the rat sciatic nerve. *J Neurosurg.* 2001;95(4): 694-699.

118. Abookasis D, Mathews MS, Lay C, Frostig RD, Tromberg BJ. Modulated imaging: a novel method for quantifying tissue chromophores in evolving cerebral ischemia. *Proc SPIE.* 2007; 6511:65110A1-65110A9.

119. Wells J, Kao C, Mariappan K, et al. Optical stimulation of neural tissue in vivo. *Opt Lett.* 2005;30(5):504-506.

120. Wells J, Kao C, Konrad P, et al. Biophysical mechanisms of transient optical stimulation of peripheral nerve. *Biophys J.* 2007; 93(7):2567-2580.

121. Wells J, Kao C, Jansen ED, Konrad P, Mahadevan-Jansen A. Application of infrared light for in vivo neural stimulation. *J Biomed Opt.* 2005;10(6):064003.

122. Callaway EM, Katz LC. Photostimulation using caged glutamate reveals functional circuitry in living brain slices. *Proc Natl Acad Sci U S A.* 1993;90:7661-7665.

123. Banghart M, Borges K, Isacoff E, Trauner D, Kramer RH. Light activated ion channels for remote control of neuronal firing. *Nat Neurosci.* 2004;7:1381-1386.

124. Nagel G, Szellas T, Huhn W, et al. Channelrhodopsin-2, a directly light-gated cation-selective membrane channel. *Proc Natl Acad Sci.* 2003;100:13940-13945.

125. Zhang F, Aravanis AM, Adamantidis A, de Lecea L, Deisseroth K. Circuit-breakers: optical technologies for probing neural signals and systems. *Nat Rev Neurosci.* 2007;8(8):577-581.

126. Taga G, Homae F, Watanabe H. Effects of source-detector distance of near infrared spectroscopy on the measurement of the cortical hemodynamic response in infants. *Neuroimage.* 2007;38(3): 452-460 [Epub ahead of print].

Laser/Light Applications in Anesthesiology

Julie A. Gayle, Elizabeth A. M. Frost, Clifford Gevirtz, Sajay B. Churi, and Alan D. Kaye

Outline

- Lasers in surgery and medicine have evolved into a specialized area with increasing use and innovative techniques requiring anesthesia providers to be familiar with the historical, technical, and procedural aspects of laser applications.
- Lasers applications in surgery include a variety of procedures with various laser types and specific anesthetic considerations.
- Currently, anesthesia providers commonly encounter use of lasers in many procedures including airway surgery, cutaneous and cosmetic surgeries and various urologic procedures.
- Development of an anesthetic plan that is safe and satisfactory to the surgeon and patient necessitates knowledge of the procedure and patient characteristics.
- Use of lasers for procedures in pediatric patients include dental procedures, dermatologic and laryngeal surgery each having special anesthetic considerations.
- In obstetrics and gynecology, monitored anesthesia care is used for procedures using lasers ranging from laser conization to in utero coagulation of placental vascular anastomosis for twin-to-twin transfusion syndrome.
- With the use of lasers in the operating becoming more common in recent years, awareness and adherence against health hazards to both the patient and personnel is essential.
- Laser safety includes vigilance on the part of the anesthesia provider to prevent laser induced fires, avoid eye injury and burns, as well as, prevent electrical hazards.

Introduction

- Laser applications for surgery are widespread and include excisions of dermatologic lesions, treatment of laryngeal lesions, pediatric dentistry and treatment of prostatic hypertrophy.
- Procedures involving lasers and the airway represent a special challenge to the anesthesia provider including risk of airway fire, aspiration, injury, and inadequate ventilation and oxygenation.
- Use of laser in cosmetic and cutaneous procedures is generally well tolerated with monitored anesthesia care supplemented with topical or local anesthesia.
- Laser use in prosthetic reduction surgery is common and often patients are elderly presenting with multiple co-morbidities influencing choice of anesthetic technique.
- Anesthesia for procedures involving laser use in specialized patient populations such as pediatrics and obstetrics requires the anesthesia provider to be familiar with the procedure and special needs of the patient.
- As laser technology continues to evolve in the fields of medicine, surgery, and dentistry, benefits to the patient as it relates to anesthesia are apparent in some areas and require further study in others.
- Laser safety programs are required nationally in all hospitals and office based surgical facilities using lasers.

History

The medical application vand uses of the laser have increased greatly over the past 40 years. Currently lasers are used for cauterization, tumor ablation, bloodless surgery and generally where destruction of a pathologic process within a small

J.A. Gayle (✉)
Department of Anesthesiology, Louisiana Health Sciences Center, New Orleans, LA, USA
e-mail: jgayle477@cox.net

K. Nouri (ed.), *Lasers in Dermatology and Medicine*,
DOI: 10.1007/978-0-85729-281-0_47, © Springer-Verlag London Limited 2011

area is indicated. Cooperation between physicists, engineers and physicians has led to the application of lasers in medicine. It is a prime example of the value of clinical application of basic science discoveries.

The safe use of any new medical instrument such as the laser requires that personnel be aware of the background principles and hazards involved. Laser is a form of electromagnetic radiation and strict adherence to safeguards against health hazards is essential.

Laser

Laser is an acronym for Light Amplification of Stimulated Emission of Radiation. The precursor of laser was Maser, a term coined by Nobel laureate, CH Townes, Microwave Amplification by Stimulated Emission of Radiation. In 1958, work was extended from microwaves to the visible light spectrum and led to the construction of the first ruby laser by Bell Telephone Laboratories. The output of early lasers was not well controlled until the technique of "Q" switching permitted all the energy of radiation to be stored in the laser and then released in pulses. Use of lasers in space technology led to further developments that have been incorporated into operating room lasers. In essence, a laser beam which is defined by wavelength, duration, energy and width of spot focused optics to direct a beam to a biological target. This effort results in ionizing radiation in situ, mechanical shock waves and vaporization of tissues by heat. The beam acts both as a scalpel and to coagulate blood vessels.

Characteristics

Lasers can be generated from solids, liquids or gases with resultant radiation of different wavelengths and biomedical properties. The materiasl used to generate the laser defines depth of vaporization and damage to tissues Table 1. Recently, fiber based lasers and distal chip flexible endoscopy have been added to facilitate a new type of surgery, especially in office based laryngeal procedures.[1]

Table 1 Some currently used laser sources

Laser Sources	
Solids	Gases
Ruby (red beam)	Carbon dioxide (invisible beam)
Neodymium-glass	Helium-neon (red beam)
Yttrium-aluminum-garnet (YAG)	Argon (blue-green beam)
Neodymium YAG	Krypton
Erbium YAG	Nitrogen

Atoms that can be excited to emit light waves are contained in the laser in long narrow tubes with mirrors at either end. External energy is provided initially to excite some of the atoms. The light wave emitted by these few atoms is amplified by stimulating other atoms to emit. A beam of wave is produced which develops tremendous energy by reflection from the mirrors. Finally, the radiation wave emerges from the partially reflective mirror as an intense directional beam of light. Laser beams are unique compared to other light wave beams because all other light or radiation is comprised of wave emissions from individual atoms independently of other excited atoms.

Laser characteristics include:

1. A near single frequency of low band-width, i.e., an almost pure monochromatic beam.
2. Precisely defined wave fronts. The point of impact can be the same as the wavelength.
3. Enormous intensity and a high frequency of temporal and spatial coherence.
4. A high plane of polarization and tremendous electromagnetic field strength.

Applications

Lasers have achieved many uses in medicine, mainly in surgery. They can be used to excise melanomas, tumors, dermatologic scars (tattoos, port wine stains) and also for cosmetic facial enhancement.[2] As noted above, the new lasers are well suited for treatment of laryngeal epithelial diseases such as dysplasia and papillomatosis.[1] Carbon dioxide lasers have been used successfully in the treatment of anogenital warts in children.[3] In pediatric dentistry erbium lasers have been found effective for both dental and soft tissue treatments.[4] Retinopathy of prematurity is amenable to diode laser therapy.[5] Other applications have been in prostatic surgery and for complex eye surgery as in vitrectomy, retinal detachment and posterior capsulotomy.[6] Perhaps one of the more innovative uses has been in the in utero coagulation of placental vascular anastomosis in the twin- to-twin transfusion syndrome.[7] Other diagnostic uses include the application of laser spectroscopy to microanalytic techniques, Papanicolau smears and immunofluorescent techniques.

Because lasers are a source of coherent and monochromatic radiation that can be focused accurately with high intensity and essentially no blood loss, that are used in procedures that require precision. The laser accomplishes tissue excision by vaporization and at the same time seals small blood vessels. The use or the operating microscope ensures a bloodless operation with controlled depth of tissue removal. The carbon dioxide laser as an example emits an invisible wave of 10.6 µm which is absorbed within 0.2 cm of tissue surface.

Laser radiographs appear superior to conventional x rays and may be used in breast tumor imaging and occlusion of hemangiomas. An argon laser counter can determine a complete blood count and calculate derived parameters. A further use may be in caries prevention in dentistry.

Laser fiberoptics have been developed for operating room use. A further application is as an effective tool for mass communication in examination of patient records, test results and for teaching purposes. A helium- neon laser beam communication system has been used for central monitoring in an operating suite.

Laser Surgery Involving the Airway

Indications and Contraindications

- Nd-YAG lasers may be used for debulking of tumors of the trachea, main-stem bronchi and upper airway by transmitting energy via fiberoptic cable through the suction port of a fiberoptic bronchoscope
- Procedures in and around the vocal cords and oropharynx may require the precision of the CO_2 laser
- Patients with underlying cardiopulmonary disease may be unable to tolerate desaturation, hypoxemia, and hypercarbia associated with low concentrations of oxygen and interruptions in ventilation during laser surgery of the airway

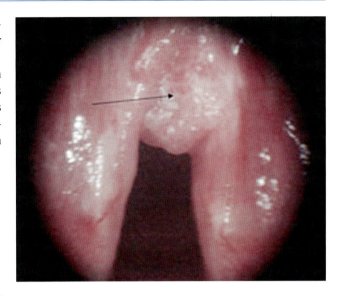

Fig. 1 Papilloma of the vocal cords

There are many types of lasers, each with specific indications. Neodymium-doped yttrium aluminum gradient (Nd-YAG) laser is the most powerful laser. It allows for a tissue penetration between 2 and 6 mm and is used for tissue debulking, particularly in the trachea, main-stem bronchi, and upper airway. The energy may be transmitted through a fiberoptic cable placed down the suction port of a fiberoptic bronchoscope. The Nd-YAG laser can be used in "contact mode" to treat a tumor mass, such as a papilloma (Fig. 1). Alternatively, the CO_2 laser has very little tissue penetration and can be used where great precision is needed. One advantage of the CO_2 laser in airway surgery is that the beam is absorbed by water, so minimal heat is dispersed to surrounding tissues. The CO_2 laser is primarily used for procedures in the oropharynx and in and around the vocal cords. The helium-neon laser (He-Ne) produces an intense red light and can be used for aiming the CO_2 and Nd-YAG lasers. It has a very low power and poses no danger to OR personnel or the patient.[8]

Because lasers are capable of igniting airway fires, use of high concentrations of oxygen and nitrous oxide is dangerous. Some patients with cardiopulmonary disease may not tolerate low concentrations of oxygen (at or just above room air) and the resultant desaturation and hypoxemia. In addition, interruptions in ventilation frequently result in hypercarbia and may result in arrhythmias. Prior to induction of anesthesia and surgery, a thorough history and physical help to identify patients who are at risk for complications during laser surgery of the airway and associated manipulations of oxygenation and ventilation.

Techniques

- Patients with pathologic conditions involving the airway (i.e., mediastinal masses, tracheal stenosis) may be difficult to ventilate and/or intubate during induction of anesthesia
- Co-morbidities such as chronic obstructive pulmonary disease and coronary artery disease are present in many patients presenting for laser surgery of the airway and should be medically optimized pre-operatively
- Airway management for laser surgery of the larynx includes endotracheal intubation, intermittent apneic ventilation, and jet ventilation
- Short-acting opioids such as remifentanil or alfentanil in combination with a sedative-hypnotic (i.e., propofol) typically provide adequate depth of anesthesia for laser surgery of the airway and rapid emergence at the conclusion of surgery
- Post-operative pain control can generally be achieved with shorter acting opioids such as fentanyl and titrated to pain relief

Pre-operative Management

Pre-operative management of patients requiring laser surgery for masses or tumors of the trachea, main-stem bronchi and upper airway involves careful attention to airway management. Airway compromise should be anticipated and a clear backup plan devised before the induction of general anesthesia. Patients with lesions in the mediastinum may be difficult to ventilate and/or intubate. Stridor suggests existing narrowing of the airway which may also compromise airway management. Inspiratory stridor indicates a supraglottic lesion, whereas, expiratory stridor suggests subglottic narrowing. Communication with the surgeon and careful planning are imperative during induction of anesthesia in this patient population. Furthermore, many patients presenting for laser surgery for lesions involving the airway are elderly and have a history of tobacco use. A history of chronic obstructive pulmonary disease suggests a need for a chest x-ray to rule out active pulmonary processes. Prior to induction, wheezing should be treated with bronchodilators. Coronary artery disease should be suspected in those at risk (age >65 years, male, family history, tobacco use, high cholesterol, hypertension, diabetes mellitus, obesity, and sedentary lifestyle.) Adrenergic response to airway manipulation should be anticipated and treated with beta blockade to decrease the risk of myocardial ischemia.[9]

Description of Technique

Laser surgery of the vocal cords requires the cords be immobile during laser firing. Adequate muscle relaxation is therefore important. The CO_2 laser is generally used because of its ability to precisely vaporize tissue. The Nd:YAG laser coagulates deeper lesions and is used for tumor debulking.

Airway management for laser surgery of the larynx includes endotracheal intubation, intermittent apneic technique, and jet ventilation.

Endotracheal intubation with a small-diameter endotracheal tube (5.0–6.0 mm) or microlaryngeal tube allows for visualization of the larynx. The lowest possible FiO_2 (less than or equal to 0.3 or 0.4) that assures adequate oxygenation is desirable. Nitrous oxide and a high FiO_2 support combustion and should be avoided. Other precautions to prevent airway fires include filling the cuff with methylene blue normal saline and using a special laser endotracheal tube such as a Mallinkrodt Laser-Flex® or Xomed Laser Shield®. It should be noted that laser endotracheal tubes do not provide 100% protection for all laser types (Table 2).

Intermittent apnea technique allows tracheal extubation after a period of hyperventilation. The laser may be used

Table 2 Characteristics of endotracheal tubes used during laser surgery of the airway

Type of tube	Non-reflective	Combustible	Kink resistant
Polyvinyl chloride	+	++	–
Red rubber	+	++	+
Silicone rubber	+	+	–
Metal	–	–	+

Adapted from Morgan et al.[10]

during the time the patient is extubated for approximately 1–5 min prior to desaturation. A pulse oximeter must be accurate and always available. A disadvantage of this technique includes increased risk of airway edema and trauma.

Jet ventilation allows for ventilation without an endotracheal tube such as in treatment of some supraglottic and subglottic lesions. A ventilating laryngoscope is commonly used for supraglottic lesions. The jet flow should be aligned with the trachea and complete exhalation should be allowed prior to the next jet ventilation. By triggering the jet between laser firing, the vocal cords remain immobile. Complete muscle relaxation is essential with the use of jet ventilation. Complications include pneumothorax, barotrauma, and gastric distension.

Standard induction techniques may be used depending on the co-morbidities of the patient (i.e., rapid sequence intubation for those at risk for aspiration.) In general, minimal post-operative discomfort implies decreased need for narcotics intra-operatively. Short-acting opioids such as remifentanil (0.1–0.25 mcg/kg/min) or alfentanil (0.25–0.1 mcg/kg/min) may be used in combination with propofol (100–150 mcg/kg/min) to maintain adequate anesthetic depth while allowing for rapid emergence. As previously mentioned, adequate neuromuscular blockade is especially important in surgery involving the vocal cords.

In most cases, full recovery of airway reflexes should be obtained prior to extubation. In special circumstances, such as vocal cord surgery, the surgeon may request a smooth emergence involving deep extubation. In either case, gastric decompression prior to extubation is prudent, especially following the use of jet ventilation.

Post-operative Management

Use of short acting opioids such as intravenous fentanyl (25–50 mcg) as needed for pain control in the post-operative is usually adequate. Depending on the nature and invasiveness of the surgical procedure, longer acting narcotics such as morphine or dilaudid may be necessary to make the patient comfortable. There is risk of pneumothorax and barotrauma with jet ventilation. If suspected, a chest x-ray should be obtained.

Adverse Events

- Factors contributing to the risk of airway fire during laser surgery include energy level of the laser, the gas environment of the airway, and the type of endotracheal tube
- A safe gas mixture of 25–30% oxygen and avoidance of nitrous oxide decreases the risk of airway fire during laser surgery
- Laser-resistant endotracheal tubes are designed to prevent fires associated with laser use
- The anesthesiologist and all members of the operating room team should remain vigilant in recognizing the early signs of airway fire (i.e., unexpected flash, flame, smoke, odors, discolorations of the breathing circuit)
- In the event of an airway fire, the endotracheal tube should be removed immediately and the flow of gases stopped followed by removal of burning materials and saline or water poured into the airway

Side Effects/Complications

The most serious complication of laser airway surgery is fire. Airway fire may occur when an endotracheal tube is ignited. Several factors contribute to the likelihood of airway fire including the energy level of the laser, the gas environment of the airway, and the type of endotracheal tube. Oxygen and nitrous oxide both support combustion thus pose a fire hazard. If the patient is being ventilated with oxygen or nitrous oxide, the endotracheal tube emits a blow-torch type of flame that results in severe injury to the trachea, lungs, and surrounding tissue. Endotracheal tubes made of polyvinyl chloride, silicone, and red rubber have oxygen flammability indices of 26%. Wrapping the endotracheal tube with reflective tape still imposes a hazard in that kinking of the tube may occur, gaps may be present, and non-laser resistant tape may be inadvertently used.

Prevention and Treatment of Side Effects/Complications

The prevention of airway fires involving laser use begins with communication amongst the anesthesiologist, surgeon, and all members of the operating room team. Precautions should be taken to minimize the risk of an oxygen rich environment

that would support ignition and combustion. To prevent fires associated with endotracheal tubes and laser use, laser-resistant endotracheal tubes have been developed. It is best to use an endotracheal tube that is designed to be resistant to a specific laser that may be used in surgery (e.g., CO_2, Nd:YAG, Ar, Er:YAG, KTP). The tracheal cuff of the laser tube should be filled with saline and colored with an indicator dye such as methylene blue to alert the surgeon if he contacts the endotracheal tube. To minimize the risk of ignition, a safe gas mixture during laser surgery involving the airway is oxygen/air or oxygen/helium to achieve an oxygen concentration 25–30% or minimal oxygen concentration required to avoid hypoxia. Nitrous oxide should be avoided. Surgical drapes should be arranged to reduce the accumulation of oxidizers under the drapes. Gauze and sponges should be moistened prior to use near an ignition source.

The energy level of the laser is controlled by the surgeon and activation of the laser should be preceded by adequate notice. Safe use of laser in airway surgery includes intermittent and noncontinous mode at moderate power (10–15 W.) In addition, allowing time for heat dispersal and packing of adjacent tissues with moist gauze helps reduce the risk of airway fire.[11] Precautions that should be taken to minimize the risk of airway fire include:

1. Intubation with a laser resistant endotracheal tube resistant to the specific type of laser to be used
2. Filling the endotracheal tube cuff with saline or an indicator dye such as methylene blue
3. Requesting the surgeon to give adequate notice prior to activating the laser
4. Reducing the concentration of oxygen to the minimum avoiding hypoxia
5. Discontinuing use of nitrous oxide
6. Waiting a few minutes after reducing the oxygen concentration before allowing laser activation

The anesthesiologist and members of the operating room team must be vigilant in recognizing the early warning signs of fire. Examples include unexpected flash, flame, smoke or heat, unusual sounds or odors, discoloration of the drapes or breathing circuit. If a fire occurs involving the airway, the anesthesiologist should immediately remove the endotracheal tube and stop the flow of all gases (Table 3). All flammable and burning materials should be removed from the

Table 3 Airway fire protocol for fires of the airway or breathing circuit[11]

1. Remove the endotracheal tube
2. Stop the flow of all gases
3. Remove flammable and burning materials from the airway
4. Pour saline or water into the patient's airway

airway and saline or water poured into the airway. Once the airway or breathing circuit is extinguished, mask ventilation should be established avoiding oxygen and nitrous oxide if possible. The removed endotracheal tube should be examined for fragments that might be left in the airway and bronchoscopy (rigid preferred) considered to assess injury and remove any debris. The patient's status and plan for ongoing care such as admission to the intensive care unit, serial chest x-rays, arterial blood gases must be reassessed.[11]

Anesthesia for Cutaneous and Cosmetic Laser Surgery

Indications and Contraindications

- Cosmetic laser surgery is frequently used to minimize the signs of aging in areas such as periorbital and perioral creases
- Laser skin resurfacing can successfully treat scars related to acne and trauma, as well as, pre-cancerous lesions

Laser skin resurfacing is used to treat a variety of skin conditions including acne scars, traumatic scars, and pre-cancerous lesions such as actinic keratosis. Cosmetic laser surgery utilizes a controlled burn to the facial skin to reduce the signs of aging, especially in the periorbital and perioral creases where previous cosmetic techniques were lacking.

Many cosmetic procedures utilizing lasers are perfomed in an office-based setting under local or topical anesthesia sometimes with monitored anesthesia care. Therefore, patients with pre-existing medical conditions preventing safe administration of sedation and/or anesthesia should probably undergo elective procedures in a hospital setting rather than an office-based environment.[12]

Techniques

- Topical and/or local anesthesia supplemented with intravenous sedation generally provides adequate anesthesia for facial laser resurfacing
- A lidocaine/tetracaine-based peel for minimal to moderately painful cutaneous laser procedures has been used successfully

Pre-operative Management

Full face laser resurfacing is painful and can be stressful to the patient. Local anesthesia is often inadequate and must be supplemented with intravenous sedation, regional nerve blocks, topical anesthetics, and/or general anesthesia. Patients presenting with chronic medical problems such as hypertension, cardiovascular and/or pulmonary disease should be evaluated and treated for these problems prior to the procedure.

Description of Technique

Usually, CO_2 or erbium:yag lasers are used for laser skin resurfacing (Fig. 2). Anesthetic technique should be chosen keeping in mind that a tremendous amount of heat is delivered to the skin surface resulting in a deep thermal injury and pain.[12] General anesthesia, regional nerve blocks with local infiltration and/or intravenous sedation may be used. Combinations of the intravenous sedation (e.g., propofol, ketamine, midazolam, opioids) with topical anesthesia (e.g., EMLA cream-eutectic mixture of local anesthetics) have been successful for laser skin resurfacing in the ambulatory setting.[14]

A novel topical anesthetic compound using lidocaine/tetracaine-based peel has been used successfully for minimally to moderately painful cutaneous laser procedures. In a study of 20 patients undergoing full-face single-pass CO_2 laser resurfacing, topical lidocaine/tetracaine-based cream was found to provide safe and effective dermal anesthesia.[15]

Post-operative Management

Patients undergoing full face laser resurfacing receive potent narcotics in a short time and should have adequate recovery time prior to discharge. Oral analgesics are generally

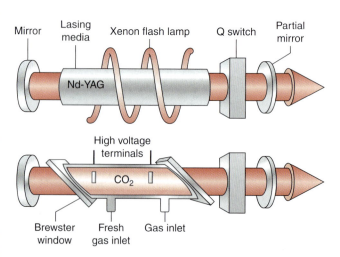

Fig. 2 Generic laser hardware[13]

Laser/Light Applications in Anesthesiology

adequate for management of pain following the procedure. Post operative nausea and vomiting should be treated with anti-emetics (e.g., ondansetron).

Adverse Events

- Laser-specific eyewear for the patient and operating room personnel are necessary to provide protection from ocular hazards during cosmetic laser surgery
- A smoke evacuation system is used to remove carbon particles, DNA, microils, and toxic fumes from the operating room environment

Ocular hazards require laser-specific eyewear for the patient and operating room personnel. Protection from fire and reflectivity hazards include: fire-retardant draping, moist draping, water basin and fire extinguisher available. Alcohol containing solutions and plastic and rubber instruments should be avoided. Also, oxygen sources and metal or reflective materials should be avoided. Fire-resistant endotracheal tubes decrease the possibility of tube breach or ignition. Furthermore, release of carbon particles, DNA, microils, and toxic fumes accompany laser destruction of cells. Utilizing a smoke evacuation system 2 cm from the plume and wearing high-filtration masks protect the patient and medical personnel. [9]

Anesthesia for Urologic Procedures Involving Laser Use

Indications and Contraindications

- Laser techniques for resection of the prostate allow for minimal use of irrigating solutions compared to classic transurethral resection of the prostate (TURP)
- Transurethral resection of the prostate with the Holmium:yttrium-aluminum-garnet and potassium-titanyl-phosphate lasers are associated with almost no absorption of irrigant and minimal blood loss

With an aging population comes an increasing incidence of bladder outlet obstruction and patients in need of prostatic reduction surgery. Advances in laser techniques for resection of the prostate have several proposed advantages over traditional transurethral resection. Classic transurethral resection of the prostate for patients with benign prostatic hypertrophy involves use of large amounts of irrigating solutions predisposing the patient to "TURP syndrome." Subarachnoid block for classic transurethral resection of the prostate allows the anesthesiologist to monitor for mental status changes associated with electrolyte abnormalities due to absorption of large amounts of irrigating fluids. In an effort to reduce peri-operative morbidity, alternatives to conventional electorcautery have been explored. The Holmium:yttrium-aluminum-garnet and potassium-titanyl-phosphate lasers allow for transurethral resection of the prostate with almost no absorption of irrigant and minimal blood loss. [16]

Techniques

- Patients undergoing TURP are often elderly with co-existing cardiovascular and pulmonary disease
- New laser technology using less irrigation fluid reduces the incidence of systemic complications associated with TURP syndrome
- KTP laser is used to treat BPH (benign prostatic hypertrophy) and allows for an almost bloodless procedure using less irrigation solution than conventional techniques

Pre-operative Management

Most patients presenting for TURP have obstructive symptoms and are elderly. Co-morbidities increase risk of cardiovascular and pulmonary complications in the peri-operative period. Preexisting medical problems including coronary artery disease, peripheral vascular disease, cerebrovascular disease, chronic obstructive pulmonary disease, and renal impairment should be evaluated and treated in the preoperative period. [9]

Anesthetic Management

While general anesthesia makes it more difficult to recognize the early manifestations of TURP syndrome (e.g., altered mental status), anticoagulants and degenerative spinal changes may prevent or make difficult use of regional anesthesia.

Holmium laser technique decreases the amount of irrigation solution required and avoids the osmotic complications associated with absorption of large quantities of glycine, mannitol, and sorbitol. By decreasing the risk of TURP syndrome, the anesthesiologist may choose among several anesthetic techniques (e.g., general, neuroaxial, local and monitored anesthesia care) and tailor the anesthetic plan to an individual patient's needs.

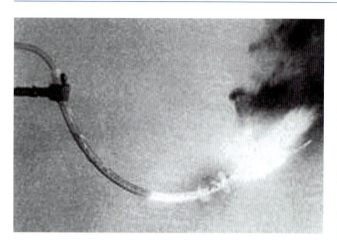

Fig. 3 Blowtorch effect of gases flowing through endotracheal tube

KTP laser is the most recent advancement in laser treatment of BPH.(Fig. 3) This technology allows for an almost bloodless procedure, fewer blood transfusions, and less absorption of the irrigant.[16]

Post-operative Management

Patients undergoing classic transurethral resection of the prostate under subarachnoid block may encounter urinary retention due to blockade of the parasympathetic fibers that control detrusor contraction and bladder neck relaxation. Delays in the recovery room and delays in discharge to home are some disadvantages of spinal anesthesia in the postoperative setting.[9] Development of new laser technology using less irrigation fluid reduces the incidence of the TURP syndrome (Table 4). The systemic complications including fluid overload, hyponatremia, and hemolysis are reduced.

Adverse Events

- Longer procedure times are associated with use of the Holmium and KTP lasers requiring longer durations of anesthesia
- As with most new technologies and procedures, KTP and Holmium lasers for prostate surgery are associated with learning curve and acquisition of skills by the surgeon

Both the Holmium laser and KTP laser have longer procedure times requiring the patient to be anesthetized for a longer time period. Holmium laser prostate surgery is technically demanding and requires a longer learning curve. However, KTP laser procedure is less technically demanding and easier to learn.[16]

Table 4 Signs and symptoms of TURP syndrome

1. Headache
2. Restlessness
3. Confusion
4. Cyanosis
5. Dyspnea
6. Arrhythmias
7. Hypotension
8. Seizures

Anesthesia for Laser Use in Special Patient Populations

Pediatrics

Indications and Contraindications

- Lasers are used for a wide variety of procedures in the pediatric population including removal of laryngeal papillomatosis and anogenital warts
- Erbium lasers are used for dental and soft tissue treatments
- Diode laser therapy is used in treatment of retinopathy of prematurity

Lasers are frequently used in certain types of procedures and surgeries involving pediatric patients. Lasers have been successfully used for removal of anogenital warts, laryngeal papillomatosis, and excision of port wine stains. Diode laser therapy for retinopathy of prematurity and erbium lasers for dental and soft tissue treatments are other indications for laser use in the pediatric patient.

Techniques

- Standard pre-operative fasting guidelines apply in the healthy pediatric patient for elective laser surgery
- Oral midazolam provides adequate pre-medication in patients older than 1 year prior to induction of anesthesia
- Pulsed dye laser treatment is commonly used to treat port wine stain (PWS) associated with Sturge Weber syndrome
- General anesthesia combined with local anesthetic filtration is commonly used for laser surgery in pediatric patients

- Addressing post-operative pain in the pediatric patient can be challenging and difficult to assess
- It is generally comforting to the child to have the parents at the bedside as he or she regains consciousness

Pre-operative Management

Factors such as age, weight, and existing medical conditions deserve special consideration in formulating the anesthetic plan prior to surgery. Regarding pre-operative fasting, standard guidelines apply for pediatric patients presenting for elective laser surgery. Clear liquids may be given until 2 h before surgery. Breast milk should be stopped 4 h prior and formula 6 h prior to surgery. Solids should be discontinued 6 h before surgery. Recommendations vary somewhat and are for healthy pediatric patients without increased risk of aspiration or decreased gastric emptying.[17]

Pre-medication is generally not necessary for patients under 1 year of age. Beyond 1 year up to 10 years, oral midazolam 0.5 mg/kg to a maximum of 15 mg provides adequate anxiolysis. Intravenous doses of commonly used pediatric drugs such as atropine and midazolam are below in table Table 5.

Description of Technique

The anesthetic plan is determined by the procedure, the requirement to stay immobile, the age of the patient, any preexisting conditions and nay special needs of the patient. Anesthetic exposures are often multiple, especially in port wine stain treatments. Regarding cosmetic concerns related to the port wine stain (PWS) and/or the child with Sturge Weber syndrome, pulsed dye laser treatment is commonly used.[18] There are no definitive numbers of treatments used in this therapy although 10–20 are commonly needed. Usually about 50–100 shots are tolerated at a time. The initial parameters for the vascular specific pulsed dye laser utilize a wavelength of 595 nm and pulse duration of 450 µs. This minimizes the spread of heat from the lesion and allows for selective destruction of capillary sized blood vessels. It is important to treat the PWS due to the negative psychosocial impact for affected children. Moreover, it is a simple procedure with minimal risk and a satisfactory cosmetic result.[18] Treatment should be started as early as possible, even in small infants as the PWS grows with the child and hence will require more sessions for removal. Each laser flash has a relatively small spot size and thus larger lesions require more shots. Also, PWS seem to be more susceptible to fading when therapy is begun early. However, the treatment is painful and infants usually require at the least sedation and often general anesthesia. Older children may be managed after application of EMLA® cream. Refractory pediatric glaucoma may also complicate Sturge Weber syndrome (SWS) and Kirwan et al. have investigated the efficacy and complications of diode laser cyclophotocoagulation (cyclodiode.)[19] Some appropriate pediatric dosages are listed in Table 5.

Many surgeons prefer to work with small patients under general anesthesia, while others prefer conscious sedation when possible. General anesthetic techniques provide many advantages such as immobility, and variables such as $PaCO_2$, blood pressure, and intracranial pressure are more easily controlled to optimize operative conditions. Combined techniques utilizing general anesthesia with local anesthetic infiltration are commonly employed. Remifentanil and fentanyl have commonly been used during conscious sedation. They may be administered by bolus or infusion techniques. Propofol infusion is also appropriate. Several anesthetic challenges exist in the patient with SWS. A prone position is often required to treat PWS of the leg. Intubation may prove difficult due to angiomas of the mouth and upper airway.[20] Placement of a supraglottic airway may be beneficial. Initial sedation with oral midazolam may be indicated, followed by EMLA® cream applied to the PWS and secured with plastic tape. A propofol infusion would then allow 30 min of flash lamp pulsed dye laser therapy, prompt awakening and discharge to home with oral acetaminophen.

Table 5 Selected pediatric drug dosages

Drug	Comment	Dosage (pertain to IV administration if not specified otherwise)
Atropine	IV	0.01–0.02 mg/kg
Vecuronium	Intubation (IV)	0.05–0.1 mg/kg
Midazolam	Sedation	0.3–0.5 mg/kg
Epinephrine	IV bolus	0.01 mg/kg
Fentanyl	Anesthetic adjunct (IV)	1–5 µg/kg
	Main anesthetic (IV)	50–100 µg/kg
Propofol	Induction (IV)	2–3 mg/kg
Ondansetron	IV	0.1 mg/kg
Phenytoin	Slowly IV	5–20 mg/kg
Sodium pentothal	Induction (IV)	1–2 mg/kg

Adapted from Morgan et al.[10]

Post-operative Management

Pain assessment in the pediatric patient can sometimes be challenging due to their inability to communicate effectively with the care giver. Irritability and crying may be attributed

Post-operative Management

Laser conization of the cervix under local anesthesia results in minimal discomfort for most women post-operatively. Oral analgesics such as acetaminophen or ketorolac are acceptable choices. Post operative nausea and vomiting can be treated with anti-emetics such as raglan or zofran. Monitoring for post operative bleeding is appropriate.

In the parturient following fetoscopic laser coagulation, management in the post-operative period involves monitoring mother for bleeding and pre-term labor. Tocolytic agents may be needed after consultation with an obstetrician.[9]

Adverse Events

- Peroneal nerve injury is a complication of the lithotomy position manifested by foot drop and loss of sensation over the dorsum of the foot
- Monitoring for pre-term labor and bleeding in the parturient post-operatively is imperative and may involve consultation of an obstetrician

A complication following gynecological and obstetrical procedures involving laser is peroneal nerve injury secondary to the lithotomy position manifested by foot drop and loss of sensation over the dorsum of the foot. Vigilance during positioning and during the surgery is the best ways to prevent this injury. Post operative nausea and vomiting should be anticipated and prophylaxis given prior to emergence in those at risk.[9] Bleeding and premature labor are risks of surgery in the parturient, particularly involving in utero procedures. Involvement of the obstetrician in the peri-operative care of these patients is important.

Future Directions of Laser Applications and Anesthesia

Further clinical research in the field of laser applications will have implications on anesthesia as laser technology evolves. For example, it is believed that pulsed angiolysis lasers are a platform technology for future innovations in management of not only laryngeal disease, but other areas in which superficial mucosa is diseased (i.e., Barrett's esophagus and granulation in the nose and ear.)[26] Furthermore, where there has already been advancements in laser technology such as in prostate surgery, the benefits of broadening anesthetic options still requires documentation and further study Yet another area of innovation is in the field of dentistry. Lasers are currently used for contouring the gums, treating mouth ulcers, and setting bonding materials. Although use of lasers in dentistry is not without a need for anesthesia, research continues to determine the effectiveness and safety of laser use in hard-tissue such as cavity removal.

Special Considerations

Safety Concerns Involving Use of Lasers in the Or

Laser Safety Program

Development of a laser safety program is a national requirement for all hospitals and for office based surgical facilities using lasers. The laser can ignite any combustible material and thus is a fire hazard. Any tissue that the laser focuses is vaporized, whether diseased or healthy. Also, contact with the laser, like all radiation, should be avoided. There is no known acceptable of safe dose. There may be biological effects from scattered or reflected radiation. The long term effects on the genetic system are unknown as are the effects during pregnancy.

Issues critical to safety include:

1. Area control is essential. Lasers should be in isolated low traffic areas, locked in cabinets and used only by authorized and trained personnel.
2. Adequate ventilation and scavenging systems should be able to remove all by-products as the dangers of inhalation or dissemination of viral, bacterial or tumor tissue has not been determined.
3. A good suction system should be available to remove smoke and vaporized tissue which might disseminate particles that might be inhaled by operating room personnel or the patient.
4. Surfaces in the room should be minimally reflective.
5. Warning signs and light alarms should be posted at entrances.
6. A laser safety officer should head up the safety program, which should include plans for emergency treatment of laser radiation and education programs.
7. Eye protection is essential. The lens of the eye can focus the laser beam and cause retinal burns. Eye safety is afforded by goggles with high optical density and specificity for the laser wavelength in use. The goggles must fit the forehead and enclose the globe. Although the carbon dioxide beam is invisible, a tracer light is incorporated to allow the surgeon to select the target area. The axis of the visible tracer and laser beam should be aligned prior to use.

8. Skin exposure may cause acute or chronic burns. Protection is afforded by using sterile gloves.
9. Other areas should be draped with cloth as laser beams undergo scattering and can be reflected. Hair, scrubbing solutions, and some anesthetic agents may be fire hazards (N_2O, O_2 support combustion).
10. Electrical hazards exist as the initial excitation of the atoms requires high energy currents and circuits which add to the existing hazards of electrical apparatus in the operating room.
11. An understanding of laser measure and knowledge is necessary for controlled use. Energy density is defined by the total energy (joules) and spot size (cm^2) but this may not adequately account for the pulse duration of the beam or the degree of biologic effect.

Patient Protection

Laser hazards to the patient arise from damage to normal tissue or from fires. The eyes should be covered with wet gauze. If a misdirected or reflected beam strikes unprotected tissue, it too is vaporized. Currently available endotracheal tubes are not flammable. Cuffs should be inflated with saline. Oil based lubricants should be avoided.

Danger to OR Personnel from Laser Use

The misuse or misfiring of a laser may cause damage to other personnel in the operating room. Eye damage is of particular concern. The site of ocular damage for any given laser depends upon its output wavelength. Laser light in the visible and near infrared spectrum from 400 to 1,400 nm constitutes the so-called *"retinal hazard region"* and can cause damage to the retina, while wavelengths outside this region (i.e., ultraviolet and far infrared spectrum) are absorbed by the anterior segment of the eye causing damage to the cornea and to the lens. The extent of ocular damage is determined by the laser irradiance, exposure duration, and size of the beam. As laser retinal burns may be painless and the damaging beam sometimes invisible, maximal care should be taken to provide protection for all persons in the laser suite including the patient, laser operator, operative assistants, anesthesiology personnel and observers.

Specific hazards may involve certain laser types:

- Exposure to the invisible **carbon dioxide laser** beam (10,600 nm) can be detected by a burning pain at the site of exposure on the cornea or sclera.
- Exposure to a visible laser beam can be detected by a bright color flash of the emitted wavelength and an after-image of its complementary color (e.g., a green 532 nm laser light would produce a green flash followed by a red after-image).
- When the retina is affected, there may be difficulty in detecting blue or green colors secondary to cone damage, and pigmentation of the retina may be detected.
- Exposure to the **Q-switched Nd:YAG laser** beam (1,064 nm) is especially hazardous and may initially go undetected because the beam is invisible and the retina lacks pain sensory nerves. Visual disorientation due to retinal damage may not be apparent to the operator until considerable thermal damage has occurred.

Protective Eyewear

Protective eyewear in the form of goggle, glasses, and shields provides the principal means to ensure against ocular injury, and must be worn at all times during laser operation (Fig. 5). *Laser safety eyewear* (LSE) is designed to reduce the amount of incident light of specific wavelength(s) to safe levels, while transmitting sufficient light for good vision. In accordance with the ANSI Z136.3 (1988) guidelines, each laser requires a specific type of protective eyewear, and factors that must be considered when selecting LSE include: laser wavelength and peak irradiance, optical density (OD), visual transmittance, field of view, effects on color vision, absence of irreversible bleaching of the filter, comfort, and impact resistance. Failure to address these factors may result in serious eye injury. As LSE often look alike in style and color, it is important to specifically check both the http://www.dermweb.com/laser/eyesafety_colour_code.htmlwavelength and OD imprinted on all LSE prior to laser use, especially in multi-wavelength facilities where

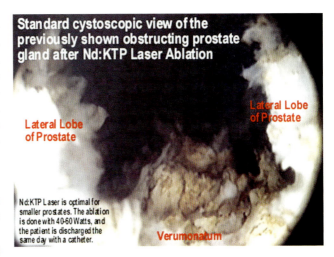

Fig. 5 View of prostate gland after Nd:KTP laser ablation

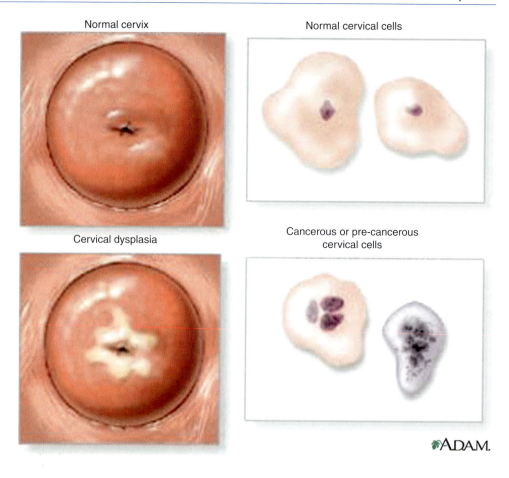

Fig. 6 Normal cervix versus cervix with dysplasia

more than one laser may be located in the same room (e.g., where urology and gynecology share the same operating room).

The integrity of LSE must be inspected on a regular basis (e.g., annually) since small cracks or loose fitting filters may transmit laser light directly to the eye. With the enormous expansion of laser use in medicine, industry and research, every facility should formulate and adhere to specific safety policies that appropriately address eye protection.

Clinical Considerations of Low Light Situations and Safety Glasses

It is also important to determine the impact of wearing LSE on the ability of the anesthesiologist to read the monitoring waveforms as well as the dials on the anesthesia in low light situations (i.e., darken rooms) before embarking on a case. The choice of waveform color can be changed in new monitors and thought needs to be given this to avoid a critical loss of vital monitoring data (Figs. 6–7).

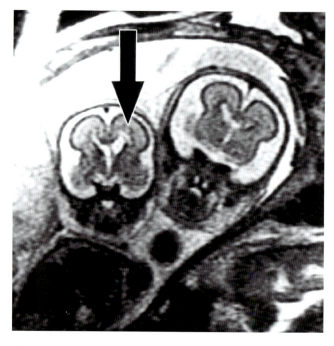

Fig. 7 Twenty four gestational week old monochorionic twin fetus with periventricular white matter injury[27]

Conclusion

With advancements in the field of laser technology, applications of lasers in medicine and surgery have become widespread and common place. Innovations in clinical uses of laser in many fields such as otolaryngology, plastic and dermatologic surgery and urologic surgery have demanded a familiarity with laser technology and safety by the anesthesiologist. In some cases, previously invasive surgeries with major blood loss have now become meticulous and practically bloodless procedures. In other cases, surgeries that in the past required general anesthesia or total intravenous anesthesia are currently performed under monitored anesthesia care with local anesthesia.

Patient populations under going laser surgery range from the fetus in utero to the elderly. Therefore, the anesthesiologist must be cognizant of many variables such as age, underlying medical conditions, and potential complications that may arise in the peri-operative period for all procedures or surgeries involving laser use.

Future directions in laser applications in anesthesia continue to evolve as different areas of medicine and surgery take advantage of innovations in laser technology. Realizing the benefits to the patient of increasing use of lasers in surgery and adaptations in the anesthetic plan deserves further study.

References

1. Zeitels SM, Burns JA. Office based laryngeal surgery with 532-nm pulsed- potassium-titanyl-phosphate laser. *Curr Opin Otolaryngol Head Neck Surg*. 2007;15(6):394-400.
2. Alexiades-Armenakas MR, Dover JS, Arndt KA. The spectrum of laser skin resurfacing: nonablative, fractional, and ablative laser resurfacing. *J Am Acad Dermatol*. 2008;58(5):719-737.
3. Collet-Villette AM, Gaudy-Marquests C, Grob JJ, Richard MA. Carbon dioxide laser therapy for anogenital warts in children. *Ann Dermatol Vénéréol*. 2007;134(11):829-832.
4. Genovese MD, Olivi G. Laser in paediatric dentistry: patient acceptance of hard and soft tissue therapy. *Eur J Paediatr Dent*. 2008; 9(1):13-17.
5. Ferrer Novella C, Gonzalez Viejo I, Oro Fraile J, et al. New anaesthetic techniques in diode laser treatment of retinopathy of prematurity. *An Pediatr (Barc)*. 2008;68(6):576-580.
6. Subash M, Horgan SE. Nd YAG laser capsulotomy in the prone position under general anesthesia ophthalmic. *Ophthalmic Surg Lasers Imaging*. 2008;39(3):257-259.
7. Middeldorp JM, Lopriore E, Sueters M, et al. Twin-to-twin transfusion syndrome after 26 weeks of gestation: is there a role for fetoscopic laser surgery? *BJOG*. 2007;114(6):694-698.

8. Barash PG, Cullen BF, Stoelting RK. *Electrical and Fire Safety. Clinical Anesthesia*. 5th ed. Philadelphia: Lippincott Williams & Wilkins; 2006:150-151.
9. Jaffe RA, Samuels SI. *Anesthesiologist's Manual of Surgical Procedures*. 3rd ed. Philadelphia: Lippincott Williams & Wilkins; 2004.
10. Morgan GE Jr, Mikhail MS, Murray MJ, Larson CP Jr. Pediatric anesthesia. In: *Clinical Anesthesiology*. 3rd ed. New York: Lange Medical Books/McGraw-Hill; 2002:849-874.
11. American Society of Anesthesiologists Task Force on Operating Room Fires, Caplan RA, Barker SJ, et al. Practice advisory for the prevention and management of operating room fires. *Anesthesiology*. 2008;108(5):786-801.
12. Kilmer SL, Chotzen V, Zelickson BD, et al. Full-face laser resurfacing using a supplemental topical anesthesia protocol. *Arch Dermatol*. 2003;139:1279-1283.
13. Lasers in Anesthesia. *Miller's Anesthesia*, 6th ed. Churchill Livingstone; 2005;2573-2587.
14. Ramos-Zabala A, Perez-Mencia MT, Fernandez-Garcia R, Cascales-Nunez MR. Anesthesia technique for outpatient facial laser resurfacing. *Lasers Surg Med*. 2004;34(3):269-272.
15. Alster TS, Lupton JR. Evaluation of a novel anesthetic agent for cutaneous laser resurfacing: a randomized comparison study. *Dermatol Surg*. 2002;28(3):1004-1006.
16. Hanson RA, Zornow MH, Conlin MJ, Brambrink AM. Laser resection of the prostate: implications for anesthesia. *Anesth Analg*. 2007;105(2):475-479.
17. American Society of Anesthesiologists Task Force on Preoperative Fasting, Warner MA, Caplan RA, et al. Practice guidelines for preoperative fastingand the use of pharmacologic agents to reduce the risk of pulmonary aspiration: application to healthy patients undergoing elective procedures. *Anesthesiology*. 1999;90:896-905.
18. Leaute-Labreze C, Boralevi F, Pedespan JM, et al. Pulsed dye laser for Sturge-Weber syndrome. *Arch Dis Child*. 2002;87(5):434-435.
19. Zimmerman TJ, Kooner KS. *Clinical Pathways in Glaucoma*. New York: Thieme; 2001:422.
20. Batra RK, Gulaya V, Madan R, et al. Anaesthesia and the Sturge-Weber syndrome. *Can J Anaesth*. 1994;41(2):133-136.
21. Boker AM. Bilateral tension pneumothorax and pneumoperitoneum during laser pediatric bronchoscopy-case report and literature review. *Middle East J Anesthesiol*. 2008;19(5):1069-1078.
22. Aqil M, Ulhaq A, Arafat A, et al. Venous air embolism during the use of a Nd YAG laser. *Anaesthesia*. 2008;63(9):1006-1009.
23. Alexiades-Armenakas MR. The spectrum of laser skin resurfacing: nonablative, fractional, and ablative laser resurfacing. *J Am Acad Dermatol*. 2008;58(5):719-737. quiz 738-740.
24. Morimoto Y, Yoshimura M, Orita H, et al. Anesthesia management for fetoscopic treatment of twin-to-twin transfusion syndrome. *Masui*. 2008;57(6):719-724.
25. Rossi AC, Kaufman MA, Bornick PW, Quintero RA. General vs local anesthesia for the percutaneous treatment of twin-twin transfusion syndrome. *Am J Obstet Gynecol*. 2008;199(2):137.
26. Zeitels SM, Burns JA. Laser applications in laryngology: past, present, and future. *Otolaryngol Clin North Am*. 2006;39(1):159-172.
27. Coakley FV et al. Fetal MRI: a developing technique for the developing patient. *Am J Roentgenol*. 2004;182(1):243-252.

Index

A

Ablative decomposition, 193
Ablative device, 337
Ablative fractional photothermolysis (aFP)
    clinical course, treatment, 140–141
    photoaging improvement, 140, 142
    tissue vaporization, 138–139
    wound healing, 140
Ablative laser, children
    indications and contraindications, 353
    intra operative management, 355
    preoperative management, 354–355
Acne and milia, 374
Acne scar, 337
Acne vulgaris
    AAD, 187
    blue light therapy, 189–190
    components, 187
    1,540 Er:glass laser, 189
    inflammation reduction curve, 248
    IPL, 190
    KTP laser, 188
    1,320 ND:YAG, 189
    1,450-nm diode laser, 189
    oxyhemoglobin, 188
    P. acnes, 247
    photodynamic therapy, 191
    prevalence, 187
    pulsed dye lasers, 188
    red/blue light combinations therapy, 190
    sebaceous glands, 188
    treatment efficacy, 248, 249
Actinic keratosis (AK)
    NMSCs, 246–247
    non-pigmented lesions, 289, 291, 294
Adipose tissue
    CO_2 laser, 199
    focused ultrasound system, 199, 201
    light and laser based treatments, 199, 200
    liposuction, 201–202
    Nd:YAG laser, 199
Age-related macular degeneration (ARMD), 440, 441
Alpha bisabolol, 361
American Academy of Dermatology (AAD)
    acne, 187
    ethical behavior, 379
    governing bodies and professional organizations, 25
    laser usage, 30–31
    online resources, 410, 411
    procedural skills, 27
American Medical Association (AMA), 379

American Osteopathic College of Dermatology (AOCD), 379
American Society for Aesthetic Plastic Surgery (ASAPS), 91, 388
American Society for Dermatologic Surgery (ASDS)
    governing bodies and professional organizations, 25
    laser usage, 30–31
    procedural skills, 27
American Society for Laser Medicine
        and Surgery (ASLMS), 25, 379, 411
American Society of Dermatologic Society, 383
American Society of Dermatologic Surgeons, 411
American Society of Dermatologic Surgery
    (ASDS), 379
Aminolevulinic acid (ALA), 418
    actinic keratoses treatment, 225–226
    Aktilite device, 223
    Blu-U device, 222
    contraindications, 224
    heme biosynthetic pathway, 221
    MAL-PDT session, 222
    PDT, 533, 534
    photoaging, 224
    porphyrin fluorescence and hematoxylin, 223, 224
    porphyrins, 221
    post-operative management, 226
    pre-operative management, 225
    prevention and treatment, 227
    side effects/complications, 227
Androgenetic alopecia, 283
Anesthesia safety, 311, 312
Anesthesiology
    airway
        co-morbidities, 599
        endotracheal intubation, 600
        indications and contraindications, 599
        intermittent apnea technique, 600
        post-operative management, 600
        pre-operative management, 600
        side effects/complications, 601–602
    carbon dioxide lasers, 598
    clinical research, 608
    cutaneous and cosmetic laser surgery, 602–603
    fiberoptics, laser, 599
    laser beam, characteristics and sources, 598
    laser safety program, 608–609
    laser types, specific hazards, 609
    medical instrument, 598
    obstetrics and gynecology
        bleeding and premature labor, 607
        conization, laser, 606, 607
        fetoscopic laser coagulation, 606
        indications and contraindications, 606

K. Nouri (ed.), *Lasers in Dermatology and Medicine*,
DOI: 10.1007/978-0-85729-281-0, © Springer-Verlag London Limited 2011

peroneal nerve injury, 607
pre-operative management, 606
pathologic process, 597–598
patient protection, 609
pediatrics
complications, 606
drug dosages, 605
indications and contraindications, 604
laryngospasm, 606
post-operative management, 605–606
pre-operative management, 604, 605
propofol infusion, 605
PWS, 605
protective eyewear, 609–610
radiographs, 598–599
retinal hazard region, 609
urology, 603–604
Antibiotic prophylaxis, 542
Anti-inflammatory agents, 361
Anti-vascular endothelial growth factors (anti-VEGF), 440
Anxiety disorder, 395
Argon fluoride (AFl) laser, 426
Argon laser
adverse events, 440
indications
choroidal neovascular membrane, 437–438
photocoagulation, focal, 437, 438
PRP, 436–437
technique
choroidal neovascular membrane, 440
photocoagulation, focal, 438–440
PRP, 438–439
uses, 440
Argon laser trabeculoplasty (ALT), 447
indications and contraindications, 453
side effects/complications, 454
techniques, 453, 454
Arnica montana, 371
Atrophic scar
ablative laser resurfacing, 49
definition, 48
fractional resurfacing, 49–50
nonablative laser resurfacing, 49
tatoos, 315, 316, 318

B
Bare/urologic fibers, 546
Basal cell carcinoma (BCC), 289, 291–293
BDD. *See* Body dysmorphic disorder
Beam propagation
absorption coefficient, 11
chromophores, 11
dermis and epidermis, 9
fluence attenuation, 10
laser light and biological tissue interaction, 9–10
light wavelength dependent optical penetration depth, 10
poikilodermatous, 10
skin optical properties, 9
Benign prostatic hyperplasia (BPH)
complication, 566–567
HoLAP and HoLRP, 565
HoLEP, 565
holmium laser resection and enucleation, 566
indications and contraindications, 565–566
KTP laser, 564, 565
medical intervention, 564
optical penetration depths, 564

PVP, 564
treatment, 564, 565, 567
Best corrected visual acuity (BCVA), 431
Bipolar disorder, 392, 393
Bleeding, 466
Body dysmorphic disorder (BDD), 322
major depression, 390
preoccupations, 389
questionnaire, 390
repetitive behaviors, 389, 390
resources, 391
Body dysmorphic disorder questionnaire (BDDQ), 390
Bone ablation process, 475
Borderline personality disorder, 393–394
Bovine mucopolysaccharide-cartilage complex (MCC), 362
Bowen's disease, 224–225
BPH. *See* Benign prostatic hyperplasia
Bruising, 326

C
Caféau lait macules (CALMs), 70–71
Candela®, 346
Capacitance coupling, 541
Capillary malformations, port wine stains/nevus flammeus
alexandrite and Nd:YAG treatments, 37, 38
hypertrophic violaceous PWS, 37, 38
PDL treatment, adverse effect, 39
pink macular PWS, 37
PWS treatment, 36–37
Carbon dioxide (CO_2) laser
ablation, tissue, 556
clinical and histologic benefits, 106
collagen fibers, 106
dissection and hemostasis, 545
Er:YAG laser, 107–109
gynecologic laparoscopic applications, 544
incision, excision and vaporization of tissues, 554–555
intermittent evacuation, 545
isotretinoin, 107
laser–tissue interaction., 108
modality, breast treatment, 556
Omniguide® fiber, 544
parameters, 542, 543
skin tone and wrinkle severity, 106, 107
waveguides, 544–545, 555
wavelength, 544
Cardiology and cardiothoracic surgery
acute myocardial infarction, 575
aorto-ostial lesions, 577
calcified lesions, 575–576
clinical complications, 580
clinical history, 573
clinical trials, 573
contraindications, 575
coronary allograft vasculopathy, 577–580
excimer laser, 573, 574
indications, cardiovascular medicine, 573, 574
left main disease, 575, 576
renal artery interventions, 580
saphenous vein grafts lesions, 577
stent restenosis, 577, 578
stroke, 580
thrombus, 575
TMLR, 577
total occlusions, 576–577

Index

undilatable/uncrossable lesions, 575
venous system, 580
Cataract, 453
Cellulite
Alma Accent RF System, 204
FDA, 202
IPL, 202, 203
light emitting diode, 203
light sources and massage, 203
VelaSmooth™, 203, 204
Charge coupled device (CCD), 403
Children
ablative laser
indications and contraindications, 353–354
intra operative management, 355
preoperative management, 354–355
adverse events, 350–351
dermatologic condition, 345, 346
HOI, 348–349
KTP, 350
pediatric skin lesion, 355
pigmented lesion
café-au-lait macules, 352
CMN, 353
melanin and lentigines, 351
nevus spilus, 352
tattoos, 352–353
port wine stain
hemangioma, 347
post-treatment purpura, 346, 347
predictive factors, 347
trigeminal nerve, 348
vascular malformation, 346
quasi continuous laser, 350
vascular laser therapy, 349–350
vascular lesion, 345, 346
Choanal atresia, 513, 514
Choroidal neovascular membrane
adverse events, 440
indications, 437–438
technique and uses, 440
Chronic periodontal disease, 480
Clinically significant macular edema (CSME), 437
Closed-angle glaucoma (CAG), 448
Cochrane Database Systematic Reviews, 533
Cognitive-behavioral therapy (CBT), 390
Cold ablation, 193
Complementary metal oxide semiconductor (CMOS), 403
Confocal laser scanning microscopy (CM), 420
Congenital melanocytic nevi (CMN), 353
Contact dermatitis, 374
Contact/fiber optic method, 546
Corneal collagen cross-linking (CXL), 432
Corneal damage, 453
Corneal ectasia, 431
Corneal haze, 431
Corticoids, 361
Cryocautery, 526
Cryogen spray cooling (CSC), 341
Cutting technique, 553, 554
Cyclophotocoagulation, 447

D
Dentistry
American Dental Laser, 464
anti-bacterial techniques

general pre-operative management, 481
indications and contraindications, 479–480
peri-implantitis treatment, 482, 483
periodontal pocket debridement, 481
post-operative management, 482–483
root canal decontamination, 481–482
side effects and complications, 483
continuous-wave emission mode, 464
erbium, chromium YSGG laser, 464
laser perceptions, 465
light dynamics, 465–466
LLLT
caries detection, 485
composite resin curing, 485
general pre-operative management, 487
indications and contraindications, 484
PAD, 485–486
photobiostimulation, 484
tooth whitening, 486
market penetration, 466
oral hard tissue
general pre-operative management, 474
indications and contraindications, 473–474
management, 474, 475
modification, 476–477
post-operative management, 478
side effects and complications, 478–479
surgical excision of bone, 477–478
tooth cavity preparation/caries removal, 475, 476
oral soft tissue
advantage, 469
general pre-operative management, 468
gingival tissue, upper left incisor, 469
gingival tissue, upper right incisor, 469, 470
immediate post-laser treatment, 469, 470
indications and contraindications, 466–467
laminate veneers/crowns, 468
pathological tissue resection, 470, 471
post-operative management, 470–471
restorative treatment, 3 months, 469, 470
side effects and complications, 471, 472
soft tissue management, 468, 469
trauma, 469
Dermal pigmented lesions
drug induced pigmentation, 74–75
melanocytic nevi, 72–73
melasma and post-inflammatory hyperpigmentation, 73–74
Nevus of Ota, 73
Dermatofibroma (DF), 293, 295
Derm Net website, 411
Dermo-epidermal junction (DEJ), 133
Diabetic Retinopathy Study (DRS), 436
Diffuse lamellar keratitis, 432
Digital nerve blocks, 333
Digital photography
advantages, 399
camera types
compact/subcompact, 400–401
SLR, 400
digital media, 403
equipment, 399, 400
flash, 402
image submission, publication, 404
imaging skill, 407
lenses

macro/close-up, 401–402
wide-angle zoom, 401
mega-pixel, 403
shooting techniques and tips
photographic technique, 405
pre and postoperative facial photography, 405–406
standard procedures, 404
surgical photography, 406
white balance, 402–403
Digital single-lens-reflex (DSLR), 400
Diode laser
adverse events, 443
indications, 441–442
technique, 442–443
uses, 444
1,450 nm Diode lasers, 169–170, 189
Diomed® laser, 549
Documentation consent. *See* Medicolegal issues
Dorsal root entry zone (DREZ) lesions, 591
Dyspigmentation, 371–372

E

Early Treatment Diabetic Retinopathy Study (ETDRS), 436
Ecchymoses. *See* Bruising
Ectropion, 374
Edema, 369–370
Education, laser patient. *See* Laser patient
ELA-Max. *See* LMX–4 cream
Electrocautery, 552
Electrosurgical devices, 540, 541
eMedicine, 411
Endolaser
adverse events, 445
indications and techniques, 444
uses, 445
Endoscopic cyclophotocoagulation (ECP), 458, 459
Enoxolone, 361
Epidermal nevi (EN), 353
Epithelial defect, 431
1,540 nm Erbium glass laser, 170, 189
Erythema, 197, 369–370
Erythroxylon coca, 329
Ethical behavior
advertisement, 381
contraindications, 381
economics, 380
elective procedures, 379
interest, 380–381
physician and patient discussion, 380
training, 380
unethical conduct, 381
Ethnic skin
acne scar, 337
laser assisted hair reduction, 340
photorejuvenation
fractional device, 338
IPL and LED, 339
532 nm laser, 338
1,064 nm laser, 338–339
pre and post laser cooling, 341
skin tightening
infrared, 340
radiofrequency, 339
tattoos, 341
test spot, 342
vascular lesion, 340–341

Eutectic mixture of local anesthetics (EMLA) cream, 330, 354
Excited dimers, 193
External auditory canal (EAC), 507
Eyelid swelling, 326
Eye protection, 497
Eye safety
corneal eye shield
placement in adult, 310, 311
placement in child, 310
size, 309, 310
tray set up, 309
different wavelengths, 309
protection, eyewear types, 309

F

Facial nerve blocks, 333
Factitial dermatoses, 322
Flashlamp-pumped dye (FLPD) laser, 341. *See also*
Pulsed dye lasers
Fluorescence guided resection (FGR), 590
5-Fluorouracil (5-FU) therapy, 372, 373
Focal argon laser photocoagulation
adverse events, 440
indications, 437, 438
technique, 438–440
uses, 440
Food and Drug Administration (FDA), 425
hair reduction, 99
hair removal concept definition, 92
Fractional device
dermis, 19
first generation, 119
photorejuvenation, 338
photothermolysis, acne scar, 337
Fractional photothermolysis (FP), 315
adverse events and clinical pitfalls
antibiotic prophylaxis, 143, 144
bulk heat generation, tissue, 141
scarring effect, 142–143
aFP (*see* Ablative fractional photothermolysis)
average power, FP laser system, 127
bulk heating precaution procedure, 128
3-dimensional pattern, generation, MTZ, 126
home-use dermatology devices, 144–145
nFP (*see* Non-ablative fractional photothermolysis)
nFP and FP devices, 123, 125
pulse duration, 127
resurfacing modalities, 125–126
selective photothermolysis, 123–124
SMAS, 130
stamping and rolling technique, 127
thermal damage patterns, factors, 129
Frequency doubled double-pulse neodymium:
YAG (FREDDY) laser, 562

G

Generic laser hardware, 602
Glaucoma. *See also* Ophthalmology
clinical triad, 449
definition, 448
diagnosis, 447, 449
management, lasers, 450
medications, 447
multifactorial optic neuropathy, 448
OAGs and CAGs, 448
POAG, 448

Index

Glottic carcinoma, 499
Glycyrrhetinic acid. *See* Enoxolone
Graphics interchange format (GIF), 404
Guide number (GN), 402
Gynecology
   CO_2 laser, 524
   endometriosis, 524
   HPV
      classification, 524
      incidence and prevalence, 524–525
      risk factors, 524
      tissue tropism and clinical infections, 525
   myoma coagulation/myolysis, 523
   vulva, vagina, and cervix
      cervical disease treatment, 527–528
      endometrial ablation, 532
      endometriosis and adhesiolysis, 533
      indications and contraindications, 525–526
      intrauterine and intra-abdominal laser
        procedure, 532
      leiomyoma, 532–533
      photodynamic therapy, 533–534
      post-operative management, 530–531
      preoperative management, 527
      side effects/complications, 531–532
      vaginal disease treatment, 528
      vulvar disease treatment, 528–530

H

Hair growth
   "biostimulation," 281
   LLLT, 280
      Hairmax Lasercomb™, 282
      helium neon laser, 282
      mitochondrial transport chain, 281
      mitochondria structure, 281
      Sunetics® International, 283
Hair removal
   ASAPS, 91
   FDA, 92
   indications/contraindications, 92, 94
   laser and intense pulsed light systems, 92, 93
   "permanent hair reduction," 92
   prevention and treatment, 99
   side effects/complications, 98–99
   skin types, 99–100
   superpulses, 92
   techniques
      intense pulsed light, 96–98
      long-pulsed 755 nm alexandrite laser, 95
      long-pulsed 694 nm ruby laser, 95
      800 nm diode laser, 95–96
      1,064 nm Nd:YAG laser, 96
      nonpigmented hair, 98
      post-operative management, 98
      pre-operative management, 94
      radiofrequency combinations, 98
   TRT, 92
Hair transplantation
   CO_2 lasers
      "biological glue," 278
      electrical hazard, 280
      erbium laser, 279
      laser recipient *vs.* steel created sites, 278, 279
      pathology, 279
      risk inherence, 279

FDA approval, 280
   follicular unit transplantation, 277
   International Society of Hair Restoration Surgery, 278
   laser applications, 278
   pros and cons, 280
Heat generation
   LTI molecular basis, 13–14
   SPT
      extreme localized heating, 11–12
      Q switched Nd YAG laser, 12
      thermal relaxation time, 12–13
Heating, reaction types and effects
   photochemical effects
      biostimulation, 16
      excimer laser, 16
      luminescence, definition, 15
      photodisruption/photodecomposition, 16
      photodynamic reactions, 16
      plasma induced ablation, 16–17
      PpIX fluorescence, 16
   photomechanical effects, 15
   photothermal effects, 14–15
Hemangiomas of infancy (HOI), 348–349
Hemorrhoidectomy, 556
Hereditary hemorrhagic telangiectasias (HHT), 513, 514
Herpes simplex virus (HSV), 374
Histrionic personality disorder, 394
Holmium laser enucleation of the prostate (HoLEP), 565
Holmium laser resection of the prostate (HoLRP), 565
Holmium laser vaporization of the prostate (HoLAP), 565
Human immunodeficiency virus (HIV), 367
Human papilloma virus (HPV), 367
   classification, 524
      incidence and prevalence, 524–525
      risk factors, 524
      tissue tropism and clinical infections, 525
Hyaluronic acid, 362
Hydroquinone, 363
Hyperthermia, 590
Hypertrichosis, 373
Hypertrophic scar, 315–318
Hyphema, 453
Hypopharyngeal carcinoma, 499
Hypopigmentation, 314, 316. *See also* Vitiligo

I

Idiopathic central serous chorioretinopathy (ICSC), 441
Idiopathic polypoidal choroidal vasculopathy (IPCV), 441
Imiquimod cream, 363
Infantile hemangioma, 316–318
Infectious keratitis, 432
Infiltrative anesthesia
   anesthetic agents, 331, 332
   bupivacaine and etidocaine, 331
   nerve block, 332–333
   non-ablative rejuvenation, 332
   pigmented lesions and hair removal, 331–332
   tattoos, 331–332
   tumescent anesthesia, 332
Inflammatory linear verrucous epidermal nevus
      (ILVEN), 353
Informed consent. *See* Medicolegal issues
Infrahyoid epiglottic cancers, 499
Infrared tightening, 340
Institutional board review (IRB), 381
Intense pulse light (IPL)

adverse reactions, 217
benign vascular lesions
   hemangiomas, 211, 212
   POC, 211–212
   PWS, 212–213
   reticular leg veins, 209–210
   telangiectasias, 210–211
device for acne, 190
hair removal, 216
indications, 209
leg vein treatment, 58–59
non-ablative photorejuvenation
   botulinum A, 215
   lumenis, 214, 215
   murine model, 214
   photodynamic therapy, 215
   sun exposure, UV damage, 213
non-coherent filtered flash lamp, 207
photorejuvenation, 339
photothermolysis, 207, 217
pigmented lesions, 213
scars, 215–216
sources, 112–113, 171, 172
spot size, 208
vascular treatment, 36
wavelength and pulse duration, 208
Interface debris, 431
Internet website
expansive source, 412
medical resources, 409
quality evaluation, 409–410
Intra-axial brain tumors, 589–590
Intralase®, 426
Intralesional corticosteroids and 5-FU, 48, 50
Intramedullary tumors, 588
Intraocular lens (IOL), 432
Intraocular pressure (IOP). *See* Ophthalmology
Intrinsic signal optical imaging (ISOI), 586
Investigational Device Exemption (IDE), 381

J
Journal of American Academy of Dermatology (JAAD), 381, 411

K
Keloid scar, 315–318
KTP laser. *See* Potassium titanyl phosphate laser

L
Laparoscopic cholecystectomy, 540
Laryngeal mask airway (LMA), 312
Laser-assisted subepithelial keratectomy (LASEK), 425
Laser assisted vascular anastomosis, 588–589
Laser discectomy, 588
Laser Eustachian tuboplasty (LETP), 507
Laser injury, laparoscopic surgery, 550–551
Laser in-situ keratomileusis (LASIK)
ablation and reshaping, 426
excimer laser, 427, 428
femtosecond laser unit, 426, 427
flap folds, 428
microkeratomes, 426
stromal hydration, 427
wave-front guided, 428–430
Laser iridotomy
alternate route for aqueous, 450
complications, 453

definition, 447
indications and contraindications, 451
post-operative management, 452
pre-operative management, 451–452
q-switched Nd:YAG and the argon laser, 452
side effects, 452
surgical iridectomies, 450
Laser parameters, 543, 544, 552
Laser patient
color, 326
delegating procedure, 323
education
   adverse event, 327
   bruising, 326
   counseling, 323–325
   downtime, 327
   erosion, 326
   hives and blisters, 326–327
   laser treatment, 325
   presenting complaints, 323
   procedure-related problems, 327
   redness and swelling, 326
selection
   body dysmorphic disorder, 322
   dissatisfied patient, 322
   problem identification, 322, 323
   procedure, performance, 323
   psychiatric illness and factitial dermatoses, 322
   reasonable patient finding, 321
tanned, 326
Laser peripheral iridoplasty, 447
Laser practice
common mistake, 415
delegate and nondelegate procedures, 415
device cost, 414
energy based device integration, 413–414
evidence based review, 414
laser/light treatment, 415
marketing, 414–415
peer review, 414
rent *vs.* lease *vs.* purchase, 414
Laser retractors, 553
Laser safety. *See also* Anesthesia safety; Eye safety
administrative controls, 27–28
anesthesia, 497
ASLMS, 25
eye and skin protection, 28–29
governing bodies and professional organizations, 25–26
laser-specific endotracheal tube, 496, 497
laser usage
   ASDS and AAD, 30–31
   Board of Medicine, 31
   state regulation, 31
   Texas Board, 32
non-beam hazards, 29–30
patient, surgeon and surgical staff, 496
practice guidelines, 26
procedural skills, 26–27
protective equipment, 28
protocol, 497
warming signs and labels, 28
Laser safety eyewear (LSE), 609, 610
Lasers and lights, pigmented lesions treatment
CALMs, 70–71
dermal pigmented lesions (*see* Dermal pigmented lesions)
epidemiology, 64

Index 619

epidermal lesions, 71, 72
epidermal pigmented lesions, 69
highly pigment selective lasers, 67–69
laser-tissue interactions (*see* Laser-tissue interactions, pigmented skin)
lentigines, 70
pigment nonselective lasers, 66–67
prevention and treatment, 79
Q-switched and pulsed lasers and light sources, 65–66
ruby laser radiation, 64
side effects/complications, 78–79
techniques
  anesthesia, 76
  patient evaluation, 75–76
  pigmented lesion, 77
  post-operative management, 78
  Q-switched laser, 77
  safety measures, 76–77
  "suntans," 78
Laser surgery
anesthesia
  adverse effects, 333, 334
  classification and mechanism, 329, 330
  conscious sedation, 334
  Erythroxylon coca, 329
  evolution, 329
  infiltrative anesthesia (*see* Infiltrative anesthesia)
  lidocaine, 329
  novacaine, 329
  pediatric patients, 334
  pregnancy, 334
  topical anesthesia, 330–331
fractionated treatment, 417–418
history, 417
in vivo optical microscopy, 420–421
LLLT, 419–420
photodynamic therapy, 418–419
PTB, 418
1,319/1,320 nm Laser systems, 167–169
Laser-tissue interactions
beam profiles, top hat *vs.* Gaussian, 6
dermis compact
  carbonization, 20
  hyperosmolar solutions, 20
  optical properties change, real-time, 19–20
  photon recycling, 20
  photothermal responses, 20–21
  polarizing lamp, 21
  scatter limited therapy, 21
  selective cell targeting, 21
  spot diameter, 19
laser beam
  focus, 17–18
  target vacuum, 18
light, 1–2
light device
  CO_2 lasers, 5
  erbium YAG lasers, 5
  laser tissue interactions, 4
  light sources, 3
  Q switched alexandrite laser, 5
  total light dose (fluence), 4
  types, 2–4
optical damping, 19
photothermal-photochemical conversion, 17, 18
pigmented skin

epidermal melanocytes activation, 65, 66
  melanin biosynthesis, 64–65
  melanin, oxyhemoglobin and water, 64–65
  Q-switched ruby laser irradiation, 65, 66
pixilated injury, 18–19
pulse profiles, square *vs.* spiky, 6
radiofrequency (RF) technology
  beam propagation (*see* Beam propagation)
  electrode deployment, 9
  heat conduction, chromophore, 17
  heat generation (*see* Heat generation)
  reaction types and effects
    (*see* Heating, reaction types and effects)
  "synergy," 9
wavelength ranges
  absorption coefficients, 6, 7
  cutaneous surgery, 6
  far infrared systems, 8–9
  MIR-lasers and deeply penetrating halogen lamps, 8
  near IR (II), 7–8
  red and near IR (I), 7
  user controllable temperature change, IPL, 7
Laser trabeculoplasty, 447, 450
ALT, 454
biologic theory, 454
indications and contraindications, 455
mechanical theory, 454
patient position, slit lamp-mounted laser, 455, 456
post-operative management, 456
pre-operative management, 455
repopulation theory, 454
side effects/complications, 456–457
SLT, 454
LASIK. *See* Laser in-situ keratomileusis
Leg veins
argon lasers, 54
cavitation, 56
classifications, 53
clinical endpoints, 59
complications, 60
contraindications, 55
diode lasers, 57
epidermal cooling techniques, 56
erythematous dermatitis, 54
indications, 55
IPL, 58–59
KTP laser, 56
long pulsed dye laser, 56
long pulsed 755 nm alexandrite laser, 56–57
Nd:YAG lasers, 55, 57–58
oxyhemoglobin, 55
postoperative results, 59
sclerotherapy, 60
varicose and spider veins, 53
Zimmer air-cooling device, 60
Leukotrichia, 373
Light-emitting diode (LED), 339
definition, 232
dome-type LED, 232, 234
vs. lasers/IPLs, 232, 235
light production, 232, 233
phototherapy
  acne vulgaris, 247–249
  applications, 260
  clinical efficacy, 245
  'colorology,' 261

continuous wave, 262
contraindications, 257–258
dose recommendation, 262
eye protection, 256
FDA, 261
history, 231–232
incident power density, 263
intensity, definition, 261–262
light-tissue interaction (*see* Light-tissue interaction)
'NASA LED,' 258
NASA technology, 261
new wavelength discovery, 258–259
NMSCs and actinic keratosis, 246–247
Omnilux® revive™, 261
'on-board' chips, 259
optical hazards, 256–257
PAT, 245
PDT (*see* Photodynamic therapy)
peer-reviewed literature/peer-reviewed journals, 263
'photobath,' 259
photon intensities, 259
platelet-rich plasma (PRP), 256
psoriasis, 255
safe handling guidelines, 256
side effects, 257
skin rejuvenation (*see* Skin rejuvenation)
'toy' systems, 245–246
'white papers,' 246
wound healing (*see* Wound healing)
substrates and colours, 232, 234
usage
flashlamp, 234
flat panel arrays, 235
laser and IPL, 232
'set-it-and-forget-it' microprocessor-controlled technology, 236
Light gated ion channels, 592–593
Light-tissue interaction
beam, temporal profile, 242–243
dosimetry
bioeffects, 241
energy density (ED), 240, 241
photothermal damage, 242
Grotthus-Draper Law, 236
membrane-located transport mechanisms, 239
optical density (OD), 236
oxyhemoglobin absorption curve, 237
photon density (PD)
Arndt-Schultz law, 240
bioeffects, 239, 240
definition, 239
LED array, 240, 241
photon intensity, 236
photoreception, 239
photospectrogram, 237, 238
photothermal and athermal reactions, 236–238
photothermolysis, 237
Propionibacterium acnes, 238
Lipomas, 588
Liposuction
external ultrasound, 201–202
internal ultrasound, 202
635 nm laser, 201
1,064 nm laser, 201
Liquefied fat, 553, 554
LLLT. *See* Low level laser therapy
LMX–4 cream, 330–331

Low level laser therapy (LLLT), 280
caries detection, 485
composite resin curing, 485
general pre-operative management, 487
Hairmax Lasercomb™, 282
helium neon laser, 282
indications and contraindications, 484
mitochondrial transport chain, 281
mitochondria structure, 281
PAD, 485–486
photobiomodulation, 556, 557
reported effects, clinical dentistry, 484
stimulatory effects, 484
Sunetics® International, 283
tooth whitening, 486
Low level light therapy, 419–420

M

Macular Photocoagulation Study (MPS), 438
Medicolegal issues
clinical outcome, 384–385
informed consent elements, 384
laser therapy, 384
nonverbal protocol function, 383
patient and physician objectives, 383
pediatric patient, 384
quality assurance, 385
Melanocytic lesions
dysplastic nevi, 297
dermal papillae, 298, 301
dermoscopic and RCM mosaic image, 298, 301
epidermal and symmetrical architecture, 298
melanocytic nests, 300, 301
lentigo simplex, 297–299
malignant melanoma, 297–298
atypical cobblestone pattern, 300, 303
cellular-level resolution, 300
cerebriform nests, 303
dermo-epidermal junction, 300
epidermis and dermis, 300, 302
follicular aperture and dendrites, 300, 304
"melanin dust," 300
non nucleated cells, 300, 304
pigmented melanomas, 300, 302
pleomorphic cells, 303
RCM, disadvantage, 304
RCM features, 301
melanocytic nevi, 297–299
Meningiomas, 589
Menorrhagia, 532
Methylaminolevulinate (MAL)
Aktilite device, 223
BCC treatment, 226
contraindications, 224
MAL-PDT session, 223
non-melanoma skin cancer, 222
porphyrin fluorescence and hematoxylin, 223, 224
post-operative management, 226
pre-operative management, 225
prevention and treatment, 226
side effects/complications, 226
Minimally invasive surgery
argon laser, 545–546
CO_2 laser
dissection and hemostasis, 545
gynecologic laparoscopic applications, 544

Index 621

intermittent evacuation, 545
Omniguide® fiber, 544
parameters, 542, 543
waveguides, 544–545
wavelength, 544
"conventional" devices, 549, 550
diode laser technology, 548–549
fiber capable lasers, 543
holmium laser, 548
KTP laser
laserscope, 547
parameters, 542, 543
persistent bleeding, 548
pure lime green light, 547
wavelength, 547, 548
laparoscopic surgery, 542, 543
lithotripsy devices, 549
Nd:YAG laser
energy, 546
parameters, 542, 544
sculpted fibers, 547
vaporization, tumors, 547
wavelength, 546
trocar placement, 550
Monoamine oxidase inhibitors (MAO) inhibitors, 392
Mood disorder
bipolar disorder, 392
major depression, 391–392
Moses effect, 548
Mucopolysaccharide-cartilage complex (MCC), 362
Multiphoton microscopy (MPM), 420
Mycosis fungoides (MF), 289, 291, 293

N

Narcissistic personality disorder, 394
National Institute of Health (NIH), 411
1,064 nm Nd:YAG lasers, 166–168
Neodymium:yttrium-aluminum-garnet
(Nd:YAG) laser, 35
energy, 546
1,320 nm length, 189
parameters, 542, 544
photocoagulation, 554, 555
sculpted fibers, 547
vaporization, tumors, 547
wavelength, 546
Neurology and neurosurgery
ISOI, 586, 587
neurophotonics, 583–584
neurotherapeutic applications
cerebrovascular, 588–589
neuroendoscopic and pediatric applications, 591
neuro-oncologic, 589–590
peripheral nerve applications, 591
spinal, 588
stereotactic and functional, 590–591
NIRS and photon migration
Beer's law technique, 585
diffusion process, 585
elastic scattering, 584
frequency domain, 585
molar extinction coefficients, 584
noninvasive monitoring, chromophores, 584
time domain, 585–586
OCT, 586–588
optical technologies

neural control, 592–593
spatial domain imaging, 591, 592
Nominal Hazard Zone (NHZ), 28
Non-ablative fractional photothermolysis (nFP)
DEJ, 133
dermal remodeling, 132–133
energy dependent response, 133–134
MEND, definition, 132
MTZs depth and diameter, 130–131
photoaging treatment, 136–137
pigment removal, MENDs shuttle process, 132–133
PIH, 134–135
scarring, clinical improvement, 138
skin histology, nFP device, 131
skin histology, nFP treatment, 131–132
small blood vessels coagulation, 133
thulium laser, 135–136
Non-ablative laser skin resurfacing
device, radiofrequency, 117
1,450 nm diode laser, 115–116
1,540 nm erbium:glass laser, 116–117
indications and contraindications, 111
IPL source, 112–113
1,320 nm Nd:YAG laser, 114–115
PDL, 112–113
postoperative management, 117
preoperative management, 112
prevention and treatment, 117
1,064 nm Q-switched Nd:YAG laser, 113–114
side effects/complications, 117
Non-invasive rejuvenation/skin tightening
dyschromias, 175
limiting factors, 175
1,064 Nm Nd:YAG laser, 184–185
skin laxity, deep stratum photoaging
animal hide contraction, 181–184
deep reticular dermis, 181
"flashlamps," 181
skin contraction, 181–183
"stamping technique," 182
trans-cooling and post cooling pulse, 181
skin strata, 175
superficial stratum, 185
Titan and 5 Nd:YAG, 175, 180
Titan, 3 Nd:YAG and 5 IPL, 175, 180
Titan 3 Nd:YAG laser, 175, 178–179
Titan treatment, 175–178
Non-melanoma skin cancers (NMSCs), 246–247
Normal-mode ruby laser (NMRL), 73
Novacaine, 329

O

Obsessive–compulsive personality disorder (OCPD), 394–395
Ocular damage, 367
Online resources
expansive source, 412
medical resources, 409
patient websites, 411–412
physicians websites, 410–411
quality evaluation, 409, 410
Open-angle glaucoma (OAG), 448
Open surgical procedures, 551–552
Operative site and surgical retractors, 552–553
Ophthalmology. *See also* Visual refraction
ALT (*see* Argon laser trabeculoplasty)
anterior segment anatomy and physiology, 448

aqueous humor, 448
argon laser (*see* Argon laser)
CAG, pupillary block, 448, 449
clinical treatment, 449–450
cyclodialysis clefts, 458
cyclophotocoagulation, 457–459
diagnosis, 449
diode laser
    adverse events, 443
    indications, 441–442
    technique, 442–443
    uses, 444
endolaser, vitreoretinal surgery
    adverse events, 445
    indications and techniques, 444
    uses, 445
endoscopic cyclophotocoagulation, 458, 459
glaucoma, 450
goniophotocoagulation, 458
goniopuncture, 458, 459
iridotomy
    alternate route for aqueous, 450
    complications, 453
    indications and contraindications, 451
    post-operative management, 452
    pre-operative management, 451–452
    q-switched Nd:YAG and the argon laser, 452
    side effects, 452
    surgical iridectomies, 450
laser sclerostomy, 458
laser trabeculoplasty, 454–457
OAG, 448, 449
PDT
    adverse events, 441
    indications, 440–442
    technique and uses, 441
pharmacotherapy, 445
posterior segment applications, 435–436
subconjunctival sutures cut, 458
symptoms, 449
xenon arc photocoagulator treatment, 435
Optical coherence tomography (OCT), 421, 440
    imaging, visualization, and quantification capabilities, 588
    reflection method, 586–587
    spectral domain system, 586, 587
    three-dimensional information, 587
Optical penetration depth (OPD)
    MTZ, 135
    nFP lasers, 127
    in water, lasers, 126
Oral hard tissue
    general pre-operative management, 474
    indications and contraindications, 473–474
    management, 474, 475
    modification, 476–477
    post-operative management, 478
    side effects and complications, 478–479
    surgical excision of bone, 477–478
    tooth cavity preparation/caries removal, 475, 476
Oral soft tissue
    advantage, 469
    general pre-operative management, 468
    gingival tissue, upper left incisor, 469
    gingival tissue, upper right incisor, 469, 470
    immediate post-laser treatment, 469, 470
    indications and contraindications, 466–467
    laminate veneers/crowns, 468

pathological tissue resection, 470, 471
post-operative management, 470–471
restorative treatment, 3 months, 469, 470
side effects and complications, 471, 472
soft tissue management, 468, 469
trauma, 469
Otolaryngology
argon laser, 496
CO_2 lasers, 495
giant pulse laser/Q-switching, 495
historical aspects, 495
holmium:YAG and erbium:YAG laser, 496
KTP(Nd:YAG) laser, 495
laryngology
    complications, 505, 506
    devices, 503
    endoscopic examination, 498
    glottic carcinoma, 503–504
    hemangiomas and vascular malformations, 500–501
    hypopharyngeal carcinoma, 504
    laryngomalacia, 501, 504–505
    larynx anatomy, 502
    malignancy, 499–500
    micromanipulator coupled surgical laser, 498
    papillomas, 500, 504, 505
    polyps, 500
    post-operative management, 505–506
    pre-operative management, 502
    Reinke's edema, 501
    safety, 506
    Steiner's work, 498
    supraglottic carcinoma, 504
    suspension laryngoscopy, 502, 503
    TLM, 501
    vocal cord paralysis, 501, 505
laser safety
    anesthesia, 497
    laser-specific endotracheal tube, 496, 497
    patient, surgeon and surgical staff, 496
    protocol, 497
oropharyngeal
    indications and contraindications, 510–511
    PDT, 512
    post-operative management, 512
    pre-operative management, 511
    RF ablation, 511
    side effects/complications, 512
    T1 and T2 oral tumors, 511
otology
    applications, 510
    audiometric analysis, 508
    cholesteatoma, 507, 508
    conductive hearing loss, 507
    Eustachian tube dysfunction, 507
    myringotomy, 508
    otosclerosis, 507
    post-operative management, 509–510
    pre-operative management and laser selection, 507–508
    side effects/complications, 510
    stapedectomy, 507–509
    stapedotomy, 507
    treatment, EAC, 507
    tympanoplasty, 508–509
    tympanostomy, 508
pediatric otolaryngology
    choanal atresia, 514–515
    congenital subglottic stenosis, 515

laryngomalacia, 515, 516
laser myringotomy, 517
pre- and post-operative management, 516
side effects/complications, 517
subglottic hemangioma, 515, 516
subglottic stenosis, 515
vallecular cyst, 515
rhinology, 513–514

P
Pain, 369
Palliative therapy, 499–500
Pan-retinal photocoagulation (PRP)
adverse events, 440
indications, 436–437
technique, 438–439
uses, 440
Papilloma, 599
Para-aminobenzoic acid (PABA), 331
Paradoxical tattoo darkening, 375
Pars plana vitrectomy (PPV), 440
PDL. *See* Pulsed dye lasers
Penetrating keratoplasty (PKP), 432
Percutaneous laser disc decompression (PLDD), 548
Personality disorders
borderline, 393–394
clusters, 392–393
histrionic, 394
narcissistic, 394
obsessive–compulsive, 394–395
Photo-activated disinfection (PAD), 485–486
Photobiomodulation, 556–557
Photobiostimulation. *See* Low level laser therapy
Photochemical tissue bonding (PTB), 418
Photoderm™, 207
Photodisruption, 427
Photodynamic therapy (PDT)
acne vulgaris, 228
actinic keratoses, 221
adverse events, 441
ALA (*see* Aminolevulinic acid)
basal cell carcinoma, 221
BPH, 567
endogenous PDT, 244–245
exogenous PDT, 243–244
gynecology, 533–534
indications, 440–442
MAL (*see* Methylaminolevulinate)
neurology and neurosurgery, 590
otolaryngology, 512
photosensitizer/photosensitizer precursor, 221
research issues, 418–419
technique and uses, 441
Photoepilation, 373
Photoimmunotargeting (PIT), 419
Photokeratomileusis (PKM), 425
Photon absorption therapy (PAT), 245
Photorefractive keratectomy (PRK), 425
Photorejuvenation, 338–339, 417
Photoselective vaporization of the prostate (PVP), 565
Photosensitizers (PS), 418, 419
Photothermal laser nerve stimulation, 592
Pigmented lesions, 373–374
Pigmented non-melanocytic lesions
DF, 293, 295
pigmented basal cell carcinoma, 293, 295
pigmented mammary Paget disease, 293, 295, 297

seborrheic keratosis, 293, 295–297
Pituitary tumors, 589
Plasma resurfacing. *See* Plasma skin regeneration
Plasma skin regeneration (PSR)
basal cell layer, 151
clinical improvements, 153, 154
coblation, 153
CO_2 lasers, 156
EMLA cream, 154
epidermis vaporization, 149
eyelid laxity and periorbital rhytides, 154
FDA, 160
finite element analysis, 151, 152
Fitzpatrick skin types I–IV, 151
Gaussian distribution, 150
indications and contraindications, 154–155
"lunch hour" procedure, 149
nonablative resurfacing, 160
Portrait® PSR system, 150, 153
postoperative management
desquamation, 158
facial rhytides, 156, 159
healing time, high energy treatment, 156
healing time, low energy PSR1 treatment, 156, 157
periorbital rhytides, 156, 158
petrolatum-based ointment, 156
postoperative erythema, 156
preoperative management, 155
prevention and treatment, 159
pulse energy effects, 151, 152
relative downtime *vs.* resurfacing modalities, 153, 154
side effects/complications, 159
single and double pass procedures, 155
skin tightening and textural improvement, 159
thermal effects, 151
treatment protocols, 151–153
turquoise blue non-contact target ring, 155
Plateau iris, 453
Platelet-derived growth factors (PDGF), 45
Poikiloderma of Civatte (POC), 211–212
Port-wine stain (PWS)
anesthesiology, 605
children
post-treatment purpura, 346, 347
predictive factors, 347
trigeminal nerve, 348
vascular malformation, 346
IPL, 212–213
Post inflammatory hyperpigmentation (PIH), 134–135
Post-resurfacing leucoderma and striae, 194
Potassium titanyl phosphate (KTP) laser
acne, 188
laserscope, 547
laser treatment, children, 350
leg vein treatment, 56
parameters, 542, 543
persistent bleeding, 548
pure lime green light, 547
wavelength, 547, 548
Power density, 542
Presumed ocular histoplasmosis syndrome (POHS), 438, 441
Prevention and treatment, laser complications
commonly used lasers, 364
cooling, 366–367
crusting and vesiculation, 370
dermatologic laser therapy, 365, 368
dyspigmentation, 371–372

erythema and edema, 369–370
laser mechanics, 366
operating room, safety, 367
pain, 369
patient factor, 368
photoepilation, 373
pigmented lesions, 373–374
professional error, 367–368
purpura, 370, 371
resurfacing, 374–375
scarring, 372–373
tattoos, 375
vascular lesions, 375
Primary open-angle glaucoma (POAG), 448
Procaine. *See* Novacaine
Proliferative diabetic retinopathy (PDR), 436
Protoporphyrin IX (PpIX), 419
Psoriasis
excimer lasers, 193–194
Fitzpatrick skin type, first dose determination, 196
indications and contraindications, 195, 196
molecular pathogenesis, 198
risks and benefits, 196
subsequent dose determination, 196
PSR. *See* Plasma skin regeneration
Psychiatric illness, 322
Psychological condition
anxiety disorder, 395
BDD (*see* Body dysmorphic disorder)
body image dissatisfaction, 387, 388
evaluation factors, 389
mood disorder
bipolar disorder, 392, 393
major depression, 391–392
patient evaluation, 388, 389
personality disorders
borderline, 393–394
clusters, 392–393
histrionic, 394
narcissistic, 394
obsessive–compulsive, 394–395
psychological complication, 388, 396
PubMed, 411
Pulsed dye lasers (PDLs)
acne, 188
anesthesia safety, 311, 312
definition, 366
disadvantage, 165
duct stone management, 555
hypertrophic scars and keloidal lesion treatment, 165
purpura, 166
rejuvenation, 166, 167
resurfacing, 112–113
selective photothermolysis, 165
skin biopsies, 165
sub-surfacing, 164
treatment, vascular, 35
type III procollagen, 166
vascular lesions, 341
Punctate inner choroidopathy (PIC), 441
Purpura, 370–371

Q
Q-switched laser, 166, 167
1,064 nm Q-switched neodymium:YAG laser, 113–114
Quantitative light-induced fluorescence (QLF), 485
Quasi continuous laser, 350

R
Radio frequency (RF), 339
Reactive oxygen species (ROS), 418
Reasonable expectations patients, 321
Reflectance-mode confocal microscopy (RCM)
anucleated polygonal corneocytes, 288–289
applications
biopsy guide, 305
dermoscopy-RCM correlation, 304–305
margin assessment and surgery
adjunct, 305, 306
treatment response, 305, 306
dermis, 288
epidermis, 288
history, 286
in vivo imaging, advantages, 286
limitations and potential solutions, 306–307
non-invasive imaging techniques, 286
non-pigmented lesions
AK, 289, 291, 294
BCC, 289, 291–293
MF, 289, 291, 293
oral cavity neoplasm, 289, 293
SCC, 289, 291, 295
skin neoplasm, 291
normal skin, objective lens, 289, 290
pigmented lesions
melanocytic lesions (*see* Melanocytic lesions)
pigmented non-melanocytic lesions
(*see* Pigmented non-melanocytic lesions)
principles
laser light, 286
melanin, 287
optical fibre, 287
pinhole resolution, 287
skin movement, 288
Resurfacing
ablative laser skin resurfacing
CO_2 laser (*see* Carbon dioxide laser)
indications and contraindications, 104–105
postinflammatory hyperpigmention, 110–111
postoperative management, 109
preoperative management, 105–106
prevention and treatment, 109–110
side effects and complications, 109, 110
fractional laser technology, 120
fractional photothermolysis, 118–119
non-ablative laser skin resurfacing
1,450 nm diode laser, 115–116
1,540 nm erbium:glass laser, 116–117
indications and contraindications, 111
IPL source, 112–113
1,320 nm Nd:YAG laser, 114–115
PDL, 112–113
postoperative management, 117
preoperative management, 112
prevention and treatment, 117
1,064 nm Q-switched Nd:YAG laser, 113–114
radiofrequency device, 117
side effects/complications, 117
procedures history, 103–104
Reticulate erythema, 373
Retinoic acid, 363
Returns on investment (ROI), 413
Risk, benefit and alternatives (RBA), 383, 384

Index

S

Safety. *See also* Eye safety; Laser safety; Laser-tissue interactions
anesthesia (*see* Anesthesia safety)
corneal eye shield
placement in adult, 310, 311
placement in child, 310
size, 309, 310
tray set up, 309
hair protection
surgical lubricant, eyebrows, 310, 312
surgical lubricant, eyelashes, 310, 312
tongue depressor, 310, 312
Sapphire tip technology, 547
Scars, 372–373
category, etiology, 315
hypertrophic, keloid and atrophic
ablative lasers, 315
baseline and melasma, 316, 320
coagulation, 316
erythema, thickness and pruritus, 315
hemangioma, 316–318
hypopigmentation and textural change, 316, 318
non-ablative fractional erbium treatments, 316, 317
resolution, atrophic scar, 316, 319
ruby laser treatments, 316, 317
skin type II, moderate acne scarring, 316, 319
indications and contraindications, 46–47
techniques
ablative laser resurfacing, 49
fractional resurfacing, 49–50
intralesional corticosteroid, 48
nonablative laser resurfacing, 49
post-operative management, 48
pre-operative management, 47–48
wound healing process, hypertrophic scars, 45–46
Seasonal affective disorder (SAD), 391
Selective laser trabeculoplasty (SLT), 447
Selective photothermolysis (SPT)
extreme localized heating, 11–12
Q switched Nd YAG laser, 12
thermal relaxation time, 12–13
Selective serotonin reuptake inhibitors (SSRIs), 390
Silicone gel, 363
Silicone ointment, 362
Single lens reflex (SLR), 400
Skin laxity, deep stratum photoaging
animal hide contraction, 181–184
deep reticular dermis, 181
"flashlamps," 181
skin contraction, 181–183
"stamping technique," 182
trans-cooling and post cooling pulse, 181
Skin protection, 497
Skin rejuvenation
5-ALA, 250
extracellular matrix (ECM), 248
fractionated/fractional technology, 249
IR/red light, 250, 251
nonablative resurfacing, 249
Skin's stratum corneum, 330
Smoke evacuation, 497
SmoothBeam laser, 169
Spatial frequency domain imaging (SFDI) system, 585, 586
Squalene oil, 362
Squamous cell carcinoma (SCC)
non-pigmented lesions, 289, 291, 295
oropharyngeal, 510, 512

Stall out phenomenon, 478
Sub-surfacing lasers
ablative laser resurfacing systems, 162
adverse events, 172
classifications, 161, 164
erythema, 162, 163
IPL sources, 171, 172
mid-infrared lasers
1,450 nm diode lasers, 169–170
1,540 nm erbium glass laser, 170
1,319/1,320 nm laser systems, 167–169
1,064 nm Nd:YAG lasers, 166–168
Q-switched laser, 166, 167
pigmentary dyschromias and vascular change, 163
post-treatment hypopigmentation, 162, 163
vascular lasers
KTP lasers, 164, 165
PDL (*see* Pulsed dye lasers)
Superficial musculoaponeurotic system (SMAS), 130
Supraglottic carcinoma, 499

T

Tagged image file format (TIFF), 404
Tattoo
allergenicity, 84–85
carbon dioxide lasers, 86
definition, 83
dermatologic uses, lasers, 86
freedom–2 ink technology, 89
historical perspectives, 83–84
ink color, tattoo removal, 88
Q-switched alexandrite laser, 87
Q-switched Nd:YAG laser, 87
removal, laser treatment, 85–86
amateur and multicolor, 313
complications, 314, 316
cosmetic, 313–314
dark skin types, 314, 315
scarring, 313
ruby laser, Q-switched, 87
tattooing techniques, 84
Tetracaine gel, 331
Textural change, 372
Thermal relaxation time (TRT), 92, 207, 208, 366
Thulium fiber laser, 567
Time domain photon migration, 585–586
Time-resolved spectroscopy (TRS). *See*
Time domain photon migration
Tissue cooling effects, 133
Tissue splatter and pinpoint bleeding, 373–374
Transforming growth factor Beta (TGF-β), 45
Trans myocardial laser revascularization (TMLR), 577
Transoral laser laryngeal microsurgery, 499
Transoral laser microsurgery (TLM), 501, 503
large granulomas formation, 506
tracheotomy post operation, 506
Transpupillary thermotherapy (TTT), 443
Transurethral resection of the prostate (TURP) syndrome, 603, 604
Triamcinolone (TAC), 50, 373

U

Ultraviolet-A light (UVA), 432
Urology
BPH
complication, 566–567
HoLAP and HoLRP, 565
HoLEP, 565

626 Index

Holmium laser resection and enucleation, 566
indications and contraindications, 565–566
KTP laser, 564, 565
medical intervention, 564
optical penetration depths, 564
PVP, 564
treatment, 564, 565, 567
laser lithotripsy
adverse event, 563
coumarin laser, 562
erbium laser, 564
fiber development, 563, 564
holmium laser, 562, 563
indications and contraindications, 562, 563
ruby laser, 561–562
technical specifications, 562
laser-tissue interaction mechanism, 561, 562
strictures
erbium:YAG laser, 568
Ho:YAG laser, 568–569
indications/contraindications, 568
laser tissue welding techniques, 569
laser urethrotomy/ureterotomy, 568
types, 567
ureteral and urethral strictures, 568
Urticarial-like plaque, 373
Uvulopalatopharyngoplasty (UPPP), 510–511

V
Vascular lesions
alexandrite laser, 35
combination pdl and Nd:YAG laser, 36
epidermal temperature control, 34
ethnic skin, 340–341
frequency-doubled Nd:YAG, 35
IPL, 36
laser treatment options
capillary malformations (*see* Capillary
malformations, port wine stains/nevus flammeus)
hemangiomas, 39
spider angiomas, 39–40
telangiectasias, 40–41
vascular anomalies, 41–42
venous lakes, 41–42
non-coherent pulsed light devices, 33, 34
PDL, 35
pulse duration, 34
reticulated purpura, 375
selective photothermolysis, 33–34
Verrucae vulgaris (VV), 350
Vestibular schwannomas, 589
Virgin angioma, 324
Visual refraction
complications
anatomic, 430–431
healing/infection/inflammation, 431–432
refractive, 431
CXL, 432
surface ablation
advantage, 426
LASEK, 426
LASIK (*see* Laser in-situ keratomileusis)
PRK, 425, 426
Vitamin C, 363
Vitiligo
erythema, 197
excimer lasers, 194
first dose determination, 197

grafting techniques, 198
indications and contraindications, 195
subsequent dose determination, 197
Vitreoretinal surgery. *See* Endolaser
Vulvar intraepithelial neoplasia (VIN), 534

W
Water-based gel filters, 207
Wave-front guided LASIK
ablation *vs.* risk of keratectasia, 430
ocular aberrations, 428
WaveScan®, 428, 429
WaveScan®, 428, 429
Wildberry extract and kojic acid, 363
Wound dressing/care
ablative laser, 359
cosmetic effects, 363
laser procedure, 359
postoperative treatment
(0–48 h), 360–361
(1–2 week), 362
(3–4 week), 362
(72 h to 1 week), 362
(greater than 4 week), 362–363
(Please insert greater than symbol)
schedule and indications, 360
topical agents ("open" technique), 360
scarring, 363
thermal injury, 359
Wound healing
acute wounds, 267
vs. chronic ulcers, 269
dye-enhanced tissue welding, 270
growth factors, 270
laser-assisted tissue bonding, 269, 271
lasers *vs.* conventional methods, 270–271
laser systems and parameters, optimal wound
bonding, 272
tissue soldering, 270
tissue welding, 269–270
chronic wounds, 273
advantages, 274
Ca influx and mitosis rate, 272
low intensity laser therapy, 274
United States, 267
cutaneous wound healing phases, 267
laser-assisted wound healing, 274
"laser welding," 269
light wavelength
'biostimulation,' 252
cytochrome-c oxidase, 253
dermal and epidermal cell, action potentials, 253, 254
Er:YAG laser ablation, 255
facial electric spark burn injury, 254
HeNe laser, 252
mesenchymal cell, 255
'quasi-wounding,' 254
PAT, 250
process phases, 251
stages, 251–252
tissue repair
classification, 267
inflammatory phase, 268
proliferative phase, 268–269
remodeling phase, 269

Z
Zenker's diverticulum, 511